Master Techniques in Orthopaedic Surgery®

Sports Medicine

SECOND EDITION

MASTER TECHNIQUES IN ORTHOPAEDIC SURGERY

Editor-in-Chief
Bernard F. Morrey, MD

Founding Editor
Roby C. Thompson Jr, MD

Volume Editors
Relevant Surgical Exposures, 2nd Edition
Bernard F. Morrey, MD
Matthew C. Morrey, MD

The Hand, 3rd Edition
Steven D. Maschke, MD
Thomas J. Graham, MD
Peter J. Evans, MD

The Wrist, 3rd Edition
Richard H. Gelberman, MD

The Elbow
Bernard F. Morrey, MD

The Shoulder
Edward V. Craig, MD

The Spine, 3rd Edition
Thomas L. Zdeblick, MD
Todd J. Albert, MD

The Hip, 3rd Edition
Daniel J. Berry, MD
William Maloney, MD

Reconstructive Knee Surgery, 4th Edition
Darren L. Johnson, MD

Knee Arthroplasty, 4th Edition
Mark W. Pagnano, MD
Arlen D. Hanssen, MD

The Foot and Ankle, 3rd Edition
Harold B. Kitaoka, MD

Fractures, 3rd Edition
Donald A. Wiss, MD

Pediatrics, 2nd Edition
David L. Skaggs, MD
Mininder Kocher, MD, MPH

Soft Tissue Surgery, 2nd Edition
Steven L. Moran, MD
S. Andrew Sems, MD

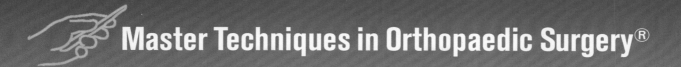

Master Techniques in Orthopaedic Surgery®

Sports Medicine

SECOND EDITION

Editors

Freddie H. Fu, MD, DSci (Hon), DPs (Hon)
Distinguished Service Professor
University of Pittsburgh
David Silver Professor and Chairman
Department of Orthopaedic Surgery
University of Pittsburgh School of Medicine
Head Team Physician
University of Pittsburgh Athletic Department
Pittsburgh, Pennsylvania

Bryson P. Lesniak, MD
Associate Professor
Division of Sports Medicine
Department of Orthopedic Surgery
University of Pittsburgh Medical Center
Team Physician, University of Pittsburgh
Head Team Physician, Carnegie Mellon University
Pittsburgh, Pennsylvania

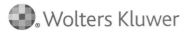. Wolters Kluwer

Philadelphia • Baltimore • New York • London
Buenos Aires • Hong Kong • Sydney • Tokyo

Acquisitions Editor: Brian Brown
Product Development Editor: Stacy Sebring
Editorial Coordinator: Dave Murphy
Marketing Manager: Phylis Hintner
Production Project Manager: Joan Sinclair
Design Coordinator: Stephen Druding
Manufacturing Coordinator: Beth Welsh
Prepress Vendor: SPi Global

Second Edition

Library of Congress Cataloging-in-Publication Data
Names: Fu, Freddie H., editor. | Lesniak, Bryson P., editor.
Title: Sports medicine / editors, Freddie H. Fu, Bryson P. Lesniak.
Other titles: Sports medicine (Fu) | Master techniques in orthopaedic surgery.
Description: 2nd edition. | Philadelphia : Wolters Kluwer, [2020] | Series: Master techniques in orthopaedic surgery | Includes bibliographical references and index.
Identifiers: LCCN 2019018446 | ISBN 9781496375179 (hardback)
Subjects: | MESH: Athletic Injuries—surgery | Orthopedic Procedures—methods | Sports Medicine
Classification: LCC RD97 | NLM QT 261 | DDC 617.1/027—dc23 LC record available at https://lccn.loc.gov/2019018446

CCS0619

Contributors

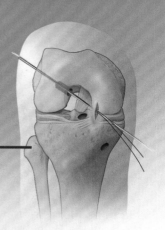

Christopher S. Ahmad, MD
Professor and Chief of Sports Medicine
Department of Orthopedic Surgery
Columbia University Medical Center
New York, New York

Craig C. Akoh, MD
Sports Medicine Fellow
Department of Orthopedics and Rehabilitation
School of Medicine and Public Health
University of Wisconsin
Madison, Wisconsin

Marcio B. V. Albers, MD
Research Fellow
Department of Orthopaedic Surgery
University of Pittsburgh Medical Center
Pittsburgh, Pennsylvania

Frank J. Alexander, MS, ATC
Physician Extender
Department of Orthopaedic Surgery
Columbia University Medical Center
New York, New York

Answorth A. Allen, MD
Orthopaedic Surgery Attending
Hospital for Special Surgery
Professor of Clinical Orthopaedic Surgery
Weill Cornell Medical College
Head Orthopaedic Surgeon
New York Knicks
New York, New York

Christina Allen, MD
Professor of Orthopaedic Surgery
Department of Orthopaedic Surgery
University of California, San Francisco
San Francisco, California

Annunziato Amendola, MD
Chief of Sports Medicine
Department of Orthopaedics
Duke University Medical Center
Professor of Orthopaedics
Department of Orthopaedics
Duke University Hospital
Durham, North Carolina

Robert A. Arciero, MD
Professor
Department of Orthopaedic Surgery
University of Connecticut Health Center
Farmington, Connecticut

Justin W. Arner, MD
Resident
Department of Orthopaedic Surgery
University of Pittsburgh
Pittsburgh, Pennsylvania

Geoffrey S. Baer, MD, PhD
Associate Professor
Department of Orthopedics and Rehabilitation
Head Team Physician
University of Wisconsin–Madison
Madison, Wisconsin

Champ L. Baker III, MD
Staff Physician
Orthopaedic Surgery
Hughston Clinic
Columbus, Georgia

Neil Bakshi, MD
Resident
Department of Orthopedic Surgery
University of Michigan
Orthopedic Surgery House Officer
Department of Orthopedic Surgery
University of Michigan Health System
Ann Arbor, Michigan

Michael G. Baraga, MD
Assistant Professor
Department of Orthopaedic Surgery
University of Miami Miller School of Medicine
Miami, Florida
Assistant Professor
University of Miami Sports Medicine Institute
Lennar Foundation Medical Center
Coral Gables, Florida

Asheesh Bedi, MD
Associate Professor, Harold and Helen W. Gehring Early
    Career
Professor of Orthopaedic Surgery
Department of Orthopaedic Surgery
University of Michigan
Chief, Sports Medicine and Shoulder Surgery
Department of Orthopaedic Surgery
MedSport, University of Michigan
Ann Arbor, Michigan

Matthew H. Blake, MD
Assistant Professor
Orthopaedic Surgery
University of South Dakota
Vermillion, South Dakota
Director of Sports Medicine
Orthopedic Surgery
Avera McKennan Hospital & University Health Center
Sioux Falls, South Dakota

Jeremy M. Burnham, MD
Orthopaedic Surgery Sports Medicine Fellow
UPMC Rooney Sports Complex
University of Pittsburgh
Pittsburgh, Pennsylvania
Sports Medicine and Orthopaedic Surgeon
Orthopaedic Surgery
Bone & Joint Clinic of Baton Rouge
Baton Rouge, Louisiana

Taylor Cabe, BA
Research Assistant
Orthopedic Surgery, Office of Mark C. Drakos Foot and
    Ankle Service
Hospital for Special Surgery
New York, New York

Abigail L. Campbell, MD, MSc
Resident
NYU Langone Orthopedic Surgery
NYU Langone Health
New York, New York

Jonathan E. Campbell, MD
Assistant Professor of Orthopaedic Surgery
Orthopaedic Surgery
Medical College of Wisconsin
Mequon Health Center
Mequon, Wisconsin

Caitlin Chambers, MD
Fellow, Sports Medicine
Orthopedic Surgery
University of California, San Francisco
San Francisco, California

Monique C. Chambers, MD, MSL
Orthopaedic Surgery Resident
Department of Orthopaedic Surgery
Baylor College of Medicine
Houston, Texas

Zaira S. Chaudhry, MPH
Medical Student
Geisinger Commonwealth School of Medicine
Geisinger Health System
Danville, Pennsylvania
Research Fellow
Orthopaedic Surgery—Sports Medicine
Rothman Institute
Philadelphia, Pennsylvania

Josh Chisem, MD
Resident
Department of Orthopaedic Surgery
Hospital for Special Surgery
New York, New York

Steven B. Cohen, MD
Director of Sports Medicine Research
Professor
Department of Orthopaedic Surgery
Rothman Institute/The Sidney Kimmel Medical
    College
Thomas Jefferson University
Philadelphia, Pennsylvania

Brian J. Cole, MD, MBA
Professor
Orthopedic Surgery
Midwest Orthopedics at Rush
Associate Chairman
Orthopedic Surgery
Rush University Medical Center
Chicago, Illinois

Philip N. Collis, MD
Assistant Professor of Orthopaedic Surgery
University of Kentucky
Bowling Green, Kentucky

Eileen Colliton, MD
Resident
Department of Orthopaedic Surgery
Tufts Medical Center
Boston, Massachusetts

Andrew J. Cosgarea, MD
Professor
Department of Orthopaedic Surgery
Johns Hopkins University
Chief
Division of Sports Medicine
Johns Hopkins Hospital
Baltimore, Maryland

James B. Cowan, MD
Medicine Fellow
Orthopaedic Surgery Sports
Department of Orthopaedic Surgery
Stanford Hospital and Clinics
Redwood City, California

S. Joseph de Groot Jr, MD
Resident
Department of Orthopaedic Surgery
University of Pittsburgh Medical Center
Pittsburgh, Pennsylvania

Peter A. J. de Leeuw, MD, PhD
Orthopaedic Surgeon
Department of Orthopaedic Surgery
Flevo Hospital
Almere, The Netherlands

Matthew J. Deasey, MD
Resident
Department of Orthopaedic Surgery
University of Virginia
Charlottesville, Virginia

Malcolm E. Dombrowski, MD
Orthopaedic Resident–Clinician Scientist Track
Department of Orthopaedic Surgery
University of Pittsburgh School of Medicine
Pittsburgh, Pennsylvania

Mark C. Drakos, MD
Associate Professor
Department of Orthopedic Surgery
Weill Cornell Medical College
New York, New York
Assistant Orthopedic Surgery Attending
Foot and Ankle Service
Hospital for Special Surgery
Uniondale, New York

Kyle R. Duchman, MD
Orthopaedic Sports Medicine
Fellow Physician
Department of Orthopaedic Surgery
Duke University
Durham, North Carolina
Visiting Associate
Department of Orthopaedic Surgery and Rehabilitation
University of Iowa
Iowa City, Iowa

Robin H. Dunn, MD
Resident
Department of Orthopedics
University of Colorado
Aurora, Colorado

Hayley E. Ennis, MD
Orthopedic Resident
Department of Orthopedic Surgery
University of Miami
Orthopedic Resident
Orthopedic Surgery
Jackson Memorial Hospital
Miami, Florida

Peter D. Fabricant, MD, MPH
Assistant Professor of Orthopaedic Surgery
Department of Orthopaedic Surgery
Weill Cornell Medical College
Attending Orthopaedic Surgeon
Division of Pediatric Orthopaedic Surgery
Hospital for Special Surgery
New York, New York

Brian T. Feeley, MD
Associate Professor in Residence
Sports Medicine & Shoulder Surgery
Department of Orthopedic Surgery
University of California, San Francisco
San Francisco, California

Nicole A. Friel, MD
Orthopedic Surgeon
Department Sports Medicine Orthopedics
Shriners Hospital for Children, Northern California
Sacramento, California

Erik M. Fritz, MD
Resident
Department of Orthopaedic Surgery
University of Minnesota
Resident
Department of Orthopaedic Surgery
University of Minnesota Medical Center
Minneapolis, Minnesota

Freddie H. Fu, MD, DSci (Hon), DPs (Hon)
Distinguished Service Professor
University of Pittsburgh
David Silver Professor and Chairman
Department of Orthopaedic Surgery
University of Pittsburgh School of Medicine
Head Team Physician
University of Pittsburgh Athletic Department
Pittsburgh, Pennsylvania

Itai Gans, MD
Chief Resident
Department of Orthopaedic Surgery
The Johns Hopkins Hospital
Baltimore, Maryland

Alan Getgood, MPhil, MD, FRCS (Tr&Orth)
Assistant Professor
Division of Orthopaedics
Department of Surgery
Western University
Consultant Orthopaedic Surgeon
Fowler Kennedy Sport Medicine Clinic
London, Ontario, Canada

Guillem Gonzalez-Lomas, MD
Assistant Professor
Department of Orthopedic Surgery
NYU Langone Health
New York, New York

Daniel Grande, PhD
Associate Professor and Director,
    Orthopedic Lab
Department of Orthopaedic Surgery
Feinstein Institute for Medical Research
Associate Professor
Department of Orthopaedic Surgery
Northwell Health System
Manhasset, New York

Max R. Greenky, MD
Orthopaedic Surgery Resident
Department of Orthopaedic Surgery
Thomas Jefferson University
Orthopaedic Surgery Resident
Department of Orthopaedic Surgery
Rothman Institute
Philadelphia, Pennsylvania

C. Thomas Haytmanek Jr, MD
Orthopaedic Surgeon
The Steadman Clinic
Steadman Philippon Research Institute
Orthopaedic Surgeon
Department of Surgery
Vail Health
Vail, Colorado

Justin J. Hicks, MD
Resident Physician
Orthopaedic Surgery
Washington University in St. Louis
Resident Physician
Orthopaedic Surgery
Barnes Jewish Hospital
St. Louis, Missouri

MaCalus V. Hogan, MD, MBA
Vice Chairman of Education and Residency Program
Director, Associate Professor
Department of Orthopaedic Surgery and Bioengineering
University of Pittsburgh
Chief
Division of Foot and Ankle Surgery
University of Pittsburgh Medical Center
Mercy Hospital
Pittsburgh, Pennsylvania

Jonathan D. Hughes, MD
Orthopedic Surgery Resident
Department of Orthopedic Surgery
Texas A&M College of Medicine–Baylor Scott & White
    Medical Center
Orthopaedic Surgery Resident
Department of Orthopaedic Surgery
Baylor Scott & White Medical Center–Temple
Temple, Texas

Zaamin B. Hussain, MA, MB BChir
Medical Doctor
Surgical Emergency Unit
Oxford University Hospitals
Oxford, United Kingdom

Darren L. Johnson, MD
Professor
Department of Orthopedic Surgery
University of Kentucky
Chief, Sports Medicine
Department of Orthopaedic Surgery
University of Kentucky
Lexington, Kentucky

Stephanie M. Jones, BA
Clinical Science Research Fellow
Foot and Ankle Injury Research Group
University of Pittsburgh
Pittsburgh, Pennsylvania

Scott G. Kaar, MD
Associate Professor
Department of Orthopaedic Surgery
Saint Louis University
St. Louis, Missouri

Patrick W. Kane, MD
Orthopaedic Surgeon
Department of Orthopaedics
Beebe Healthcare
Lewes, Delaware

Lee D. Kaplan, MD
Director
University of Miami Sports Medicine Institute
Petra and Stephen Levin Endowed Chair in Sports Medicine
University of Miami Sports Medicine Institute
University of Miami Miller School of Medicine
Coral Gables, Florida

Moin Khan, MD, MSc, FRCSC
Assistant Professor
Division of Orthopaedic Surgery
Department of Sports Medicine & Shoulder Surgery
McMaster University
Staff Physician
Department of Surgery
St. Joseph's Healthcare Hamilton
Hamilton, Ontario, Canada

Christopher Kim, MD, FRCS
Instructor
Department of Orthopaedic Surgery
Saint Louis University
St. Louis, Missouri

Hubert Kim, MD, PhD
Professor and Vice Chair
Department of Orthopedic Surgery
University of California, San Francisco
San Francisco, California

Jacob M. Kirsch, MD
Orthopedic Resident
Department of Orthopedic Surgery
University of Michigan
Ann Arbor, Michigan

Mininder S. Kocher, MD, MPH
Professor
Department of Orthopaedic Surgery
Harvard Medical School
Associate Director, Division of Sports Medicine
Orthopaedic Surgery
Boston Children's Hospital
Boston, Massachusetts

Marcin Kowalczuk, MD, FRCSC
Orthopaedic Surgeon
Department of Surgery
Lakeridge Health Ajax and Pickering Hospital
Ajax, Ontario, Canada

Joseph J. Kromka, MD
Resident
Department of Orthopedic Surgery
University of Pittsburgh Medical Center
Orthopaedic Surgery Resident
Foot and Ankle Injury Research Group
Department of Orthopaedic Surgery
University of Pittsburgh
Pittsburgh, Pennsylvania

Eric J. Kropf, MD
Associate Professor
Department of Orthopaedic Surgery
Lewis Katz SOM/Temple University
Chair
Department of Orthopedic Surgery and Sports Medicine
Temple University
Philadelphia, Pennsylvania

Bradley Kruckeberg, MD
Orthopedic Resident
Department of Orthopedic Surgery
Mayo Clinic
Rochester, Minnesota

Alexander S. Kuczmarski, MS
Medical Student
Department of Orthopaedic Surgery
The Warren Alpert Medical School of Brown University
Providence, Rhode Island

Drew A. Lansdown, MD
Assistant Professor in Residence
Sports Medicine & Shoulder Surgery
Orthopedic Surgery
University of California, San Francisco
San Francisco, California

Robert F. LaPrade, MD, PhD
Adjunct Professor
Department of Orthopaedic Surgery
University of Minnesota
Minneapolis, Minnesota
Chief Medical Officer
Steadman Philippon Research Institute
Vail Health Hospital
Vail, Colorado

Christopher M. Larson, MD
Program Director–FV/MOSMI Sports Medicine
    Fellowship
Twin Cities Orthopedics
Edina, Minnesota

George F. LeBus, MD
Physician
Orthopaedic Surgery
Texas Health Physicians Group Orthopaedic Specialty
    Associates
Fort Worth, Texas

Simon Lee, MD
House Officer
Orthopedic Surgery
University of Michigan
Ann Arbor, Michigan

Bryson P. Lesniak, MD
Associate Professor
Division of Sports Medicine
Department of Orthopedic Surgery
University of Pittsburgh Medical Center
Team Physician, University of Pittsburgh
Head Team Physician, Carnegie Mellon University
Pittsburgh, Pennsylvania

Ryan T. Li, MD
Sports Medicine Fellow
Department of Orthopaedic Surgery
University of Pittsburgh Medical Center
Pittsburgh, Pennsylvania

Albert Lin, MD
Associate Professor
Department of Orthopaedic Surgery
University of Pittsburgh
Associate Chief of Sports Medicine
Department of Orthopaedic Surgery
University of Pittsburgh Medical Center
Pittsburgh, Pennsylvania

C. Benjamin Ma, MD
Professor in Residence
Chief, Sports Medicine & Shoulder Surgery
Department of Orthopedic Surgery
University of California, San Francisco
San Francisco, California

Arthur R. McDowell, BS
Basic Science Research Fellow
Foot and Ankle Injury Research Group
Department of Orthopaedic Surgery
University of Pittsburgh School of Medicine
Pittsburgh, Pennsylvania

W. Scott McGuffin, MD, FRCSC
Clinical Fellow
Fowler Kennedy Sport Medicine Clinic
Western University
London, Ontario, Canada

Mitchell B. Meghpara, MD
Sports Medicine Fellow
Department of Orthopedic Surgery
University of Pittsburgh
Pittsburgh, Pennsylvania

Kellie K. Middleton, MD, MPH
Surgical Resident
Department of Orthopaedic Surgery
University of Pittsburgh Medical Center
Pittsburgh, Pennsylvania
Fellow
Orthopaedic Surgery Sports
Hospital for Special Surgery
New York, New York

Mark D. Miller, MD
S. Ward Casscells Professor
Department of Orthopaedic Surgery
University of Virginia
Charlottesville, Virginia

Peter J. Millett, MD, MSc
Director of Shoulder Surgery
Shoulder, Knee, Elbow and Sports Medicine
Orthopaedic Surgery at The Steadman Clinic
Center for Outcomes-Based Orthopaedic Research
Steadman Philippon Research Institute
Vail, Colorado

Emily Monroe, MD
Fellow, Sports Medicine
Department of Orthopedic Surgery
University of California, San Francisco
San Francisco, California

Bernard F. Morrey, MD
Professor
Orthopedic Surgery
Mayo Clinic
Rochester, Minnesota
University of Texas Health Center
Professor
San Antonio, Texas

Mark Morrey, MD, MSc
Associate Professor
Department of Orthopedic Surgery
Mayo Clinic
Rochester, Minnesota

Kyle Muckenhirn, BA
Research Assistant
Department of Biomedical Engineering
Steadman Philippon Research Institute
Vail, Colorado

Conor I. Murphy, MD
Resident Physician
Department of Orthopedic Surgery
University of Pittsburgh Medical Center
Pittsburgh, Pennsylvania

Volker Musahl, MD
Associate Professor
Department of Orthopaedic Surgery and Bioengineering
University of Pittsburgh Medical Center
Chief of Sports Medicine and Medical Director
UPMC Rooney Sports Complex
University of Pittsburgh
Pittsburgh, Pennsylvania

Neal B. Naveen, BS
Researcher
Department of Orthopedics
Rush University Medical Center
Chicago, Illinois

Russell Nord, MD
Chairman
Orthopaedic Surgery Section
Washington Hospital
Fremont, California

Benedict U. Nwachukwu, MD, MBA
Sports Medicine Fellow
Midwest Orthopaedics at Rush
Chicago, Illinois

Brett D. Owens, MD
Professor of Orthopaedic Surgery
Department of Orthopaedic Surgery
Brown University Alpert Medical School
East Providence, Rhode Island

Thierry Pauyo, MD, FRCSC
Assistant Professor
Department of Orthopedic Surgery
McGill University
Assistant Professor
Orthopedic Surgery
Montreal Children & Shriners Hospital
Montreal, Quebec, Canada

Jonas Pogorzelski, MD, MHBA
Research Fellow
International Scholars Program
Steadman Philippon Research Institute
Vail, Colorado
Technical University of Munich
Department of Orthopaedic Sports Medicine
Munich, Germany

Christopher Potts, MD
Orthopedic Sports Medicine Surgeon
Department of Orthopedic Sports Medicine
Northside Hospital
Atlanta, Georgia

Stephen J. Rabuck, MD
Clinical Assistant Professor
Department of Orthopaedic Surgery
University of Pittsburgh School of Medicine
Clinical Assistant Professor
Department of Orthopaedic Surgery
University of Pittsburgh Medical Center
Pittsburgh, Pennsylvania

Mikel L. Reilingh, MD, PhD
Orthopaedic Surgeon
Department of Orthopaedic Surgery
St. Antonius Hospital
Utrecht, The Netherlands

Samuel I. Rosenberg, BA
Researcher
Department of Biomedical Engineering
Steadman Philippon Research Institute
Vail, Colorado

James R. Ross, MD
Associate Professor
Department of Orthopedic Surgery
College of Medicine
Florida Atlantic University
BocaCare Orthopedics–Boca Raton Regional Hospital
Boca Raton, Florida

Benjamin B. Rothrauff, MD, PhD
Postdoctoral Fellow
Department of Orthopaedic Surgery
University of Pittsburgh Medical Center
Pittsburgh, Pennsylvania

Marc R. Safran, MD
Professor
Department of Orthopaedic Surgery
Stanford University
Stanford, California
Chief
Division of Sports Medicine
Department of Orthopaedic Surgery
Stanford University
Redwood City, California

Alexander M. Satin, MD
Resident Physician
Department of Orthopaedic Surgery
Donald and Barbara Zucker School of Medicine at Hofstra/
  Northwell
Hofstra University
Resident Physician
Department of Orthopaedic Surgery
Long Island Jewish Medical Center
New Hyde Park, New York

William Schulz, BS
Medical Student
Department of Orthopaedic Surgery
University of Pittsburgh School of Medicine
Pittsburgh, Pennsylvania

Andrew Schwartz, MD
Resident
Department of Orthopaedics
Emory University
Resident
Department of Orthopaedics
Emory University Orthopaedics and Spine Hospital
Atlanta, Georgia

Jon K. Sekiya, MD
Professor
Department of Orthopaedic Surgery
University of Michigan
Ann Arbor, Michigan

Nicholas A. Sgaglione, MD
Professor and Chair
Department of Orthopedic Surgery
Northwell Health
Great Neck, New York

Humza S. Shaikh, MD
Surgical Resident
Department of Orthopaedic Surgery
University of Pittsburgh Medical Center
Pittsburgh, Pennsylvania

Jason J. Shin, MD, FRCSC
Assistant Professor
Department of Surgery
University of Saskatchewan
Saskatoon, Canada
Staff Surgeon
Department of Surgery
F.H. Wigmore Hospital
Moose Jaw, Saskatchewan, Canada

Michael Shin, MD
Orthopaedic Surgeon
Valley Orthopaedics & Sports Medicine
Spring Valley, Illinois

Mark Slabaugh, MD
Associate Professor
Department of Surgery
Uniformed Services University of the Health Sciences
Bethesda, Maryland
Chief of Sports Medicine
Department of Orthopaedics
U.S. Air Force Academy
USAFA, Colorado

Harris Slone, MD
Assistant Professor
Department of Orthopaedics
Medical University of South Carolina
Surgeon
Division of Sports Medicine
Department of Orthopaedics
MUSC Health
Charleston, South Carolina

Jeremy S. Somerson, MD
Assistant Professor of Orthopedic Surgery
Department of Orthopaedic Surgery
University of Texas Medical Branch
Galveston, Texas

Taylor M. Southworth, BS
Researcher
Department of Orthopedics
Rush University Medical Center
Chicago, Illinois

Spencer M. Stein, MD
Resident Physician
Department of Orthopaedic Surgery
Donald and Barbara Zucker School of Medicine at Hofstra/
    Northwell
Hofstra University
Hempstead, New York
Resident Physician
Department of Orthopaedic Surgery
Long Island Jewish Medical Center
New Hyde Park, New York

Miho J. Tanaka, MD
Director
Women's Sports Medicine Program
Department of Orthopaedic Surgery
Johns Hopkins Medicine
Baltimore, Maryland

Tracy M. Tauro, BS, BA
Research Assistant
Researcher
Department of Orthopedics
Rush University Medical Center
Chicago, Illinois

Ekaterina Urch, MD
Orthopaedic Surgeon
Department of Sports Medicine
The Center–Orthopedic and Neurosurgical Care and
    Research
Bend, Oregon

C. Niek van Dijk, MD, PhD
Professor
Orthopaedic Surgeon
Department of Orthopaedic Surgery
Academic Medical Center
Amsterdam, The Netherlands

Maayke van Sterkenburg, MD, PhD
Trauma Surgeon
Department of Surgery
North West Hospital Group
Alkmaar, The Netherlands

Danica Davies Vance, MD
Resident Physician
Department of Orthopaedic Surgery
Columbia University Medical Center
New York, New York

Zachary Vaughn, MD
Clinical Assistant Professor
Department of Orthopaedic Surgery & Sports Medicine
Stanford University
Los Gatos, California

Armando F. Vidal, MD
Associate Professor
Department of Orthopedic Surgery
University of Colorado School of Medicine
Denver, Colorado

Dharmesh Vyas, MD, PhD
Assistant Professor of Orthopedic Surgery
Department of Orthopaedic Surgery
University of Pittsburgh Medical Center
Pittsburgh, Pennsylvania

Megan Walters, MD
Fellow
Foot and Ankle Surgery
Department of Orthopaedics and Sports Medicine
Harborview Medical Center
University of Washington
Seattle, Washington

Juntian Wang, MD
Resident
Department of Orthopaedic Surgery
Cedars-Sinai Medical Center
Los Angeles, California

J. Kristopher Ware, MD, DPT
Orthopedic Surgeon
Department of Orthopedic Surgery
Orthopedic Associates of Hartford/Hartford Hospital
Hartford, Connecticut

Jeffrey C. Wera, MD
Resident Physician
Orthopaedic Surgery and Sports Medicine
Lewis Katz School of Medicine at Temple University
Philadelphia, Pennsylvania

Robin Vereeke West, MD
Associate Professor
Department of Orthopaedics
Georgetown University Medical Center
Washington, District of Columbia
Chairman, Inova Sports Medicine
Inova Medical Group Orthopaedics and Sports Medicine
Inova Fairfax Hospital and Inova Loudoun Hospital
Fairfax, Virginia

Megan R. Wolf, MD
Resident
Department of Orthopaedic Surgery
University of Connecticut Health Center
Farmington, Connecticut

Vonda Joy Wright, MD, MS, FAOA
Chief of Sports Medicine
Northside Hospital Orthopedic Institute
Northside Hospital System
Alpharetta, Georgia

Frank B. Wydra, MD
Resident
Department of Orthopedics
University of Colorado School of Medicine
Resident
Department of Orthopedics
University of Colorado Hospital
Aurora, Colorado

John Xerogeanes, MD
Chief of Sports Medicine
Professor of Orthopaedic Surgery
Emory University School of Medicine
Head Orthopaedist and Team Physician
Georgia Tech, Emory University, Agnes Scott College and
    the Atlanta Dream Basketball Club
Medical Director Atlanta Hawks Basketball Club
Team Orthopaedist, Atlanta Braves
Atlanta, Georgia

Alan Yong Yan, MD
Assistant Professor
Department of Orthopedic Surgery
University of Pittsburgh Medical Center
Attending
Foot and Ankle Division
Mercy Hospital
Pittsburgh, Pennsylvania

M. Christopher Yonz, MD
Orthopaedic Surgeon
Summit Sports Medicine and Orthopaedic Surgery
Southeast Georgia Health System
St. Marys, Georgia

Jason P. Zlotnicki, MD
Orthopaedic Surgery Resident
Orthopaedic Surgery
University of Pittsburgh Medical Center
Pittsburgh, Pennsylvania

Series Preface

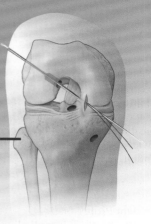

Since its inception in 1994, the *Master Techniques in Orthopaedic Surgery* series has become the gold standard for both physicians in training and experienced surgeons. Its exceptional success may be traced to the leadership of the original series editor, Roby Thompson, whose clarity of thought and focused vision sought "to provide direct, detailed access to techniques preferred by orthopedic surgeons who are recognized by their colleagues as 'masters' in their specialty," as he stated in his series preface. It is personally very rewarding to hear testimonials from both residents and practicing orthopedic surgeons on the value of these volumes to their training and practice.

A key element of the success of the series is its format. The effectiveness of the format is reflected by the fact that it is now being replicated by others. An essential feature is the standardized presentation of information replete with tips and pearls shared by experts with years of experience.

Abundant color photographs and drawings guide the reader through the procedures step-by-step.

The second key to the success of the *Master Techniques* series rests in the reputation and experience of our volume editors. The editors are truly dedicated "masters" with a commitment to share their rich experience through these texts. We feel a great debt of gratitude to them and a real responsibility to maintain and enhance the reputation of the *Master Techniques* series that has developed over the years. We are proud of the progress made in formulating the third edition volumes and are particularly pleased with the expanded content of this series. Six new volumes will soon be available covering topics that are exciting and relevant to a broad cross section of our profession. While we are in the process of carefully expanding *Master Techniques* topics and editors, we are committed to the now-classic format.

The first of the new volumes is *Relevant Surgical Exposures*, which I have had the honor of editing. The second new volume is *Essential Procedures in Pediatrics*. Subsequent new topics to be introduced are *Soft Tissue Reconstruction*, *Management of Peripheral Nerve Dysfunction*, *Advanced Reconstructive Techniques in the Joint*, and finally *Essential Procedures in Sports Medicine*. The full library thus will consist of 16 useful and relevant titles.

I am pleased to have accepted the position of series editor, feeling so strongly about the value of this series to educate the orthopedic surgeon in the full array of expert surgical procedures. The true worth of this endeavor will continue to be measured by the ever-increasing success and critical acceptance of the series. I remain indebted to Dr. Thompson for his inaugural vision and leadership, as well as to the *Master Techniques* volume editors and numerous contributors who have been true to the series style and vision. As I indicated in the preface to the second edition of *The Hip* volume, the words of William Mayo are especially relevant to characterize the ultimate goal of this endeavor: "The best interest of the patient is the only interest to be considered." We are confident that the information in the expanded *Master Techniques* offers the surgeon an opportunity to realize the patient-centric view of our surgical practice.

Bernard F. Morrey, MD

Preface

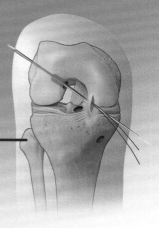

This is the second edition of the *Master Techniques in Orthopedic Surgery* series dedicated to sports medicine and provides the orthopedic surgeon with a comprehensive overview of current pathology and treatment in field of sports medicine. We have included new advances and novel approaches in the areas of shoulder, elbow, hip, knee, ankle, and foot to provide a comprehensive update of the first edition.

Since the publication of the first edition of this text, there has been continued innovation and evolution of surgical techniques in sports medicine. Tremendous efforts have been made in improving outcomes in the treatment of musculoskeletal injuries with the use of minimally invasive arthroscopic techniques and advanced rehabilitation protocols.

Our "masters" in the field of sports medicine have once again shared their approaches to common and uncommon procedures in an expanded collection of 59 chapters that represent the current standard of care for musculoskeletal injuries.

Bryson P. Lesniak, MD
Associate Professor
Division of Sports Medicine
Department of Orthopedic Surgery
University of Pittsburgh Medical Center
Team Physician, University of Pittsburgh
Head Team Physician, Carnegie Mellon University
Pittsburgh, Pennsylvania

Freddie H. Fu, MD, DSci (Hon), DPs (Hon)
Distinguished Service Professor
University of Pittsburgh
David Silver Professor and Chairman
Department of Orthopaedic Surgery
University of Pittsburgh School of Medicine
Head Team Physician
University of Pittsburgh Athletic Department
Pittsburgh, Pennsylvania

Preface to the First Edition

This is the first of the *Master Techniques in Orthopaedic Surgery* series dedicated to sports medicine and provides the orthopedic surgeon with a comprehensive overview of current pathology and treatment in field of sports medicine including new advances and novel approaches in the areas of shoulder, hip, knee, and foot.

Over the past several years, there has been an international explosion in sports medicine research. Tremendous efforts have been made in improving outcomes in the treatment of musculoskeletal injuries with the use of minimally invasive arthroscopic techniques and advanced rehabilitation protocols.

Many well-respected "masters" in the field of sports medicine have shared in an expanded collection of 54 chapters an overview of the current standard of care for musculoskeletal injuries.

Freddie H. Fu, MD, DSci (Hon), DPs (Hon)
Distinguished Service Professor
University of Pittsburgh
David Silver Professor and Chairman
Department of Orthopaedic Surgery
University of Pittsburgh School of Medicine
Head Team Physician
University of Pittsburgh Athletic Department

Acknowledgments

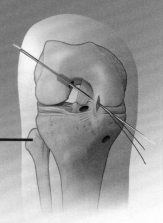

First and foremost, I would like to thank each author for her or his expertise and willingness to share it with our peers and colleagues. Further thanks to the publishing staff at Wolters Kluwer who worked tirelessly throughout the preparation of this text. I would also like to extend my gratitude to Darci Garofolo PA-C and Ruth Pesante, my clinical and administrative team, for their irreplaceable assistance with my clinical practice, which allowed me to dedicate the proper time and effort to this project.

I would also like to thank Dr. Freddie Fu for inviting me to join him in shepherding this volume of the masters' series. It is a true honor to work with Dr. Fu not only on this project but also in clinical practice.

Finally, I would be remiss to not extend my deepest thanks to my wife, Meg, and two daughters, Audrey and Addison, for enduring my hours of evening and late night work on the computer. Your patience and understanding were gracious and selfless. This endeavor was impossible without your understanding and support.

Bryson P. Lesniak, MD

My thanks to each of the contributing authors for sharing their sports medicine expertise and for the many hours spent in preparing their manuscripts.

I would also like to thank Dr. Bryson P. Lesniak for his tedious work on this project.

Finally, my thanks to Dr. Bernard F. Morrey who invited me to undertake the editorship of this volume of the masters' series and to the staff at Wolters Kluwer for their determination and diligence in bringing this one-of-a-kind book to fruition.

Freddie H. Fu, MD, DSci (Hon), DPs (Hon)

Contents

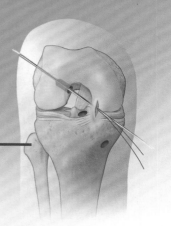

PART II Shoulder

PART III Knee

PART IV   Hip

PART V   Ankle

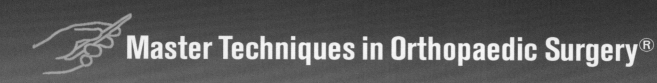

Sports Medicine

SECOND EDITION

1 Valgus Extension Overload

Danica Davies Vance, Frank J. Alexander, and Christopher S. Ahmad

ETIOLOGY

Originally described by Bennett in 1959 (1), valgus extension overload (VEO) develops in the overhead athlete from distinctive forces created at the elbow during repetitive high-velocity throwing. Three major forces across the elbow are generated: tension on the medial aspect, compression on the lateral aspect, and shear on the posterior aspect. In 1969, King et al. (2) clinically described this same condition as "medial elbow–stress syndrome" consisting of a triad of medial soft tissue insufficiency, posteromedial compartment impingement, and lateral compartment chondrosis. Wilson et al. (3) in 1983 then postulated the mechanism of VEO as a wedging effect of the olecranon in the olecranon fossa during the acceleration phase of throwing. While these early descriptions gave insight into the condition, more recent research has further elucidated the etiology.

During overhand throwing, valgus torque and rapid extension results in major forces across the elbow that are resisted by articular, ligamentous, and muscular restraints. Valgus torque is estimated to reach 64 Nm during the late cocking and early acceleration phases of throwing. The anterior bundle of the medial ulnar collateral ligament (MUCL) serves as the primary resistor to these forces and therefore is often compromised. Toward full elbow extension, the bony articulation has greater contribution to elbow stability than the MUCL, and in the posterior compartment, shear forces are developed between the posteromedial olecranon and trochlea (4). The angular velocities extending the elbow are estimated to reach 5,000 degrees/s in the acceleration phase of throwing (5). The established arm momentum generated during the acceleration phase must then be decelerated in the follow-through phase. When deceleration is poorly controlled by the dynamic muscle forces, the olecranon traumatically abuts the posterior compartment toward full extension. Thus, the olecranon is subject to injury from both valgus and extension forces, described as VEO. The repetitive forceful shearing of the olecranon within its fossa leads to posteromedial olecranon chondromalacia and osteophyte formation as shown in Figure 1-1. Posteromedial osteophytes are often observed in asymptomatic throwers, and it has been postulated that symptoms most commonly develop when the osteophyte fractures and goes onto nonunion (6).

The relationship of posteromedial impingement and valgus stability has been a focus of several biomechanical studies (7–9). Ahmad et al. (7) demonstrated in cadavers that existing MUCL insufficiency causes contact alterations in the posteromedial compartment that factor into the development of symptomatic chondrosis and osteophyte formation that manifests as VEO syndrome. This suggests that clinically, patients with symptomatic VEO with posteromedial impingement may have valgus instability, although the instability may not be the presenting symptom.

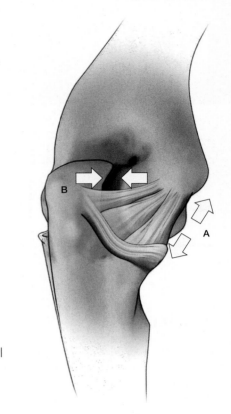

FIGURE 1-1

In the posterior compartment, the olecranon is subjected to medial shearing forces with valgus stress, which may be accentuated by increased valgus laxity. *A*, ligament tension; *B*, posterior medial contact and shear.

HISTORY

Patients will classically present with a history of repetitive overhead activity. Although VEO is most common in baseball pitchers, it has also been documented in several other sports including javelin throwing, football, tennis, and lacrosse. For isolated posteromedial impingement, elbow pain is localized to the medial aspect of the olecranon and usually occurs just after ball release during the deceleration phase of throwing. This phase of throwing is where the elbow approaches full extension. Pain during the acceleration phase should increase the suspicion for medial elbow instability that often occurs concomitantly (10). Patients may report limited extension from posterior impingement due to osteophytes or locking and catching from loose bodies. Other complaints often include difficulty warming up, fatigue, popping, and decreased performance such as loss of pitch, velocity, and accuracy. Ulnar neuritis and subluxation may occur concomitantly, and therefore, a history of numbness or paresthesias in the fourth and fifth digits should be ascertained. Additionally, a thorough history of prior MUCL or ulnar nerve injury and subsequent treatment should be obtained.

PHYSICAL EXAMINATION

Osteophytes on the posteromedial olecranon observed on imaging studies do not always cause impingement pain. Therefore, it is critical to confirm the diagnosis of symptomatic VEO using history and physical examination. The patient will exhibit tenderness and crepitus with palpation over the posterior medial olecranon. Often there will be a loss of terminal elbow extension with active range of motion (ROM).

The extension impingement test should be performed on all patients with suspected VEO. The examiner performs this test by quickly snapping the patient's partially flexed elbow into terminal extension. Reproduction of posterior or posteromedial pain that is similar to the pain felt while throwing is considered a positive exam. Simultaneous valgus load during the maneuver will typically increase the pain, while varus will diminish the pain.

The arm bar test is performed with the patient's hand placed on the examiner's shoulder with their shoulder in 90 degrees of forward elevation and full internal rotation. The examiner then pulls down on the olecranon, leveraging the elbow into extension. In the setting of posteromedial impingement, pain will be elicited.

The MUCL must be evaluated in all throwers presenting with medial elbow pain using direct palpation and the moving valgus stress test. Examination of the ulnar nerve involves assessing intrinsic muscle weakness or wasting, Tinel sign, and subluxation of the nerve.

IMAGING STUDIES

Anterior-posterior, lateral, oblique, and axillary views of the elbow may reveal posteromedial olecranon osteophytes and/or loose bodies (Fig. 1-2). Conway et al. also have described a posterior impingement view to assist in assessment of patients with suspected valgus extension syndrome (Conway AOSS Elbow Arthroscopy ICL 2009). The radiograph is a modified AP with the humerus in 40 degrees of external rotation and 140 degrees of flexion. The best imaging study overall is a CT scan with two-dimensional sagittal (Fig. 1-3) and coronal reconstructions and three-dimensional surface renderings (Fig. 1-4) to demonstrate the overall morphologic changes, loose bodies, and osteophyte fragmentation. Magnetic resonance imaging (MRI) is also informative, especially if MUCL pathology is expected. MRI can also demonstrate osteochondral damage, synovial plicae, edema, and early stress fractures that can occur in the olecranon. Stress fractures can occur in the setting of a normal MRI, and if suspected, a bone scan can be useful.

INDICATIONS/CONTRAINDICATIONS

VEO is a condition that affects throwing athletes primarily and is rare in nonthrowing athletes. An initial course of nonoperative treatment consists of activity modification with a period of rest from throwing, intra-articular cortisone injections, and nonsteroidal anti-inflammatory drugs (NSAIDs). Pitching mechanics should be evaluated, and proper instruction should be instituted to correct any flaws that may be contributing to the injury. After a period of rest, a progressive throwing program is instituted under the direct supervision of experienced physical therapists and athletic trainers. Surgical treatment is indicated for those patients who maintain symptoms despite nonoperative management and wish to return to the same level of competition.

In a report of professional baseball players who underwent olecranon debridement, 25% developed valgus instability and eventually required MUCL reconstruction. Subsequent basic science studies have demonstrated that excessive olecranon resection increases the demands on the MUCL

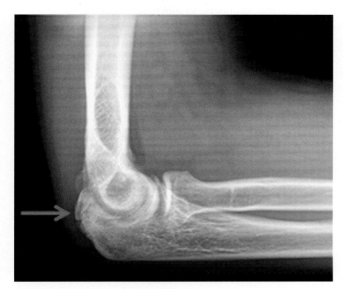

FIGURE 1-2

Lateral radiograph of the elbow demonstrating posteromedial osteophyte (red arrow).

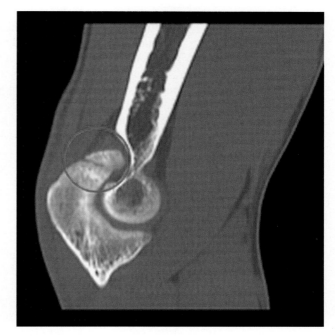

FIGURE 1-3

Sagittal CT scan clearly demarcating the posterior osteophyte in the olecranon.

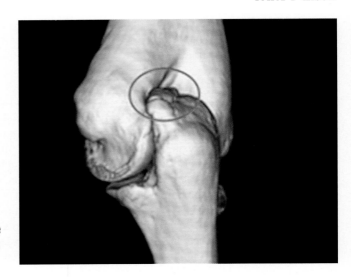

FIGURE 1-4

Three-dimensional reconstruction of the elbow showing morphology and precise location of the osteophyte.

during valgus stress and increases valgus instability (8,9). These studies, therefore, suggest that MUCL insufficiency may develop following posteromedial decompression, and consequently, current recommendations are to limit olecranon resection to osteophytes only and avoid removal of normal olecranon. It has also been demonstrated that existing MUCL insufficiency created in cadavers causes contact alterations in the posteromedial compartment that may be the cause of symptomatic chondrosis and osteophyte formation that eventually manifests as VEO syndrome (7). In addition, osteophyte formation may make the elbow clinically stable despite MUCL injury, and thus, treating the bony impingement with osteotomy may convert an asymptomatic MUCL into a painful MUCL. In summary, patients with posteromedial elbow pain should have a thorough evaluation of the MUCL, and overaggressive resection of posteromedial osteophytes should be avoided (7).

SURGERY

There are several options for anesthesia including regional, general, or a combination. Regional anesthesia optimizes postoperative pain control, reduces postoperative nausea, and facilitates patient positioning. A disadvantage is the inability to perform a thorough postoperative neurologic exam of the operative extremity. Advantages of general anesthesia include total muscle relaxation, more options for patient positioning including prone, and the ability to test nerve function at the end of the case. Disadvantages include higher risk of nausea, more postoperative pain, and longer postoperative unit stay.

Patients may be positioned in a supine, prone, or lateral decubitus position. The lateral decubitus position with a nonsterile tourniquet and arm support is the preferred position. The lateral position places the shoulder in 90 degrees of abduction, with the elbow flexed 90 degrees while suspended over an arm holder (Fig. 1-5). The arm is draped free so that it can be manipulated during surgery to improve arthroscopic access. A beanbag is used to pad the patient and hold him or her securely

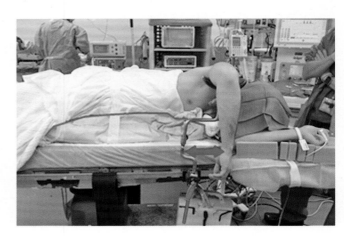

FIGURE 1-5

Lateral decubitus position. The shoulder is placed in 90 degrees of flexion and maintained over lateral arm support to allow enough room near the thorax for medial-sided work. The arm is free to allow flexion and extension. The level of the beanbag is correctly positioned (see *red line*) to avoid any interference with the trajectory of surgical instruments.

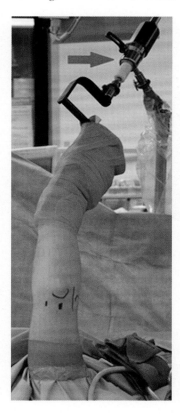

FIGURE 1-6

Alternate patient positioning for cases with concurrent open procedures. An articulating arm holder fixed to the contralateral side of the OR table (*red arrow*) suspends the arm across the body.

in place during the operation. An axillary roll is placed under the contralateral axilla to support the chest and prevent damage to the brachial plexus. In cases where open procedures are warranted, such as an ulnar nerve transposition or MUCL reconstruction, it is preferred that the patient be in the supine position with a Spider arm holder on the contralateral side. In such instances, arthroscopy precedes open procedures (Fig. 1-6).

The arm should be brought into a full 90 degrees of abduction as less abduction can cause impingement against the torso while working on the ulnar side of the elbow. Also, the arm holder should be placed close to the axilla to allow access to the anterior compartment. Advantages to the lateral position include the ability to easily manipulate the elbow, access to both anterior and posterior compartments, without the requirement of additional equipment such as a hydraulic arm holder. Disadvantages include need to reposition if conversion to an open procedure is required, such as an MCL reconstruction or ulnar nerve transposition, and limited access if the patient is obese.

PORTALS

At the start of the procedure, all relevant surface anatomy is outlined including all bony landmarks, potential portals, the ulnar nerve, and the proposed olecranon osteophyte (Figs. 1-7 and 1-8). Using the lateral soft spot (between the lateral epicondyle, radial head, and olecranon), the elbow joint is insufflated with 10 to 15 cc of normal saline.

Arthroscopy begins with establishment of the *proximal anteromedial portal* for visualization. The anterior compartment is evaluated for chondral injuries, loose bodies, synovitis, and synovial plica. The portal is located 2 cm above the medial epicondyle and approximately 1 cm anterior to the intermuscular septum. The medial antebrachial cutaneous nerve is the structure most at risk as it is located on average 2.3 mm from the cannula. The ulnar nerve is on average 12 to 23 mm from the portal. Prior transposition of the nerve or subluxation requires exposure or identification of the nerve prior to placing the portal.

The *proximal anterolateral portal* is used as a working portal to debride the anterior compartment. It is located 2 cm proximal to the lateral epicondyle and is placed directly on the anterior surface of the humerus under direct visualization (11,12). The posterior antebrachial cutaneous nerve is on average 6.1 mm away but lies in direct contact with the cannula 29% of the time (12). The radial nerve lies 4.9 mm away in extension and 9.9 mm away in flexion.

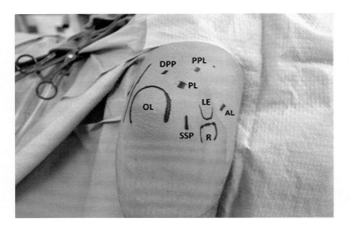

FIGURE 1-7

Posterolateral view of the elbow. OL, olecranon; R, radial head; LE, lateral epicondyle; SSP, soft spot portal; DDP, direct posterior portal; PL, posterolateral portal; PPL, proximal posterolateral portal.

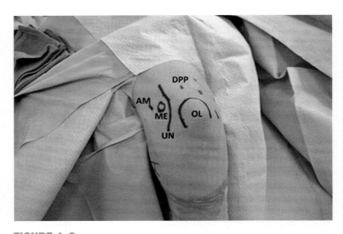

FIGURE 1-8

Posteromedial view of elbow. DDP, direct posterior portal; AM, anteromedial portal; O, olecranon; UN, ulnar nerve; ME, medial epicondyle; OL, olecranon.

The primary portals for managing posteromedial impingement from VEO are the superior posterolateral portal and the direct posterior portal. The *posterolateral portal* can be located anywhere from the tip of the olecranon to 3 cm proximal in the posterolateral gutter just off of the triceps tendon. For posteromedial debridement, we prefer to make it 1 cm proximal to the olecranon tip. The elbow is held in 30 degrees of flexion to relax the triceps while establishing the portal. It has one of the largest areas of safety. It provides excellent visualization of the entire posterior compartment and can be useful in debriding the olecranon fossa, tip of the olecranon, and lateral gutter when necessary.

The *direct posterior portal* splits the triceps in its midline 3 cm proximal to the olecranon tip. It is the workhorse portal for VEO and is used for debriding posteromedial olecranon osteophytes, removing loose bodies, and addressing any posterior chondral lesions. The *soft spot portal* is located in the center of the triangle formed by the lateral epicondyle, tip of the olecranon, and radial head. It is useful in insufflating the elbow joint and debriding posterolateral plica and osteochondritis dissecans (OCD) of the capitellum.

TECHNIQUE

After anesthesia is established, the patient is appropriately positioned, prepped, and draped. Next, all relevant anatomic landmarks are marked including all bony landmarks, potential portals, the ulnar nerve, and the proposed olecranon osteophyte. Next, 1 to 2 cc of local anesthetic is injected into each marked portal sight. An Esmarch bandage is applied, and the tourniquet is raised to exsanguinate.

At this point, the elbow is insufflated using 30 cc of normal saline introduced through an 18-gauge needle into the soft spot lateral portal (Fig. 1-9). The joint distention facilitates the introduction of the trocar but more importantly shifts the neurovascular structures further away from the bone thereby decreasing risk of nerve injury. The procedure begins with an anterior compartment arthroscopy. A superficial incision is made with an 11 blade scalpel through the skin at the proximal medial portal. Next, the soft tissues are spread with a blunt clamp to prevent injury to the neurovascular structures. A blunt-tipped trocar is introduced into the anterior compartment hugging the anterior humerus and directed toward the radiocapitellar joint (Fig. 1-10).

Diagnostic arthroscopy is performed anteriorly to look for loose bodies and thoroughly examine the articular cartilage and synovium. The anterior radiocapitellar joint is evaluated for osteochondral lesions of the capitellum and the radial head. The coronoid tip and fossa are then examined for osteophytes followed by visualization of the trochlea and any cartilage lesions present. The anterior capsule is evaluated for thickening or contracture in the context of a loss of passive extension. Of note, the radial nerve lies in close proximity to the anterolateral capsule so any debridement in this area should utilize a retractor such as a switching stick introduced through an accessory portal and/or minimal suction with the hood of the shaver to the capsule to prevent iatrogenic injury. To test

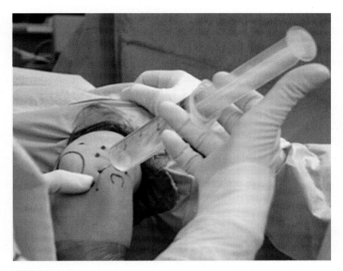

FIGURE 1-9
Joint insufflation is achieved with a 60-cc syringe through an 18-gauge needle in the soft spot portal.

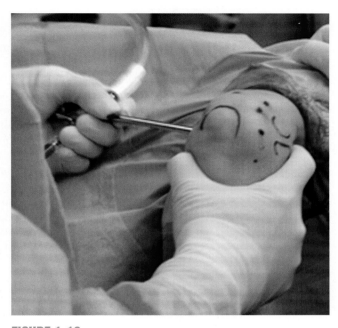

FIGURE 1-10
The anterior elbow joint is entered through the anteromedial portal with a blunt trocar and arthroscopic cannula. Counter pressure is applied to stabilize the elbow.

for MUCL insufficiency, an arthroscopic valgus stress test is performed. With the arthroscope in the proximal lateral portal visualizing the medial compartment, a valgus stress is applied manually to the elbow. A gap of 3 mm or more seen between the coronoid process and medial trochlea supports MUCL insufficiency (13).

After completion of the anterior arthroscopy, a posterolateral portal is then established with the elbow held in 30 degrees of flexion for viewing (Fig. 1-11). A direct posterior portal is then

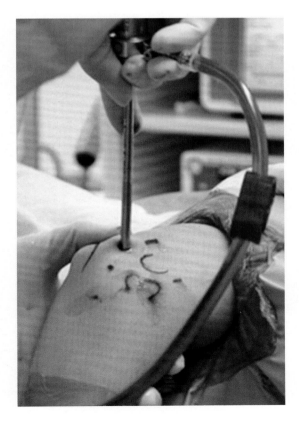

FIGURE 1-11
Establishment of the posterolateral portal.

established as a working portal. Diagnostic arthroscopy is then performed evaluating for osteo-phytes on the posteromedial aspect of the olecranon, loose bodies in the lateral gutter, and any evidence of chondromalacia. Synovial reflections, fibrous tissue, and any other extra soft tissue that obscures visualization may be removed using a cautery or a shaver. We prefer to use a 3.5-mm nonaggressive shaver for this purpose. The posterior radiocapitellar joint can also be inspected from the posterolateral portal.

The pathology of a fractured osteophyte on the posteromedial olecranon is identified with the camera in the posterolateral portal. The osteophyte may be encased in soft tissue and often requires probing and a debridement with a shaver introduced in the direct posterior portal before it can be fully appreciated. A small osteotome/elevator is inserted through the direct posterior portal to free the osteophytes, as shown in Figure 1-12. The olecranon can be further contoured with a burr and shaver (Fig. 1-13). Often, osteophytes are also present in the olecranon fossa, which are debrided as well. Once the osteophyte is removed, which may be performed using a tissue grasper (Fig. 1-14) or burr, the humeral chondral surface can be visualized more completely, and the kissing lesion of chondral abrasion opposite the osteophyte will be in direct view. For large osteophyte fragments, removal through the posterolateral portal is preferred as there are fewer layers of soft tissue between the elbow joint and skin. If a "kissing" injury is present, standard principles apply. Loose chondral flaps should be debrided, and if necessary, microfracture or Antegrade drilling can be performed. Creation of perforations 2 to 3 mm apart allows the release of bone marrow elements and induces the formation of a fibrocartilage healing response (Fig. 1-15). When olecranon contouring is com-plete (Fig. 1-16), a lateral radiograph may be obtained intraoperatively to assess adequacy of bone removal. It is imperative to recognize the position of the ulnar nerve just superficial to the capsule in the posteromedial gutter. Avoid the use of cautery and suction when the shaver is near this area of the capsule.

It is preferred to remove only the olecranon osteophytes present and to not remove any of the normal bone (8). Should there be a lack of optimal visualization, it is preferred to remove more bone from the humeral side if there is doubt whether debridement is sufficient. This is intuitive as increased posteromedial olecranon resection increases the amount of elbow valgus and subsequently the strain placed on the MUCL.

Once the arthroscopy is completed, the fluid is evacuated from the posterior cannulas, and the portals are closed with simple interrupted 4-0 nylon. If MUCL reconstruction or ulnar nerve trans-position is needed, the patient's arm is taken down from the Spider and open procedures may begin. The technique for MUCL reconstruction is addressed in Chapter 2.

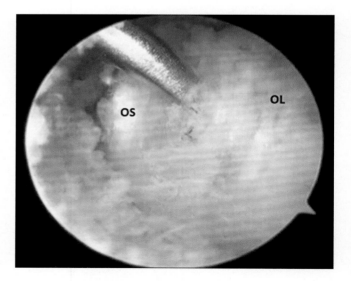

FIGURE 1-12

Osteophyte on olecranon tip with osteotome in position. OS, osteophyte; OL, olecranon.

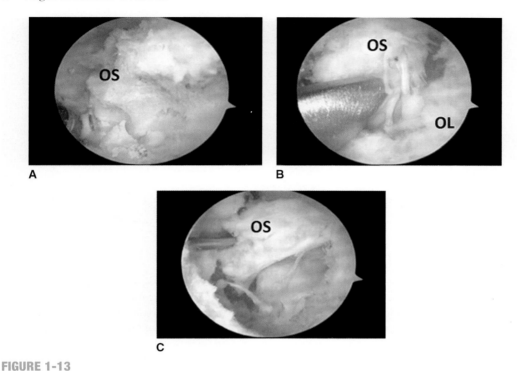

FIGURE 1-13

A, **B**, and **C** showing the use of cautery **(A)** and an elevator **(B, C)** to free the main fragment of the osteophyte (OS) from the surrounding soft tissue and normal olecranon (OL) bone.

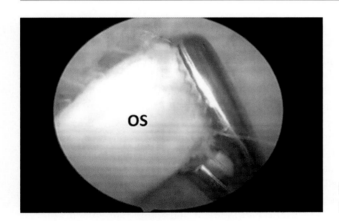

FIGURE 1-14

Removal of osteophyte. OS, osteophyte.

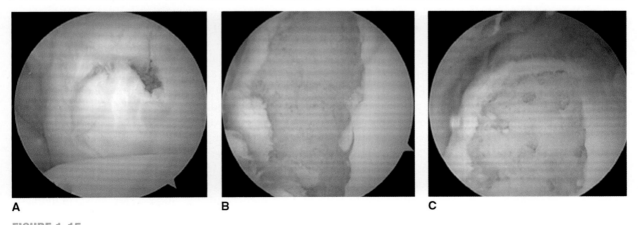

FIGURE 1-15

Debridement and microfracture of associated chondral lesion. **A:** Unstable cartilage lesion. **B:** After debridement of loose flaps. **C:** After microfracture.

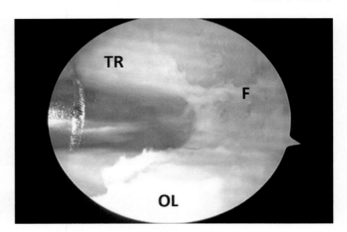

FIGURE 1-16

Contouring of the olecranon fossa to restore the anatomic fossa. OL, olecranon; TR, trochlea; F, olecranon fossa. (Photo courtesy of Dr. Christopher S. Ahmad.)

POSTOPERATIVE MANAGEMENT

The patient is placed in a compressive dressing and simple sling postoperatively. The dressing may be removed on postoperative day 1, and the patient may shower keeping the incisions dry. The sling is worn for comfort only and discontinued within 1 week. Active elbow flexion and extension exercises are initiated immediately. Emphasis is also placed on restoring flexor-pronator strength, as well maintaining rotator cuff and periscapular muscle strength to avoid shoulder injuries upon return to throwing. At 6 weeks, a progressive throwing program is begun and plyometric exercises and neuromuscular training are enhanced. Return to competition is typically allowed at 3 to 4 months postoperatively after the patient demonstrates full ROM, no pain or tenderness to stress testing and palpation, and full strength of the involved extremity.

RESULTS

With the improvement in arthroscopy equipment and a clear understanding of portal placement and proximity to neurovascular structures, elbow arthroscopy has become a reliable, safe, and effective way to treat pathology in the thrower's elbow (13–15). Good results have been reported in treating multiple pathologic conditions in the throwing elbow including loose body removal, osteophyte debridement for VEO, and OCD.

Wilson et al. (3) reported the results for five pitchers treated with open osteophyte excision after failure of nonoperative treatment, and all returned to play for at least one season at 8 to 20 months of follow-up. One patient required repeat excision within two seasons. Andrews and Timmerman (16) reported on 72 professional baseball players undergoing either open or arthroscopic elbow surgery. Posteromedial osteophytes were identified in 65% of these cases. They reported a 41% reoperation rate in the group undergoing olecranon debridement and found that 25% developed valgus instability requiring MUCL reconstruction. They concluded that the incidence of MUCL insufficiency is underestimated and that treatment focused solely on the secondary effects of MUCL insufficiency without treating the underlying MUCL pathology that may lead to unsatisfactory results.

In 2000, Reddy et al. (17) reported on the results of 187 elbow arthroscopies. The most common diagnoses were posterior impingement (51%), loose bodies (31%), and degenerative joint disease (22%). The average Figgie score improved from 27.7 to 45.4 points, with the largest increases occurring in the pain score. An excellent result was achieved in 51%, a good result in 36%, a fair result in 11%, and poor result in 4% of the patients. Forty-seven of fifty-five baseball players (85%) were able to return to the same level of competition. The complication rate was 1.6%.

Recently (2016), Park et al. (18) reviewed outcomes of adolescent baseball players with VEO who either underwent isolated arthroscopic olecranon tip resection or a staged procedure with arthroscopic olecranon tip resection, followed by MUCL reconstruction 2 weeks later. They demonstrated an overall return to play of 85% and found that at >2 years those individuals with isolated elbow arthroscopy had better outcomes then those with the additional MUCL reconstruction.

COMPLICATIONS

Elbow arthroscopy has evolved to be a safer procedure through a better understanding of the neurovascular structures about the elbow and avoiding them during portal placement and intra-articular work on or near the capsule. However, there still remains a real risk of serious nerve injury especially to the inexperienced elbow arthroscopist.

Nerve injury is the most devastating reported complication of elbow arthroscopy (14,15,19,20). Injury can be caused by direct laceration from a knife penetrated deep to the dermis, from the cannula trocar, overly aggressive debridement from a shaver, or getting wrapped in a burr. Other possible causes of nerve injury include fluid extravasation, direct infiltration with local anesthetic, and direct compression from cannulas or instruments (21). As noted previously, some portals described in the literature place the neurovascular structures at a higher relative risk than other portals. For this reason, to minimize the risk of neurovascular insult, we have chosen the portals as outlined above, incise only through the skin, spread the soft tissues with a straight hemostat, use blunt trocars to enter the elbow joint, and use retractors especially when working adjacent to the ulnar nerve.

It must also be mentioned that elbow arthroscopy inherently carries the risks of any arthroscopy or orthopaedic intervention about a joint. These include infection, articular cartilage injury, synovial fistula formation, instrument breakage, and tourniquet-related complications. Finally, the patient's compliance with postoperative physical therapy is crucial, and they are advised if they do not comply with the postoperative program they risk failure of the surgery or elbow stiffness.

Complications specific to olecranon debridement for VEO included missed MUCL injury and overaggressive olecranon resection. As previously mentioned, existing MUCL injury may become symptomatic after the recovery from the arthroscopic debridement. It is critical to remove only the osteophyte and not the normal olecranon. Removal of the normal olecranon can increase valgus angulation of the elbow and increase MUCL strain during valgus loading and contribute to MUCL pathology (8,9). It is recommended to council all patients who elect arthroscopic posteromedial decompression of the possibility of developing MUCL injury and symptoms. In addition, care should be taken to avoid injury to the ulnar nerve that lies near this area in the cubital tunnel. The use of arthroscopic soft tissue retractors is extremely helpful when working in the medial gutter to protect the ulnar nerve.

REFERENCES

1. Bennett GE. Elbow and shoulder lesions of baseball players. *Am J Surg.* 1959;98:484–492.
2. King J, Brelsford HJ, Tullos HS. Analysis of the pitching arm of the professional baseball pitcher. *Clin Orthop Relat Res.* 1969;67:116–123.
3. Wilson FD, Andrews JR, Blackburn TA, et al. Valgus extension overload in the pitching elbow. *Am J Sports Med.* 1983;11(2):83–88.
4. Morrey BF, An KN. Articular and ligamentous contributions to the stability of the elbow joint. *Am J Sports Med.* 1983;11(5):315–319.
5. Pappas AM, Zawacki RM, Sullivan TJ. Biomechanics of baseball pitching. A preliminary report. *Am J Sports Med.* 1985;13(4):216–222.
6. O'Driscoll SW. Valgus extension overload and plica. In: Levine WN, ed. *The Athlete's Elbow.* Rosemont, IL: American Academy of Orthopaedic Surgeons; 2008:71–83.
7. Ahmad CS, Park MC, Elattrache NS. Elbow medial ulnar collateral ligament insufficiency alters posteromedial olecranon contact. *Am J Sports Med.* 2004;32(7):1607–1612.
8. Kamineni S, ElAttrache NS, O'Driscoll SW, et al. Medial collateral ligament strain with partial posteromedial olecranon resection. A biomechanical study. *J Bone Joint Surg Am.* 2004;86-A(11):2424–2430.
9. Kamineni S, Hirahara H, Pomianowski S, et al. Partial posteromedial olecranon resection: a kinematic study. *J Bone Joint Surg Am.* 2003;85-A(6):1005–1011.
10. Conway JE, Jobe FW, Glousman RE, et al. Medial instability of the elbow in throwing athletes. Treatment by repair or reconstruction of the ulnar collateral ligament. *J Bone Joint Surg Am.* 1992;74(1):67–83.
11. Field LD, Altchek DW, Warren RF, et al. Arthroscopic anatomy of the lateral elbow: a comparison of three portals. *Arthroscopy.* 1994;10(6):602–607.
12. Stothers K, Day B, Regan WR. Arthroscopy of the elbow: anatomy, portal sites, and a description of the proximal lateral portal. *Arthroscopy.* 1995;11(4):449–457.
13. Field LD, Altchek DW. Evaluation of the arthroscopic valgus instability test of the elbow. *Am J Sports Med.* 1996;24(2):177–181.
14. Andrews JR, Carson WG. Arthroscopy of the elbow. *Arthroscopy.* 1985;1(2):97–107.
15. O'Driscoll SW, Morrey BF. Arthroscopy of the elbow. Diagnostic and therapeutic benefits and hazards. *J Bone Joint Surg Am.* 1992;74(1):84–94.
16. Andrews JR, Timmerman, LA. Outcome of elbow surgery in professional baseball players. *Am J Sports Med.* 1995;23(4):407–413.
17. Reddy AS, Kvitne RS, Yocum LA, et al. Arthroscopy of the elbow: a long-term clinical review. *Arthroscopy.* 2000;16(6):588–594.

18. Park JY, Yoo HY, Chung SW, et al. Valgus extension overload syndrome in adolescent baseball players: clinical characteristics and surgical outcomes. *J Shoulder Elbow Surg.* 2016;25(12):2048–2056.
19. Haapaniemi T, Berggren, M, Adolfsson L. Complete transection of the median and radial nerves during arthroscopic release of post-traumatic elbow contracture. *Arthroscopy.* 1999;15(7):784–787.
20. Thomas MA, Fast A, Shapiro D. Radial nerve damage as a complication of elbow arthroscopy. *Clin Orthop Relat Res.* 1987;215:130–131.
21. Walcott GD, Savoie FH, Field LD. Arthroscopy of the elbow: setup, portals, and diagnostic technique. In: Altcheck DW, Andrews JR, eds. *The Athlete's Elbow.* Philadelphia, PA: Lippincott Williams & Wilkins; 2001:249–273.

2 Ulnar Collateral Ligament Reconstruction

Ekaterina Urch

INTRODUCTION

The medial structures of the elbow are subjected to extraordinarily high forces in the overhead athlete (1), and the anterior bundle of the ulnar collateral ligament (UCL) is the main restraint to these valgus forces in the flexed, throwing position (2,3). UCL insufficiency in a baseball pitcher was once considered to be a career-ending diagnosis. In 1974, Dr. Frank Jobe introduced the UCL reconstruction of the elbow, commonly referred to as Tommy John surgery. Since the first UCL reconstruction procedure, this surgical technique has afforded countless athletes the opportunity to return to their preinjury level of play with predictable outcomes.

Despite the numerous different variations of the Tommy John procedure described since the original surgery performed by Dr. Jobe, the primary goal of the procedure remains to restore medial elbow stability in the overhead athlete. The insufficient UCL should be reconstructed using a free tendon autograft using stable fixation and tensioned at an isometric point. In Dr. Jobe's own words, "the goal is to put a good piece of collagen in the right orientation."

INDICATIONS

Athletes failing conservative treatment or those with full-thickness tears who wish to quickly return to their preinjury level of play are candidates for surgical treatment. Historically, literature has shown that direct repair of the UCL results in significantly worse outcomes in professional athletes when compared to reconstruction (4,5). Other studies, however, suggested that direct repair of the UCL may be indicated in the few patients with acute avulsion injuries, especially in young, nonprofessional athletes (6). More recently, Dugas (7) introduced a novel UCL repair construct using suture anchors to augment the soft tissue repair and demonstrated equivalent biomechanical properties when compared to the gold standard reconstruction (8). Although clinical data are still pending, this repair construct may be a viable treatment option for some high-level throwing athletes with avulsion-type injuries of the UCL. Indeed, as the age of athletes diagnosed with UCL injuries continues to drop, the role of UCL repair may see a rise in popularity over the next decade (9). Nonetheless, the operative management of choice for a chronically injured, attenuated UCL remains to be reconstruction using an ipsilateral palmaris tendon autograft. Alternative graft options include the gracilis tendon or contralateral palmaris tendon.

CONTRAINDICATIONS

Elbow UCL reconstruction is contraindicated in athletes with asymptomatic tears. This type of situation is most often seen in athletes who self-limit the valgus demand on their elbow or those who do not wish to continue throwing. For example, UCL injury in a nonthrowing athlete or one with lower elbow demands, such as a football player, may be treated successfully with conservative management (10). Additionally, UCL reconstruction is contraindicated in patients who are unable or unwilling to complete the extensive rehabilitation postoperatively.

Relative contraindications include young athletes with medial elbow pain. In skeletally immature athletes, the injury usually involves the apophysis. However, in situations where the UCL is also involved, conservative management is preferred due to the close proximity of the UCL origin to the medial epicondyle physis (11). Finally, patients with evidence of ulnohumeral or radiocapitellar arthritis who choose to proceed with UCL reconstruction must be counseled on the possibility of persisting or worsening pain following surgery.

PREOPERATIVE PREPARATION

The diagnosis of valgus instability of the elbow due to UCL insufficiency is largely clinical and is heavily based upon a careful history and thorough physical examination. Additional information from imaging studies is a valuable adjunct in the decision-making algorithm but should never be the primary driver in the process.

History

The majority of elbow throwing injuries occur during the acceleration phase of throwing where high valgus forces are countered by rapid elbow extension. Unsurprisingly, athletes usually present with medial elbow pain in the late cocking or acceleration phases of repetitive overhand throwing activities. History of the injury may reveal a single event during a pitch associated with sharp pain and/or a "pop" in the medial elbow leading to the inability to continue pitching. Alternatively, the athlete may report a gradual onset of medial-sided elbow pain with throwing followed by significant pain after a strenuous throwing load with unsuccessful attempts to throw above 50% to 75% of maximum velocity. Changes in pitch velocity, accuracy, and stamina are hallmarks of medial elbow instability and are important details to obtain from the patient's history. Finally, neurologic complaints of paresthesias or radicular symptoms in the ulnar nerve distribution should be elicited and documented.

Physical Examination

A complete physical examination of the elbow includes range of motion testing, palpation of the bony landmarks as well as the UCL and flexor-pronator tendon origin, and forearm and elbow muscle strength testing. Tenderness over the UCL or flexor-pronator muscle unit is indicative of local inflammation. Pain with resisted wrist flexion or pronation or a defect in the tendinous origin of the flexor-pronator mass may be indicative of flexor-pronator injury rather than UCL instability. Flexor-pronator mass injury can be further evaluated with the temporal pressure test. The athlete is asked to apply firm pressure to the ipsilateral temporal region of the head using the thumb, middle, and index fingers. Reproducible pain in the medial elbow is a positive test and indicates muscular injury. The presence or absence of a palmaris longus tendon should be noted for future surgical planning (Fig. 2-1).

Valgus instability is tested with several exam maneuvers, including the valgus stress test performed with the elbow in 25 to 30 degrees of flexion and the forearm in full supination. The "milking maneuver" is a sensitive test for UCL damage and is performed by grasping the athlete's thumb with the arm in the cocked position (90-degree shoulder abduction and 90-degree elbow flexion) and applying a valgus stress by pulling down on the thumb (12). Reproduction of the athlete's pain is a positive result and indicates UCL injury. Finally, the "bounce home test" can be used to evaluate for posterior elbow impingement and valgus extension overload. The athlete is asked to sharply move his or her elbow from flexion into full extension, repeating the movement in rapid succession to create a whip-like effect on the elbow in extension. Pain in the posterior compartment is consistent with posterior impingement from a posteromedial olecranon osteophyte or olecranon fossa overgrowth.

All athletes should have a detailed neurovascular assessment with careful attention paid to ulnar nerve motor and sensory function. Palpation of the ulnar nerve proximal and distal to the epicondyle should be performed, and a gentle anterior force applied proximally as the elbow is brought into flexion will assess if the nerve will sublux over the medial epicondyle out of the cubital tunnel. A Tinel sign is also elicited over the cubital tunnel. Medial elbow instability due to UCL insufficiency has been shown to cause ulnar nerve symptoms in as many as 41% of overhead athletes (13,14). Traction on the nerve with repetitive medial joint space widening or abrasion by posteromedial

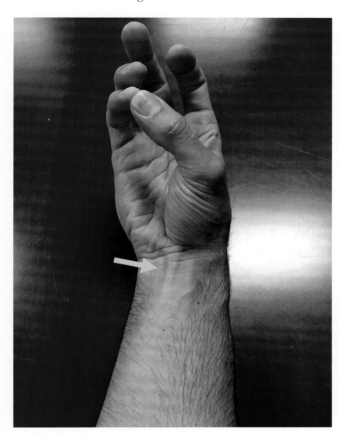

FIGURE 2-1

Evaluation for the presence of the palmaris longus tendon. The patient holds the forearm on full supination and the wrist in neutral. The thumb and small finger are adducted together to meet in the midline of the palm. The palmaris longus tendon (*yellow arrow*), if present, is the predominant structure in the center of the wrist, ulnar to the flexor carpi radialis tendon.

osteophytes may cause paresthesias that affect the player's ability to perform. If clinical evidence of ulnar neuritis is present, a baseline electromyography test (EMG) is a helpful diagnostic tool and may be performed prior to operative intervention.

Imaging

Standard AP, lateral, oblique, and cubital tunnel views should be attained for each patient. These are evaluated for the presence of arthritic changes, bony UCL avulsions, spurring or calcification within the ligament, and posteromedial or marginal osteophytes. Bilateral valgus stress radiographs can be helpful to identify medial joint line gapping. Joint space widening >0.5 mm compared to the unaffected side has been shown to be diagnostic for a complete or high-grade partial tear of the UCL (15). However, other studies have found that a small amount of opening in pitchers may be a normal adaptation, making stress radiography a less reliable modality for diagnosing UCL injury (16). It is also important to note that the presence of increased medial laxity on clinical or radiographic examination without pain or instability does not justify surgical intervention.

Magnetic resonance imaging (MRI) is helpful in better defining soft tissue anatomy and identifying injured structures. Abnormalities such as a high-signal intensity within the UCL on fat-suppressed T2-weighted coronal images as well as a thin and redundant contour without obvious discontinuity are suggestive of a high-grade partial tear. Additionally, MRI can help identify other pathology such as intra-articular loose bodies, osteochondral lesions, and edema within the flexor-pronator mass. Literature has shown that MRI without intra-articular contrast can reliably detect a full-thickness tear of the UCL (17). Historically, however, standard MRI without intra-articular contrast has been shown to be much less accurate in identifying partial-thickness tears of the UCL with reported sensitivity as being as low as 14% (18). As such, despite recent advances in MR technology, the current gold standard for diagnosing UCL injuries is MR arthrography (19).

Along with important findings such as contrast extravasation into or around the ligament, ligamentous laxity or wavy fibers, and fiber disruption, the T-sign seen on the coronal view of an MR arthrogram is a critical clue for identifying partial-thickness tears. This sign occurs when injected contrast tracks from the joint line distally along the cortical margin of the sublime tubercle but is contained under the superficial fibers of a partially torn UCL. It is important to note that some contrast tracking along the UCL may be normal as the ligament has been found to attach, on average, 2.8 mm distal to the articular surface of the ulna (20).

Dynamic ultrasound (US) imaging of the UCL is an additional imaging modality that has gained recent popularity and has been shown to be a reliable diagnostic tool for UCL pathology (21). Anatomic abnormalities such as increased ligament thickness, calcifications, and joint line gapping with valgus stress are easily identified on US by an experienced technician. Stress US has been shown to have 96% sensitivity and 81% specificity for identifying UCL tears (22). Furthermore, the authors found that when done in conjunction with stress US, the sensitivity and specificity of MRI for identifying UCL tears increased from 74% and 92% to 90% and 100%, respectively. It is evident that US imaging of the UCL could be a helpful addition to the workup of UCL injuries. It is important to note, however, that the efficacy of this modality is limited by the proficiency of the operator at both performing and interpreting the test.

SURGICAL TECHNIQUE

The patient is positioned supine with the operative extremity on a hand table attachment. General endotracheal anesthesia is used without regional blockade of the brachial plexus. This is done to allow for accurate postoperative evaluation of ulnar nerve function. A nonsterile tourniquet is used, taking care to ensure that the tourniquet is placed as far proximally on the arm as possible.

A 10-cm curvilinear incision, centered over the medial epicondyle, is made from the distal portion of the intramuscular septum on the humerus to 2 cm distal to the sublime tubercle (Fig. 2-2). Dissection is carried out through the subcutaneous tissue using Metzenbaum scissors. Care is taken to identify and preserve the branches of the medial antebrachial cutaneous nerve. The intermuscular septum is identified and incised just proximal to the apex of the medial epicondyle, and the muscle mass is dissected anteriorly to expose the anterior cortex. The apex of the medial epicondyle is located, and electrocautery is used to mark the center of the UCL insertion. The sublime tubercle is identified distally, and the fascia overlying the flexor pronator mass is incised longitudinally in line with the two identified points (Fig. 2-3). A small periosteal elevator is used to bluntly split the deep muscle fibers, exposing the underlying UCL. The ulnar nerve runs at the posterior border of the UCL in this location. Using either a scalpel or a small elevator, the anterior edge of the ulnar nerve is carefully

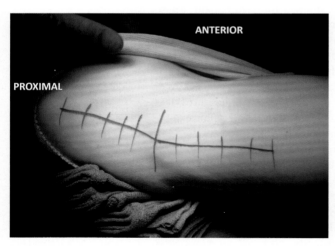

FIGURE 2-2

The surgical incision is centered over the medial epicondyle and runs from the palpable intermuscular septum proximally to 2 cm distal to the sublime tubercle on the forearm. In muscular patients, the incision may need to be extended for optimal exposure.

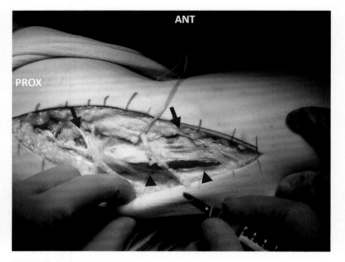

FIGURE 2-3

The branches of the medial antebrachial cutaneous nerve (MABC) are preserved during soft tissue dissection (*arrows*). The posterior one third of the fascia overlying the flexor pronator mass is split longitudinally (*arrowheads*).

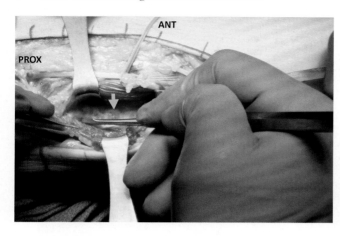

FIGURE 2-4

The ulnar nerve, running along the posterior border of the ulnar collateral ligament (*arrow*), is dissected off of the ligament using a small periosteal elevator.

dissected off of the UCL, freeing up its anterior edge (Fig. 2-4). This allows for safe retraction of the nerve when exposing the ligament's entire footprint on the sublime tubercle. If there is clinical evidence of ulnar nerve compression, the nerve is circumferentially released and transposed.

The center of the sublime tubercle is identified and marked with electrocautery. The medial ulnar ridge is a palpable structure just distal to the tubercle and can be used to localize the center of the tubercle. The UCL is longitudinally incised from the sublime tubercle to the humeral insertion, exposing the ulnotrochlear joint (Fig. 2-5). The ulnar and humeral insertions of the ligament are left intact, and the stability of the medial elbow is tested using a valgus load. Insufficiency of the UCL will result in joint space gapping. A 55-degree V-drill guide is placed just distal to the marked center of the tubercle and at least 5 mm from the joint line. Aiming slightly distal to avoid joint penetration, a 3.5-mm drill with an auto depth stop is used to make two convergent tunnels anterior and posterior to the center of the tubercle. The V-guide produces a 6.5-mm bone bridge between the apertures of the two tunnels. The two tunnels are connected using a small curved curette (Fig. 2-6).

The humeral socket is drilled at the anatomic footprint of UCL insertion using a 4.5-mm drill with a depth stop of 15 mm. The tunnel is directed proximally toward the epicondylar attachment of the intermuscular septum (Fig. 2-7A and B). Care must be taken to avoid penetrating the posterior cortex of the epicondyle. To accommodate three strands of the graft, a large (#2) straight curette is used to enlarge the tunnel to a diameter of 5.0 mm. An adjustable C-guide is used to drill the two exit tunnels connecting to the epicondylar socket. The peg end of the guide is placed into the humeral socket, while the drill end of the guide is positioned on the superior aspect of the epicondyle in line with the epicondylar ridge. A 3.5-mm drill is used to make the first exit tunnel connecting to the blind epicondylar socket (Fig. 2-7C). The C-guide is then redirected anteriorly through a split in the

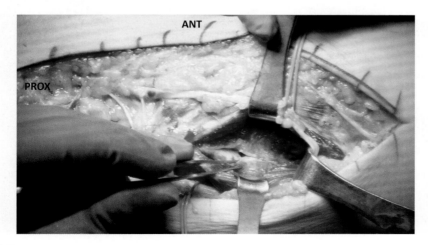

FIGURE 2-5

The ligament is longitudinally incised from its insertion to the sublime tubercle, exposing the ulnotrochlear joint.

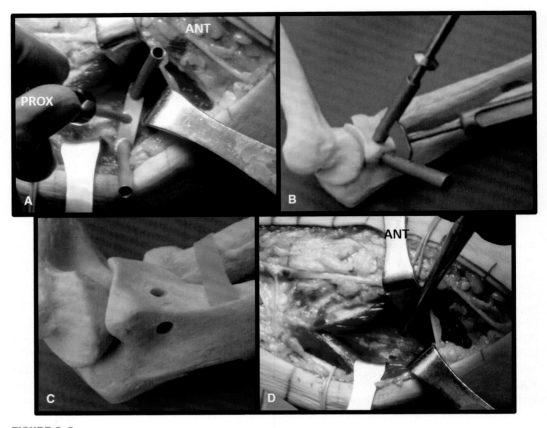

FIGURE 2-6

The 55-degree V-drill guide is used to drill two convergent tunnels just distal to the center of the sublime tubercle **(A, B)**. The two tunnels **(C)** are connected using a small curved curette **(D)**.

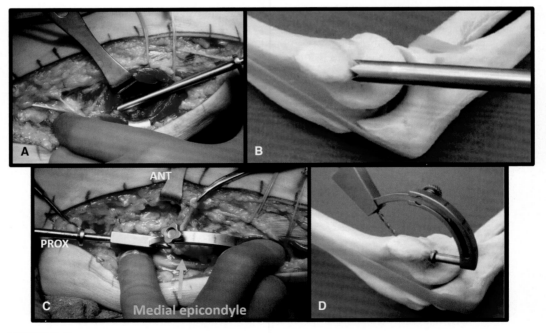

FIGURE 2-7

A 4.5-mm drill with a depth stop of 15 mm is used to drill the docking tunnel in the medial epicondyle **(A)**. The tunnel is drilled in line with the apex of the medial epicondyle, taking care not to penetrate the posterior cortex **(B)**. The two exit tunnels are drilled with the help of a C-drill guide, making the epicondylar ridge tunnel with a 3.5-mm drill **(C)** and the anterior tunnel with a 2.0-mm drill **(D)**.

pronator muscle mass (Fig. 2-7D). A 2.0-mm drill is used to make the anterior exit tunnel. Care is taken to maintain an 8- to 10-mm bone bridge between the two exit tunnels.

The wound is irrigated, and attention is turned to harvesting the tendon graft. The preferred graft is the ipsilateral palmaris longus tendon. Alternatively, the contralateral palmaris longus or gracilis tendon can be used if an ipsilateral palmaris is not available.

The presence of a palmaris longus is confirmed preoperatively with the patient awake. In the operating room, the tendon is identified visually and by palpation. A 2-cm transverse incision is made at the level of the distal flexor crease of the wrist, and the tendon is identified and isolated using a clamp. Holding the tendon under tension, a second 2-cm transverse incision is made over the tendon approximately 7.5 cm proximal in the forearm. In a similar fashion, a third transverse incision is made 15 cm proximal to the flexor crease, at the level of the musculotendinous junction. The more proximal incision should allow visualization of the musculotendinous junction and ensure continuity of the tendon from the muscle to its insertion in the distal incision (Fig. 2-8). The tendon is transected in the distal incision and pulled sequentially through the subsequent proximal incisions to the musculotendinous junction. The free end of the tendon is whip stitched using a #0 nonabsorbable suture. Prior to graft harvest, the length of the graft is confirmed to be at least 15 cm.

The whip-stitched end of the graft is passed posterior to anterior through the ulnar tunnel. A looped suture can be used to facilitate graft passage (Fig. 2-9A). The whip-stitched (anterior) limb of the graft is docked into the humeral tunnel, and the suture limbs are passed through the anterior (2.0 mm) exit hole. This represents reconstruction of the anterior limb of the anterior bundle.

Next, the posterior limb of the graft is approximated to the epicondyle and marked at 1 cm proximal to the aperture of the humeral socket (Fig. 2-9B). This ensures that 1 cm of the graft will be docked into the epicondyle, leaving roughly 5 mm of additional space for tensioning. The graft is cycled several times to ensure an isometric point is identified and marked. A whip stitch is placed at this mark leaving the distal tail of the graft free. The suture is passed through the humeral socket and out of the epicondylar (3.5 mm) exit tunnel. As the tendon is pulled into the tunnel, the free end of the graft doubles onto itself, creating a 3-ply graft (Fig. 2-9C).

With the elbow held at 60 degrees of flexion and neutral rotation without any valgus load, the two ends of the graft are docked into the tunnel and the graft is tensioned. Isometry is checked and the two suture limbs are tied over the medial epicondyle bone bridge. The elbow is passively ranged to confirm isometry of the graft. Any laxity in the graft can be reduced by placing absorbable, figure-of-8 sutures between the anterior and posterior limbs. Finally, the doubled free edge of the posterior limb is tagged with a whip stitch, passed through the ulnar tunnel posterior to anterior, and sutured to the anterior limb of the graft. This reinforces the posterior limb of the UCL and completes the 3-ply reconstruction (Fig. 2-10).

If ample tissue of the UCL remains, the longitudinal split can be closed over the tendon autograft, incorporating the entire reconstruction into one UCL unit. Alternatively, the entire construct is sutured together with three #0 nonabsorbable sutures (Fig. 2-11). The wound is irrigated, and the flexor-pronator fascia is closed with interrupted absorbable sutures. The skin incisions are closed in a standard fashion. The elbow is splinted in 75 degrees of flexion and neutral forearm rotation prior to emergence from anesthesia. Immobilization is discontinued after 7 to 10 days once the sutures are removed.

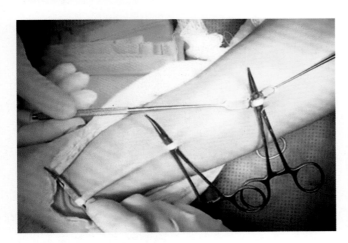

FIGURE 2-8

The palmaris longus is harvested using three 2-cm incisions. Prior to graft resection, tension is pulled through the tendon via the three separate incisions, confirming continuity of the structure from its myotendinous junction proximally to its insertion on the palmar fascia distally.

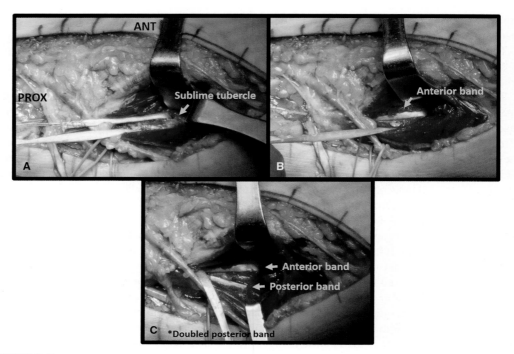

FIGURE 2-9

The graft is passed through the ulnar tunnel posterior to anterior **(A)**. The anterior limb is docked into the humeral tunnel, reconstructing the anterior band of the ligament **(B)**. The posterior limb of the graft is whip stitched and docked in to the humerus via the epicondylar exit tunnel, reconstructing the posterior band. The graft is doubled over, creating the third limb for the 3-ply reconstruction **(C)**.

FIGURE 2-10

The anterior and posterior suture limbs are tied over the epicondylar bony bridge, securing the graft. The doubled limb of the posterior band is whip stitched, passed through the ulnar tunnel posterior to anterior, and sutured to the anterior band. This completes the 3-ply reconstruction.

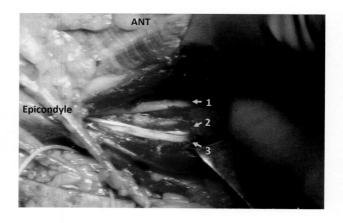

FIGURE 2-11

The final construct, after cerclage sutures were placed around all three strands, further tensioning the construct.

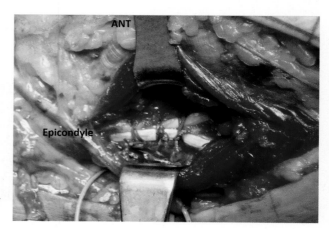

PEARLS AND PITFALLS

During soft tissue exposure, careful superficial dissection should be carried out in order to identify and protect branches of the medial antebrachial cutaneous nerve. Injury to these structures can cause numbness, pain, and neuroma formation.

In harvesting the palmaris tendon graft, the two most common reasons for erroneous harvest of the median nerve are (a) failure to confirm the presence of the tendon preoperatively and (b) harvesting the graft through one incision. Harvesting the graft through three incisions minimizes this risk by allowing the surgeon to easily identify the tendon prior to resection. In patients with well-developed forearm musculature, closing the fascia over the palmaris tendon defect in the proximal-most incision will prevent muscle herniation—a postsurgical manifestation that can lead to significant morbidity for the patient and may require additional surgery.

The medial ulnar ridge is a consistently reliable landmark that can be used to identify the isometric point of the UCL at the sublime tubercle. This is especially helpful in revision cases when the bony anatomy is often distorted. Once identified, when drilling the ulnar tunnels, it is important to keep in mind that the ulnar articular surface is concave. Drilling the tunnels directly perpendicular to the bone and too close to the joint can lead to articular surface penetration. Additionally, when drilling both the ulnar and humeral tunnels, close attention should be paid to the width of the bony bridge as an insufficient bridge can lead to fixation failure. One should aim for a 6- to 7-mm bridge on the ulna and an 8- to 10-mm bridge on the humerus. If the medial epicondyle bony bridge is violated during suture fixation, or in a revision case when it is important to minimize the amount of drill holes in the epicondyle to avoid fracture, a suture button can be used for humeral fixation (Fig. 2-12). This is also useful in patients whose anatomy, either due to excessive musculature or an overlying venous plexus, precludes a direct approach to the anterior aspect of the medial epicondyle.

POSTOPERATIVE MANAGEMENT

Differences between individual patients should be taken into consideration during the rehabilitation program. Not all athletes progress in a linear fashion or at the same rate. In general, the goal is to return the athlete to the preinjury level of competition approximately 12 months after UCL reconstruction.

Full, active shoulder and wrist motion along with gripping exercises are allowed while immobilized and continued in the early postoperative period. Elbow flexion and extension is allowed after immobilization is discontinued. Full elbow range of motion should be achieved by 4 to 6 weeks, at which point light resistance exercises for elbow and wrist muscle strengthening are initiated.

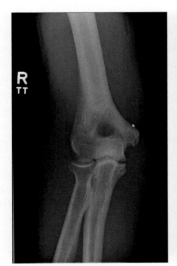 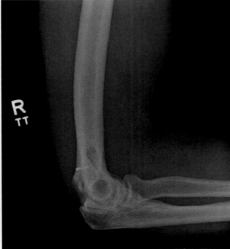

FIGURE 2-12

Radiographs of a patient who had undergone revision UCL reconstruction using suture button fixation. This was done to preserve the residual bony architecture of the epicondyle.

Positions of valgus stress with resistance training are avoided for 4 months. The importance of a total-body conditioning program including core muscle strengthening, cardiovascular training, and periscapular and rotator cuff strengthening cannot be understated. This should begin early in the postoperative period (with adherence to limitations on valgus stress at the elbow) and continued throughout the player's progression.

An easy throwing (tossing) program with no wind up is initiated 3 to 4 months postoperatively if the patient has no swelling and full, pain-free elbow range of motion. After 4 to 6 months, throwing days can be alternated with exercise days. Throwing distances may be gradually increased at 2- to 3-week intervals provided there is no swelling or discomfort during the previous level of the throwing program. After 6 months, easy wind up on flat ground is introduced into the program. At 7 to 8 months postoperatively, supervised throwing off of a mound is allowed at 50% intensity. Proper throwing mechanics are critical when introducing this phase of the program and throughout the rehabilitation period. During months 8 and 9, pitchers can increase to 70% speed while throwing off of a mound.

Over the final 2 to 3 months, focus on proper throwing mechanics and a total-body conditioning program continues. Pitchers gradually increase throwing intensity in bullpens to eventually simulate a game situation. Throwing in competition is allowed at 12 months postoperatively if the player has full shoulder and elbow range of motion, has normal upper extremity strength, has trunk stability, and is pain-free when throwing. Rhythm, proprioception, and accuracy are the last skills to return and may take several more months. Professional pitchers may require more than 18 months in order to return to full, preinjury levels of competition, whereas position players or other overhead athletes may have a shorter recovery (23).

COMPLICATIONS

The most common complication following UCL reconstruction is ulnar nerve neuropraxia, which usually resolves over the course of several months (24). Reported rates of this complication have been high as 16% though these data are associated with older surgical techniques in which transposition of the ulnar nerve was regularly performed (25). Outcomes studies involving the docking technique have shown a significant decline in postoperative neuropraxia secondary to limited handling of the nerve (13,26). Ulnar nerve neurolysis should only be considered when symptoms of persistent ulnar neuropathy are present or when pathology in the posterior compartment requires exposure through the cubital tunnel. Other reported complications are rare and include medial epicondyle avulsion fractures, wound complications, and stiffness (24).

RESULTS

In the first series of long-term results following UCL reconstruction, Conway et al. (27) reported good to excellent results in 80% of patients. Of the 56 patients who underwent reconstruction, 38 were able to return to their preinjury level of play including professional pitching. Over the past several decades, the reported outcomes following primary UCL reconstruction have remained favorable. Recently, a large case series evaluating the clinical outcomes in 743 athletes undergoing UCL reconstructions found that 83% of athletes were able to return to the same or higher level of competition after surgery (25). In the same study, the average time from surgery to competition was 11.6 months. Other studies have found excellent functional outcomes in 90% of patients following the docking technique with a trend toward greater rate of return to play when compared to the Jobe modification technique (13,26,28). The DANE TJ modification method has also shown to have excellent outcomes with 86% of athletes returning to preinjury level of play (29).

Recent literature has reported revision rates ranging from 3.9% to as high as 15% in professional pitchers (30,31). Revision surgery is associated with difficult exposure, altered anatomy, and higher complication rates. Although primary UCL reconstruction can be expected to produce excellent results, the success of revision UCL reconstruction is significantly lower with studies reporting return-to-sport rates ranging from only 33% to 65% with complication rates reported to be as high as 40% (32,33).

CONCLUSION

As new operative strategies continue to evolve, it is possible that the rate of complications associated with graft failure will continue to improve. Nonetheless, since the first procedure in 1974 performed by Dr. Jobe, UCL reconstruction has provided consistent and predictable results. As such, it continues to be the workhorse treatment strategy for elite overhead athletes with UCL insufficiency wishing to return to the same level of play.

ACKNOWLEDGMENT

This chapter was built on the strong foundation provided by Neal S. ElAttrache, MD in the first edition.

REFERENCES

1. Werner SL, Fleisig GS, Dillman CJ, et al. Biomechanics of the elbow during baseball pitching. *J Orthop Sports Phys Ther.* 1993;17(6):274–278.
2. Davidson PA, Pink M, Perry J, et al. Functional anatomy of the flexor pronator muscle group in relation to the medial collateral ligament of the elbow. *Am J Sports Med.* 1995;23(2):245–250.
3. Morrey BF, An KN. Articular and ligamentous contributions to the stability of the elbow joint. *Am J Sports Med.* 1983;11(5):315–319.
4. Andrews JR, Timmerman LA. Outcome of elbow surgery in professional baseball players. *Am J Sports Med.* 1995;23(4):407–413.
5. Cain EL Jr, Dugas JR, Wolf RS, et al. Elbow injuries in throwing athletes: a current concepts review. *Am J Sports Med.* 2003;31(4):621–635.
6. Savoie FH III, Trenhaile SW, Roberts J, et al. Primary repair of ulnar collateral ligament injuries of the elbow in young athletes: a case series of injuries to the proximal and distal ends of the ligament. *Am J Sports Med.* 2008;36(6):1066–1072.
7. Dugas JR. Ulnar collateral ligament repair: an old idea with a new wrinkle. *Am J Orthop (Belle Mead, NJ).* 2016;45(3):124–127.
8. Dugas JR, Walters BL, Beason DP, et al. Biomechanical comparison of ulnar collateral ligament repair with internal bracing versus modified Jobe reconstruction. *Am J Sports Med.* 2016;44(3):735–741.
9. Erickson BJ, Nwachukwu BU, Rosas S, et al. Trends in medial ulnar collateral ligament reconstruction in the United States: a retrospective review of a large private-payer database from 2007 to 2011. *Am J Sports Med.* 2015;43(7):1770–1774.
10. Dodson CC, Slenker N, Cohen SB, et al. Ulnar collateral ligament injuries of the elbow in professional football quarterbacks. *J Shoulder Elbow Surg.* 2010;19(8):1276–1280.
11. Wei AS, Khana S, Limpisvasti O, et al. Clinical and magnetic resonance imaging findings associated with Little League elbow. *J Pediatr Orthop.* 2010;30(7):715–719.
12. Cain EL Jr, Dugas JR. History and examination of the thrower's elbow. *Clin Sports Med.* 2004;23(4):553–566, viii.
13. Erickson BJ, Bach BR, Jr, Cohen MS, et al. Ulnar collateral ligament reconstruction: the rush experience. *Orthop J Sports Med.* 2016;4(1):2325967115626876.
14. Thompson WH, Jobe FW, Yocum LA, et al. Ulnar collateral ligament reconstruction in athletes: muscle-splitting approach without transposition of the ulnar nerve. *J Shoulder Elbow Surg.* 2001;10(2):152–157.
15. Rijke AM, Goitz HT, McCue FC, et al. Stress radiography of the medial elbow ligaments. *Radiology.* 1994;191(1):213–216.
16. Ellenbecker TS, Mattalino AJ, Elam EA, et al. Medial elbow joint laxity in professional baseball pitchers. A bilateral comparison using stress radiography. *Am J Sports Med.* 1998;26(3):420–424.
17. Fowler KA, Chung CB. Normal MR imaging anatomy of the elbow. *Magn Reson Imaging Clin N Am.* 2004;12(2):191–206, v.
18. Timmerman LA, Andrews JR. Undersurface tear of the ulnar collateral ligament in baseball players. A newly recognized lesion. *Am J Sports Med.* 1994;22(1):33–36.
19. Joyner PW, Bruce J, Hess R, et al. Magnetic resonance imaging-based classification for ulnar collateral ligament injuries of the elbow. *J Shoulder Elbow Surg.* 2016;25(10):1710–1716.
20. Dugas JR, Ostrander RV, Cain EL, et al. Anatomy of the anterior bundle of the ulnar collateral ligament. *J Shoulder Elbow Surg.* 2007;16(5):657–660.
21. Ciccotti MG, Atanda A Jr, Nazarian LN, et al. Stress sonography of the ulnar collateral ligament of the elbow in professional baseball pitchers: a 10-year study. *Am J Sports Med.* 2014;42(3):544–551.
22. Roedl JB, Gonzalez FM, Zoga AC, et al. Potential utility of a combined approach with US and MR arthrography to image medial elbow pain in baseball players. *Radiology.* 2016;279(3):827–837.
23. Jobe FW, Stark H, Lombardo SJ. Reconstruction of the ulnar collateral ligament in athletes. *J Bone Joint Surg Am.* 1986;68(8):1158–1163.
24. Bruce JR, Andrews JR. Ulnar collateral ligament injuries in the throwing athlete. *J Am Acad Orthop Surg.* 2014;22(5):315–325.
25. Cain EL Jr, Andrews JR, Dugas JR, et al. Outcome of ulnar collateral ligament reconstruction of the elbow in 1281 athletes: results in 743 athletes with minimum 2-year follow-up. *Am J Sports Med.* 2010;38(12):2426–2434.
26. Bowers AL, Dines JS, Dines DM, et al. Elbow medial ulnar collateral ligament reconstruction: clinical relevance and the docking technique. *J Shoulder Elbow Surg.* 2010;19(2 suppl):110–117.
27. Conway JE, Jobe FW, Glousman RE, et al. Medial instability of the elbow in throwing athletes. Treatment by repair or reconstruction of the ulnar collateral ligament. *J Bone Joint Surg Am.* 1992;74(1):67–83.
28. Watson JN, McQueen P, Hutchinson MR. A systematic review of ulnar collateral ligament reconstruction techniques. *Am J Sports Med.* 2014;42(10):2510–2516.
29. Dines JS, ElAttrache NS, Conway JE, et al. Clinical outcomes of the DANE TJ technique to treat ulnar collateral ligament insufficiency of the elbow. *Am J Sports Med.* 2007;35(12):2039–2044.
30. Erickson BJ, Gupta AK, Harris JD, et al. Rate of return to pitching and performance after Tommy John surgery in Major League Baseball pitchers. *Am J Sports Med.* 2014;42(3):536–543.
31. Wilson AT, Pidgeon TS, Morrell NT, et al. Trends in revision elbow ulnar collateral ligament reconstruction in professional baseball pitchers. *J Hand Surg [Am].* 2015;40(11):2249–2254.
32. Dines JS, Yocum LA, Frank JB, et al. Revision surgery for failed elbow medial collateral ligament reconstruction. *Am J Sports Med.* 2008;36(6):1061–1065.
33. Marshall NE, Keller RA, Lynch JR, et al. Pitching performance and longevity after revision ulnar collateral ligament reconstruction in Major League Baseball pitchers. *Am J Sports Med.* 2015;43(5):1051–1056.

3 Posterolateral Rotatory Instability

James B. Cowan, Russell Nord, and Marc R. Safran

BACKGROUND, ANATOMY, AND ETIOLOGY

Posterolateral rotatory instability (PLRI) of the elbow was first described by Osborne and Cottrell (1). The pathoetiology and diagnosis was further elucidated and popularized by O'Driscoll et al. in 1991 (2). PLRI is defined by subluxation of the proximal radius from the distal humerus resulting in a posteriorly subluxated radial head. This differs from a radial head dislocation because the proximal radioulnar joint remains intact. It also differs from acute elbow dislocation because PLRI describes a chronic lateral-sided rotatory instability, whereas in an elbow dislocation, the lateral structures (and occasionally medial structures) are disrupted.

The lateral side of the elbow is supported by four structures: the lateral ulnar collateral ligament (LUCL), radial collateral ligament (RCL), annular ligament, and accessory radial collateral ligament (Fig. 3-1). The LUCL originates on the lateral epicondyle and inserts on the ulnar supinator tubercle and crest. The RCL originates on the lateral epicondyle and inserts on the annular ligament. The annular ligament both originates and inserts on the proximal ulna, enveloping the proximal radius (3). The accessory RCL runs from the inferior portion of the annular ligament to the supinator crest of the ulna (4). Other authors have failed to find discrete ligamentous structures on cadaveric specimens and have instead suggested that one confluent capsule or "conjoint ligament" with various thickenings provides stability to the lateral side of the elbow (5). The overlying muscles and underlying bony architecture also contribute to both dynamic and static stability.

O'Driscoll and colleagues initially implicated the LUCL as the essential anatomic lesion leading to PLRI (2). However, this has been challenged as the importance of the RCL and overlying musculature of the common extensors have also been shown to play an important role in lateral-sided elbow stability (5–7). Seki et al. (8) demonstrated that the lateral ligament complex functions as a Y-shaped structure, with disruption of the anterior band leading to significant laxity to varus torque

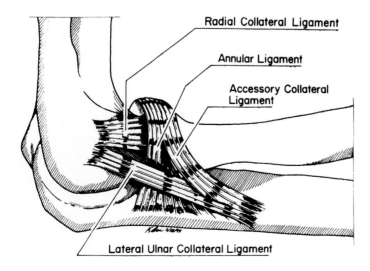

FIGURE 3-1

Ligamentous anatomy of the lateral aspect of the elbow. Note the lateral ulnar collateral ligament, radial collateral ligament, accessory radial collateral ligament, and annular ligament.

and further sectioning of the posterior band resulting in gross instability. This suggests that isolated distal RCL or LUCL injury (the anterior and posterior arms of the "Y") may not result in PLRI, whereas a proximal injury of the lateral epicondyle (the base of the "Y") will disrupt the function of the other two arms and can result in PLRI.

The etiology of PLRI is typically posttraumatic. PLRI is most commonly a late sequela of elbow dislocation or subluxation, when the lateral-sided structures are stretched or torn and fail to heal with nonoperative treatment (9). It may also result from posttraumatic conditions such as coronoid insufficiency or gradual stretching of the lateral structures from cubitus varus after a pediatric supra-condylar humerus fracture malunion (10,11). PLRI may also be iatrogenic. It has been described after radial head resection where there was likely an unrecognized LUCL injury, after multiple steroid injections for lateral epicondylitis in a series of three middle-aged females, and as a conse-quence of overly aggressive surgery for lateral epicondylitis (12–14).

DIAGNOSIS

The diagnosis of PLRI can be elusive. Patients will often present with vague symptoms, though they may note catching, snapping, recurrent instability, or apprehension (9,15). For example, the patient may note locking or catching when turning the car steering wheel, with the forearm going into supination.

The gold standard diagnostic examination for PLRI is the pivot shift maneuver (Fig. 3-2). However, its usefulness in the office and without anesthesia is limited as patients will often guard against subluxation. In such situations, the examiner may only appreciate apprehension or patient discomfort in an awake patient. In one study of eight patients with PLRI, only three had a positive pivot shift test while awake, whereas all eight had a positive pivot shift test under anesthesia (16).

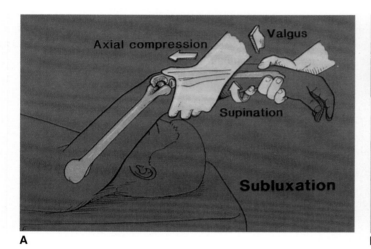

A

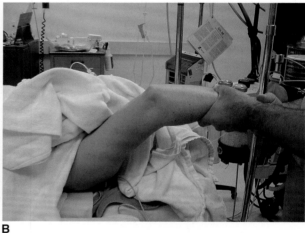

B

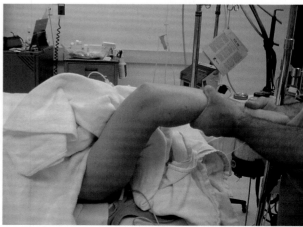

C

FIGURE 3-2

Pivot shift maneuver of the elbow to assess for posterolateral rotatory laxity and instability. **A:** The patient is supine with the arm in full forward elevation. The extended elbow is supinated and a valgus stress applied. The radial head is subluxated posteriorly in this position when there is laxity or injury to the posterolateral ligamentous structures **(B)**. As an axial load is applied, the elbow is flexed, and there is usually a clunk associated with reduction of the radial head **(C)**. This usually occurs at 40 degrees of elbow flexion but may occur in greater degrees of flexion with more ligamentous laxity or injury. In the awake patient, the patient may be apprehensive not allow completion of this maneuver. (Reprinted from O'Driscoll SW, Morrey BF. Surgical reconstruction of the lateral collateral ligament. In: Morrey BF, ed. *Master Techniques in Orthopaedic Surgery: The Elbow*. 2nd Ed. Philadelphia, PA: Lippincott Williams & Wilkins; 2002. Fig. 15-3B, with permission.)

The pivot shift test is most reliable when done under anesthesia when the subluxation can be better appreciated. The pivot shift test is most easily performed with the patient supine, the affected limb overhead, the forearm in full supination, and the shoulder in full forward elevation. The elbow begins in extension and an axial load with valgus is applied, resulting in posterior subluxation of the radial head, which is often recognized by a prominence of the radial head and a dimple just proximal to it (Fig. 3-2). The elbow is slowly flexed as the axial load and valgus force are applied. As the elbow is flexed, at approximately 40 degrees, the triceps becomes taut and reduces the radial head, which is felt as a clunk by the examiner. With greater degrees of laxity of the posterolateral structures of the elbow, greater degrees of elbow flexion are necessary to produce the reduction. Other tests performed in the awake patient may suggest a preliminary diagnosis of PLRI, including palpation for posterior radial head subluxation, the chair test, the push-up test, and the tabletop test. We have found that simply supinating the forearm gently with the elbow at 90 degrees of flexion may lead to a palpable posterior subluxation of the radial head. Regan has shown the efficacy of the chair and push-up tests for the diagnosis of PLRI (16). In both of these tests, the elbow is positioned and loaded in a fashion similar to the pivot shift test. For the chair test (chair sign), the patient is seated in a chair with arms, and the patient puts his or her hands on those arms with the elbows at 90 degrees, forearms supinated, and arms abducted slightly beyond shoulder width (Fig. 3-3). The patient then rises from the chair using only the upper extremities for power. Apprehension, reluctance to fully extend the elbows, or subluxation is considered a positive test. When the forearms are pronated and the test repeated, the patient's symptoms should disappear. For the push-up test (active floor push-up sign), the patient is prone on the floor in the push-up position with the elbows at 90 degrees, forearms supinated, and the arms abducted slightly greater than shoulder width (Fig. 3-4). A push-up is then performed, and apprehension with terminal extension, guarding, or dislocation is considered a positive test. In the aforementioned study, the chair test and the push-up test were both positive in seven of eight patients with PLRI (16).

Another test that may be performed is the tabletop relocation test (17). This test involves the patient leaning on the edge of a table and doing a one-arm press-up with the forearm in full supination. A positive test is noted with patient apprehension or frank subluxation of the radial head. The test is then repeated with the examiner's thumb stabilizing the radial head to prevent subluxation or apprehension. We do not routinely use this test as we have not found it to be more sensitive or specific compared with the aforementioned clinical tests.

For any patient with a possible diagnosis of PLRI, we routinely obtain elbow radiographs to rule out lateral epicondylar avulsion or pathology of the radial head or capitellum. We have not

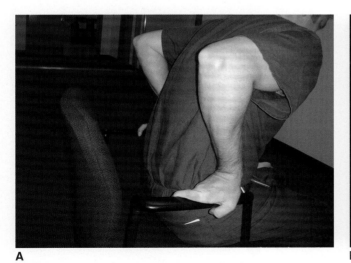
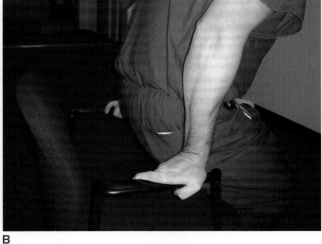

A   **B**

FIGURE 3-3

Chair test—another sign of posterolateral rotatory instability is pain, apprehension, or inability to use one's hands to raise from a chair. With the arms in supination, shoulder width apart, and the elbows flexed, the patient attempts to get out of the chair using the arms. Inability to do this or clunking as they arise, may be consistent with PLRI.

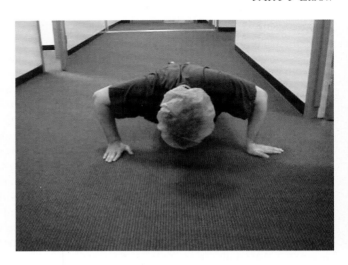

FIGURE 3-4

Push-up test—another sign of posterolateral rotatory instability is pain, apprehension, or inability to use one's hands to perform a push-up with the arms supinated, shoulder width apart, and the elbows flexed. As the patient attempts to push-up, he or she may have apprehension, pain, or clunking, which may be consistent with PLRI.

found stress radiographs, performed with a varus and posterolateral force, to be helpful in the awake patient due to guarding. However, stress radiographs under anesthesia may be useful to document and confirm PLRI of the elbow.

We recommend preoperative MRI on all patients with a preliminary diagnosis of PLRI (Fig. 3-5). While some authors believe that MRI is not sensitive enough to identify LUCL injuries, our experience has been similar to those who have found MRI to be reliable in evaluating the LUCL (18,19). Hackl et al. (20) found that on MRI, sagittal radiocapitellar incongruity of >2 mm and axial ulnohumeral incongruity >1 mm were highly suspicious for PLRI.

In an effort to combine both physical examination and imaging modalities for the evaluation of PLRI, Camp et al. conducted a cadaver study to evaluate whether ultrasound could accurately assess increasing degrees of PLRI of the elbow both at rest and during manual posterolateral rotatory stress testing (21). While acknowledging the limits of a cadaver study and the need for additional clinical studies, the authors concluded that this test may be a useful adjunct to the standard history, examination, and static imaging used to evaluate a patient who may have PLRI.

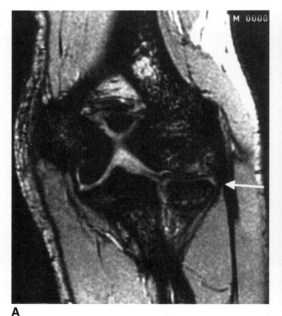
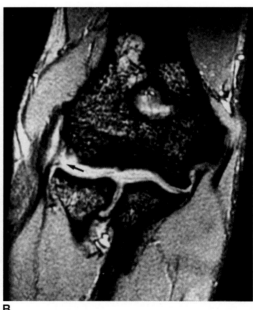

A   B

FIGURE 3-5

(A) is an MRI of a patient with an intact lateral collateral ligament complex, while **(B)** is an MRI of a patient with PLRI. Note the injury to the lateral collateral ligament complex.

TREATMENT AND SURGICAL INDICATIONS

Unlike an acute elbow dislocation, which can often be effectively managed nonoperatively, there is no accepted and effective nonoperative treatment of PLRI other than symptomatic management and activity modification. However, repair of the lateral ligament complex is often possible in the acute setting. We have encountered the need to repair the lateral ligament complex acutely when we operate on an acutely dislocated elbow for another reason such as radial head or capitellar fracture, persistent instability despite reduction, and lateral epicondylar avulsion. In this setting, we perform a suture anchor repair with one or two anchors in the lateral epicondyle with either a Krackow- or Bunnell-type stitch in the avulsed ligamentous sleeve (Fig. 3-6).

In the chronic setting, we typically advocate treating PLRI with reconstruction rather than repair. This recommendation is in concordance with a retrospective study comparing the outcomes in 12 PLRI patients treated with direct repair with the outcomes in 32 PLRI patients treated with autograft tendon reconstruction (22). In this series, while only 7/12 patients treated with repair were satisfied with their outcome, 27/32 patients in the reconstruction group were satisfied. Caution must be taken when interpreting this study and its results, as this was neither a randomized nor a prospective study.

While the pathophysiology of PLRI may not relate solely to LUCL incompetence, the current reconstructive strategies all focus on LUCL reconstruction. A variety of different autograft and allograft options have been used for LUCL reconstruction, but we recommend using the ipsilateral palmaris autograft when available. This may be harvested through a 1-cm incision at the distal volar wrist crease using a standard tendon stripper. If this is not available, the contralateral palmaris is the next choice. Our third option is a hamstring autograft—either gracilis or semitendinosus. A soft tissue allograft, such as a semitendinosus, gracilis, or tibialis tendon, is favored by some surgeons. These grafts are of adequate size, match the native ligament size well, and fit nicely through bone tunnels of modest diameter. The graft must be approximately 20 cm in length.

Our operative technique is similar to that originally described (9,23). Prior to sterile prepping, an exam under anesthesia is performed on both elbows, including a pivot shift test and medial and lateral stability testing (23). The patient is positioned supine with the upper extremity on a hand table. The forearm is pronated to minimize risk to the posterior interosseous nerve during the approach. The medial and lateral sides of the elbow are identified to avoid confusion. The lateral side of the elbow is approached via an 8- to 10-cm incision beginning 3 cm proximal to the lateral epicondyle and terminating over the anterior border of the anconeus (Fig. 3-7). Dissection is carried through Kocher interval between the extensor carpi ulnaris (innervated by the posterior interosseous nerve) and the anconeus (innervated by the radial nerve). Proximally, the anconeus and distal triceps may be reflected off the lateral supracondylar ridge and lateral epicondyle to improve exposure. Distally, the extensor carpi ulnaris is elevated off the annular ligament and reflected anteriorly. The distal

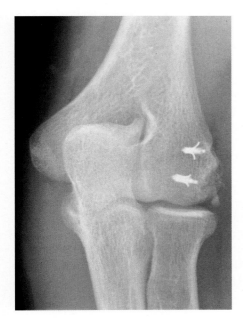

FIGURE 3-6

Radiograph of a 16-year-old male who spontaneously reduced an elbow dislocation following a snowboarding accident. His elbow was unstable to examination awake and under anesthesia. He underwent primary repair of his proximal avulsion of the lateral collateral ligamentous complex using suture anchors.

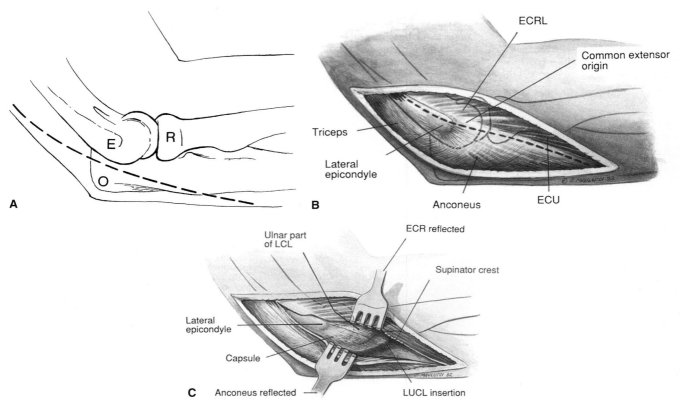

FIGURE 3-7

Incision for open repair or reconstruction of the LUCL complex—the Kocher approach. **(A)** is a schematic representation of the incision, while **(B)** demonstrates the Kocher interval for the fascial incision along the supracondylar ridge of the distal humerus and continuing distally between the anconeus and extensor carpi ulnaris. Deeper dissection **(C)** demonstrates the triceps and anconeus elevated from the humerus, exposing the lateral distal humerus and proximal ulna. The common extensor tendinous origin is reflected to expose the capsule and attenuated capsuloligamentous structures. O, olecranon; E, lateral epicondyle; R, radial head. (Reprinted from O'Driscoll SW, Morrey BF. Surgical reconstruction of the lateral collateral ligament. In: Morrey BF, ed. *Master Techniques in Orthopaedic Surgery: The Elbow*. 2nd Ed. Philadelphia, PA: Lippincott Williams & Wilkins; 2002. Figs. 15-5B, 15-6B, and 15-7B, with permission.)

anconeus may also be reflected posteriorly to reveal the distal attachment of the lateral ligaments at the supinator crest of the ulna. The origin of the common extensors is elevated off the anterior aspect of the lateral epicondyle, revealing the lateral ligamentous complex. The lateral ligamentous complex and anterior capsule must be protected while elevating the common extensors. This is best accomplished by beginning the dissection distally, where the interval between muscle and capsule is more easily defined, and dissecting with a Freer or periosteal elevator rather than a knife to prevent inadvertent migration out of this interval.

At this point, a stretching or disruption of the lateral ligamentous complex is usually appreciated. If it is unclear, a pivot shift test should clearly illustrate a subluxating radial head. An attempt should be made to preserve all lateral tissue that is present. If very robust, a repair or imbrication can be attempted, although we are very selective with this choice given the aforementioned literature that argues against it (22). Otherwise, the tissue can be used to augment the reconstruction and provide additional collagen for healing.

As the ligament complex typically fails proximally, if primary repair is selected, the lateral ligament complex should be reattached to the inferior and posterior portion of the lateral epicondyle. Either suture anchor(s) or transosseous sutures may be employed. We prefer a double-loaded anchor rather than transosseous sutures as it eliminates the risks associated with a bone bridge. The limbs of the sutures are utilized to repair the remaining ligament with a Krackow stitch. If there is any laxity to the capsule, a capsular plication is performed anteriorly and/or posteriorly using imbricating horizontal mattress sutures. Postoperatively, the elbow is splinted in 60 to 90 degrees of flexion with the forearm in pronation.

If reconstruction is elected, the capsule should be incised anterior to the lateral ligamentous complex, so the joint can be inspected for loose bodies or articular damage. This incision is later closed in an imbricated fashion.

Next, two 3.5-mm drill holes are placed in the ulna. One of these drill holes is into the supinator tubercle just distal to the lateral capsular attachment, and the second is placed 1 to 1.5 cm posterior to the first. These two holes should be oriented so that the line between them is perpendicular to the long axis of the soon-to-be reconstructed LUCL (Fig. 3-8). The two holes in the ulna are connected by channeling with a curved awl or curette, taking care to maintain as robust a bony bridge as possible. Recent biomechanical cadaver studies have found that the location of the ulnar tunnels may not be as critical as the location of the humeral tunnel, as long as at least one ulnar tunnel is at the level of, or distal to, the radial head-neck junction (24,25).

The next step is to determine the isometric point on the humeral side. A suture is passed through the tunnel formed by the two ulnar holes and clamped. This clamp is placed on candidate locations on the humerus, and the elbow is taken through a range of motion. If the suture remains taught throughout the range of motion, the isometric point has been identified (Fig. 3-9). While one study found the isometric point of the LUCL to be approximately 2 mm proximal to the center of the capitellum when viewed on lateral x-ray, another study was unable to identify a single point of perfect isometry but found the humeral center of rotation to be the most isometric point (25,26).

A 4.5-mm drill hole is placed just proximal and anterior to the isometric point so that its distal aspect, over which the reconstructed LUCL will be draped, is at the isometric point. If this hole is too posterior, the graft will remain lax in extension, where PLRI typically occurs. This drill hole should be angled medially and proximally. A motorized bur is then used to dilate this hole to 5 to 6 mm in size. A second humeral hole is created just posterior to the supracondylar ridge, 1.5 cm proximal to the first hole using a 3.5-mm drill. Curved curettes or awls are used to make a tunnel by connecting the two holes, once again taking care to maintain the bone bridge. A third, and final, humeral hole is drilled 1 to 1.5 cm distal to the second hole. It is connected to the first hole (the hole at the humeral isometric point) by a tunnel using curved curettes or curved awls (Fig. 3-10). Posterior holes are used for the nonisometric humeral holes because the posterior humeral bone is stronger than the anterior bone.

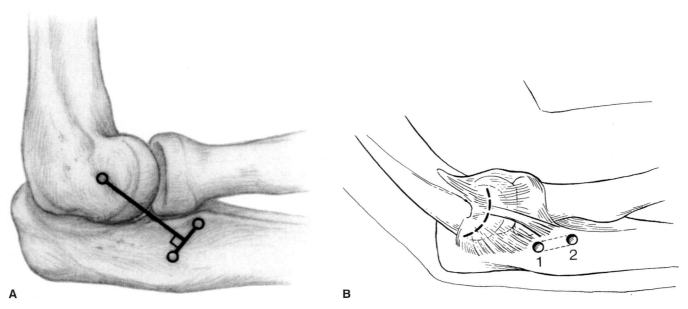

A

B

FIGURE 3-8

Ulnar tunnel for LUCL reconstruction made by connecting two drill holes made at the crista supinatoris, perpendicular to the line of the proposed LUCL ligament **(A)**. Capsular incision is also demonstrated for identification of humeral tunnel **(B)**. *1* and *2* represent where the 2 tunnels would be located relative to capsular incision. (Reprinted from O'Driscoll SW, Morrey BF. Surgical reconstruction of the lateral collateral ligament. In: Morrey BF, ed. *Master Techniques in Orthopaedic Surgery: The Elbow.* 2nd Ed. Philadelphia, PA: Lippincott Williams & Wilkins; 2002. Figs. 15-8B and 15-8C, with permission.)

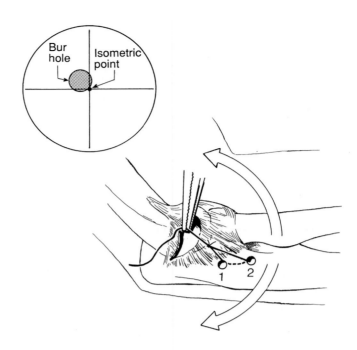

FIGURE 3-9

Identification of the isometric point on the distal humerus for LUCL reconstruction and relative tunnel position to this isometric point slightly proximal and posterior. *1* and *2* represent the two adjoining tunnels in the proximal ulna/crista supinatoris. (Reprinted from O'Driscoll SW, Morrey BF. Surgical reconstruction of the lateral collateral ligament. In: Morrey BF, ed. *Master Techniques in Orthopaedic Surgery: The Elbow.* 1st Ed. New York: Raven Press; 1994. Fig. 8B, with permission.)

A passing suture is sewn into one end of the graft, leaving a curved needle on the end of the suture. This facilitates graft passage. The graft is then passed through the ulnar tunnel from anterior to posterior. Next, the graft is passed into the isometric hole in the humerus and out the proximal hole in the humerus. The graft is then run along the posterior humeral cortex, into the distal/posterior hole and finally emerging out the isometric hole (Fig. 3-11). A curved 22-gauge wire can also be used to assist in graft passage.

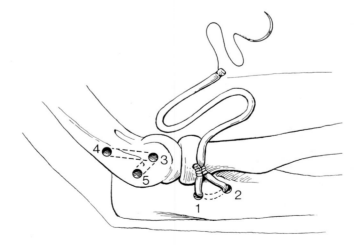

FIGURE 3-10

Humeral tunnels made in a "Y" fashion to allow for passage of the graft in a "figure-of-8" pattern. Hole 3 is made at the isometric point on the lateral epicondyles, and holes 4 and 5 are made and connected with hole 3 to complete the "Y" configuration of distal humeral tunnels. The graft, first passed through the ulnar tunnel, is brought in hole 3 and out hole 4. Usually the suture in the tendon is passed using a needle or a looped suture or wire. (Reprinted from O'Driscoll SW, Morrey BF. Surgical reconstruction of the lateral collateral ligament. In: Morrey BF, ed. *Master Techniques in Orthopaedic Surgery: The Elbow.* 2nd Ed. Philadelphia, PA: Lippincott Williams & Wilkins; 2002. Fig. 15-10B, with permission.)

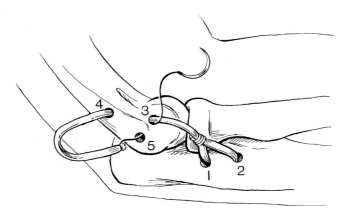

FIGURE 3-11

Graft being passed through the humeral tunnels. The graft being brought in hole 3 and out hole 4 is brought back in hole 5 with a suture, needle, or wire, to exit out the isometric point (hole 3). (Reprinted from O'Driscoll SW, Morrey BF. Surgical reconstruction of the lateral collateral ligament. In: Morrey BF, ed. *Master Techniques in Orthopaedic Surgery: The Elbow.* 2nd Ed. Philadelphia, PA: Lippincott Williams & Wilkins; 2002. Fig. 15-11B, with permission.)

The graft is then tensioned with the elbow in 30 to 40 degrees of flexion and the forearm fully pronated, with a gentle valgus load. The end of the graft is then sutured to itself with the tension maintained (Fig. 3-12). Care is taken to remove any slack from all segments of the graft's figure-of-8 path. Further tensioning is achieved by pulling the graft anteriorly and suturing it to the capsule (Fig. 3-13A). Even greater tension within the graft may be generated by suturing limbs of the figure-of-8 to one another, thus reducing the size of the distal loop of the figure-of-8 (Fig. 3-13B). The capsule is then closed and the soft tissue closed in layers.

Rather than the classic figure-of-8 graft, other constructs may be used for the reconstruction. A recent biomechanical cadaver study comparing three reconstruction methods (single-bundle LUCL reconstruction, single-bundle LUCL reconstruction with RCL augmentation, and dual reconstruction of both the LUCL and RCL) found no significant differences between posterolateral rotatory stability of the elbow over a full range of motion following (27). While we have not had a failure of the ulnar or humeral tunnels, if this was to occur, an Endobutton (Smith and Nephew, Andover, MA) or a similar suspensory fixation device could be used as salvage fixation, by relying on the opposite cortex of the ulna or humerus while bringing the soft tissue into the bone for biologic fixation. However, when drilling for the Endobutton in the humerus, one should aim anteriorly to avoid the ulnar nerve on the medial side of the humerus.

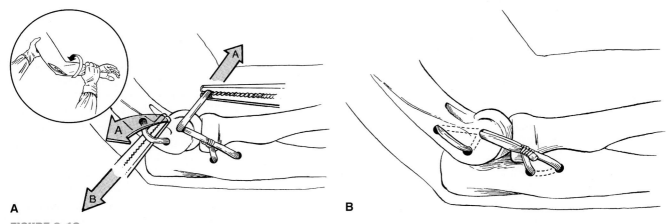

A   **B**

FIGURE 3-12

Graft being tensioned and then sutured to itself. The free limb of the graft is pulled with the elbow flexed 30 to 40 degrees with the forearm in full pronation to tension the graft **(A)**. The graft is then sutured to itself **(B)**. (Reprinted from O'Driscoll SW, Morrey BF. Surgical reconstruction of the lateral collateral ligament. In: Morrey BF, ed. *Master Techniques in Orthopaedic Surgery: The Elbow.* 2nd Ed. Philadelphia, PA: Lippincott Williams & Wilkins; 2002. Figs. 15-12B and 15-13B, with permission.)

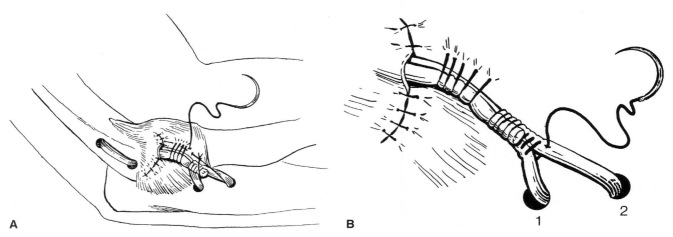

FIGURE 3-13

Graft being sutured to the capsule and native LUCL complex **(A)** and tensioning further by suturing the limbs of the graft to each other. This closes the figure-of-8 and tightens the overall construct **(B)**. (Reprinted from O'Driscoll SW, Morrey BF. Surgical reconstruction of the lateral collateral ligament. In: Morrey BF, ed. *Master Techniques in Orthopaedic Surgery: The Elbow*. 2nd Ed. Philadelphia, PA: Lippincott Williams & Wilkins; 2002. Figs. 15-15B and 15-16B, with permission.)

Lastly, rather than using a figure-of-8 construct, interference screws in blind tunnels can be used on either or both the humeral and ulnar sides. This results in a double-stranded rather than triple-stranded LUCL reconstruction, but this can be compensated for by starting with a slightly larger-sized graft. Using this technique, the capsule is closed and plicated in a similar fashion as in the figure-of-8 construct.

REHABILITATION

There is no evidence-based consensus for postoperative rehabilitation following surgery for PLRI (28). However, regardless of the method of repair or reconstruction, the elbow must be protected postoperatively. The elbow should be splinted at 90 degrees of flexion with the forearm in full pronation. This splint is removed 1 week postoperatively and exchanged for a hinged brace with a 30-degree extension block. Full range of motion is begun at 6 weeks postoperatively. The brace is used until the patient is 3 months out from surgery, at which point, a gradual strengthening program is begun. Full recovery and return to sport is anticipated at 6 to 9 months depending on the patient, the recovery, and the sport to which they return. One risk of this regimen is the possibility of a mild (<10 degrees) flexion contracture. However, this contracture may serve a protective role as it would keep the patient out of a position of PLRI.

RESULTS

The results of LUCL reconstruction for PLRI are generally good in terms of both objective stability and subjective patient outcome (Table 3-1). Anakwenze et al. (29) completed a systematic review of eight studies including 130 patients to examine the outcomes of LUCL reconstruction for PLRI of the elbow. There was one level II prospective cohort study, one level III retrospective cohort study, and six level IV case series studies. The mean patient age was 38.1 years, the mean time between symptom onset and surgical intervention was 55.7 weeks, and the mean follow-up was 44.5 months. Although the reporting and outcomes varied among included studies, postoperative pivot shift test was negative in 92% of patients (72/78 patients in fives studies), 98% of patients were satisfied (50/51 patients in five studies), and 91% had Mayo Elbow Performance Score (MEPS) that were considered excellent or good (43/47 patients in three studies). The overall complication rate was 11% (8/76) with recurrent laxity or instability occurring in 8% (6/76) of patients. Overall, this review was limited by the quality of the included studies and the heterogeneity of the included patient populations, surgical techniques, and reported outcomes.

TABLE 3-1 Results after Ligament Reconstruction of the LUCL

Author	Year	Mean Follow-Up (months)	Outcome
Lee and Teo (30)	2003	24	6/6 (100%) stable 6/6 (100%) satisfied
Olsen and Sojbjerg (31)	2003	44	14/18 (78%) stable 17/18 (94%) satisfied
Sanchez-Sotelo et al. (22)	2005	72	30/32 (94%) stable 27/32 (84%) satisfied
Savoie et al. (32)	2009	41	Significant improvement in subjective and objective Andrews-Carson scores
Jones et al. (33)	2012	85	6/8 (75%) stable 8/8 (100%) satisfied
Lin et al. (34)	2012	49	13/14 (93%) stable 13/14 (93%) satisfied
Kim et al. (35)	2016	23	13/13 (100%) stable 12/13 (92%) excellent MEPS score

REFERENCES

1. Osborne G, Cotterill P. Recurrent dislocation of the elbow. *J Bone Joint Surg Br.* 1966;48(2):340–346.
2. O'Driscoll SW, Bell DF, Morrey BF. Posterolateral rotatory instability of the elbow. *J Bone Joint Surg Am.* 1991;73(3):440–446.
3. Mehta JA, Bain GI. Posterolateral rotatory instability of the elbow. *J Am Acad Orthop Surg.* 2004;12(6):405–415.
4. Morrey BF, An KN. Functional anatomy of the ligaments of the elbow. *Clin Orthop Relat Res.* 1985;(201):84–90.
5. Cohen MS, Hastings H II. Rotatory instability of the elbow. The anatomy and role of the lateral stabilizers. *J Bone Joint Surg Am.* 1997;79(2):225–233.
6. Dunning CE, Zarzour ZD, Patterson SD, et al. Ligamentous stabilizers against posterolateral rotatory instability of the elbow. *J Bone Joint Surg Am.* 2001;83-a(12):1823–1828.
7. McAdams TR, Masters GW, Srivastava S. The effect of arthroscopic sectioning of the lateral ligament complex of the elbow on posterolateral rotatory stability. *J Shoulder Elbow Surg.* 2005;14(3):298–301.
8. Seki A, Olsen BS, Jensen SL, et al. Functional anatomy of the lateral collateral ligament complex of the elbow: configuration of Y and its role. *J Shoulder Elbow Surg.* 2002;11(1):53–59.
9. Nestor BJ, O'Driscoll SW, Morrey BF. Ligamentous reconstruction for posterolateral rotatory instability of the elbow. *J Bone Joint Surg Am.* 1992;74(8):1235–1241.
10. Okazaki M, Takayama S, Seki A, et al. Posterolateral rotatory instability of the elbow with insufficient coronoid process of the ulna: a report of 3 patients. *J Hand Surg [Am].* 2007;32(2):236–239.
11. O'Driscoll SW, Spinner RJ, McKee MD, et al. Tardy posterolateral rotatory instability of the elbow due to cubitus varus. *J Bone Joint Surg Am.* 2001;83-a(9):1358–1369.
12. Morrey BF. Reoperation for failed surgical treatment of refractory lateral epicondylitis. *J Shoulder Elbow Surg.* 1992;1(1):47–55.
13. Hall JA, McKee MD. Posterolateral rotatory instability of the elbow following radial head resection. *J Bone Joint Surg Am.* 2005;87(7):1571–1579.
14. Kalainov DM, Cohen MS. Posterolateral rotatory instability of the elbow in association with lateral epicondylitis. A report of three cases. *J Bone Joint Surg Am.* 2005;87(5):1120–1125.
15. Charalambous CP, Stanley JK. Posterolateral rotatory instability of the elbow. *J Bone Joint Surg Br.* 2008;90(3):272–279.
16. Regan W, Lapner PC. Prospective evaluation of two diagnostic apprehension signs for posterolateral instability of the elbow. *J Shoulder Elbow Surg.* 2006;15(3):344–346.
17. Arvind CH, Hargreaves DG. Tabletop relocation test: a new clinical test for posterolateral rotatory instability of the elbow. *J Shoulder Elbow Surg.* 2006;15(6):707–708.
18. Potter HG, Weiland AJ, Schatz JA, et al. Posterolateral rotatory instability of the elbow: usefulness of MR imaging in diagnosis. *Radiology.* 1997;204(1):185–189.
19. Terada N, Yamada H, Toyama Y. The appearance of the lateral ulnar collateral ligament on magnetic resonance imaging. *J Shoulder Elbow Surg.* 2004;13(2):214–216.
20. Hackl M, Wegmann K, Ries C, et al. Reliability of magnetic resonance imaging signs of posterolateral rotatory instability of the elbow. *J Hand Surg [Am].* 2015;40(7):1428–1433.
21. Camp CL, O'Driscoll SW, Wempe MK, et al. The sonographic posterolateral rotatory stress test for elbow instability: a cadaveric validation study. *PM R* 2017;9(3):275–282.
22. Sanchez-Sotelo J, Morrey BF, O'Driscoll SW. Ligamentous repair and reconstruction for posterolateral rotatory instability of the elbow. *J Bone Joint Surg Br.* 2005;87(1):54–61.
23. Rightmire E, Safran MR. Posterolateral Instability of the Elbow. In: Cole B, Sekiya J, eds. *Surgical Techniques of the Shoulder, Elbow and Knee in Sports Medicine.* New York: Elsevier; 2008:371–378.
24. Kim HM, Andrews CR, Roush EP, et al. Effect of ulnar tunnel location on elbow stability in double-strand lateral collateral ligament reconstruction. *J Shoulder Elbow Surg.* 2017;26(3):409–415.
25. Alaia MJ, Shearin JW, Kremenic IJ, et al. Restoring isometry in lateral ulnar collateral ligament reconstruction. *J Hand Surg [Am].* 2015;40(7):1421–1427.
26. Moritomo H, Murase T, Arimitsu S, et al. The in vivo isometric point of the lateral ligament of the elbow. *J Bone Joint Surg Am.* 2007;89(9):2011–2017.
27. Dargel J, Boomkamp E, Wegmann K, et al. Reconstruction of the lateral ulnar collateral ligament of the elbow: a comparative biomechanical study. *Knee Surg Sports Traumatol Arthrosc.* 2017;25(3):943–948.

28. Reuter S, Proier P, Imhoff A, et al. Rehabilitation, clinical outcome and return to sporting activities after posterolateral elbow instability: a systematic review. *Eur J Phys Rehabil Med.* 2016.
29. Anakwenze OA, Kwon D, O'Donnell E, et al. Surgical treatment of posterolateral rotatory instability of the elbow. *Arthroscopy.* 2014;30(7):866–871.
30. Lee BP, Teo LH. Surgical reconstruction for posterolateral rotatory instability of the elbow. *J ShoulderElbow Surg.* 2003;12(5):476–479.
31. Olsen BS, Sojbjerg JO. The treatment of recurrent posterolateral instability of the elbow. *J Bone Joint Surg Br.* 2003;85(3):342–346.
32. Savoie FH 3rd, Field LD, Gurley DJ. Arthroscopic and open radial ulnohumeral ligament reconstruction for posterolateral rotatory instability of the elbow. *Hand Clin.* 2009;25(3):323–329.
33. Jones KJ, Dodson CC, Osbahr DC, et al. The docking technique for lateral ulnar collateral ligament reconstruction: surgical technique and clinical outcomes. *J Shoulder Elbow Surg.* 2012;21(3):389–395.
34. Lin KY, Shen PH, Lee CH, et al. Functional outcomes of surgical reconstruction for posterolateral rotatory instability of the elbow. *Injury.* 2012;43(10):1657–1661.
35. Kim JW, Yi Y, Kim TK, et al. Arthroscopic lateral collateral ligament repair. *J Bone Joint Surg Am.* 2016;98(15):1268–1276.

4 Arthroscopic Management of Elbow Osteochondritis Dissecans Lesions

Guillem Gonzalez-Lomas and Abigail L. Campbell

INTRODUCTION

The incidence of sport-specific injuries in young athletes has increased with earlier and more rigorous young athlete participation in sports. The radiocapitellar compartment of the young athlete's elbow withstands significant stresses during repetitive activities (such as throwing) or during sports that convert the elbow joint into a weight-bearing joint (such as gymnastics) (1). Specifically, lateral compartment compression can lead to Panner diseases (osteochondrosis) in the very young, preadolescent (6–10-year-old) patient or capitellar osteochondritis dissecans (OCD) in the adolescent or young adult (2–5). OCD may in turn generate loose bodies. This chapter describes Panner disease and OCD and describes a treatment algorithm, including detailing their arthroscopic management.

PANNER DISEASE

In 1927, Hans Jessen Panner described "osteochondrosis" of the capitellum, remarking on its similarities to Legg-Calvé-Perthes of the hip (6). Like other osteochondroses, it consists of noninflammatory disordered endochondral ossification. Its specific etiology and relationship to OCD remain debatable. It is generally accepted, however, that abnormal radiocapitellar compressive forces during a period of vulnerability predispose children to this pathology (2,5,7). Etiologically, it may result from the combination of an avascular insult (likely related to the capitellum's predominantly end-artery supply) and repetitive microtrauma (8).

Epidemiology

Panner disease predominantly affects males younger than age 10 (9). Young boys tend to be predisposed to it for two reasons. One, compared to girls, they have a delayed appearance and maturation of their secondary ossification centers. Two, boys traditionally are more prone to trauma from more aggressive early childhood activities they select (7). This may change as more girls become involved in higher-risk athletic activities at younger ages. Although Panner's can be confused with OCD, and the age of onset may overlap, it distinguishes itself by three epidemiologic characteristics. One, Panner disease does not share the strict association with repetitive throwing that OCD does. Two, it is usually self-limiting. And three, it resolves without any long-term sequelae.

Presentation

Patients with Panner disease will initially present complaining of pain and stiffness in the elbow, relieved by rest. On physical exam, they will have poorly localized tenderness over the lateral elbow. Radiographs will initially show fissuring, lucencies, fragmentation, and irregularity of the capitellum (shown in Fig. 4-1), particularly near or at the chondral surface. Subsequent films, taken at 3 to 5 months, will demonstrate larger radiolucent areas followed by reossification of the bony epiphysis with a corresponding resolution of symptoms. In 1 to 2 years, the epiphysis regains its contour, usually without flattening (4). It should be noted that, as in Legg-Calvé-Perthes, radiographs often lag behind

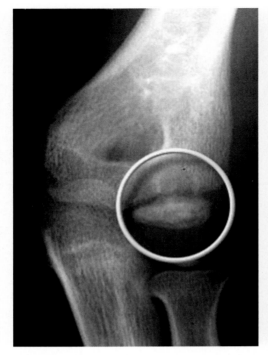

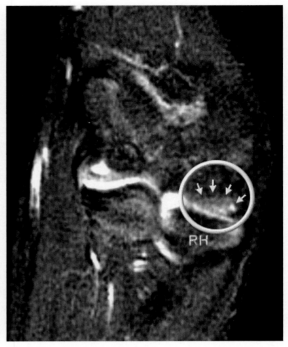

FIGURE 4-1

Panner disease. AP radiograph of the left elbow demonstrating fragmentation and lucency of the capitellum (*circle*) near the chondral surface.

FIGURE 4-2

Panner disease, as seen on T2-weighted MRI. *Circle* surrounds Panner lesion, demarcated by *small arrows*, opposite radial head (RH). Notice the more typical finding of edema adjacent to the capitellar chondral surface, rather than deeper in the subchondral bone as in OCD.

clinical symptoms. MRI can also document the extent of the lesion. Typically, edema is localized to the chondral surface with less involvement of the subchondral bone, as compared to OCD (Fig. 4-2).

Treatment

Treatment involves complete rest from the activity in question and administering modalities such as ice and anti-inflammatory medication. The elbow may occasionally need to be immobilized for a brief period to control symptoms. Symptoms usually resolve within 6 to 8 weeks, although they occasionally persist for months, and activities should be reinstituted progressively and as tolerated. The condition has excellent long-term prognosis, although in some patients there may be a slight residual flexion contracture.

OSTEOCHONDRITIS DISSECANS

OCD of the capitellum is a noninflammatory degeneration of subchondral bone occurring in the context of repetitive trauma to the lateral compartment of the elbow (10,11). The prevalence of capitellar OCD in youth baseball players has been recently estimated to be 2.1% to 3.4%. Panner disease and OCD may represent two different stages of the same disorder (4). The two conditions, however, do differ in certain characteristics: age of onset, etiology, and natural history. One, while Panner disease affects children under 10, OCD victimizes older athletes between ages 11 and 15 (12). Two, unlike Panner disease, OCD is thought to be directly linked to repetitive trauma. Three, OCD is not always self-limiting. If left unaddressed, it results in profound destruction of the capitellum (12).

Etiology

The etiology of capitellar OCD lesions is multifactorial, with anatomy, physeal immaturity, loading pattern, and vascular anatomy all contributing to the pathophysiology of this disease.

OCD is associated with repetitive and excessive compressive forces generated by either large valgus stresses on the elbow during throwing or racket swinging or from constant axial compressive loads on the elbow such as those endured by gymnasts (12–14). Specific activities predispose patients to the condition. In the case of baseball players, throwing sliders and breaking pitches, throwing more than 600 pitches per season, and increased age of the athlete increase the risk of developing OCD (14). Repetitive shear loading has been shown to occur across the radiocapitellar joint during late cocking and early acceleration phases of throwing (15,16). In female gymnasts, overtraining involving excessive handstand maneuvers creating repetitive axial loading has been linked to OCD (17,18). Kajiyama et al. recently demonstrated a difference in pattern of OCD between gymnasts and baseball players; the lesions were more anterior on the capitellum in baseball players due to the loading pattern of throwing compared to gymnastics (19).

Other risk factors include genetic predisposition and the tenuous end-artery vascular supply to the capitellum. In the young adult population, the capitellum is supplied by two end arteries coursing from posterior to anterior, which are branches of the radial recurrent and interosseous recurrent arteries (Fig. 4-3) (20). As a result of the longitudinal blood supply to the capitellar epiphyseal plate and minimal collateral circulation in the area, blood flow to the capitellum may be disrupted by both repetitive microtrauma resulting in an avascular state and a single traumatic event leading to posttraumatic subchondral bone bruises (21,22).

Presentation

Patients with OCD will initially present complaining of pain and stiffness in the elbow, relieved by rest. If left unaddressed, the symptoms may progress to "locking" or "catching" due to intra-articular loose bodies. Physical examination tends to be remarkable for poorly localized lateral elbow tenderness over the radiocapitellar joint. Loss of range of motion with a 15- to 20-degree flexion contracture is common. Loss of extension is more common than loss of flexion. Radiocapitellar joint provocative maneuvers include the active radiocapitellar compression test (Fig. 4-4). A positive test elicits pain in the lateral compartment of the elbow when the patient pronates and supinates the forearm with the arm in extension.

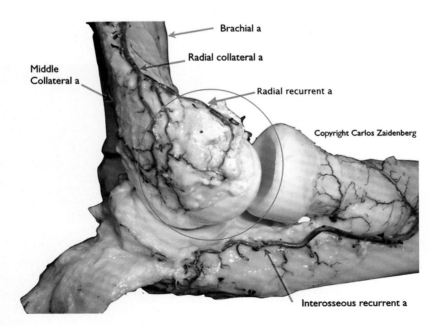

FIGURE 4-3

Capitellar blood supply. In the young adult population (under age 20), the *radial recurrent and interosseous recurrent arteries* give off branches that course from posterior to anterior and supply the capitellum (inside *red circle*). This end-artery blood supply makes the capitellum susceptible to an avascular insult. From Eygendaal D, et al. Osteochondritis dissecans of the elbow: state of the art. *J ISAKOS.* 2017;2(1):47–57, with permission.

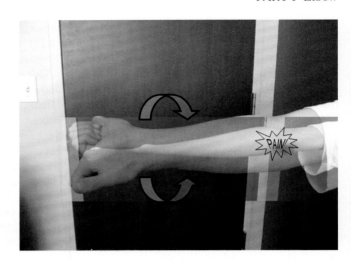

FIGURE 4-4

Radiocapitellar compression test. Pain in lateral elbow when the extended arm is pronated and supinated.

Imaging

Anterior-posterior in full extension, anterior-posterior in 45 degrees of flexion, and lateral views of the elbow should be obtained. Radiographs may be negative early in the disease process. It is critical to note the stage of closure at the capitellar physis. As the condition progresses, flattening and sclerosis of the capitellum, fissuring, or fragmentation will become apparent. Irregular areas of lucency and intra-articular loose bodies also appear. The anterolaterally located capitellar lesion of OCD is best seen on an AP at 45-degree elbow flexion (Fig. 4-5).

In suspected OCD, an MRI should always be obtained as plain radiographs can miss up to one third of diagnoses (23). It will detect bony edema early in early disease stages (24). An MRI arthrogram can further delineate the extent of the injury by demonstrating any detached fragments from subchondral bone (Fig. 4-6). Peiss et al. felt that fragment enhancement (seen in Fig. 4-7B) (as

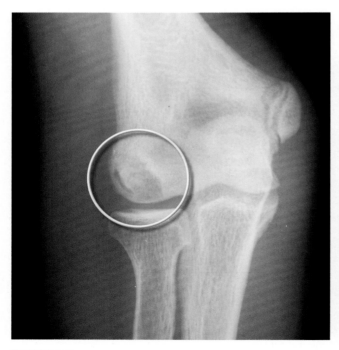

FIGURE 4-5

AP radiograph at 45-degree flexion. OCD lesion (*circle*) is seen more clearly with the elbow flexed to 45 degrees.

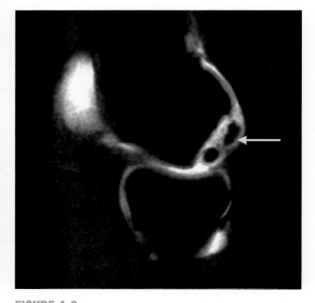

FIGURE 4-6

MR arthrogram showing contrast surrounding unstable OCD fragment (*arrow*).

opposed to the perifragment enhancement seen in Fig. 4-6) denotes viability and may be a reasonable indication for nonoperative treatment (25). The authors hypothesize that enhancement of the fragment-subchondral bone interface is caused by vascular granulation tissue, indicating instability and requiring operative intervention. Of note, it is critically important to distinguish "pseudolesions," an anatomic variation appearing on the posteroinferior junction of the articular and nonarticular portions of the capitellum, from OCD, which almost always present on the anterolateral aspect (26).

Ultrasound has also been shown to have a high positive predictive value for identifying capitellar OCD from irregular capitellar articular contour. This imaging modality, however, relies on user experience requiring dedicated training (11).

Management

Management of OCD lesions is based primarily on the status and stability of the overlying cartilage. The size and location of the lesion and the patency of the capitellar physis also influence decision-making (27–29). In order to guide treatment, detailed classification systems based on radiographic (30,31) and arthroscopic (27) findings have been described (32,33). We have chosen to simplify these algorithms into a succinct, three-stage classification that provides a template for management. Table 4-1 illustrates the classification.

Stage 1

In Stage 1, the osteochondral fragment is intact, stable, and nondisplaced. Radiographs are often negative. Signal on MRI is variable, typically abnormal on T1 and normal on T2, although T2 signal may also be abnormal. Figure 4-7A and B shows a Stage 1 lesion coronal image with abnormal signal on both T1 and T2. Arthroscopically, the articular cartilage is intact with a general preservation of subchondral stability. This stage is best treated nonoperatively. Figure 4-7C and D shows 6-month follow-up coronal T1 and T2 images from the same patient as in Figure 4-7A and B after conservative treatment. MRI demonstrates clear reconstitution of the subchondral bone. If symptoms return, additional rest is mandated. With persistently refractory symptoms, pitchers may have to change positions and gymnasts may have to change sports. Lesions that progress to Stage 2 should be treated accordingly.

Stage 2

In Stage 2, the osteochondral fragment is partially separated as documented both radiographically and arthroscopically. Radiographs will demonstrate fissuring, lucencies, and fragmentation. On MRI, both T1 and T2 sequences will show an abnormal signal and a margin around the fragment, denoting its instability (Fig. 4-8). CT scan may also reveal the partially separated

---

TABLE 4-1 Classification and Treatment of Capitellar Osteochondritis Dissecans Lesions

Stability	Stage	MRI Findings	Arthroscopic Findings	Treatment
Stable	I	Normal XR T1 abnormal T2 normal	Intact articular cartilage Subchondral bone edema but structurally sound	1. Hinged elbow brace: 3–6 wk 2. PT 3. NSAIDs 4. Follow-up XR and or MRI at 3–6 mo
Unstable	II	Abnormal XR T1/T2 abnormal contrast shows margin around lesion	Partially detached fragment Cartilage fracture Subchondral bone collapse **Lateral buttress involved:** poorer prognosis	1. *Acute:* Consider fragment fixation, but higher success treating as chronic (below) 2. *Chronic:* a. **<6–7-mm lateral buttress involved/radial head does not engage:** Fragment removal + microfracture/drilling b. **>6–7-mm lateral buttress involved/head engages:** Removal + osteochondral autograft/synthetic graft
	III	Loose bodies	Completely detached-Loose bodies	1. Loose body removal 2. Treat as Stage II
		Associated radial head OCD	Any of the above	1. **<30% radial head involvement:** Treat as Stage II 2. **>30%:** No osteochondral grafting; microfracture drilling ok

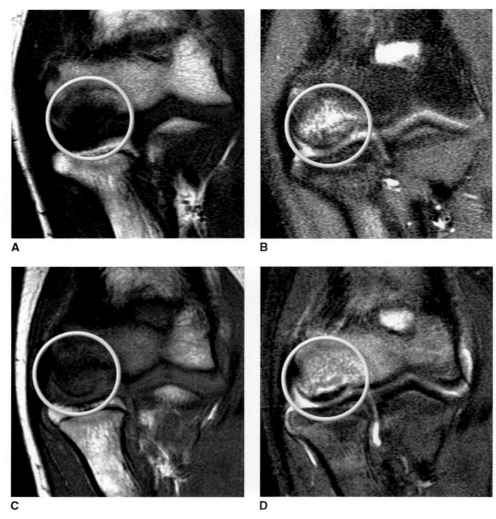

FIGURE 4-7

Stage 1 OCD lesion progress. Stable, intact, nondisplaced fragment (*circles*) with abnormal signal on coronal slices in **(A)** T1 and T2 sequences **(B)**. After 6 months of conservative management, T1 **(C)** and T2 **(D)** sequences show reconstitution of subchondral bone in the area of the lesion. The patient was symptom-free at the 6-month follow-up.

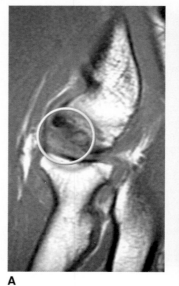
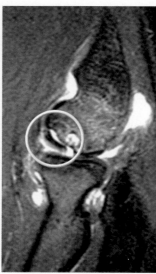

FIGURE 4-8

Stage 2 OCD lesion as seen on MRI. **(A)** T1 and **(B)** T2 sequences showing a margin around the OCD fragment (*circles*) denoting its instability.

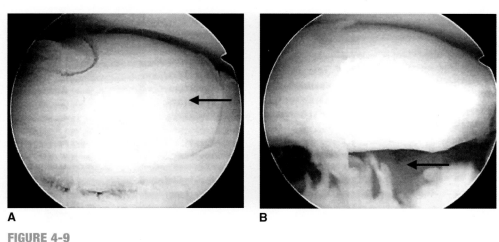

A   B

FIGURE 4-9

Stage 2 OCD lesion as seen arthroscopically. **A:** *Arrow* points to osteochondral fragment located at its donor site. **B:** *Arrow* points to space between osteochondral fragment and bone, denoting fractured cartilage and instability.

fragment. Arthroscopically, the cartilage is fractured and the subchondral bone is unstable and partially displaced (Fig. 4-9). When an unstable lesion is identified, conservative treatment should be bypassed. It warrants prompt surgical intervention in order to return the athlete to their sport or activities of daily living as soon as possible. In Stage 2 lesions, the size and location of the lesion govern treatment. For smaller lesions, debridement is an option. Patients typically have immediate relief of symptoms, but their long-term natural history includes arthritis. Fragment fixation has been advocated by some for this stage, although questions linger concerning the long-term healing potential of fixed fragments and clinical results of the procedure (30,31,34,35). Finally, osteochondral autografts or synthetic grafts can address large, radial head-engaging defects involving the lateral buttress of the capitellum. If the decision rests between fixation and osteochondral restoration, our preference is for osteochondral or synthetic plug grafting as this has generated more reliable results.

SIZE. Takahara et al. (36) differentiated between small (<5% of the capitellum on an anterior-posterior radiograph of the elbow, <60-degree angle formed by lines drawn along the borders of the lesion on a lateral radiograph), moderate (5%–70%), and large (>70%, >90 degrees) lesions. They concluded that large lesions should be addressed operatively. This same group demonstrated that debridement alone has been associated with poorer outcomes than when accompanied by reconstruction procedure in lesions in which more than 50% of the capitellar surface is involved (30). Shimada et al. (37) suggested that smaller lesions (<1 cm^2) can be treated with debridement, chondroplasty, and possibly microfracture or drilling as described by Bradley and Dandy (38). Larger lesions (>1 cm^2) should be treated with osteochondral autografts. Costal osteochondral autograft transplantation is a recent technique described for lateral lesions >15-mm diameter with promising short-term results. This technique, however, is technically demanding and carries the risk of serious complications (39,40).

LOCATION. In our opinion, the location of the lesion may be more important than size in guiding treatment. Extension of the lesion into the lateral margin of the capitellum, as described by ElAttrache and co-author (41) and Ruch et al. (42), is associated with a potentially poorer prognosis. The lateral column of the capitellum supports large compressive forces when the elbow is stressed in valgus or with axial loading. When the lateral column is intact, a defect treated with microfracture alone is relatively protected and fibrocartilage healing may occur. Lesions that do not involve a significant portion of the lateral buttress of the capitellum and do not engage the radial head during arthroscopic observation (pronation and supination with the elbow in extension) have been successfully treated with microfracture or subchondral drilling. If intact cartilage cap is present, retrograde drilling is recommended. Antegrade drilling or microfracture can be utilized when the cartilage has been disrupted. Figure 4-10 shows an OCD lesion with a predominantly intact lateral column.

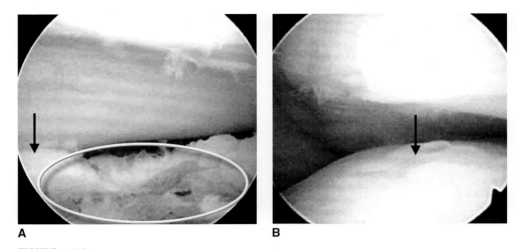

FIGURE 4-10

OCD lesion with intact lateral column. **A:** OCD lesion (*oval*) adjacent to significant portion of intact lateral column (*arrow*). **B:** Lateral column (*arrow*) supports RH and does not permit engagement with defect.

Conversely, lateral column involvement of more than about 6 to 7 mm cannot be dealt with acceptably by microfracture. In this case, the absence of a lateral buttress forestalls fibrocartilage healing, by subjecting the defect to increased radiocapitellar forces. Furthermore, engagement of the radial head in the defect also compromises healing and may lead to accelerated radiocapitellar arthrosis. For these larger, engaging defects or those that extend substantially into the lateral buttress (over 6–7 mm) (Fig. 4-11), we recommend removal of the loose fragment and osteochondral restoration by means of mosaicplasty or osteochondral autograft transplantation (OATS). In the case of early partially detached fragments, the detached portion (usually central) should be debrided from central to lateral. Once stable osteochondral borders have been obtained, the lesion is carefully evaluated arthroscopically to ascertain how much of the lateral column is involved and if the radial head engages with the defect. Chappell and ElAttrache reported that lesions >1 cm^2 (average 1.32 cm^2) and no lateral column involvement were treated successfully with microfracture while those involving the lateral column did well with osteochondral grafting. Fragment fixation is an option as well, but we have had superior and more consistent results with grafting (41). When fixation is feasible, fixation with bioabsorbable pins has been associated with high union rates in large unstable lesions (43).

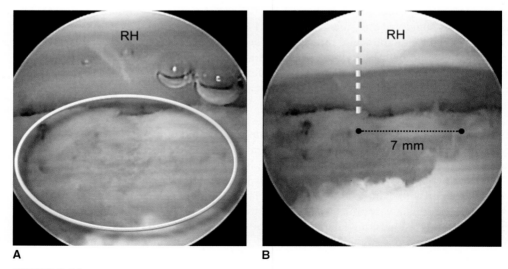

FIGURE 4-11

Lesion extends into lateral column. **A:** OCD lesion (*circle*). **B:** *White dotted line* denotes ulnar margin of lateral column. Lesion extends 7 mm into lateral column (*black dotted line*) and allows RH to engage.

Stage 3

In Stage 3, the fragment is fully displaced and has become or is imminently becoming a loose body. Figure 4-12 shows an example of a Stage 3 lesion on MRI (A,B) and arthroscopically (C,D). Patients may present with mechanical symptoms related to loose bodies, such as locking. In this stage, debridement, drilling, or osteochondral replacement is indicated. If the loose osteochondral piece is shown to be acutely displaced in a patient with previously documented OCD, one can attempt to fix it to its donor site. Results of fixation are, however, inconsistent. Chronically present loose bodies (documented by serial XR or MRI) should be removed and the donor bed debrided in preparation for one of the aforementioned treatment options, following the same algorithm. These patients will often be unable to return to sports, and the long-term prognosis usually includes radiocapitellar arthrosis.

Radial Head Involvement

Radial head involvement, in addition to capitellar pathology, indicates advanced disease and does not generally occur in athletes. If the radial lesion is <30% of the radial head, then treatment of the capitellar OCD should proceed as delineated above. For radial lesions >30%, treatment of the capitellar lesion should be limited to debridement, drilling, and microfracture (9). Severe radiocapitellar degenerative arthritis is a relative contraindication to mosaicplasty.

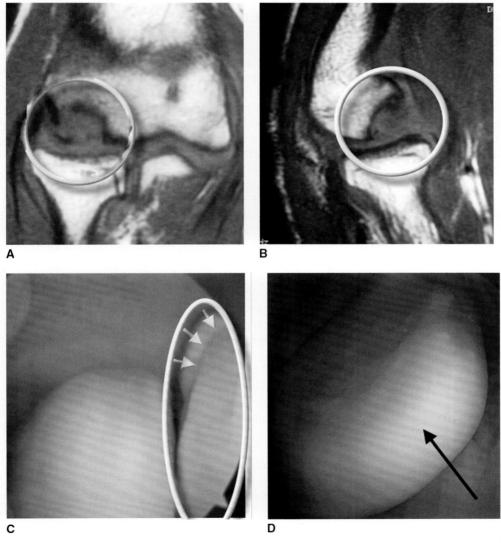

FIGURE 4-12

Stage 3 OCD lesion. T1 coronal **(A)** and T1 sagittal **(B)** MRI showing unroofed OCD lesion. **C:** Arthroscopic image showing OCD lesion (*oval*) with no overlying cartilage. *Small arrows* demarcate edge of lesion. **D:** The loose body osteochondral fragment (*arrow*) is found in the joint.

Radiocapitellar Plica

A comorbid condition that may be found in throwing athletes at the time of arthroscopy for OCD includes posterolateral elbow impingement caused by a thickened radiocapitellar plica (44–46). The plica can cause chondromalacic changes on the radial head and capitellum (44). Symptoms may include painful clicking or catching and effusions and can overlap with those from the OCD lesion. If there is snapping, it often occurs at >90 degrees of elbow flexion with the forearm in pronation (44,46). If found during arthroscopic inspection, the plica should be resected. Kim et al. reported excellent results after plica debridement in throwing athletes and golfers (45).

Outcomes

Nonoperative Treatment

Nonoperative treatment is indicated for Stage 1 OCD with a stable lesion and in patients with open capitellar growth plates. Takahara et al. retrospectively reviewed 106 cases of capitellar OCD with an average 7-year follow-up (30,31). They found that stable lesions, which healed completely with nonoperative treatment, had the following three common characteristics at initial presentation: one, an open capitellar growth plate; two, localized flattening or radiolucency of the subchondral bone; and, three, good elbow motion.

Nonoperative treatment mandates complete cessation of elbow use including activities such as throwing, gymnastics, arm wrestling, push-ups, and weight lifting. The arm may be immobilized, but for no more than 3 weeks (33). Gentle range of motion should be instituted immediately after this period of immobilization if this treatment route is chosen. Progressive physical therapy should begin as symptoms abate. Follow-up radiographs and MRIs should be obtained at 2- to 3-month intervals to track progress. At 4 to 5 months, an interval throwing program can be initiated based on satisfactory clinical and radiographic findings. Return to sport usually can be expected around 6 months and should be governed primarily by the patient's clinical response, since radiographic changes often lag behind the clinical symptoms by months or even years (47,48).

REST. Takahara et al. noted that repetitive forces on existing OCD lesions led to an increase in lesion size (36,48). Therefore, cessation of repetitive stress on the elbow needs to be categorically emphasized to the athlete's parents, trainers, and coaches. They need to be reminded that this is a potentially sport-ending injury, with degenerative arthritis as a possible outcome. Highlighting this, the incidence of residual capitellar deformity in high-level pitchers is, in fact, very low (49). This may suggest that athletes who develop a degenerative elbow from failed OCD treatment do not go on to play high-level baseball.

STAGE. Early-stage OCD responds better to nonoperative treatment than advanced stage, so identifying the disease promptly can have a significant impact on prognosis. Matsuura et al. (50) found that 91% of early-stage OCD but only 53% of advanced-stage OCD improved after nonoperative treatment.

STABILITY. Stability of the fragment also affects the final outcome. If the fragment is stable, Mitsunaga et al. showed that <50% of those lesions will go on to become unstable in the long term (51). However, Takahara et al. demonstrated that those fragments that do become unstable have a low rate of healing (30).

PATIENT AGE AND GROWTH PLATE STATUS. Age has not been correlated with likelihood of healing (42,47). Mihara et al. noted, however, a significant correlation between open capitellar growth plates and healing. In their study, 94% of early-stage patients with open growth plates healed, while the rate in those with closed growth plates was only 71% (29).

Operative Treatment

Failure of conservative treatment for early-stage, stable lesions, or the diagnosis of an advanced-stage, unstable lesion, are indications for pursuing operative treatment. The ultimate goals of surgery are to eliminate mechanical symptoms and stimulate a healing response. Takahara et al. found that unstable lesions that did well with surgery compared to elbow rest had the following common findings at initial presentation: one, a closed capitellar growth plate; two, radiographic fragmentation; and, three, restriction of elbow motion >20 degrees (31). Patients with closed capitellar physes did significantly better with surgery than with elbow rest. In larger lesions, they also noted better results with reconstruction of the articular surface than with simple fragment fixation.

Arthroscopic loose body removal and debridement have been reported to provide reliable pain relief and improved motion when <50% of capitellar surface area is affected without involvement of the lateral capitellum, though largely these patients did not return to preinjury levels of sport (27,52,53).

Microfracture and drilling have been associated with reproducible results in shallow OCD not involving the lateral capitellum. MRI follow-up of microfracture has demonstrated fibro-cartilage growth and restoration of articular congruity in 80% of patients as well as high rates of return to sport (54,55). Bojanic et al. reported symptom resolution in three adolescent gymnasts 5 months after arthroscopic debridement and microfracture of lesions around Stage 2 (56). They remained symptom-free 1 year postoperatively. Using microfracture in 11 athletes with an average age of 15, Chappell and ElAttrache obtained excellent results at 3-year follow-up with a return to previous level in all 11 (41). The size of the OCD lesions ranged from 7 × 6 mm to 17 × 15 mm.

For larger lesions involving >50% of the articular surface or lateral capitellum or column, initial outcomes were mixed, but more recent studies utilizing larger bone plug diameter have reported more reliable pain relief, union, and return to sport rates (57,58). Using OATS, Iwasaki obtained good or excellent results in seven out of eight teenaged baseball players with OCD. Yamamoto et al. found that six of nine adolescents with Grade 3 and eight of nine with Grade 4 OCD returned to competitive baseball after an OATS procedure (59). Chappell and ElAttrache treated five baseball players with OCD using OATS (41). All five returned to competitive baseball and were still playing 5 years postoperatively. The authors recommended the procedure particularly when more than 6 to 7 mm of the lateral column is involved, and the radial head is seen to be engaging with the lesion with a careful arthroscopic examination during supination/pronation and flexion/extension of the forearm.

Surgical Techniques

Arthroscopic Positioning

Elbow arthroscopy can proceed with the patient either supine, prone, or in the lateral decubitus position. We use the supine position because it facilitates general anesthesia and provides an easy conversion to an open procedure if needed (Fig. 4-13). Structures may lie in a more anatomic orientation in this position as well. In the supine position, the elbow is positioned at 90 degrees of elbow flexion and 90 degrees of shoulder abduction with the hand suspended from a pulley, using

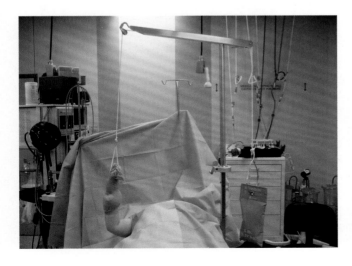

FIGURE 4-13

Supine position.

5 lb of traction. The lateral position gives improved posterior compartment access. The prone position also gives good posterior compartment access and does not require traction. General anesthesia provides complete muscle relaxation and obviates the need for a regional block that may prevent diagnosing a postoperative neurologic problem. A tourniquet may or may not be used.

Arthroscopic Technique

2.9- and 4.0-mm, 30-degree arthroscopes, burrs, and shavers should be available. The elbow is distended with 30 to 50 mL of saline through the direct lateral portal. Standard arthroscopic portals are created, and a diagnostic arthroscopy to evaluate for the presence of loose bodies, osteophytes, and chondral damage is performed, usually with the arthroscope in the anteromedial portal and working instrumentation in the anterolateral portal. In throwers, a valgus stress test with the elbow flexed to 70 degrees can be performed during the diagnostic portion of the procedure. A 1- to 2-mm opening of the ulnohumeral joint denotes laxity of the ulnar collateral ligament, although clinical correlation is mandatory. Once the initial arthroscopic examination is complete, a midlateral portal (lateral soft spot) is created in line with the lateral epicondylar ridge and entered with the arthroscope. The radial head, capitellum, trochlear notch, and trochlear ridge are best seen through this portal. Care should be taken to avoid the posterior antebrachial cutaneous nerve, at risk near this portal. A working portal is created adjacent and slightly ulnar to the midlateral portal. Carefully placed dual direct lateral portals have been shown to not damage lateral ligamentous structures and provide superior exposure to the capitellum (60). Patients with OCD and lateral compartment symptoms will occasionally also have a thickened radiocapitellar plica (Fig. 4-14). If found, the plica should be resected.

The OCD lesion is evaluated and graded. If unstable and loose, the lesion is prepared by removing any loose fragments, shaving loose fragments of cartilage down to subchondral bone, and establishing healthy cartilage borders (Fig. 4-15). The size of the lesions is determined by a calibrated probe. If osteochondral grafting is planned, the portals must allow access to the required 4- to 6-mm instruments. At this point, depending on the indication, one of the following procedures can be performed: abrasion chondroplasty, drilling, microfracture, fixation of large fragments, and osteochondral autograft transfer (mosaicplasty).

Microfracture and Subchondral Drilling

The indications for microfracture or subchondral drilling are similar: early-stage lesions with cartilage fibrillation and fissuring and small Stage 2 lesions with exposed bone that do not significantly involve the lateral column of the capitellum. The lesion bed is prepared as stated above (Fig. 4-15). Detached fragments or loose bodies are removed. With the arthroscope in the direct lateral portal,

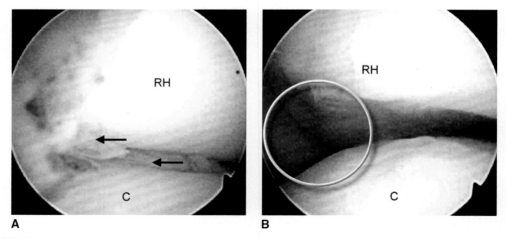

A   **B**

FIGURE 4-14

Radiocapitellar plica. **A:** *Arrows* point to radiocapitellar plica, which may cause abrasion of RH and capitellar (C) chondral surfaces. **B:** *Postplica resection:* *Circle* demarcates region formerly occupied by plica, now cleared.

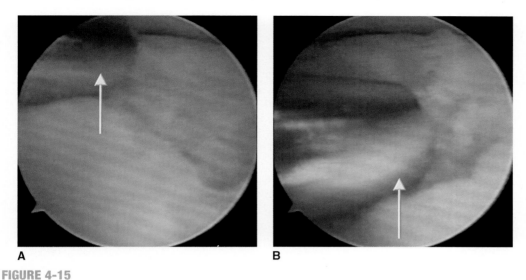

FIGURE 4-15

(A) OCD lesion is debrided with shaver (*arrow*) to **(B)** stable borders.

a 0.062-in Kirschner wire is inserted through the accessory lateral portal and used to perforate the lesion (Fig. 4-16A). Multiple holes are made in the lesion (Fig. 4-16B). Marrow elements released from the holes induce a fibrocartilage healing response.

If microfracture is selected, a similar approach can be employed using microfracture awls instead of pins.

Mosaicplasty

Mosaicplasty (OATS) has been recently applied in the context of elbow OCD lesions. In this procedure, small-sized cylindrical osteochondral grafts are obtained from the lateral periphery or trochlear edge of the femoral condyles and transplanted to prepared osteochondral defects (61). Mosaicplasty is indicated when a large capitellar lesion engages the radial head, as observed while rotating the extended arm during arthroscopy or when there is significant (over 6–7 mm) lateral column involvement (Fig. 4-17A). Radial head degeneration and severe deformities of the capitellum are relative contraindications.

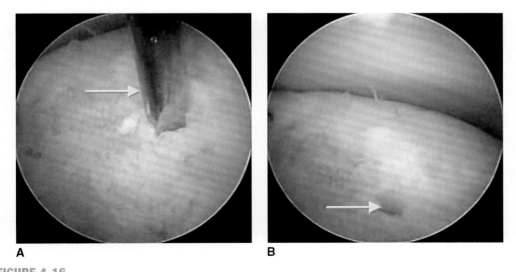

FIGURE 4-16

Microfracture technique. **A:** A 0.062-in Kirschner wire (*arrow*) is inserted through the accessory midlateral portal and used to perforate the lesion. **B:** Holes (*arrow*) in the lesion allow marrow elements to induce a fibrocartilage healing response.

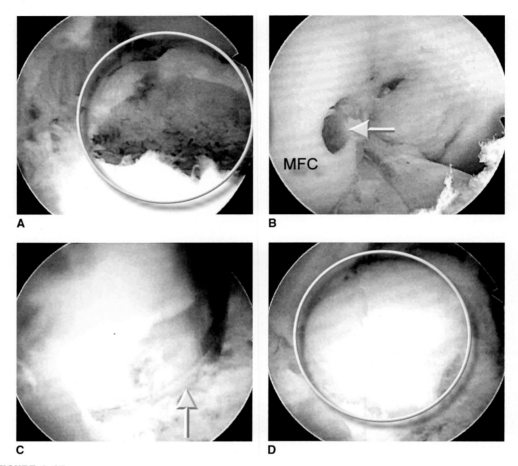

FIGURE 4-17

Osteochondral plug reconstruction of capitellar OCD defect extending into lateral column. **A:** OCD defect extending into lateral column of the capitellum (*circle*). **B:** *Arrow* points to donor site for osteochondral plug (6 mm in diameter, 1 cm in depth), harvested from medial trochlea of the knee, on lateral aspect of MFC. **C:** *Arrow* points to implantation of osteochondral plug using inserter. **D:** *Circle* demarcates osteochondral plug, postimplantation.

A midlateral working portal is used to establish healthy, stable cartilage borders. In the case of a partially detached fragment, the detached area is first evaluated. Often, the detached region is located centrally. In this situation, the senior author (NSE) recommends debriding the partially detached portion beginning centrally and proceeding laterally, toward the lateral column. Debridement proceeds until an area of bony integrity, consisting of an osseous connection between the fragment and the subchondral bone, is encountered, if there is one present. The extent of posterolateral column involvement is then determined (Fig. 4-17A), and an arthroscopic evaluation (consisting of supination and pronation of the extended forearm) of radial head engagement in the defect is performed. If more than 6 to 7 mm of the lateral column is involved or the radial head engages in the defect, osteochondral grafting proceeds. The goal should be to restore a bony buttress to prevent radial head subluxation into the defect, not necessarily replace every millimeter of the lesion.

If osteochondral grafting is elected, the elbow is then flexed 90 to 100 degrees, and a spinal needle is introduced through the anconeus to gauge the feasibility of a perfectly perpendicular approach to the lesion. The incision is widened to provide access for a 4- to 6-mm-diameter plug, so that it is in line with the perpendicular path delineated by the needle. After bluntly spreading the soft tissue to avoid neurovascular structures, the recipient site is then drilled as perpendicular to the chondral surface as possible creating a tunnel of the necessary diameter. At this point, the knee, which has been prepped, undergoes an arthroscopic harvest of an identically sized chondral plug from the intercondylar notch. The arthroscope is placed into an anterolateral portal. Instrumentation is inserted through an anteromedial portal. Using the harvesting instrumentation, a 6 mm in diameter, 1 cm in depth plug is harvested from the trochlear edge off the medial femoral condyle (MFC) (Fig. 4-17B). Usually, one plug is sufficient because of the small size of the capitellar lesions. The plug is introduced into the recipient site and impacted flush with the surrounding cartilage (Fig. 4-17C and D). The goal should be to reconstitute the lateral buttress (Fig. 4-18A and B) so that the radial head does not engage the defect. The process of osteochondral grafting is repeated until the lateral column integrity is adequately restored. If some corners of the lesion cannot be fully replaced, they are treated with drilling or microfracture (Fig. 4-18C and D). If autograft is unavailable, allograft or synthetic scaffolding can be used.

Fragment Fixation

Fragment fixation has been performed in patients with unstable, partially open OCD lesions through arthroscopic or open approaches (34). This requires sufficient area for fixation device. A recent meta-analysis found lower return to sport rates following fixation than either debridement or OATS (62). Our recommendation at this time remains excision and drilling or grafting for partially detached lesions.

Postoperative Management

Postoperatively, all patients should be protected for 2 to 3 weeks with a long arm cast or hinged brace. Active motion should not be started until bony union is seen on radiographs. Gentle resistance exercises are initiated at 3 months, progressing to greater resistance at 4 months. For throwing

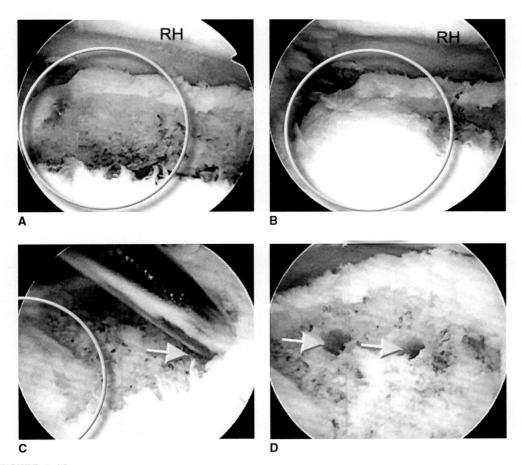

FIGURE 4-18

Lateral buttress of the capitellum reconstructed with osteochondral autograft. **A:** OCD lesion extending into lateral column of the capitellum (*circle*); during arthroscopic exam (pronation/supination in extension), RH engages defect. **B:** Osteochondral plug (*circle*) placed in lateral aspect of the capitellum, reconstituting lateral buttress. RH no longer engages. **C:** *Circle* surrounds osteochondral plug, *arrow* points to remaining OCD lesion addressed with microfracture using 0.0062-in Kirschner wire. **D:** Postmicrofracture: *Arrows* point to holes allowing release of marrow elements.

athletes, a throwing program is started at 5 months. Full effort return to sport is usually achieved 6 months after surgery. Athletes that have undergone simple debridement and drilling or microfracture can usually return 1 to 2 months sooner depending on their rehabilitation progress.

Return to Sport

Return to sports has been variable. Historically, gymnasts have had inferior outcomes compared to throwers, perhaps related to significantly increased axial loads borne by their elbows. Jackson et al. treated 10 female gymnasts with removal of loose bodies and drilling after failure of nonoperative treatment (3). Only one returned to sport. They concluded that while surgery for lesions refractory to conservative treatment may improve symptoms, a return to gymnastics is unlikely. A meta-analysis recently analyzed 492 athletes treated for capitellar OCD. Lesion size or grade was not specified as well as type of sport. Nevertheless, this study comprised the largest group of capitellar OCDs. Comparing OATS to debridement to fragment fixation, the authors reported highest rates of return to sport in OATS (94%), followed by debridement (71%), then fixation (64%). However, lesion size was not described (62). Microfracture in 236 elbows of mean age 14.5 years had a 71% rate of return to previous level of sport and 87% return to any level of sport at mean 4.2 months postoperatively. Ninety-two patients treated with fragment fixation had a 64% rate of returning to prior level of sport and 68% to any level at mean 5.9 months postoperatively. Osteochondral autograft transfer (knee and rib included) was performed in 164 patients, 94% returned to previous level of sport and 95% to any level at mean 5.9 months postoperatively. Matsuura et al. recently reported that OATS for unstable capitellar lesions had better radiographic and functional outcomes as well as return to play rates in central lesions compared to lateral lesions (63). Overall this meta-analysis reports reasonably high rates of return to sport with the assumption that the operative techniques were selected appropriately.

Prognosis

Prognosis for OCD of the capitellum is good when diagnosed early at Stage 1. Unfortunately, most cases are diagnosed at Stage 2. While surgery will usually alleviate symptoms and allow a return to play, these patients have a less favorable long-term outcome. Longitudinal studies have documented that 50% of radiocapitellar OCD patients will go on to eventually develop osteoarthritis (64). Nevertheless, newer techniques, including osteochondral grafting (mosaicplasty), may mitigate the onset of long-term degenerative joint disease. Ultimately, prevention is the best treatment. For throwers, pitch counts should be monitored and kept under 600/wk. Players or gymnasts should never pitch or practice when in pain and should never be medicated to play.

CONCLUSION

Young throwers and gymnasts are at risk for Panner disease and OCD as performance demands and expectations escalate. For Panner disease and early OCD, nonoperative treatment, consisting primarily of strict activity cessation, forms the mainstay of management. Advanced OCD lesions require operative intervention, which is feasible arthroscopically with reliable outcomes. The size and location of the lesion as well as its functional relationship to the radial head help guide management. As always, prevention, by monitoring and limiting pitch counts and excessive training and educating athletes, parents, and coaches on early warning signs, provides the most reproducible solution for these potentially sport-ending conditions.

ACKNOWLEDGMENT

This chapter was built on the strong foundation provided by Neal S. ElAttrache, MD in the first edition.

REFERENCES

1. Brown R, Blazina ME, Kerlan RK, et al. Osteochondritis of the capitellum. *J Sports Med.* 1974;2(1):27–46.
2. Douglas G, Rang M. The role of trauma in the pathogenesis of the osteochondroses. *Clin Orthop Relat Res.* 1981;(158):28–32.
3. Jackson DW, Silvino N, Reiman P. Osteochondritis in the female gymnast's elbow. *Arthroscopy.* 1989;5(2):129–136.

4. Ruch DS, Poehling GG. Arthroscopic treatment of Panner's disease. *Clin Sports Med.* 1991;10(3):629–636.

5. Singer KM, Roy SP. Osteochondrosis of the humeral capitellum. *Am J Sports Med.* 1984;12(5):351–360.

6. Panner H. An affection of the capitulum humeri resembling Calve-Perthes disease of the hip. *Acta Radiol.* 1927;8:617–618.

7. Duthie RB, Houghton GR. Constitutional aspects of the osteochondroses. *Clin Orthop Relat Res.* 1981;158:19–27.

8. Yamaguchi K, Sweet FA, Bindra R, et al. The extraosseous and intraosseous arterial anatomy of the adult elbow. *J Bone Joint Surg Am.* 1997;79(11):1653–1662.

9. Kobayashi K, Burton KJ, Rodner C, et al. Lateral compression injuries in the pediatric elbow: Panner's disease and osteochondritis dissecans of the capitellum. *J Am Acad Orthop Surg.* 2004;12(4):246–254.

10. Matsuura T, Suzue N, Iwame T, et al. Prevalence of osteochondritis dissecans of the capitellum in young baseball players: results based on ultrasonographic findings. *Orthop J Sports Med.* 2014;2:2325967114545298.

11. Kida Y, Morihara T, Kotoura Y, et al. Prevalence and clinical characteristics of osteochondritis dissecans of the humeral capitellum among adolescent baseball players. *Am J Sports Med.* 2014;42:1963–1971.

12. Voloshin I, Schena A. Elbow injuries. In: Schepsis AA, Busconi BD, eds. *Sports Medicine.* Philadelphia, PA: Lippincott Williams & Wilkins; 2006.

13. Lord J, Winell JJ. Overuse injuries in pediatric athletes. *Curr Opin Pediatr.* 2004;16(1):47–50.

14. Lyman S, Fleisig G, Waterbor J, et al. Longitudinal study of elbow and shoulder pain in youth baseball pitchers. *Med Sci Sports Exerc.* 2001;33(11):1803–1810.

15. Tis JE, et al. Short-term results of arthroscopic treatment of osteochondritis dissecans in skeletally immature patients. *J Pediatr Orthop.* 2012;32(3):226–231.

16. Kosaka M, et al. Outcomes and failure factors in surgical treatment for osteochondritis dissecans of the capitellum. *J Pediatr Orthop.* 2013;33(7):719–724.

17. Caine D, et al. Does repetitive physical loading inhibit radial growth in female gymnasts? *Clin J Sport Med.* 1997;7(4): 302–308.

18. Caine DJ, Nassar L. Gymnastics injuries. *Med Sport Sci.* 2005;48:18–58.

19. Kajiyama S, Muroi S, Sugaya H, et al. Osteochondritis dissecans of the humeral capitellum in young athletes: comparison between baseball players and gymnasts. *Orthop J Sports Med.* 2017;5:2325967117692513.

20. Haraldsson S. On osteochondrosis deformas juvenilis capituli humeri including investigation of intra-osseous vasculature in distal humerus. *Acta Orthop Scand Suppl.* 1959;38:1–232.

21. Krappel FA, Bauer E, Harland U. Are bone bruises a possible cause of osteochondritis dissecans of the capitellum? A case report and review of the literature. *Arch Orthop Trauma Surg.* 2005;125(8):545–549.

22. Yang Z, Wang Y, Gilula LA, et al. Microcirculation of the distal humeral epiphyseal cartilage: implications for post-traumatic growth deformities. *J Hand Surg [Am].* 1998;23(1):165–172.

23. Kijowski R, De Smet AA. Radiography of the elbow for evaluation of patients with osteochondritis dissecans of the capitellum. *Skelet Radiol.* 2005;34(5):266–271.

24. Griffith JF, Roebuck DJ, Cheng JCY, et al. Acute elbow trauma in children: spectrum of injury revealed by MR imaging not apparent on radiographs. *Am J Roentgenol.* 2001;176(1):53–60.

25. Peiss J, Adam G, Casser R, et al. Gadopentetate-dimeglumine-enhanced MR imaging of osteonecrosis and osteochondritis dissecans of the elbow: initial experience. *Skeletal Radiol.* 1995;24(1):17–20.

26. Rosenberg ZS, Beltran J, Cheung YY. Pseudodefect of the capitellum: potential MR imaging pitfall. *Radiology.* 1994;191(3):821–823.

27. Baumgarten TE, Andrews JR, Satterwhite YE. The arthroscopic classification and treatment of osteochondritis dissecans of the capitellum. *Am J Sports Med.* 1998;26(4):520–523.

28. DiFelice GS, Meunier M, Paletta GJ. Elbow injury in the adolescent athlete. In: Andrews J, Altchek D, eds. *The Athlete's Elbow.* Philadelphia, PA: Lippincott Williams & Wilkins; 2001:231–248.

29. Mihara, K., Tsutsui H, Nishinaka N, et al. Nonoperative treatment for osteochondritis dissecans of the capitellum. *Am J Sports Med.* 2009;37(2):298–304.

30. Takahara M, Mura N, Sasaki J, et al. Classification, treatment, and outcome of osteochondritis dissecans of the humeral capitellum. *J Bone Joint Surg Am.* 2007;89(6):1205–1214.

31. Takahara M, Mura N, Sasaki J, et al. Classification, treatment, and outcome of osteochondritis dissecans of the humeral capitellum. Surgical technique. *J Bone Joint Surg Am.* 2008;90(suppl 2 pt 1):47–62.

32. Petrie RBJ. Osteochondritis dissecans of the humeral capitellum. In: De Lee J, Miller DD, eds. *Orthopaedic Sports Medicine: Principles and Practice.* Philadelphia, PA: W.B. Saunders; 2003.

33. Bradley JP, Petrie RS. Osteochondritis dissecans of the humeral capitellum. Diagnosis and treatment . *Clin Sports Med.* 2001;20(3):565–590.

34. Larsen MW, Pietrzak WS, DeLee JC. Fixation of osteochondritis dissecans lesions using poly(L-lactic acid)/poly(glycolic acid) copolymer bioabsorbable screws. *Am J Sports Med.* 2005;33(1):68–76.

35. Kuwahata Y. Inoue G. Osteochondritis dissecans of the elbow managed by Herbert screw fixation. *Orthopedics.* 1998;21(4):449–451.

36. Takahara M, Shundo M, Kondo M, et al. Nonoperative treatment of osteochondritis dissecans of the humeral capitellum. *Am J Sports Med.* 1999;27(6):728–732.

37. Shimada K, Yoshida T, Nakata K, et al. Reconstruction with an osteochondral autograft for advanced osteochondritis dissecans of the elbow. *Clin Orthop Relat Res.* 2005;435:140–147.

38. Bradley J, Dandy DJ. Results of drilling osteochondritis dissecans before skeletal maturity. *J Bone Joint Surg Br.* 1989;71(4):642–644.

39. Nishinaka N, et al. Costal osteochondral autograft for reconstruction of advanced-stage osteochondritis dissecans of the capitellum. *J Shoulder Elbow Surg.* 2014;23(12):1888-1897.

40. Shimada K, et al. Cylindrical costal osteochondral autograft for reconstruction of large defects of the capitellum due to osteochondritis dissecans. *J Bone Joint Surg Am.* 2012;94(11):992.

41. Chappell JD, ElAttrache NS. *Clinical outcome of arthroscopic treatment of OCD lesions of the capitellum.* Paper presented at American Orthopaedic Society for Sports Medicine. Orlando, FL, 2008.

42. Ruch DS, Cory JW, Poehling GG. The arthroscopic management of osteochondritis dissecans of the adolescent elbow. *Arthroscopy.* 1998;14(8):797–803.

43. Hennrikus WP, et al. Internal fixation of unstable in situ osteochondritis dissecans lesions of the capitellum. *J Pediatr Orthop.* 2015;35(5):467–473.

44. Antuna SA, O'Driscoll SW. Snapping plicae associated with radiocapitellar chondromalacia. *Arthroscopy.* 2001;17(5):491–495.
45. Kim DH, Gambardella RA, Elattrache NS, et al. Arthroscopic treatment of posterolateral elbow impingement from lateral synovial plicae in throwing athletes and golfers. *Am J Sports Med.* 2006;34(3):438–444.
46. Steinert AF, Goebel S, Rucker A, et al. Snapping elbow caused by hypertrophic synovial plica in the radiohumeral joint: a report of three cases and review of literature. *Arch Orthop Trauma Surg.* 2010;130(3):347–351.
47. Takahara M, Mura N, Sasaki J, et al. Long term outcome of osteochondritis dissecans of the humeral capitellum. *Clin Orthop Relat Res.* 1999;363:108–115.
48. Takahara M, Shundo M, Kondo M, et al. Early detection of osteochondritis dissecans of the capitellum in young baseball players. Report of three cases. *J Bone Joint Surg Am.* 1998;80(6):892–897.
49. Mihara K. Osteoarthritic elbow caused by sports [in Japanese]. *Rinsho Seikei Geka.* 2000;35:1243–1249.
50. Matsuura T, Kashiwaguchi S, Iwase T, et al. Conservative treatment for osteochondrosis of the humeral capitellum. *Am J Sports Med.* 2008;36(5):868–872.
51. Mitsunaga MM, Adishian DA, Bianco AJ Jr. Osteochondritis dissecans of the capitellum. *J Trauma.* 1982;22(1):53–55.
52. Byrd JW, Jones KS. Arthroscopic surgery for isolated capitellar osteochondritis dissecans in adolescent baseball players: minimum three-year follow-up. *Am J Sports Med.* 2002;30(4):474–478.
53. Brownlow HC, O'Connor-Read LM, Perko M. Arthroscopic treatment of osteochondritis dissecans of the capitellum. *Knee Surg Sports Traumatol Arthrosc.* 2006;14(2):198–202.
54. Churchill RW, Munoz J, Ahmad CS. Osteochondritis dissecans of the elbow. *Curr Rev Musculoskelet Med.* 2016;9(2):232–239.
55. Bojanić I, Smoljanović T, Dokuzović S. Osteochondritis dissecans of the elbow: excellent results in teenage athletes treated by arthroscopic debridement and microfracture. *Croat Med J.* 2012;53(1):40–47.
56. Bojanic I, Ivkovic A, Boric I. Arthroscopy and microfracture technique in the treatment of osteochondritis dissecans of the humeral capitellum: report of three adolescent gymnasts. *Knee Surg Sports Traumatol Arthrosc.* 2006;14(5):491–496.
57. Lyons ML, et al. Osteochondral autograft plug transfer for treatment of osteochondritis dissecans of the capitellum in adolescent athletes. *J Shoulder Elbow Surg.* 2015;24(7):1098–1105.
58. Maruyama M, et al. Outcomes of an open autologous osteochondral plug graft for capitellar osteochondritis dissecans: time to return to sports. *Am J Sports Med.* 2014;42(9):2122–2127.
59. Yamamoto Y, Ishibashi Y, Tsuda E, et al. Osteochondral autograft transplantation for osteochondritis dissecans of the elbow in juvenile baseball players: minimum 2-year follow-up. *Am J Sports Med.* 2006;34(5):714–720.
60. Davis JT. Dual direct lateral portals for treatment of osteochondritis dissecans of the capitellum: an anatomic study. *Arthroscopy.* 2007;23(7):723–728.
61. Iwasaki N, Kato H, Ishikawa J, et al. Autologous osteochondral mosaicplasty for capitellar osteochondritis dissecans in teenaged patients. *Am J Sports Med.* 2006;34(8):1233–1239.
62. Westermann RW, et al. Return to sport after operative management of osteochondritis dissecans of the capitellum: a systematic review and meta-analysis. *Orthop J Sports Med.* 2016;4(6):2325967116654651.
63. Matsuura T, et al. Comparison of clinical and radiographic outcomes between central and lateral lesions after osteochondral autograft transplantation for osteochondritis dissecans of the humeral capitellum. *Am J Sports Med.* 2017;45(14):3331–3339.
64. Bauer M, Jonsson K, Josefsson PO, et al. Osteochondritis dissecans of the elbow. A long-term follow-up study. *Clin Orthop Relat Res.* 1992;2(284):156–160.

5 Distal Biceps Tendon Rupture in the Athlete

Mark Morrey and Bernard F. Morrey

Once thought to be an uncommon injury, avulsion of the distal biceps tendon from the radial tuberosity is being seen in increasing numbers in both competitive and recreational athletes. In general, it is of interest that the injury occurs almost exclusively in males, usually those with heavy lifting requirements of work or avocation.

PATHOLOGY

The distal biceps tendon complex may be injured at the musculotendinous junction, by a disruption of the tendon itself in continuity, or a complete or partial tear or avulsion (Fig. 5-1). The anatomy of the tendon is such that it spirals 90 degrees from proximal to distal placing the long head in a posterior and proximal position relative to the distally inserted short head (Fig. 5-2). The lesion can involve the long head or short head of the tendon independently (Fig. 5-3), but by far the most common lesion is the avulsion of the conjoined heads from the tuberosity, and this is the only lesion that will be dealt with in this chapter.

Of the tears from the radial tuberosity, approximately 95% are complete ruptures whereas about 5% are partial tears. Both conditions, along with delayed reconstruction, will be addressed in this chapter.

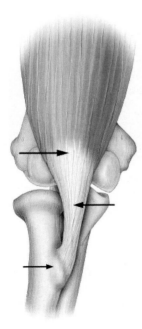

FIGURE 5-1

The biceps mechanism may be injured at the muscle/tendinous junction, intratendinous, or at the tuberosity.

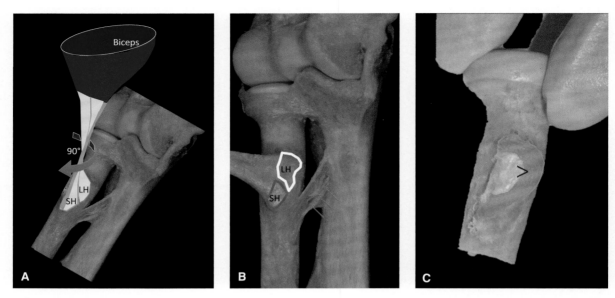

FIGURE 5-2

The distal biceps tendon spirals from proximal to distal toward its insertion point on the radial tuberosity **(A)**. The anatomy is such that the short head (*SH*) is inserted anterior and distal to the long head (*LH*) **(B)** in a crescentic attachment **(C)** just medial to the apex of the tuberosity (>). *Arrows* represent the proximal oblique cord in **(B)**.

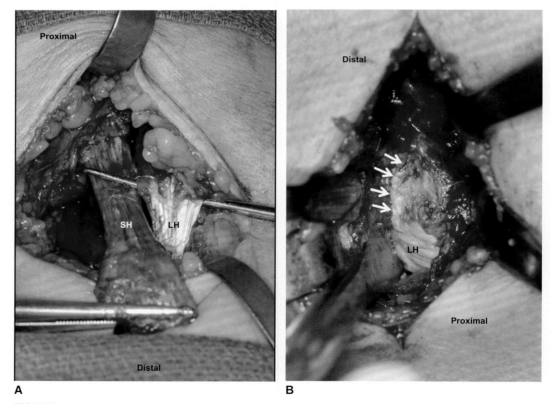

FIGURE 5-3

A distal biceps tendon rupture of the short head (*SH*) only. In **(A)**, the long head (*LH*) of the biceps is seen elevated by the instrument and short head emerging from the wound and discontinuous from the long head of the biceps. In **(B)**, the long head can be seen attached proximally and short head is absent from its normal crescentic insertion on the distal portion of the tuberosity (*arrows*).

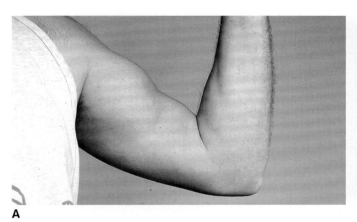
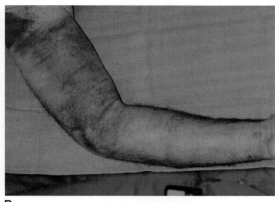

A   **B**

FIGURE 5-4

In most instances, proximal retraction is diagnostic **(A)**. Ecchymosis is uncommon. In this instance, this competitive athlete had been on high-dose aspirin at the time of injury **(B)**.

THE DIAGNOSIS

Complete rupture is easy to diagnose in most instances due to retraction of the distal biceps muscle belly with elbow flexion. The history is that of eccentric loading during flexion. Hematoma formation is variable, as is the location of the pain (Fig. 5-4).

Imaging

The physical examination alone with an absent biceps hook test can be reliably used in most instances of complete rupture (1). If the diagnosis is in question, there has been a significant improvement in the ability to diagnose the injury, especially incomplete rupture, with an MRI. By placing the arm overhead, the course of the biceps tendon may be brought in plane thus allowing a more accurate assessment of the pathology. This position was described by Giuffre and Moss (2) and is termed the "flexion abduction supination 'FABS'" view (Fig. 5-5). This is of particular value for surgical planning in instances of partial or chronic ruptures where scarring may involve adjacent neurovascular structures.

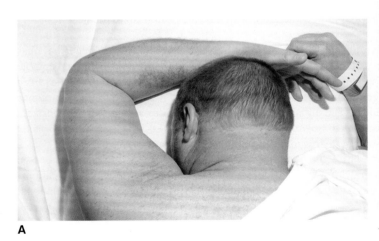
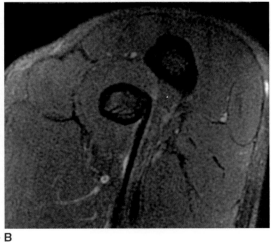

A   **B**

FIGURE 5-5

The FABS view **(A)** brings the entire tendon and its attachment into profile with MRI **(B)**. An example of a distal biceps tendon rupture as viewed on FABS MRI. **C:** This sagittal shows the recoil affect (→) of the biceps tendon **(D)**, and FABS view the extensive scarring (^) down to the tuberosity adjacent to the brachialis tendon (#), which obliterates the tunnel down to the tuberosity and must be excavated at the time of surgery.

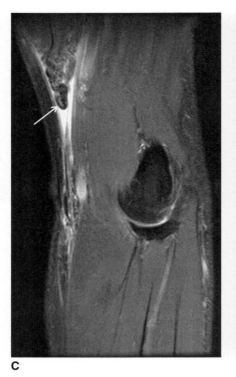 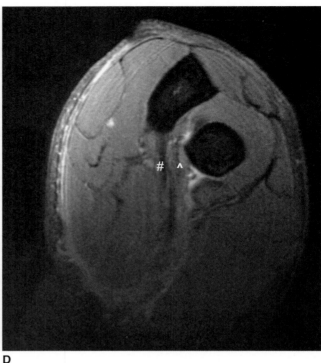

C   D

FIGURE 5-5 (*Continued*)

INDICATIONS/CONTRAINDICATIONS

In our judgment, there is little question that in the athlete, distal biceps tendon rupture should be repaired as soon as possible (3–7). There have been several studies, including our own, attempting to estimate and evaluate both subjective and objective dysfunction following the nonrepaired biceps tendon. These studies have generally shown reasonable function under most circumstances with minimal pain. However, with excessive exertion, the patients do have pain and lack endurance; hence the need for reconstruction in some patients if the repair is not performed acutely. The average age of patients with the injury is approximately 55, and virtually every report has documented the almost exclusive occurrence in males. In our practice at Mayo, we have treated only two females from among over 100 with this diagnosis, both with partial ruptures. Usually, the patient is involved with heavy labor or athletic activity, which further emphasizes the need for early definitive treatment.

Delayed reattachment is difficult because the tendon retracts and scars. If this has occurred, reattachment or embedding the biceps tendon into the brachialis is easy but not considered acceptable today as it does nothing to restore supination power. Reconstruction for selected patients has been effective in recent years but is technically demanding (8) and typically is referred to those surgeons with experience with this procedure. The author prefers to use an Achilles allograft for reconstruction if the native tendon is of insufficient quality to accept a minimum of 4 Krackow sutures spaced approximately 5 to 8 mm apart within the residual tendon or tendon stump of at least 2½ cm before the myotendinous junction. Secondarily, if the tendon will not reach the tuberosity in flexion of >90 degrees, an Achilles tendon allograft may be considered as described herein. Fortunately, patients can be repaired in flexion of up to 90 degrees without concern for residual motion loss or functional deficits (9).

Contraindications

Reattachment is contraindicated in patients who do not have significant functional impairment. This is not very applicable in the athlete but might be considered in a sedentary patient—but rarely does such an individual sustain this injury. Attempts to reattach this tendon if there has been a delay of over 3 weeks require careful thought as the tendon typically is retracted into the biceps muscle and the tendon tract is scarred. If the delay is prolonged, there may not be adequate length to reach to the radial tuberosity (6). Furthermore, the tract of the tendon to the tuberosity will have scarred and become obliterated, making the surgery much more difficult with a higher complication rate (10).

Surgical Considerations

The surgeon has two interrelated technical considerations when addressing these patients. The first is the selection of either a one- or two-incision technique. The second is the mode of fixation. In this chapter, we will deal with three types of fixation that, with their variations, reflect virtually all of the approaches used today: bone tunnel, suture anchor, and endo button.

The surgical approach is clearly the preference of the surgeon. Surgical procedures have been described using a modified Henry approach (5,11) or through a two-incision approach described by Boyd and Anderson (12). The advantage of the anterior Henry approach is that it is felt to be less likely to create ectopic bone, although recent studies have challenged this notion (13,14). The disadvantage is that it puts the radial nerve at jeopardy (5,7,11). However, it must be emphasized that the two-incision approach currently used is *NOT* that described by Boyd and Anderson. The advantage of the two-incision technique is that it lessens and virtually eliminates the likelihood of injury to the radial nerve (6). The original Boyd-Anderson approach exposes the ulna, and hence can be associated with ectopic bone (15). Through the years, we have employed the Mayo modification of the Boyd-Anderson approach, which does *NOT* expose the ulna, and hence is associated with very little ectopic bone (10).

The author continues to use the two-incision technique with excellent results and minimal complications (10). This technique allows for anatomic positioning of the tendon and restoration of the cam effect of the radial tuberosity. Several studies have shown that the two-incision technique allows for more anatomic placement of the tendon over a one-incision technique and that supination strength is slightly greater with anatomic restoration of the tendon (16–20). Nevertheless, it is recognized that the one-incision technique is also popular with the thought that it lessens the likelihood of ectopic bone formation. Although this has not been demonstrated to be the case, the complication of ectopic bone has motivated many to use a single anterior approach (13). Furthermore, the training of the individual surgeon on a particular technique is of considerable importance to achieving optimal results, and surgeons should do the approach with which they feel most comfortable. The direct exposure is correlated with the mode of fixation. An anterior approach can be used for the endo button or the suture anchor. For bone tunnels, a two-incision technique is required.

PREOPERATIVE PLANNING

If the injury is more than 4 weeks since onset, be prepared to perform a more detailed dissection in the antecubital space with careful review of the MRI to avoid neurovascular structures. If the tendon has retracted, direct reattachment to the tuberosity with the elbow flexed up to 90 degrees is preferred. If this is not possible, restoration of length with an Achilles tendon allograft is preferred. The patient must be prepared for these eventualities.

TECHNIQUE

Complete Rupture—Immediate Reattachment

Incision

The arm is prepped and draped with the patient supine. A sandbag may be placed under the shoulder to allow the arm to comfortably be brought across the chest. Under a general anesthesia, a single 3- to 4-cm transverse incision in the antecubital crease is employed (Fig. 5-6).

TENDON PREPARATION. By digital palpation or limited dissection, the tendon is identified, dissected free of soft tissue, and is delivered from the wound (Fig. 5-7). The end of the tendon tends to be bulbous and is trimmed in order to allow it to fit well into the tuberosity. After the tendon has been trimmed, two heavy nonabsorbable sutures are placed through the torn portion entering the end of the tendon. Typically, we utilize a locking stitch (Krakow) in which two different colors or

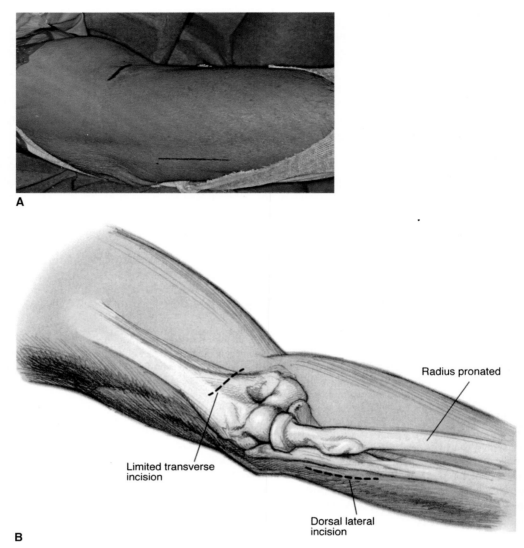

A

B

Radius pronated

Limited transverse
incision

Dorsal lateral
incision

FIGURE 5-6

The two-incision technique employs a simple 4-cm transverse incision in the antecubital space **(A)** and a 5- to
7-cm incision over the posterior aspect of the proximal forearm **(B)**.

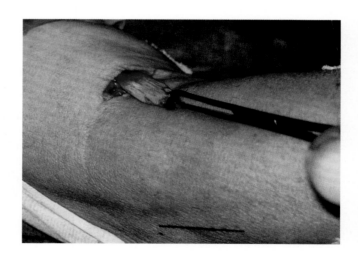

FIGURE 5-7

The tendon is identified by digital
palpation and delivered through the
skin incision revealing a bulbous
degenerative process at the site of
disruption.

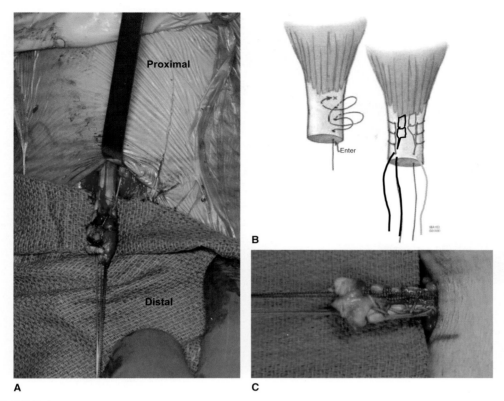

FIGURE 5-8

A–C: Two nonabsorbable sutures are inserted in a Krackow fashion **(A,B)** and emerging from the ends of the long and short head of the biceps, respectively **(C)**.

lengths in order to differentiate the long head and short head of the biceps tendon. This allows for anatomic restoration of the long head of the biceps more proximally and posteriorly with the short head being inserted more distally and anterior as the tendon spirals down toward the tuberosity (Fig. 5-8).

Forearm Incision

A curved clamp is then introduced into the tunnel previously occupied by the biceps tendon (Fig. 5-9). It is directed by palpation to and then past the tuberosity between the radius and ulna. Rotation of the forearm confirms proper position of the instrument on the ulnar side of the radius. A lead suture is grasped by the curved hemostat and is advanced until it punctures the muscle and subcutaneous tissues of the dorsal aspect of the forearm. An incision is then made over the site of prominence splitting the common extensor and incising the supinator muscle (Fig. 5-10).

Tuberosity Identity and Preparation

With full forearm pronation, the tuberosity is then identified and cleaned of tendon or bursal remnants. A high-speed burr is used to excavate the cancellous bone from just posterior to the apex of the tuberosity (Fig. 5-11). A trough in this location allows for preservation of the cam effect of the apex of the tuberosity. After an adequate orifice of 10 to 12 mm × 7 to 8 mm has been made to receive the tendon, the forearm is partially segmented and three drill holes are placed on the radial side of the tuberosity and excavated to allow for suture passage (Fig. 5-12). Allowing the forearm to supinate slightly brings this margin of the radial tuberosity into better alignment. The holes should be placed in such a way as to leave sufficient bone to avoid osseous rupture or pullout of the sutures (Fig. 5-13).

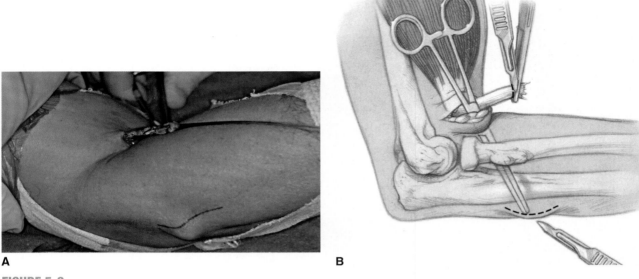

A

B

FIGURE 5-9

The curved hemostat is passed between the radial tuberosity and the ulna **(A)** to emerge through the common extensor muscle mass and tent the skin on the proximal posterolateral aspect of the forearm **(B)**.

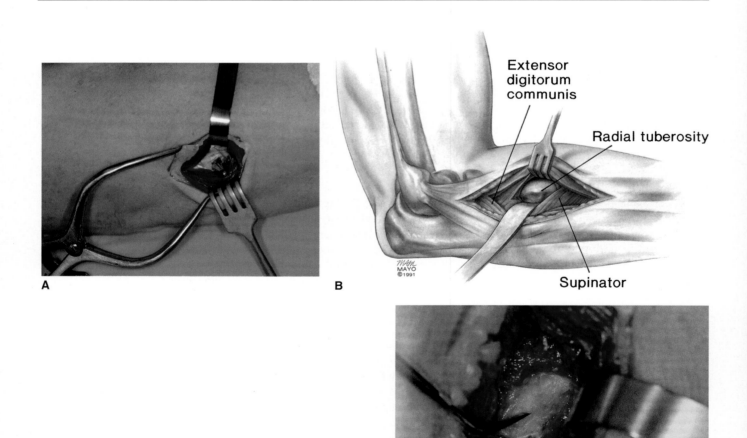

A

B

Extensor
digitorum
communis

Radial tuberosity

Supinator

FIGURE 5-10

A–C: An incision is made over this prominence, the muscle is split, the forearm is fully pronated, and the tuberosity is exposed.

C

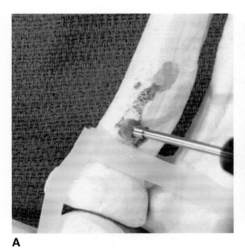

A

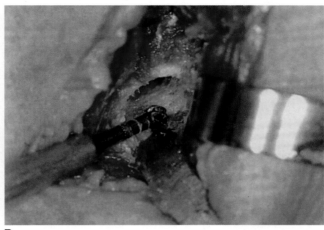

B

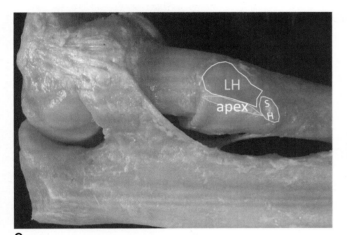

C

FIGURE 5-11

The radial tuberosity is excavated just posterior to its apex (**A**—sawbones and **B**—intraoperative view) using a high-speed bur in order to preserve the cam effect of the tuberosity and provide anatomic positioning of the long head (*LH*) and short head (*SH*) of the tendon represented in *blue* and *orange*, respectively (**C**).

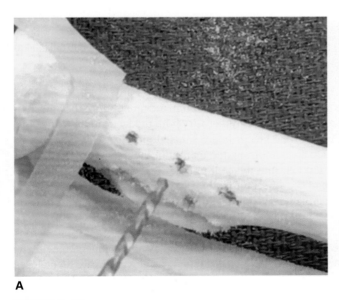

A

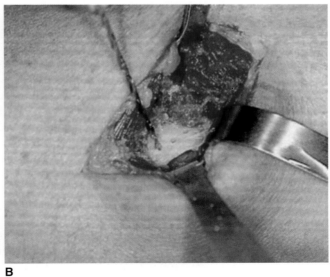

B

FIGURE 5-12

A,B: Drill holes (**A**—sawbone and **B**—in patient) are placed 5 to 7 mm from the edge of the trough and 7 to 10 mm apart by slightly supinating from the maximally pronated position after trough preparation. The holes are excavated (**C**) to allow for easy passage of the suture needle (**D**).

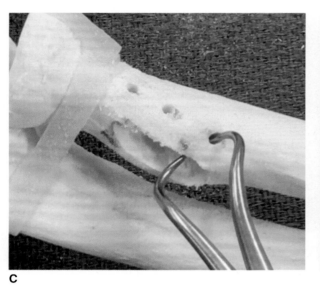
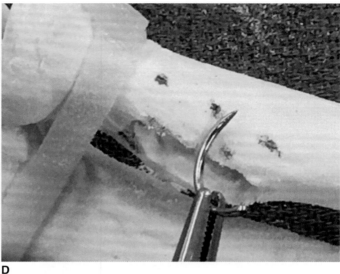

C   D

FIGURE 5-12 (*Continued*)

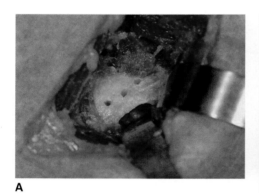
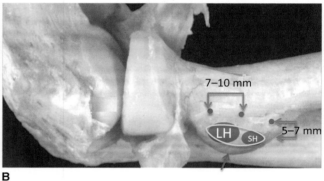

A   B

FIGURE 5-13

A,B: Intraoperative drill holes **(A)** and diagram **(B)** show the relative position of the trough to the anatomic position of the tendons and in reference to the drill holes (*dots*) and apex (*arrow*) of the tuberosity.

REATTACHMENT OF THE TENDON. The tendon is then brought through the tunnel from the antecubital space (Fig. 5-14) and drawn past the ulnar side of the tuberosity with the lead suture (Fig. 5-15) in its anatomic location with the long head of the biceps being situated more proximally and posteriorly. The sutures are threaded into each of the holes at the margin of the tuberosity. One suture is brought into the proximal and distal, and two into the central hole (Fig. 5-16) corresponding to the anatomic locations of the long head and short head of the biceps. The biceps tendon is threaded into the tuberosity; once again, this is facilitated by slightly supinating the forearm. With the arm remaining in less than full pronation, the sutures are tied (Fig. 5-17).

CLOSURE. Pronation and supination are gently tested to assure that there is no impingement with the ulna. Extension is assessed to determine tautness for the biceps repair. The incisions are then closed in a routine fashion. At the proximal forearm, the fascia over the split muscle is closed with a 2-0 absorbable suture and a subcutaneous and skin suture of choice is used. In the antecubital space, the tissues are allowed to resume their former position, and the remainder of the wound is closed in layers as desired.

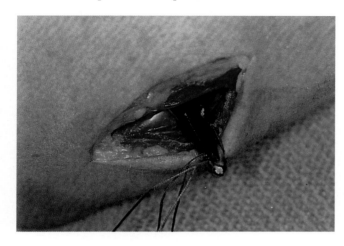

FIGURE 5-14

The sutures are grasped again with a curved hemostat and introduced through the tunnel of the biceps tendon to emerge through the forearm incision.

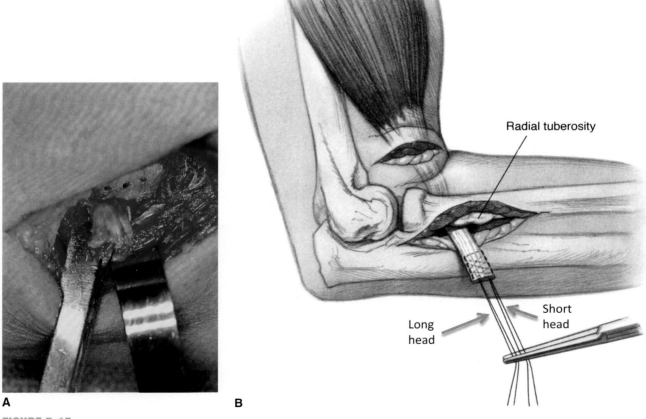

A   **B**

FIGURE 5-15

A,B: The tendon is then pulled through the lateral wound while maintaining its anatomic orientation with the long head proximal and short head distal.

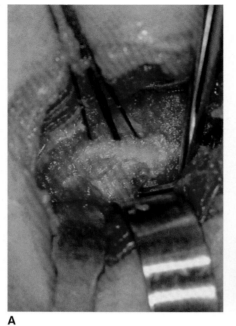
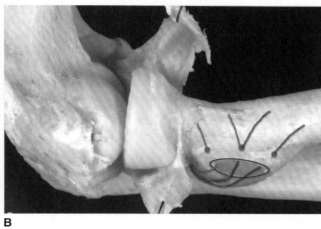

A **B**

FIGURE 5-16

A: The distal aspect of the biceps tendon is threaded into the excavated portion of the radial tuberosity. **B:** The sutures are brought through the three holes with the center hole receiving one arm of each of the sutures and maintaining the anatomic orientation of the long and short heads.

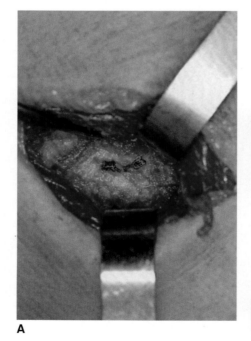
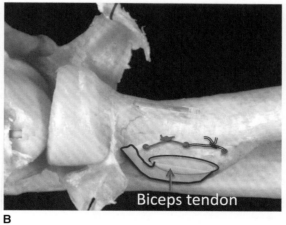

A **B**

FIGURE 5-17

A,B: The sutures are tied while the forearm is allowed to supinate slightly to facilitate this process.

ANTERIOR APPROACHES/SUTURE ANCHORS

Suture anchors employ a Henry or modified Henry skin incision, and a detailed understanding of the neurovascular anatomy is essential to avoiding complications (Fig. 5-18). The lacertus fibrosis can be found medially as it becomes continuous with the medial forearm fascia, which, if intact, prevents significant proximal migration of the tendon (Fig. 5-19). The lateral antebrachial cutaneous nerve is identified at the lateral margin of the biceps muscle and protected. The radial nerve lies just lateral and parallel to the lateral antebrachial cutaneous nerve, and full supination allows for lateral displacement of the nerve, which should be protected as it enters the supinator muscle (Fig. 5-20). The fascia is split and the recurrent radial artery is ligated, allowing exposure of the tuberosity (Fig. 5-21).

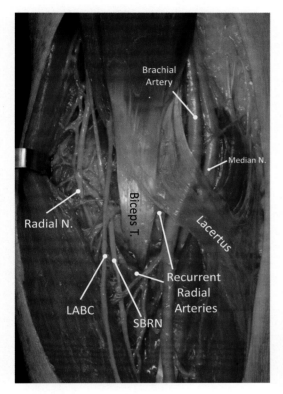

FIGURE 5-18

Anatomy and neurovascular structures at risk during an anterior approach to the biceps. The lateral antebrachial cutaneous (LABC) nerve is the most commonly injured nerve during this approach due to overzealous retraction and can be found exiting just lateral to the biceps tendon proximally and is the terminal branch of the musculocutaneous nerve. The radial nerve lies just deep and slightly lateral to the LABC in a roughly parallel course to it. Radial recurrent arteries must be ligated for hemostasis. SBRN, superficial branch of the radial nerve.

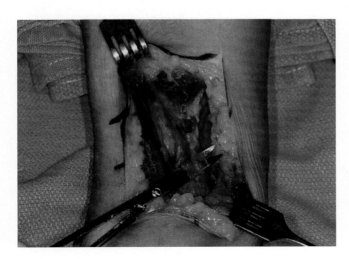

FIGURE 5-19

A Henry anterior exposure identifying the tendon and lacertus fibrosis. The extent of this exposure is surgeon preference.

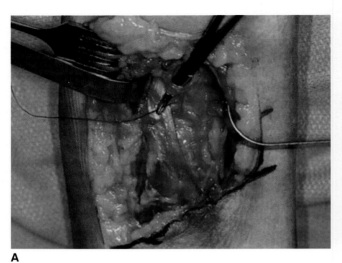

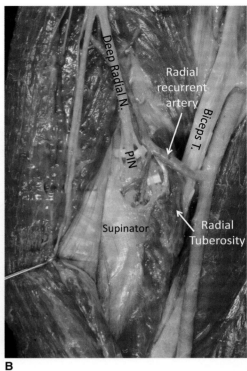

A

B

The deep radial nerve is identified emerging from the interval between the brachialis and brachioradialis **(A)**, and the more proximal braches of the radial recurrent artery are ligated. The deep anatomic dissection in **(B)** illustrates the course of the biceps tendon and proximity of the radial recurrent artery and PIN to the attachment site of the biceps tendon to the tuberosity.

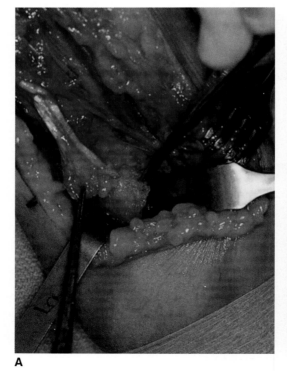

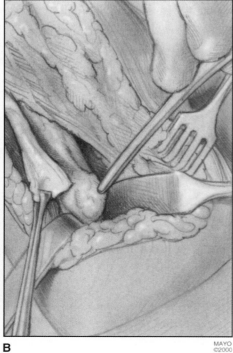

A

B

A,B: The tuberosity is exposed.

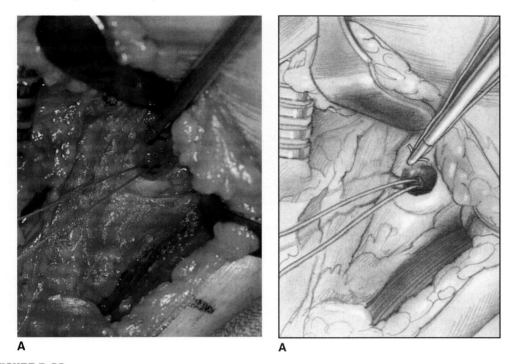

FIGURE 5-22

A,B: The tuberosity is excavated, and two suture anchors are embedded in the tuberosity.

If a suture anchor is used, the tuberosity is excavated and two anchors are embedded in the base of the excavated bone (Fig. 5-22).

The sutures are passed through the end of the tendon and threaded proximally while the tendon is being teased distally into the prepared tuberosity bed (Fig. 5-23). The sutures are tied with the forearm in neutral rotation.

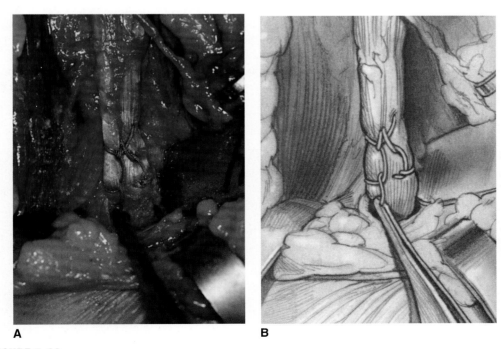

FIGURE 5-23

A crisscross or Krackow stitch is used to secure the tendon, which is then advanced into the tuberosity **(A)** as demonstrated in the drawing **(B)** and radiographically **(C)**.

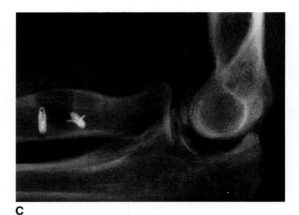

FIGURE 5-23 (*Continued*)   **C**

Endo Button

The endo button technique (ACUFEX, Smith & Nephew, Andover, MA) was described by Bain et al. (21) in 2000 and enjoys some popularity. The reason for this is that it clearly offers the most secure immediate fixation of any of the described techniques to date (22).

Technique

1. The bicipital tuberosity is exposed as described for the suture anchor technique above (see Figs. 5-17–5-21).
2. The forearm is fully extended and placed in maximum supination. An elliptical cortical window approximately 6 × 12 mm is made in the most medial portion of the tuberosity. Note: Either a burr or an adequate sized drill bit may be used for this step.
3. The contralateral cortical window is achieved drilling a 2-mm guide wire, protected by a drill guide, through the tuberosity and penetrating the opposite cortex (Fig. 5-24).
4. The opposite cortex is opened with a 4.5-mm drill in order to allow the passage of the endo button (Fig. 5-25).
5. The degenerated tendon is trimmed as noted previously. The endo button is secured according to surgeon preference and connected to the tendon with a running locked stitch. A gap of 2 to 3 mm is maintained between the end of the tendon and the endo button (Fig. 5-26). This allows the endo button to tilt through the defect and engage the opposite cortex of the radius.

   Note: We prefer a No. 5 nonabsorbable suture for this step. A fiber wire or other suitable nonabsorbable suture may also be employed. Either a Bunnell or Krackow stitch may be used in the tendon according to the surgeon's preference.

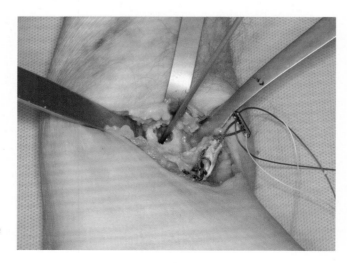

FIGURE 5-24

Endo button. A 2-mm pin is drilled into the cortex opposite to the tuberosity.

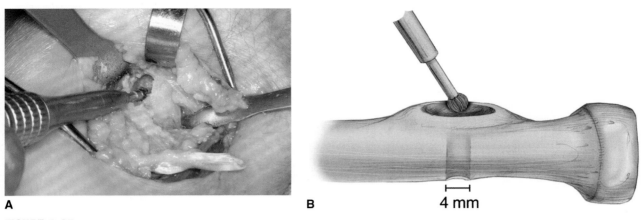

A   B   4 mm

FIGURE 5-25

The opening is enlarged at the entrance of the tuberosity with a 4.5-mm drill bit or a burr **(A,B)**.

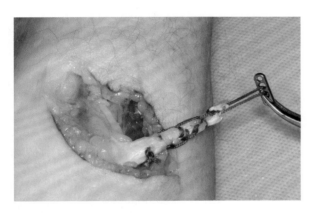

FIGURE 5-26

A running locked stitch begins proximally and includes the endo button. Care is taken to allow 4 to 5 mm space between the tendon and button for its deployment through the window in the radial cortex.

6. Two sutures of different colors are placed at either end of the endo button. These sutures should be strong enough as tension is applied to pull the endo button through the hole created in the radius for this purpose. Both sutures are threaded through a single large Keith-type needle (Fig. 5-27).

7. The forearm is flexed to 90 degrees and maximally supinated. The needle is then passed through the prepared bicipital tuberosity, through the defect in the opposite cortex, and then through the skin of the dorsal forearm (Fig. 5-28).

   Note: The needle is directed in a more ulnar direction, but it should not touch the ulna. This lessens the likelihood of injury to the posterior interosseous nerve.

8. Using the color code, the lead suture is tensioned to deliver the endo button through the radial defect. Tension is then placed on the trailing suture in order to flip the end button and prevent it from passing back through the dorsal surface of the radius (Fig. 5-29).

   Note: Intraoperative confirmation can be done with fluoroscopy (Fig. 5-30). The sutures are then pulled through the skin, and closure is routine.

Incomplete Distal Biceps Tendon Rupture

This is a relatively uncommon problem (23). The important features are that the tendon once partially torn, in the author's experience, does not heal, and hence surgery will be required (23). This is especially true in the athlete. The second major point is that remnants of the tendon cannot be sutured to bone but rather the partial rupture must be completed surgically, the degenerative tissue trimmed, and then the tendon reattached into the tuberosity. The one important feature from a technical standpoint is since the tendon still is attached to the tuberosity, one can potentially retrieve the tendon by

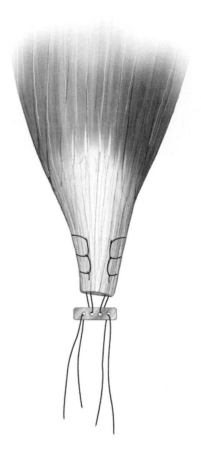

FIGURE 5-27

Lead sutures of opposite colors are threaded through each marginal hole and through the eye of a Keith needle.

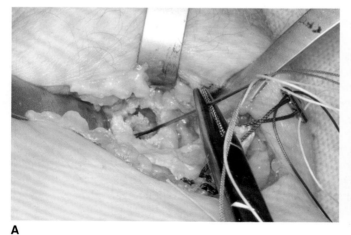

A

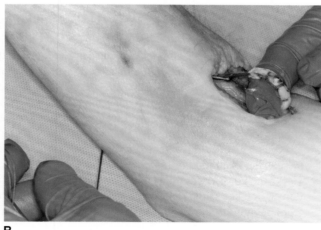

B

FIGURE 5-28

In 90 degrees of flexion, the needle is passed through the tuberosity **(A)**, out the opposite cortex, and penetrates the skin **(B)**.

the single dorsal incision over the forearm as is described below. Otherwise, any of the techniques above are used to reattach the tendon once the remaining fibers have been surgically released.

Surgical Technique: Partial Tendon Rupture

POSITION. As in many of the previous techniques, we employ the supine position with the arm brought across the chest.

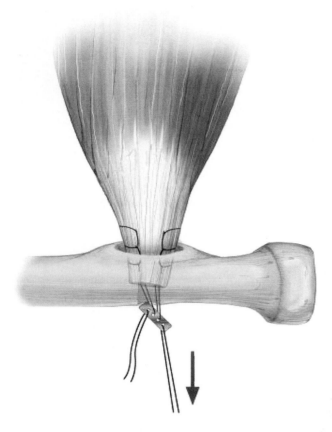

FIGURE 5-29

The button is deployed first by pulling on the lead suture, purple, and secured by pulling on the white "flip" suture.

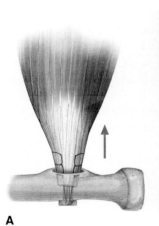

A

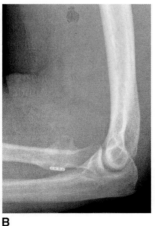

B

FIGURE 5-30

Proper development **(A)** confirmed by radiograph **(B)**.

INCISION

1. A 5-cm incision is made over the forearm similar to the second incision that is made in the two-incision technique. This is located 5 to 7 cm from the lateral epicondyle (Fig. 5-31).
2. The author prefers to palpate the interval between the anconeus and the extensor carpi ulnaris to assure that this incision is well anterior to the ulna (Fig. 5-32).
3. The extensor muscle mass and supinator are split until the tuberosity is palpated.
4. In most instances, the remaining fibers are those most proximal in the wound. A No. 0 nonabsorbable suture is placed in the tendon to prevent its retraction, and the remaining fibers of the biceps tendon are released from the tuberosity (Fig. 5-33).
5. The soft tissue is cleared from the tuberosity, and the arm is brought into maximum pronation.

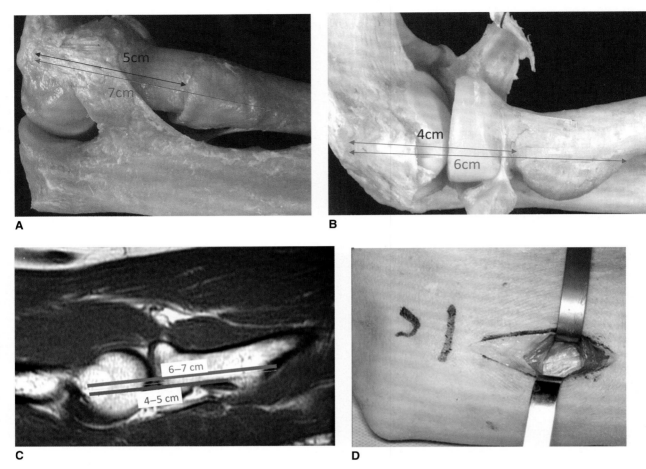

FIGURE 5-31

There is individual variability in the position of the tuberosity referable to the lateral epicondyle with the average apex lying 5 to 6 cm distal to the epicondyle as seen in cadaveric specimens **(A,B)** and MRI **(C)**. A 5-cm incision is made beginning just distal to the joint and centered over the tuberosity for a direct approach to the biceps with the arm at 90 degrees and full pronation **(D)**.

> Note: Bursal reactive tissue is commonly encountered with this step and may be quite extensive (Fig. 5-34).

6. The biceps tendon should be able to be brought fully into the wound sufficiently to allow first the trimming of the degenerative end and second placement of the sutures as noted in the steps above (Fig. 5-35). At this juncture, the preparation of the tuberosity is as shown above for the two-incision technique (Fig. 5-36). The placement of the sutures and the securing of the tendon are identical.

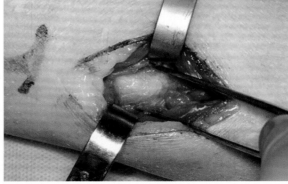

FIGURE 5-32

Palpation with the arm in free pronation provides the location of the radial tuberosity.

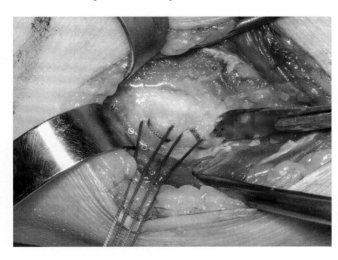

FIGURE 5-33

Two No. 0 sutures are placed in the portion of the tendon still attached to the tuberosity.

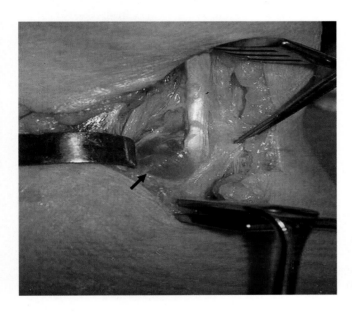

FIGURE 5-34

In some instances, extensive reaction occurs around the distal tendinous attachment, as shown by *arrow*.

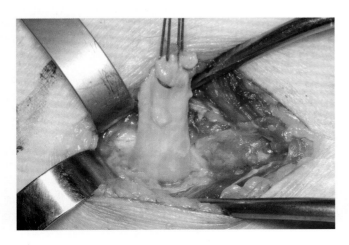

FIGURE 5-35

The tendon is released and drawn into the wound.

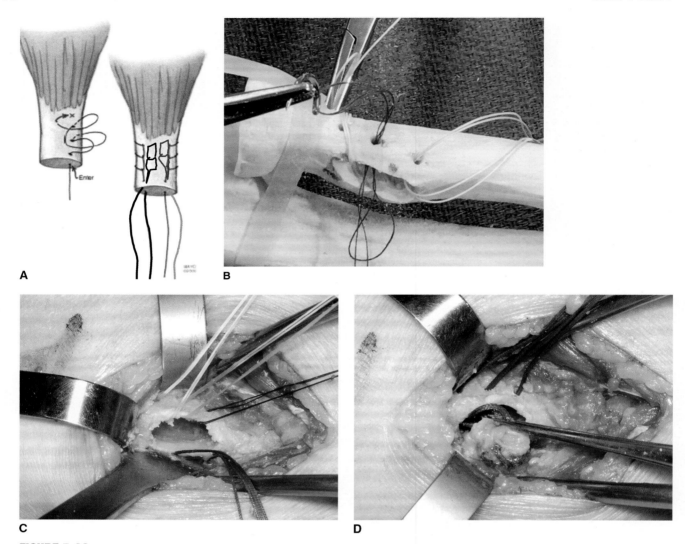

FIGURE 5-36

Two Krackow locking sutures are placed in the distal tendon after trimming **(A)**. Shuttle sutures are placed through the holes into the excavated cavity **(B,C)** and the tendon is docked into the trough **(D)**.

RESULTS

The results of virtually all of the reattachment techniques have been exceptionally good. In general, patients may be advised that there is a 90% chance of restoring more than 90% of normal function. In the majority of instances, patients will have essentially a normal elbow. The two reasons to prevent this is the development of ectopic bone or a radial nerve palsy (4,24–26).

DELAYED RECONSTRUCTION

Frequency of delayed reconstruction appears to be slightly increasing in recent years. However, we have discontinued preserving the fleck of calcaneus on the Achilles graft and simply embed the allograft tendon as noted below.

When the tendon has retracted to the point that it cannot be reattached directly to the tuberosity, augmentation with an Achilles tendon allograft is our technique of choice. Of note, and as noted above, if the host tendon can be attached with the elbow at 90 degrees, this is preferable to reconstruction. The 90-degree contracture will stretch out to near normal extension with time and function is excellent (9).

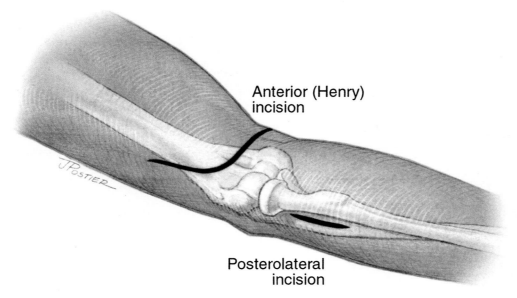

FIGURE 5-37

The two-incision technique is used and employs a Henry-type incision in the antecubital space and a 4-cm incision over the posterolateral aspect of the proximal forearm. The anterior incision is extended as needed to expose the biceps muscle.

Technique: Achilles Tendon Allograft

1. The exposure is more extensive as the biceps muscle belly must be exposed (Fig. 5-37).
2. After it is determined that the biceps tendon is inadequate for reattachment (Fig. 5-38), the tuberosity is exposed by blunt and sharp dissection as needed, and the curved hemostat identifies the site of the forearm incision (Fig. 5-39).
3. The tuberosity is exposed and excavated as described above (Fig. 5-40).
4. A No. 5 nonabsorbable suture is placed in the allograft tendon as in the acute rupture.

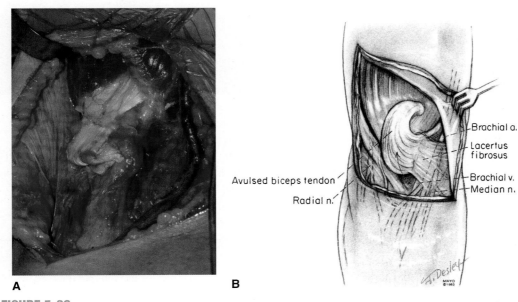

A   **B**

FIGURE 5-38

The tendon usually has recoiled (**A**—patient example and **B**—drawing) and is of variable length, but the biceps stump is adequate to secure to the tendon allograft.

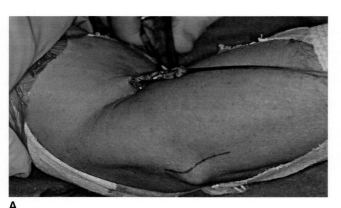

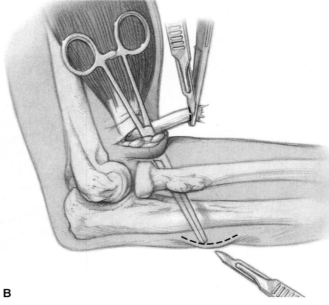

A   **B**

FIGURE 5-39

A,B: A more detailed dissection in the anticubital space is required to identify the radial tuberosity. Then, a curved hemostat is passed between the radial tuberosity and the ulna to emerge through the common extensor muscle mass and tent the skin on the proximal posterolateral aspect of the forearm as is done for acute injuries.

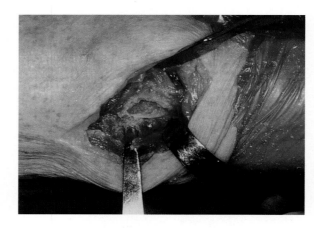

FIGURE 5-40

The exposure and preparation of the tuberosity is identified to that described above for acute injuries.

5. The tendon is then threaded from the anterior exposure into the forearm incision (Fig. 5-41).
6. This is inserted into the tuberosity and secured through the holes in the tuberosity (Fig. 5-42).
7. With the elbow at about 80 to 90 degrees of flexion, the Achilles fascia is secured around its margin to the biceps muscle, which has been retracted distally as much as possible to develop appropriate resting tension (Fig. 5-43).

POSTOPERATIVE MANAGEMENT

Acute Repair

The patient is placed in a posterior splint with the elbow in 90 degrees of flexion and the forearm in neutral rotation. This is kept in place for 3 to 7 days.

At 1 week or less, the posterior splint is removed and gentle passive flexion is allowed. Active extension to 30 degrees is allowed and encouraged from the 1st week after surgery. Full extension is allowed as tolerated and generally attained by the 3rd week. Four weeks after surgery, the patient

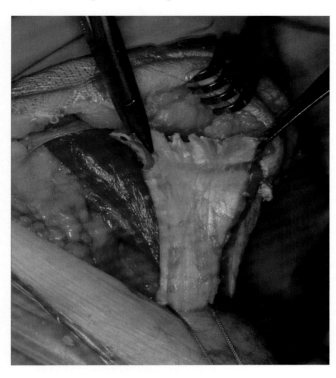

FIGURE 5-41

The Achilles tendon allograft is inserted from the anterior incision to emerge through the forearm incision.

is allowed to flex and extend against gravity as able. At 6 weeks, a gentle flexion strengthening program is allowed starting with 1 kg. Activity as tolerated is permitted at 3 months. Full activity without restriction is allowed 6 months after surgery.

Note: This program is also effective if elbow flexion is required for reattachment. The time frame is adjusted according to patient progress.

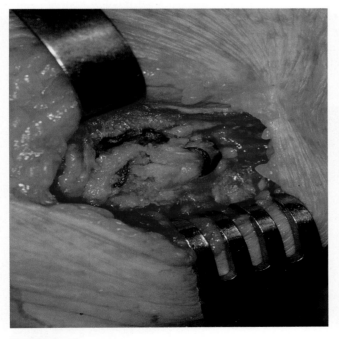

FIGURE 5-42

The tendon is inserted into the tuberosity and secured with sutures placed through the margin of the tuberosity in the acute injury.

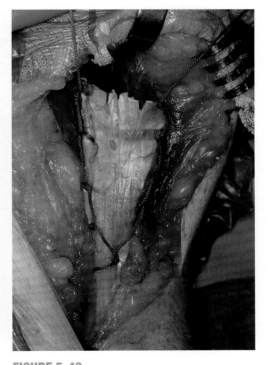

FIGURE 5-43

With the elbow at 80 to 90 degrees of flexion, the biceps muscle is "enveloped" with the Achilles fascia.

Allograft Reconstruction

The program is delayed somewhat when an allograft is used. The patient is protected for 3 weeks. Passive assisted motion is begun at 3 and continued to 6 weeks. Full extension is avoided until the 6th week. Active motion for activities of daily living is allowed at 6 to 12 weeks. Activity as tolerated progresses from the 4th to the 8th month.

RESULTS

Regardless of technique, the results of immediate reattachment of the tendon are very good. Studies have shown virtually 100% improvement for restoration of flexion and supination strength (3–6,8). Loss of motion is not seen, and we have observed only one rerupture after an acute repair. Although popular, the clinical experience with suture anchors is limited. To date, what data are available reveal no problems from several combined sources (24,27–30). Laboratory studies, however, reveal a statistically significant ($p < 0.01$) greater initial strength with the transosseous holes than suture anchor. The endo button technique has been shown to provide the best, most secure initial fixation of any of these techniques but may not restore the cam effect and true anatomy of the insertion. Nevertheless, clinically all techniques described are reported as effective, and one randomized controlled trial shows no difference between the two approaches (14).

COMPLICATIONS

There are two major complications associated with this procedure: radial nerve injury and ectopic bone formation. Rerupture is uncommon. Radial nerve injury has been reported and may be seen as often as 5% after distal biceps tendon reattachment through anterior modified Henry approach (8,12). Ectopic bone is a recognized complication of both approaches; however, the two-incision technique is more often associated with bridging between the proximal radius and ulna (Fig. 5-44) with limited forearm rotation. This, however, can be minimized or avoided not by exposing the periosteal surface of the ulna with the forearm incision (Fig. 5-45) but rather splitting the muscle fibers as the tuberosity is exposed and avoiding muscle damage (Fig. 5-46) (11).

If a synostosis occurs, it significantly limits function. Between 3 and 6 months, the osseous bar may be resected. The exposure is generally through the previously used forearm incision. Care should be taken during the exposure to avoid excessive retraction on the supinator muscle, which may injure the posterior interosseous nerve. Occasionally, the reattached biceps tendon itself is involved in the ectopic bone. In this instance, the tendon may be released during the ectopic bone removal (Fig. 5-47) and is then reattached at the end of the excision.

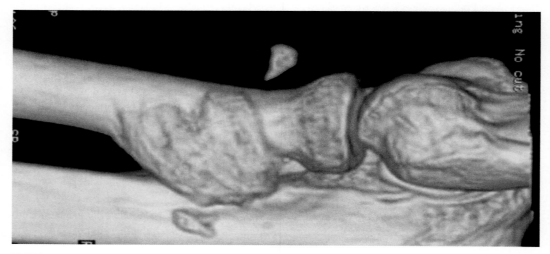

FIGURE 5-44

Ectopic bone bridging the proximal ulna and radius. The exposure of the radial tuberosity was across the periosteal surface of the ulna.

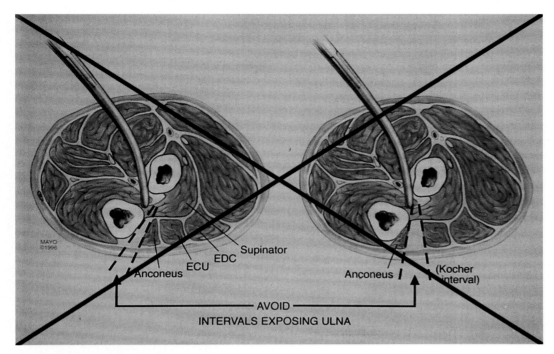

FIGURE 5-45

The forearm incision should not be through Kocher interval or otherwise expose the periosteal surface of the proximal ulna.

MAYO EXPERIENCE

Our original experience was quite favorable with virtual 100% return of function in 90% of patients (Morrey). More recently, assessment of nine patients who were not treated revealed a mean flexion torque of 26 nm compared to the uninjured torque of 41 (37% reduction). Supination torque was 4.5 in the involved and 8.3 in the uninvolved (46% reduction) (31). The Mayo experience was further reported with a focus on complications after 88 procedures by Kelly et al. Overall, the satisfactory rate was over 90%. One rerupture occurred in a patient requiring active use with wheelchair transfer

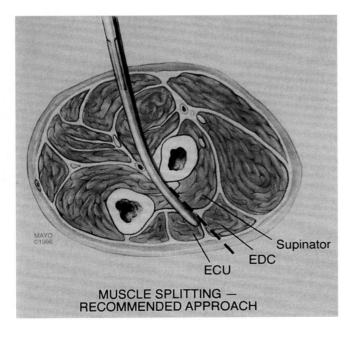

FIGURE 5-46

The forearm incision is a muscle-splitting approach.

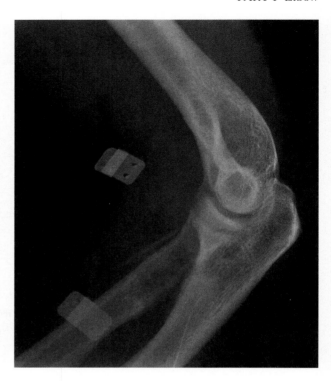

FIGURE 5-47

Removal of the ectopic bone restores functional forearm rotation in most patients. In this instance (Fig. 5-42), the tendon insertion was involved and required reattachment.

the day after surgery. No synostosis occurred after 74 Mayo modified two-incision approaches. Of note is that the rate of complication doubles ($p < 0.05$) if a delay to repair is >21 days (2).

We have also recently reviewed our experience with resecting the osseous bridging in 12 cases referred to Mayo for management. In this sample, at a mean of 6.7 years after surgery, all 12 were pain free with excellent strength and averaged 122 degrees of pronation and supination (32).

REFERENCES

1. O'Driscoll SW, Goncalves LB, Dietz P. The hook test for distal biceps tendon avulsion. *Am J Sports Med.* 2007;35(11):1865–1869.
2. Giuffre BM, Moss MJ. Optimal position for MRI of the distal biceps brachii tendon: flexed abducted supinated view. *AJR Am J Roentgenol.* 2004;182:994–996.
3. Agins HJ, Chess JL, Hoekstra DV, et al. Rupture of the distal insertion of the biceps brachii tendon. *Clin Orthop.* 1988;234:34.
4. Baker BE, Bierwagen D. Rupture of the distal tendon of the biceps brachii. *J Bone Joint Surg.* 1985;67A:414.
5. Louis DS, Hankin FM, Eckenrode JF, et al. Distal biceps brachii tendon avulsion: a simplified method of operative repair. *Am J Sports Med.* 1986;14:234.
6. Morrey BF, Askew LJ, An KN, et al. Rupture of the distal biceps tendon: biomechanical assessment of different treatment options. *J Bone Joint Surg.* 1985;67A:418.
7. Norman WH. Repair of avulsion of insertion of biceps brachii tendon. *Clin Orthop.* 1985;193:189.
8. Hovelius L, Josefsson G. Rupture of the distal biceps tendon. *Acta Orthop Scand.* 1977;48:280.
9. Morrey ME, Abdel MP, Sanchez-Sotelo J, et al. Primary repair of retracted distal biceps tendon ruptures in extreme flexion. *J Shoulder Elbow Surg.* 2014;23:679–685.
10. Kelly EW, Morrey BF, O'Driscoll SH. Complications of repair of the distal biceps tendon with modified two-incision technique. *J Bone Joint Surg.* 2000;82A:1575.
11. Dobbie RP. Avulsion of the lower biceps brachii tendon: analysis of 51 previously reported cases. *Am J Surg.* 1941;51:661.
12. Boyd HB, Anderson MD. A method for reinsertion of the distal biceps brachii tendon. *J Bone Joint Surg.* 1961;43A:1041.
13. Amin NH, Volpi A, Lynch TS, et al. Complications of distal biceps tendon repair: a meta-analysis of single-incision versus double-incision surgical technique. *Orthop J Sports Med.* 2016;4(10):2325967116668137.
14. Grewal R, Athwal GS, MacDermid JC, et al. Single versus double-incision technique for the repair of acute distal biceps tendon ruptures: a randomized clinical trial. *J Bone Joint Surg Am.* 2012;94:1166–1174. Available at: http://dx.doi.org/10.2106/JBJS.K.00436
15. Failla JM, Amadio PC, Morrey BF, et al. Proximal radioulnar synostosis after repair of distal biceps brachii rupture by the two-incision technique: report of four cases. *Clin Orthop.* 1990;253:133.
16. Forthman CL, Zimmerman RM, Sullivan MJ, et al. Cross-sectional anatomy of the bicipital tuberosity and biceps brachii tendon insertion: relevance to anatomic tendon repair. *J Shoulder Elbow Surg.* 2008;17:522–526. Available at: http://dx.doi.org/10.1016/j.jse.2007.11.002
17. Hasan SA, Cordell CL, Rauls RB, et al. Two-incision versus one-incision repair for distal biceps tendon rupture: a cadaveric study. *J Shoulder Elbow Surg.* 2012;21:935–941. Available at: http:// dx.doi.org/10.1016/j.jse.2011.04.027

18. Jobin CM, Kippe MA, Gardner TR, et al. Distal biceps tendon repair: a cadaveric analysis of suture anchor and interference screw restoration of the anatomic footprint. *Am J Sports Med.* 2009;37:2214–2221. Available at: http://dx.doi.org/10.1177/0363546509337451

19. Prud'homme-Foster M, Louati H, Pollock JW, Papp S. Proper placement of the distal biceps tendon during repair improves supination strength—a biomechanical analysis. *J Shoulder Elbow Surg.* 2015;24:527–532. Available at: http://dx.doi.org/10.1016/j.jse.2014.09.039

20. Schmidt CC, Weir DM, Wong AS, et al. The effect of biceps reattachment site. *J Shoulder Elbow Surg.* 2010;19:1157–1165. Available at: http://dx.doi.org/10.1016/j.jse.2010.05.027

21. Bain GI, Prem H, Heptinstall RJ, et al. Repair of distal biceps tendon rupture: a new technique using the endo button. *J Shoulder Elbow Surg.* 2000;9(2):120–126.

22. Greenberg JA, Fernandez JJ, Wang T, et al. Endo button-assisted repair of distal biceps tendon ruptures. *J Shoulder Elbow Surg.* 2003;12(5):484–490.

23. Bourne MH, Morrey BF. Partial rupture of the distal biceps tendon. *Clin Orthop.* 1991;271:143.

24. Lintner S, Fishcer T. Repair of the distal biceps tendon using suture anchors and an anterior approach. *Clin Orthop.* 1996;322:116–119.

25. Mazzocca AD, Spang JT, Arciero RA. Distal biceps rupture. *Orthop Clin North Am.* 2008;39(2):237–249, vii.

26. Schmidt A, Johann K, Kunz M. Operative treatment of ruptures of distal tendon of biceps muscle with a minimally invasive technique using suture anchors—clinical results. *Z Orthop Ihre Grenzgeb.* 2006;144(6):614–618.

27. Brunner F, Gelpke H, Hotz T, et al. Distal biceps tendon ruptures—experiences with soft tissue preserving reinsertion by bone anchors. *Swiss Surg.* 1999;5(4):186–190.

28. Strauch RJ, Michelson H, Rosenwasser MP. Repair of rupture of the distal tendon of the biceps brachii. Review of the literature and report of three cases treated with a single anterior incision and suture anchors. *Am J Orthop.* 1997;26(2):151–156.

29. Verhaven E, Huylebroek J, Van Nieuwenhuysen W, et al. Surgical treatment of acute biceps tendon ruptures with a suture anchor. *Acta Orthop Belgica.* 1993;59(4):426–429.

30. Woods DA, Hoy G, Shimmin A. A safe technique for distal biceps repair using a suture anchor and a limited anterior approach. *Injury.* 1999;30(4):233–237.

31. Nesterenko S, Domire ZJ, Morrey BF, et al. Elbow strength and endurance in patients with a ruptured distal biceps tendon. *J Shoulder Elbow Surg.* 2010;19(2):184–189.

32. Jost B, Morrey BF, Adams RA, et al. Ectopic bone excision following distal biceps tendon repair. *Am JBJS.* 2009, unpublished data.

6 Triceps Tendon Repair and Reconstruction in the Athlete

Jeremy S. Somerson and Bernard F. Morrey

Injuries to the distal triceps are rare. Recent literature has provided greater insight into the anatomy of the triceps tendon (1) as well as biomechanical stability and expected outcomes after surgical repair (2–9). Distal triceps ruptures occur most frequently in serious power lifters and body builders (10–12), football players, and other athletic endeavors. Also, anabolic steroids used as a strength enhancement have been implicated as a risk factor. The injury has much more variation in the pathoanatomy than distal biceps injury, with the failure occurring at the central tendinous attachment with or without osseous avulsion (13) at the musculotendinous fixation or even in the muscle belly itself (12,14–17). The important characteristic of this tendon injury is that an immediate repair is the treatment of choice; however, unlike the biceps tendon, the duration of recovery is more prolonged. Unlike injuries to the distal biceps, which often result in restored function in 6 months, triceps ruptures may take a full year to completely recover.

ANATOMY

Reports of partial ruptures (18–20) of the distal triceps have led to interest in defining the discrete insertion sites of the heads of the triceps. Madsen (21) identified a discrete deep tendon corresponding to the medial head of the triceps but noted that the three heads of the triceps blended on histologic examination to form a single tendinous insertion. More recently, Barco (1) noted a plane of cleavage between the deep muscular insertion of the medial head and the tendinous insertion of the long and lateral heads (Fig. 6-1). This demonstrated discrete insertion sites at the footprint of the olecranon including the posterior capsule at the deepest layer, the medial head above this, and the long/lateral heads at the most superficial level. Knowledge of this arrangement can be of value in understanding the clinical presentation as well as directing a surgical strategy. This arrangement does explain why those with the most common injury, an isolated avulsion of the superficial tendinous portion, may present with modest extension strength due to an intact deep medial head insertion.

DIAGNOSIS

The diagnosis of tendon injury is usually not difficult, although missed injuries have been reported (22). Dimpling of the skin proximal to the olecranon may be present (Fig. 6-2A). The problem in making a decision regarding intervention is that some residual strength is almost always present. This is because the anconeus and its attachment to the lateral triceps aponeurosis are rarely included in the injury. An associated ulnar nerve stretch has also been reported (with this injury in a power lifter) (10,23).

Today, imaging modalities have significantly improved our ability to diagnose triceps injury and to characterize the extent of the pathology (24,25). The radiograph showing an avulsion of the osseous attachment, or Dunn-Kusnezov sign, is pathognomonic for distal triceps rupture; a systematic review of triceps tendon ruptures showed this sign to be positive in 61% to 88% of published cases (26) (Fig. 6-2B). Today, MR imaging can and should be used to confirm the diagnosis especially if any doubt exists (Fig. 6-3). The common central slip ruptures do well if repaired acutely but do less well if repaired or reconstructed at a later date. Ultrasound has also been reported as a sensitive and specific test for differentiating partial from complete ruptures (27).

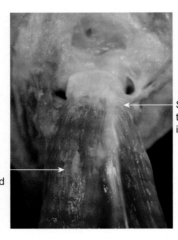

Superficial tendinous insertion

Deep medial muscular head of the triceps mechanism

A

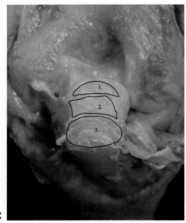

Superficial tendinous insertion

Deep medial muscular head insertion

B

FIGURE 6-1

A: The triceps mechanism has been resected in the midhumerus and reflected proximally revealing the distinct medial muscular and the central tendinous components.
B: The medial head is dissected free of the superficial tendinous portion, and the two heads are separated.
C: Complete resection of soft tissue attachment to the olecranon reveals the respective footprints of the component parts. (Modified from Barco R, Sánchez P, Morrey ME, et al. The distal triceps tendon insertional anatomy—implications for surgery. *JSES Open Access.* 2017;1(2):98–103. doi:10.1016/j.jses.2017.05.002.)

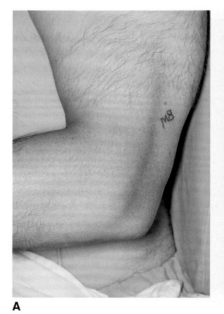

Footprint of:
1. Capsular insertion
2. Deep muscular (medial) insertion
3. Superficial tendinous insertion

C

A   **B**

FIGURE 6-2

The clinical finding of a dimple or deficiency at the site of attachment is a valuable but uncommon finding **(A)**. An x-ray with bone fleck *(white arrow)* signifying triceps avulsion is pathognomonic for rupture **(B)**.

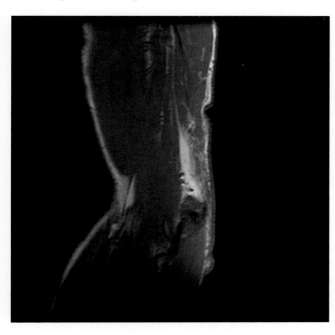

FIGURE 6-3
The MRI is quite effective in
demonstrating triceps disruption.

Acute Rupture/Repair

Indications

1. An acute rupture exhibiting functional extension weakness or fatigue pain and weakness in a patient who requires extension strength (this includes almost everybody)
2. Failure to regain extensor strength after several weeks of nonoperative management
3. Persistent pain, even if strength is not a major complaint

Contraindications

1. Few, if the patient is symptomatic and if the diagnosis has been accurately made
2. Willingness to perform rehabilitation
3. Ongoing or generalized enthesopathy and morbidity that will not be addressed by triceps reconstitution

Surgical Technique

1. Position: The patient is placed supine on the operating table. The arm is prepped and draped, but the tourniquet is not inflated.
2. Incision: A straight posterior skin incision is made and centered just medial to the tip of the olecranon (Fig. 6-4). The dissection carries through the triceps fascia, and the defect is identified. In most instances, the avulsion is from the central tendinous attachment to the olecranon. The triceps disruption is mobilized.

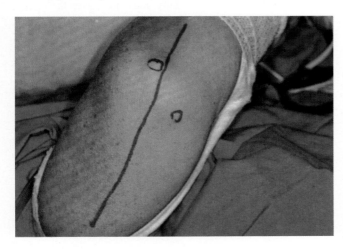

FIGURE 6-4
Midline incision showing tip of
olecranon and medial epicondyle.

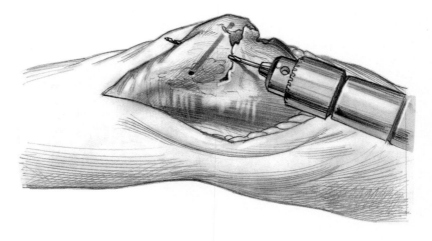

dp936431-018-0

FIGURE 6-5

Cruciate drill holes are placed in the olecranon.

3. Cruciate drill holes are placed in the proximal ulna (Fig. 6-5).
4. A no. 5 nonabsorbable suture is introduced from distal to proximal and enters the torn portion of the tendon at its torn surface.
5. A running locked type of stitch is then placed with three to four passes on each side of the mid-tendinous portion of the triceps tendon.
6. The suture is then brought back through the opposite cruciate hole (Fig. 6-6). This results in a very firm and adequate repair, but a second transverse drill hole may be placed and a second direct suture if there is any question about the security of the attachment. Note: The precise site of disruption is roughened with a rongeur to enhance healing.
7. Sutures are tied at the margin of the subcutaneous border of the ulna with the elbow in approximately 20 to 30 degrees of extension.
8. The arm is elevated, and an anterior splint is applied with the elbow in approximately 30 degrees of flexion.

Postoperative Management

The elbow is maintained in the anterior splint for approximately 4 to 5 days after which gentle passive assisted flexion to 60 degrees is allowed. At 3 weeks, flexion is allowed to 90 degrees. At the end of 3 weeks, flexion past 90 degrees is encouraged and allowed by active assist. Passively, assisted extension occurs with gravity and with the opposite extremity. At 4 to 6 weeks, active flexion and extension is allowed, but no forced extension is permitted for an additional 4 weeks. At 10 weeks, routine daily activities are permitted, but no extension force >10 lbs is permitted. After 3 months, if there is no pain, the patient can gradually resume full daily activities. Over the next 3 months, full extension activity and strength exercises are allowed.

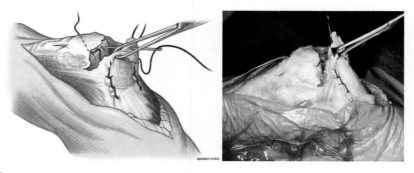

dp936431-019-0

FIGURE 6-6

A Krackow stitch secures the tendon as the suture is being brought back across the olecranon. Note: The tissue is handled with an Allis clamp to avoid crush injury.

Reconstruction

We have regularly performed two reconstructive procedures for chronic dysfunction (28). One is the so-called anconeus slide, in which the anconeus is identified at Kocher interval between the superior margin of the anconeus and the extensor carpi ulnaris (Fig. 6-7). The anconeus is elevated from the lateral bed of the ulna, and importantly, the humeral attachment of the anconeus is released. The entire mechanism is then displaced from lateral to medial and is centralized over the olecranon. This maneuver is used in those in whom there is inadequate tendinous tissue of the central tendon to perform a direct attachment, but there is still an anconeus mechanism, which is in continuity.

Note: Our observation has been that while this may be an effective means for restoring some extension strength in patients with total elbow arthroplasty, it is less reliable for the athlete who needs as much extension strength as possible (29). For this reason, we would typically not recommend the anconeus slide in the athlete.

Indications for Triceps Reconstruction

1. Failure of an acute repair
2. Weakness that has become a major limitation of one's sporting activities or occupation
3. No improvement over the prior 3 months
4. Note: Pain is rarely a major factor but is commonly present

Contraindications

1. Unclear or unreasonable expectations
2. Inability or unwillingness to participate in the postoperative program or to accept the period of postoperative recovery

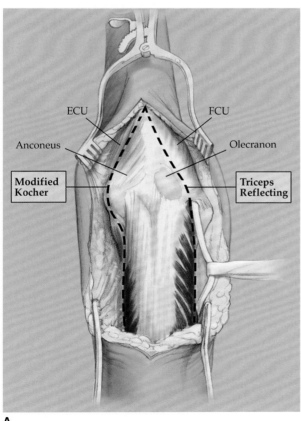
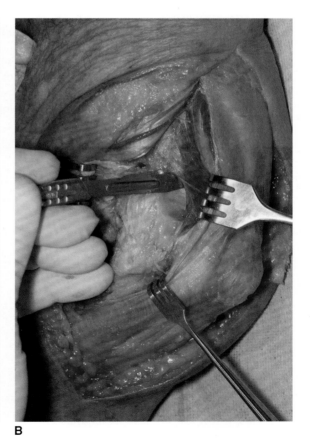

A   B

FIGURE 6-7

A: The anconeus is an extension of the extensor mechanism laterally. **B:** It can be readily mobilized by elevating the ulnar and humeral attachments.

Techniques

Anconeus rotational reconstruction—not typically performed in the athlete but is described here for completeness.

1. Position and incision. The positioning, prepping, draping, and initial skin incision are as described above.
2. If the residual tendon is contracted and cannot be advanced to bone (Fig. 6-8) and if the anconeus is present, the interval (Kocher) between the anconeus and extensor carpi ulnaris is identified.
3. Kocher interval is entered, and the anconeus is mobilized from its humeral attachment (Fig. 6-9). Ideally, the translocated muscle is left intact distally, and the proximal fascial attachment to the triceps is preserved.
4. The muscle is elevated from the ulna and rotated medially. The proximal ulna is cleaned of soft tissue and prepared with cruciate drill holes as for the acute repair.
5. With the elbow in about 30 degrees of flexion, a no. 5 nonabsorbable suture is used to secure the rotated anconeus/triceps mechanism (Fig. 6-10).
6. An additional suture is placed in the original remnant of tendon and rotated in the residual triceps attachment.

Aftercare. This is similar to that of the acute rupture described above.

Achilles Tendon Allograft

If the defect is massive or in most athletes, an Achilles tendon allograft reconstruction is employed (Fig. 6-11).

Note: The calcaneus is no longer employed unless the olecranon was resorbed. This is seen after elbow replacement but rare in the athlete.

1. Positioning and incision are as for the acute injury.
2. Care is taken to dissect and mobilize the triceps sufficiently to ensure the maximum possible excursion.
3. The proximal ulna is prepared by creating a groove on the subcutaneous border of the olecranon (Fig. 6-12).
4. The tendon is placed in the groove (Fig. 6-13A) and secured with two to three no. 5 nonabsorbable sutures placed through transverse drill holes (Fig. 6-13B).
5. After the distal attachment has been secured, the triceps is brought as far distally as possible according to the dictates of the pathology. The central portion of the triceps, which contains the

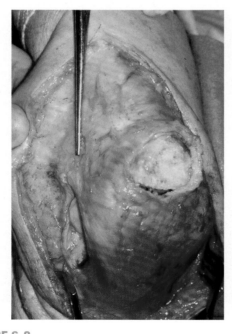

FIGURE 6-8

Large defect at the central attachment of the triceps in patient with total elbow arthroplasty.

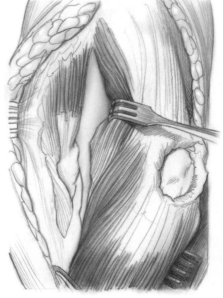

dp936431-020-0

FIGURE 6-9

The anconeus is mobilized to cover the proximal ulna leaving its distal attachment intact.

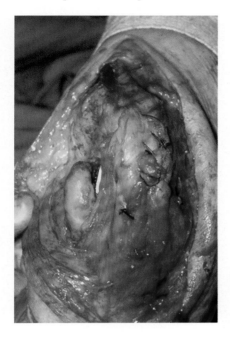

FIGURE 6-10

It is secured to the ulna through drill holes in the olecranon process.

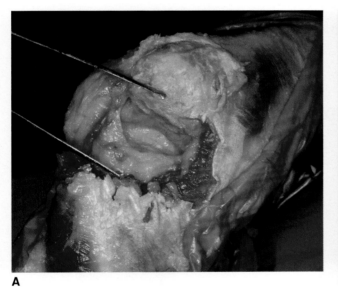

A

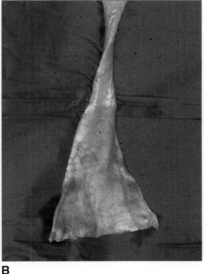

B

FIGURE 6-11

A: Large defect in the triceps does not allow direct repair to bone. Violation of the anconeus attachment precludes anconeus rotation as a solution. **B:** Achilles tendon allograft with the calcaneus resected is an excellent tissue for reconstruction.

residual triceps tendon, is secured with a locked stitch, and the triceps is then attached to the allograft tendon graft in the midline as far distally in the allograft as possible with the elbow in about 20 degrees of extension (Fig. 6-14).

6. Once this tension has been secured, the remainder of the proximal portion of the Achilles graft is used to envelope the triceps musculature (Fig. 6-15). An absorbable no. 0 suture is used as a running stitch to further secure the allograft to the triceps musculature.

Postoperative Management

This is similar to the acute repair; however, we delay efforts to regain strength allowing only sedentary stretching and unloaded extension for up to 3 months. The recovery period is dictated by the features of the case. Caution is advised.

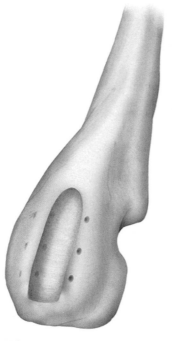

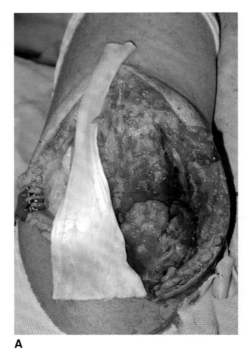

A

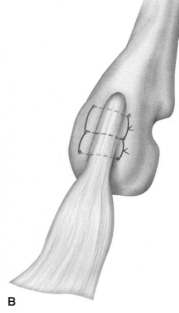

B

FIGURE 6-12

A trough is created in the proximal ulna to receive the triceps tendon.

FIGURE 6-13

A,B: The distal aspect of the triceps graft is placed in the groove created in the olecranon **(A)** and is securely attached to the proximal ulna with a no. 5 nonabsorbable suture **(B)**.

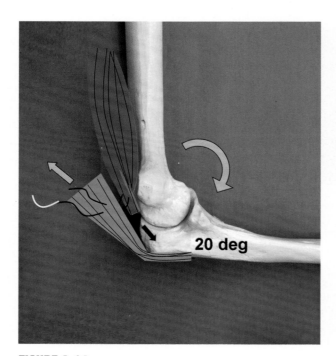

FIGURE 6-14

The residual tendon of the triceps is mobilized and displaced distally. This is stabilized to the graft with a no. 5 nonabsorbable stitch.

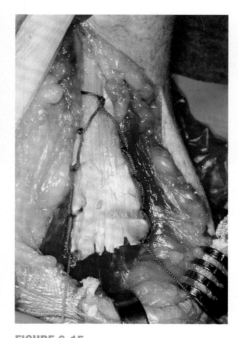

FIGURE 6-15

The triceps allograft is enveloped around the triceps and secured at the margins with a running locked stitch.

RESULTS AND COMPLICATIONS

Until recently, the majority of publications regarding the distal triceps repair were small series and case reports (10,11,16,23,30–33). More recent literature has provided insights into expected outcomes and complications (3–9,34). In a series of 184 surgically treated distal triceps ruptures, Mirzayan et al. (8) reported 7 cases of retear (4%) and 11 cases of reoperation (6%). In addition to the 7 retears, the reoperations included 2 surgeries for infection, 1 for postoperative stiffness and 1 for subcutaneous suture removal. No preoperative or postoperative outcome scores were reported, but a higher retear rate was reported among patients who underwent fixation using a transosseous technique compared to a suture anchor technique.

Other recent multicenter studies have shown retear rates ranging from 4% to 7%, with no differences noted comparing suture anchor and transosseous techniques (4,5). A biomechanical study comparing transosseous and knotless suture anchor repair showed greater load to yield using a suture anchor repair, although it is unknown whether the difference carries clinical relevance to justify the added cost (2).

We reported outcomes from 23 distal triceps repairs at the Mayo Clinic, of which 14 were acute repairs and 9 were chronic reconstructive procedures (35). Of these, 8 were considered partial, principally involving the central tendinous attachment. After treatment, isokinetic strength studied in 10 revealed an average of 82% of the "normal" opposite extremity; endurance was 99% of normal. Subjectively, 90% were satisfied with their outcome. Final motion averaged 10 to 135 degrees. The time to recovery was somewhat prolonged, with a mean recovery period over 6 months; some patients who underwent reconstruction for chronic injury continued to improve more than a year after surgery. In the Mayo experience, there were no permanent complications. Transient ulnar nerve palsy, rerupture, persistent weakness, and discomfort are recognized as potential problems with surgery or with the pathology.

CASE PRESENTATION

A 28-year-old football professional tight end ruptured the central slip of his triceps tendon while shielding a block by extending his elbow against resistance. A failed effort at suture anchor repair (Fig. 6-16A) prompted further assessment and required a reoperation (Fig. 6-16B). Since his career depended on "normal" function, a reconstructive procedure with an Achilles graft was performed (Fig. 6-16C). He returned for a successful season after this surgery.

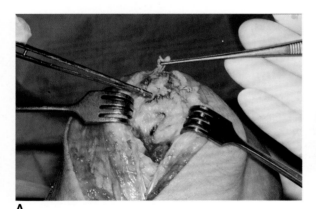
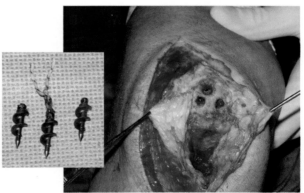

A

B

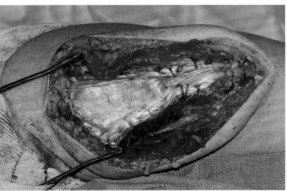

C

FIGURE 6-16

The suture anchor repair failed causing a painful bursitis and weakness **(A)**. The anchors were removed; the debridement resulted in triceps tissue loss **(B)**. An Achilles tendon allograft was successfully applied as described above **(C)**.

REFERENCES

1. Barco R, Sánchez P, Morrey ME, et al. The distal triceps tendon insertional anatomy—implications for surgery. *JSES Open Access.* 2017;1(2):98–103. doi:10.1016/j.jses.2017.05.002.

2. Clark J, Obopilwe E, Rizzi A, et al. Distal triceps knotless anatomic footprint repair is superior to transosseous cruciate repair: a biomechanical comparison. *Arthroscopy.* 2014;30(10):1254–1260. doi:10.1016/j.arthro.2014.07.005.

3. Dunn JC, Kusnezov N, Fares A, et al. Outcomes of triceps rupture in the US military: minimum 2-year follow-up. *Hand (N Y).* 2017. doi:10.1177/1558944717745499.

4. Giannicola G, Bullitta G, Rotini R, et al. Results of primary repair of distal triceps tendon ruptures in a general population. *Bone Joint J.* 2018;100-B(5):610–616. doi:10.1302/0301-620X.100B5.BJJ-2017-1057.R2.

5. Horneff JG, Aleem A, Nicholson T, et al. Functional outcomes of distal triceps tendon repair comparing transosseous bone tunnels with suture anchor constructs. *J Shoulder Elbow Surg.* 2017;26(12):2213–2219. doi:10.1016/j.jse.2017.08.006.

6. Kokkalis ZT, Mavrogenis AF, Spyridonos S, et al. Triceps brachii distal tendon reattachment with a double-row technique. *Orthopedics.* 2013;36(2):110–116. doi:10.3928/01477447-20130122-03.

7. Kose O, Kilicaslan OF, Guler F, et al. Functional outcomes and complications after surgical repair of triceps tendon rupture. *Eur J Orthop Surg Traumatol.* 2015;25(7):1131–1139. doi:10.1007/s00590-015-1669-3.

8. Mirzayan R, Acevedo DC, Sodl JF, et al. Operative management of acute triceps tendon ruptures: review of 184 cases. *Am J Sports Med.* 2018;46:1451–1458. doi:10.1177/0363546518757426.

9. Neumann H, Schulz A-P, Breer S, et al. Traumatic rupture of the distal triceps tendon (a series of 7 cases). *Open Orthop J.* 2015;9:536–541. doi:10.2174/1874325001509010536.

10. Herrick RT, Herrick S. Ruptured triceps in a powerlifter presenting as cubital tunnel syndrome. A case report. *Am J Sports Med.* 1987;15(5):514–516. doi:10.1177/036354658701500517.

11. Louis DS, Peck D. Triceps avulsion fracture in a weightlifter. *Orthopedics.* 1992;15(2):207–208.

12. Sherman OH, Snyder SJ, Fox JM. Triceps tendon avulsion in a professional body builder. A case report. *Am J Sports Med.* 1984;12(4):328–329. doi:10.1177/036354658401200415.

13. Farrar EL, Lippert FG. Avulsion of the triceps tendon. *Clin Orthop Relat Res.* 1981;(161):242–246.

14. Aso K, Torisu T. Muscle belly tear of the triceps. *Am J Sports Med.* 1984;12(6):485–487. doi:10.1177/036354658401200614.

15. Match RM, Corrylos EV. Bilateral avulsion fracture of the triceps tendon insertion from skiing with osteogenesis imperfecta tarda. A case report. *Am J Sports Med.* 1983;11(2):99–102. doi:10.1177/036354658301100210.

16. Tarsney FF. Rupture and avulsion of the triceps. *Clin Orthop Relat Res.* 1972;83:177–183.

17. Wagner JR, Cooney WP. Rupture of the triceps muscle at the musculotendinous junction: a case report. *J Hand Surg [Am].* 1997;22(2):341–343. doi:10.1016/S0363-5023(97)80175-X.

18. Downey R, Jacobson JA, Fessell DP, et al. Sonography of partial-thickness tears of the distal triceps brachii tendon. *J Ultrasound Med.* 2011;30(10):1351–1356.

19. Heikenfeld R, Listringhaus R, Godolias G. Endoscopic repair of tears of the superficial layer of the distal triceps tendon. *Arthroscopy.* 2014;30(7):785–789. doi:10.1016/j.arthro.2014.03.005.

20. Khiami F, Tavassoli S, De Ridder Baeur L, et al. Distal partial ruptures of triceps brachii tendon in an athlete. *Orthop Traumatol Surg Res.* 2012;98(2):242–246. doi:10.1016/j.otsr.2011.09.022.

21. Madsen M, Marx RG, Millett PJ, et al. Surgical anatomy of the triceps brachii tendon: anatomical study and clinical correlation. *Am J Sports Med.* 2006;34(11):1839–1843. doi:10.1177/0363546506288752.

22. Sharma S, Singh R, Goel T, et al. Missed diagnosis of triceps tendon rupture: a case report and review of literature. *J Orthop Surg (Hong Kong).* 2005;13(3):307–309. doi:10.1177/230949900501300317.

23. Duchow J, Kelm J, Kohn D. Acute ulnar nerve compression syndrome in a powerlifter with triceps tendon rupture—a case report. *Int J Sports Med.* 2000;21(4):308–310. doi:10.1055/s-2000-9468.

24. Fritz RC, Steinbach LS. Magnetic resonance imaging of the musculoskeletal system: part 3. The elbow. *Clin Orthop Relat Res.* 1996;(324):321–339.

25. Zionts LE, Vachon LA. Demonstration of avulsion of the triceps tendon in an adolescent by magnetic resonance imaging. *Am J Orthop.* 1997;26(7):489–490.

26. Dunn JC, Kusnezov N, Fares A, et al. Triceps tendon ruptures: a systematic review. *Hand (N Y).* 2017;12(5):431–438. doi:10.1177/1558944716677338.

27. Tagliafico A, Gandolfo N, Michaud J, et al. Ultrasound demonstration of distal triceps tendon tears. *Eur J Radiol.* 2012;81(6):1207–1210. doi:10.1016/j.ejrad.2011.03.012.

28. Sanchez-Sotelo J, Morrey BF, Adams RA, et al. Reconstruction of chronic ruptures of the distal biceps tendon with use of an Achilles tendon allograft. *J Bone Joint Surg Am.* 2002;84(6):999–1005.

29. Celli A. Triceps insufficiency following total elbow arthroplasty. *J Bone Joint Surg Am.* 2005;87(9):1957. doi:10.2106/JBJS.D.02423.

30. Bach BR, Warren RF, Wickiewicz TL. Triceps rupture. A case report and literature review. *Am J Sports Med.* 1987;15(3):285–289. doi:10.1177/036354658701500319.

31. Clayton ML, Thirupathi RG. Rupture of the triceps tendon with olecranon bursitis. A case report with a new method of repair. *Clin Orthop Relat Res.* 1984;(184):183–185.

32. Inhofe PD, Moneim MS. Late presentation of triceps rupture. A case report and review of the literature. *Am J Orthop.* 1996;25(11):790–792.

33. Pantazopoulos T, Exarchou E, Stavrou Z, et al. Avulsion of the triceps tendon. *J Trauma.* 1975;15(9):827–829.

34. Balazs GC, Brelin AM, Dworak TC, et al. Outcomes and complications of triceps tendon repair following acute rupture in American military personnel. *Injury.* 2016;47(10):2247–2251. doi:10.1016/j.injury.2016.07.061.

35. van Riet RP, Morrey BF, Ho E, et al. Surgical treatment of distal triceps ruptures. *J Bone Joint Surg Am.* 2003;85(10):1961–1967.

7 Proximal Biceps Injury: Open versus Arthroscopic Tenodesis

Jason J. Shin, Thierry Pauyo, and Albert Lin

INDICATIONS

Despite considerable biomechanical and clinical research, there is lack of consensus among orthopedic surgeons on the functional role of the long head of the biceps tendon (LHBT). Although some consider the LHBT to play a significant role in glenohumeral stability, others consider it to be a vestigial anatomic structure (1,2). Regardless of its function, the LHBT is richly supplied by a network of sensory and sympathetic innervation and is widely recognized as a source of shoulder pain and disability (3,4).

Proximal biceps pathology has multiple etiologies including inflammation, degeneration, overuse, trauma, and instability. Primary biceps tendinopathy is rare, and close to 95% of biceps tendinitis, tears, and degeneration are related to secondary causes. Furthermore, gross and microscopic studies have demonstrated that as part of the degenerative process, tenosynovitis can progress to cellular infiltration and fibrosis of the tendon. This cascade can also lead to scarring and adhesion development within the bicipital groove. Eventually, progression of tendinosis may result in spontaneous tendon rupture (4).

Making an accurate diagnosis of LHB tendinopathy is often challenging owing to the nearby proximity of neighboring structures in the shoulder such as the rotator cuff, superior labrum, or acromioclavicular joint, which may be potential primary pain generators. Thus, a thorough understanding of shoulder anatomy is critical to successfully diagnose and treat LHBT pathology.

The typical history of patients with proximal biceps pathology includes anterior shoulder pain that may or may not radiate to the biceps muscle. Younger, active individuals may complain of discomfort with repetitive overhead activities. In the older patient population, LHB tendinopathy is often associated with rotator cuff tears. In cases of subscapularis involvement, biceps instability with concomitant snapping may be noted.

During the physical examination, patients may have tenderness over the LHB in the intertubercular groove that moves laterally with external rotation. Additionally, the biceps can be palpated for tenderness just adjacent to the distal edge of the pectoralis major tendon. Other provocative special tests include O'Brien, Speed, and Yergason. Although clinical tests are well established, few studies have corroborated their sensitivity, reliability, or accuracy. Because physical exam findings are nonspecific for LHB pathology, a constellation of thorough history and physical exam findings is critical in making an accurate diagnosis (3).

Patients with biceps tendinitis are generally treated nonoperatively as a first-line treatment with rest, cessation of provocative activities, antiinflammatory medications and are prescribed a course of physical therapy. The structured physical therapy may also be addressed toward other pathologies present in the shoulder while focusing on range of motion, scapular kinesis, and periscapular strengthening. Little is known about the natural history of biceps tendinopathy, thus predicting an

TABLE 7-1 Indications for Biceps Tenodesis (Absolute and Relative)
More than 25% partial thickness biceps tear Tenosynovitis Any subluxation of the biceps tendon from the bicipital groove SLAP > 35 years old Failed SLAP repair Patients in which the risk of cosmetic deformity from tenotomy would be deemed unacceptable Work compensation

individual's clinical course is difficult. Consequently, there is insufficient evidence to guide the duration of nonsurgical management of LHB tendinopathy, and the length of conservative management should be individualized to each patient.

An additional nonsurgical modality includes corticosteroid injection into the bicipital groove, which can be both diagnostic and therapeutic. However, to avoid injecting the tendon itself and to improve accuracy, it is best performed under ultrasound guidance. Patients with concomitant pathology who are not surgical candidates may also benefit from glenohumeral joint and subacromial space injections.

In patients with biceps-related dysfunction who have failed conservative therapy, surgical treatment of the LHBT is recommended (Table 7-1). In appropriately indicated patients, both biceps tenotomy and tenodesis have been proven to provide symptomatic relief with high patient satisfaction (5,6). Advantages of tenotomy include technical ease of procedure, decreased surgical time, lack of implant cost, and no postoperative immobilization. However, the potential disadvantages of biceps cramping, decreased supination strength and endurance as well as cosmetic deformity, may warrant performing proximal bicep tenotomy in older sedentary patients.

CONTRAINDICATIONS

Biceps tenodesis is contraindicated in patients who are unwilling or unable to follow postoperative restrictions or rehabilitation protocols. Additional absolute contraindications to biceps tenodesis include active infection, patients who are unfit for surgery and administration of anesthetics.

PREOPERATIVE PREPARATION

A thorough history and physical examination is necessary to identify associated shoulder pathology. Often there is concomitant pathology as biceps disease in isolation is less common. It is important for the surgeon to identify and discuss treatment options with the patients of all the potential pain and dysfunction generators. This will enable the patient to make an informed decision and potentially lead to a more optimal outcome.

Plain radiographs are seldom useful in identifying LHBT tendinopathy. However, they are routinely obtained to rule out other causes of shoulder pain such as subacromial spurs, calcific tendonitis, avulsions, fractures, glenohumeral dislocation, and arthritis. Radiographs of the bicipital groove can be obtained by performing a Fisk view. This view is obtained by orienting the x-ray beam in line with the groove and along the axis of the humeral shaft and enables the evaluation of the width and medial wall angle of the sulcus and osteophytes. In our clinical practice, a Fisk view radiograph is rarely obtained.

Magnetic resonance imaging (MRI) provides valuable information concerning the LHBT as well as other structures in the shoulder. The standard MRI in multiple planes is well suited to identify inflammation, soft tissue tears as well as bicep subluxation (Fig. 7-1). The addition of intraarticular contrast is helpful when evaluating for labral pathology. When labral pathology is suspected, we routinely obtain magnetic resonance arthrogram.

SURGICAL TECHNIQUE

Anesthesia

Preoperatively, after discussing with the anesthesiologist and the surgeon, the patient may elect to have an ultrasound-guided interscalene nerve block. The surgery is then performed under sedation or general anesthesia. Depending on surgeon preference, the patient is positioned in a beach chair or lateral decubitus position with all susceptible neurovascular structures and bony prominences well protected.

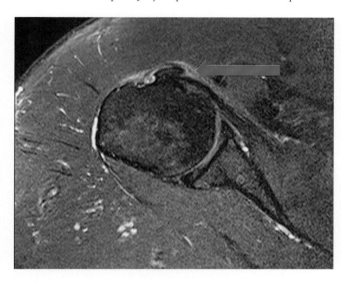

FIGURE 7-1

T2 axial shoulder MRI demonstrating long head of the biceps tendon that is dislocated medially out of the groove lying between the superficial and deep layers of subscapularis (*red arrow*).

After a surgical time-out, every case starts with examination of the shoulders under anesthesia. The patient is prepped and draped in a sterile fashion and after marking the anatomic landmarks of the shoulder, a posterior viewing portal is established. After introducing the arthroscope into the glenohumeral joint, an anterior working portal is established with a cannula through the rotator interval. When planning to perform an arthroscopic tenodesis, establishing the anterior portal more laterally is recommended as the patient's head can interfere with anchor insertion. A systematic diagnostic arthroscopy is then carried out to assess the capsule, rotator cuff, and articular cartilage. Because only a portion of the LHB tendon is visualized within the joint, a probe should be utilized to pull the biceps tendon into the joint to visualize the distal component. Additionally, the labrum is palpated to assess for potential tears. Certain biceps pathologies may be more suitable for an intraarticular arthroscopic tenodesis such as biceps dislocations and chronic tenosynovitis that have minimal tearing or deneageration within the intraarticular portion. Significant tearing or degeneration of the intraarticular biceps may be more appropriate for a more distal technique such as an arthroscopic-assisted subpectoral tenodesis.

All Arthroscopic Intraarticular Biceps Tenodesis

After the decision is made to proceed with an arthroscopic tenodesis, while viewing from the posterior portal, a radiofrequency device is brought into the joint through the anterior portal and is used to clear the soft tissue from the intraarticular portion of the bicipital groove. To assist with visualizing the biceps groove, the shoulder can be positioned in 30 degrees of forward elevation from the plane of the patient's body while a manual posterior translation is applied to the humeral head externally. A 70-degree arthroscope can also be used to improve visualization of the bicipital groove. An arthroscopic bur is then used to gently abrade the cortex to a bleeding surface in preparation for the tenodesis.

A closed loop end suture (FiberSnare; Arthrex, Naples, FL) is first introduced into the joint through the anterior portal and passed under or over the tendon. A retriever is then used to retrieve the looped end of the suture around the tendon. The free end is then passed through the loop end as a cinch knot around the tendon. The free end of the suture is then loaded into a self-retrieving shoulder suture passer (Scorpion; Arthrex, Naples, FL). The suture is penetrated through the center point on the biceps tendon with a racking type stitch to gain control of the tendon. (Fig. 7-2A and B). Using arthroscopic scissors, the tendon is cut at its origin near the labral insertion. The remaining biceps stump can be debrided with a shaver or radiofrequency device down to a stable, smooth edge on the superior labrum. The suture is then preloaded onto the islet of abiocomposite, fully threaded, knotless anchor (Bio-SwiveLock 4.75 mm; Arthrex, Naples, FL). At the projected site of tenodesis—along the articular margin of the humerus at the superior aspect of the groove—a bone socket is prepared with an awl. After tensioning the suture, the anchor and the tendon are fixed into the humerus (Fig. 7-3A and B). The suture limbs are cut, and the remaining limb of the biceps is cut flush against the tenodesis site.

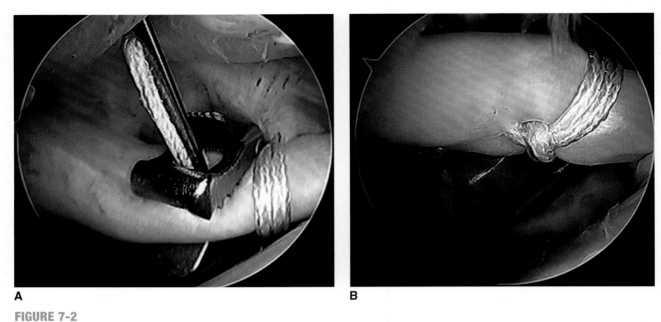

FIGURE 7-2

A: Suture is penetrated through the tendon. **B:** Control of the tendon is achieved prior to releasing it from the superior labral attachment.

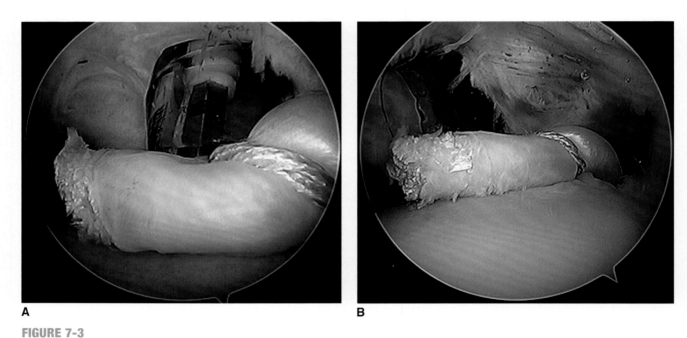

FIGURE 7-3

A: The tendon is tenodesed at the top of the biceps groove using an anchor fixation. **B:** Completed tenodesis after cutting the suture.

Open Subpectoral Biceps Tenodesis

An alternative to arthroscopic biceps tenodesis is the open subpectoral technique, which has been the focus of recent studies. Proponents of the subpectoral technique state that bicipital groove pain is better addressed by removing the tendon from its groove. Like the arthroscopic technique, the procedure starts with a complete diagnostic arthroscopy, and the biceps is released arthroscopically at its origin, on the superior glenoid. After concomitant pathologies are addressed, arthroscopic instruments are removed and attention is turned to the open portion of the procedure.

The arm is positioned in 90 degrees of abduction and 90 degrees of external rotation. Approximately, a 2 to 3 cm longitudinal skin incision is made in the axilla, centered over the inferior border of the pectoralis major tendon. Hemostasis is achieved with electrocautery. Dissection is carried out to the level of the fascia overlying the pectoralis major. The inferior portion of the pectoralis muscle tendon is identified, and the fascia is incised on the inferior border in a proximal and distal fashion in line with the muscle fibers (Fig. 7-4A). A Hohmann retractor is placed along the lateral border of the humerus to retract the pectoralis tendon superolaterally, and the arthroscopically tenotomized biceps tendon comes into view (Fig. 7-4B and C). The diseased tendon is retrieved from the wound.

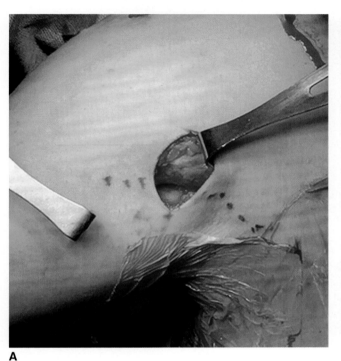

A

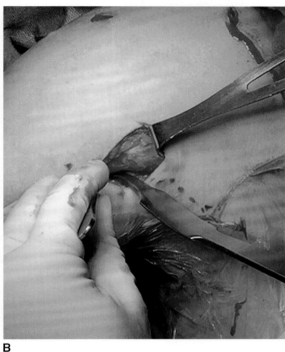

B

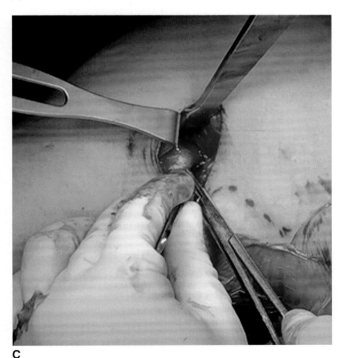

C

FIGURE 7-4

A: Inferior border of the pectoralis major tendon is visualized. **B:** Hohmann retraction is inserted to retract the pectoralis tendon superolaterally. **C:** The long head of the biceps tendon is retrieved border.

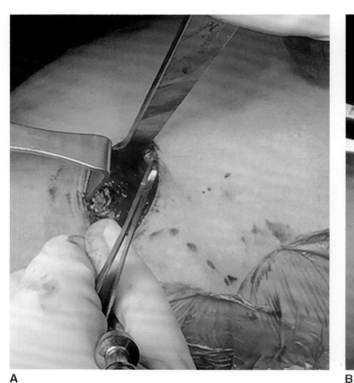 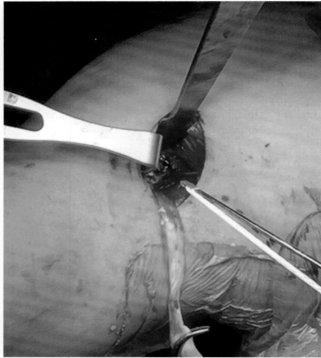

A   **B**

FIGURE 7-5

A: Biceps tenodesis site is visualized and marked with electrocautery. **B:** A unicortical button loaded with two sutures is being docked into the hole in the humerus.

The inferior aspect of the bicipital groove is marked with electrocautery (Fig. 7-5A), and the cortical bed is prepared with an osteotome to initiate healing. A 3.2-mm unicortical hole is drilled perpendicularly through the anterior cortex. Aunicortical button (Proximal Biceps Tenodesis Button; Arthrex, Naples, FL), preloaded with two sutures, is positioned into the hole and is deployed by a flipping mechanism (Fig. 7-5B). A piercing suture grasper is used to pass through the tendon (1 cm from the muculotendinous junction) on one side of the tendon, and a single limb of suture is partly pulled through (Fig. 7-6A). A loop is created and the end of the suture, at the same side used to make the loop, is passed through the loop, thereby creating a lasso-loop stitch (Fig. 7-6B) (7). The opposite limb of the same suture is then passed through the tendon slightly proximal in simple fashion on the same side of the tendon. The steps are repeated on the other side of the tendon using the other suture, ending up with four suture limbs that have been passed through the tendon (Fig. 7-6C). By pulling on the sliding limb of each suture, the lasso-loop stitch is brought down onto the humerus with a docking technique (Fig. 7-7A). The sutures limbs are tied and the excess tendon is removed to complete the procedure (Fig. 7-7B).

After thoroughly irrigating the wound with copious normal saline, the wound is closed in layers. The subcutaneous tissue is closed using an absorbable 2-0 suture and subcuticular layer with an absorbable 4-0 suture.

PEARLS AND PITFALLS

- It is important to have a thorough discussion with the patient regarding goals and expectation of surgery, as well as postoperative restrictions. The patient may present with preconceived notions and/or specific preference for biceps management, whether tenotomy versus tenodesis (open or arthroscopic).
- During diagnostic arthroscopy, it is critical to pull the intertubercular portion of the biceps tendon into the joint to look for distal inflammation, which may not otherwise be visualized.
- Fluid management (pump pressure) during concomitant procedure (i.e., rotator cuff repair, sub-acromial decompression) can limit soft tissue extravasation, which will make dissection easier when performing open subpectoral biceps tenodesis.

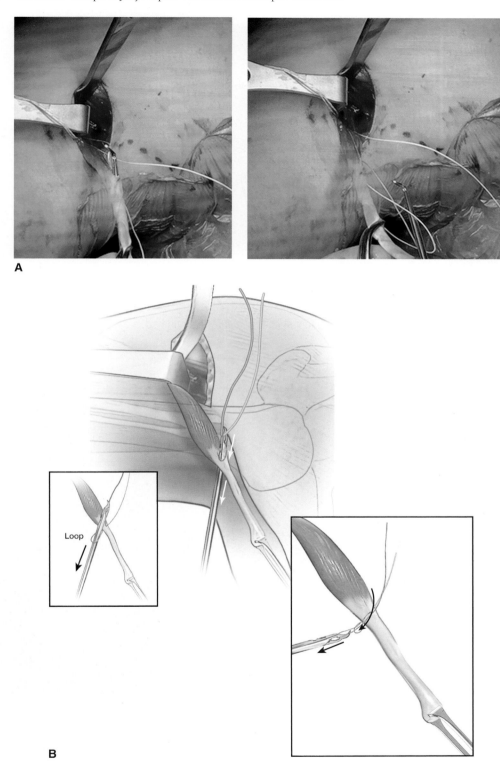

FIGURE 7-6

A: A piercing suture grasper is passed through the tendon. **B:** Lasso-loop stitch is created.

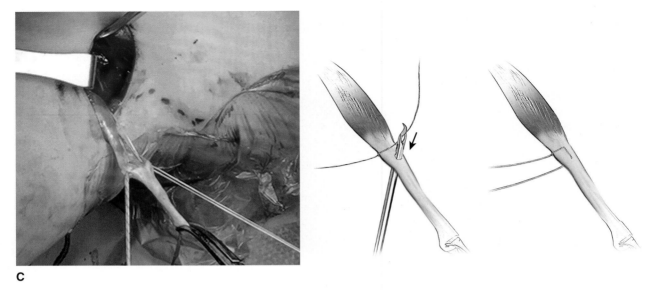

C

FIGURE 7-6 (*Continued*)
C: Lasso-loop is created on the opposite side of the tendon, and four strands of sutures are retrieved.

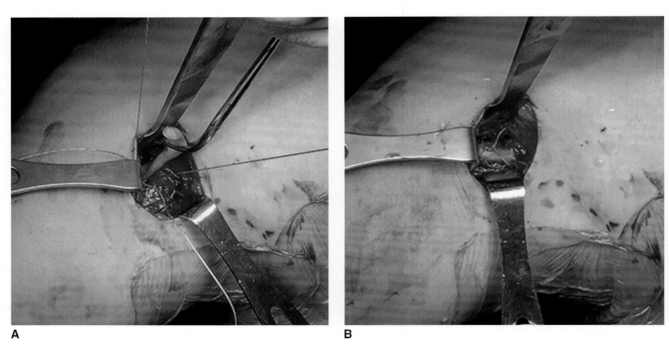

A   **B**

FIGURE 7-7
A: Tendon is brought down to bone by pulling on the sliding limb of each suture. **B:** Completed tenodesis after tying and cutting the sutures.

- Appropriate tensioning of the tendon during fixation to the humerus will avoid distal retraction and popeye deformity.
- During open subpectoral biceps tenodesis, staying inferior to the pectoral fascia and not going through inferior muscle fibers with lateral retractors will create an avascular plane.
- During open subpectoral biceps tenodesis, avoid placing medial retractors on the humerus to prevent neurovascular injuries.

POSTOPERATIVE MANAGEMENT

Given that patients often have associated shoulder pathologies and additional procedures performed, rehabilitation is often dictated by concomitant surgery, including rotator cuff repair. Total sling immobilization for isolated tenodesis is typically 3 weeks. Pendulums may begin at the first postoperative visit in 10 days. Early passive range-of-motion exercises of the hand, wrist, elbow, and shoulder are permitted at 3 weeks after sling removal, but active shoulder and elbow motion is limited until 6 weeks postoperative to protect the tenodesis. Stiffness is uncommon following biceps tenodesis (unlike SLAP repair in older patients and open rotator cuff surgery). After 6 weeks, active ROM is started and low-resistance strengthening is initiated at 8 weeks. Formal therapy is not typically necessary after 3 months postoperative, and patients can continue to work on strengthening and motion with a home exercise program. Return to full, unrestricted activities can occur as early as 3 months postoperatively.

COMPLICATIONS

Overall, complications of biceps tenodesis are rare. One study of 353 patients reported a 2.0% complication rate following open subpectoral biceps tenodesis (8). One patient in that study developed musculocutaneous neuropathy. By using careful technique as well as having in-depth knowledge of the shoulder anatomy, brachial plexus injuries can be avoided. During open subpectoral biceps tenodesis, Dickens et al. demonstrated that musculocutaneous, radial nerve, and deep brachial artery are within 1 cm of a medial retractor (9). Sharp medial retractors should not be utilized to avoid neurovascular injuries.

There have been case reports of humeral fracture after subpectoral biceps tenodesis. One case involved a middle-age patient who suffered a spiral humerus fracture after returning to pitching at 10 months after surgery (10). In two other reported cases of low mechanism injury, one involved a fall at 6 months and another occurred while picking up a bag 4 months postoperatively (11). In all three of these cases, patients had biceps tenodesis secured with an 8-mm diameter interference screws. Biomechanical studies have demonstrated that eccentric positioning of screws can decrease the torsional strength of the humerus (12). By placing smaller, concentrically placed holes, surgeons can minimize disrupting the structural integrity of the humerus.

Persistent pain and refractory tenosynovitis have been described following intraarticular, arthroscopic tenodesis. Advocates of open subpectoral tenodesis state that the quality of remaining tendon in the bicipital groove can significantly affect the success of the procedure (4). However, true biceps-related complications after arthroscopic tenodesis are rare. One study of 1,083 patients treated with arthroscopic proximal biceps tenodesis at the articular margin of the humeral head reported a revision rate of 0.4% for biceps-related issues (13). Moreover, in the same study, there were no reported incidences of infection, fracture or neurovascular injuries. In rare situations where patients have persistent symptoms of groove pain after arthroscopic tenodesis, open subpectoral technique is a viable revision option.

Other described complications include failure of the tenodesis to heal as well as attritional rupture at the bone-tendon interface, which can result in distal tendon retraction. In such cases, the patient may present with cosmetic deformity. However, most studies demonstrate that patient reported that outcomes and functional results of biceps tenotomy and tenodesis are comparable (5,6,14).

RESULTS

Interpreting comparative outcome studies can be challenging due to lack of homogeneous patient population, and typically biceps tenodesis is often only one component of multiple pathologies that are surgically treated simultaneously in the shoulder. Additionally, the surgical techniques and implants utilized vary between studies, which make direct comparison even more challenging. Nevertheless, satisfactory results have been consistently reported regardless of surgical approach and fixation technique (13,15,16).

In a comparative study of open versus arthroscopic biceps tenodesis, which included 82 patients, Werner et al. (16) reported excellent clinical and functional results in both groups. Between the two tenodesis methods, no differences were noted at a minimum 2 years postoperatively with respect to validated outcome measures, range of motion and strength (16). In another study comparing open and arthroscopic tenodesis, Duchman et al. (15) reported no difference in biceps apex difference or strength at minimum 1-year follow-up. The authors reported a single clinical failure that identified at 9 weeks postoperatively in a patient who underwent arthroscopic tenodesis, leading to an overall failure rate of 2.2% (15). Interestingly, although not statistically significant, bicipital groove tenderness was present in 20.0% and 10.0% of patients after undergoing open and arthroscopic tenodesis, respectively.

In a recent systematic review of 16 studies that included 476 patients, 98% had good to excellent outcome. Three failures of fixation were noted following arthroscopic tenodesis and two failures after open tenodesis. The authors did not identify any differences in outcome or complications between the two approaches (17).

Given the overall, consistently good to excellent clinical results with few complications, the approach to LHB tenodesis can be dictated by concomitant pathology, including rotator cuff or labral pathology. Ultimately, the choice of technique is at the discretion of the surgeon.

REFERENCES

1. Rodosky MW, Harner CD, Fu FH. The role of the long head of the biceps muscle and superior glenoid labrum in anterior stability of the shoulder. *Am J Sports Med.* 1994;22(1):121–130.
2. Yamaguchi K, Riew KD, Galatz LM, et al. Biceps activity during shoulder motion: an electromyographic analysis. *Clin Orthop.* 1997;(336):122–129.
3. Nho SJ, Strauss EJ, Lenart BA, et al. Long head of the biceps tendinopathy: diagnosis and management. *J Am Acad Orthop Surg.* 2010;18(11):645–656.
4. Mellano CR, Shin JJ, Yanke AB, et al. Disorders of the long head of the biceps tendon. *Instr Course Lect.* 2015;64:567–576.
5. Friedman JL, FitzPatrick JL, Rylander LS, et al. Biceps tenotomy versus tenodesis in active patients younger than 55 years: is there a difference in strength and outcomes? *Orthop J Sports Med.* 2015;3(2):2325967115570848.
6. Lee H-J, Jeong J-Y, Kim C-K, et al. Surgical treatment of lesions of the long head of the biceps brachii tendon with rotator cuff tear: a prospective randomized clinical trial comparing the clinical results of tenotomy and tenodesis. *J Shoulder Elbow Surg.* 2016;25(7):1107–1114.
7. Lafosse L, Van Raebroeckx A, Brzoska R. A new technique to improve tissue grip: "the lasso-loop stitch". *Arthroscopy.* 2006;22(11):1246.e1–1246.e3.
8. Nho SJ, Reiff SN, Verma NN, et al. Complications associated with subpectoral biceps tenodesis: low rates of incidence following surgery. *J Shoulder Elbow Surg.* 2010;19(5):764–768.
9. Dickens JF, Kilcoyne KG, Tintle SM, et al. Subpectoral biceps tenodesis: an anatomic study and evaluation of at-risk structures. *Am J Sports Med.* 2012;40(10):2337–2341.
10. Dein EJ, Huri G, Gordon JC, et al. A humerus fracture in a baseball pitcher after biceps tenodesis. *Am J Sports Med.* 2014;42(4):877–879.
11. Sears BW, Spencer EE, Getz CL. Humeral fracture following subpectoral biceps tenodesis in 2 active, healthy patients. *J Shoulder Elbow Surg.* 2011;20(6):e7–e11.
12. Euler SA, Smith SD, Williams BT, et al. Biomechanical analysis of subpectoral biceps tenodesis: effect of screw malpositioning on proximal humeral strength. *Am J Sports Med.* 2015;43(1):69–74.
13. Brady PC, Narbona P, Adams CR, et al. Arthroscopic proximal biceps tenodesis at the articular margin: evaluation of outcomes, complications, and revision rate. *Arthroscopy.* 2015;31(3):470–476.
14. Koh KH, Ahn JH, Kim SM, et al. Treatment of biceps tendon lesions in the setting of rotator cuff tears: prospective cohort study of tenotomy versus tenodesis. *Am J Sports Med.* 2010;38(8):1584–1590.
15. Duchman KR, DeMik DE, Uribe B, et al. Open versus arthroscopic biceps tenodesis: a comparison of functional outcomes. *Iowa Orthop J.* 2016;36:79–87.
16. Werner BC, Evans CL, Holzgrefe RE, et al. Arthroscopic suprapectoral and open subpectoral biceps tenodesis: a comparison of minimum 2-year clinical outcomes. *Am J Sports Med.* 2014;42(11):2583–2590.
17. Abraham VT, Tan BHM, Kumar VP. Systematic review of biceps tenodesis: arthroscopic versus open. *Arthroscopy.* 2016;32(2):365–371.

8 Internal Impingement/ SLAP Lesions

Frank B. Wydra, Robin H. Dunn, and Armando F. Vidal

INTRODUCTION

Since Walch first described the phenomenon of internal impingement of the shoulder in 1992, there has been increasing interest in the topic and in the spectrum of associated pathology. Shoulder problems in overhead athletes have been recognized for decades, especially in baseball pitchers. The physician's understanding of the condition has evolved significantly in recent years. Although the underlying cause of internal impingement remains a topic of debate, the resultant spectrum of shoulder pathology has been well characterized. This includes posterior labral tears, superior labrum anterior-to-posterior (SLAP) tears, posterior glenoid erosion, greater tuberosity cysts, and partial-thickness rotator cuff tears. There is now documentation in the literature of this spectrum of pathology in the general population, not just overhead athletes (1,2). This recognition makes the diagnosis and treatment of internal impingement all the more relevant for the orthopedic surgeon.

PATHOPHYSIOLOGY/PATHOLOGY

The underlying pathophysiology that initiates the cascade leading to the constellation of shoulder pathology seen at arthroscopy in patients with internal impingement remains controversial. Two conflicting theories exist. Are these shoulders too tight or too loose? There are multiple studies to support both theories (3–14). It is plausible that both theories are valid and can lead to posterior-superior shoulder pathology. Understanding these two theories is important in treating patients with internal impingement.

Microinstability

Jobe and colleagues have described anterior instability in the overhead athlete (7–9,12). They note that there is often a continuum of instability in the throwing athlete and that it may present as occult or subtle. These authors have documented that rotator cuff injury in throwers results from increased glenohumeral motion that arises from instability (12). A subtle increase in motion can result in impingement of the rotator cuff between the greater tuberosity and the posterosuperior glenoid, leading to the pathology seen in internal impingement. The degree and chronicity of the instability and impingement will affect the severity of injury. This is often related to the age of the athlete and how long they have been throwing or participating in overhead athletics.

Both static and dynamic stabilizers are responsible for the stability of the shoulder. Secondary or dynamic stabilizers may be fatigued with repetitive throwing or overhead motions (e.g., the serving motion in tennis and volleyball). The static stabilizers may be stretched or disrupted with a single traumatic event or, more often, through microtraumatic events associated with overhead sports. Davidson et al. noted that increases in glenohumeral motion can arise from stretching of the inferior glenohumeral ligament (IGHL) complex or labral tearing (15).

In support of the instability theory, Jobe et al. reported high rates of return to competitive play in throwers who were treated with anterior capsular labral reconstruction (7). Levitz et al. also reported favorable results when capsular laxity in throwers was addressed at time of arthroscopy (11). In their study, patients were divided into two groups based on treatment. The first group of baseball throwers underwent débridement and/or repair of labral and rotator cuff tears. The second group underwent this same treatment plus thermal capsulorrhaphy. At 30 months after surgery, 90% of the thermal capsulorrhaphy group was back to competition compared to 67% of the débridement/repair-only group.

Glenohumeral Internal Rotation Deficit

Burkhart et al. have popularized the concept of an internal rotation deficit as a cause of the pathology seen with internal impingement (4,5). They propose that internal impingement is a natural phenomenon in all shoulders during abduction and external rotation, a concept that has been supported by Walch et al. (1) and Halbrecht et al. (6). According to this theory, it is a tightening of the posteroinferior capsule that leads to the changes seen in the posterosuperior shoulder of overhead athletes. This contracture secondarily leads to hyperexternal rotation in abduction (5).

The definition of glenohumeral internal rotation deficit (GIRD) is the loss of internal rotation when comparing the symptomatic shoulder to the contralateral shoulder. It is measured with the shoulder in 90 degrees of abduction (Fig. 8-1). The IGHL complex functions as a hammock to stabilize the shoulder in abduction. It is composed of the posterior inferior glenohumeral ligament (PIGHL) and the anterior inferior glenohumeral ligament (AIGHL), which act as interdependent cables. Contracture of the PIGHL can shift the center of rotation of the glenohumeral joint posterosuperiorly with the shoulder in abduction. This allows increased external rotation as the greater tuberosity can now rotate further before contacting the posterior glenoid (Fig. 8-2). This posterosuperior

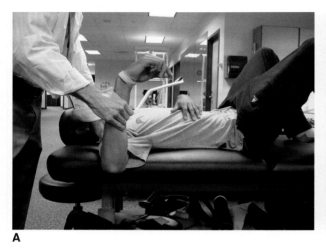
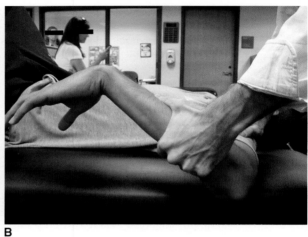

A   **B**

FIGURE 8-1

Severe GIRD in a collegiate tennis player. **A:** 0-degree internal rotation dominant shoulder. **B:** 60-degree internal rotation nondominant shoulder.

FIGURE 8-2

Reciprocal cable model of the IGHL complex. When the posterior cable shortens (contracted posterior band), the glenohumeral contact point shifts posterosuperiorly and the allowable arc of external rotation (before the greater tuberosity contacts the posterior glenoid) significantly increases (*dotted lines*). (Reprinted from Burkhart SS, Morgan CD, Kibler WB. The disabled throwing shoulder: spectrum of pathology Part I: pathoanatomy and biomechanics. *Arthroscopy.* 2003;19(4):404–420.)

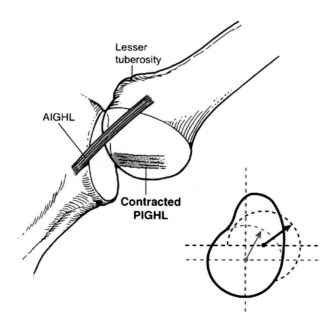

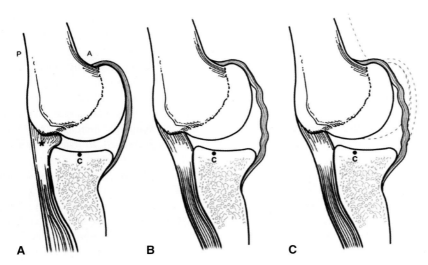

FIGURE 8-3

A: With the arm in a position of abduction and external rotation, the humeral head and the proximal humeral calcar produce a significant cam effect of the anteroinferior capsule, tensioning the capsule by virtue of the space-occupying effect. **B:** With the posterosuperior shift of the glenohumeral contact point, the space-occupying effect of the proximal humerus on the anteroinferior capsule is reduced (reduction of the cam effect). This creates a relative redundancy in the anteroinferior capsule that has probably been misinterpreted in the past as microinstability. **C:** Superimposed neutral position (*dotted line*) shows the magnitude of the capsular redundancy that occurs as a result of the shift in the glenohumeral contact point. (Reprinted from Burkhart SS, Morgan CD, Kibler WB. The disabled throwing shoulder: spectrum of pathology Part I: pathoanatomy and biomechanics. *Arthroscopy.* 2003;19(4):404–420. Copyright © 2003 Arthroscopy Association of North America, with permission.)

shift in the contact point and greater tuberosity clearance leads to a decrease in the CAM effect of the proximal humeral calcar (Fig. 8-3), which decreases tension on the anterior capsule and causes capsular redundancy. Burkhart et al. believe that this redundancy can be misinterpreted as anterior instability (5). A shoulder that abducts and excessively externally rotates is prone to overuse injury. The biceps anchor and posterosuperior labrum can fail due to shear forces via the "peel-back" mechanism. The posterosuperior rotator cuff sees both increased shear and torsional stresses, which can lead to failure of the undersurface fibers. Thus, with time, the thrower with GIRD can develop the pathologic changes seen with internal impingement.

Recent biomechanical studies by Mihata et al. have supported to the role that GIRD plays in causing the pathologic changes seen in shoulders with internal impingement (13,14). Using cadaveric shoulders, they demonstrated that both posteroinferior capsular plication and anterior capsular attenuation significantly increase contact pressures in the posterosuperior glenohumeral joint, shifting the humeral head posteriorly and increasing impingement on the supraspinatus and infraspinatus.

PREOPERATIVE PREPARATION

Physical Exam

Patients with internal impingement can have a variety of findings on physical exam. A thorough shoulder exam with comparison to the uninvolved shoulder is very important. Evaluation of range of motion, rotator cuff strength, palpation, impingement maneuvers, scapular mechanics, stability, and biceps anchor or SLAP stress tests are all part of the exam. Exam findings will vary with length and severity of symptoms.

Internal impingement may mimic subacromial impingement insofar as overhead athletes with chronic impingement frequently experience pain with external impingement maneuvers. Differentiating internal from subacromial impingement is difficult but important because outcomes from subacromial decompression in overhead athletes have historically been poor (16). In 2001, Zaslav et al. described a maneuver to differentiate internal impingement from subacromial impingement in patients with a positive Neer impingement test (17). In the internal rotation resistance strength test (IRRST), the examiner tests the patient's strength in both internal and external rotation with the shoulder abducted to 90 degrees. A significant deficit of internal compared to external rotation of the affected shoulder had sensitivity of 88%, specificity of 96%, positive predictive value of 88%, and negative predictive value of 96% in a cohort of 110 patients tested.

Overhead athletes, especially throwers, develop specific adaptations in range of motion. As mentioned previously, GIRD has been associated with internal impingement (4,5,18). Forward flexion and abduction are often normal or near normal. Rotation should be assessed with the shoulder in adduction and in 90 degrees of abduction and should be compared with the contralateral side. In abduction, these patients—especially baseball pitchers—often have substantially increased external rotation. Simultaneously, internal rotation in abduction is significantly decreased. In many instances, the loss of internal rotation is greater than the gain in external rotation. It is important to compare motion to the uninvolved shoulder. A 20-degree difference in total arc of motion associated with a >20-degree loss of internal rotation between shoulders (20 degrees of GIRD) is considered pathologic (5).

Evaluation of scapular mechanics is essential for any patient with shoulder pain, especially the overhead athlete. Burkhart et al. have described the SICK scapula syndrome (*S*capular malposition, *I*nferior medial border prominence, *C*oracoid pain and malposition, and dys*K*inesis of scapular movement) and its relation to shoulder dysfunction (19). Excessive scapular protraction, evidenced by prominent medial or inferomedial scapular border on exam, increases glenohumeral angulation, posterior compression, and the peel-back effect. Restoring proper scapular mechanics is one of the primary goals in rehabilitation of the overhead athlete.

Assessing shoulder stability is a key component of the exam, and many of the provocative maneuvers for internal impingement are variations on tests for glenohumeral instability. These patients usually do not have gross instability on exam. Instead, they experience pain. With the patient supine, the apprehension, relocation, and load-and-shift tests can all be performed. The apprehension test is considered positive for internal impingement if it elicits pain rather than apprehension. The relocation test, first described by Jobe et al., is positive if the patient experiences posterior shoulder pain when placed in an abducted and maximally externally rotated position followed by relief with posteriorly directed force on the shoulder (2,15). Of note, the pain is different from the feeling of apprehension and anterior shoulder pain in patients with anterior instability.

Rotator cuff strength is usually normal but may be decreased or painful with inflammation or high-grade partial-thickness tears. Patients sometimes have posterior joint line or bicipital tenderness with palpation. SLAP or biceps anchor provocative tests, including the Active Compression (O'Brien) test, the Biceps Load II test, the Dynamic Labral Shear (O'Driscoll) test, and Speed test, may also elicit pain. There is significant controversy regarding the utility of many of the physical exam maneuvers to detect SLAP tears (20). However, given the high frequency of superior labral pathology in this population, some combination of tests to load the biceps and superior labrum is warranted.

Imaging

The radiographic evaluation of suspected internal impingement begins with standard plain radiographic views of the shoulder, including AP, axillary, and scapular Y views. In addition, West Point and Stryker notch views can be helpful. There are four radiographic findings that have been associated with internal impingement. These include the following:

1. Exostosis from the posteroinferior glenoid (Bennett lesion),
2. Sclerotic changes of the greater tuberosity,
3. Posterior humeral head osteochondral lesions, and
4. Rounding of the posterior glenoid rim (21).

Although these findings can be seen especially in patients with long-standing internal impingement, it is important to note that plain radiographs are often unremarkable.

Magnetic resonance imaging (MRI) is central in evaluating shoulder pain in overhead athletes. Standard coronal, sagittal, and axial cuts can be supplemented with coronal and sagittal oblique reformats to fully assess the rotator cuff (22). Previously, many authors would have recommended using magnetic resonance arthrography to evaluate suspected labral pathology (23–29). This has recently evolved, as the image quality obtained with more powerful MRI scanners (3 Tesla) shows remarkable detail without the need for arthrography. In addition to standard positioning, it can be helpful to obtain MRI scanning with the shoulder in an abducted and externally rotated (ABER) position (30,31). This puts the shoulder in the position that recreates the impingement and approximates the sites of pathology, including the undersurface of the supraspinatus and infraspinatus, the humeral head, and the posterosuperior labrum.

MRI findings in patients with internal impingement are very similar to those seen during arthroscopy. These include the following:

- Labral tears, including SLAP lesions and posterior lesions;
- Partial-thickness, articular-sided rotator cuff tears of the supraspinatus, and anterior portion of the infraspinatus;
- Thickened posterior IGHL;
- Cystic changes in the posterosuperior portion of the humeral head;
- Bennett lesions; and
- Posterosuperior glenoid erosion (22).

Internal impingement in the ABER position is not necessarily pathologic, and when pathologic findings exist, they can be asymptomatic. For instance, Halbrecht et al. performed MRI on both shoulders in 10 asymptomatic collegiate baseball players in the ABER position. They noted contact between the rotator cuff and posterosuperior glenoid in all shoulders, which they concluded is a normal occurrence in all shoulders placed in that position (6). However, there were pathologic findings that were found exclusively in the throwing shoulders, including rotator cuff tendinosis, labral tears, and paralabral cysts. Other authors have also documented such pathologic findings on MRI in asymptomatic overhead athletes (32,33). The surgeon must be cautious to correlate findings on history and physical exam with pathology found on radiographic studies.

INDICATIONS

Patients presenting with internal impingement must be evaluated on a case-by-case basis. As with the majority of overuse injuries, the initial approach to the patient with internal impingement should be conservative. Rest, ice, and a short course of oral nonsteroidal anti-inflammatory medication can all be beneficial in internal impingement. Physical therapy should focus on both stretching and strengthening. Sleeper stretches (Fig. 8-4) and cross-chest adduction stretches have been shown to improve the GIRD by stretching the posterior capsule. Tyler et al. reported that, after a 7-week program of internal rotation and posterior capsule stretches, patients with symptomatic internal impingement experienced significant symptom improvement and gained an average of 26 degrees of internal rotation (GIRD improved from 35 to 9 degrees) (34). Strengthening exercises should focus on the rotator cuff and periscapular musculature. Burkhart et al. reported a 100% return to sport rate with a scapular exercise program in athletes with SICK scapula syndrome (19).

If an extensive trial of nonoperative treatment, including physical therapy, fails to relieve symptoms or allow return to play, then surgical intervention may be considered. Since several authors

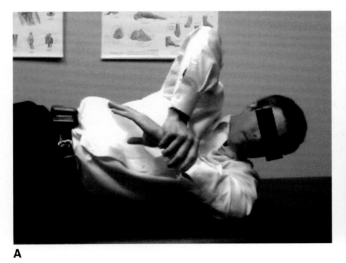
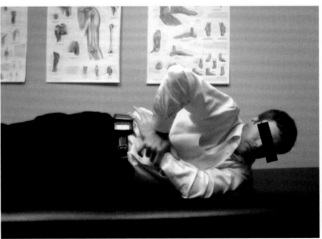

A   **B**

FIGURE 8-4

Dedicated posterior inferior capsular stretches. **A:** Sleeper stretch. **B:** Rollover sleeper stretch.

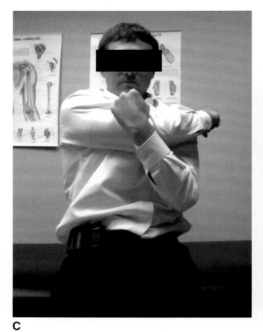

C

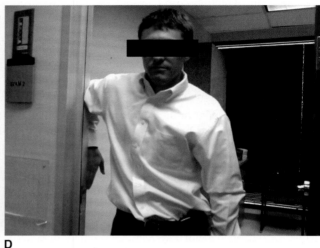

D

FIGURE 8-4 (*Continued*)

C: Cross-arm stretch. **D:** Doorway stretch.

have documented pathologic findings in asymptomatic individuals (6), and because of the variety of pathology seen in internal impingement, the surgeon must carefully correlate the patient's symptoms, physical exam, and imaging findings in order to address the true pathology with surgery.

CONTRAINDICATIONS

Patients need to exhaust a comprehensive physical therapy regimen before being considered for surgery. General contraindications to arthroscopic procedures include active infection, or significant patient medical comorbidities should preclude such patients. Concomitant pathology such as arthritis may preclude some patients from such surgeries as successful outcomes are diminished.

TECHNIQUE

Key components of this procedure are the examination under anesthesia (EUA) and the diagnostic arthroscopy. It is important to perform a thorough EUA and to compare findings to the uninvolved shoulder. Particular attention should focus on range of motion, especially GIRD, and instability, including the presence of a sulcus sign.

A thorough diagnostic arthroscopy should be performed on every patient undergoing surgery for internal impingement. Many of these patients have concomitant pathology, and all sites of injury must be identified at arthroscopy. Particular attention should be paid to the articular surface of the rotator cuff, posterosuperior glenoid and labrum, anterior capsulolabral complex, and the humeral head. The surgeon should also examine the subacromial space looking for bursitis. If significant bursitis is present, then simple bursectomy without acromioplasty is warranted. Many authors have documented the poor return to play results with acromioplasty in athletes (16).

Rotator Cuff

Rotator cuff pathology is probably the most common finding in internal impingement. Most often, the site of pathology is the articular surface of the posterior supraspinatus and anterior infraspinatus—the sites of impingement between the greater tuberosity and the posterosuperior glenoid. Fraying or partial tears can be seen at the musculotendinous junction or at the insertion of the rotator cuff on the greater tuberosity. Tears at the musculotendinous junction are almost always minor and respond well to débridement alone. Tears at the rotator cuff footprint are seen more often in the older overhead athlete as chronic internal impingement varies widely in severity. For partial-thickness tears, simple débridement is preferred in the high-level thrower. For very high-grade partial tears and full-thickness tears, repair should be considered with caution.

High-grade partial tears can be repaired with either a PASTA (partial articular-sided tendon avulsion) repair technique, which involves repairing the tear with anchors and suture through the rotator cuff while preserving the insertion site, or completion of the tear and standard arthroscopic repair.

It should be noted that results for return to play in overhead athletes undergoing rotator cuff repair are generally poor (35). This may be due to the age of the patient and the severity of the injury. The results of débridement alone for partial-thickness rotator cuff tears are more favorable, but these may represent less significant injuries (36,37). When appropriate, rotator cuff débridement should be favored over repair in high-level overhead athletes.

PASTA Technique

In the PASTA repair technique, suture anchors are placed transtendinous. Standard anterior and posterior portals are made. A thorough diagnostic arthroscopy is performed, and the degree of pathology is determined. A subacromial bursectomy is then performed prior to suture anchor placement in order to visualize and prevent damage to sutures later in the procedure. After bursectomy, a working cannula is placed in the lateral portal in the subacromial space for later suture retrieval and knot tying. Next, the arthroscope is returned to the glenohumeral joint via the posterior portal. Working with a shaver through the anterior portal, the exposed portion of the greater tuberosity footprint is débrided to a bleeding bed (Fig. 8-5). Anchors (usually only one or two double-loaded anchors are needed) are then placed through the tendon into the footprint on the humeral head (Fig. 8-6A). More recently, we've been using a Swivelock (Arthrex, Naples, FL) anchor loaded with

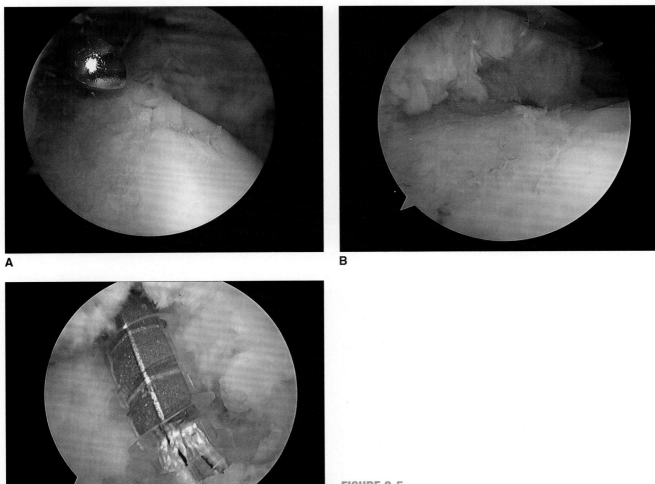

A

B

C

FIGURE 8-5

PASTA repair. **A:** Preparation of footprint. **B:** Footprint débrided down to bleeding bed. **C:** Transtendinous placement of suture anchor in footprint.

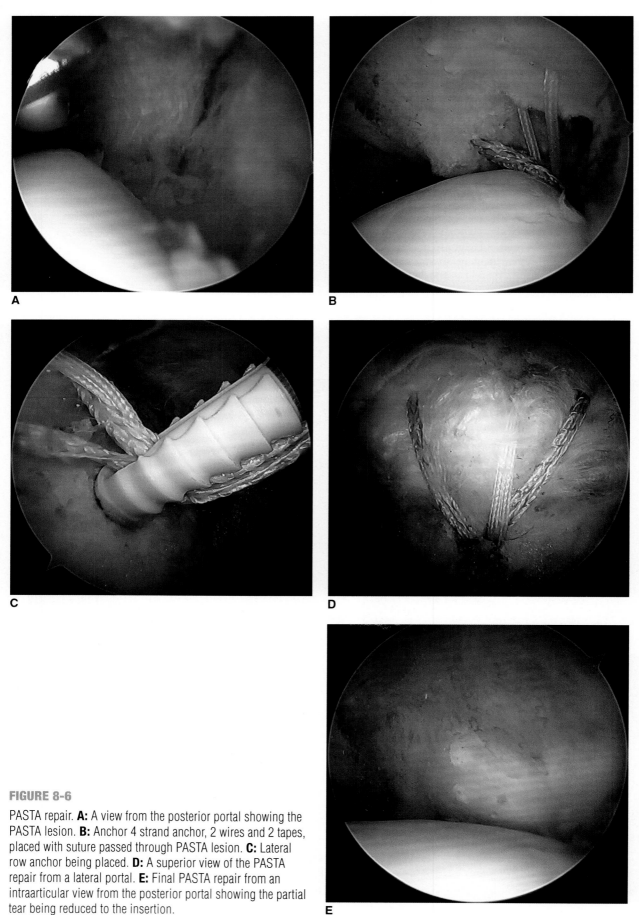

FIGURE 8-6

PASTA repair. **A:** A view from the posterior portal showing the PASTA lesion. **B:** Anchor 4 strand anchor, 2 wires and 2 tapes, placed with suture passed through PASTA lesion. **C:** Lateral row anchor being placed. **D:** A superior view of the PASTA repair from a lateral portal. **E:** Final PASTA repair from an intraarticular view from the posterior portal showing the partial tear being reduced to the insertion.

one standard suture and one tape suture. Suture passage is performed with a shuttling technique using a PDS suture, which is percutaneously placed through the rotator cuff using an 18-gauge spinal needle. The spinal needle is placed percutaneously through the rotator cuff medial to the edge of the tear. A 1-0 PDS suture is then shuttled through the spinal needle into the joint. This is retrieved through the anterior portal paired with one of the sutures from the anchor and shuttled. This process is repeated until all sutures from the anchors are passed through the rotator cuff in a horizontal mattress fashion with the 2 wire sutures centrally in a mattress fashion and the tapes at the most anterior and posterior extents (Fig. 8-6A). The arthroscope is then placed back in the subacromial space. As stated before, it is critical that a thorough subacromial bursectomy was performed prior to anchor placement so that the sutures can be visualized for knot tying. Performing a bursectomy after the sutures have been passed risks damaging the sutures. The two Fiberwires are retrieved through the lateral cannula and tied down securely on the rotator cuff using arthroscopic knot tying techniques. Once those are secured, a lateral row knotless anchor is placed securing appropriate tension on all four strands. The surgeon must be vigilant about tensioning the tape sutures, as they are thicker and more difficult to glide through the loop of the anchor (Fig. 8-6B). The view from the lateral portal should show adequate tissue covering the humeral head (Fig. 8-6C). The arthroscope is then placed back into the joint to inspect the repair. The previously exposed footprint should now be covered with tendon from the repair (Fig. 8-6D).

Tear Completion with Standard Repair

In order to use standard single- or double-row repair techniques for partial-thickness rotator cuff tears, the tear must be completed with either a shaver or knife. Once the tear has been completed and the ends of the rotator cuff débrided, a thorough subacromial decompression with or without acromioplasty is completed. Two cannulas are then placed into the subacromial space. One is placed directly lateral to the acromion, and the second is placed just off the anterolateral corner. The greater tuberosity is then débrided to a bleeding bed. The arthroscope is placed in the lateral cannula for viewing. The suture anchor(s) can be placed through the anterolateral cannula or through percutaneous stab incisions. The sutures are retrieved out through one of the nonworking portals/stab incisions for suture management. This will keep the sutures out of the way while subsequently passing separate suture through the tendon. There are various antegrade and retrograde passers for passing suture through the rotator cuff. The repair can be completed with either a single- or double-row technique depending on surgeon preference, although most of these tears are small enough that a single row will suffice. Arthroscopic knots are tied through the anterolateral cannula while continuing to view through the lateral cannula.

SLAP Tears

Snyder type II SLAP tears have long been associated with overhead athletes (5,38). Because the SLAP tear in these patients often extends posteriorly from the biceps anchor, we prefer to use the lateral position, which offers excellent visualization of the posterior labrum. Using a standard posterior viewing portal and anterior working portal, the superior labrum is examined. A probe is used to test the stability of the anchor. If the biceps is stable and there is only fraying present, then a débridement alone will suffice. If there is a true type II SLAP tear with instability of the biceps anchor, then it should be repaired (Fig. 8-7). If a repair is to be completed, the labrum and glenoid must be prepared prior to suture anchor placement. The labrum should be elevated off of the superior glenoid. This is usually complete by the injury itself but can also be completed with an arthroscopic elevator. Any fraying of the labrum should be gently débrided using a shaver. Using either the shaver in burr mode or a small round burr, we prepare the glenoid by débriding the bone to a bleeding bed to promote healing of the labral repair. We then place small (6.5 mm) screw-in cannulas through both the anterior and the posterior portals. As a general point, we try to avoid any sutures anterior to the biceps anchor. Additionally, care should be taken to try to avoid capturing the posterosuperior capsule in the suture to avoid stiffness and pain. Either single-loaded traditional suture anchors or knotless anchors are utilized posterior to the biceps anchor. The anchors are placed transtendinous through a portal of Wilmington, just off the acromial edge. For knotless fixation, a cannula is necessary to manage the sutures and avoid a tissue bridge. Traditional fixation with knots can be performed without the need for a transtendinous cannula. We prefer using the Spectrum suture passer (Linvatec) to pass a 1-0 PDS through the labrum and then shuttling the suture from the anchor through the

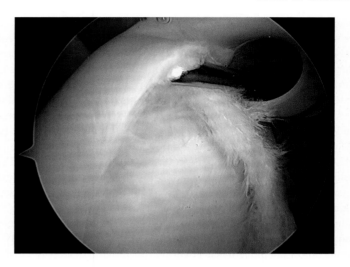

FIGURE 8-7

SLAP repair. Type II SLAP tear.

labrum. As noted above, this should be as pure a labral stitch as possible with avoidance of capturing the adjacent capsule in the suture loop. Typically, this is easiest to accomplish by viewing from the anterior portal and working through the posterior portal. The anchors are placed percutaneously just off the rim of the glenoid (Fig. 8-8A). The sutures are passed and tied through the posterior cannula (Fig. 8-8B). Care should be taken to avoid overtensioning the biceps anchor (Fig. 8-8C).

Posteroinferior Capsulotomy

Patients with severe GIRD that does not respond to stretching may be candidates for a selective posteroinferior capsulotomy (5). These athletes tend to have long-standing symptoms and be older, elite pitchers with chronic shoulder problems. As with all patients with internal impingement, they often have associated intraarticular pathology (e.g., type II SLAP tears, partial-thickness rotator cuff tears). Burkhart et al. have described a technique of releasing the thickened and contracted posterior capsule in the area of the PIGHL (5). By selectively performing a capsulotomy in this region, they report an immediate 65-degree increase in internal rotation. This can be done using a hooked

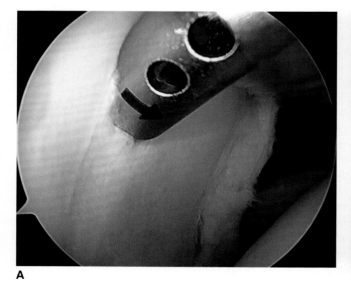

A

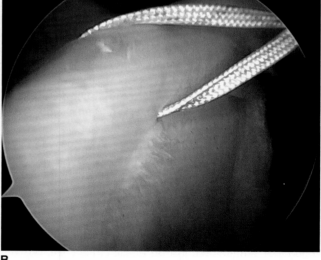

B

FIGURE 8-8

SLAP repair. **A:** Placement of suture anchor guide through Wilmington portal. **B:** Suture passed around the superior labrum.

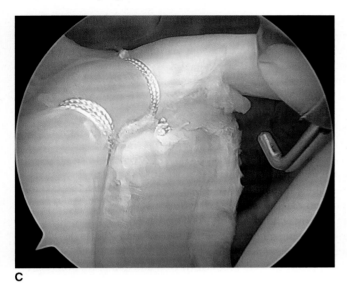

FIGURE 8-8 (*Continued*)
C: SLAP tear after final repair taking care to avoid overtensioning the biceps anchor.

electrocautery device (Fig. 8-9). The tissue can be 6 mm thick or more in these patients (normal: 1–2.5 mm). An immediate postoperative stretching protocol focusing on the posterior inferior capsule through stretches like sleeper stretches must be started to maintain the gain in motion and prevent the capsulotomy from closing down (39).

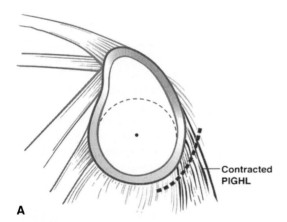

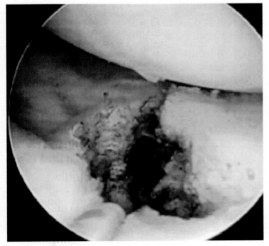

FIGURE 8-9

Selective posteroinferior capsulotomy. **A:** The capsular contracture is located in the posteroinferior quadrant of the capsule in the zone of the posterior band of the IGHL complex. The capsulotomy is made ¼ in away from the labrum from the 9 or 3 o' clock position to the 6 o' clock position. **B:** On arthroscopic inspection after the capsulotomy is made, note how thick the capsule in this zone has become. (Reprinted from Burkhart SS, Morgan CD, Kibler WB. The disabled throwing shoulder: spectrum of pathology Part I: pathoanatomy and biomechanics. *Arthroscopy.* 2003;19(4):404–420. Copyright © 2003 Arthroscopy Association of North America, with permission.)

PEARLS AND PITFALLS

- Whether beach chair or lateral decubitus positioning, choose a position that the surgeon is comfortable with and can address all pathology.
- Limit acromioplasty in athletes currently involved in overhead activities.
- Favor débridement over repair for partial-thickness rotator cuff tears in elite level overhead athletes.
- Avoid overtensioning the biceps anchor or capturing the posterior-superior capsule when performing SLAP repairs.

POSTOPERATIVE MANAGEMENT

Postoperative management will depend on the extent of surgery. For labral repairs, the authors limit patients to Codman exercises and gentle passive range of motion (PROM) within a pain-free range for 4 weeks. The patients should avoid extension and external rotation past neutral. They are encouraged to start scapular stabilization exercises.

After 4 weeks, therapy is advanced to PROM to 90 degrees of flexion and abduction, 60 degrees of internal rotation, and 30 degrees of external rotation and extension. Light weight can be added to pendulum exercises and they begin light band work. Once comfortable, patients can start active-assisted ROM (AAROM).

At the 6-week mark, they can advance to full ROM. Isotonic rotator cuff strengthening is initiated with light weight working up to 6 to 8 lbs. Proprioception exercises are introduced.

At 8 weeks, biceps strengthening is started. Isokinetic rotator cuff exercises are added to their regimen. At 12 weeks, throwers can begin light tennis ball tossing as they work on their mechanics. An interval throwing program is initiated at the 14- to 16-week mark. Return to sport is variable and if influenced by the sport, position, hand dominance, and extent of the surgery. For nonthrowers or nondominant shoulders—anticipation of return to sport by 4 to 6 months is reasonable. In the dominant shoulder of a high-level thrower, return to unrestricted throwing can take 9 to 12 months.

The postoperative rehabilitation of rotator cuff repair is slightly different and generally slower. Sling immobilization is used at all times except while at therapy for the first 4 weeks. PROM can be initiated in the first 4 weeks up to 90 degrees of flexion and abduction and 30 degrees of extension, internal and external rotation. ROM is advanced at 4 weeks and submaximal isometric rotator cuff strengthening is started. At 6 weeks, patients have no ROM restrictions, and they begin isotonic rotator cuff strengthening and proprioception exercises. Core rotator cuff exercises are initiated at 8 weeks. Light tennis ball throwing is allowed at the 14-week mark. Interval throwing program starts at 4 months and throwers can return to sport when they complete isokinetic testing and the interval throwing program and have no pain.

COMPLICATIONS

Muto's retrospective review of 25 patients showed no retear in their cohort of rotator cuff repairs in overhead athletes. They also reported zero infections (40). Katz et al. performed a retrospective review and found 40 patients who presented with pain and stiffness following a SLAP repair. Of these, 21 patients had a revision surgery, which range from biceps tenodesis/tenotomy, revision SLAP repair, labral or glenohumeral joint débridement, subacromial decompression, rotator cuff repair, and total shoulder arthroplasty (41). Further studies support either a biceps tenotomy/tenodesis are viable options for patients with persistent pain following a SLAP repair (42).

RESULTS

Rotator Cuff Tears

Previously, there were concerns that overhead athletes did not respond well to rotator cuff repair, especially full-thickness tears (35,43). In a 2005 case series, for instance, Ide et al. reported the outcomes of arthroscopic transtendinous repair technique in a group of 17 Japanese patients with PASTA lesions, 6 of whom were overhead athletes (44). At mean follow-up of 39 months, the average University of California at Los Angeles (UCLA) shoulder scores improved from 17.3 to 32.9 ($p < 0.01$)

and average Japanese Orthopedic Association (JOA) scores from 68.4 to 94.8 ($p < 0.01$). Of the six overhead throwing athletes, two were able to return to the same level of competitive sport (badminton, tennis), three returned at a lower level (two baseball, one volleyball), and one was unable to return to sport (baseball). The average time they were able to return to sport was 8.4 months (range 6–12 months). A recent study by Muto et al. examining outcomes in 25 nonprofessional overhead athletes following rotator cuff repair provided more favorable outcomes. Most of their patients were baseball players and volleyball players. They showed statistically significant improvements of both the UCLA shoulder scale and the JOA shoulder scores, and 88% of the patients were able to return to their preoperative activity level (40).

There have been several studies examining the differences between the two techniques for rotator cuff repair previously described: the transtendinous PASTA repair technique versus tear completion with traditional repair. In 2012, Shin published the results of a randomized controlled trial comparing these two techniques in group of 48 nonathlete Korean patients with partial articular-sided rotator cuff tears that were >50% of the tendon thickness (45). The author reported good clinical outcomes in both groups, with 92% of patients in each group reporting satisfaction with surgery at a mean of 31 months follow-up. However, the patients treated with tear completion and standard repair demonstrated less pain and faster recovery of shoulder function and range of motion, as measured by the American Shoulder and Elbow Surgeons (ASES) and constant shoulder scores, than the transtendinous technique. MRIs of the surgical shoulders at 6-month follow-up demonstrated full integrity of all patients in the transtendinous repair group and 22 of 24 patients in the completion and standard repair group.

SLAP Tears

The outcomes from repair of type II SLAP tears are generally positive in young patients with regard to improvements in pain, function, and patient satisfaction. For overhead athletes, however, the rate of return to sport is less favorable. For instance, in 2013, Park et al. published the outcomes of a case series of 24 elite overhead athletes who underwent arthroscopic repair of isolated type II SLAP lesions (46). Overall, these patients experienced significant improvement in pain and function, as measured by visual analog scales for pain and satisfaction as well as ASES scores. However, at a mean of 45.8 months after surgery, only 12 (50%) of the 24 athletes were able to return to sport. A systematic review of outcomes after type II SLAP repair published in 2012 by Sayde et al. provided slightly more favorable results regarding return to sport for athletes, but overhead athletes fared worse than other athletes. The authors reviewed a total of 14 studies, including 506 athletes (198 overhead athletes, 81 baseball players). Again, patient satisfaction with clinical outcome was generally favorable, with 83% rating their pain and function as "good to excellent." Overall, 73% of the athletes were able to return to their prior level of play, but only 63% of the overhead athletes returned to their previous level.

CONCLUSION

Internal shoulder impingement and SLAP tears are common pathologies that affect overhead athletes. Recent attention to these entities has led to surgical techniques and rehabilitation protocols that have shown to be quite effective in improving symptoms and restoring shoulder function. Overhead athletes undergoing surgical intervention, however, have not been able to return to their prior level of sport as often as other athletes. As such, they represent a particular challenge to the shoulder surgeon that warrants further investigation and innovation.

REFERENCES

1. Walch G, Boileau P, Noel E, et al. Impingement of the deep surface of the supraspinatus tendon on the posterosuperior glenoid rim: an arthroscopic study. *J Shoulder Elbow Surg.* 1992;1(5):238–245. doi:10.1016/S1058-2746(09)80065-7.
2. Jobe CM. Posterior superior glenoid impingement: expanded spectrum. *Arthroscopy.* 1995;11(5):530–536. doi:10.1016/0749-8063(95)90128-0.
3. Kibler WB, Chandler TJ. Range of motion in junior tennis players participating in an injury risk modification program. *J Sci Med Sport.* 2003;6(1):51–62. doi:10.1016/S1440-2440(03)80008-7.
4. Burkhart SS, Morgan CD, Kibler WB. Shoulder injuries in overhead athletes. The "dead arm" revisited. *Clin Sports Med.* 2000;19(1):125–158. doi:10.1016/s0278-5919(05)70300-8.
5. Burkhart SS, Morgan CD, Kibler BW. The disabled throwing shoulder: spectrum of pathology part I: pathoanatomy and biomechanics. *Arthroscopy.* 2003;19(4):404–420. doi:10.1053/jars.2003.50128.

6. Halbrecht JL, Tirman P, Atkin D. Internal impingement of the shoulder: comparison of findings between the throwing and nonthrowing shoulders of college baseball players. *Arthroscopy.* 1999;15(3):253–258. doi:10.1016/S0749-8063(99)70030-7.

7. Jobe FW, Giangarra CE, Kvitne RS, et al. Anterior capsulolabral reconstruction of the shoulder in athletes in overhand sports. *Am J Sports Med.* 1991;19(5):428–434. https://doi.org/10.1177/036354659101900502

8. Jobe FW, Kvitne RS, Giangarra CE. Shoulder pain in the overhand or throwing athlete. The relationship of anterior instability and rotator cuff impingement. *Orthop Rev.* 1989;18(9):963–975. http://www.ncbi.nlm.nih.gov/pubmed/2797861

9. Kvitne RS, Jobe FW. The diagnosis and treatment of anterior instability in the throwing athlete. *Clin Orthop Relat Res.* 1993;(291):107–123. doi:10.1097/00003086-199306000-00013.

10. Kvitne RS, Jobe FW, Jobe CM. Shoulder instability in the overhand or throwing athlete. *Clin Sports Med.* 1995;14(4):917–935. Available at: http://sfx.scholarsportal.info/western?sid=OVID:medline&id=pmid:8582006&id=doi:&issn=0278-5919&isbn=&volume=14&issue=4&spage=917&pages=917-35&date=1995&title=Clinics+in+Sports+Medicine&atitle=Shoulder+instability+in+the+overhand+or+throwing+athlete.&aulas

11. Levitz CL, Dugas J, Andrews JR. The use of arthroscopic thermal capsulorrhaphy to treat internal impingement in baseball players. *Arthroscopy.* 2001;17(6):573–577. doi:10.1053/jars.2001.24853.

12. Paley KJ, Jobe FW, Pink MM, et al. Arthroscopic findings in the overhand throwing athlete: evidence for posterior internal impingement of the rotator cuff. *Arthroscopy.* 2000;16(1):35–40. doi:10.1016/S0749-8063(00)90125-7.

13. Mihata T, Gates J, McGarry MH, et al. Effect of posterior shoulder tightness on internal impingement in a cadaveric model of throwing. *Knee Surg Sports Traumatol Arthrosc.* 2013;23(2):548–554. doi:10.1007/s00167-013-2381-7.

14. Mihata T, McGarry MH, Neo M, et al. Effect of anterior capsular laxity on horizontal abduction and forceful internal impingement in a cadaveric model of the throwing shoulder. *Am J Sports Med.* 2015;43(7):1758–1763. doi:10.1177/0363546515582025.

15. Davidson PA, Elattrache NS, Jobe CM, et al. Rotator cuff and posterior-superior glenoid labrum injury associated with increased glenohumeral motion: a new site of impingement. *J Shoulder Elbow Surg.* 1995;4(5):384–390. doi:10.1016/S1058-2746(95)80023-9.

16. Tibone JE, Jobe FW, Kerlan RK, et al. Shoulder impingement syndrome in athletes treated by an anterior acromioplasty. *Clin Orthop Relat Res.* 1985;198:134–140.

17. Zaslav KR. Internal rotation resistance strength test: a new diagnostic test to differentiate intra-articular pathology from outlet (Neer) impingement syndrome in the shoulder. *J Shoulder Elbow Surg.* 2001;10(1):23–27. doi:10.1067/mse.2001.111960.

18. Myers JB. Glenohumeral range of motion deficits and posterior shoulder tightness in throwers with pathologic internal impingement. *Am J Sports Med.* 2005;34(3):385–391. doi:10.1177/0363546505281804.

19. Burkhart SS, Morgan CD, Kibler WB The disabled throwing shoulder: spectrum of pathology part III: the SICK scapula, scapular dyskinesis, the kinetic chain, and rehabilitation. *Arthroscopy.* 2003;19(6):641–661. doi:10.1016/S0749-8063(03)00389-X.

20. Cook C, Beaty S, Kissenberth MJ, et al. Diagnostic accuracy of five orthopedic clinical tests for diagnosis of superior labrum anterior posterior (SLAP) lesions. *J Shoulder Elbow Surg.* 2012;21(1):13–22. doi:10.1016/j.jse.2011.07.012.

21. Heyworth BE, Williams RJ 3rd. Internal impingement of the shoulder. *Am J Sport Med.* 2009;37(5):1024–1037. doi:0363546508324966 [pii]\r10.1177/0363546508324966.

22. Roy EA, Cheyne I, Andrews GT, et al. Beyond the cuff: MR imaging of labroligamentous injuries in the athletic shoulder. *Radiology.* 2016;279(1):328. doi:10.1148/radiol.2016164008.

23. Chandnani VP, Deberardino A, Gagliardi A, et al. Glenohumeral ligaments and shoulder capsular mechanism: evaluation with MR arthrography. *Radiology.* 1995;196:27–32. doi:10.1148/radiology.196.1.7784579.

24. Chandnani VP, Yeager TD, DeBerardino T, et al. Glenoid labral tears: prospective evaluation with MRI imaging, MR arthrography, and CT arthrography. *AJR Am J Roentgenol.* 1993;161(6):1229–1235. doi:10.2214/ajr.161.6.8249731.

25. Palmer WE, Brown JH, Rosenthal DI. Labral-ligamentous complex of the shoulder: evaluation with MR arthrography. *Radiology.* 1994;190(3):645–651. doi:10.1148/radiology.190.3.8115604.

26. Palmer WE, Caslowitz PL. Anterior shoulder instability: diagnostic criteria determined from prospective analysis of 121 MR arthrograms. *Radiology.* 1995;197(3):819–825. doi:10.1148/radiology.197.3.7480762.

27. Tirman PF, Bost FW, Garvin GJ, et al. Posterosuperior glenoid impingement of the shoulder: findings at MR imaging and MR arthrography with arthroscopic correlation. *Radiology.* 1994;193(2):431–436. doi:10.1148/radiology.193.2.7972758.

28. Tirman PF, Palmer WE, Feller JF. MR arthrography of the shoulder. *Magn Reson Imaging Clin N Am.* 1997;5(4):811–839.

29. Tirman PF, Stauffer AE, Crues JV, et al. Saline magnetic resonance arthrography in the evaluation of glenohumeral instability. *Arthroscopy.* 1993;9(5):550–559. doi:10.1016/S0749-8063(05)80403-7.

30. Tirman PF, Bost FW, Steinbach LS, et al. MR arthrographic depiction of tears of the rotator cuff: benefit of abduction and external rotation of the arm. *Radiology.* 1994;192(3):851–856. doi:10.1148/radiology.192.3.8058959.

31. Fessa CK, Peduto A, Linklater J, et al. Posterosuperior glenoid internal impingement of the shoulder in the overhead athlete: pathogenesis, clinical features and MR imaging findings. *J Med Imaging Radiat Oncol.* 2015;59(2):182–187. doi:10.1111/1754-9485.12276.

32. Connor PM, Banks DM, Tyson AB, et al. Magnetic resonance imaging of the asymptomatic shoulder of overhead athletes: a 5-year follow-up study. *Am J Sports Med.* 2003;31(5):724–727. doi:10.1177/03635465030310051501.

33. Miniaci A, Mascia AT, Salonen DC, et al. Magnetic resonance imaging of the shoulder in asymptomatic professional baseball pitchers. *Am J Sports Med.* 2002;30(1):66–73. doi:10.1177/03635465020300012501.

34. Tyler TF, Nicholas SJ, Lee SJ, et al. Correction of posterior shoulder tightness is associated with symptom resolution in patients with internal impingement. *Am J Sports Med.* 2010;38(1):114–119. doi:10.1177/0363546509346050.

35. Tibone JE, Elrod B, Jobe FW, et al. Surgical treatment of tears of the rotator cuff in athletes. *J Bone Joint Surg Am.* 1986;68(6):887–891.

36. Sonnery-Cottet B, Edwards TB, Noel E, et al. Results of arthroscopic treatment of posterosuperior glenoid impingement in tennis players. *Am J Sports Med.* 2002;30(2):227–232. Available at: http://www.ncbi.nlm.nih.gov/pubmed/11912093

37. Reynolds SB, Dugas JR, Cain EL, et al. Débridement of small partial-thickness rotator cuff tears in elite overhead throwers. *Clin Orthop Relat Res.* 2008;466:614–621. doi:10.1007/s11999-007-0107-1.

38. Abrams GD, Safran MR. Diagnosis and management of superior labrum anterior posterior lesions in overhead athletes. *Br J Sports Med.* 2010;44(5):311–318. doi:10.1136/bjsm.2009.070458.

39. Bey MJ, Hunter SA, Kilambi N, et al. Structural and mechanical properties of the glenohumeral joint posterior capsule. *J Shoulder Elbow Surg.* 2005;14(2):201–206. doi:10.1016/j.jse.2004.06.016.

40. Muto T, Inui H, Ninomiya H, et al. Characteristics and clinical outcomes in overhead sports athletes after rotator cuff repair. *J Sports Med (Hindawi Publ Corp)*. 2017;2017:5476293. doi:10.1155/2017/5476293.
41. Katz LM, Hsu S, Miller SL, et al. Poor outcomes after SLAP repair: descriptive analysis and prognosis. *Arthroscopy*. 2009;25(8):849–855. doi:10.1016/j.arthro.2009.02.022.
42. Erickson J, Lavery K, Monica J, et al. Surgical treatment of symptomatic superior labrum anterior-posterior tears in patients older than 40 years. *Am J Sports Med*. 2015;43(5):1274–1282. doi:10.1177/0363546514536874.
43. Mazoué CG, Andrews JR. Repair of full-thickness rotator cuff tears in professional baseball players. *Am J Sports Med*. 2006;34(2):182–189. doi:10.1177/0363546505279916.
44. Ide J, Maeda S, Takagi K. Arthroscopic transtendon repair of partial-thickness articular-side tears of the rotator cuff. *Am J Sports Med*. 2005;33(11):1672–1679. doi:10.1177/0363546505277141.
45. Shin SJ. A comparison of 2 repair techniques for partial-thickness articular-sided rotator cuff tears. *Arthroscopy*. 2012;28(1):25–33. doi:10.1016/j.arthro.2011.07.005.
46. Park JY, Chung SW, Jeon SH, et al. Clinical and radiological outcomes of type 2 superior labral anterior posterior repairs in elite overhead athletes. *Am J Sports Med*. 2013;41(6):1372–1379. doi:10.1177/0363546513485361.

9 Arthroscopic Anterior Stabilization

Drew A. Lansdown, Caitlin Chambers, Brian T. Feeley, and C. Benjamin Ma

INTRODUCTION

Anterior shoulder instability is one of the most common injuries of the shoulder and accounts for one-third of all emergency visits related to the shoulder, with an estimated incidence of 23.9 dislocations per 100,000 person-years (1). Arthroscopic stabilization has become the most prevalent treatment for anterior shoulder instability, with 84% of anterior stabilization cases from a large national database performed arthroscopically (2). With advancements in modern suture anchor technology, improvements in arthroscopic techniques, and proper patient selection, the long-term outcomes for arthroscopic stabilization are now comparable to the previous gold standard of open stabilization (2–6). The arthroscopic approach allows better preservation of motion, particularly external rotation (7), and avoids the potential complications of open surgery including subscapularis tendon disruption. An arthroscopic procedure allows for a thorough inspection of potential associated injuries to the superior and posterior labrum. Arthroscopic stabilization has been shown to allow for better rates of return to play at the same level of competition, range of motion, and subjective satisfaction with shoulder function in competitive athletes (4,8). Further advantages of an arthroscopic procedure include lower levels of postoperative pain, improved recovery time, and cosmesis (9,10).

For many patients with anterior shoulder instability, the optimal surgical treatment is therefore arthroscopic stabilization, though there are several injury-specific and patient-specific factors that may influence the likelihood of success with arthroscopic anterior stabilization. Results after arthroscopic anterior stabilization can be optimized with an understanding of appropriate indications, preoperative planning, and certain technical steps, as discussed in this chapter.

INDICATIONS AND CONTRAINDICATIONS

The indications for arthroscopic treatment of anterior shoulder instability (Table 9-1) include patients who have had more than one traumatic dislocation with minimal glenoid bone loss and those patients who continue to have symptoms of instability despite a trial of physical therapy. Arthroscopic anterior stabilization may also be considered following a first-time dislocation in competitive athletes, contact athletes, or active patients ≤ 30 years old (11). Reported recurrence rates after first-time dislocation range from 19% to 88%, with significantly greater risk for redislocation in males and younger patients, particularly ≤ 20 years old (12). The rate of recurrent anterior instability may be >80% in patients younger than 20 years of age (13) and <50% for patients over 30 years of age for those treated nonoperatively (14). While the rate of recurrence was previously felt to be higher for contact athletes treated with arthroscopic rather than open stabilization (15,16), appropriate use of evidence-based surgical indications and modern arthroscopic techniques reduces recurrence rates to approximate those seen in the general population after open or arthroscopic stabilization, with increased rate of return to sport in arthroscopic stabilization (4,17).

As arthroscopic techniques continue to improve, the indications for arthroscopic rather than open stabilization have expanded with several relative indications for arthroscopic stabilization. Some surgeons will consider revision arthroscopic stabilization or arthroscopic treatment of a humeral

TABLE 9-1 Surgical Indications for Anterior Shoulder Stabilization

Absolute Indications for Arthroscopic Anterior Stabilization
Recurrent anterior instability with no/minimal glenoid bone loss with:

- Presence of a Bankart lesion on MRI
- Normal laxity on physical exam
- Well-developed inferior glenohumeral ligament complex

Relative Indications for Arthroscopic Anterior Stabilization
First-time dislocation in patient ≤ 30 years old or competitive/contact athlete
Recurrent instability after prior arthroscopic anterior stabilization in the absence of glenoid bone loss

Relative Indication for Arthroscopic Remplissage in Conjunction with Anterior Stabilization
Engaging or off-track Hill-Sachs lesion in the setting of minimal (<10%) glenoid bone loss

Relative Indications for Open Stabilization or Bony Augmentation
Critical glenoid bone loss (>25% generally, may consider >13.5% in high-demand/contact athletes)
Off-track Hill-Sachs with advanced glenoid bone loss
Anterior capsular deficiency/redundancy, or generalized ligamentous laxity
HAGL lesion
Recurrent instability after prior arthroscopic anterior stabilization in the absence of glenoid bone loss
Instability severity index score ≥4 out of 10

Contraindications to Arthroscopic or Open Stabilization
Voluntary dislocator
Multidirectional instability without thorough attempt at physical therapy
Unable to participate in postoperative rehabilitation

avulsion of the glenohumeral ligament (HAGL) lesion, though these conditions may also be treated in an open fashion (18,19). A significant Hill-Sachs lesion in the setting of minimal glenoid bone loss (<10%) may be treated with an arthroscopic anterior stabilization and an arthroscopic remplissage (20,21).

Open Bankart repair with capsular shift may be more appropriate for patients who have failed prior arthroscopic stabilization, anterior capsular deficiency or redundancy, generalized ligamentous laxity, or multidirectional instability with failure of nonoperative treatment (22). To help identify the best treatment method for each individual patient's circumstance, the instability severity index score (ISIS) (Table 9-2) is decision tool that may be used to appropriately account for the various risk factors. For patients with preoperative scores of ≥4 out of 10, recurrence rates are as high as 70% with an arthroscopic anterior stabilization procedure alone (23–25).

Advanced bone loss is a contraindication for arthroscopic anterior stabilization. Critical bone loss was first described as 25% loss of the anterior glenoid and is a clear indication for bony augmentation (Latarjet, distal tibia allograft, or iliac crest bone graft) procedure given failure rates of over 70% with arthroscopic anterior stabilization alone (26). More recent literature, however, suggests that even as little as 13.5% to 20% glenoid bone loss may result in increased recurrence rates and

TABLE 9-2 Instability Severity Index Score

Prognostic Factor		Points
Age at surgery	≤20 y	2
	>20	0
Degree of sport participation (preoperative)	Competitive	2
	Recreational or none	0
Type of sport (preoperative)	Contact or overhead	1
	Other	0
Shoulder hyperlaxity	Anterior or inferior shoulder hyperlaxity	1
	Normal laxity	0
Hill-Sachs lesion (AP radiograph)	Visible in external rotation	2
	Not visible in external rotation	0
Glenoid loss of contour (AP radiograph)	Loss of contour	2
	Normal contour	0
Total points		_____ /10

inferior subjective outcomes after arthroscopic stabilization alone (27,28). Utilization of a remplissage procedure to fill in the humeral head defect with posterior capsule and infraspinatus tendon is generally recommended for Hill-Sachs lesions occupying 20% of the humeral head diameter, while open techniques such as bone grafting, humeral head resurfacing, or arthroplasty options are indicated for Hill-Sachs lesions >40% of the diameter (29).

The glenoid track concept highlights the importance of considering bipolar bone loss, allows for a measurement that accounts for both glenoid and humeral-sided bone loss, and can help select the appropriate surgical approach (30). For this measurement, the width of the glenoid contact area, or "track," on the articular surface of the humeral head is equal to 84% of the intact glenoid width. With decreasing glenoid width due to bone loss, this track on the humeral head is narrowed proportionately. When the medial margin of a Hill-Sachs lesion extends outside of the area of the glenoid track, the Hill-Sachs lesion overrides and engages the edge of the glenoid, and the lesions are said to be "off-track." This concept highlights the interaction of bipolar lesions and the importance of humeral bone loss location. This concept has been validated clinically for the purposes of predicting failure after arthroscopic Bankart repair, demonstrating 75% positive predictive value of MRI-based off-track measurements as compared to only 44% positive predictive value for glenoid bone loss >20% (31).

Absolute contraindications for undergoing arthroscopic or open surgical stabilization include recurrent voluntary dislocators and patients who are poorly motivated or unable to comply with the postoperative rehabilitation program.

PREOPERATIVE PREPARATION

History

As with any orthopedic problem, the first step toward a diagnosis is a thorough history. For anterior shoulder instability, the mechanism of injury should be obtained to determine if the injury was of high energy or low energy. Patients with lower-energy dislocations may have a component of excess laxity and should be evaluated accordingly. The patient is asked if the shoulder subluxated or truly dislocated and whether he or she reduced the shoulder on the own or if it required anesthesia to achieve reduction. Clearly, the most important question to ask is if this dislocation was the first dislocation, and if not, how many previous dislocations have occurred on the affected shoulder.

Examination

Physical examination of the shoulder begins with visual inspection of the shoulder girdle. The contour of the deltoid should be evaluated to assess for an axillary nerve injury, which is an uncommon but reported complication following a shoulder dislocation. Range of motion is assessed and is typically normal, though patients may self-limit external rotation to avoid the position of apprehension. Isometric testing of the rotator cuff is performed. A rotator cuff tear is unlikely in a young patient with anterior instability; however, there is increasing frequency of rotator cuff tears as the patient ages. The apprehension sign, which is performed by bringing the arm into the abduction and external rotation position, is typically quite positive following a recent dislocation. The relocation test, which consists of applying a posterior-directed force on the shoulder while abducting and externally rotation the arm, is likewise positive in most patients with anterior instability. In a positive test, the patient feels more comfortable with this additional pressure placed anteriorly than in the apprehension position alone.

A load and shift test can be performed in the office setting as well, but it may be difficult for the patient to relax enough to determine the correct amount of instability. The sulcus sign is performed by pulling down on the arm with the patient in a seated position. When positive, there is increased translation between the acromion and the humeral head, suggesting laxity in the rotator interval. In patients with suspected multidirectional instability, the sulcus sign is usually positive. Other joints should be evaluated for signs of generalized ligamentous with the Beighton mobility score, which awards one point for hyperextension of each elbow and knee >10 degrees, small finger >90 degrees, apposition of each thumb to the volar forearm, and ability to place the palms flat on the floor with knees in full extension, for a possible total of 9 (32). These patients with generalized laxity are at increased risk of recurrent instability after stabilization (33,34). The Gagey hyperabduction sign indicates inferior capsular laxity and involves passive abduction of the arm (35). Normal passive abduction is 90 degrees, while passive abduction past 105 degrees indicates inferior capsular laxity.

Imaging

We typically obtain a true AP view of the shoulder in external and internal rotation, an axillary view, a West Point lateral view, a scapular-Y view, and a Stryker notch view (Fig. 9-1). Bony Bankart

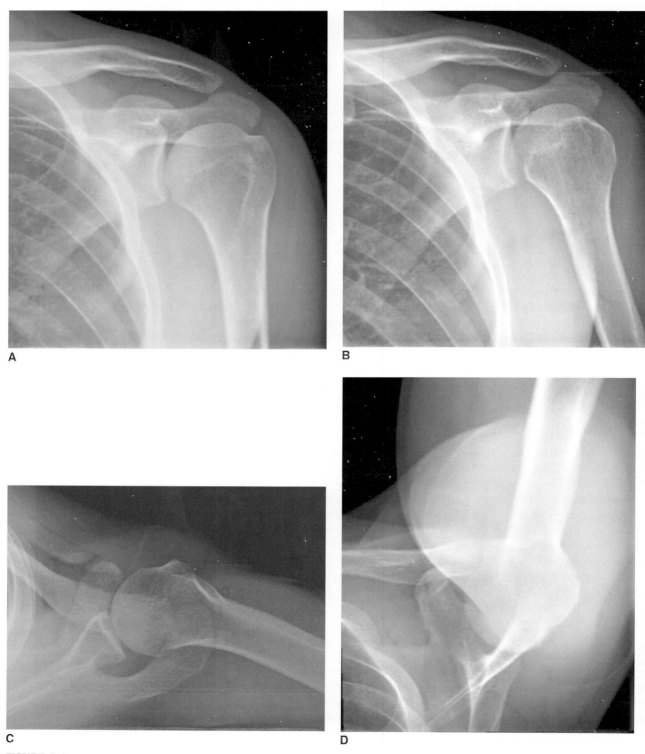

A   **B**

C   **D**

FIGURE 9-1

Five radiographic views of the shoulder are obtained to evaluate the bony anatomy, including **(A)** AP view of the glenohumeral joint in external rotation; **(B)** AP view of the glenohumeral joint in internal rotation; **(C)** an axillary lateral view; **(D)** West Point lateral view;

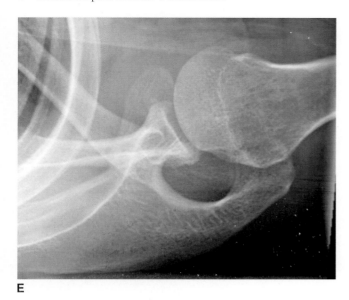

E

FIGURE 9-1 (*Continued*)
(E) Stryker notch view.

lesions are best assessed by evaluating the contour of the anterior-inferior glenoid the West Point lateral view. A Hill-Sachs lesion is best seen on the Stryker notch view.

Magnetic resonance imaging (MRI) allows for the best visualization of anterior labral tears (Fig. 9-2). It is particularly useful in determining concomitant pathology such as superior labral tears, biceps lesions, and posterior labral tears. It is also helpful in determining if the instability is due to a Bankart lesion or a HAGL lesion, which may alter the operative plan. Arthroscopically confirmed HAGL lesions are present in 7.5% to 9.3% of primary instability cases and occur more commonly in males injured during sporting events (36). HAGL lesions can occur in isolation but more commonly are associated with additional pathology such as labral injury, glenoid bone loss, and rotator cuff injury. If unrecognized or untreated, HAGL lesions can cause recurrent postoperative instability. In the older patient, rotator cuff disruption may also be seen in association with shoulder dislocation. In our institution, we use contrast-enhanced MR arthrograms for shoulder dislocations more than 3 weeks old to evaluate labral pathology, but other radiologists find it as accurate to perform noncontrast MRI to evaluate shoulder labral pathology (37,38). Contrast is not needed in the acute evaluation of shoulder instability due to the presence of hemarthrosis.

CT scan with three-dimensional reconstruction is useful in cases of concerning glenoid or humeral bone loss. This technique provides three-dimensional reconstruction of the glenoid with humeral subtraction for unobstructed en face view of the glenoid and allows for humeral and glenoid rotation to provide a full understanding of the amount and location of bipolar bone loss. In a study of shoulder surgeons, Bishop et al. demonstrated that three-dimensional CT reconstructions are the most reproducible method for determining glenoid bone loss (39).

Several techniques have been described to quantify glenoid bone loss. The Pico method (63) utilizes a bilateral shoulder CT scan with 3D reconstruction to create a best-fit circle along the inferior rim of the healthy glenoid, then transpose this circle onto the affected glenoid. The area of the circle (A) and the area of the bone defect represented by the missing portion of the circle (D) are calculated, with bone loss expressed as a percentage [Bone loss = $100 \times (A/D)$]. Alternatively, unilateral MRI or 3D CT scan can be used to quantify glenoid bone loss as the area missing from a best-fit circle aligned with the inferior glenoid (41,42). The presence of off-track bipolar lesions can also be determined utilizing CT scan or MRI to calculate the glenoid track width (84% of remaining glenoid width) in comparison to the medial extent of the Hill-Sachs lesion as measured from the rotator cuff insertion (30).

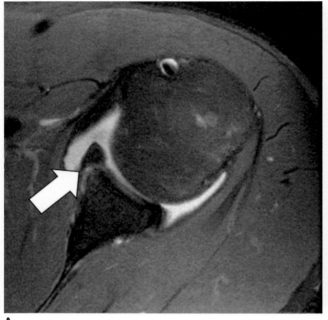

A

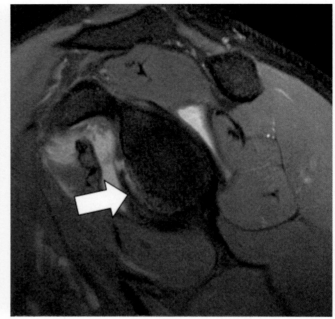

B

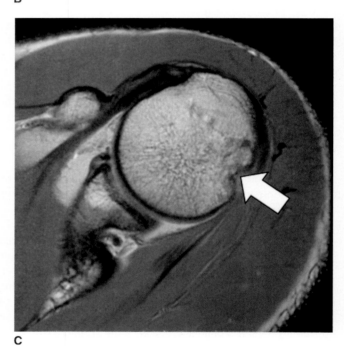

C

FIGURE 9-2

Preoperative noncontrast magnetic resonance images are shown for a patient with recurrent anterior instability, demonstrating an anterior labral tear (*arrow*) on **(A)** the axial fat-suppressed T2-weighted image and **(B)** the sagittal oblique fat-suppressed T2-weight image. There is a Hill-Sachs lesion on the posterior aspect of the humeral head (*arrow*) on **(C)** the axial proton density–weighted image.

TECHNIQUE

Anesthesia and Positioning

Most patients receive an interscalene nerve block and general anesthesia. The interscalene block is helpful in limiting intraoperative narcotics and decreases postoperative pain and nausea.

Exam Under Anesthesia

Prior to any incision, and before the arm is placed into the arm holder or traction device, it is critical to perform an examination of the shoulder under anesthesia. The examination should be performed on both shoulders to assess asymmetry in the exam compared to the contralateral side. Range of motion is recorded as well. Exam under anesthesia should confirm grade 2 to 3+ anterior instability without any posterior or inferior translation. In some cases of inferior laxity, however, there will be some degree of inferior subluxation, and this should be accounted for in the capsular plication.

Patient Positioning

The procedure can be performed in either the beach chair or lateral decubitus position, and this decision is largely surgeon dependent. With the beach chair position, the surgeon can more readily convert to an open procedure if needed, though posterior and inferior glenoid access may be more challenging. The lateral decubitus position can allow for better visualization, easier placement of anchors at the posterior and inferior aspects of the glenoid, and has been identified in one systematic review as potentially associated with lower rates of recurrent instability (43). For both positions, the patient is first anesthetized supine on a full-length beanbag.

Beach Chair Positioning

The patient is placed in the beach chair position (Fig. 9-3), and the beanbag is inflated to secure the patient in the upright position. The beanbag must be properly folded to leave the entire medial border of the scapula free. This setup allows excellent control of the head and body during the procedure and is easy to adapt for people of any body habitus. Once the beanbag is inflated, the patient and the beanbag are brought laterally to the edge of the bed, allowing complete exposure of the shoulder to the medial border of the scapula. The arm is prepped and draped in the usual sterile fashion. An arm holder is used for both arthroscopic and open stabilizations. It is extremely useful to provide traction during the stabilization procedure. A strap is placed around the upper arm to facilitate lateral humeral distraction during the procedure for circumferential access to the glenoid.

Lateral Decubitus Positioning

The patient is placed in the lateral decubitus position. The down leg is padded to protect the peroneal nerve. The traction device is attached to the bed on the anterior side when the patient is placed lateral. Proper configuration of the traction device allows for intraoperative visualization, and the top beam should be at the level of the humeral head, aiming toward the axilla. The patient is placed in the lateral position and held securely with the beanbag with the operative scapula free from the beanbag. The patient is rolled back toward the surgeon by 10 to 20 degrees to aid in distraction. The arm is prepped and draped in the usual sterile fashion. A well-padded arm sleeve is placed on the arm to allow for distraction, and a strap is placed over the proximal arm to allow for lateral distraction. For shoulder stabilization, the arm will be in approximately 40 degrees of abduction and 10 to 20 degrees of forward flexion with 10 lbs of traction applied.

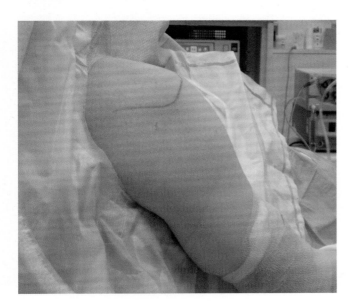

FIGURE 9-3

Beach chair positioning for anterior stabilization. The posterior portal is placed more medially and inferiorly compared to a rotator cuff repair. The arm is draped free, and the body is positioned off the bed so as to allow free motion with the arthroscope.

Portal Placement

There are typically three to four portals used for anterior stabilization of the shoulder. The primary viewing portal is made posteriorly in line with the glenohumeral joint. For the beach chair position, this portal is located in the soft spot of the glenohumeral joint, 2 cm distal and medial to the posterolateral tip of the acromion. In the lateral position, the posterior portal will be more lateral and superior relative to the soft spot, in line with the lateral border of the acromion. There are two anterior portals, and these must be carefully placed in order to facilitate the remainder of the procedure. The anteroinferior portal is placed with an outside-in technique with a spinal needle. It is placed in the rotator interval, just above the subscapularis tendon and laterally enough to facilitate placement of anchors at a 45-degree angle to the glenoid. The anterosuperior portal is placed in the superior aspect of the rotator interval, just anterior to the biceps tendon, with a skin incision located high, just in front of the clavicle. This portal is also localized with a spinal needle, and an 11 blade is used along the path of the spinal needle to create the trajectory into the joint, taking care not to cut the biceps tendon. A switching stick is then inserted, followed by progressive dilation and cannula placement. This facilitates suture management and can be utilized for anchor placement if a superior labrum anterior to posterior (SLAP) tear repair is necessary. We typically use a 7- to 8-mm clear cannula so that all instrumentation can be managed via either anterior portal. Additional posterior portals may facilitate suture passing and anchor placement if the labral injury extends posterior to the 6 o'clock position. A posterior working portal can be established approximately 3 cm inferior to the posterolateral corner of the acromion. A posterior-inferior portal, for anchor placement in the posterior-inferior glenoid and suture passage through the posterior-inferior labrum, is established 3 to 4 cm inferior and 1 to 2 cm lateral to the posterolateral acromion corner.

Diagnostic Arthroscopy

In cases where we suspect that an open procedure is necessary, we routinely perform a diagnostic arthroscopy to evaluate the status of the entire glenohumeral joint. The injury is classified based on the type of lesion that is found on the anteroinferior glenoid. A Bankart lesion is a disruption of the labrum off the glenoid rim, with or without disruption of the glenohumeral ligaments (Fig. 9-4). A Perthes lesion occurs when there is a periosteal avulsion of the labrum together with the glenohumeral ligaments off the glenoid neck. If the labrum scars medially following this injury, it is termed an ALPSA lesion (anterior labrum periosteal sleeve avulsion).

Complete evaluation of the anterior injury is achieved by moving the arthroscope to the anterosuperior portal. This portal may also be used for viewing while mobilizing the anteroinferior injury

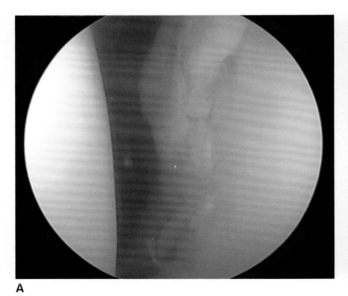
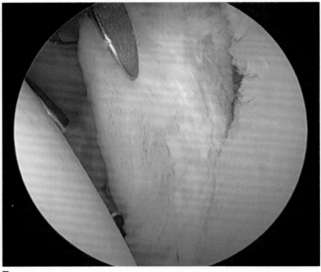

A   **B**

FIGURE 9-4

Diagnostic arthroscopy shows the anterior–inferior labral injury **(A)**, viewing through a posterior portal with a 30-degree arthroscope in the beach chair position.After mobilization with labral elevator, the labrum can be reduced to its anatomic position with a grasper **(B)**.

with instruments through the standard anterior portal. In high-energy injuries, there can be concomitant injuries to the superior labrum or posterior labrum as well, and these should be critically evaluated in any shoulder stabilization procedure.

The glenohumeral ligaments are often injured in cases of recurrent shoulder instability and should be carefully evaluated during the arthroscopy. With a probe, the insertion sites of the IGHL and the MGHL should be checked on the inferior labrum to determine whether they have been disrupted or whether they have scarred in medially along the glenoid neck. The humeral insertion site should be carefully evaluated to assess for the presence of a HAGL lesion. Visualization of this insertion point can be facilitated by use of a 70-degree arthroscope when needed.

Finally, the chondral surfaces of the humeral head and glenoid should be carefully evaluated. Chondral defects of the anterior glenoid rim (GLAD lesions—glenoid labrum articular disruptions) typically cause pain and feelings of subluxation but without frank dislocation. The humeral head is evaluated to determine the size of the Hill-Sachs lesion. A Hill-Sachs lesion that is >30% of the humeral sphere may require bone grafting or remplissage procedure.

Mobilization of the Labrum Off the Glenoid Neck

In a majority of cases, the labrum has scarred medially along the glenoid neck, and adequate mobilization of the labrum may be difficult. A 30-degree tissue elevator is advanced through the anteroinferior portal carefully up to the junction of the glenoid neck and labrum and used to create a tissue plane between the labrum and neck. Start at the superior aspect of the Bankart lesion and work down toward the inferior extent of the lesion. It is often helpful to look down on this lesion by placing the arthroscope in the anterosuperior portal during this aspect of the procedure. Work the release medially with the use of an electrocautery device and the elevator until the labrum is completely free and detached from the glenoid neck. An adequate release is confirmed with visualization of the subscapularis muscle behind the freed labral tissue.

Decortication of the Glenoid Neck

Decortication of the glenoid neck is performed with the arthroscopic shaver placed in the anteroinferior portal. This step is critical for developing a healing bed for the labrum along the glenoid neck. A 3.5- or 4-mm standard or bone-cutting shaver is used with the blades facing toward the neck of the glenoid, and it is done until bleeding has been achieved. It is important to protect the free labrum from inadvertent damage from the shaver. A meniscal rasp or a 4-mm burr can be used alternatively, although a shaver is adequate in most cases.

Capsulolabral Plication and Anchor Placement

Numerous anchor types are available to successfully perform an arthroscopic anterior stabilization procedure, including all-suture anchors, bioabsorbable anchors, and metal anchors. Our preference is to use single-loaded all-suture anchors given their pull-out strength and limited footprint in the glenoid. The repair begins at the posterior-most extent of the injury and proceeds in an anterosuperior direction. If the injury extends past the 6 o'clock position, the initial anchor is placed through the posterior-inferior portal. If not, the initial anchor is placed through the anteroinferior portal. The drill guide is inserted and placed at the glenoid articular margin at an angle of at least 45 degrees relative to the glenoid. Placement of the anchor too medial on the glenoid neck will result in malreduction of the labrum. Too shallow of an angle can cause disruption of the articular cartilage. If the anteroinferior portal does not allow for an optimal angle, a percutaneous, trans-subscapularis portal may be used for anchor insertion. A spinal needle is used to localize the trajectory, and a sharp-tipped drill guide trocar is inserted through the subscapularis tendon. No cannula is used to minimize disruption of the subscapularis.

A suture relay device or a suture lasso device is inserted to pierce the capsule at a level below the inferior extension of the labral tear in order to advance the capsule superiorly (Fig. 9-5). Our preference is to pierce the capsule and labrum separately if there is capsular redundancy, and the placement through capsule begins approximately 1 cm off the glenoid and 8 to 10 mm inferior to the extension of the tear. The suture or shuttling device is advanced into the joint and retrieved with a grasper through the accessory portal. One limb of suture from the anchor is shuttled through the labrum and capsule, and then, both suture limbs are pulled through the same cannula to allow for knot tying. If the initial pass through capsulolabral tissue is too superior, a poly-dioxanone (PDS)

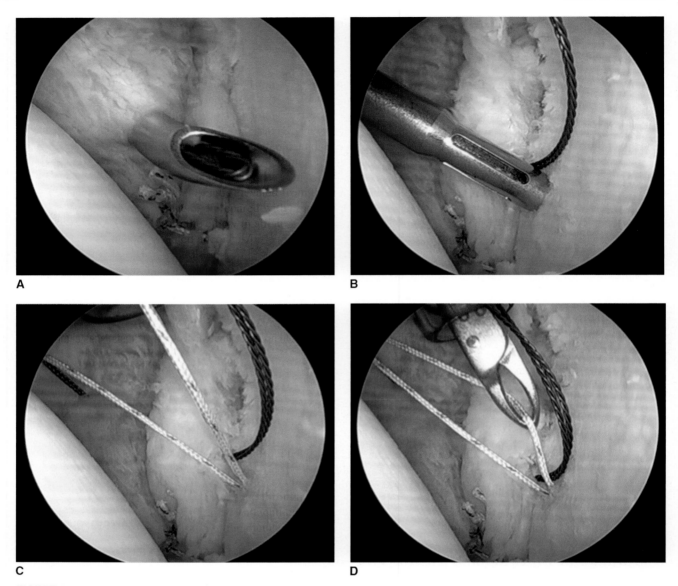

FIGURE 9-5

A suture lasso is placed through the capsule in a separate pass **(A)**, followed by placement around the labrum. Next, the drill trocar **(B)** for anchor insertion is placed at the glenoid face. With the suture anchor in place, the suture lasso is seen passing through capsule and around the labrum **(C)**. A suture limb is then shuttled **(D)** and tied to restore the capsulolabral tissue to its anatomic position at the glenoid rim.

suture may be shuttled through and used as a traction suture. The suture around this capsulolabral tissue may then be used to mobilize the torn labrum more superiorly while an even more inferior pass is made through the capsulolabral tissue at the anterior-inferior glenoid.

Stable Knot Tying

The suture limb through the capsule and labrum serves as the post for the arthroscopic knot, as this configuration will allow for the knot to sit away from the articular surface and push the capsulo-labral tissue toward the glenoid. The choice of arthroscopic knot is based on surgeons' preference. The most important aspect of arthroscopic knot tying is the use of a knot that the surgeon can reproducibly secure without difficulty. There are many knot-tying techniques, although we prefer an alternating half-hitch knot. Both sutures are retrieved through the same cannula. The limb that runs through the labrum and capsule acts as the post and is shortened accordingly. Two simple

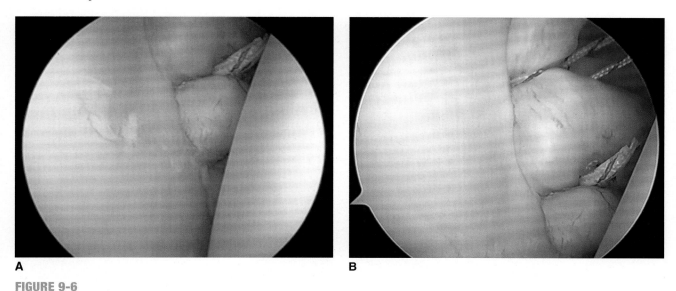

A   B

FIGURE 9-6

The capsulolabral repair is completed, demonstrating anchor placement at the 5 o'clock position **(A)** and restoration of the labrum to its anatomic position **(B)** at the anterior glenoid.

sutures are thrown in the same direction, and the post is pulled upon until the knot advances down to the level of the labrum. If the anchor was correctly placed, this reduces the capsule and labrum to the glenoid rim (Fig. 9-6). A knot pusher is then advanced, and the knot is secured with the knot medial to the repair so as not to put the knot on the articular surface. We place a total of six knots for each suture anchor, and a suture cutter is used to cut the ends. Recent advances in implant technology allows for the use of knotless anchors. Our current preference is to tie knots for shoulder stabilization procedures as this technique allows for the most secure and reproducible method for setting tension at the labral repair. For most Bankart repairs, two to four suture anchors are necessary for a complete repair. They should be separated by at least 4 to 5 mm. In general, all anchors should be positioned below the equator of the glenoid, which is marked by the upper border of the subscapularis tendon.

Remplissage

In cases with a large (>20%), engaging Hill-Sachs lesion or a Hill-Sachs lesion that is off-track, it may be beneficial to use a soft tissue augmentation to decrease this defect. The remplissage (French for "to fill") technique utilizes the posterior capsule or infraspinatus to fill defect and to transform this into an extra-articular defect (Fig. 9-7). Our preference is to perform this prior to the anterior labral repair as this sequence provides the best visualization of the Hill-Sachs lesion. The arm is externally rotated, and the arthroscope is placed in the anterosuperior portal. External rotation can allow more working space over the posterior shoulder. A switching stick is placed in the posterior portal, and a 7.5-mm cannula is inserted over the switching stick. A 5-mm corkscrew anchor, either metal or polyetheretherketone (PEEK), is then placed into the defect. This may be inserted through the cannula if the angle is appropriate or percutaneously through an accessory posterolateral portal established with spinal needle localization and in line with the Hill-Sachs defect. A straight penetrator is advanced into the joint through the posterior capsule and infraspinatus tendon. A suture limb is delivered to the penetrator with a knot pusher if needed. This process is then repeated with the corresponding suture limb to allow for a mattress-type suture configuration. Based on the defect size, we will use either one or two mattress sutures. The sutures are then tied down blindly through the percutaneous incision with a knot pusher and alternating half hitches. This will then allow a mattress-type suture through the infraspinatus tendon. The limbs are then tied down blindly in the subdeltoid space to tenodese the infraspinatus into the defect. The filing of the Hill-Sachs lesion is confirmed by viewing through both the anterosuperior portal and posterior portal.

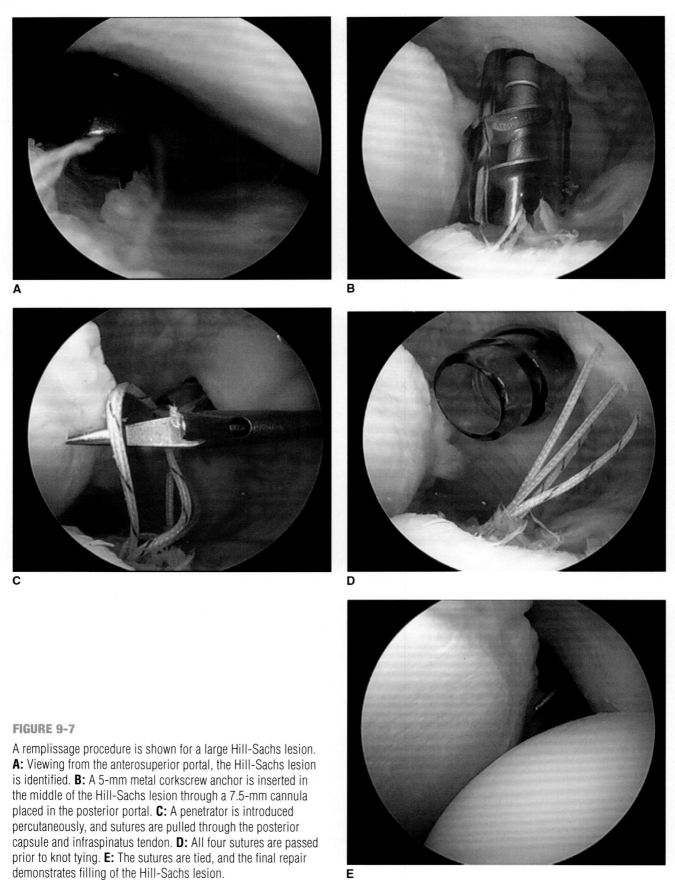

FIGURE 9-7

A remplissage procedure is shown for a large Hill-Sachs lesion. **A:** Viewing from the anterosuperior portal, the Hill-Sachs lesion is identified. **B:** A 5-mm metal corkscrew anchor is inserted in the middle of the Hill-Sachs lesion through a 7.5-mm cannula placed in the posterior portal. **C:** A penetrator is introduced percutaneously, and sutures are pulled through the posterior capsule and infraspinatus tendon. **D:** All four sutures are passed prior to knot tying. **E:** The sutures are tied, and the final repair demonstrates filling of the Hill-Sachs lesion.

PEARLS AND PITFALLS

Pearls

1. Recognize bipolar bone loss both preoperatively and intraoperatively to allow for appropriate surgical decision-making.
2. Mobilization of the labrum off the glenoid neck will allow for the restoration of the labrum to its anatomic position.
3. Decortication of the glenoid neck provides a fresh healing surface for the labral repair.
4. Accurate and safe placement of the suture anchors with appropriate utilization of accessory or percutaneous portals as needed will allow for complete treatment of the labral injury.
5. Capsulolabral fixation with adequate passes through tissue and multiple points of suture fixation allow for a stable repair construct.
6. Perform a remplissage to assist in stabilization as needed for large or off-track Hill-Sachs lesions.
7. Stable knot tying.

Pitfalls

1. Inadequate recognition of the severity of glenoid bone loss, a HAGL lesion, or significant Hill-Sachs lesion may lead to failure of arthroscopic repair.
2. Incomplete mobilization of the labrum may lead to a medialized repair that will not adequately restore stability to the shoulder.
3. Improper anchor trajectories can cause damage to the glenoid articular cartilage.

POSTOPERATIVE MANAGEMENT

Arthroscopic stabilization is performed on an outpatient basis, and the patients are placed in a sling postoperatively. Pain medication and anti-inflammatories are given for pain relief. During the first 3 weeks, passive range of motion exercises are initiated with a goal and limit of 30-degree abduction, no external rotation, 30-degree forward flexion, and 60-degree internal rotation. Abduction and forward flexion are increased to 90 degrees from 3 to 6 weeks. After 6 weeks, range of motion limits are removed and strengthening is commenced. Return to sports usually occurs at approximately 6 months.

COMPLICATIONS

Complications after arthroscopic anterior stabilization are rare, with the primary complication being recurrent instability as discussed below. Infection is reported at <1% of cases for shoulder arthroscopy (44). Complications may also be associated with patient positioning, including decreased cerebrovascular perfusion in the beach chair position and down-leg neuropraxia in the lateral position (44). Neural injuries in the operative extremity are also unlikely, with most reports being neuropraxias that resolve with observation alone (5).

RESULTS

Timing of arthroscopic anterior stabilization continues to be a controversial topic. Dickens et al. evaluated in-season return to play compared to surgical stabilization for a cohort of collegiate contact athletes. Nonoperative treatment allowed for 60% of athletes to complete the following season without recurrence, while surgical stabilization resulted in 90% of athletes completing the following season (45). For first-time dislocators under the age of 25 years, surgical stabilization after the initial dislocation may lead to decreased likelihood of recurrence relative to following multiple dislocations (46,47). Recurrent dislocators also have greater incidence of intra-articular pathology that may contribute to inferior results (48). In younger patients, arthroscopic stabilization may be reasonable after a first dislocation given these findings.

With refinements in arthroscopic techniques and advancements in suture anchor technology, the results of arthroscopic anterior stabilization surgery have improved with outcomes approaching those seen in open stabilization procedures. Mohtadi et al. conducted a randomized clinical trial to compare arthroscopic versus open stabilization in 162 patients (5). There were no differences between the groups for the Western Ontario Shoulder Instability (WOSI) score or American Shoulder and Elbow Surgeons (ASES) score at up to 2 years after surgery, and there were no differences with regard to shoulder range of motion. For arthroscopic stabilization, the mean WOSI score was 81.9 points and mean ASES score was 91.4 points. The rate of recurrent instability was 11% in the open group, which was significantly lower than 23% in the arthroscopic group ($p = 0.05$). After arthroscopic stabilization, 87% of patients have long-term stability at the shoulder (49). In a series of 153 Division 1 collegiate football players, Robins et al. reported return to play rates of 82% after anterior stabilization surgery with a 10% rate for recurrent instability (50). Multiple systematic reviews have been published to compare results of arthroscopic and open anterior stabilization (6,49,51–57). Chalmers et al. reviewed eight meta-analyses on the topic with a key finding that meta-analyses published after 2008 demonstrated no difference in failure rates or outcomes between these approaches (51). This observation suggests that improvements in suture anchors and surgical technique may have narrowed the difference between arthroscopic and open anterior stabilization results.

The presence of humeral head bone loss is an important finding that may increase the risk of failure for arthroscopic repair (5,58,59). The significance of a Hill-Sachs lesion can be determined with the glenoid track method, the depth of the lesion, and dynamic assessment at the time of arthroscopy. For larger lesions (off track, >20%, engaging on exam), a remplissage may be considered as part of the treatment algorithm. Buza et al. identified the recurrence rate for instability after remplissage in addition to arthroscopic anterior stabilization to be 5.4% in this high-risk group (21). A potential concern, since this procedure involves tenodesis of the infraspinatus tendon, is restriction in range of motion, with approximately 10-degree loss of external rotation at the side (60). This deficit may be especially problematic in throwing athletes, with 65% of throwers reporting difficulty throwing after arthroscopic stabilization and remplissage (61).

Certain factors are associated with an increased risk of failure after arthroscopic stabilization and should be considered carefully prior to proceeding with an arthroscopic stabilization. Patients who are under the age of 25, male, and have a Hill-Sachs lesion visible on shoulder radiographs were identified by Mohtadi et al. at being at higher risk for recurrent instability with arthroscopic stabilization (5). Glenoid bone loss also confers increased risk of failure of soft tissue stabilization procedures (62). Critical bone loss has been defined as 20% to 25% loss, though more recently, Shaha et al. described inferior WOSI scores in military patients with 13.5% glenoid bone loss after arthroscopic stabilization (27). Shin et al. has also reported bone loss >17.3% as the optimal cutoff for defining clinically important glenoid bone loss (28). The roles for open stabilization and bony augmentation will be further clarified with improved assessments of bone loss and refinements in surgical indications.

SUMMARY

Arthroscopic anterior stabilization provides a minimally invasive method for restoring shoulder function in patients who are frequently young and active. With the use of current suture anchors and arthroscopic techniques, surgeons can achieve results that at least approach those of open stabilization procedures. In a subset of patients, including younger male patients, contact athletes, and those with glenoid or humeral-sided bone loss, alternative procedures, including open stabilization or bony augmentation, should be considered. A thorough preoperative and intraoperative assessment of the shoulder will allow surgeons to identify associated pathology, including Hill-Sachs lesions, SLAP tears, posterior labral injuries, and multidirectional instability, that may necessitate additional surgical intervention at the time of arthroscopic stabilization. Arthroscopic anterior stabilization can result in a stable shoulder with excellent functional outcomes and high rates of return to sport.

REFERENCES

1. Zacchilli MA, Owens BD. Epidemiology of shoulder dislocations presenting to emergency departments in the United States. *J Bone Joint Surg Am.* 2010;92(3):542–549.
2. Zhang AL, Montgomery SR, Ngo SS, et al. Arthroscopic versus open shoulder stabilization: current practice patterns in the United States. *Arthroscopy.* 2014;30(4):436–443.
3. Aboalata M, Plath JE, Seppel G, et al. Results of arthroscopic Bankart repair for anterior-inferior shoulder instability at 13-year follow-up. *Am J Sports Med.* 2017;45(4):782–787.
4. Blonna D, Bellato E, Caranzano F, et al. Arthroscopic Bankart repair versus open Bristow-Latarjet for shoulder instability: a matched-pair multicenter study focused on return to sport. *Am J Sports Med.* 2016;44(12):3198–3205.

5. Mohtadi NG, Chan DS, Hollinshead RM, et al. A randomized clinical trial comparing open and arthroscopic stabilization for recurrent traumatic anterior shoulder instability: two-year follow-up with disease-specific quality-of-life outcomes. *J Bone Joint Surg Am.* 2014;96(5):353–360.
6. Petrera M, Patella V, Patella S, et al. A meta-analysis of open versus arthroscopic Bankart repair using suture anchors. *Knee Surg Sports Traumatol Arthrosc.* 2010;18(12):1742–1747.
7. Hohmann E, Tetsworth K, Glatt V. Open versus arthroscopic surgical treatment for anterior shoulder dislocation: a comparative systematic review and meta-analysis over the past 20 years. *J Shoulder Elbow Surg.* 2017;26(10):1873–1880.
8. Ialenti MN, Mulvihill JD, Feinstein M, et al. Return to play following shoulder stabilization: a systematic review and meta-analysis. *Orthop J Sports Med.* 2017;5(9):2325967117726055.
9. Fabbriciani C, Milano G, Demontis A, et al. Arthroscopic versus open treatment of Bankart lesion of the shoulder: a prospective randomized study. *Arthroscopy.* 2004;20(5):456–462.
10. Green MR, Christensen KP. Arthroscopic versus open Bankart procedures: a comparison of early morbidity and complications. *Arthroscopy.* 1993;9(4):371–374.
11. Bottoni CR, Wilckens JH, DeBerardino TM, et al. A prospective, randomized evaluation of arthroscopic stabilization versus nonoperative treatment in patients with acute, traumatic, first-time shoulder dislocations. *Am J Sports Med.* 2002;30(4):576–580.
12. Wasserstein DN, Sheth U, Colbenson K, et al. The true recurrence rate and factors predicting recurrent instability after nonsurgical management of traumatic primary anterior shoulder dislocation: a systematic review. *Arthroscopy.* 2016;32(12):2616–2625.
13. Rowe CR, Zarins B, Ciullo JV. Recurrent anterior dislocation of the shoulder after surgical repair. Apparent causes of failure and treatment. *J Bone Joint Surg Am.* 1984;66(2):159–168.
14. Robinson CM, Dobson RJ. Anterior instability of the shoulder after trauma. *J Bone Joint Surg Br.* 2004;86(4):469–479.
15. Cho NS, Hwang JC, Rhee YG. Arthroscopic stabilization in anterior shoulder instability: collision athletes versus noncollision athletes. *Arthroscopy.* 2006;22(9):947–953.
16. Pagnani MJ, Dome DC. Surgical treatment of traumatic anterior shoulder instability in American football players. *J Bone Joint Surg Am.* 2002;84-A(5):711–715.
17. Leroux TS, Saltzman BM, Meyer M, et al. The influence of evidence-based surgical indications and techniques on failure rates after arthroscopic shoulder stabilization in the contact or collision athlete with anterior shoulder instability. *Am J Sports Med.* 2017;45(5):1218–1225.
18. Richards DP, Burkhart SS. Arthroscopic humeral avulsion of the glenohumeral ligaments (HAGL) repair. *Arthroscopy.* 2004;20(suppl 2):134–141.
19. Spang JT, Karas SG. The HAGL lesion: an arthroscopic technique for repair of humeral avulsion of the glenohumeral ligaments. *Arthroscopy.* 2005;21(4):498–502.
20. Brilakis E, Mataragas E, Deligeorgis A, et al. Midterm outcomes of arthroscopic remplissage for the management of recurrent anterior shoulder instability. *Knee Surg Sports Traumatol Arthrosc.* 2016;24(2):593–600.
21. Buza JA, Iyengar JJ, Anakwenze OA, et al. Arthroscopic Hill-Sachs remplissage: a systematic review. *JBJS.* 2014;96(7):549–555.
22. Johnson SM, Robinson CM. Shoulder instability in patients with joint hyperlaxity. *J Bone Joint Surg Am.* 2010;92(6):1545–1557.
23. Balg F, Boileau P. The instability severity index score. A simple pre-operative score to select patients for arthroscopic or open shoulder stabilisation. *J Bone Joint Surg Br.* 2007;89(11):1470–1477.
24. Phadnis J, Arnold C, Elmorsy A, et al. Utility of the instability severity index score in predicting failure after arthroscopic anterior stabilization of the shoulder. *Am J Sports Med.* 2015;43(8):1983–1988.
25. Rouleau DM, Hebert-Davies J, Djahangiri A, et al. Validation of the instability shoulder index score in a multicenter reliability study in 114 consecutive cases. *Am J Sports Med.* 2013;41(2):278–282.
26. Burkhart SS, Debeer JF, Tehrany AM, et al. Quantifying glenoid bone loss arthroscopically in shoulder instability. *Arthroscopy.* 2002;18(5):488–491.
27. Shaha JS, Cook JB, Song DJ, et al. Redefining "critical" bone loss in shoulder instability: functional outcomes worsen with "subcritical" bone loss. *Am J Sports Med.* 2015;43(7):1719–1725.
28. Shin S-J, Kim RG, Jeon YS, et al. Critical value of anterior glenoid bone loss that leads to recurrent glenohumeral instability after arthroscopic Bankart repair. *Am J Sports Med.* 2017;0363546517697963.
29. Longo UG, Loppini M, Rizzello G, et al. Remplissage, humeral osteochondral grafts, weber osteotomy, and shoulder arthroplasty for the management of humeral bone defects in shoulder instability: systematic review and quantitative synthesis of the literature. *Arthroscopy.* 2014;30(12):1650–1666.
30. Yamamoto N, Itoi E, Abe H, et al. Contact between the glenoid and the humeral head in abduction, external rotation, and horizontal extension: a new concept of glenoid track. *J Shoulder Elbow Surg.* 2007;16(5):649–656.
31. Shaha JS, Cook JB, Rowles DJ, et al. Clinical validation of the glenoid track concept in anterior glenohumeral instability. *J Bone Joint Surg Am.* 2016;98(22):1918–1923.
32. Beighton P, Solomon L, Soskolne CL. Articular mobility in an African population. *Ann Rheum Dis.* 1973;32(5):413–418.
33. Robinson CM, Howes J, Murdoch H, et al. Functional outcome and risk of recurrent instability after primary traumatic anterior shoulder dislocation in young patients. *JBJS.* 2006;88(11):2326–2336.
34. Salomonsson B, Von Heine A, Dahlborn M, et al. Bony Bankart is a positive predictive factor after primary shoulder dislocation. *Knee Surg Sports Traumatol Arthrosc.* 2010;18(10):1425–1431.
35. Gagey O, Gagey N. The hyperabduction test. *Bone Joint J.* 2001;83(1):69–74.
36. Bozzo A, Oitment C, Thornley P, et al. Humeral avulsion of the glenohumeral ligament: indications for surgical treatment and outcomes—a systematic review. *Orthop J Sports Med.* 2017;5(8):2325967117723329.
37. Connell DA, Potter HG. Magnetic resonance evaluation of the labral capsular ligamentous complex: a pictorial review. *Australas Radiol.* 1999;43(4):419–426.
38. Connell DA, Potter HG, Wickiewicz TL, et al. Noncontrast magnetic resonance imaging of superior labral lesions. 102 cases confirmed at arthroscopic surgery. *Am J Sports Med.* 1999;27(2):208–213.
39. Bishop JY, Jones GL, Rerko MA, et al. 3-D CT is the most reliable imaging modality when quantifying glenoid bone loss. *Clin Orthop Relat Res.* 2013;471(4):1251–1256.
40. Baudi P, Righi P, Bolognesi D, et al. How to identify and calculate glenoid bone deficit. *Chir Organi Mov.* 2005;90(2):145–152.
41. Huijsmans PE, Haen PS, Kidd M, et al. Quantification of a glenoid defect with three-dimensional computed tomography and magnetic resonance imaging: a cadaveric study. *J Shoulder Elbow Surg.* 2007;16(6):803–809.

42. Sugaya H, Moriishi J, Dohi M, et al. Glenoid rim morphology in recurrent anterior glenohumeral instability. *J Bone Joint Surg Am.* 2003;85-A(5):878–884.

43. Frank RM, Saccomanno MF, McDonald LS, et al. Outcomes of arthroscopic anterior shoulder instability in the beach chair versus lateral decubitus position: a systematic review and meta-regression analysis. *Arthroscopy.* 2014;30(10):1349–1365.

44. Weber SC, Abrams JS, Nottage WM. Complications associated with arthroscopic shoulder surgery. *Arthroscopy.* 2002;18(2):88–95.

45. Dickens JF, Rue JP, Cameron KL, et al. Successful return to sport after arthroscopic shoulder stabilization versus non-operative management in contact athletes with anterior shoulder instability: a prospective multicenter study. *Am J Sports Med.* 2017;45(11):2540–2546.

46. Gigis I, Heikenfeld R, Kapinas A, et al. Arthroscopic versus conservative treatment of first anterior dislocation of the shoulder in adolescents. *J Pediatr Orthop.* 2014;34(4):421–425.

47. Polyzois I, Dattani R, Gupta R, et al. Traumatic first time shoulder dislocation: surgery vs non-operative treatment. *Arch Bone Joint Surg.* 2016;4(2):104–108.

48. Shin S-J, Ko YW, Lee J. Intra-articular lesions and their relation to arthroscopic stabilization failure in young patients with first-time and recurrent shoulder dislocations. *J Shoulder Elbow Surg.* 2016;25(11):1756–1763.

49. Harris JD, Gupta AK, Mall NA, et al. Long-term outcomes after Bankart shoulder stabilization. *Arthroscopy.* 2013;29(5):920–933.

50. Robins RJ, Daruwalla JH, Gamradt SC, et al. Return to play after shoulder instability surgery in National Collegiate Athletic Association Division I Intercollegiate Football Athletes. *Am J Sports Med.* 2017;45(10):2329–2335.

51. Chalmers PN, Mascarenhas R, Leroux T, et al. Do arthroscopic and open stabilization techniques restore equivalent stability to the shoulder in the setting of anterior glenohumeral instability? A systematic review of overlapping meta-analyses. *Arthroscopy.* 2015;31(2):355–363.

52. Freedman KB, Smith AP, Romeo AA, et al. Open Bankart repair versus arthroscopic repair with transglenoid sutures or bioabsorbable tacks for recurrent anterior instability of the shoulder: a 6-month study. *Am J Sports Med.* 2004;32(6):1520–1527.

53. Hobby J, Griffin D, Dunbar M, et al. Is arthroscopic surgery for stabilisation of chronic shoulder instability as effective as open surgery? *Bone Joint J.* 2007;89(9):1188–1196.

54. Lenters TR, Franta AK, Wolf FM, et al. Arthroscopic compared with open repairs for recurrent anterior shoulder instability: a systematic review and meta-analysis of the literature. *JBJS.* 2007;89(2):244–254.

55. Mohtadi NG, Bitar IJ, Sasyniuk TM, et al. Arthroscopic versus open repair for traumatic anterior shoulder instability: a meta-analysis. *Arthroscopy.* 2005;21(6):652–658.

56. Ng C, Bialocerkowski A, Hinman R. Effectiveness of arthroscopic versus open surgical stabilisation for the management of traumatic anterior glenohumeral instability. *Int J Evid Based Healthc.* 2007;5(2):182–207.

57. Pulavarti RS, Symes TH, Rangan A. Surgical interventions for anterior shoulder instability in adults. *Cochrane Database Syst Rev.* 2009(4):CD005077.

58. Boileau P, Villalba M, Hery JY, et al. Risk factors for recurrence of shoulder instability after arthroscopic Bankart repair. *J Bone Joint Surg Am.* 2006;88(8):1755–1763.

59. Ozturk BY, Maak TG, Fabricant P, et al. Return to sports after arthroscopic anterior stabilization in patients aged younger than 25 years. *Arthroscopy.* 2013;29(12):1922–1931.

60. Merolla G, Paladini P, Di Napoli G, et al. Outcomes of arthroscopic Hill-Sachs remplissage and anterior Bankart repair: a retrospective controlled study including ultrasound evaluation of posterior capsulotenodesis and infraspinatus strength assessment. *Am J Sports Med.* 2015;43(2):407–414.

61. Garcia GH, Wu H-H, Liu JN, et al. Outcomes of the remplissage procedure and its effects on return to sports: average 5-year follow-up. *Am J Sports Med.* 2016;44(5):1124–1130.

62. Burkhart SS, De Beer JF. Traumatic glenohumeral bone defects and their relationship to failure of arthroscopic Bankart repairs: significance of the inverted-pear glenoid and the humeral engaging Hill-Sachs lesion. *Arthroscopy.* 2000;16(7):677–694.

63. Magarelli N, Milano G, Sergio P, et al. Intra-observer and interobserver reliability of the 'Pico' computed tomography method for quantification of glenoid bone defect in anterior shoulder instability. *Skeletal Radiol.* 2009;38(11):1071–1075.

10 Posterior Shoulder Stabilization

Drew A. Lansdown, Emily Monroe, Brian T. Feeley, and C. Benjamin Ma

INTRODUCTION

Glenohumeral posterior instability is significantly less common than its anterior counterpart. In most large series, posterior instability accounts approximately 10% of all patients with glenohumeral instability (1–4). However, recent studies in specific populations report up to 24% prevalence in a consecutive series of young active patients undergoing stabilization surgery (5). In a recent multicenter evaluation of the characteristics of posterior labral injuries, most patients were young, male, and participated in contact sports with football being most frequent. The spectrum of disease can range from the locked posterior dislocation to recurrent subluxation events. The etiology of recurrent posterior instability can be from a single isolated traumatic event, repeated microtraumatic stress as seen in offensive linemen, or atraumatic associated with ligamentous laxity. In many cases of posterior instability, there is a component of inferior laxity or multidirectional instability. Anatomic considerations for posterior instability include soft tissue abnormalities, such as a thin or patulous posterior capsule and abnormal version of the glenoid and humeral head.

INDICATIONS AND CONTRAINDICATIONS

Posterior stabilization is indicated in the younger patient with isolated posterior instability following a trial of physical therapy that has not relieved the feelings of pain and instability. The patient should not have global instability and should have a history of an identifiable traumatic event or recurrent lesser traumatic events. Excessive glenoid retroversion is not a contraindication but should be evaluated properly as it will alter the intraoperative plan considerably. Patients with multidirectional instability are generally not considered candidates for surgery, although those who have failed physical therapy and continue to have primarily posterior-inferior instability may benefit from a posterior capsular shift. The decision on whether to perform an open or arthroscopic posterior stabilization is usually determined based on the need to perform a capsular plication. Those patients who require an isolated labral repair are better managed with an arthroscopic posterior stabilization. Patients who have failed arthroscopic management, patients who have excessive posterior laxity on exam, and those with poor capsular tissue when evaluated arthroscopically should be considered for open posterior stabilization. Patients who voluntarily sublux their shoulder posteriorly with their arm at their side by selective muscle activation should not undergo posterior stabilization. Patients with a psychiatric history, active infection, inability to comply with postoperative immobilization and therapy, and secondary gain are not candidates for surgery.

PREOPERATIVE PREPARATION

History

A thorough history and physical exam is important in the evaluation of suspected posterior instability. Patients typically have a traumatic event where the arm was positioned below shoulder level. There is often a posteriorly directed blow to an arm extended or flexed at the elbow. Other patients report repeated minor traumatic events with the arm positioned in a similar manner. Unlike anterior instability where the primary concern is usually apprehension, patients with posterior instability often present with vague activity–related posterior shoulder pain, clicking, or popping. Patients often complain of difficulty pushing open heavy doors or other similar motions.

Physical Examination

The physical examination should document range of motion and must include a complete instability exam. It is vitally important to determine if the posterior instability is isolated or due to a more global instability pattern. Care must be taken to attempt to elucidate signs of multidirectional instability and generalized laxity. The sulcus test can be performed with the arm adducted and in neutral rotation to assess for inferior component of instability generally indicative of more generalized laxity (6). Patients with hyper flexibility of the elbows, wrists, and laxity of the contralateral shoulder should raise the possibility of global laxity, and any surgical procedure should commence only after a complete trial of physical therapy has failed (7).

Isolated posterior instability can be elicited in the office setting. The load and shift test is performed by flexing the arm to 90 degrees, flexing the elbow to 90 degrees, and applying a posterior-directed force while stabilizing the scapula with the other hand. The patient may complain of pain, or subluxation may be evident on exam. The jerk test is performed with an axial posterior load onto an arm flexed at 90 degrees, adducted, and internally rotated; it is positive with reproduction of the instability sensation (Fig. 10-1). It is important to confirm with the patient that the pain felt during this exam is indeed the same pain that is limiting activities as athletes may have multiple causes of shoulder pain. If the load and shift exam does not reproduce the pain experienced by the patient, alternative sources of pathology should be thoroughly explored.

Imaging

Imaging of the shoulder begins with radiographs. An instability series should be obtained, including an AP of the glenohumeral joint in internal rotation, a West Point axillary view, and a scapular Y view. Plain radiographs are usually normal but can identify a reverse Hill-Sachs lesion and can identify bone loss in the posterior glenoid. Magnetic resonance imaging (MRI) is routinely performed at our institution and provides excellent resolution for visualizing the posterior labrum (Fig. 10-2). When evaluating a more chronic injury, we prefer the addition of a gadolinium arthrogram to better delineate labral pathology, glenoid morphology, and capsular volume. Increased glenoid retroversion and findings of glenoid dysplasia are common findings in those with posterior instability (8). Greater posterior capsular volume can be suggestive of posterior or multidirectional instability; however, the reproducibility of measurement methods is limited reliability (8). In cases of suspected bone loss or bony abnormalities, a computerized tomography scan with reconstructions is quite beneficial in surgical planning and can allow for three-dimensional modeling of the glenoid to better appreciate the magnitude of bone loss.

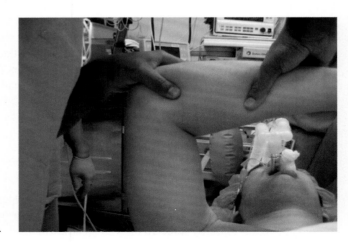

FIGURE 10-1

Jerk test. The "jerk test" is performed with an axial posterior load onto an arm flexed at 90 degrees, adducted, and internally rotated. It is positive with reproduction of the instability sensation.

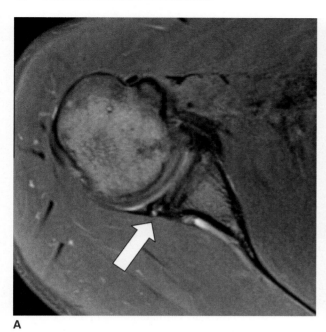
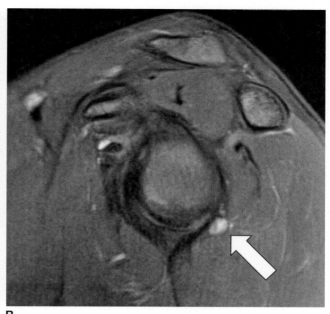

A   B

FIGURE 10-2

A: A fat-suppressed, proton density–weighted axial MRI shows **(A)** posterior labral tear (*arrow*). **B:** On the sagittal oblique image, a labral cyst (*arrow*) is noted adjacent to the posterior labral disruption.

TECHNIQUE

Anesthesia

Our preference is for patients to receive an interscalene nerve block and general anesthesia. The interscalene block is helpful in limiting intraoperative narcotics and decreases postoperative pain and nausea.

Exam Under Anesthesia

Prior to any incision, and before the arm is placed into the arm holder or traction device, it is critical to perform an examination of the shoulder under anesthesia. The examination should be performed on both shoulders to assess asymmetry in the exam compared to the contralateral side. Range of motion is recorded as well. Exam under anesthesia should confirm grade 2 to 3+ posterior instability without any anterior or inferior translation. In some cases of more extensive injury, there will be anterior-inferior instability, and this finding should be noted and addressed surgically.

Patient Positioning

The procedure can be performed in either the beach chair or lateral decubitus position, and this decision is largely surgeon dependent. With the beach chair position, the surgeon can more readily convert to an open procedure if needed, though posterior and inferior glenoid access may be more challenging. The lateral decubitus position can allow for better visualization, easier placement of anchors at the posterior and inferior aspects of the glenoid. For both positions, the patient is first anesthetized supine on a full-length beanbag.

Beach Chair Positioning

The patient is placed in the beach chair position, and the beanbag is inflated to secure the patient in the upright position (Fig. 10-3). The beanbag must be properly folded to leave the entire medial border of the scapula free. This setup allows excellent control of the head and body during the procedure and is easy to adapt for people of any body habitus. Once the beanbag is inflated, the patient and the beanbag are brought laterally to the edge of the bed, allowing complete exposure of the shoulder to the medial border of the scapula. The arm is prepped and draped in the usual sterile fashion. An arm holder is used for both arthroscopic and open stabilizations. It is extremely useful to provide distal traction during the stabilization procedure. A strap is placed around the upper arm to facilitate lateral distraction during the procedure for circumferential access to the glenoid.

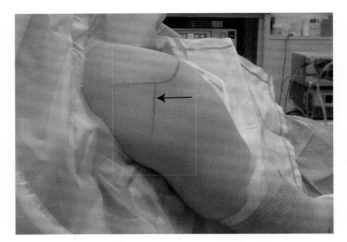

FIGURE 10-3

Patient positioning and surface anatomy. The patient is placed in a beach chair position with the beanbag medial to the medial scapula border. The posterior surface anatomy is marked along the proper portal position (*arrow*).

Lateral Decubitus Positioning

The patient is placed in the lateral decubitus position with the down leg padded to protect the peroneal nerve and an axillary roll placed to protect the axillary nerve. The patient is held securely with the beanbag with the operative scapula free from the beanbag. The patient is rolled back toward the surgeon by 10 to 20 degrees to aid in distraction. The traction device is attached to the bed on the anterior side when the patient is placed lateral. Proper configuration of the traction device allows for intraoperative visualization, and the top beam should be at the level of the humeral head. The arm is prepped and draped in the usual sterile fashion. A well-padded arm sleeve is placed on the arm to allow for distraction, and a strap is placed over the proximal arm to allow for lateral distraction. For shoulder stabilization, the arm will be in approximately 40 degrees of abduction and 10 to 20 degrees of forward flexion with 10 lbs of traction applied.

Portal Placement

The procedure begins with establishing a posterior portal at the soft spot of the glenohumeral joint. This portal is, in general, located 2 cm inferior and 2 cm medial to the posterolateral corner of the acromion. In the lateral position, the portal is often moved slightly higher and more lateral to improve the trajectory into the joint. The 30-degree arthroscope is introduced into the joint, and a thorough diagnostic examination is performed (Fig. 10-4). An anterior portal is established

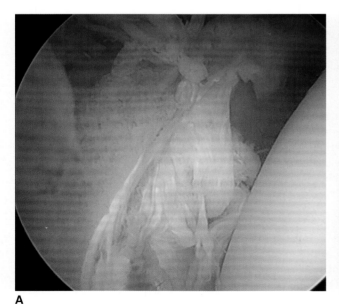

A

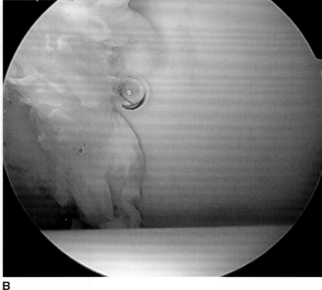

B

FIGURE 10-4

A posterior labral tear is seen through **(A)** posterior viewing portal and **(B)** anterosuperior portal at time of diagnostic arthroscopy, prior to debridement and preparation for repair.

with spinal needle localization in the rotator interval. An arthroscopic probe is used to determine the extent of labral injury. Depending on the location of the lesion, Wissinger rods are used to move the arthroscope to the anterior portal while maintaining the posterior portal location. A 7- to 8-mm cannula is inserted into the posterior cannula to allow for instrument passage. An anterior superolateral portal may be established immediately behind the biceps tendon to allow for viewing while using the standard anterior portal as a working portal for repair. This portal is also established through spinal needle localization, and the arthroscope may be switched to this portal with a Wissinger rod.

Labral Debridement and Glenoid Preparation

Using a combination of a 4-mm motorized shaver and radiofrequency (RF) ablation device, frayed labrum is gently debrided. The labrum may be scarred medially along the glenoid neck. In these cases, a labral elevator is used to elevate to allow for return to its anatomic position (Fig. 10-5). The bony surface of the glenoid is prepared with a combination of a bone-cutting shaver, rasp, or burr, taking care to not injure the remaining labral tissue during this step. The goal is to remove fibrous tissue from the glenoid rim and provide bleeding bone to enhance healing potential of the labrum.

Anchor Placement and Suture Passage

The repair begins at the inferior-most extent of the injury to allow for the repair to reestablish the posterior band of the inferior glenohumeral ligament. We prefer to use all-suture anchors due to their small footprint in the glenoid and excellent pullout strength. Other options, including bio-composite anchors and knotless suture anchors, are also available and can be used with excellent results (9).

A 7 o'clock portal may be established with spinal needle localization to allow for posterior-inferior anchor insertion. This portal is located 4 to 5 cm inferior to the posterolateral corner of the acromion, and a spinal needle is used to ensure appropriate placement and trajectory. This portal passes through the teres minor tendon and is approximately 3 cm from the suprascapular nerve and 4 cm from the axillary nerve (10). The portal is created by making the skin incision but avoid advancing the blade. A switching stick is used to avoid injury to the axillary and nerve, and the cannula can be then inserted over the switching stick. The trocar and drill guide for the anchor can also be inserted percutaneously along this path; however, it is easier to put it through the cannula when multiple anchors are needed. The trocar is malleted gently into bone to ensure it is seated, the pilot hole is drilled, and the anchor is inserted.

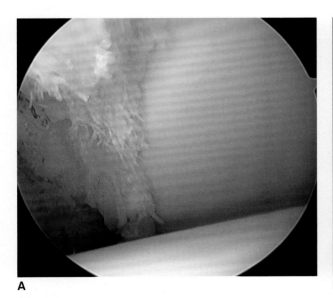
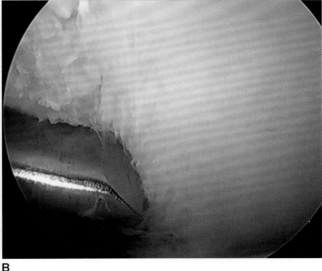

A   **B**

FIGURE 10-5

Fraying of the posterior labrum and synovitis are debrided, leaving **(A)** the prepared posterior labrum prior to repair. **(B)** A labral elevator is used to mobilize the posterior labrum prior to repair.

A curved suture passage device with a passing suture is used through the posterior portal to pass sutures through the capsule and labral tissue (Fig. 10-6). For a left shoulder, a left 45-degree suture lasso is used, and for a right shoulder, a right 45-degree suture lasso is used. The suture lasso is advanced through the posterior portal and passed gently through the posterior labrum at the level of, or just inferior to, the anchor. Again, care is taken not to damage the posterior glenoid cartilage surface. In cases with minor posterior capsular laxity, the lasso can be advanced through the posterior capsule approximately 1 cm lateral to the labrum, then underneath the labrum itself (Fig. 10-6). This will effectively reduce the posterior capsular volume. As the posterior capsule is continuous along the posterior glenoid, different from the anterior capsule where there is a sublabral foramen, the posterior capsule cannot be tightened up by shifting the capsule superiorly commonly done with the anterior capsule. The posterior capsule is tightened up with labral plication with the repair. The monofilament suture is passed into the joint, retrieved with one of the sutures from the anchor, and the suture from the anchor is then passed through the labral tissue.

Both limbs of the suture are then retrieved through the posterior cannula. The suture through the labral tissue serves as the post for the knot to place the knot off the articular surface. The choice of arthroscopic knot is based on surgeon preference. The most important aspect of arthroscopic knot tying

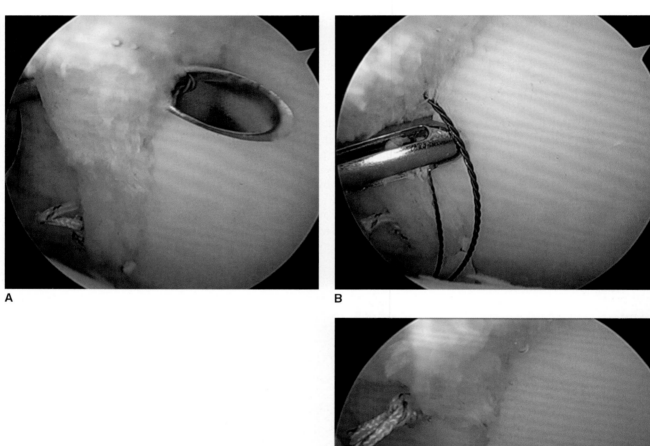

A   **B**

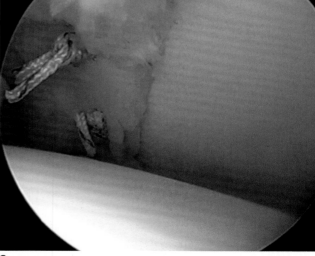

FIGURE 10-6

While viewing from the anterosuperior portal, **(A)** a suture lasso is passed around the torn posterior labrum. **(B)** The drill trocar is inserted through the posterior portal to place the all-suture anchor, followed by suture shuttling and knot tying to **(C)** reapproximate the posterior labrum.

C

is the use of a knot that the surgeon can reproducibly secure without difficulty. We prefer an alternating half-hitch knot. Two simple sutures are thrown, and the post is pulled upon until the knot advances down to the level of the labrum. If the anchor was correctly placed, this reduces the labrum to the glenoid rim. A knot pusher is then advanced, and the knot is secured with the knot medial to the repair so as not to put the knot on the articular surface. We place a total of six knots for each suture anchor.

A total of two to four anchors are placed for most posterior repairs, dependent upon the extent of the labral injury. The repair proceeds in the superior direction. At the completion of the repair, a probe is used to test the stability of the repair.

Open Posterior Stabilization

In cases where open posterior stabilization is to be performed, the diagnostic arthroscopy is performed quickly, the instruments are removed, and the open procedure is started. A vertical skin incision is planned, parallel to the glenohumeral joint. The line for the glenohumeral joint usually is directly posterior to the AC joint. The incision is started at the level of the scapular spine superiorly, incorporates the posterior arthroscopic portal, and is continued distally for approximately 7 to 9 cm to the axillary crease.

The dissection is sharply taken down to the level of the deltoid fascia, and skin flaps are elevated medially and laterally. The deltoid fascia is split in line with its fibers that typically run slightly medial to lateral. This split should be directly posterior to the glenohumeral joint. Once the entire deltoid is spilt, deep retractors are placed, exposing the infraspinatus superiorly and the teres minor inferiorly. Internal rotation of the shoulder generally facilitates identification of the infraspinatus and teres minor (Fig. 10-7). There is typically a heavy layer of fascia covering these muscles, and the infraspinatus is identified as the bipennate muscle with a yellow strip of fat that runs between its two heads. The fascia is incised longitudinally in this area from the lateral tendinous portion to the medial aspect of the wound. The suprascapular nerve runs medially, approximately 1.5 cm from the glenoid, so dissection should stop short of this point. The infraspinatus is carefully elevated off the capsule with a Cobb elevator and sharp dissection. Care should be taken to preserve the capsule in order to facilitate repair and capsulorrhaphy at the end of the procedure. At this point, it is important to expose the entire posterior capsule. This is most readily facilitated with thorough blunt dissection of the infraspinatus off the capsule and placement of curved retractors superiorly and inferiorly over the glenohumeral joint (Fig. 10-8).

Capsulotomy

The capsular incision is usually performed with a T-shaped medial incision. A medial based capsulorrhaphy is used more commonly for posterior stabilization as it is not easy to detach and repair the infraspinatus tendon. The tendon is quite short, and it is more difficult to repair well. A Bovie device

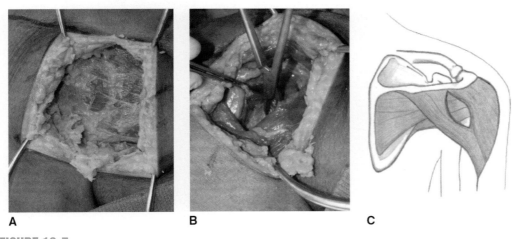

A   B   C

FIGURE 10-7

A: Following the longitudinal incision, the deltoid muscle is identified. Gelpi retractors are placed in the skin to facilitate exposure. **B:** The deltoid is splint in line with its fibers, exposing the infraspinatus deep to the deltoid. **C:** Deltoid split demonstrating exposure to the infraspinatus.

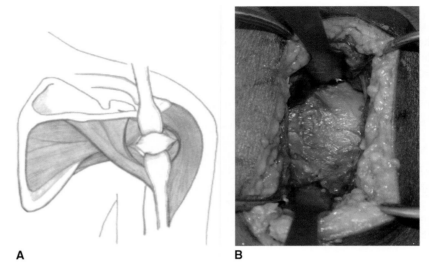

FIGURE 10-8

A: Split of the infraspinatus along the fat stripe, exposing the capsule deep to the rotator cuff muscle. **B:** Once the capsule is exposed, deep retractors are placed on either side of the humeral head in order to facilitate exposure of the capsule and labrum.

or marking pen is used to mark the capsulotomy incision site. The vertical incision is placed just lateral to the capsular attachment on the glenoid, and the longitudinal incision is placed at the equator of the glenohumeral joint. The flaps are tagged with suture and retracted superiorly and inferiorly to expose the joint (Fig. 10-9).

Labral Repair

In many cases, the posterior labrum will be intact. However, in some cases, the initial arthroscopy will have determined that a labral repair is necessary in addition to a capsulorrhaphy. The injured labrum is elevated and mobilized free of the glenoid. The glenoid neck is roughened to provide a bleeding surface. The hole for the anchor is placed at the cartilage border, and the anchor is placed.

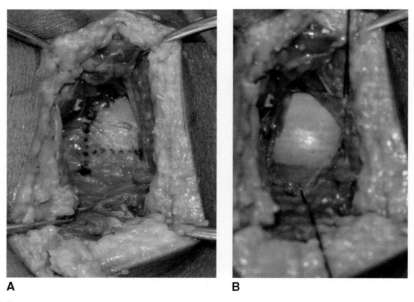

FIGURE 10-9

A: With the capsule exposed, a medial T-shaped incision is planned. The longitudinal incision is just lateral to the glenoid and labral rim, and the transverse incision is planned with the incision along the inferior one-third of the humeral head. **B:** Capsulotomy has been performed, and the leading edges of the capsule have been tagged.

Nonabsorbable suture is placed around the labrum, and the labrum is secured to the glenoid rim. The knot is tied so that it does not interfere with the glenohumeral articulation. We typically place two to three anchors for a posterior repair (Fig. 10-10).

Capsulorrhaphy

The arm is placed in 20 degrees of abduction, and a medially based capsular shift is performed. The inferior flap is advanced superiorly to the superior border of the glenoid and labrum. It is reapproximated to the capsulolabral complex. The superior flap is then folded inferiorly, effectively augmenting the superior flap. The longitudinal incision is imbricated with nonabsorbable suture to reinforce the repair (Fig. 10-11).

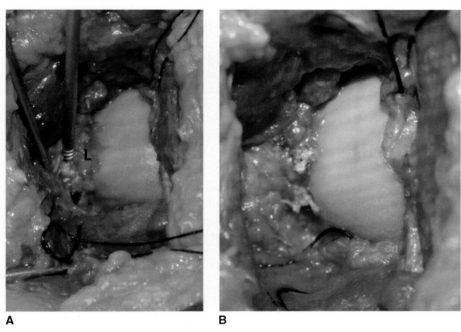

A   B

FIGURE 10-10

A: Placement of anchors at the bony insertion of the glenoid after the labrum (L) has been elevated. **B:** Two anchors placed in the labrum, reattaching the labrum to bone.

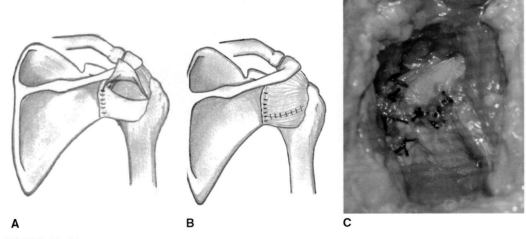

A   B   C

FIGURE 10-11

A: The capsular closure is performed by bringing the inferior limb superiorly and attaching it to the medial capsulotomy with interrupted sutures. **B:** The superior limb is then pulled inferiorly to decrease the space in the capsule. **C:** Completed capsulotomy with the final longitudinal and transverse sutures.

Augmentation

In rare cases such as revision surgery for posterior instability, a very thin patulous capsule, it may be necessary to augment the capsulorrhaphy. Soft tissue augmentation of the capsular repair can be performed by vertically incising the infraspinatus and securing it to the capsule with use of the capsule repair sutures. Alternatively, an Achilles tendon allograft can be used to augment the posterior capsule, although long-term data utilizing this in clinical practice are not available.

Bone Loss/Retroversion

Posterior instability resulting from excessive glenoid retroversion is rare but is important to identify preoperatively as soft tissue procedures alone may result in continued posterior instability (11). After the posterior glenoid has been exposed, a burr is used to abrade the posterior cortex of the glenoid and provide a fresh bed of bleeding bone. Ipsilateral iliac crest, distal tibial allograft, or preformed allograft bone block from femoral head specimens may be used (12–14). The graft should measure approximately 4 × 2.5 cm. The graft and glenoid neck are predrilled prior to capsule repair, and the capsule is interposed between the bone block and the glenoid rim. The bone block is placed on the posteroinferior quadrant of the glenoid using bicortical screws parallel to the articular surface (Fig. 10-12). Alternatively, a glenoid-opening wedge osteotomy can be performed in those patients with excessive (>10 degrees) glenoid retroversion (15,16). However, this operation is technically difficult with the proximity of the suprascapular nerve, and bony fixation can be challenging.

Closure

The wound is closed in layers, with a running 2-0 vicryl used to loosely close the infraspinatus fascia and the deltoid fascia. The skin is closed with 2-0 vicryl in the deep dermal layer and a running 2-0 Prolene subcuticular stitch. Sterile dressings are applied, and the patient is placed in an abduction orthosis that maintains slight abduction and neutral rotation. Drains are not typically used.

Arthroscopic Posterior Bone Block Procedure

Advances in surgical techniques also allow for performing a posterior bony augmentation procedure arthroscopically (17). This can avoid a posterior incision and allow for preservation of the rotator cuff tendons. A 2 × 1 × 1-cm bone block is harvested from the anterior iliac crest, and two 3.2-mm pilot holes are drilled and tapped in the center of the graft. Three primary portals are utilized for preparation and graft passage: the standard posterior portal ("A" portal), a posterosuperior trans-infraspinatus portal ("B" portal), and a rotator interval portal anteriorly ("E" portal). While viewing from the anterior portal, the capsule and labrum are mobilized off the glenoid neck with an elevator and RF device. This dissection is continued until the infraspinatus and teres minor muscle fibers are visible. A bur is used to debride the glenoid rim back to a flat, bleeding surface. The A portal is enlarged to 2 to 3 cm, and a double-barrel cannula is used to pass the graft through the posterior

FIGURE 10-12

A: Axillary lateral demonstrating significant bone loss along the posterior rim of the glenoid. **B:** Schematic of iliac crest bone graft used to augment the posterior glenoid. The bone graft is secured with 4.5-mm partially threaded cancellous screws to compress the graft to the posterior glenoid.

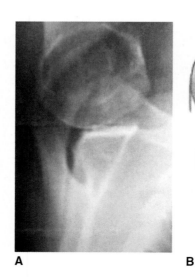
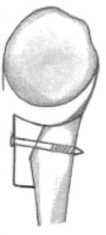

A   **B**

muscle split and capsulotomy. The cancellous surface of the bone block is positioned next to the glenoid rim, and the block is fixed provisionally with two 1.48-mm K-wires. The graft is then fixed with two 3.5-mm partially threaded screws. The inferior screw is fixed first, and the graft is rotated if needed prior to final fixation of the superior screw. If there is remaining capsule or labrum that would benefit from repair, this tissue is fixed to the periphery of the bone block with suture anchor fixation.

PEARLS AND PITFALLS

Pearls

1. Complete mobilization of the injured posterior labrum will allow for anatomic repair to the glenoid rim.
2. The familiarity with accessory portals and percutaneous paths for anchor insertion enables the surgeon to access all quadrants of the glenoid for instrumentation and repair.
3. Preparation of the glenoid rim creates a fresh bony surface to enhance labral healing.
4. Stable knot tying or use of knotless suture anchors provides for secure capsulolabral fixation.
5. Capsulorrhaphy is performed with plication of the capsule, not by superior shift as seen for anterior stabilization surgery.

Pitfalls

1. Inadequate preoperative planning or incomplete diagnostic exam may lead to the failure to recognize specific factors, such as glenoid bone loss or excessive glenoid retroversion, that predispose patients to higher failure rates after arthroscopic posterior stabilization.
2. Improper angle trajectory may lead to chondral damage at the glenoid or humeral head.

POSTOPERATIVE MANAGEMENT

Physical therapy is reviewed preoperatively to counsel the patient on the postoperative precautions to protect the repair. We typically will place the patient in a gunslinger sling to immobilize the arm in external rotation and avoid internal rotation. Passive abduction and forward flexion is allowed daily out of the sling with limits of forward flexion to 120 degrees and internal rotation to 30 degrees. The sling is worn for a majority of the time until postoperative week 6. After week 6, active and passive range of motion is initiated with a goal of 90% of expected range of motion by week 12. Progressive resistance exercises and strengthening exercises for the rotator cuff and scapular stabilizing muscles are added after range of motion improves. Patients can expect return to full activities at 7 to 9 months following surgery in most cases.

COMPLICATIONS

Complications after posterior instability surgery remain unlikely but are important to consider. As discussed in the Results section, one of the primary risks with arthroscopic and open posterior stabilization is recurrent instability, in the range of 8% to 19% (18). Infection is reported at <1% of cases for shoulder arthroscopy (19). Complications may also be associated with patient positioning, including decreased cerebrovascular perfusion in the beach chair position and down-leg neuropraxia in the lateral position (19).

RESULTS

With the evolution in techniques and instrumentation, posterior shoulder instability can reliably be addressed with arthroscopic stabilization. In a prospective study of 183 athletes and 200 shoulders with posterior instability, Bradley et al. reported excellent results at a mean of 36 months after surgical treatment (6). Postoperative American Shoulder and Elbow Surgeons (ASES) scores averaged 85.1 points and return to play rates of >90%. DeLong et al. performed a meta-analysis for outcomes after posterior stabilization procedures and included 27 studies on arthroscopic stabilization (18). These studies comprised 817 shoulders in 773 patients with an average age of 24.5 years. The rate of recurrent instability was 8.1% overall, with the lowest rate (5.1%) seen in contact athletes and highest rate (12.1%) seen in throwing athletes. The mean postoperative ASES score for studies that reported this outcome was 89.7 points. Return to sport was 91.8%, with satisfactory range of motion in 90.4% of patients and overall satisfaction rate of 93.8%.

The outcomes following open posterior shoulder stabilization in general have been quite good. Most studies report good to excellent results in 75% to 90% of patients, with recurrence rates between 7% and 30% (20–24). Bottoni et al. reported on 31 patients who underwent posterior stabilization, 12 of which were open procedures (20). All patients suffered a traumatic event causing their posterior instability. At an average follow-up of 40 months, there was one recurrence each in the open and arthroscopic group. Eleven of the twelve patients (91%) who underwent open posterior stabilization rated their outcome as good or excellent. Wolf et al. described the largest series to date of open posterior shoulder stabilizations (24). At an average of 7.6 years, 32 of 44 (72%) rated their outcomes as good to excellent, and the recurrence rate was 13%. The outcomes following posterior bone block augmentation are promising as well (11). A recent study retrospectively reviewed 21 shoulders that underwent glenoid augmentation at a mean of 6 years. All patients reported their subjective outcomes as good or excellent, and 15 of the 21 patients returned to their preinjury level of sports. Three patients were considered failures, two with posterior apprehension, and one with recurrent posterior instability.

DeLong et al. reviewed 26 level 4 studies, including 321 shoulders treated with open posterior stabilization, in their meta-analysis (18). The recurrence rate was 19.4% with patient satisfaction of 86.1% and return to sport rates of 66.4%. While these rates are inferior to those reported in arthroscopic stabilization, these studies were noncomparative and those patients with open procedures may have had different pathology compared to patients treated arthroscopically. The advantages of arthroscopic posterior stabilization include minimizing disruption to the posterior rotator cuff and deltoid, which may also be responsible for these observed differences. Further high-level studies are needed on this topic to clarify surgical indications and treatment recommendations.

Wellmann et al. has reported initial results with the arthroscopic posterior bone block technique in addition to posterior capsular repair (25). A total of 24 shoulders were evaluated at 26 months after surgery. The recurrence rate was 12.5% (3/24 shoulders), which is similar to prior reports from open posterior bone block procedures. The Western Ontario Shoulder Instability (WOSI) score improved to 66% postoperatively, and the Rowe score improved by 25 points. Hardware removal was frequently performed (16/24 shoulders) due to irritation from the screws. This early report shows that the arthroscopic posterior bone block technique may provide results that are in line with open bone block procedures, though further research is needed to clarify the role of this newer procedure.

SUMMARY

Recurrent posterior instability is much less common than anterior shoulder instability. The diagnosis can be elusive, but a thorough history and physical examination combined with the appropriate imaging modalities should lead to an accurate diagnosis in a majority of cases. In those patients who do not improve with a trial of physical therapy, posterior stabilization offers a treatment option with reliable outcomes. Whether to proceed with arthroscopic or open stabilization is based on the patients' symptoms, exam under anesthesia, and diagnostic arthroscopy, though the current literature and technical limitations support arthroscopic treatment. Isolated labral tears or labral tears with minimal capsular laxity can be treated arthroscopically. The posterior approach to the shoulder is straightforward and provides excellent access to the posterior glenohumeral joint. Repair of the labrum in combination with a posterior capsulorrhaphy will restore stability to the shoulder.

REFERENCES

1. Blomquist J, Solheim E, Liavaag S, et al. Shoulder instability surgery in Norway: the first report from a multicenter register, with 1-year follow-up. *Acta Orthop.* 2012;83(2):165–170.
2. Krøner K, Lind T, Jensen J. The epidemiology of shoulder dislocations. *Arch Orthop Trauma Surg.* 1989;108(5):288–290.
3. Owens BD, Campbell SE, Cameron KL. Risk factors for posterior shoulder instability in young athletes. *Am J Sports Med.* 2013;41(11):2645–2649.
4. Owens BD, Duffey ML, Nelson BJ, et al. The incidence and characteristics of shoulder instability at the United States Military Academy. *Am J Sports Med.* 2007;35(7):1168–1173.
5. Song DJ, Cook JB, Krul KP, et al. High frequency of posterior and combined shoulder instability in young active patients. *J Shoulder Elbow Surg.* 2015;24(2):186–190.
6. Bradley JP, McClincy MP, Arner JW, et al. Arthroscopic capsulolabral reconstruction for posterior instability of the shoulder: a prospective study of 200 shoulders. *Am J Sports Med.* 2013;41(9):2005–2014.
7. Beighton P, Solomon L, Soskolne CL. Articular mobility in an African population. *Ann Rheum Dis.* 1973;32(5):413–418.

8. Galvin JW, Parada SA, Li X, et al. Critical findings on magnetic resonance arthrograms in posterior shoulder instability compared with an age-matched controlled cohort. *Am J Sports Med.* 2016;44(12):3222–3229.

9. Mazzocca AD, Chowaniec D, Cote MP, et al. Biomechanical evaluation of classic solid and novel all-soft suture anchors for glenoid labral repair. *Arthroscopy.* 2012;28(5):642–648.

10. Davidson PA, Rivenburgh DW. The 7-o'clock posteroinferior portal for shoulder arthroscopy. *Am J Sports Med.* 2002;30(5):693–696.

11. Servien E, Walch G, Cortes ZE, et al. Posterior bone block procedure for posterior shoulder instability. *Knee Surg Sports Traumatol Arthrosc.* 2007;15(9):1130–1136.

12. Barbier O, Ollat D, Marchaland J-P, et al. Iliac bone-block autograft for posterior shoulder instability. *Orthop Traumatol Surg Res.* 2009;95(2):100–107.

13. Millett PJ, Schoenahl J-Y, Register B, et al. Reconstruction of posterior glenoid deficiency using distal tibial osteoarticular allograft. *Knee Surg Sports Traumatol Arthrosc.* 2013;21(2):445–449.

14. Smucny M, Miniaci A. A new option for glenoid reconstruction in recurrent anterior shoulder instability. *Am J Orthop.* 2017;46(4):199–202.

15. Graichen H, Koydl P, Zichner L. Effectiveness of glenoid osteotomy in atraumatic posterior instability of the shoulder associated with excessive retroversion and flatness of the glenoid. *Int Orthop.* 1999;23(2):95–99.

16. Hawkins RH. Glenoid osteotomy for recurrent posterior subluxation of the shoulder: assessment by computed axial tomography. *J Shoulder Elbow Surg.* 1996;5(5):393–400.

17. Schwartz DG, Goebel S, Piper K, et al. Arthroscopic posterior bone block augmentation in posterior shoulder instability. *J Shoulder Elbow Surg.* 2013;22(8):1092–1101.

18. DeLong JM, Jiang K, Bradley JP. Posterior instability of the shoulder: a systematic review and meta-analysis of clinical outcomes. *Am J Sports Med.* 2015;43(7):1805–1817.

19. Weber SC, Abrams JS, Nottage WM. Complications associated with arthroscopic shoulder surgery. *Arthroscopy.* 2002;18(2):88–95.

20. Bottoni CR, Franks BR, Moore JH, et al. Operative stabilization of posterior shoulder instability. *Am J Sports Med.* 2005;33(7):996–1002.

21. Fronek J, Warren R, Bowen M. Posterior subluxation of the glenohumeral joint. *JBJS.* 1989;71(2):205–216.

22. Tibone J, Ting A. Capsulorrhaphy with a staple for recurrent posterior subluxation of the shoulder. *JBJS.* 1990;72(7):999–1002.

23. Tibone JE, Bradley JP. The treatment of posterior subluxation in athletes. *Clin Orthop Relat Res.* 1993;291:124–137.

24. Wolf BR, Strickland S, Williams RJ, et al. Open posterior stabilization for recurrent posterior glenohumeral instability. *J Shoulder Elbow Surg.* 2005;14(2):157–164.

25. Wellmann M, Pastor MF, Ettinger M, et al. Arthroscopic posterior bone block stabilization-early results of an effective procedure for the recurrent posterior instability. *Knee Surg Sports Traumatol Arthrosc.* 2018;26(1):292–298.

11 Open Anterior Shoulder Stabilization

Champ L. Baker III

INDICATIONS

Anterior shoulder instability is a common problem among contact and collision athletes. Several studies have detailed high rates of recurrence in young, active individuals following anterior shoulder dislocation (1–4). Surgical treatment is typically recommended in these individuals secondary to high rates of recurrence and risk of progressive bone loss and additional pathology with subsequent events. Nonoperative management may be initially attempted, especially in season; however, the athlete remains at risk for a subsequent instability event (5,6). In one study, 33 of 45 collegiate athletes (73%) were able to return to their sport for either all of part of the season after sustaining an anterior subluxation or dislocation. Of those athletes who returned, 21 of 33 (64%) had subsequent recurrent instability (5). Older, less active individuals who have persistent symptoms after appropriate conservative treatment may also be candidates for operative treatment for recurrent anterior shoulder instability.

Several surgical techniques have been described for the management of anterior shoulder instability including arthroscopic Bankart repair, open anterior capsulorrhaphy, and bone block procedures. Open anatomic anterior stabilization procedures have historically been considered the gold standard in the treatment of anterior instability; however, as arthroscopic techniques have continued to improve and evolve, recent studies have demonstrated similar outcomes between the two approaches (7). Appropriate patient selection is critical for optimal outcomes. Balg and Boileau (8) prospectively reviewed their series of 131 patients with recurrent anterior instability treated with an arthroscopic Bankart repair. Six risk factors were associated with failure: patient age <20 years, competitive sports participation, involvement in a contact or forced overhead sport, shoulder hyperlaxity, the presence of a Hill-Sachs lesion on an AP radiograph in external rotation, and loss of normal glenoid contour on an AP radiograph. The authors developed the instability severity index score as a score from 0 to 10 representing these risk factors with a score of 0 indicating no risk factors. Patients with a score of ≤6 were found to have a recurrence rate of 10%. Patients with a score of >6 had a recurrence rate of 70% with an arthroscopic technique. An open stabilization procedure was recommended by the authors for these high-risk patients (8).

Open anterior stabilization should be considered over arthroscopic management in contact and collision athletes especially in the presence of bone loss, patients with multiple dislocations with potentially poor-quality capsulolabral tissue, and patients who have failed a prior technically well-done arthroscopic repair (9,10). Select glenoid fractures and the presence of a HAGL lesion are also relative indications for open repair based upon the treating surgeon's experience and ability. The presence of significant glenoid bone defects, Hill-Sachs lesions, or bipolar bone loss has demonstrated significantly higher failure rates after arthroscopic procedures (11). Open anterior stabilization procedures with Bankart repair and capsular shift have demonstrated good success even in the presence of glenoid defects up to 25% (10,12,13).

CONTRAINDICATIONS

Although there have been reports detailing success in treating patients with open capsular repair even in the presence of significant bone defects, the presence of glenoid bone loss >25% should be addressed with a bone block augmentation procedure. In the overhead throwing athlete, restoration of motion and preservation of external rotation are of utmost importance. Arthroscopic stabilization should be considered in this group of patients over open techniques to minimize potential motion loss. If an open procedure is performed, the use of a subscapularis split and horizontal capsulotomy has been shown to minimize range of motion loss and effectively return a cohort of overhead athletes back to sport (14).

PREOPERATIVE PREPARATION

A careful and thorough preoperative evaluation including history, physical examination, advanced imaging, and examination under anesthesia is critical to choose the appropriate surgical procedure in the patient with recurrent, anterior glenohumeral instability. A detailed history includes initial injury mechanism consisting of arm position, degree of trauma, and need for formal reduction. Onset of symptoms without significant trauma suggests a multidirectional instability component. The clinician should note the number and frequency of episodes. Increasing frequency with minimal trauma or during sleep suggests significant bone loss. Bilateral shoulders should be inspected for atrophy, active and passive range of motion, strength testing, and provocative maneuvers. Increased passive abduction beyond 90 degrees is suggestive of hyperlaxity of the inferior capsule. A large sulcus sign recreating symptoms reflects multidirectional instability. A sulcus sign persisting in external rotation indicates rotator interval insufficiency. Positive apprehension in abduction and external rotation combined with a positive relocation test is diagnostic of anterior shoulder instability. Load and shift testing assesses anteroposterior laxity of the shoulder. The arm position that recreates symptoms should be noted. Symptomatology in shoulder flexion, adduction, and internal rotation should raise suspicion for posterior shoulder instability that can be further evaluated with jerk and Kim tests. Instability symptoms in midrange abduction should raise suspicion for bone loss. Rotator cuff integrity should be assessed, in particular the subscapularis with belly press and bear hug maneuvers.

Plain radiographs include AP, axillary, and Y outlet views (Fig. 11-1). Additional radiographs include a Stryker notch view to evaluate for a Hill-Sachs lesion and a West Point view for improved visualization of the anterior glenoid rim. MRI is useful to identify the variety of pathologies produced from instability events including Bankart lesions, HAGL lesions, ALPSA lesions, associated rotator cuff injuries, posterior labral tears, and SLAP tears. If there is concern for significant bone loss by clinical history or if any bone loss is visualized on radiographs, then a CT scan should be obtained. A three-dimensional (3D) CT reconstruction with humeral head subtraction helps to quantify glenoid bone loss. The CT scan can also quantify bipolar bone loss with the concept of the glenoid track (15). The glenoid track is the area on the humeral head in contact with the glenoid as

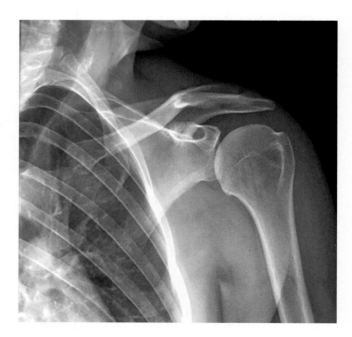

FIGURE 11-1

AP radiograph of the left shoulder demonstrating loss of normal glenoid contour.

the shoulder elevates in a position of abduction and external rotation. The width of the glenoid track decreases with progressive glenoid bone loss. If the entire Hill-Sachs lesion lies within the glenoid track, it is considered on track and will not engage. If the Hill-Sachs lesion extends medially beyond the medial margin of the glenoid track, it is considered off track and is at high risk for engagement and dislocation (15,16).

TECHNIQUE

Prior to transport to the operative suite, the correct shoulder is marked and identified by the operating surgeon. An interscalene block is administered. After induction of general anesthesia, an examination under anesthesia with the patient supine is performed of both the operative and unaffected shoulders. Anterior, posterior, and inferior glenohumeral translation is graded according to the criteria of Altchek et al. (17) The head of the bed is elevated approximately 30 degrees, and pillows are placed underneath the thighs to keep the knees and hips in a slightly flexed position. Two folded surgical towels are placed behind the scapula for support. The entire upper extremity is then prepped and draped in standard fashion with the arm free. A well-padded and well-draped Mayo stand is used for arm support. Bony landmarks of the clavicle and coracoid process are palpated and outlined with a marking pen.

The incision is placed directly over the deltopectoral groove starting adjacent to the coracoid process and progressing distally. Two Gelpi self-retaining retractors are inserted to place tension on the tissues while exposing the fascia. Thick skin flaps are developed. After identification of the fat stripe localizing the deltopectoral interval, the cephalic vein is located and mobilized laterally with the deltoid (Fig. 11-2). The deltopectoral interval is developed with a combination of blunt

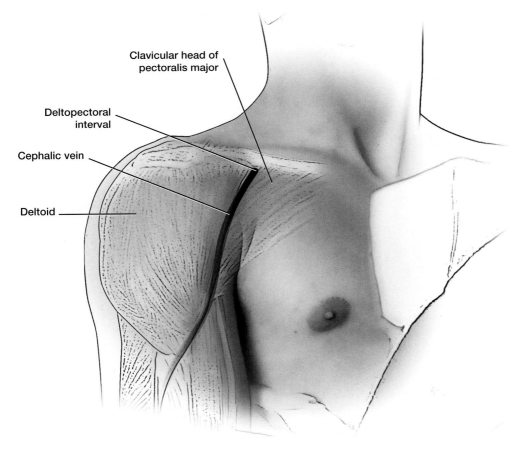

FIGURE 11-2

Deltopectoral interval with cephalic vein marking interval.

digital dissection and use of Bovie electrocautery. The Gelpi retractors are adjusted and placed in the interval as the exposure progresses. The falciform ligament of the pectoralis major is divided to allow further exposure inferiorly. The subdeltoid plane is bluntly developed thoroughly to improve deltoid mobilization laterally. A pointed Hohmann retractor is placed on top of the coracoacromial ligament for visualization superiorly. There is typically a group of vessels at the level of the coracoid process going across to the medial aspect of the deltoid that should be ligated to allow complete opening of the deltopectoral interval. From its attachment site of the palpable coracoid process, the white tendinous stripe of the short head of the biceps and the more lateral red muscular stripe of the short head are identified. The clavipectoral fascia is incised with Bovie electrocautery just lateral to the short head of the conjoined tendon. This incision is made proximally from adjacent to the coracoid to distally at the level of the pectoralis insertion. The surgeon then places an index finger underneath the conjoint tendon medially along the anterior surface of the subscapularis tendon to sweep downward to palpate and localize the axillary nerve. A Kolbel self-retaining retractor is then placed medially to retract the conjoint tendon and laterally to retract the deltoid. Care is taken to protect the musculocutaneous nerve when placing the medial Kolbel blade and to avoid excessive traction. The Kolbel retractor handle is then secured with a towel clip to Coban wrapped around the patient's brachium.

The subscapularis is now thoroughly exposed with the arm externally rotated approximately 65 degrees (Fig. 11-3). At the subscapularis inferior border, the anterior humeral circumflex artery and its venae comitantes are localized. Laterally, the tendinous attachment on the lesser tuberosity is palpated. The rotator interval defines the superior border of the subscapularis. A subscapularis

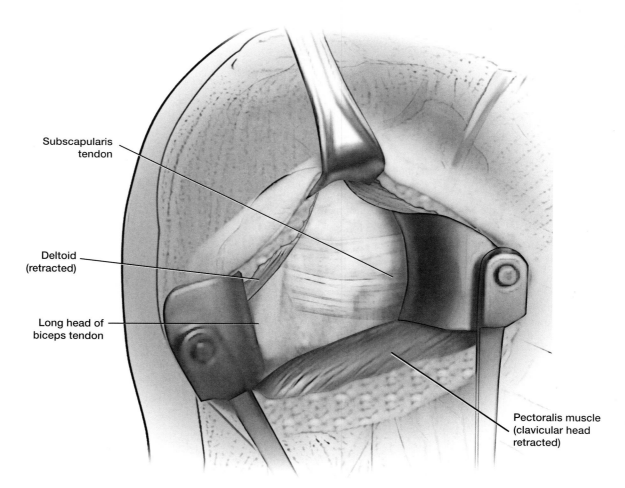

Subscapularis
tendon

Deltoid
(retracted)

Long head of
biceps tendon

Pectoralis muscle
(clavicular head
retracted)

FIGURE 11-3

Subscapularis is exposed completely.

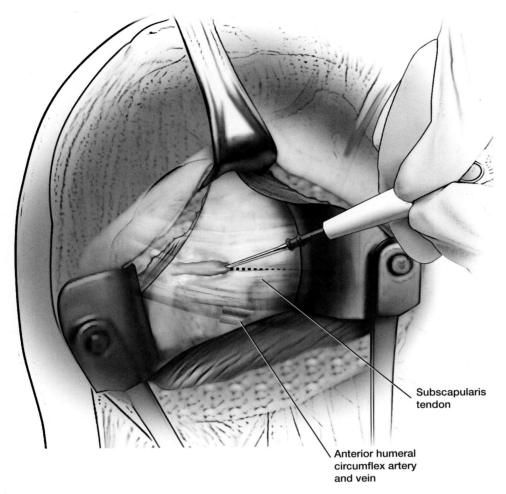

Subscapularis
tendon

Anterior humeral
circumflex artery
and vein

FIGURE 11-4

Transverse incision made in the subscapularis at the junction between superior two thirds and inferior one third.

split approach is then performed as initially described by Montgomery and Jobe (14). A transverse incision is made in the subscapularis in line with its fibers with electrocautery between the upper two thirds and lower one third of the tendon (Fig. 11-4). Care is taken not to inadvertently penetrate too deeply and incise the capsule at this stage. This split incision is taken from the insertion laterally to overlying the glenoid neck medially. The subscapularis is carefully dissected from the underlying capsule with the use of Freer and key elevators. It is easier to start the separation more medially where the subscapularis and glenohumeral capsule have a more anatomic, natural separation. Once the overlying subscapularis has been completely separated from the capsule, Gelpi self-retaining retractors are placed between the superior and inferior subscapularis components. A three-pronged pitchfork retractor is placed medially along the anterior glenoid neck to complete the exposure of the capsule. The capsule is then incised horizontally in line with the previous subscapularis split just superior to the thickening of the anterior band of the inferior glenohumeral ligament (Fig. 11-5). Care is taken not to go too deep and injure the anterior labrum. Traction sutures are placed with braided No. 2 suture in the superior and inferior capsular limbs. A ringed Fukuda retractor is then placed intra-articularly between the posterior glenoid and humeral head for final exposure. The anterior glenoid rim is inspected for the presence of a Bankart lesion. The anteroinferior capsulolabrum is dissected free, elevated, and mobilized from the anterior glenoid rim. The anterior glenoid rim and neck are prepared to a bleeding bed with the use of a small round burr with care taken not to remove too much bone. Typically, three biocomposite suture anchors loaded with braided No. 2 suture are placed on the anterior glenoid rim as far laterally as possible (Fig. 11-6). These anchors are placed

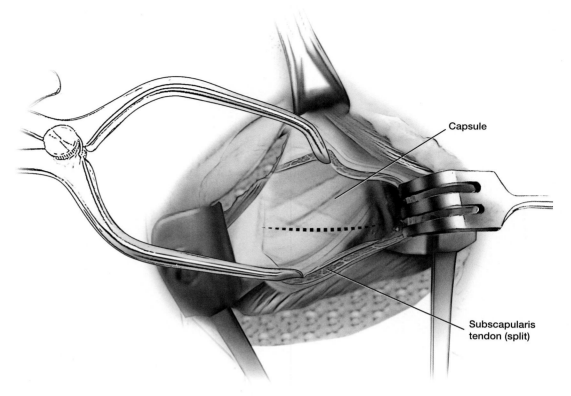

FIGURE 11-5

A horizontal capsulotomy exposes the Bankart lesion.

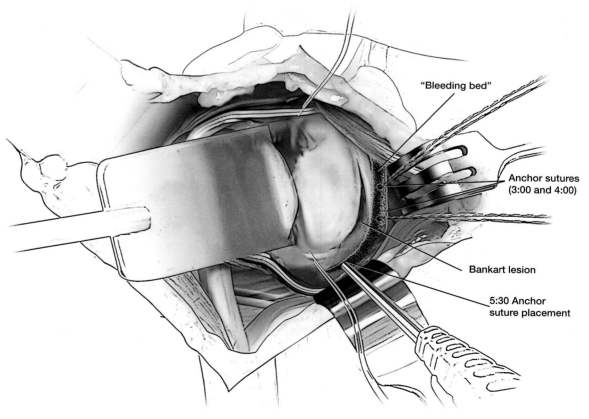

FIGURE 11-6

Typically, three suture anchors are placed along the lateral glenoid rim.

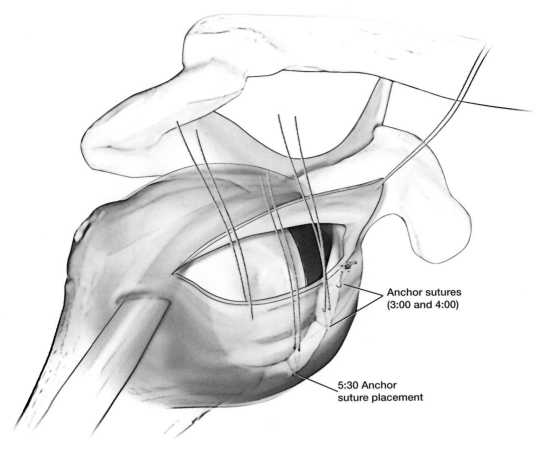

Anchor sutures
(3:00 and 4:00)

5:30 Anchor
suture placement

FIGURE 11-7

Sutures from the inferior and middle anchor are passed through the inferior capsular limb in mattress fashion.
Sutures from the superior anchor are passed through the superior capsular limb.

at the 5:30, 4 o'clock, and 3 o'clock positions for a right shoulder. A double-loaded suture anchor is utilized for the most inferior anchor, while the remaining anchors are single loaded. Starting with the most inferior anchor, sutures are loaded onto a Davis Tonsil needle as they are passed underneath the labrum and through the inferior capsular limb in horizontal mattress fashion. Tension is placed on the traction sutures in the inferior capsular limb to help shift the tissue in a superior direction. Care is taken to shift the capsule superiorly but not medially to prevent restriction of external rotation. Sutures are passed with the arm in approximately 45 degrees of abduction and 45 degrees of external rotation. After both sets of sutures from the inferior anchor are placed, the sutures from the middle anchor are passed similarly in the inferior capsular limb. The sutures from the 3-o'clock anchor are then passed through the superior capsular limb again in horizontal mattress fashion (Fig. 11-7). Finally, the sutures from the middle anchor, after having been passed through the inferior capsular limb, are then passed through the superior capsular limb so as to shift the superior capsular flap inferiorly to overlap and reinforce the inferior capsular limb. Sutures are then sequentially tied starting inferiorly (Fig. 11-8). The lateral portion of the capsule is closed with another No. 2 braided suture completing the repair.

The wound is irrigated. The subscapularis split is closed with No. 0 absorbable sutures. The deltopectoral interval is closed loosely with a No. 2-0 absorbable suture, followed by closure of the subcutaneous layer with No. 2-0 absorbable sutures, and subcuticular closure with a running No. 3-0 absorbable suture. Adhesive skin strips are applied followed by application of a sterile dressing and placement of an abduction sling.

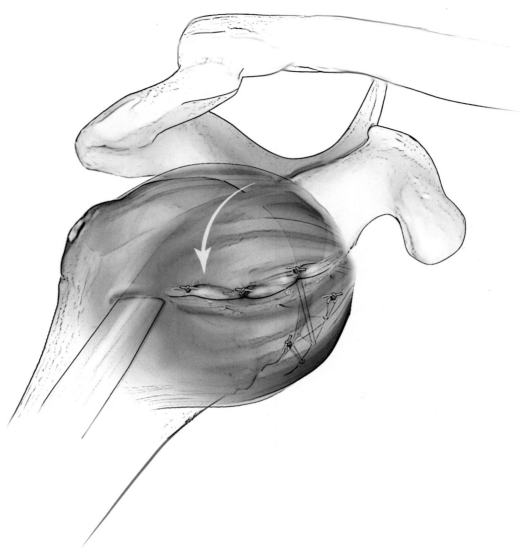

FIGURE 11-8

The superior capsular limb is shifted inferiorly completing the repair and capsular closure.

PEARLS AND PITFALLS

Increasing number and frequency of instability episodes, symptoms in midrange abduction, and episodes during sleep should raise the possibility of the presence of substantial osseous defects on the humeral or glenoid side that can be confirmed with appropriate imaging. Large glenoid defects are best treated with bone block procedures to decrease recurrence. The presence of a large symptomatic sulcus sign indicates the presence of a definitive inferior component to the instability requiring an inferior capsular shift in addition to repair of any anterior labral pathology.

Gill et al. (18) in an early report on their results of the open Bankart procedure noted that treatment of anterior shoulder instability is a balance between minimizing loss of glenohumeral motion and gaining glenohumeral stability. Choice of surgical stabilization should be individualized to minimize complications, restore stability, and return a functional range of motion. Use of a horizontal capsulotomy versus a vertical capsulotomy along the glenoid rim can help prevent excessive overtightening of the capsule medially and resultant restriction of external rotation that can be severely detrimental to the overhead athlete. A subscapularis spilt versus a complete or upper subscapularis takedown may allow for earlier restoration of range of motion. Care should be made during the capsular repair to have the arm approximately in a position of 45-degree abduction and external rotation to help prevent overconstraint of the joint.

Neurovascular complications may be minimized with a thorough knowledge of the anatomy, attention to surgical detail, and appropriate exposure with retractors. Dissection through the delto-pectoral interval should be done medial to the cephalic vein as most of its tributaries enter laterally. The anterior humeral circumflex artery and its venae comitantes are found at the inferior border of the subscapularis. Care should be taken not to dissect too inferiorly. External rotation of the arm for subscapularis exposure helps to protect the axillary nerve. Overzealous retraction on the conjoint tendon may cause injury to the musculocutaneous nerve.

POSTOPERATIVE MANAGEMENT

Patients are placed into an abduction pillow sling for 4 weeks after surgery. Sling may be removed for dressing, showering, and exercises. Immediately, the patient may perform elbow and wrist range of motion exercises and gentle pendulum (Codman) exercises several times daily. Formal physical therapy starts at 1 week after surgery for passive shoulder elevation limited to 90 and 25 degrees of external rotation in adduction. After sling is discontinued at 4 weeks, active and active assisted range of motion shoulder exercises are instituted with limitations of external rotation to 45 degrees until 8 weeks after surgery. Passive range of motion in other planes continues to tolerance. Deltoid and rotator cuff isometric exercises begin at approximately 6 weeks postoperatively. Periscapular strengthening is also instituted at this time. The goal is normalization of range of motion by 12 weeks after surgery. Strengthening is advanced as tolerated with progression to bands and followed by light weights. Introduction of plyometrics, sport-specific exercises, and advanced conditioning start at 12 weeks postoperatively with continued scapular rehabilitation. Return to athletic competition and contact sports is typically at 6 months after surgery.

COMPLICATIONS

Recurrence of instability after open Bankart repair is the most frequently reported complication. Recurrence may be secondary to an incorrect diagnosis such as the failure to recognize and appropriately address the presence of a posterior or multidirectional component of the instability pattern. An inadequately performed surgery that leaves residual Bankart lesions or does not correct anterior capsular redundancy can also lead to recurrence. Substantial glenoid or humeral bone defects can also compromise results (19). Postoperative episodes of subluxation and dislocation may occur after new traumatic events or atraumatically. The published rates of recurrence after open Bankart repair are generally <10% in midterm follow-up, although some studies have reported higher failure rates (Table 11-1).

Ho et al. (31) in a review of neurologic complications after anterior shoulder instability surgery at one institution noted an overall incidence of 8.2%. Neurologic injuries may include difficult

TABLE 11-1 Rates of Recurrence after Open Bankart Repair		
Author	**Number of Shoulders**	**Recurrence Rate**
Uhorchak et al. (20)	66	23%
Mohtadi et al. (21)	79	11%
Montgomery and Jobe (14)	31	3%
Wirth et al. (22)	142	3%
Magnusson et al. (23)	47	17%
Gill et al. (18)	60	5%
Thomas and Matsen (24)	39	2%
Pagnani and Dome (25)	58	3%
Cole et al. (26)	22	9%
Rhee et al. (27)	32	12%
Rowe et al. (28)	145	3%
Karlsson et al. (29)	48	10%
Bottoni et al. (30)	29	7%

to localize sensory disturbances, more diffuse brachial plexopathies with motor and sensory components, or defined incomplete cord or peripheral nerve lesions including the axillary or musculocutaneous nerves. The most common mechanism for neurologic injury is traction. Overall risk is minimized with careful patient positioning with the cervical spine in neutral alignment, avoidance of excessive humeral distraction, and careful placement and use of retractors. Specifically, the musculocutaneous nerve variably enters the conjoint tendon 5 to 8 cm inferior to the coracoid and may be injured by improper retractor placement or excessive medial traction. The axillary nerve may be found an average of 3 mm from the inferior capsule and is at risk for injury (32). Although rare, some authors have noted injury to the axillary nerve (31,33). Palpation of the nerve intraoperatively with the tug test and placement of the arm in external rotation may further minimize iatrogenic injury to the axillary nerve. McFarland et al. (34) noted that a subscapularis splitting approach to open Bankart repair with placement of a retractor for the inferior portion of the subscapularis may obviate the need for nerve exploration or palpation.

After an open Bankart procedure, loss of external rotation may be expected as a result of the labral repair and tightening of the anteroinferior capsule to prevent recurrence of instability (18,22,25). Repair should be completed with the shoulder in a position of 30 to 45 degrees of abduction and 30 to 45 degrees of external rotation to prevent excessive overconstraint and loss of motion. Significant loss of external rotation, particularly in overhead athletes, may result in a poor outcome with failure to return to activities despite a stable shoulder. The overall shoulder function should not be compromised to achieve a stable joint (14). The surgeon should be cognizant of the amount of capsular shift required to correct the pathology encountered for each individual patient.

Glenohumeral arthrosis has been well described as a complication following nonanatomic procedures to address anterior shoulder instability (35). An excessively tight anatomic anterior capsulorrhaphy that restricts external rotation may also result in increases in shear and compressive forces at the articular surface leading to degenerative changes (36). Rosenberg et al. (37) noted a relationship between degenerative radiographic changes and restriction of external rotation with the arm abducted and length of follow-up. Other authors have noted increasing incidence of osteoarthritis with longer follow-up studies (38–40). Degenerative changes may also result from improper placement of suture anchors on the articular surface.

The majority of descriptions of open Bankart repair techniques include a takedown and repair of the subscapularis tendon. Postoperative subscapularis insufficiency can occur despite meticulous attention toward repair. Sachs et al. (41) noted in their series of 30 patients a 23% incidence of an incompetent subscapularis at follow-up with only 57% reporting good to excellent results. In those 77% of patients with an intact subscapularis, there were 91% good to excellent results found. The authors noted that postoperative subscapularis function was the most important factor in determining the patient's perception of success (41). Although perhaps more technically demanding for exposure, a subscapularis split approach may allow for a more aggressive rehabilitation and return of motion (14).

RESULTS

In a classic report on the Bankart procedure, Rowe et al. (28) detailed their results and surgical findings in a series of 145 patients with anterior shoulder instability treated with a standard technique. Exposure and repair were accomplished with a coracoid osteotomy, subscapularis takedown, and vertical capsulotomy just lateral to the glenoid rim. The lateral capsular flap was sutured directly to the anterior glenoid rim and reinforced with the medial flap. At an average follow-up of 6 years, there were five recurrences of instability for a recurrence rate of 3.5%. By Rowe evaluation, there were 97% good or excellent results. Seventy-five of seventy-seven patients (97%) who were involved in athletics were able to return to sport. The authors noted in 85% of cases the presence of a Bankart lesion with disruption of the capsule at the anterior glenoid rim to be the most significant and frequently found lesion. Gill et al. (18) presented their outcomes of a series of 60 shoulders in 56 patients treated with a modified Bankart procedure at an average of 12 years follow-up. After a complete subscapularis takedown and separation from the capsule, a vertical capsulotomy was performed at the level of the glenoid rim with the arm in a position of external rotation approximately half the range of contralateral extremity to minimize the risk of overtightening the capsule during repair. Mattress sutures around the labrum are passed through the lateral capsular flap to anchor the lateral capsule down. The medial capsular flap is then imbricated over this repair. With this technique, three patients (5%) had recurrent instability with a mean loss of 12 degrees of external rotation. Forty-six of forty-seven patients were able to return to their preoperative level of sporting activity. Ninety-three percent of patients had a good or excellent result based upon their novel scoring system. The authors noted a direct association between range of motion and quality of results and cautioned against overtightening the repair. Thomas and Matsen (24) reported on their experience of an anatomic repair in 39 shoulders with traumatic shoulder instability at an average of 5.5 years follow-up. The subscapularis and capsule were elevated en masse from the lateral attachment on the humerus for exposure. The avulsed capsule medially is reattached to the glenoid to complete the repair. At final evaluation by Rowe scores, there were 97% good or excellent results with one episode of instability postoperatively (2%). Thirty-five patients (90%) had no limitations in work or sporting activities. Wirth et al. (22) reported on 142 shoulders with recurrent anterior instability treated with a capsular imbrication procedure. The upper two thirds of the subscapularis were reflected medially exposing the capsule. The capsule was divided midway between the glenoid rim and humerus. The medial capsulolabral injury was repaired followed by a double breasting imbrication of the capsule to decrease overall capsular volume. At an average of 5 years after surgery, 132 shoulders (93%) had a good or excellent result by Rowe criteria. Five shoulders (3.5%) had symptoms of recurrent instability at final evaluation. Sixty-three of seventy patients (90%) returned to sporting activity in some capacity. Montgomery and Jobe (14) reported on their results of a modified anterior capsulolabral reconstruction in a series of 31 overhead athletes at an average of 27 months follow-up. Repair of the Bankart lesion was performed through a subscapularis split and horizontal capsulotomy. At final evaluation, 25 of 31 patients (81%) had returned to their prior level of competitive sports. By Rowe evaluation, there were 30 (91%) good or excellent results with one (3%) failure of recurrent instability. Only two patients lost motion >5 degrees. Pagnani and Dome (25) reported on 58 American football players at an average follow-up of 37 months. Repair of the Bankart lesion was performed through a takedown of the subscapularis and transverse capsulotomy. A T-plasty capsular shift was performed in 16 patients to address capsular laxity. Two athletes (3%) sustained a repeat subluxation after surgery. Fifty-two players (90%) returned to American football for at least 1 year postoperatively. By Rowe evaluation, there were 55 (95%) good or excellent results. There was an average loss of external rotation of 9 degrees with the arm at the side and an average loss of 8 degrees of external rotation with the arm in 90 degrees of abduction.

Open Bankart repair has also provided good results in a revision setting. Sisto (42) reported on 30 patients treated with an open repair after failure of an arthroscopic Bankart procedure. At an average follow-up of 46 months, mean modified Rowe scores improved significantly from 25 to 84 postoperatively with overall 87% good to excellent results. Twenty-six of thirty patients (87%) returned to their previous level of sporting activity without recurrence of instability symptoms. There was an average of 8 degrees loss of external rotation versus the contralateral shoulder. Similarly, Nevaiser et al. (43) reported on 30 patients who underwent a revision open Bankart repair at an average follow-up of 10.2 years. There were no recurrent episodes of instability and no significant motion losses reported. Twenty-two of twenty-three patients were able to return to sports. Mean Rowe score was 87 with 28 of 30 patients (93%) having a good or excellent result.

REFERENCES

1. Hovelius L. Anterior dislocation of the shoulder in teenagers and young adults. Five year prognosis. *J Bone Joint Surg Am.* 1987;69:393–399.
2. Robinson CM, Howes J, Murdoch H, et al. Functional outcome and risk of recurrent instability after primary traumatic shoulder dislocation in young patients. *J Bone Joint Surg Am.* 2006;88:2326–2336.
3. Bottoni CR, Wilckens JH, DeBarardino TM, et al. A prospective, randomized evaluation of arthroscopic stabilization versus nonoperative treatment in patients with acute, traumatic, first-time shoulder dislocations. *Am J Sports Med.* 2002;30:576–580.
4. Arciero RA, Wheeler JH, Ryan JB, et al. Arthroscopic Bankart repair versus nonoperative treatment for acute, initial anterior shoulder dislocations. *Am J Sports Med.* 1994;22:589–594.
5. Dickens JF, Owens BD, Cameron KL, et al. Return to play and recurrent instability after in-season anterior shoulder instability: a prospective multicenter study. *Am J Sports Med.* 2014;42:2842–2850.
6. Buss DD, Lynch GP, Meyer CP, et al. Nonoperative management for in-season athletes with anterior shoulder instability. *Am J Sports Med.* 2004;32:1430–1433.
7. Chalmers PN, Mascarenhas R, Leroux T, et al. Do arthroscopic and open stabilization techniques restore equivalent stability to the shoulder in the setting of anterior glenohumeral instability? A systemic review of overlapping meta-analyses. *Arthroscopy.* 2015;31:355–363.

8. Balg F, Boileau P. The instability severity index score. A simple preoperative score to select patients for arthroscopic or open shoulder stabilization. *J Bone Joint Surg Br.* 2007;89:1470–1477.

9. Williams AA, Arciero RA. Arthroscopic and open stabilization techniques for anterior instability in the contact athlete. *Oper Tech Sports Med.* 2016;24:278–285.

10. Delos D, Moran C, Warren RF. Open Bankart repair in contact athletes: why and how. *Oper Tech Sports Med.* 2013;21:220–224.

11. Burkhart SS, DeBeer JF. Traumatic glenohumeral bone defects and their relationship to failures of arthroscopic Bankart repairs: significance of the inverted-pear glenoid and the humeral engaging Hill-Sachs lesion. *Arthroscopy.* 2000;16:677–694.

12. Bigliani LU, Newton PM, Steinmann SP, et al. Glenoid rim lesions associated with recurrent anterior dislocation of the shoulder. *Am J Sports Med.* 1998;26:41–45.

13. Pagnani MJ. Open capsular repair without bone block for recurrent anterior shoulder instability in patients with and without bony defects of the glenoid and/or humeral head. *Am J Sports Med.* 2008;36:1805–1812.

14. Montgomery WH III, Jobe FW. Functional outcomes in athletes after modified anterior capsulolabral reconstruction. *Am J Sports Med.* 1994;22:352–358.

15. Yamamoto N, Etoi E, Abe H, et al. Contact between the glenoid and the humeral head in abduction, external rotation, and horizontal extension: a new concept of glenoid track. *J Shoulder Elbow Surg.* 2007;16:649–656.

16. Di Giacomo G, Etoi E, Burkhart SS. Evolving concept of bipolar bone loss and the Hill-Sachs lesion: from "engaging/non-engaging" lesion to "on-track/off-track" lesion. *Arthroscopy.* 2014;30:90–98.

17. Altchek DW, Warren RF, Skyhar MJ, et al. T-plasty modification of the Bankart procedure for multidirectional instability of the anterior and inferior types. *J Bone Joint Surg Am.* 1991;73:105–112.

18. Gill TJ, Micheli LJ, Gebhard F, et al. Bankart repair for anterior instability of the shoulder: long-term outcome. *J Bone Joint Surg Am.* 1997;79:850–857.

19. Millett PJ, Clavert P, Warner JJP. Open operative treatment for anterior shoulder instability: when and why? *J Bone Joint Surg Am.* 2005;87:419–432.

20. Uhorchak JM, Arciero RA, Huggard D, et al. Recurrent shoulder instability after reconstruction in athletes involved in collision and contact sports. *Am J Sports Med.* 2000;28:794–799.

21. Mohtadi NGH, Chan DS, Hollinshead RM, et al. A randomized clinical trial comparing open and arthroscopic stabilization for recurrent traumatic anterior shoulder instability. *J Bone Joint Surg Am.* 2014;96:353–360.

22. Wirth MA, Blatter G, Rockwood CA. The capsular imbrication procedure for recurrent anterior instability of the shoulder. *J Bone Joint Surg Am.* 1996;78:246–259.

23. Magnusson L, Kartus J, Ejerhed L, et al. Revisiting the open Bankart experience: a four- to nine-year follow-up. *Am J Sports Med.* 2002;30:778–782.

24. Thomas SC, Matsen FA III. An approach to the repair of avulsion of the glenohumeral ligaments in the management of traumatic anterior glenohumeral instability. *J Bone Joint Surg Am.* 1989;71:506–513.

25. Pagnani MJ, Dome DC. Surgical treatment of traumatic anterior shoulder instability in American football players. *J Bone Joint Surg Am.* 2002;84:711–715.

26. Cole BJ, L'Insalata J, Irrgang J, et al. Comparison of arthroscopic and open anterior shoulder stabilization: a two- to six-year follow-up study. *J Bone Joint Surg Am.* 2000;82:1108–1114.

27. Rhee YG, Ha JH, Cho NS. Anterior shoulder stabilization in collision athletes: arthroscopic versus open Bankart repair. *Am J Sports Med.* 2006;34:979–985.

28. Rowe CR, Patel D, Southmayd WW. The Bankart procedure: a long-term end-result study. *J Bone Joint Surg Am.* 1978;60:1–16.

29. Karlsson J, Magnusson L, Ejerhed L, et al. Comparison of open and arthroscopic stabilization for recurrent shoulder dislocation in patients with a Bankart lesion. *Am J Sports Med.* 2001;29:538–542.

30. Bottoni CR, Smith EL, Berkowitz MJ, et al. Arthroscopic versus open shoulder stabilization for recurrent anterior instability: a prospective randomized clinical trial. *Am J Sports Med.* 2006;34:1730–1737.

31. Ho E, Cofield RH, Balm MR, et al. Neurological complications of surgery for anterior shoulder instability. *J Shoulder Elbow Surg.* 1999;8:266–270.

32. Bryan WJ, Schauder K, Tullos HS. The axillary nerve and its relationship to common sports medicine shoulder procedures. *Am J Sports Med.* 1986;14:113–116.

33. Neer CS II, Foster CR. Inferior capsular shift for involuntary inferior and multidirectional instability of the shoulder: a preliminary report. *J Bone Joint Surg Am.* 1980;62:897–908.

34. McFarland EG, Caicedo JC, Kim TK, et al. Prevention of axillary nerve injury in anterior shoulder reconstructions: use of a subscapularis muscle-splitting technique and a review of the literature. *Am J Sports Med.* 2002;30:601–606.

35. Hawkins RJ, Angelo RL. Glenohumeral osteoarthrosis: a late complication of the Putti-Platt repair. *J Bone Joint Surg Am.* 1990;72:1193–1197.

36. Ahmad CS, Wang VM, Sugalski MT, et al. Biomechanics of shoulder capsulorrhaphy procedures. *J Shoulder Elbow Surg.* 2005;14(suppl S):12S–18S.

37. Rosenberg BN, Richmond JC, Levine WN. Long-term follow up of Bankart reconstruction. Incidence of late degenerative glenohumeral arthrosis. *Am J Sports Med.* 1995;23:538–544.

38. Pelet S, Jolles BM, Farron A. Bankart repair for recurrent anterior glenohumeral instability: results at twenty-nine years follow-up. *J Shoulder Elbow Surg.* 2006;15:203–207.

39. Fabre T, Abi-Chahla ML, Billaud A, et al. Long-term results with Bankart procedure: a 26-year follow-up study of 50 cases. *J Shoulder Elbow Surg.* 2010;19:318–323.

40. Moroder P, Odorizzi M, Pizzinini S, et al. Open Bankart repair for the treatment of anterior shoulder instability without substantial osseous glenoid defects: results after a minimum follow-up of twenty years. *J Bone Joint Surg Am.* 2015;97:1398–1405.

41. Sachs RA, Williams B, Stone ML, et al. Open Bankart repair: correlation of results with postoperative subscapularis function. *Am J Sports Med.* 2005;33:1458–1462.

42. Sisto DJ. Revision of failed arthroscopic Bankart repairs. *Am J Sports Med.* 2007;35:537–541.

43. Neviaser AS, Benke MT, Nevaiser RJ. Open Bankart repair for revision of failed prior stabilization: outcome analysis at a mean of more than 10 years. *J Shoulder Elbow Surg.* 2015;24:897–901.

12 Latarjet Procedure

Jeffrey C. Wera and Eric J. Kropf

INTRODUCTION

The shoulder is the most commonly dislocated major joint in the body with an annual incidence of 24 cases per 100,000 reported in 2010 (1). Anteroinferior instability, being the most common pattern, accounts for over 90% of cases (2). Nearly half of all anterior shoulder dislocations occur in persons aged 15 to 29 years with the incidence being three times higher in males (1). Recurrence rates have been reported as high as 96% in young athletes treated nonoperatively (2,3). Arthroscopic capsulolabral repair, which represents first-line surgical management for a majority of patients, has also been associated with recurrent instability rates ranging from 10.8% to 21.1% (4). Young age (<22 years), male gender, competitive-level sporting activity, and glenohumeral bone loss have been identified as risk factors that predispose patients to recurrent anterior shoulder instability after nonoperative management and/or arthroscopic repair (4).

Bony defects of the anteroinferior aspect of the glenoid can occur acutely or gradually over time with recurrent episodes of instability. Glenoid bone loss has been reported in up to 22% of initial dislocations (5) and up to 86% in cases of recurrent instability (6). Unaddressed glenoid bone loss is a known risk factor to failure after arthroscopic soft tissue stabilization. Inferior glenoid bone loss from recurrent instability results in an inverted pear-shaped glenoid. In a cohort of 194 patients with recurrent anterior shoulder instability, Burkhart and De Beer (7) found that capsulolabral repair alone in the setting of an inverted pear glenoid led to a 67% failure rate and 89% recurrent instability in contact athletes treated with soft tissue stabilization alone (8).

Recent emphasis has shifted to effectively quantifying critical bone loss values. Cadaveric studies have demonstrated glenoid bone loss of 19% to 21% compromises range of motion (ROM) and stability after soft tissue repair (9,10). Glenoid bone loss of >25% has been demonstrated to be predictive of a 75% failure rate after arthroscopic Bankart repair in patients with excessive external rotation (>90 degrees) (11). It is generally accepted that with >20% to 25% glenoid defect, bone augmentation procedures should be strongly considered (12). However, recent research has also shown inferior clinical outcomes after arthroscopic soft tissue stabilization even in cases of "subcritical" bone loss as little as 13.5% (13).

The role of humeral-sided bone loss is less well defined, but many patients will present with a concomitant Hill-Sachs deformity (14). Glenoid bone loss coupled with a humeral-sided bone lesion can increase the risk of engagement and subsequent instability (15). Bipolar bone loss has additive deleterious effects on shoulder stability. As anterior glenoid bone loss increases, the glenoid track decreases in width making it more likely that the medial aspect of the Hill-Sachs lesions engages resulting in instability. As glenoid bone loss increases, smaller Hill-Sachs lesions become increasingly clinically relevant (16).

Effective surgical management of shoulder instability must account for and address the full extent of pathology. Soft tissue stabilization alone is appropriate for the majority of patients without significant bone loss. However, as bone loss increases, a soft tissue procedure alone is likely to result in an unacceptably high rate of recurrent instability and inferior patient outcomes. Bony augmentation procedure such as Latarjet coracoid transfer may be indicated.

In 1954, Latarjet first described a coracoid bone block technique for recurrent anterior shoulder dislocation (17). In 1958, Helfet (18) published results using a similar procedure that he attributed to his mentor Rowley Bristow. The original Bristow procedure harvests the distal 1-cm of coracoid and sutures it to the anterior aspect of the scapular neck through a vertically orientated subscapularis split. Over the decades, the Bristow procedure has endured several modifications (19–21) evolving to more closely mirror the procedure originally described by Latarjet.

With the Latarjet procedure, three mechanisms known as the "triple-block" effect contribute to glenohumeral stability. Firstly, the osseous coracoid graft extends the articular arc of the glenoid increasing the arc of motion required before potential dislocation. Secondly, the conjoined tendon provides a dynamic "sling effect" resisting anterior translation of the humeral head when the arm is abducted and externally rotated. Lastly, the conjoined tendon with its attachment to the transferred coracoid travels over the subscapularis tendon creating a tenodesis effect reinforcing a deficient anteroinferior capsule.

INDICATIONS

Indications for open coracoid transfer remain controversial. Patient age, activity level, and degree of bone loss are key factors. Generally, >20% glenoid bone loss or a large "engaging" Hill-Sachs is an appropriate indication for coracoid transfer. The threshold for a bony procedure should be lower in settings of bipolar bone loss. Also, patients who have failed well-performed arthroscopic or open soft tissue repair may be candidates for bony reconstruction.

The instability severity index score (ISIS) was developed to predict potential for recurrent instability and the need for more extensive procedures. ISIS evaluates risk factors such as age, sports participation, hyperlaxity, and glenoid and humeral head bone loss. A score of >6 predicts an unacceptably high recurrence rate of 70% following soft tissue stabilization (22). As a result, Balg and Boileau recommend Latarjet procedure as the index treatment with an ISIS score >6. Bessière et al. (23) similarly found Latarjet was more reliable than arthroscopic Bankart repair with less recurrent instability and significantly better Rowe scores at 6-year follow-up. The authors now recommend open Latarjet as the index procedure in patients with ISIS scores of 4 or greater.

CONTRAINDICATIONS

Patients with voluntary instability, multidirectional instability associated with generalized ligament laxity, soft tissue loss, and instability associated with paresis of the deltoid and rotator cuff are not good surgical candidates for open coracoid transfer and are contraindicated for the procedure. Although rare, associated coracoid fracture is a contraindication.

PREOPERATIVE PREPARATION

History

A detailed history should be obtained including age at time of first instability event, number of dislocations, chronicity, traumatic or atraumatic etiology, high- or low-energy mechanism, subluxation or dislocation, and if reduction required sedation or could be easily reduced (24). All prior treatments including any period of immobilization or physical therapy, and previous operative interventions, activity level/contact sports, and patient expectations should be reviewed and discussed (25).

The history may suggest glenoid bone loss when associated with initial high-energy mechanism. Recurrent instability with activities of daily living, instability at low abduction angles (20–60 degrees), subsequent subluxation or dislocation with minor or no trauma and instability in sleep all should raise concern for bone loss (26).

Examination

A focused physical examination is undertaken including inspection, palpation, ROM testing, evaluation of motor strength, neurovascular status, and provocative tests. The contralateral shoulder is examined to determine the patient's baseline laxity and motion. Beighton's criteria are also evaluated (24).

Provocative maneuvers should be performed to detect and confirm the presence of anterior instability (27–29). The apprehension test is performed with the patient supine bringing the arm into 90 degrees of abduction with elbow flexed to 90 degrees. An external rotational force is placed simultaneously as the examiner uses his other hand applying an anteriorly directed force to the humeral head. Fear of impending instability is a positive result (24). Apprehension in midranges of abduction and lesser amounts of external rotation may be indicative of more significant glenoid bone loss (26).

The relocation test is performed by changing the force applied from anterior to posterior depressing the humeral head and should provide relief of the patient's symptoms.

The anterior load and shift test is also performed with the patient supine. The arm is abducted to 20 degrees with slight flexion in the plane of the scapula, and the humeral head is centered within the glenoid fossa. An anteriorly directed force is applied to the proximal humerus. This can be done with arm in neutral, 45 and 90 degrees of abduction to assess the laxity of the superior, middle, and inferior glenohumeral ligament (SGHL, MGHL, and IGHL), respectively (30,31).

Imaging

Radiography

Evaluation begins with standardized plain radiographs including glenohumeral anteroposterior (AP) (Grashey), lateral outlet (scapular Y), and axillary lateral or Bernageau glenoid profile views. In the setting of chronic instability, a poorly defined anteroinferior glenoid contour suggests bone loss (12). Other views such as the apical oblique view described by Garth et al., the Didiée view, or West Point view can be used to better assess glenoid bone loss (32–34). To evaluate a potential Hill-Sachs lesion, an AP radiograph with the arm in internal rotation and Stryker notch views should be obtained (34). Radiographs are an excellent screening tool but are typically not sufficient to accurately define glenoid shape and quantify glenoid bone loss.

Computed Tomography

Undetected glenoid bone loss is the leading cause of recurrent instability after surgical stabilization (7,35). If glenoid bone loss is suspected based on radiographs or the history and physical exam suggests recurrent or minimally provoked shoulder instability, computed tomography (CT) should be obtained. While some studies have demonstrated the use of sagittal MRI images to be equivalently accurate (36–38), CT scan with three-dimensional (3D) reconstructions remain the gold standard for defining the orientation and degree of glenoid bone loss and size and configuration of a Hill-Sachs lesion (12,39–41).

Several methods have been described that attempt to quantify the amount of glenoid bone loss (12). Commonly employed is the "best-fit circle" method on the sagittal oblique imaging with humeral head subtraction. The surface area of the anterior rim defect is quantified as the percentage of total surface area from a best-fit circle superimposed on the inferior two-thirds of the glenoid rim (42) (Fig. 12-1). Another method involves measuring the AP distance from the bare area, which can typically be approximated on CT scan (42). The distance from the posterior aspect of the glenoid rim to the bare spot (B) and from the bare spot to the anterior glenoid edge (A) is measured. The percent bone loss is calculated by $([B - A]/2B) \times 100\%$ (43).

Magnetic Resonance Imaging

Magnetic resonance imaging (MRI) and magnetic resonance arthrogram (MRA) may be useful in clinical situations where the diagnosis is unclear. MRI is preferred to evaluate tissue injuries to the

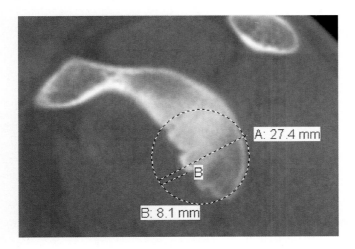

FIGURE 12-1

CT scan, left shoulder, sagittal plane of patient with recurrent anterior instability. Using the "best-fit circle" technique, anterior glenoid bone loss is estimated to be 30% (B/A; 8.1 mm/27.4 mm).

shoulder including labral damage, rotator cuff injuries, and capsular avulsions. Anterior periosteal sleeve avulsion (ALPSA) or a humeral avulsion of glenohumeral ligament (HAGL) lesions will result in high rates of recurrent instability if left untreated (44,45). For that reason, we recommend MRI for all first-time shoulder dislocations.

SURGICAL TECHNIQUE

Patient Positioning

The patient is positioned in a beach-chair position with the arm draped free to allow intraoperative abduction and external rotation. The operative arm is secured to a mechanical arm-holding device, which is used for positioning throughout the case. A padded Mayo stand may also be utilized in place of pneumatic arm positioner if unavailable.

A standard deltopectoral approach is carried out through a 4- to 6-cm midaxillary skin incision centered over the coracoid process with extension to the axillary fold (Fig. 12-2). Dissection is carried down through the skin and subcutaneous tissue to the level of the clavipectoral fascia. The cephalic vein is identified and retracted laterally and any crossing branches are ligated. The delto-pectoral fascia is incised in line with the skin incision.

Coracoid Graft Harvest

Once down to the level of the coracoid, it is important to obtain adequate exposure for visualization of surrounding structures. The coracoclavicular (CC) ligaments are located superiorly and proximally and should be maintained throughout the case. Soft tissue release up to the base of the CC ligaments will allow for approximately 20- to 30-mm graft. The coracoacromial ligament (CAL) is identified laterally with the shoulder abducted and externally rotated. Incise the CAL approximately 1-cm from its coracoid insertion preserving the cuff of tissue for later incorporation into the capsular reconstruction. The arm is then adducted and internally rotated, and the pectoralis minor is released sharply from the medial aspect of the coracoid (Fig. 12-3). A periosteal elevator is used to remove any remaining soft tissue from the inferior coracoid surface. The surgeon should be able to pass an instrument or finger along the undersurface of the coracoid without difficulty. The elevator is then positioned inferiorly and medially to the coracoid to protect the musculocutaneous nerve, axillary

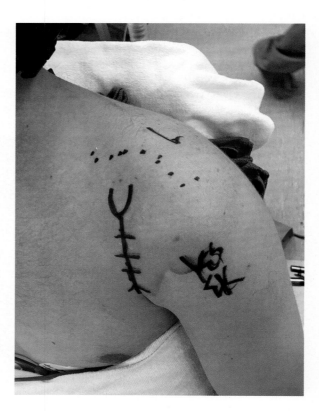

FIGURE 12-2

A standard deltopectoral approach is carried out through a 4- to 6-cm midaxillary skin incision centered over the coracoid process with extension to the axillary fold.

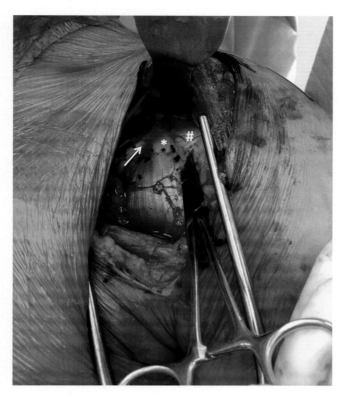

FIGURE 12-3

Soft tissue attachments onto the coracoid process (*). The *arrow* denotes the pectoralis minor, the conjoined tendon is outlined with surgical marker, and the # indicates the CAL in relation to the coracoid process.

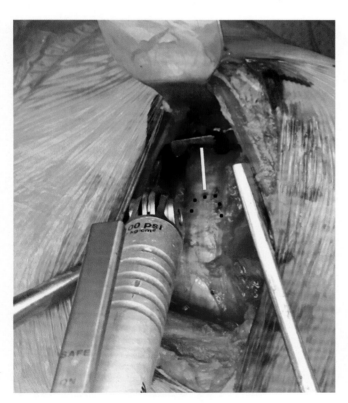

FIGURE 12-4

Oscillating saw positioned at the base of the coracoid process resulting in a graft approximately 20- to 30-mm.

nerve, and brachial plexus. Harvest the coracoid graft in the medial to lateral direction at the base of the CC ligaments using a 90-degree oscillating saw (Fig. 12-4). The osteotomy is then completed with an osteotome. It is important to perform the osteotomy perpendicularly to the coracoid process in order to avoid iatrogenic glenoid fracture.

With toothed forceps or nonpenetrating clamp, grasp the coracoid graft. Remove any remaining coracohumeral ligament attachments, which can be large and must be divided. Care should be taken not to disturb the blood supply to the graft, which enters at the medial aspect of the conjoined tendon. Release any remaining tissue from the distal end of the coracoid as well as the posterior aspect of the conjoined tendon to allow for more excursion, and ensure adequate translation to the glenoid to prevent tension on the musculocutaneous nerve. With an oscillating saw, decorticate the posterior aspect of the coracoid along the long axis to expose a broad, flat cancellous bed to optimize graft healing to the glenoid margin. Typically, there will be a small spike of bone at the base of the osteotomized coracoid-scapula junction. This bone should be excised to better match the articular arc of the glenoid. The coracoid graft is now ready for transfer and is placed under the pectoralis major and retracted exposing the subscapularis muscle.

Glenoid Exposure and Preparation

With the arm abducted and externally rotated, expose and identify the superior and inferior borders of the subscapularis. The subscapularis split should be performed at the distal third of the muscle belly at the junction of the superior two-thirds and the inferior one-third (Fig. 12-5). The subscapularis is then bluntly split longitudinally in line with its fibers with aid of a sponge. With the muscle fibers opened perpendicularly, the sponge is then slid under the subscapularis superomedially, and a Hohmann retractor is placed into the subscapularis fossa. In this manner, the muscle is separated from the underlying anterior glenohumeral capsule. The subscapularis split is then extended laterally to the level of the lesser tuberosity to allow for visualization of the glenohumeral joint line and capsule (Fig. 12-6). A single prong blunt tip Gelpi self-retaining retractor is placed to retract the subscapularis. A blunt Bennett retractor is placed on the inferior aspect of the subscapularis and inferior glenoid neck and can aid in visualization as well. Capsulotomy can be performed in variable manner based on surgeon preference and patient anatomy/pathology.

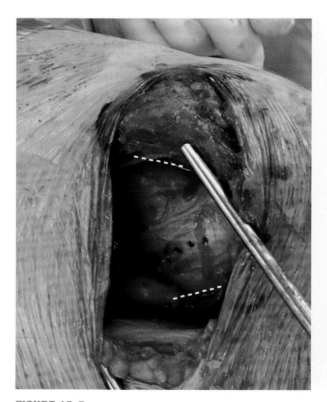

FIGURE 12-5

Surgical marking demonstrating the distal third of the muscle belly at the junction of the superior two-thirds and the inferior one-third of the subscapularis.

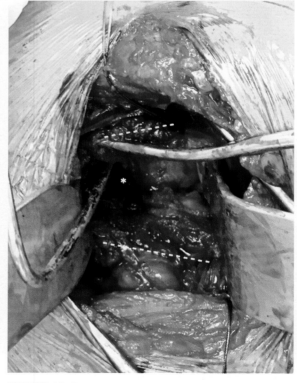

FIGURE 12-6

Self-retraining retractor is seen here retracting subscapularis. The *asterisk* denotes the glenoid bone loss.

Typically, a vertical glenoid-based capsulotomy is performed and allows for later capsular repair. A T-shaped capsulotomy can be performed if significant scarring is encountered. The glenohumeral joint is entered, and the capsulotomy is extended inferiorly down to the 6-o'clock position on the glenoid. The anteroinferior glenoid labrum and periosteum are dissected from the glenoid neck. The Hohmann retractor is repositioned and placed as medial as possible along the scapular neck. With the arm adducted, a humeral head retractor is placed into the joint, and the entire anterior glenoid now completely exposed. An osteotome, high-speed burr, or curette can be used to decorticate the anterior glenoid with the goal of obtaining a bleeding, flat bed of bone on which the coracoid graft can be placed.

Coracoid Graft Transfer and Fixation

The primary objective of coracoid transfer is to increase the glenoid articular surface and in turn, the safe arc of motion. Appropriate positioning of the coracoid graft is essential to achieve a balance of stability and motion. The optimal position lies between 3- and 5-o'clock on the glenoid (right shoulder) flush to or just medial (1–2 mm) to the native glenoid. Excessive medialization of the graft fails to improve stability, whereas excessive lateralization has been associated with an increased rate of postoperative arthritis (19). The graft can be positioned with the posterior surface flush to the native glenoid, or the graft can be rotated and the medial surface affixed to the native glenoid ("congruent arc technique"). The coracoid is typically wider in a medial-lateral than anterior-posterior direction. As a result, the "congruent arc technique" can better restore the glenoid width in cases of severe bone loss. However, the trade-off is that the area of screw placement is decreased and fracture of the coracoid or loss of fixation can occur, particularly in cases where the coracoid is very small.

Once the desired orientation has been determined, the graft is positioned superoinferiorly along the glenoid neck with the decorticated surface of the coracoid sitting flush to the articular surface. The graft is provisionally held in place with Kirschner wires to ensure proper positioning of the graft. Definitive fixation is achieved with two fully threaded self-tapping, self-drilling cortical screws placed approximately 1-cm apart via standard lag technique. Of note, both screws are tightened sequentially using a "two-finger" technique to prevent rotation or fracture of the coracoid graft. Care should be taken to ensure the graft lies parallel to the anterior border of the glenoid. Careful planning should avoid lateral overhang, but if necessary, a high-speed burr can be used to trim the graft prior to capsular repair.

Capsular and Subscapularis Repair

In cases of recurrent instability, the quality of anterior capsular tissue can be variable. If healthy, high-quality tissue is present, with the arm adducted and externally rotated, the capsule is repaired directly to the native glenoid with suture anchors. This prevents direct articulation with the coracoid graft rendering it extracapsular. If capsular deficiency exists or the tissue cannot be translated to the glenoid without excessive tension, the native capsule is repaired directly to the CAL with no. 2 nonabsorbable sutures. The subscapularis split is then repaired with no. 0 absorbable suture. When the repair of the capsule and subscapularis is completed, the conjoined tendon will be seen exiting between the upper and lower segments of the previously split subscapularis (Fig. 12-7). The conjoined tendon now acts as a dynamic anterior soft tissue sling as the arm is brought into the high-risk position of abduction and external rotation. Additional stability is obtained from the inferior third of the subscapularis tendon providing a buttress to anterior translation and the added articular arc from the coracoid graft (46,47).

The wound is then copiously irrigated and closed in a layered fashion. The deltopectoral interval is closed using interrupted 0 Vicryl (Ethicon). The subcutaneous tissue is closed with buried 2-0 Vicryl (Ethicon) followed by a running 4-0 Monocryl subcuticular stitch (Ethicon). After dressing the wound with sterile dressings, a shoulder immobilizer and sling is applied.

Classic Latarjet versus Congruent Arc Techniques

In the original description of the Latarjet procedure, the coracoid is secured to the glenoid neck with the lateral aspect of the coracoid flush with the glenoid articular surface. Typically, approximately 1 cm of the CAL is left on the coracoid graft for later augmentation of the capsular repair. This technique is commonly employed in Europe, hence the designation as "European Latarjet." The

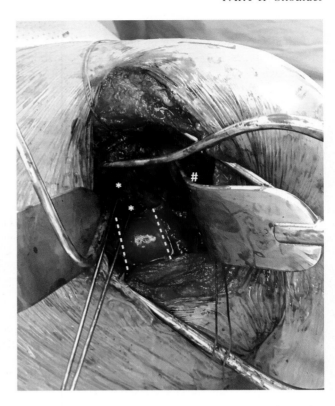

FIGURE 12-7

With humeral head retracted (#), the coracoid graft is provisionally held in place with two Kirschner wires (*). The conjoined tendon (*dashed lines*) is seen here with the arm in adducted positioning. It provides a dynamic "sling effect" resisting anterior translation of the humeral head when the arm is abducted and externally rotated.

congruent arc modification was described by De Beer and Roberts (48) and has been popularized by Burkhart et al. (49) The coracoid is rotated 90 degrees, so that the inferior aspect of the coracoid is oriented flush to the glenoid face. This modification, popularly used in the United States, provides an improved match in the radius of curvature of the glenoid rim with graft (50) and optimizes glenohumeral contact pressures when compared with the traditional Latarjet technique (51). This approach potentially allows the surgeon to address a greater glenoid deficit as the coracoid graft is typically wider than it is thick. With this approach, the CAL is often excised and the capsular repair is reattached to the native glenoid with suture anchors making the graft an extra-articular structure.

POSTOPERATIVE MANAGEMENT

Rehabilitation guidelines should encourage progressive mobilization while optimizing healing at coracoid transfer site and protecting the subscapularis repair. A shoulder immobilizer is used for the first 4 weeks after surgery. Active internal rotation and passive external rotation are avoided. Pendulum exercises are begun immediately. The patient is permitted to perform gentle passive, active, and active-assisted shoulder ROM in the scapular plane as well as external rotation (0–30 degrees) and forward flexion (0–90 degrees) during this time.

Active and active-assisted ROM is emphasized starting at 6 weeks to reestablish full ROM. Once full, painless ROM is obtained and there is evidence of osseous healing on radiographs, strengthening is permitted. Sport-specific exercises are begun around 16 to 20 weeks. Return to contact sports or heavy labor activities is typically allowed at 24 weeks.

RESULTS

Many studies have shown the Latarjet to be effective in restoring glenohumeral stability. In a prospective study of 118 patients, Hovelius et al. (52) found a 3.4% rate of recurrent dislocation and a 10% rate of subluxation at 15.2 years follow-up. Ninety-eight percent of patients were satisfied or very satisfied at the final follow-up. Mizuno et al. (53) reported a postoperative rate of recurrence of 5.9% in 68 patients at 20-years follow-up. Dumont et al. (19) reported only one recurrent dislocation in a cohort of 63 shoulders, with 58 patients returning to sports.

In a systematic review of 10 studies, Bhatia et al. (54) reported recurrent anterior instability rates ranging from 0% to 8% with 90% of patients reporting good to excellent satisfaction at the final follow-up. Similarly, in a large systematic review, Griesser et al. (55) found that the overall mean rate of recurrent dislocation was 2.9% and subluxation rate of 5.8% in 1,904 shoulders. An et al. (56) performed a metaanalysis of 376 patients that underwent the Latarjet procedure versus 416 shoulders treated with Bankart repair. The Latarjet cohort reported a postoperative recurrent instability rate of 11.6% compared with 21.1% in the Bankart repair.

Despite its effectiveness in restoring glenohumeral stability, complications are not uncommon. Short-term complications include infection, hematoma, graft failure, malpositioning, nonunion/malunion, and hardware complications. Longer-term complication rates have been reported as high as 30% (55). Most commonly patients report decreased external rotation and later glenohumeral arthritis. Griesser et al. (55) found the mean loss of external rotation was 13 degrees in their systematic review of 1,904 shoulders. Hovelius et al. (57) reported a mean loss of 7.4 degrees of external rotation in adduction and 8 degrees in abduction. Fourteen percent of patients exhibited moderate to severe arthropathy and mild arthropathy in another 35% of patients. Conversely, Allain et al. (46) demonstrated that only 8.4% of their patients progressed to either grade 3 or 4 end-stage arthritis. Mizuno et al. (53) reported that while arthritis developed in 23.5% of their cohort, no cases of end-stage arthritis were seen. Hovelius (56) noted 9% moderate to severe arthrosis at 10-year follow-up in 247 first-time anterior shoulder dislocations. Longitudinal literature supports the notion that the initial dislocation may predispose patients to end-stage osteoarthritis, so the impact (positive or negative) of the Latarjet procedure is challenging to determine.

SUMMARY

Recurrent anterior shoulder instability can be attributed to many causes, but bone loss of both the glenoid and humeral head can be a major contributing factor. Obtaining a thorough history and physical examination is necessary to diagnose and determine an appropriate treatment plan. Defining bone loss in the setting of instability with advanced imaging is critical when planning any stabilization procedure. Soft tissue stabilization procedures in the setting of significant bone loss are associated with unacceptably high failure rates, necessitating a bony augmentation procedure.

The Latarjet procedure has consistently restored glenohumeral stability in both cadaveric and clinical studies. While the Latarjet is a reliable stabilizing procedure, surgeons should be aware of complications related to the procedure in order to take appropriate intraoperative precautions and better tailor communication with patients.

REFERENCES

1. Zacchilli MA, Owens BD. Epidemiology of shoulder dislocations presenting to emergency departments in the United States. *J Bone Joint Surg Am.* 2010;92:542–549.
2. Levy DM, Cole BJ, Rach BR Jr. History of surgical intervention of anterior shoulder instability. *J Shoulder Elbow Surg.* 2016;25:139–150.
3. Chahal J, Marks PH, MacDonald PB, et al. Anatomic Bankart repair compared with nonoperative treatment and/or arthroscopic lavage for first-time traumatic shoulder dislocation. *Arthroscopy.* 2012;28:565–575.
4. McHale KJ, Sanchez G, Lavery KP, et al. Latarjet technique for treatment of anterior shoulder instability with glenoid bone loss. *Arthrosc Tech.* 2017;16:791–799.
5. Taylor DC, Arciero RA. Pathologic changes associated with shoulder dislocations: arthroscopic and physical examination findings in first-time, traumatic anterior dislocations. *Am J Sports Med.* 1997;25:306–311.
6. Piasecki DP, Verma NN, Romeo AA, et al. Glenoid bone deficiency in recurrent anterior shoulder instability: diagnosis and management. *J Am Acad Orthop Surg.* 2009;17:482–493.
7. Burkhart SS, De Beer JF. Traumatic glenohumeral bone defects and their relationship to failure of arthroscopic Bankart repairs: significance of the inverted-pear glenoid and the humeral engaging Hill-Sachs lesion. *Arthroscopy.* 2000;16:677–694.
8. Wiesel BB, Gartsman GM, Press CM, et al. What went wrong and what was done about it: pitfalls in the treatment of common shoulder surgery. *J Bone Joint Surg Am.* 2013;95:2061–2070.
9. Lo I, Parten PM, Burkhart SS. The inverted pear glenoid: an indicator of significant glenoid bone loss. *Arthroscopy.* 2004;20:169–174.
10. Itoi E, Lee SB, Berglund LJ, et al. The effect of a glenoid defect on anteroinferior stability of the shoulder after Bankart repair: a cadaveric study. *J Bone Joint Surg Am.* 2000;82:35–46.
11. Boileau P, Villalba M, Hery JY, et al. Risk factors for recurrence of shoulder instability after arthroscopic Bankart repair. *J Bone Joint Surg Am.* 2006;88:1755–1763.
12. Streubel PN, Krych AJ, Simone JP, et al. Anterior glenohumeral instability: a pathology-based surgical treatment strategy. *J Am Acad Orthop Surg.* 2014;22:283–294.

13. Shaha JS, Cook JB, Song DJ, et al. Redefining "Critical" bone loss in shoulder instability: functional outcomes worsen with "Subcritical" bone loss. *Am J Sports Med.* 2015;43:1719–1725.

14. Rowe CR. Acute and recurrent anterior dislocations of the shoulder. *Orthop Clin North Am.* 1980;11:253–270.

15. Provencher MT, Frank RM, Leclere LE, et al. The Hill-Sachs lesion: diagnosis, classification, and management. *J Am Acad Orthop Surg.* 2012;20:242–252.

16. Yamamoto N, Itoi E, Abe H, et al. Contact between the glenoid and the humeral head in abduction, external rotation, and horizontal extension: a new concept of glenoid track. *J Shoulder Elbow Surg.* 2007;16:649–656.

17. Latarjet M. Treatment of recurrent dislocation of the shoulder. *Lyon Chir.* 1954;49:994–997.

18. Helfet AJ. Coracoid transplantation for recurring dislocation of the shoulder. *J Shoulder Elbow Surg.* 1958;40:198–202.

19. Collins HR, Wilde AH. Shoulder instability in athletics. *Orthop Clin North Am.* 1973;4:759–774.

20. Lombardo SJ, Kerlan RK, Jobe FW, et al. The modified Bristow procedure for recurrent dislocation of the shoulder. *J Bone Joint Surg Am.* 1976;58:256–261.

21. May VR Jr. A modified Bristow operation for anterior recurrent dislocation of the shoulder. *J Bone Joint Surg Am.* 1970;52:1010–1016.

22. Balg F, Boileau P. The instability severity index score. A simple pre-operative score to select patients for arthroscopic or open shoulder stabilisation. *J Bone Joint Surg Br.* 2007;89:1470–1477.

23. Bessière C, Trojani C, Carles M, et al. The open Latarjet procedure is more reliable in terms of shoulder stability that arthroscopic Bankart repair. *Clin Orthop Rel Res.* 2014;472:2345–2351.

24. Dumont G, Russell R, Robertson W. Anterior shoulder instability: a review of pathoanatomy, diagnosis and treatment. *Curr Rev Musculoskelet Med.* 2011;4:200–207.

25. Davis D, Abboud J. Operative management options for traumatic anterior shoulder instability in patients younger than 30 years. *Orthopedics.* 2015;9:570–576.

26. Owens BD, Burns TC, DeBerardino TM. Examination and classification of instability. In: Provencher M, Romeo A, eds. *Shoulder Instability: A Comprehensive Approach.* Philadelphia, PA: Elsevier Saunders; 2011.

27. van Kampen DA, van den Berg T, van der Woude HJ, et al. Diagnostic value of patient characteristics, history, and six clinical tests for traumatic anterior shoulder instability. *J Shoulder Elbow Surg.* 2013;10:1310–1319.

28. Hegedus EJ, Goode AP, Cook CE, et al. Which physical examination tests provide clinicians with the most value when examining the shoulder? Update of a systematic review with meta-analysis of individual tests. *Br J Sports Med.* 2012;46:964–978.

29. Farber AJ, Castillo R, Clough M, et al. Clinical assessment of three common tests for traumatic anterior shoulder instability. *J Bone Joint Surg Am.* 2006;88:1467–1474.

30. Gerber C, Ganz R. Clinical assessment of instability of the shoulder: with special reference to anterior and posterior drawer tests. *J Bone Joint Surg Br.* 1984;66:551–556.

31. Gagey OJ, Gagey N. The hyperabduction test. *J Bone Joint Surg Br.* 2001;83:69–74.

32. Garth WP Jr, Slappey CE, Ochs CW. Roentgenographic demonstration of instability of the shoulder: the apical oblique projection. A technical note. *J Bone Joint Surg Am.* 1984;66:1450–1453.

33. Pavlov H, Warren RF, Weiss CB Jr, et al. The roentgenographic evaluation of anterior shoulder instability. *Clin Orthop Relat Res.* 1985;194:153–158.

34. Rokous JR, Feagin JA, Abbott HG. Modified axillary roentgenogram: a useful adjunct in the diagnosis of recurrent instability of the shoulder. *Clin Orthop Relat Res.* 1972;82:84–86.

35. Tauber M, Resch H, Forstner R, et al. Reasons for failure after surgical repair of anterior shoulder instability. *J Shoulder Elbow Surg.* 2004;13:279–285.

36. Huijsmans PE, Haen PS, Kidd M, et al. Quantification of a glenoid defect with three-dimensional computed tomography and magnetic resonance imaging: a cadaveric study. *J Shoulder Elbow Surg.* 2007;16:803–809.

37. Gyftopoulos S, Hasan S, Bencardino J, et al. Diagnostic accuracy of MRI in the measurement of glenoid bone loss. *Am J Roentgenol.* 2012;199:873–878.

38. Lee RK, Griffith JF, Tong MM, et al. Glenoid bone loss: assessment with MR imaging. *Radiology.* 2013;267:496–502.

39. Chuang TY, Adams CR, Burkhart SS. Use of preoperative three-dimensional computed tomography to quantify glenoid bone loss in shoulder instability. *Arthroscopy.* 2008;24:376–382.

40. Rerko MA, Pan X, Donaldson C, et al. Comparison of various imaging techniques to quantify glenoid bone loss in shoulder instability. *J Shoulder Elbow Surg.* 2013;22:528–534.

41. Provencher MT, Bhatia S, Ghodadra NS, et al. Recurrent shoulder instability: current concepts for evaluation and management of glenoid bone loss. *J Bone Joint Surg Am.* 2010;92:133–151.

42. Sugaya H, Moriishi J, Dohi M, et al. Glenoid rim morphology in recurrent anterior glenohumeral instability. *J Bone Joint Surg Am.* 2003;85:878–884.

43. Burkhart SS, De Beer JF, Tehrany AM, et al. Quantifying glenoid bone loss arthroscopically in shoulder instability. *Arthroscopy.* 2002;18:488–491.

44. Ozbaydar M, Elhassan B, Diller D, et al. Results of arthroscopic capsulolabral repair: Bankart lesion versus anterior labroligamentous periosteal sleeve avulsion lesion. *Arthroscopy.* 2008;24:1277–1283.

45. Kim DS, Yoon YS, Yi CH. Prevalence comparison of accompanying lesions between primary and recurrent anterior dislocation in the shoulder. *Am J Sports Med.* 2010;38:2071–2076.

46. Allain J, Goutallier D, Glorion C. Long-term results of the Latarjet procedure for the treatment of anterior instability of the shoulder. *J Bone Joint Surg Am.* 1998;80:841–852.

47. Yamamoto N, Muraki T, An KN, et al. The stabilizing mechanism of the Latarjet procedure: a cadaveric study. *J Bone Joint Surg Am.* 2013;95:1390–1397.

48. De Beer JF, Roberts C. Glenoid bone defects: open Latarjet with congruent arc modification. *Orthop Clin North Am.* 2010;41:407–415.

49. Burkhart SS, De Beer JF, Barth JR, et al. Results of modified Latarjet reconstruction in patients with anteroinferior instability and significant bone loss. *Arthroscopy.* 2007;23:1033–1041.

50. Armitage MS, Elkinson I, Giles JW, et al. An anatomic, computed tomographic assessment of the coracoid process with special reference to the congruent-arc Latarjet procedure. *Arthroscopy.* 2011;27:1485–1489.

51. Ghodadra N, Gupta A, Romeo AA, et al. Normalization of glenohumeral articular contact pressures after Latarjet or iliac crest bone-grafting. *J Bone Joint Surg Am.* 2010;92:1478–1489.

52. Hovelius L, Sandstrom B, Sundgren K, et al. One hundred eighteen Bristow-Latarjet repairs for recurrent anterior dislocation of the shoulder prospectively followed for fifteen years: study I—clinical results. *J Shoulder Elbow Surg.* 2004;13:509–516.

53. Mizuno N, Denard PJ, Raiss P, et al. Long-term results of the Latarjet procedure for anterior instability of the shoulder. *J Shoulder Elbow Surg.* 2014;23:1691–1699.
54. Bhatia S, Frank RM, Ghodadra NS, et al. The outcomes and surgical techniques of the Latarjet procedure. *Arthroscopy.* 2014;30:227–235.
55. Griesser MJ, Harris JD, McCoy BW, et al. Complications and re-operations after Bristow-Latarjet shoulder stabilization: a systematic review. *J Shoulder Elbow Surg.* 2013;22:286–292.
56. An VV, Sivakumar BS, Phan K, et al. A systematic review and meta-analysis of clinical and patient-reported outcomes following two procedures for recurrent traumatic anterior instability of the shoulder: Latarjet procedure vs. Bankart repair. *J Shoulder Elbow Surg.* 2016;25:853–863.
57. Hovelius L, Sandström B, Saebö M. One hundred eighteen Bristow-Latarjet repairs for recurrent anterior dislocation of the shoulder prospectively followed for fifteen years: study II. The evolution of dislocation arthropathy. *J Shoulder Elbow Surg.* 2006;15:279–289.

13 HAGL: Arthroscopic/Open

Megan R. Wolf and Robert A. Arciero

INTRODUCTION

Humeral avulsion of the glenohumeral ligament (HAGL) lesions is an important but less common cause of recurrent instability in the shoulder after injury. Typically, in the pathology of shoulder instability, either a capsulolabral avulsion of the anteroinferior portion of the inferior glenohumeral ligament (IGHL), the so-called Bankart lesion, or capsular laxity is observed.

Although reports of Bankart lesions accounting for anterior shoulder instability are seen in 45% to 100% of cases, the glenohumeral ligaments can fail at the humeral insertion site (1). These HAGL lesions have been reported in 1% to 9% of patients with recurrent shoulder instability (2–4). Bokor et al. (2) reviewed 547 shoulders for the cause of instability and found HAGL lesions in 7.5% of patients. They further found that in looking at their failed recurrent instability procedures, at revision surgery the incidence of an HAGL lesion was 18.2%. Another study (5) found that only 50% of patients who were found to have an HAGL lesion had detectable pathology on magnetic resonance imaging (MRI).

To diagnose an HAGL lesion, one needs a high suspicion, an understanding of the anatomy of the ligaments, and an understanding of its mechanisms of injury. Approximately 66% of HAGL lesions in the literature had other associated abnormalities at the time of arthroscopy (6). HAGL lesions have been associated with rotator cuff tears, Bankart lesions (i.e., a floating IGHL), Hill-Sachs lesions, and labral tears (5). Because of the associated pathology seen with HAGL lesions, a thorough arthroscopic inspection of the shoulder should include the axillary pouch and the IGHL attachment to the humeral neck to avoid missing the lesions (7,8). Bach et al. (7) state that in the absence of capsular laxity and glenoid pathology, a disruption of the lateral capsule (i.e., HAGL lesion) must be excluded. Failure to diagnose the HAGL lesion could lead to persistent instability and pain.

Nicola has been credited with describing the first known HAGL defect after an anterior shoulder dislocation (9). In a clinical and cadaveric study, he found that, unlike a Bankart defect that occurs with the arm in a hyperabducted position with impaction, the HAGL lesion was most likely to occur with the arm in both the hyperabducted and externally rotated positions (2,9).

Shoulder dislocations are associated with various structural abnormalities, depending on the age of the patient. Younger patients are more likely to disrupt the anterior labral-ligamentous attachment to the glenoid. Older patients are more likely to disrupt the anterior capsular attachment to the humerus (HAGL lesion) and may disrupt the subscapularis tendon. In fact, older patients with anterior dislocations may be misdiagnosed with an axillary nerve neurapraxia or a rotator cuff tear if they cannot abduct their arm (10,11). The difference in pathology due to age may be secondary to a weakening of the rotator cuff and weakening of the capsular attachment to the humerus. This results in a higher likelihood that the capsular-humeral interface fails rather than the capsular-glenoid interface (10,12).

The reported incidence of HAGL lesions has increased with shoulder arthroscopy. Therefore, it could be a site for ligament failure more commonly than previously believed (2,8). Trauma has been shown to contribute to HAGL lesions in over 94% of reported cases in the literature (13,14), but there has been one reported case of an HAGL lesion after a repetitive microtrauma from overhead throwing (15). Warner first described a combined Bankart and HAGL lesion, the so-called floating AIGHL. He treated it with an open repair and had excellent results (16).

Anatomy

The inferior glenohumeral ligament (IGHL) has two bands, the anterior inferior glenohumeral ligament (AIGHL) and the posterior inferior glenohumeral ligament (PIGHL). The IGHL also has an axillary pouch that spans between the AIGHL and the PIGHL (17) (Fig. 13-1). In the right shoulder, the AIGHL extends from the 2:00 to 4:00 position and the PIGHL extends from the 7:00 to 9:00 position. The IGHL complex attaches to the medial humerus just under the cartilage of the humeral head. Two configurations have been identified. One is a collar-like attachment, where the entire IGHL complex inserts just below the anatomical neck of the humerus. The other is a V-shaped attachment, where the AIGHL and PIGHL attach at the margins of the humeral neck cartilage surface and the interposing pouch inserts more distally on the neck of the humerus (7,17). The IGHL is the primary restraint to anterior shoulder dislocation with the arm at 90 degrees of abduction and external rotation (18). Other stabilizing structures include static stabilizers (the labrum) and dynamic stabilizers (the subscapularis muscle) with the arm at zero degrees of abduction (4).

History and Physical Examination

Although no specific historical feature will indicate the presence of an HAGL lesion, the senior author has observed a higher preponderance of this lesion in wrestlers. In this mechanism, the wrestler almost always reports a combination of hyperabduction and external rotation.

As with all examinations, inspection of the shoulder should be performed first. One should look for signs of ecchymoses, swelling, or skin deformity that can be associated with acute shoulder dislocations. Range of motion should be evaluated and clearly noted in flexion, external rotation with the arm at the side, external rotation in abduction, and internal rotation. Especially with external rotation in abduction, the point of shoulder apprehension should be carefully noted. The feeling of apprehension at small degrees of external rotation and more so with the arm at the side are clues to the severity of the instability. Rotator cuff strength should be tested. Older patients may be misdiagnosed with an axillary nerve neurapraxia or rotator cuff tear if they cannot abduct their arm (10,11). Biceps pathology is evaluated with the Speeds test (biceps tendon pathology) and the O'Brien test (superior labral tears). The subscapularis muscle, often involved in older patients with anterior shoulder dislocations, is tested using the lift-off test, belly-press test, and bear-hug test.

Although no specific clinical test can differentiate an HAGL lesion from a Bankart lesion (19), shoulder stability special tests should be performed. Specific clinical examinations for shoulder stability include the apprehension and relocation tests, assessing anterior shoulder instability, the posterior jerk test assessing posterior shoulder instability, and the load-and-shift test. The latter gives the examiner a sense for how "loose" the shoulder or capsule is in the anterior and posterior directions. A grade 1, 2, or 3 is given to the load-and-shift test based on the examiner's ability to bring the humeral head to the glenoid rim, over the glenoid rim but with a spontaneous reduction, or over the glenoid rim without a reduction, respectively. The load-and-shift is tested in the anterior, anteroinferior, and posterior directions.

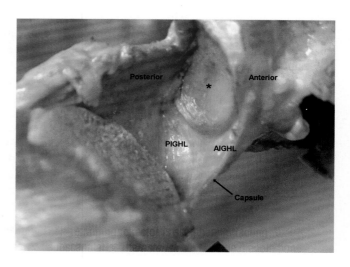

FIGURE 13-1

Anatomic specimen showing the IGHL with a resected part of humeral head (*asterisk*, glenoid).

Imaging

The bony humeral avulsion of the glenohumeral ligament, or BHAGL, lesion was first described by Bach et al. (7). They found a bony fragment avulsed from the medial aspect of the humeral neck that was the cause of recurrent dislocations (Fig. 13-2). The bony fragment in a BHAGL lesion is best visualized with a Garth view of the shoulder, which is a 15-degree oblique x-ray in the anterior plane of the shoulder (20). However, in order to distinguish a BHAGL from a bony Bankart lesion, a West Point axillary lateral view is recommended (5). Other studies, in addition, have shown that scalloping of the medial humeral neck on the anteroposterior x-ray view can be consistent with an HAGL defect, even without seeing any calcification in the soft tissues (2).

CT arthrography can be useful in identifying a BHAGL lesion. Typically, the linear bony density representing the BHAGL is seen posterior to the MGHL and contrast extravasation is seen anterior to the BHAGL (20).

The imaging diagnosis of HAGL lesions is typically seen on MRI examination; however, the diagnosis of HAGL lesions is missed in 50% of cases based on imaging studies alone (5). The MRI diagnosis of an HAGL lesion is best seen on the fat-suppressed T2-weighted images in the coronal oblique and sagittal oblique planes (5). The MRI arthrogram characteristics of an HAGL lesion include (a) increased signal intensity and increased thickness of the inferior capsule, (b) extravasation of the contrast material or the joint effusion along the medial humeral neck, and (c) conversion of the normal U-shaped axillary pouch to a J-shaped structure (5,21) (Fig. 13-3). Posterior or reverse HAGL lesions ("RHAGL") have also been described (Fig. 13-4). MRI can also lead to the false-positive diagnosis of HAGL lesions. Therefore, the recommendation from Melvin et al. (22) was that an HAGL diagnosis be reserved for arthroscopy. This also shows the difficulty in distinguishing HAGL lesions from other IGHL abnormalities. Interestingly, when an HAGL lesion is associated with a tear of the subscapularis tendon, MRI is especially useful in making that diagnosis (3).

Classification

Injury to the IGHL typically occurs in three possible locations—failure at the glenoid, failure at the humerus, or an intrasubstance tear. In addition, one could have an injury to the AIGHL or PIGHL in each of the locations described above. Lastly, when the failure occurs at the humerus, it could either

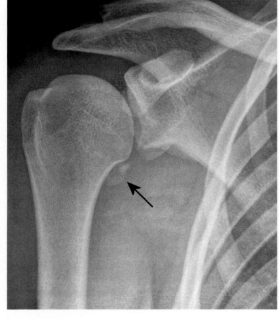

FIGURE 13-2

A calcification is noted inferiorly that represents a BHAGL lesion (*black arrow*).

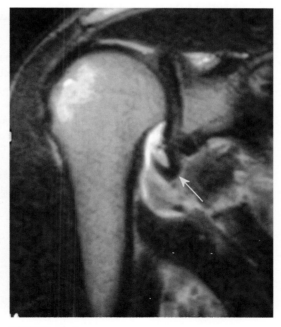

FIGURE 13-3

MRI depicting an HAGL lesion. The *white arrow* shows the avulsed capsule.

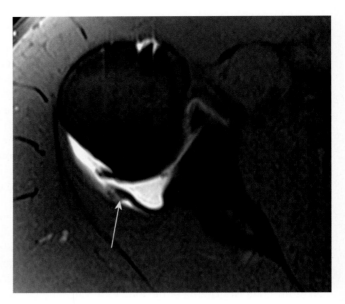

FIGURE 13-4

MRI depicting a posterior lateral avulsion of the IGHL (i.e., reverse HAGL lesion). The *white arrow* points to the avulsed capsule.

be a pure ligamentous tear or a piece of the medial cortex of the humerus could avulse off with the ligament, producing a bony HAGL (BHAGL).

Bui-Mansfield et al. (6) proposed a classification scheme derived from the terminology in the literature combined with the anatomic sites of rupture of the IGHL. They found six forms of HAGL lesions based on the involvement of the anterior or posterior band of the IGHL, the presence or absence of a bony avulsion, and whether or not a labral tear was also identified in the injury pattern. The anterior band was involved in 97% of the HAGL lesions. The strict avulsion of the IGHL from the humerus could either be purely ligamentous—anterior HAGL (AHAGL)—or with a bony lesion, BHAGL. The last is a floating HAGL where both the humeral and the glenoid sides of the IGHL complex are torn. The same nomenclature exists for the PIGHL. Table 13-1 lists the frequency of HAGL lesions based on their anatomic locations.

TREATMENT OPTIONS

Nonoperative Treatment

The conservative treatment of HAGL lesions depends on the associated pathology found in the shoulder. If truly an isolated defect, treatment includes a sling immobilizer for 4 weeks followed by a shoulder-strengthening program (20); however, isolated HAGL lesions are rare. Approximately 66% of HAGL lesions were found to have associated shoulder pathology found at the time of arthroscopy (6). Wolf et al. (4) identified that the incidence of an HAGL lesion was 9.3% and that of a Bankart lesion 73.5% and that generalized capsular laxity was seen in 17.2% of 64 shoulders

TABLE 13-1 Frequency of HAGL Lesions Based on Anatomic Location	
AHAGL	55%
Anterior BHAGL	17%
Floating AIGHL	21%
PHAGL	3%
Posterior BHAGL	0%
Floating PIGHL	4%

AIGHL, anterior inferior glenohumeral ligament; BHAGL, bony humeral avulsion of the glenohumeral ligament; PIGHL, posterior inferior glenohumeral ligament.
Source: Reprinted from Bui-Mansfield LT, Banks KP, Taylor DC. Humeral avulsion of the glenohumeral ligaments: the HAGL lesion. *Am J Sports Med.* 2007;35(11):1960–1966. Copyright © 2007 SAGE Publications, with permission.

with anterior shoulder instability prospectively evaluated with arthroscopy. The failure to diagnose an HAGL defect and its associated pathology could lead to persistent instability and pain.

Operative Treatment

The surgical diagnosis and/or treatment of HAGL lesions can be done either open or arthroscopically. The HAGL lesion, as seen on an open dissection, is below the level of the subscapularis muscle, in the inferior pouch of the shoulder. It is a thickened, rolled edge in the capsular defect (2). On open shoulder dissection, the HAGL lesion may be difficult to diagnose because, if the plane between the subscapularis and capsule is inadvertently entered, this may lead to a false-positive diagnosis of an HAGL lesion. Along the same lines, this could also lead to a false-negative diagnosis of an HAGL lesion if the surgeon thinks that he or she dissected through the capsule. Furthermore, if one leaves the deep portion of the subscapularis muscle/tendon over the capsule, this may hide the presence of an HAGL lesion (4).

Arthroscopy may be the most accurate method for evaluating the IGHL ligaments and documenting an HAGL lesion. The HAGL lesion can be seen at the inferior aspect of the shoulder, in the axillary recess (Fig. 13-5). With the arthroscope in the posterior portal, one may need a 70-degree scope to formally evaluate the IGHL complex. On the other hand, with the arthroscope in the anterosuperior portal, one could use a standard 30-degree scope for the diagnosis (Fig. 13-6). In all cases of shoulder arthroscopy, the capsular attachment of the IGHL to the humerus should be documented (23). The cardinal sign of an HAGL lesion at arthroscopy is the visualization of the fibers of the subscapularis

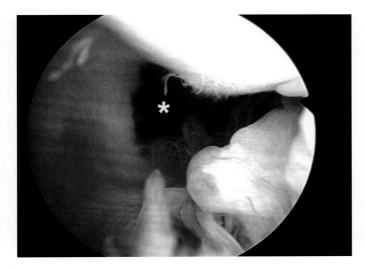

FIGURE 13-5

Arthroscopic inferior axillary view in a left shoulder showing HAGL lesion (*asterisk*, HAGL lesion).

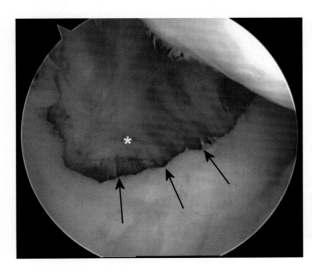

FIGURE 13-6

HAGL lesion with subscapularis exposed. Avulsed leading edge of IGHL (*black arrows*). Right shoulder viewed with arthroscope in ASP (*asterisk*, subscapularis muscle).

muscle through the rent in the inferior capsule (4,23) (Fig. 13-6). Another sign of an HAGL lesion at arthroscopy is disruption of the wave formed by the reflection of the inferior capsule onto the humeral neck (2).

TECHNIQUE

Arthroscopic HAGL Repair

The patient is placed into the lateral decubitus position with proper padding. An examination under anesthesia is documented in the lateral position. The arm is placed into lateral traction in 50 degrees of abduction and 15 degrees of forward flexion with 5 to 10 lb of weight. A standard posterior arthroscopy portal is made, taking care to avoid entering the joint medially relative to the glenoid and inferiorly along the posterior labrum. Most HAGL lesions can be viewed from this position with the arthroscope in the axillary pouch (Fig. 13-5). A second portal is made high in the rotator interval (anterosuperior portal—ASP), and a full diagnostic arthroscopy is performed. The arthroscope is then placed into the ASP, and the posterior diagnostic arthroscopy is completed. Viewing from the anterior portal during arthroscopy is important in making the diagnosis of an AHAGL or a PHAGL lesion (19,24).

The humeral insertion of the IGHL is best visualized from the ASP portal with a 30-degree scope. If a combined HAGL defect and Bankart defect occur, the HAGL defect is repaired first prior to the Bankart to avoid overtensioning the capsule medially on the glenoid without leaving enough excursion to repair the lateral HAGL lesion.

From a second midanterior portal traditionally placed just superior to the leading edge of the subscapularis tendon, a grasper is used to assess the mobility of the HAGL defect. A burr is used from the midanterior portal to create a bleeding bony bed at the anatomic HAGL insertion site on the humerus. At this time, the HAGL insertion on the humerus may be better observed with a 70-degree arthroscope viewing from the ASP (Fig. 13-7). The correct path for suture anchor placement onto the medial humeral neck is determined under direct visualization using an 18-gauge spinal needle and may be placed in a percutaneous fashion through the subscapularis. The trocar for the suture anchor is then placed along this path, and a 3.0-mm bioabsorbable anchor is placed (Fig. 13-8A and B). One limb of the suture is retrieved through the posterior portal and the other limb is left through the insertion trocar. From the midanterior portal, a suture-passing device is used to thread a monofilament suture through the detached lateral capsule of the HAGL lesion. The limb of the monofilament suture is retrieved through the posterior portal, and using proper suture shuttling technique, the suture limb from the anchor is shuttled back through the IGHL and out the midanterior portal (Fig. 13-9). This technique is repeated following the steps above to pass the other limb of the suture anchor through the IGHL to create a mattress suture. The sutures are tied from the midanterior portal (Fig. 13-10).

FIGURE 13-7

Arthroscopic probe marking anchor placement (*arrow*). Right shoulder viewed with arthroscope in ASP and the probe is through the midanterior portal.

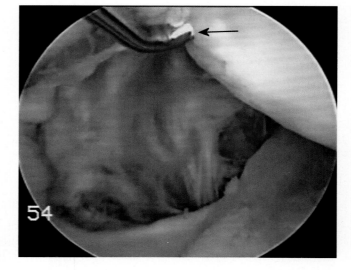

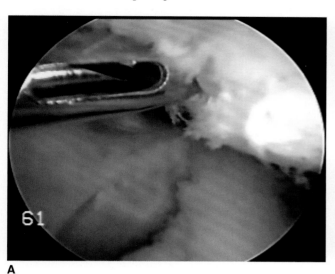

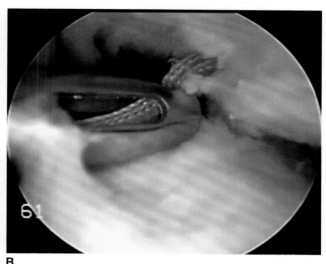

A   **B**

FIGURE 13-8

A: Drilling for placement of anchor along neck of humerus. Right shoulder viewed with arthroscope in ASP. **B:** First anchor is placed along neck of humerus. Right shoulder viewed with arthroscope in ASP.

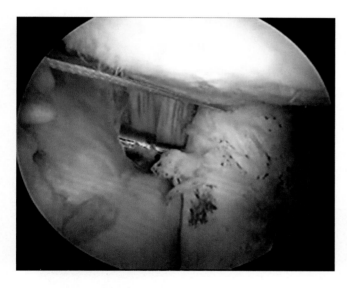

FIGURE 13-9

The suture from the first anchor is shuttled through the HAGL lesion. Right shoulder viewed with arthroscope in ASP.

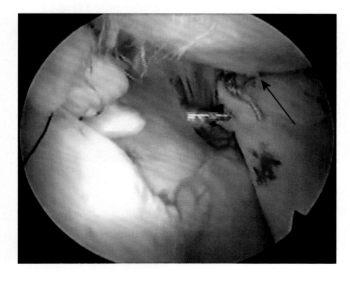

FIGURE 13-10

The first inferior anchor sutures are tied in a mattress-type fashion (*arrow*). Right shoulder viewed with arthroscope in ASP.

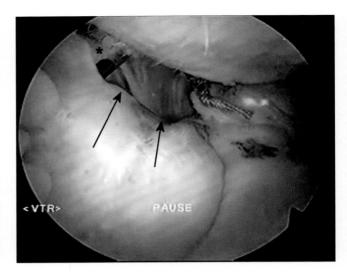

FIGURE 13-11

The second more proximal anchor is being placed. The *black arrows* point to the remaining HAGL defect to be repaired. The *asterisk* shows the anchor trocar.

To continue the repair anteriorly, a transsubscapularis portal is made (accessory low anterior portal, 5:00) for anchor placement. The anchor trocar is inserted into this pathway, and another anchor is placed at the humeral attachment of the IGHL (Fig. 13-11). To allow for the proper angle of anchor placement, rotation of the arm may be necessary. Using a suture-passing device from the accessory posterolateral 7:00 portal, the previous suture shuttling technique is repeated as stated above, and each limb of the suture anchor is shuttled through the IGHL in a mattress-type fashion and tied through the midanterior portal (Fig. 13-12A and B).

Mini Open HAGL Repair

The arthroscopic technique can be challenging due to the limited exposure along the anteroinferior pouch and humeral neck. If that is the case, a technique has been described by the senior author that spares the superior 50% of the subscapularis tendon with a limited open exposure (1).

The patient is placed into the beach chair position with all bony prominences and head carefully secured. The surgical extremity is draped free and supported by a padded Mayo stand. A 3- to 4-cm skin incision is made from the axillary fold to the coracoid process. The deltopectoral interval is

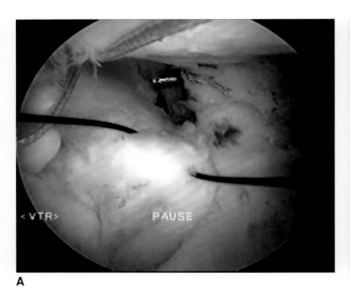

A

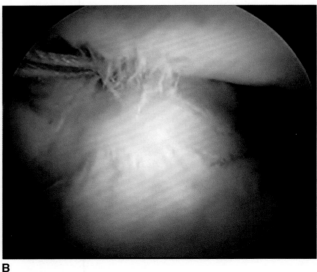

B

FIGURE 13-12

A: An absorbable suture (*dark blue*) is seen through the HAGL lesion. It is used to shuttle the nonabsorbable suture from the anchor.
B: HAGL lesion repaired.

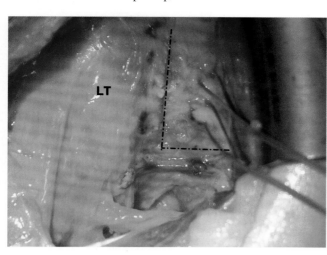

FIGURE 13-13

The open repair incision in the subscapularis muscle. The "L"-shaped incision spares the upper proximal tendinous portion of subscapularis. Tag stitches have been placed in the subscapularis muscle. The *dotted line* shows the orientation of the incision. LT, lesser tuberosity.

opened, and the cephalic vein is retracted laterally. The clavipectoral fascia is then opened to but not through the coracoacromial ligament.

The subscapularis tendon and anterior humeral circumflex vessels are now exposed. An L-shaped incision is made at the lower half of the subscapularis tendon. The vertical part of the incision is made 1.5 cm medial to the lesser tuberosity and started at the inferior half of the subscapularis tendon (Fig. 13-13). The incision ends just proximal to the circumflex vessels. The axillary nerve is then palpated to ensure its protection. The subscapularis tendon and muscle fibers are incised medially for 1.5 to 2 cm, thus creating the horizontal portion of the L-shaped subscapularis incision. The fleshy fibers of the inferior subscapularis are gently spread with a Cobb elevator or Metzenbaum scissors, and the L-shaped incision is lifted proximally (Fig. 13-14) exposing the HAGL defect (Fig. 13-15).

The lesion is located at the anteroinferior aspect of the glenohumeral joint from the 8:00 to 6:00 position on a right shoulder. A tag suture is placed into the leading edge of the avulsed IGHL. The cortex of the anatomic attachment site of the IGHL on the humeral neck is gently debrided to a bleeding bony bed. Suture anchors are placed into the neck of the humerus (Fig. 13-16). The sutures are passed through the HAGL lesion in a mattress-type fashion and tied (Fig. 13-17). Two anchors are typically required for this repair. Once the repair is completed, the inferior half of the subscapularis tendon is repaired anatomically back to its insertion site using nonabsorbable sutures (Fig. 13-18).

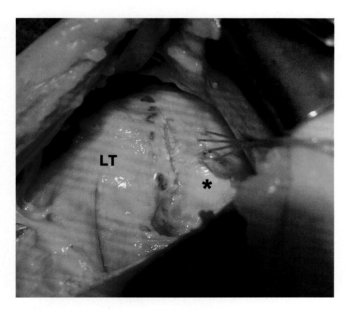

FIGURE 13-14

The lower third of subscapularis is reflected proximally. LT, lesser tuberosity; *asterisk,*"L"-shaped edge of subscapularis.

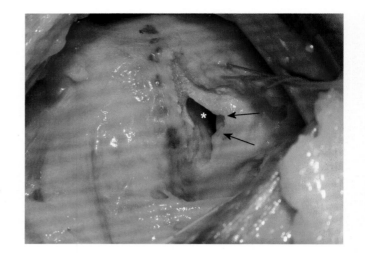

FIGURE 13-15

The HAGL defect is exposed. *Black arrows* show avulsed capsule. *Asterisk* shows defect created by HAGL. Tag stitches are in subscapularis tendon/ muscle.

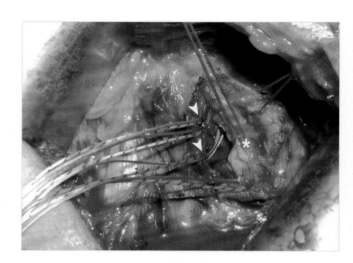

FIGURE 13-16

Suture anchors have been placed in the humeral neck (*white arrowheads*). Note single tag suture in leading edge of HAGL lesion (*white asterisk*).

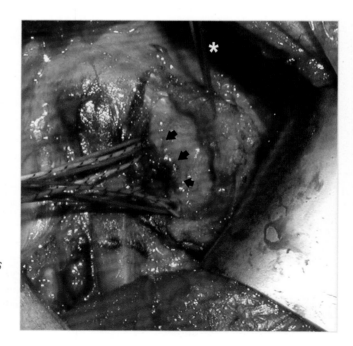

FIGURE 13-17

HAGL defect repaired. *Black arrowheads* show leading edge of HAGL lesion attached back to humeral neck. *White asterisk* shows tag suture in subscapularis.

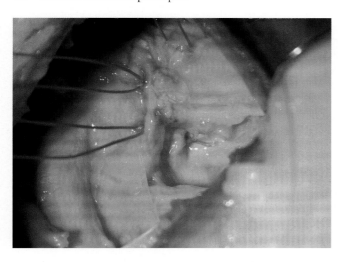

FIGURE 13-18
Lower portion of subscapularis muscle/tendon is repaired.

PEARLS AND PITFALLS

HAGL lesions may be seen in patients with recurrent anterior shoulder instability or after a failed labral repair. Therefore, one must have a high suspicion and evaluate patients for the potential of a lesion of the IGHL in the setting of anterior shoulder instability. Repair may be performed in an open or arthroscopic fashion. Although arthroscopic evaluation may better identify the presence of an HAGL lesion, the arthroscopic technique can be challenging due to the limited exposure along the anteroinferior pouch and humeral neck. Proper placement of portals, use of a 70-degree arthroscope, and percutaneous suture anchors are helpful in the evaluation and repair of the lesion arthroscopically.

POSTOPERATIVE MANAGEMENT

The postoperative course includes placing the arm into a sling in neutral or slight internal rotation for 4 weeks. During the first 3 to 4 weeks, the patient is allowed Codman exercises and supine well-arm assisted forward elevation. Isometric exercises are started within 2 to 3 weeks of surgery. At 4 to 6 weeks postoperatively, external rotation exercises are started. Progressive resistance with bands, cords, and weights is started at 6 weeks postoperatively. After 4 months postop, the patient is returned to full activity and contact sports. The main benefit of the mini open technique is that patients experience a rapid return of lift-off power and little weakness in subscapularis function.

RESULTS

The surgical treatment of HAGL defects has been successful using open or arthroscopic techniques (2,4,7,8,15,16,25). The open approaches can be subdivided into traditional subscapularis detachment techniques (2,4,7) or partial detachment techniques (1). Bach et al. (7) were the first to describe the operative treatment of the HAGL defect. They reported on two cases treated with open repair. Bokor et al. (2) reported on 41 HAGL defects that were repaired open with suture anchors or drill holes.

The advantages of all-arthroscopic technique include easier identification of the lesion, less soft tissue trauma (i.e., less injury to the subscapularis), better surgical visualization, less postoperative pain, and the ability to perform accelerated rehabilitation (19). There are a small number of published articles on arthroscopic HAGL repairs in the literature (4,23,24,26,27). Wolf et al. (4) described the repair of the HAGL defects with plication of the IGHL over the deltopectoral fascia. Kon et al. (24) reported on three arthroscopic HAGL repairs with no recurrences and documented a return to preinjury activity with 12- to 24-month follow-up. Huberty and Burkhart (26) additionally reported that at 31.8-month follow-up of six HAGL defects treated arthroscopically, no patients had sustained recurrent dislocations and all were satisfied with their repair.

CONCLUSIONS

In conclusion, HAGL lesions are an important cause of recurrent instability in the shoulder after injury. The incidence of these lesions as a cause of anterior shoulder instability is seen in 7.5% to 9.3% of cases. As there is no single clinical test that can reliably diagnose an HAGL lesion, one must have a high suspicion. The definitive diagnosis is made at surgery, and in all cases of shoulder arthroscopy, the capsular attachment of IGHL to the humeral should be documented.

REFERENCES

1. Arciero RA, Mazzocca AD. Mini-open repair technique of HAGL (humeral avulsion of the glenohumeral ligament) lesion. *Arthroscopy.* 2005;21(9):1152.
2. Bokor DJ, Conboy VB, Olson C. Anterior instability of the glenohumeral joint with humeral avulsion of the glenohumeral ligament. A review of 41 cases. *J Bone Joint Surg Br.* 1999;81(1):93–96.
3. Tirman PF, Steinbach LS, Feller JF, et al. Humeral avulsion of the anterior shoulder stabilizing structures after anterior shoulder dislocation: demonstration by MRI and MR arthrography. *Skeletal Radiol.* 1996;25(8):743–748.
4. Wolf EM, Cheng JC, Dickson K. Humeral avulsion of glenohumeral ligaments as a cause of anterior shoulder instability. *Arthroscopy.* 1995;11(5):600–607.
5. Bui-Mansfield LT, Taylor DC, Uhorchak JM, et al. Humeral avulsions of the glenohumeral ligament: imaging features and a review of the literature. *Am J Roentgenol.* 2002;179(3):649–655.
6. Bui-Mansfield LT, Banks KP, Taylor DC. Humeral avulsion of the glenohumeral ligaments: the HAGL lesion. *Am J Sports Med.* 2007;35(11):1960–1966.
7. Bach BR, Warren RF, Fronek J. Disruption of the lateral capsule of the shoulder. A cause of recurrent dislocation. *J Bone Joint Surg Br.* 1988;70(2):274–276.
8. Field LD, Bokor DJ, Savoie FH III. Humeral and glenoid detachment of the anterior inferior glenohumeral ligament: a cause of anterior shoulder instability. *J Shoulder Elbow Surg.* 1997;6(1):6–10.
9. Nicola T. Anterior dislocation of the shoulder. *J Bone Joint Surg.* 1941;26:614–616.
10. Neviaser RJ, Neviaser TJ, Neviaser JS. Anterior dislocation of the shoulder and rotator cuff rupture. *Clin Orthop Relat Res.* 1993;291:103–106.
11. Neviaser RJ, Neviaser TJ, Neviaser JS. Concurrent rupture of the rotator cuff and anterior dislocation of the shoulder in the older patient. *J Bone Joint Surg Am.* 1988;70(9):1308–1311.
12. McLaughlin H. Injuries of the shoulder and arm. In: McLaughlin H, ed. *Trauma.* Philadelphia, PA: WB Saunders; 1959:233–296.
13. Coates MH, Breidahl W. Humeral avulsion of the anterior band of the inferior glenohumeral ligament with associated subscapularis bony avulsion in skeletally immature patients. *Skeletal Radiol.* 2001;30(12):661–666.
14. Rowe CR, Zarins B, Ciullo JV. Recurrent anterior dislocation of the shoulder after surgical repair. Apparent causes of failure and treatment. *J Bone Joint Surg Am.* 1984;66(2):159–168.
15. Gehrmann RM, DeLuca PF, Bartolozzi AR. Humeral avulsion of the glenohumeral ligament caused by microtrauma to the anterior capsule in an overhand throwing athlete: a case report. *Am J Sports Med.* 2003;31(4):617–619.
16. Warner JJ, Beim GM. Combined Bankart and HAGL lesion associated with anterior shoulder instability. *Arthroscopy.* 1997;13(6):749–752.
17. O'Brien SJ, Neves MC, Arnoczky SP, et al. The anatomy and histology of the inferior glenohumeral ligament complex of the shoulder. *Am J Sports Med.* 1990;18(5):449–456.
18. Turkel SJ, Panio MW, Marshall JL, et al. Stabilizing mechanisms preventing anterior dislocation of the glenohumeral joint. *J Bone Joint Surg Am.* 1981;63(8):1208–1217.
19. Parameswaran AD, Provencher MT, Bach BR Jr, et al. Humeral avulsion of the glenohumeral ligament: injury pattern and arthroscopic repair techniques. *Orthopedics.* 2008;31(8):773–779.
20. Oberlander MA, Morgan BE, Visotsky JL. The BHAGL lesion: a new variant of anterior shoulder instability. *Arthroscopy.* 1996;12(5):627–633.
21. Stoller DW. MR arthrography of the glenohumeral joint. *Radiol Clin North Am.* 1997;35(1):97–116.
22. Melvin JS, Mackenzie JD, Nacke E, et al. MRI of HAGL lesions: four arthroscopically confirmed cases of false-positive diagnosis. *Am J Roentgenol.* 2008;191(3):730–734.
23. Spang JT, Karas SG. The HAGL lesion: an arthroscopic technique for repair of humeral avulsion of the glenohumeral ligaments. *Arthroscopy.* 2005;21(4):498–502.
24. Kon Y, Shiozaki H, Sugaya H. Arthroscopic repair of a humeral avulsion of the glenohumeral ligament lesion. *Arthroscopy.* 2005;21(5):632.
25. Schippinger G, Vasiu PS, Fankhauser F, et al. HAGL lesion occurring after successful arthroscopic Bankart repair. *Arthroscopy.* 2001;17(2):206–208.
26. Huberty DP, Burkhart SS. Arthroscopic repair of anterior humeral avulsion of the glenohumeral ligaments. *Tech Shoulder Elbow Surg.* 2006;7(4):186–190.
27. Richards DP, Burkhart SS. Arthroscopic humeral avulsion of the glenohumeral ligaments (HAGL) repair. *Arthroscopy.* 2004;20(suppl 2):134–141.

14 Arthroscopic Subacromial Decompression

Juntian Wang, Jason J. Shin, and Albert Lin

INDICATIONS

Rotator cuff impingement is a common cause of shoulder pain, especially in patients who participate in repetitive activity at or above the shoulder during work or sports. Patients typically complain of pain with overhead reaching and abduction. The described pain is classically localized to the lateral aspect of the acromion extending distally into the deltoid and can be elicited by active forward flexion and abduction. Physical examination findings such as the Neer and Hawkins signs are highly sensitive and are commonly performed but are limited by poor specificity (1,2). Resolution of pain upon forward elevation following a subacromial local anesthetic injection, or a Neer subacromial test, may help to localize the source of symptoms and aid in the diagnosis. Symptoms from subacromial impingement were originally hypothesized to occur as a result of progressive wear of the rotator cuff tendons with undersurface acromial bone spurring during shoulder elevation and abduction, thus leading to a spectrum of disease from irritation to eventual degenerative tearing (3). However, other authors have since argued that degenerative tearing of the rotator cuff may be related to intrinsic abnormalities within the tendon or subacromial bursa, perhaps making both structures prone to inflammation and degeneration (4,5). To date, the pathophysiology of rotator cuff impingement remains debated and not fully understood. Recent work investigating acromial morphology has suggested that an increased "critical shoulder angle" and lateralized acromial edge may also predispose patients to rotator cuff tearing (6).

The first-line treatment for rotator cuff impingement is usually conservative. Nonsurgical management typically involves anti-inflammatories (e.g., ice, corticosteroid subacromial injections, NSAIDs), physical therapy targeting the rotator cuff, and activity modification. Arthroscopic subacromial decompression (SAD) is a common surgical procedure indicated for treating subacromial impingement that remains refractory to nonsurgical treatment for 3 to 6 months. Although recent literature has questioned the utility of an isolated arthroscopic SAD, the procedure remains useful in situations of obvious mechanical impingement from substantial undersurface acromial bone spurs (7). As relative indications, an arthroscopic SAD may be necessary for increasing the subacromial working space when performing a rotator cuff repair and, in addition, may stimulate bony bleeding, providing a source of biologic augmentation for healing following a repair (8).

CONTRAINDICATIONS

Contraindications to an arthroscopic SAD have not been well studied in the literature. Aside from general surgical contraindications such as joint infection, it has been suggested that an arthroscopic SAD should not be performed for a massive and irreparable rotator cuff tear or rotator cuff arthropathy, where there may be a concern for disruption of a static restraint toward progressive proximal humeral head migration (4,5).

PREOPERATIVE PREPARATION

Radiographs are typically performed. A true anteroposterior view is necessary to visualize the gleno-humeral joint and assess for findings of chronic rotator cuff pathology such as a decreased acromial humeral distance. A supraspinatus outlet view best assesses acromial morphology (Fig. 14-1). An axillary lateral view allows for assessment of an os acromiale as well as overall glenohumeral joint stability. Finally, a Zanca view can evaluate the acromioclavicular (AC) joint for degenerative changes and osteolysis. Although magnetic resonance imaging (MRI) is not required, it can be helpful in assessing the condition of the rotator cuff and can show inflammatory changes around the AC joint.

TECHNIQUE

The patient is placed in an upright beach chair or lateral decubitus position, depending on surgeon preference (Figs. 14-2 and 14-3). Several landmarks are marked on the skin: acromion, clavicle, AC joint, coracoid (Fig. 14-4). Three portals are utilized: posterior, anterior, and lateral. The posterior portal is used for viewing purposes and is typically 2 to 3 cm inferomedial to the posterolateral acromial edge. The portal marks the soft spot in the triangular region bordered by the humeral head, glenoid, and acromion. The anterior portal is placed lateral and slightly cephalad to the tip of the coracoid and is used as a working portal to assess the glenohumeral joint during diagnostic arthros-copy. The lateral portal is used for instrumentation and should be placed at least 2 to 3 fingerbreadths distal from the midlateral border of the acromion. By cheating the lateral portal slightly more ante-riorly, the working space will be closer to the area of SAD and adjacent to the supraspinatus tendon, the most common area for rotator cuff tears. A more distal portal allows the best trajectory for work on the undersurface of the acromion. If the portal is too distal, then the working trajectory may be accommodated by abducting the shoulder, whereas if the portal is too proximal, then the trajectory cannot be accommodated in any fashion. If the lateral portal is more than 5 to 8 cm distal to the acromion, the axillary nerve may be at risk of being injured.

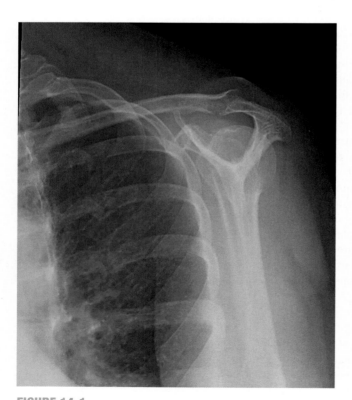

FIGURE 14-1

The supraspinatus outlet view, which assesses the acromial morphology, is shown here. The anterior acromion has a noticeable spur.

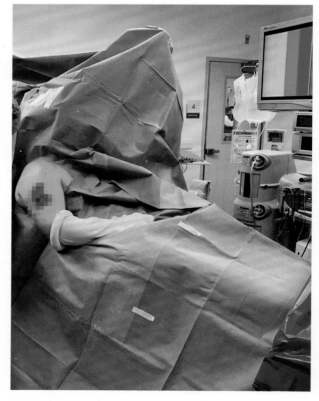

FIGURE 14-2

The patient is first placed in the upright beach-chair position.

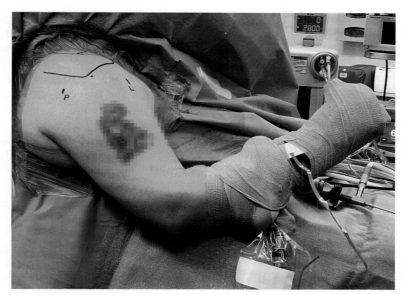

FIGURE 14-3

The forearm is then wrapped and placed in an arm holder.

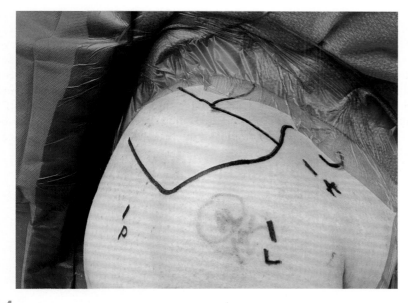

FIGURE 14-4

Portals used for arthroscopic SAD are marked on the skin. The locations of the anterior (A), lateral (L), and posterior (P) portals are shown in relationship to the coracoid, clavicle, acromion, and scapular spine, which are also marked on the skin.

The positions of the anterior and lateral portals should be confirmed when the arthroscope is inside the joint, using a spinal needle from outside-in. A 30-degree arthroscope is introduced into the joint from the posterior portal. The anterior portal is then made, and an arthroscopic trocar is introduced into the joint. Diagnostic glenohumeral arthroscopy is performed to assess the cartilage, labrum, capsuloligamentous structures, biceps, and rotator cuff. Any signs of concomitant joint pathology should be inspected at this time, and intra-articular copathologies can be treated as appropriate. The arthroscope is removed from the joint, and the arthroscopic sheath and trocar are reintroduced through the posterior portal into the subacromial space. The arthroscopic sheath and trocar should remain close to the undersurface of the acromion so the bursa remains below the entry site. At this time, it may be helpful to break up subacromial adhesions with a medial to lateral sweeping motion of the trocar under the acromion and deltoid fascia. The trocar is removed in place of the arthroscope, which should be aimed toward the coracoacromial (CA) ligament. Visualization of the CA ligament is critical as a reference to visualize the anterolateral edge of the acromion. Triangulation of a spinal needle directed toward the coracoid is used to help localize the final incision for the lateral portal.

A 4.0- or 5.0-mm arthroscopic shaver is then introduced through the lateral portal to perform a subacromial bursectomy, proceeding from anterior to posterior and lateral to medial to expose the subacromial space. The shaver should be viewed clearly from the posterior portal, and the shaver blades should be pointed away, parallel or superior to the cuff to avoid iatrogenic injury to the inferior rotator cuff tendons. When debriding tissue medially, it is not uncommon to encounter some bleeding, which can be controlled with electrocautery. The anterolateral aspect of the acromion should be exposed first to help widen the viewing and working spaces.

The shaver is removed, and an arthroscopic electrocautery ablation device is introduced through the lateral portal to debride the subacromial soft tissues (Fig. 14-5). The CA ligament can either be peeled subperiosteally or resected completely depending on surgeon preference. If there is a massive irreparable rotator cuff tear, the CA ligament should be preserved as it may help to prevent superior migration of the humerus and contribute to shoulder stability. The anterolateral edge of the acromion should be identified first with the ablator as this defines the most anterior and lateral edge of the acromioplasty. The ablation device should be used with caution to avoid going through the deltoid fascia or detaching the deltoid muscle fibers. The undersurface of the acromion is further defined with the ablation device until the entire anterior border can be visualized. The medial extent is then defined once the AC joint is visualized. Finally, the acromion is well exposed for subsequent SAD and acromioplasty.

The electrocautery ablation device is removed, and a 5.0-mm arthroscopic burr is introduced through the lateral portal to perform the SAD (Figs. 14-6–14-8). Again, the front edge of the anterolateral acromion should be resected first moving from anterior to posterior and lateral to medial. The objective of this procedure is to make the anterolateral acromion level with the midportion of the acromion in an anteroposterior plane, effectively converting the acromion into a type I acromion. Roughly 4 to 6 mm should be resected at the anterolateral edge, setting a level for the remainder of the bone resection. The burr is moved progressively and medially to match the lateral level of resection without violating the AC joint. Note that if the lateral portion of the acromion is not properly resected, then the burr will not be able to reach the medial aspect of the acromion. Once completed, the resected acromial undersurface should be level and flat.

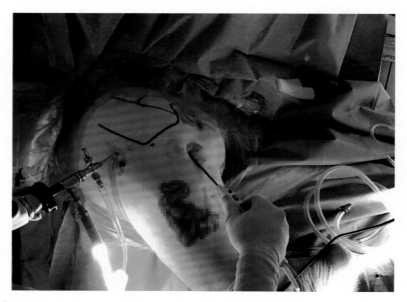

FIGURE 14-5

A radiofrequency device is introduced into the lateral portal to clean the subacromial bursa and space in preparation for subacromial decompression.

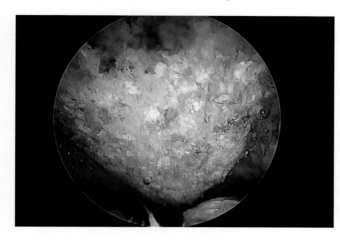

FIGURE 14-6

The unresected acromion after electrocautery ablation and debridement, prior to arthroscopic SAD, is shown here. This patient demonstrates a type III acromion.

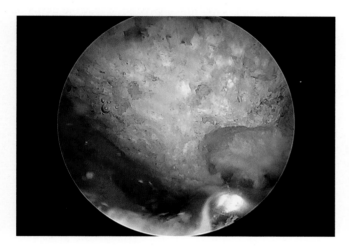

FIGURE 14-7

The lateral half of the anterior third of the acromion is resected with the 5.0-mm arthroscopic burr. The resected portion is then used as a template for the medial portion of the acromion.

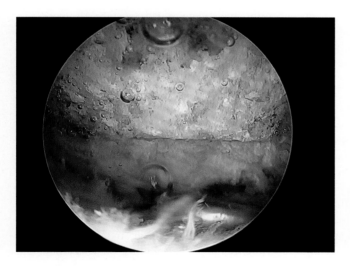

FIGURE 14-8

This image shows a completed arthroscopic SAD. The surface is flat without hidden, uneven ridges.

Alternatively, the arthroscope can be placed into the lateral portal, and the burr can be placed into the posterior portal. This "cutting-block technique" enables resection of the undersurface of the anterior acromion using the posterior undersurface as a guide to the angle of resection.

Finally, bone particles are removed with an arthroscopic shaver and suction. The arthroscope can be placed both in the lateral and posterior portals to confirm that the acromion is now smooth, flat, and flush with the rest of the acromion.

PEARLS AND PITFALLS

- Hemostasis through controlling the patient's blood pressure, intermittently increasing inflow pump pressure, and utilizing electrocautery can assist with visualization.
- Inadequate resection can be a cause of surgical failure. Complete bursectomy over the rotator cuff and the visualization of the entire undersurface of the acromion will allow for appropriate visualization of the bone spur for adequate decompression.
- Appropriate lateral portal placement is important to facilitate adequate SAD. Cheating the lateral portal more distal typically allows the best trajectory for resection. A spinal needle can be used to localize the ideal portal location prior to making an incision.
- When performing an isolated subacromial SAD, do not resect into the AC joint to avoid destabilizing the joint.
- Levering the hand can create divots in the acromion. Keep the burr parallel and directly under the acromion, and use a sweeping motion to create a smooth, flat surface.

POSTOPERATIVE MANAGEMENT

The patient is first placed in a shoulder sling. If the decompression was performed in isolation, then pendulum exercises and passive and active range-of-motion exercises for the shoulder, elbow, wrist, and hand are initiated the next day. Formal physical therapy is initiated within a week of surgery. Once full range of motion is achieved and patients can tolerate strengthening exercises, rotator cuff and periscapular strengthening is begun. Return to most activities is expected within 6 to 8 weeks, and full return to intensive activities is expected within 3 to 6 months. When concomitant procedures are performed, the therapy is adjusted appropriately.

COMPLICATIONS

Complications from an arthroscopic SAD include excessive resection of the acromion, which can result in an acromial fracture. On the opposite spectrum, inadequate resection can result in ongoing pain. Violating the AC joint may lead to instability or arthrosis. Complications such as infection, adhesive capsulitis, and disruption of the acromial branch of the thoracoacromial artery are rare but well-described complications to most arthroscopic shoulder procedures. Axillary nerve injury is exceedingly rare.

RESULTS

In a recent retrospective study, Jaeger et al. found that in patients with subacromial impingement, isolated arthroscopic SAD provided successful outcomes in 90.9% of cases with partial-thickness rotator cuff tears, 70.6% of cases with full-thickness tears, and 65.2% of cases with calcific tendinitis (9). However, Ketola et al. in a prospective randomized study showed that SAD provides no clinically important effects or cost-effectiveness over a structured exercise program alone (7). The role of SAD when combined with rotator cuff repair in treating full-thickness rotator cuff tears has also been controversial. MacDonald et al. in a prospective randomized study showed that at 2-year follow-up visits, there were no significant differences in patient-reported pain, function, and quality-of-life scores for patients who underwent rotator cuff repair with or without SAD. However, patients who underwent SAD had a lower reoperation rate (10). Gartsman et al. and Milano et al. in prospective randomized studies also showed that rotator cuff repair with or without SAD did not affect functional outcome at 2-year follow-up visits (11,12). In the most recent prospective randomized study of 114 patients by Abrams et al., there were no significant differences in functional outcomes between non-SAD and SAD groups or between subjects with different acromial features at any follow-up time point up to 2 years. Nevertheless, although not statistically significant, the investigators noted that during the follow-up period, four additional procedures were performed in the non-SAD group and one in the SAD group (8).

REFERENCES

1. MacDonald PB, Clark P, Sutherland K. An analysis of the diagnostic accuracy of the Hawkins and Neer subacromial impingement signs. *J Shoulder Elbow Surg.* 2000;9(4):299–301.
2. Çalış M, Akgün K, Birtane M, et al. Diagnostic values of clinical diagnostic tests in subacromial impingement syndrome. *Ann Rheum Dis.* 2000;59(1):44–47.
3. Neer CS. Anterior acromioplasty for the chronic impingement syndrome in the shoulder. *J Bone Joint Surg.* 1972;54:41–50.
4. Bigliani LU, Levine WN. Current concepts review: subacromial impingement syndrome. *J Bone Joint Surg.* 1997;79-A(12):1854–1868.
5. McFarland EG, Selhi HS, Keyurapan E. Clinical evaluation of impingement: what to do and what works. *J Bone Joint Surg.* 2006;88-A(2):432–441.
6. Moor BK, Wieser K, Slankamenac K, et al. Relationship of individual scapular anatomy and degenerative rotator cuff tears. *J Shoulder Elbow Surg.* 2014;23(4):536–541.
7. Ketola S, Lehtinen J, Arnala I, et al. Does arthroscopic acromioplasty provide any additional value in the treatment of shoulder impingement syndrome? A two-year randomised controlled trial. *J Bone Joint Surg.* 2009;91-B(10):1326–1334.
8. Abrams GD, Gupta AK, Hussey KE, et al. Arthroscopic repair of full-thickness rotator cuff tears with and without acromioplasty: randomized prospective trial with 2-year follow-up. *Am J Sports Med.* 2014;42(6):1296–1303.
9. Jaeger M, Berndt T, Rühmann O, et al. Patients with impingement syndrome with and without rotator cuff tears do well 20 years after arthroscopic subacromial decompression. *Arthroscopy.* 2016;32(3):409–415.
10. MacDonald P, Mcrae S, Leiter J, et al. Arthroscopic rotator cuff repair with and without acromioplasty in the treatment of full-thickness rotator cuff tears: a multicenter, randomized controlled trial. *J Bone Joint Surg.* 2011;93-A(21):1953–1960.
11. Gartsman GM, O'Connor DP. Arthroscopic rotator cuff repair with and without arthroscopic subacromial decompression: a prospective, randomized study of one-year outcomes. *J Shoulder Elbow Surg.* 2004;13(4):424–426.
12. Milano G, Grasso A, Salvatore M, et al. Arthroscopic rotator cuff repair with and without subacromial decompression: a prospective randomized study. *Arthroscopy.* 2007;23(1):81–88.

15 Arthroscopic Double-Row Rotator Cuff Repair

J. Kristopher Ware and Brett D. Owens

Arthroscopic rotator cuff repair has proven to be effective in decreasing pain and improving function (1–5). Long-term follow-up studies have shown maintenance of good to excellent outcomes in the majority of patients (1,6,7). However, imaging studies examining the structural integrity of the repaired tendons have shown variable results with retear rates in recent studies ranging from 11% to 49% (8–15). The majority of these retears occur within 3 months of repair suggesting that the mechanical stability of the repair construct likely plays a role in the rate of retear (12). Furthermore, repair integrity has been shown to correlate with outcomes, especially in regard to strength and functional outcome measures (3,8,12,15,16).

An ideal rotator cuff repair should restore the anatomic footprint of the tendon, provide solid fixation, resist gap formation, and ultimately maintain structural integrity until biologic healing can occur (17). To achieve these goals, arthroscopic rotator cuff repair has undergone an evolution in repair techniques. Traditional single-row repairs have proven successful for small tears with good tendon quality (18,19). However, for larger tears or tears with significant tendon degeneration, this technique may be less than optimal. The double-row repair was developed to improve footprint coverage and provide additional fixation to improve the resistance to failure and gap formation (20). Several studies have compared single-row and double-row techniques (21–24). Double-row repairs have been shown in cadaveric models to cover a greater percentage of the footprint, have less gap formation, higher ultimate tensile load to failure, and increased stiffness compared to single-row repairs (25–27). In addition, multiple studies have shown a lower retear rate in double-row repairs (19,22–24). Despite these benefits of double-row repair, the current literature has not shown a difference in functional outcomes associated with repair technique (19,21,28–30).

Although the double-row repair addressed some of the biomechanical disadvantages of single-row repair, it can also present new challenges, such as anchor crowding. A modification of the double-row repair using a suture bridge, also known as the transosseous equivalent technique, was developed (31). The transosseous equivalent/suture bridge double-row repair has been shown to have increased footprint contact area and pressure as well as higher ultimate load to failure compared to traditional double-row repairs (32,33). This technique also reduces the risk of anchor crowding by lateralizing the lateral row of anchors. We prefer the suture bridge double-row repair as described in this chapter for repair of rotator cuff tears >1 cm.

INDICATIONS

Multiple factors must be considered in determining the appropriate course of treatment for patients with symptomatic rotator cuff tears. These include the age and activity of the patient, complete versus incomplete tears, tear size and retraction, muscle atrophy, and degree of fatty degeneration. In the young patient with an acute traumatic tear, early repair has been shown to result in better outcomes (34), and therefore, early operative intervention is indicated. For those with an atraumatic onset of shoulder pain, the chronicity of the tear is often uncertain. Partial- and full-thickness rotator cuff tears have been shown to progress over time (35,36). Tear progression and retraction are associated with fatty infiltration of the rotator cuff muscles that may lead to a worse outcome (37). Therefore, for active patients younger than 65 years old with a full-thickness, symptomatic rotator cuff tear, we offer operative intervention if they do not respond rapidly to conservative measures. On the other hand, for older, less active patients with chronic partial- or full-thickness tears, extensive conservative treatment is our first-line approach. Physical therapy, nonsteroidal anti-inflammatories, and activity modification are initially used with the goal of symptomatic relief. In select cases, corticosteroids may be beneficial but often provide short-term relief, and repeated injections may have an adverse effect on outcomes of future rotator cuff repair (38). If the patient has continued pain and/or functional limitations after conservative treatment, we recommend arthroscopic rotator cuff repair.

CONTRAINDICATIONS

There are several contraindications to rotator cuff repair associated with high risk to the patient or low likelihood of success. Active shoulder infection, serious comorbidities that would present an unacceptable risk to undergo general anesthesia, and cuff tear arthropathy are absolute contraindications to rotator cuff repair. Additionally, advanced neurologic disorders limiting upper extremity function, hematologic disorders affecting blood clotting, and cognitive or social disorders impairing the ability to comply with postoperative restrictions are relative contraindications. Patients with adhesive capsulitis in the setting of a rotator cuff tear have traditionally been considered relative contraindications to rotator cuff repair. However, recent literature has shown acceptable outcomes in these patients when the repair is performed with a concurrent capsular release (39,40).

Risk Factors for Failure

Predicting the risk of failure after rotator cuff repair is a challenge. Although a retear rate of up to 49% has been reported (8,14), functional outcomes are good to excellent in the majority of patients (3,8,12,29). Several variables have been shown to correlate with the healing potential and risk of retear after rotator cuff repair. Characteristics of the rotator cuff tear including increased tear size, increased tear thickness, and worse tissue quality have been found to positively correlate with higher risk of retear (10,13). In addition, muscle atrophy and fatty degeneration portend worse outcomes (41). Patient variables including age (13,14,42), smoking (43), obesity (44), and workers compensation (37) are also associated with higher retear rates or worse clinical outcomes.

PREOPERATIVE PREPARATION

The first step in optimizing patient outcomes is appropriate patient selection. It has been clearly shown that rotator cuff tears can be asymptomatic, and therefore, it is important to verify that the tear seen on imaging is the source of the patient's symptoms. Pain due to a rotator cuff tear is often localized over the lateral deltoid and may radiate down to the elbow. Due to abnormal scapulohumeral mechanics, pain may also be experienced in the upper trapezius region. The pain may be described as sharp or aching and is often aggravated by overhead activities or internal rotation. Patients often complain of pain interfering with their ability to sleep.

The physical examination should include a brief cervical spine examination to rule out a radicular source of shoulder pain. The shoulder should be observed for signs of atrophy and scapulohumeral rhythm should be evaluated. Palpation should include the acromioclavicular (AC) joint, biceps, and the anterior edge of the rotator cuff with the arm held in extension and internal rotation. Additionally, it is important to evaluate shoulder range of motion (ROM) both actively and passively. Active ROM may be decreased in the presence of a large cuff tear. Passive ROM should be full, although frequently painful especially at end range of glenohumeral elevation. Limited passive ROM may be associated with severe arthritis or adhesive capsulitis. Strength of all shoulder actions should be assessed and compared to the contralateral side. Pain and weakness with resisted abduction and external rotation is common for superior rotator cuff tears.

The patient may present with a positive hornblower sign in large to massive tears. A positive empty can test, drop arm test, and impingement test help to confirm the diagnosis for superior rotator cuff tears (45). The belly press test or lift-off test should be performed to test the integrity of the subscapularis (45). In addition, Speed tests can help to identify biceps pathology although the test has limited specificity (45).

Imaging

Initial imaging should include anterior-posterior, scapular Y, and axillary radiographs. The anterior-posterior view should be inspected for signs of glenohumeral arthritis, superior migration of the humeral head, and AC joint arthrosis. The scapular Y allows visualization of acromial morphology. The axillary view will reveal the humeral head position and glenoid version.

Advanced imaging is used for both confirming the diagnosis and preparing for rotator cuff repair. Magnetic resonance imaging (MRI) is the standard for imaging rotator cuff pathology. MRI is helpful in identifying the location of the rotator cuff tear as well as size and shape. The amount of retraction of the tendon is inspected to plan for how much release may be needed to get a tension-free repair. In addition, the quality of the muscle is inspected to determine atrophy and fatty degeneration.

Multiple studies have shown similar accuracy of ultrasound compared to MRI in diagnosing full-thickness rotator cuff tears (46,47). The advantage of ultrasound is that it can be performed in the office and decreases the delay in diagnosis. However, it is less effective in determining muscle atrophy and quality, and it does not allow for clear visualization of intraarticular pathology that may need to be addressed concurrently with the rotator cuff repair.

TECHNIQUE

Positioning

We prefer to use the beach chair position for rotator cuff repairs. The patient is positioned with the trunk inclined 70 degrees. Careful attention is paid to placing the head in a neutral position to decrease risk of traction on the brachial plexus. The head rest is matched to the head position and a foam face mask is applied while the anesthetist monitors and maintains the airway. Lateral supports are placed snug against the lower thorax. The nonoperative upper extremity is supported on a padded arm holder, and the lower extremities are positioned on a wedge to allow knee flexion and support the trunk from sliding down. Compressive stocking along with sequential compression devices are applied to the lower extremities to decrease the risk of venous thrombosis. Sterile drapes are applied, and the operative upper extremity is controlled with a pneumatic arm positioning device. The arm is then placed in slight flexion and neutral rotation in preparation for the arthroscopy (Fig. 15-1).

Portals and Diagnostic Arthroscopy

The bony landmarks of the shoulder are identified and marked with a sterile marker. Care is taken to accurately palpate and mark the acromion, distal clavicle, and coracoid process. Our standard

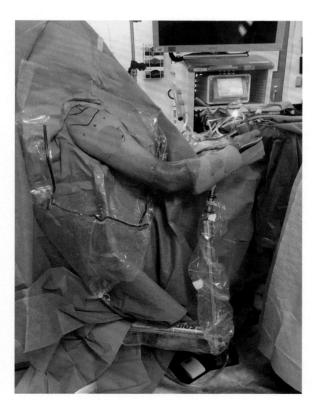

FIGURE 15-1
Beach chair setup.

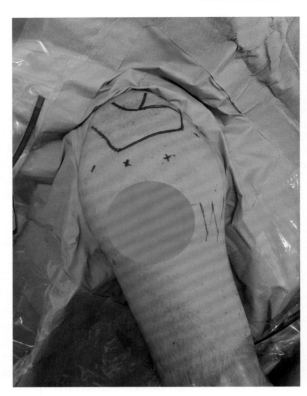

FIGURE 15-2
Portal placement.

rotator cuff repair is made with 3 or 4 portals (Fig. 15-2). The posterior portal is made at the soft spot inferior to the posterior acromion signifying the junction of the humeral head and glenoid. This is approximately 2 cm inferior and 1-2 cm medial to the posterolateral corner of the acromion. The remaining portals are made after a complete diagnostic arthroscopy and using direct visualization with a spinal needle for accurate localization. The anterior portal is made off the anterior edge of the acromion. This allows access to the joint through the rotator interval as well as easy access to the subacromial space for suture passage and management. The lateral portal is generally made just anterior to the midpoint of the lateral acromion. This is created while visualizing from the subacromial space. The accessory posterolateral portal can be added to improve visualization of the tear and preparation of the footprint. It is made midway between the lateral and posterior portals.

The diagnostic arthroscopy begins intra-articularly. The subscapularis is inspected as the arm is rotated from internal to external rotation. The articular side of the superior rotator cuff is then inspected continuing posteriorly and examining the attachment of the infraspinatus adjacent to the bare area. The pouch is also inspected ensuring continuity of the capsular attachment to the humerus and the absence of loose bodies. Next, our anterior portal is created from off the anterior edge of the acromion and a cannula is introduced. A probe is then used to check the integrity of the subscapularis, biceps tendon, and undersurface of the superior rotator cuff. If a partial-thickness cuff tear is visualized, a spinal needle can be introduced laterally and a 0 PDS suture passed through the tear. This facilitates identifying the tear location after entering the subacromial space. In addition, if there is evidence of biceps tendinopathy, we tag and cut the biceps while in the joint for later tenodesis with our medial row anchor.

The arthroscope is then transitioned to the subacromial space. A lateral portal is created and a 3.5 mm arthroscopic shaver is then introduced. Care is taken to clear the bursa overlying the superior cuff and lateral edge of tuberosity to allow clear visualization of the entire superior rotator cuff. A radiofrequency ablator is used to coagulate any bleeding vessels. A cannula is then placed in the lateral portal, and the arthroscope is transitioned into the lateral cannula to inspect the tear pattern. Using a spinal needle, an accessory posterolateral portal may be created to facilitate visualization during repair. Finally, the anterior cannula is retrieved from the rotator interval and advanced into the subacromial space. This allows for multiple viewing angles of the rotator cuff as well as multiple trajectories for suture passing. It also facilitates effective suture management.

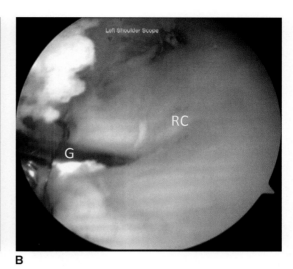

A   **B**

Arthroscope in left shoulder viewing subacromial space through posterior portal. **A:** Rotator cuff tear and footprint visualized. **B:** A grasper is introduced through the lateral portal and the rotator cuff is reduced to the footprint. H, humerus; RC, rotator cuff; G, grasper.

Decision-Making

With our portals established, the rotator cuff quality and tear pattern are carefully inspected. An arthroscopic grasper is used to check mobility of the cuff and the ability to reduce the torn tendon to the greater tuberosity (Fig. 15-3). Using a radiofrequency ablator, adhesions are released from above and below the supraspinatus and infraspinatus muscles to maximize mobility and allow a tension-free repair.

The decision of repair method is customized based on the tear pattern. As mentioned previously, we prefer a modified double-row/suture bridge technique for medium and large rotator cuff tears. The configuration and number of suture anchors is dependent on multiple factors including tear size, shape, and tissue quality, as is described below. For U-shaped and L-shaped tears, a margin convergence repair is performed prior to repairing to the tuberosity (48). We then check the trajectory of the tendon to ensure that the final repair remains collinear with the natural direction of the tendon fibers and to ensure that the repaired cuff rests flat on its footprint.

In addition to the tear morphology, the quality of the available tendon must be determined. This is partially ascertained from the preoperative MRI. Intraoperatively, the subjective quality of the tendon is determined through visual inspection and probing. With poor tendon quality, we preferentially increase the number of sutures and may use flattened tape instead of round suture to improve distribution of force through the tendon.

For medium-size tears with good tendon quality, we will typically use a three anchor construct. This involves placement of a single double-loaded medial row anchor and two lateral row anchors. For larger tears, we will use a four anchor or six anchor construct, depending on the space available, to improve footprint coverage and better distribute forces.

Footprint Preparation

A shaver is used to clear loose soft tissue from over the supraspinatus and/or infraspinatus footprint (Fig. 15-4). If a partial tear involving >50% of the tendon is identified, the remaining fibers are released. A blade rasp is then used to create a flat surface, free of soft tissue, extending to the edge of the articular surface. A microfracture awl is then used to create channels in the greater tuberosity to allow marrow elements and blood to access the tendon-bone interface (Fig. 15-5). Creating multiple channels in the footprint has been shown to enhance tendon healing (9).

Three Anchor Repair

Once the rotator cuff is mobilized and the footprint is prepared, the next step in our double-row rotator cuff repair is placement of the medial anchor. We use a spinal needle placed just off the lateral edge

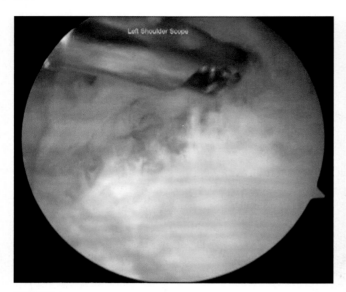

FIGURE 15-4
Footprint preparation with shaver.

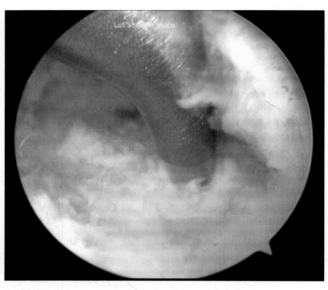

FIGURE 15-5
Channels created in greater tuberosity.

of the acromion to localize. By manipulating the arm, the trajectory of the implant can be modified allowing placement of the anchor nearly perpendicular to the footprint (Fig. 15-6). This has been shown to have higher pullout strength compared to the traditional 45-degree "dead man's angle" (49). We use a Biocomposite 5.5-mm double-loaded anchor with no. 2 suture. Figure 15-7 shows placement of the anchor at the medial margin of the footprint. Three sutures are retrieved through the anterior cannula and one through the lateral cannula. Next, the sutures are passed sequentially using a grasping device with deployable needle or a curved suture passer (Fig. 15-8). Care is taken to pass the sutures through the tendon approximately 10 mm lateral to the musculotendinous junction (50). The sutures are passed approximately 1 to 1.5 cm apart in a horizontal mattress fashion. After all the sutures are passed, we tie each pair with two consecutive half hitches to approximate the cuff to the footprint and follow with an alternate direction throw to lock the knot with a square knot. This is followed by an additional 1 to 2 throws to ensure knot security. With the four sutures tied, this creates a medial row of two horizontal mattress stitches.

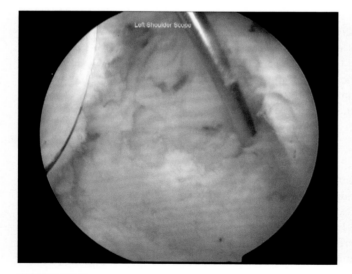

FIGURE 15-6
Percutaneous localization with spinal needle adjacent to articular margin.

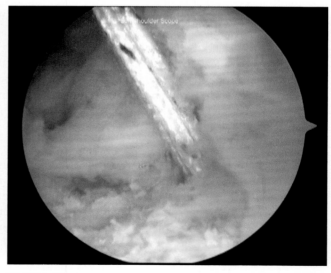

FIGURE 15-7
Placement of medial row anchor.

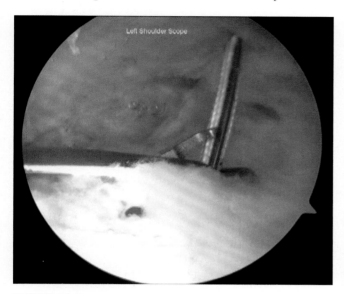

FIGURE 15-8

Suture passing with grasping deployable needle device.

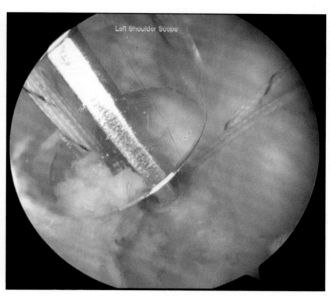

FIGURE 15-9

Placement of lateral row anchor.

For the three anchor repair, we use two lateral row anchors. The anchors are placed approximately 1 cm distal to the lateral edge of the supraspinatus footprint. We first ensure that soft tissue has been sufficiently cleared to allow visualization of the lateral edge of the greater tuberosity. The radiofrequency ablator is used to mark the location for two 4.75-mm screw in anchors (Fig. 15-9). One of the anterior and one of the posterior sutures are retrieved and placed in the first anchor. An awl is used to create the pilot hole, and the anchor is placed flush with the cortex. The sutures are then cut, and the process is repeated for the second lateral row anchor. The completed three anchor repair is shown in Figure 15-10.

Four Anchor Repair

For larger rotator cuff tears, a four or six anchor double-row repair is preferred to maximize footprint coverage and provide more points of fixation. The technique is similar to the three anchor repair, except two medial row anchors are placed. After the tendon has been mobilized and the footprint prepared, the location for the medial row anchors is selected and percutaneous placement is

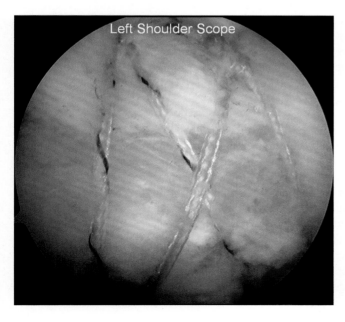

FIGURE 15-10

Completed three anchor repair.

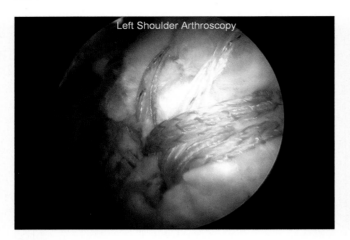

FIGURE 15-11

Four anchor flat suture repair with tied medial row.

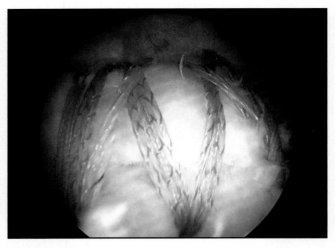

FIGURE 15-12

Completed six anchor repair.

performed. Two double-loaded anchors are placed. This allows for four horizontal mattress sutures for the medial row. The sutures are passed sequentially from posterior to anterior to prevent crossing, and each pair is tied.

As with the three anchor repair, two lateral row anchors are used to complete the repair. One tail from each horizontal mattress is delivered through a single cannula and inserted into one 4.75-mm screw in anchor. The anterior anchor is placed first, localized just off the lateral edge of the greater tuberosity. The process is repeated with the posterior anchor.

Alternatively, for patients with poor tendon quality, a broad, flat tape can be used for the repair. In this situation, we will typically load one 4.75-mm anchor with the flat suture and a second with a different color flat suture. The anchors are preloaded with a no. 2 rescue suture that allows us to tie a medial row. Once the medial row anchors are placed, we pass a suture with a loop on one end to serve as a passing suture. Using the passing suture, one flat suture and one of the rescue sutures are passed through the same hole. This is repeated for all 4 limbs of suture. The rescue sutures from each anchor are then tied creating a medial row. The flat suture tails along with the tied rescue suture tails are delivered laterally and secured in two 4.75-mm anchors as described above (Fig. 15-11).

Six Anchor Repair

With large to massive, reducible rotator cuff repairs, additional anchors may be necessary. A double-row repair with six anchors is performed similar to that of the four anchor repair. We use flat suture loaded in the anchor islet along with rescue sutures as described above. In this situation, three horizontal mattress sutures from the rescue sutures form the medial row. The tails of all sutures are delivered laterally and secured in three lateral row anchors as shown in Figure 15-12.

PEARLS AND PITFALLS

Challenges presented during rotator cuff repair can be related to aberrant portal placement, impaired visualization, failure to adequately prepare the tendon and footprint, and poor suture management. Correctly identifying the patient's anatomy prior to making portals is an essential initial step in preventing the struggle of a poorly placed portal. Care should be taken to mark the edges of the acromion accurately. With the exception of the posterior portal, a spinal needle under direct visualization is used to ensure that the portals are placed in the appropriate location and with a trajectory that will facilitate the repair. For the lateral portals, ensuring that they are adequately distal to the acromion can mitigate challenges presented by shoulder swelling.

Excellent visualization of the subacromial space is necessary to effectively repair the rotator cuff. Switching the arthroscope to the lateral or posterolateral portal can provide an improved perspective when evaluating the tissue. In addition, sufficient clearing of the subacromial bursa improves visualization and facilitates suture passage. Precise hemostasis, achieved with the use of a radiofrequency ablator, must be maintained.

Another key to a successful repair is preparation of both the footprint and releasing of adhesions to the tendon that limit its lateral mobility. The footprint should be cleared of all soft tissue to provide a well-vascularized bony bed for healing. As described, channels can be created to allow egress of marrow elements. If there is any resistance to mobilizing the tendon, the adhesions from above and below the tendon must be fully released. In some cases, an interval slide may be needed to allow a tension-free repair.

Finally, careful attention to suture management will prevent the frustration of suture tangles. The use of multiple portals allows sutures to be retrieved either anteriorly or posteriorly out of the way. We will also frequently remove and replace the cannulas with sutures parked outside the cannula tunnel, which allows for continued instrumentation through the cannula. Using a sequence of placing anchors, passing sutures, and tying either from anterior to posterior or the reverse can minimize the risk of entanglement. Additionally, tying sutures through the cannula limits the risk of creating a soft tissue bridge.

POSTOPERATIVE MANAGEMENT

Effective postoperative rehabilitation is paramount in maximizing outcomes following rotator cuff repair. The goals of early rehabilitation are focused on restoring ROM while allowing the repaired tendon to heal. As recovery progresses, the goals shift to maximizing strength and ultimately function of the upper extremity. Rehabilitation must not only include the glenohumeral joint but also to maximize function, scapulothoracic motion as well as elbow, wrist, and hand function should be addressed. We follow a standard rehabilitation protocol with the majority of our patients and will modify timelines based on the quality of tissue and size of the tear.

Phase 1 (1–4 Weeks): Protected Motion Phase

During the first 4 postoperative weeks, patients are kept in an abduction sling at all times except during physical therapy and when performing their home exercises. Patients are issued a cryotherapy device to help with postoperative inflammation and pain. Beginning on postoperative day 2, patients begin Codman pendulum exercises and active ROM for the elbow, wrist, and hand. If a concomitant biceps tenotomy or tenodesis was performed, elbow ROM is performed passively during this phase. Physical therapy is initiated within 1 week of surgery. Therapist works on gentle passive ROM and gentle glenohumeral joint mobilization. Patients are instructed on active-assisted ROM for abduction, flexion, and external rotation. These exercises are performed at least three times per day as part of their home exercise program. In addition, postural exercises and manual periscapular strengthening exercises are initiated. Physical therapy modalities to decrease pain and inflammation are used as needed. The goals of the first phase include pain control, the ability to maintain correct posture, and glenohumeral ROM of 90-degree flexion, 90-degree abduction, and 30-degree external rotation.

Phase 2 (4–8 Weeks): Active Motion Phase

Patients are progressed to phase 2 of the rehabilitation protocol when they are at or beyond 4 weeks postoperative and have achieved the goals of phase 1. At this point, patients are weaned from their sling use but instructed not to lift any objects heavier than 1 lb. The physical therapist continues to work on shoulder mobility through passive ROM and glenohumeral joint mobilization. In addition, patients begin guided active ROM in all planes. Our therapists carefully evaluate the quality of a patient's scapulohumeral mechanics and correct abnormal movement patterns. Strengthening for scapular stabilizers is progressed. In addition, home exercises are progressed to incorporate active ROM exercises and are custom tailored to the individual's motion limitations. The goals of this phase are near full ROM, minimal to no pain, and the ability to elevate arms overhead with symmetric scapulohumeral rhythm.

Phase 3 (9–12 Weeks): Strengthening

Phase 3 begins at 9 weeks if the goals of phase 2 have been achieved. This portion of the rehabilitation program is focused on progressive strengthening of the rotator cuff and periscapular muscles. Progressive resistance exercises begin with isotonic strengthening using elastic resistance and advances to include free weights. Both open and closed chain exercises are included to maximize strength gains and synergistic muscle actions. Patients are allowed and encouraged to use their operative extremity during routine activities of daily living and are only restricted from heavy or repeated use.

Phase 4 (3–5 Months): Functional Exercise

During this phase, patients continue to work on developing strength and incorporate multiplanar functional exercises into their rehabilitation. Throwing and upper extremity plyometrics are initiated. Additionally, any strength imbalances are targeted, and proper quality of motion is addressed. During this phase, the frequency of visits is often decreased, and the patient performs the majority of their rehabilitation as an independent home/gym exercise program. At the conclusion of phase 4, patients have symmetric shoulder ROM, strength, and scapulohumeral mechanics.

Phase 5 (5+ Months): Return to Work/Sports

The final phase of the rehabilitation program is customized to the individual needs of the patient. Depending on work or sports requirements, exercises can be developed that will facilitate return to a manual labor occupation and/or sports. It should be noted that most patients have returned to work by 6 weeks, but they are restricted from heavy lifting or repetitive overhead tasks until completing this phase of rehabilitation. The work and sports tasks are broken down into components, and the exercises are designed to allow successive approximation of these tasks. Patients are ultimately returned to their preinjury activities at the conclusion of this phase. We advise to refrain from contact sports for 9 months from the time of surgery.

COMPLICATIONS

Potential complications of rotator cuff repair include infection, stiffness, and failure of repair. Infections are rare, occurring in <0.1% of arthroscopic rotator cuff repairs (51,52), but can be devastating to the success of the repair. The most commonly identified organisms are *Propionibacterium acnes*, *Staphylococcus epidermidis*, and *Staphylococcus aureus* (52,53). Treatment includes irrigation and debridement, which most often can be performed arthroscopically, and intravenous antibiotics. Shoulder stiffness has been reported in 18% of rotator cuff repairs at 3 months postoperatively (54). Postoperative stiffness has been shown to correlate with preoperative stiffness (55). We therefore have patients with preoperative ROM restrictions work on aggressive ROM exercises to maximize motion before surgery. For those with a persistent capsular contracture, concomitant capsular release with rotator cuff repair has shown satisfactory outcomes (39). Finally, failure of the repair to fully heal has been reported in several studies (8,10–12,14). Despite the high frequency of recurrent tears on imaging, many patients will have improvement in their symptoms and may remain a therapeutic success (29). However, in those with persistent pain, limited function, and evidence of retear, a revision rotator cuff repair can be performed. The retear rate of revision rotator cuff repair is higher than primary repair (56). Despite this, significant improvement in pain and functional outcome measures have been demonstrated following revision rotator cuff repair (57).

RESULTS

Several studies have examined the functional outcomes of arthroscopic rotator cuff repair (1,7,11,58,59). Huijsmans et al. (59) reported on 242 shoulders at an average of 22 months after arthroscopic double-row rotator cuff repair. They found an improvement in visual analogue scale (VAS) pain score from 7.4 to 0.7 points, an average improvement on Constant score of 25.4 points, and subjective outcomes were good to excellent in 90%. They found a retear rate of 15% at final follow-up with tear rate associated with size of the initial tear and the quality of the tendon. Similarly, Kim et al. (58) showed a significant improvement in UCLA, ASES, and Constant scores at 2 years in 52 subjects with either a double-row rotator cuff repair or suture bridge technique. In addition, these early improvements in clinical outcomes are maintained at longer term follow-up. Wolf et al. (7) found 90% good to excellent results on the UCLA scoring system in 95 subjects with 4- to 10-year follow-up. Marrero et al. (1) found good to excellent outcomes in 88% of 33 shoulders, as measured by the UCLA Shoulder Score, with a minimum follow-up of 9 years. These results show that arthroscopic rotator cuff repair results in significant improvement in shoulder function with durable results on long-term follow-up.

REFERENCES

1. Marrero LG, Nelman KR, Nottage WM. Long-term follow-up of arthroscopic rotator cuff repair. *Arthroscopy.* 2011;27(7):885–888. doi:10.1016/j.arthro.2011.02.019.
2. Karas V, Hussey K, Romeo AR, et al. Comparison of subjective and objective outcomes after rotator cuff repair. *Arthroscopy.* 2013;29(11):1755–1761. doi:10.1016/j.arthro.2013.08.001.
3. Robinson HA, Lam PH, Walton JR, et al. The effect of rotator cuff repair on early overhead shoulder function: a study in 1600 consecutive rotator cuff repairs. *J Shoulder Elbow Surg.* 2016;26(1):20–29. doi:10.1016/j.jse.2016.05.022.
4. Bennett WF. Arthroscopic repair of full-thickness supraspinatus tears (small-to-medium): a prospective study with 2- to 4-year follow-up. *Arthroscopy.* 2003;19(3):249–256. doi:10.1053/jars.2003.50083.
5. Ide J, Maeda S, Takagi K. A comparison of arthroscopic and open rotator cuff repair. *Arthroscopy.* 2005;21(9):1090–1098. doi:10.1016/j.arthro.2005.05.010.
6. Millett PJ, Horan MP, Maland KE, et al. Long-term survivorship and outcomes after surgical repair of full-thickness rotator cuff tears. *J Shoulder Elbow Surg.* 2011;20(4):591–597. doi:10.1016/j.jse.2010.11.019.
7. Wolf EM, Pennington WT, Agrawal V. Arthroscopic rotator cuff repair: 4- to 10-year results. *Arthroscopy.* 2004;20(1):5–12. doi:10.1016/j.arthro.2003.11.001.
8. Boileau P, Brassart N, Watkinson DJ, et al. Arthroscopic repair of full-thickness tears of the supraspinatus: does the tendon really heal?. *J Bone Joint Surg Am.* 2005;87(6):1229–1240. doi:10.2106/JBJS.D.02035.
9. Jo CH, Shin JS, Park IW, et al. Multiple channeling improves the structural integrity of rotator cuff repair. *Am J Sports Med.* 2013;41(11):2650–2657. doi:10.1177/0363546513499138.
10. Kim IB, Kim MW. Risk factors for retear after arthroscopic repair of full-thickness rotator cuff tears using the suture bridge technique: classification system. *Arthroscopy.* 2016;32(11):2191–2200. doi:10.1016/j.arthro.2016.03.012.
11. Sugaya H, Maeda K, Matsuki K, et al. Repair integrity and functional outcomes after arthroscopic suture-bridge rotator cuff repair. *J Bone Joint Surg Am.* 2007;89-A(5):953–960. doi:10.2106/JBJS.K.00158.
12. Kluger R, Bock P, Mittlbock M, et al. Long-term survivorship of rotator cuff repairs using ultrasound and magnetic resonance imaging analysis. *Am J Sports Med.* 2011;39(10):2071–2081. doi:10.1177/0363546511406395.
13. Le BTN, Wu XL, Lam PH, et al. Factors predicting rotator cuff retears. *Am J Sports Med.* 2014;42(5):1134–1142. doi:10.1177/0363546514525336.
14. Tashjian RZ, Hollins AM, Kim H-M, et al. Factors affecting healing rates after arthroscopic double-row rotator cuff repair. *Am J Sports Med.* 2010;38(12):2435–2442. doi:10.1177/0363546510382835.
15. Lafosse L, Brozska R, Toussaint B, et al. The outcome and structural integrity of arthroscopic rotator cuff repair using the double-row suture anchor technique (SS-39). *Arthroscopy.* 2007;23(805):e20. doi:10.1016/j.arthro.2007.03.051.
16. Slabaugh MA, Nho SJ, Grumet RC, et al. Does the literature confirm superior clinical results in radiographically healed rotator cuffs after rotator cuff repair?. *Arthroscopy.* 2010;26(3):393–403. doi:10.1016/j.arthro.2009.07.023.
17. Provencher MT, Kercher JS, Galatz LM, et al. Evolution of rotator cuff repair techniques: are our patients really benefiting?. *Instr Course Lect.* 2011;60:123–136. http://www.ncbi.nlm.nih.gov/pubmed/21553768.
18. Park JY, Lhee SH, Choi JH, et al. Comparison of the clinical outcomes of single- and double-row repairs in rotator cuff tears. *Am J Sports Med.* 2008;36(7):1310–1316. doi:10.1177/0363546508315039.
19. Saridakis P, Jones G. Outcomes of single-row and double-row arthroscopic rotator cuff repair: a systematic review. *J Bone Joint Surg Am.* 2010;92(3):732–742. doi:10.2106/JBJS.I.01295.
20. Cole BJ, ElAttrache NS, Anbari A. Arthroscopic rotator cuff repairs: an anatomic and biomechanical rationale for different suture-anchor repair configurations. *Arthroscopy.* 2007;23(6):662–669. doi:10.1016/j.arthro.2007.02.018.
21. Nicholas SJ, Lee SJ, Mullaney MJ, et al. Functional outcomes after double row versus single row rotator cuff repair: a prospective randomized trial. *Orthop J Sports Med.* 2015;3(2 suppl):14–16. doi:10.1177/2325967115S00155.
22. Mascarenhas R, Chalmers PN, Sayegh ET, et al. Is double-row rotator cuff repair clinically superior to single-row rotator cuff repair: a systematic review of overlapping meta-analyses. *Arthroscopy.* 2014;30(9):1156–1165. doi:10.1016/j.arthro.2014.03.015.
23. Hein J, Reilly JM, Chae J, et al. Retear rates after arthroscopic single-row, double-row, and suture bridge rotator cuff repair at a minimum of 1 year of imaging follow-up: a systematic review. *Arthroscopy.* 2015;31(11):2274–2281. doi:10.1016/j.arthro.2015.06.004.
24. Duquin TR, Buyea C, Bisson LJ. Which method of rotator cuff repair leads to the highest rate of structural healing? A systematic review. *Am J Sports Med.* 2010;38:835–841. doi:10.1177/0363546509359679.
25. Kim DH. Biomechanical comparison of a single-row versus double-row suture anchor technique for rotator cuff repair. *Am J Sports Med.* 2005;34(3):407–414. doi:10.1177/0363546505281238.
26. Ma CB, Comerford L, Wilson J, et al. Biomechanical evaluation of arthroscopic rotator cuff repairs: double-row compared with single-row fixation. *J Bone Joint Surg Am.* 2006;88(2):403–410. doi:10.2106/JBJS.D.02887.
27. Mazzocca AD, Millett PJ, Guanche CA, et al. Arthroscopic single-row versus double- row suture anchor rotator cuff repair. *Am J Sports Med.* 2005;33(12):1861–1868. doi:10.1177/0363546505279575.
28. Franceschi F, Ruzzini L, Longo UG, et al. Equivalent clinical results of arthroscopic single-row and double-row suture anchor repair for rotator cuff tears: a randomized controlled trial. *Am J Sports Med.* 2007;35(8):1254–1260. doi:10.1177/0363546507302218.
29. Kim KC, Shin HD, Cha SM, et al. Comparison of repair integrity and functional outcomes for 3 arthroscopic suture bridge rotator cuff repair techniques. *Am J Sports Med.* 2013;41(2):271–277. doi:10.1177/0363546512468278.
30. DeHaan AM, Axelrad TW, Kaye E, et al. Does double-row rotator cuff repair improve functional outcome of patients compared with single-row technique?: a systematic review. *Am J Sports Med.* 2012;40(5):1176–1185. doi:10.1177/0363546511428866.
31. Park MC, ElAttrache NS, Ahmad CS, et al. "Transosseous-equivalent" rotator cuff repair technique. *Arthroscopy.* 2006;22(12):1–5. doi:10.1016/j.arthro.2006.07.017.
32. Park MC, ElAttrache NS, Tibone JE, et al. Part I: footprint contact characteristics for a transosseous-equivalent rotator cuff repair technique compared with a double-row repair technique. *J Shoulder Elbow Surg.* 2007;16(4):461–468. doi:10.1016/j.jse.2006.09.010.
33. Park MC, Tibone JE, ElAttrache NS, et al. Part II: biomechanical assessment for a footprint-restoring transosseous-equivalent rotator cuff repair technique compared with a double-row repair technique. *J Shoulder Elbow Surg.* 2007;16(4):469–476. doi:10.1016/j.jse.2006.09.011.
34. Bassett RW, Cofield RH. Acute tears of the rotator cuff. The timing of surgical repair. *Clin Orthop Relat Res.* 1983;(175):18–24.

35. Moosmayer S, Tariq R, Stiris M, et al. The natural history of asymptomatic rotator cuff tears. *J Bone Joint Surg Am.* 2013;95(14):1249–1255. doi:10.2106/JBJS.L.00185.

36. Keener JD, Galatz LM, Teefey SA, et al. A prospective evaluation of survivorship of asymptomatic degenerative rotator cuff tears. *J Bone Joint Surg Am.* 2015;97(2):89–98. doi:10.2106/JBJS.N.00099.

37. Oh LS, Wolf BR, Hall MP, et al. Indications for rotator cuff repair: a systematic review. *Clin Orthop Relat Res.* 2007;455(455):52–63. doi:10.1097/BLO.0b013e31802fc175.

38. Bjorkenheim JM, Paavolainen P, Ahovuo J, et al. Surgical repair of the rotator cuff and surrounding tissues. Factors influencing the results. *Clin Orthop Relat Res.* 1988;(236):148–153.

39. Cho CH, Jang HK, Bae KC, et al. Clinical outcomes of rotator cuff repair with arthroscopic capsular release and manipulation for rotator cuff tear with stiffness: a matched-pair comparative study between patients with and without stiffness. *Arthroscopy.* 2015;31(3):482–487. doi:10.1016/j.arthro.2014.09.002.

40. Park J-Y, Chung SW, Hassan Z, et al. Effect of capsular release in the treatment of shoulder stiffness concomitant with rotator cuff repair. *Am J Sports Med.* 2014;42(4):840–850. doi:10.1177/0363546513519326.

41. Fermont AJ, Wolterbeek N, Wessel RN, et al. Prognostic factors for recovery after arthroscopic rotator cuff repair: a prognostic study. *J Shoulder Elbow Surg.* 2015;24(8):1249–1256. doi:10.1016/j.jse.2015.04.013.

42. Lichtenberg S, Liem D, Magosch P, et al. Influence of tendon healing after arthroscopic rotator cuff repair on clinical outcome using single-row Mason-Allen suture technique: a prospective, MRI controlled study. *Knee Surg Sports Traumatol Arthrosc.* 2006;14(11):1200–1206. doi:10.1007/s00167-006-0132-8.

43. Neyton L, Godenèche A, Nové-Josserand L, et al. Arthroscopic suture-bridge repair for small to medium size supraspinatus tear: healing rate and retear pattern. *Arthroscopy.* 2013;29(1):10–17. doi:10.1016/j.arthro.2012.06.020.

44. Fermont AJM, Wolterbeek N, Wessel RN, et al. Prognostic factors for successful recovery after arthroscopic rotator cuff repair: a systematic literature review. *J Orthop Sports Phys Ther.* 2014;44(3):153–163. doi:10.2519/jospt.2014.4832.

45. Jain NB, Luz J, Higgins LD, et al. The diagnostic accuracy of special tests for rotator cuff tear. *Am J Phys Med Rehabil.* 2016;96:176. doi:10.1097/PHM.0000000000000566.

46. Roy J-S, Braën C, Leblond J, et al. Diagnostic accuracy of ultrasonography, MRI and MR arthrography in the characterisation of rotator cuff disorders: a systematic review and meta-analysis. *Br J Sports Med.* 2015;49(20):1316–1328. doi:10.1136/bjsports-2014-094148.

47. Lenza M, Buchbinder R, Takwoingi Y, et al. Magnetic resonance imaging, magnetic resonance arthrography and ultrasonography for assessing rotator cuff tears in people with shoulder pain for whom surgery is being considered. *Cochrane Database Syst Rev.* 2013;9(9):CD009020. doi:10.1002/14651858.CD009020.pub2.

48. Shindle MK, Nho SJ, Nam D, et al. Technique for margin convergence in rotator cuff repair. *HSS J.* 2011;7(3):208–212. doi:10.1007/s11420-011-9222-3.

49. Strauss E, Frank D, Kubiak E, et al. The effect of the angle of suture anchor insertion on fixation failure at the tendon-suture interface after rotator cuff repair: deadman's angle revisited. *Arthroscopy.* 2009;25(6):597–602. doi:10.1016/j.arthro.2008.12.021.

50. Virk MS, Bruce B, Hussey KE, et al. Biomechanical performance of medial row suture placement relative to the musculotendinous junction in transosseous equivalent suture bridge double-row rotator cuff repair. *Arthroscopy.* 2017;33(2):242–250. doi:10.1016/j.arthro.2016.06.020.

51. Owens BD, Williams AE, Wolf JM. Risk factors for surgical complications in rotator cuff repair in a veteran population. *J Shoulder Elbow Surg.* 2015;24(11):1707–1712. doi:10.1016/j.jse.2015.04.020.

52. Pauzenberger L, Grieb A, Hexel M, et al. Infections following arthroscopic rotator cuff repair: incidence, risk factors, and prophylaxis. *Knee Surg Sports Traumatol Arthrosc.* 2016;25(2):595–601. doi:10.1007/s00167-016-4202-2.

53. Vopat BG, Lee BJ, DeStefano S, et al. Risk factors for infection after rotator cuff repair. *Arthroscopy.* 2015;32(3):428–434. doi:10.1016/j.arthro.2015.08.021.

54. Chung SW, Huong CB, Kim SH, et al. Shoulder stiffness after rotator cuff repair: risk factors and influence on outcome. *Arthroscopy.* 2013;29(2):290–300. doi:10.1016/j.arthro.2012.08.023.

55. McNamara WJ, Lam PH, Murrell GAC. The relationship between shoulder stiffness and rotator cuff healing: a study of 1,533 consecutive arthroscopic rotator cuff repairs. *J Bone Joint Surg Am.* 2016;98(22):1879–1889. doi:10.2106/JBJS.15.00923.

56. Shamsudin A, Lam PH, Peters K, et al. Revision versus primary arthroscopic rotator cuff repair: a 2-year analysis of outcomes in 360 patients. *Am J Sports Med.* 2015;43(3):557–564. doi:10.1177/0363546514560729.

57. Kowalsky MS, Keener JD. Revision arthroscopic rotator cuff repair: repair integrity and clinical outcome: surgical technique. *J Bone Joint Surg Am.* 2011;93(suppl 1):62–74. doi:10.2106/JBJS.J.01173.

58. Kim KC, Shin HD, Lee WY, et al. Repair integrity and functional outcome after arthroscopic rotator cuff repair. *Am J Sports Med.* 2012;40(2):294–299. doi:10.1177/0363546511425657.

59. Huijsmans PE, Pritchard MP, Berghs BM, et al. Arthroscopic rotator cuff repair with double-row fixation. *J Bone Joint Surg Am.* 2007;89(6):1248–1257. doi:10.2106/JBJS.E.00743.

16 Multidirectional Instability

Megan R. Wolf, Eileen Colliton, and Robert A. Arciero

INTRODUCTION

The concept of multidirectional instability (MDI) was first described in 1980 by Neer and Foster (1). In this classic report, a cohort of patients with either failed surgery for instability or uncertainty in diagnosis was identified. All patients had pathologic inferior glenohumeral joint laxity combined with anterior or posterior instability, or both. These patients were treated successfully with an open inferior capsular shift, which eliminated capsular redundancy by selective capsular release and imbrication. Since this original report, there have been multiple permutations of the definition of MDI. Open and arthroscopic techniques have emerged that are designed to eliminate pathologic laxity of the glenohumeral joint without sacrificing motion. This chapter reviews our approach to the clinical evaluation and treatment of patients with MDI.

To make the diagnosis of MDI, the patient must have symptomatic, involuntary subluxation, or dislocation in more than one direction. This definition is in contrast to instability, which is a pathologic condition whereby pain or discomfort is attributable to excessive translation of the humeral head during active motion. The diagnosis and management of MDI is challenging. Part of the difficulty in diagnosing patients with MDI comes from the inconsistent definitions in the literature (2,3). Instability can be defined as subluxation or dislocation and voluntary or involuntary. Matsen popularized the acronyms TUBS (traumatic, unilateral, Bankart, surgery) and AMBRII (atraumatic, multidirectional, bilateral, rehabilitation, inferior capsular shift, interval closure) to divide instability patterns into two groups (4).

The diagnosis of MDI relies heavily upon a precise patient history and clinical examination. MDI patients are often athletic and may participate in sports that involve strenuous shoulder activity, such as swimming, gymnastics, weight lifting, or overhead sports. These patients may be aware of instability as a cause of their symptoms, or they may complain of pain or mechanical symptoms (grinding, popping, clicking) with activities. These symptoms are often experienced in the midrange positions of glenohumeral motion, such as those that occur with activities of daily living. The position of the shoulder at the time of symptom onset provides clues as to the pattern of instability that is present. Pain that occurs with the arm in a forward flexed, adducted, and internally rotated position (such as during push-ups, bench pressing, etc.) suggests posterior instability. Competitive athletes may not report pain with these maneuvers, but some patients describe the affected arm as lagging behind the contralateral arm with bench pressing. Pain with the arm overhead is usually indicative of anterior pathology. Patients with inferior instability may notice pain or paresthesias when carrying heavy objects with the arm at the side, as the shoulder allows downward traction on the brachial plexus. The condition is bilateral in approximately 20% of cases, but symptoms in both shoulders may not occur simultaneously. Thus, it is important to inquire about a history of similar symptoms in either shoulder in the past.

The physical examination of the shoulder begins with a general cervical spine evaluation. Proper examination of the shoulder requires that the entire shoulder and periscapular muscles be exposed. We start our examination of the shoulder from the back, inspecting for any evidence of atrophy or asymmetry in scapular position and motion. Many patients will exhibit pseudowinging of the scapula or will have malpositioning of the scapula with a protracted appearance when viewed posteriorly as they range through a full arc of motion. Active and passive ranges of motion are evaluated. Anterior and posterior load-shift tests determine laxity in their respective directions. They are graded as 1+, to glenoid rim; 2+, over glenoid rim with spontaneous reduction; and 3+, glenohumeral dislocation requiring manipulation to reduce. To perform this test, the arm is abducted to 90 degrees and a gentle axial load is applied to center the humeral head within the glenoid. The scapula is stabilized, and anterior and posterior translation is assessed. Anterior laxity becomes more apparent if and when the examiner attempts to translate the humeral head in an anteroinferior direction. Provocative tests such as the apprehension-relocation tests also assess anterior instability. Posterior laxity is also evaluated by positioning the arm in forward flexion, adduction, and internal rotation and applying a force directed posteriorly. It is important to flex the arm enough so that the humeral head does not impinge against the spine of the scapula because this can mask posterior translation. Inferior instability is determined by the sulcus sign. With the arm at the patient's side, downward traction is applied to the arm. In the presence of inferior capsular laxity, a dimple will form in the region between the humeral head and the lateral acromion. In a normal shoulder, this dimple disappears with maximal external rotation of the arm. A pathologic sulcus sign is one that does not diminish with humeral external rotation and signifies an incompetent rotator interval. The literature has shown a wide range of normal variants of shoulder laxity. It is not uncommon to be able to subluxate a shoulder over the glenoid rim, particularly with the examination under anesthesia. Thus, it is crucial that these clinical examination findings correlate with the patients' symptoms. Lastly, the examiner should look for other signs of generalized ligamentous laxity, as described by the Beighton score (5). These include passive elbow hyperextension, thumb to forearm apposition, metacarpophalangeal joint extension beyond 90 degrees, and the ability to flex from the standing position and place the palms on the floor.

Plain radiographs should be inspected for evidence of bony defects in the glenoid or humeral head. In many instances for the patient with MDI, these studies are normal. Indications for a CT scan include a history of dislocation requiring reduction, recurrent dislocation, apprehension at low abduction angles, recurrent dislocation following minimal provocation (e.g., washing hair), and instability at low abduction angles (e.g., reaching in front of body). Magnetic resonance imaging with intra-articular gadolinium in a patient with MDI will show a capacious inferior capsular pouch. An abduction external rotation MRI will show laxity of the inferior glenohumeral ligament. Injuries to the glenoid labrum are less common in MDI than in cases of unidirectional instability. Lim et al. reported that the inferior labrocapsular distance measured on coronal MRI in a mid-glenoid cut can potentially be used as a screening tool for MDI, with a distance >16.88 mm having 76% sensitivity and 96% specificity (6). Another study (7) showed that rotator interval measurements and joint capsule dimensions measured on MRI can also be used as potential MDI identifiers.

INDICATIONS

Nonoperative management of MDI, including physical therapy and patient education, is the first line of treatment. Many patients with MDI (65%–90% in current studies) will improve following an appropriate trial of conservative modalities, but improvement may take up to 3 months (8–10). Current literature supports nonoperative treatment utilizing the Watson MDI program, which is focused on first achieving humeral head and scapular control and then proceeding to shoulder musculature strengthening (11–13). When the Watson MDI program was compared to another rehabilitation program (the Rockwood instability program), the Watson program was statistically superior. However, significant benefit from rehabilitation can be expected after 6 months (11). The indication for surgical intervention includes patients who have persistent pain and disability, especially with activities of daily living, after a minimum of 3 to 6 months of appropriate nonoperative management.

CONTRAINDICATIONS

The classification of MDI has divided patients into groups based on whether they have voluntary or involuntary instability. It is essential to ascertain whether the patient can subluxate or dislocate his or her shoulder voluntarily. Voluntary dislocators may have a psychiatric disorder or secondary gain at the root of their instability. Habitual dislocators have instability episodes attributable to muscular imbalance. These patients often do poorly with surgical intervention. Positional dislocators are aware of activities or arm positions that will reproduce their symptoms but will avoid these positions because the feeling is uncomfortable or painful. Involuntary subluxators are not able to reproduce their symptoms and may represent the best indication for surgical intervention if nonoperative treatment fails.

PREOPERATIVE PREPARATION

The authors' preferred technique for the patient with MDI who fails nonoperative treatment is arthroscopic capsulorrhaphy. An interscalene block is administered in the preoperative holding area. After administration of a general anesthetic in the operating room, the patient is placed in the lateral

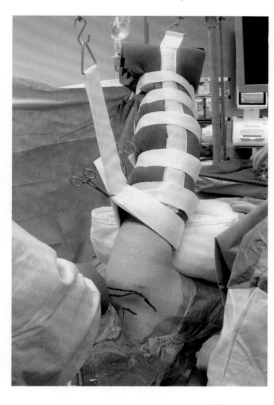

FIGURE 16-1

The operative extremity is placed in a traction sleeve in 70 degrees of abduction and 10 to 20 degrees of forward flexion with 10 to 12 lb of traction. A sterile bump is placed to in the axilla to facilitate exposure.

decubitus position with a vacuum bean bag. An examination under anesthesia is performed to reinforce the clinical findings identified on preoperative examination and imaging. The arm is then prepared and draped in a usual sterile fashion. The operative extremity is placed in a traction sleeve in 70 degrees of abduction and 10 to 20 degrees of forward flexion with 10 to 12 lb of traction. A sterile bump is placed in the axilla to facilitate exposure (Fig. 16-1). It is important to avoid an extended position of the arm as this is associated with a higher risk of neurologic injury. A posterior portal is created, and a diagnostic arthroscopy is performed. For arthroscopic stabilization cases, this portal is created 2 cm inferior to the posterolateral corner of the acromion, as this will provide a better angle of approach to the posterior and inferior labrum.

TECHNIQUE

Anterosuperior (ASP) and anteroinferior (AIP) portals are established within the rotator interval by an outside-in technique (Fig. 16-2). A spinal needle is inserted high within the rotator interval, and once its position is confirmed, a pointed switching stick is inserted immediately adjacent to this

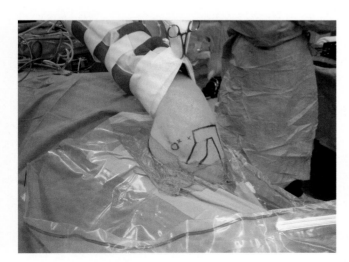

FIGURE 16-2

Lateral decubitus positioning for arthroscopic stabilization of a right shoulder. The "X's" mark the estimated positions of the ASP and AIP portals within the rotator interval.

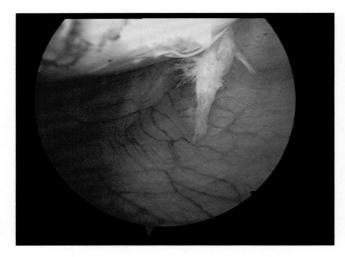

FIGURE 16-3

Inferior capsular redundancy is a hallmark of MDI.

needle. We then "park" this switching rod superior to the biceps. The AIP is created just superior to the rolled edge of the subscapularis tendon and cannulated with an 8-mm cannula. The arthroscope is brought to the ASP, placed over the switching rod. A cannula is then inserted in the posterior portal. The majority of the surgery is performed viewing with the arthroscope in the ASP. There is no "essential lesion" that produces MDI, although redundancy of the axillary pouch is present always (Fig. 16-3). This produces the so-called arthroscopic drive-through sign whereby the arthroscope is maneuvered easily between the humeral head and the glenoid at the level of the anterior band of the inferior glenohumeral ligament.

A shaver or rasp is brought through the posterior cannula to lightly debride the labrum and synovium to create a healing bed of tissue. Initially, two mattress sutures of #2 Orthocord (Depuy, Mitek) are passed posteroinferiorly. To achieve this, a 45-degree suture hook (Spectrum Suture Hook, Linvatex, Inc., Largo, FL) is inserted through the posterior portal and pierces the capsule at the 6 o'clock position, taking 1 to 1.5 cm of capsule (Fig. 16-4) and then penetrating through the labrum (Fig. 16-5). Posteriorly, it is common to use a curve-to-the-left device for right shoulders and a curve-to-the-right for left shoulders. A #0 PDS is advanced and retrieved through the AIP (Fig. 16-6A and B). One limb of the #2 Orthocord is shuttled from the AIP and back out the posterior portal (Fig. 16-7). These steps are repeated a second time, placating a portion of the capsule more anteriorly and using the PDS shuttling the second limb of the Orthocord posteriorly (Fig. 16-8A and B). The limbs of Orthocord are now tied from the posterior portal to create a horizontal mattress suture with the knot away from the articular surface (Fig. 16-9A and B). A second posteroinferior capsular plication is made at about the 5 o'clock or 4:30 position (left shoulder). For this plication, the curved suture hook can be used in either the AIP or the posterior portal, depending on which is easier. This effectively eliminates the posteroinferior pouch. Knots may be tied after each plication,

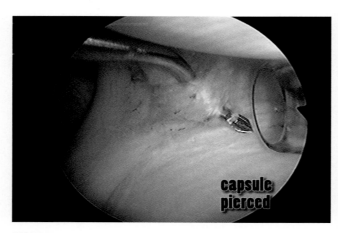

FIGURE 16-4

Spectrum suture hook penetrates capsule.

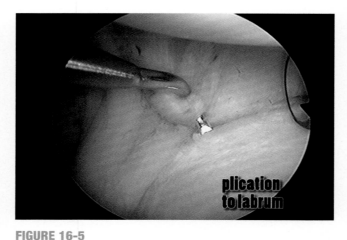

FIGURE 16-5

Suture hook is then passed through glenolabral junction to plicate with capsule. This eliminates capsular redundancy.

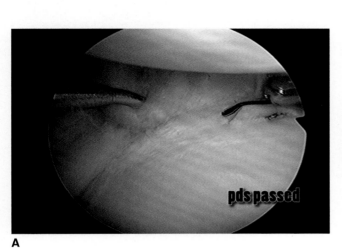

A

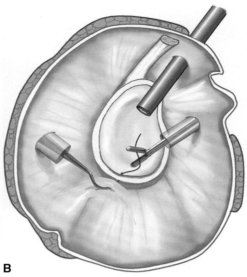

B

FIGURE 16-6

View from ASP looking at posterior cannula **(A)** and illustration **(B)** show PDS suture being passed from posterior cannula to plicate posteroinferior capsule. This will be used to shuttle nonabsorbable suture.

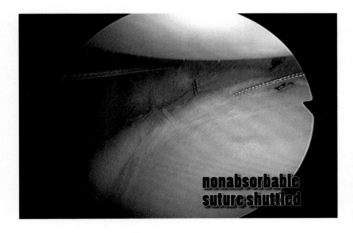

FIGURE 16-7

Nonabsorbable suture has been shuttled to create first limb of a horizontal mattress suture.

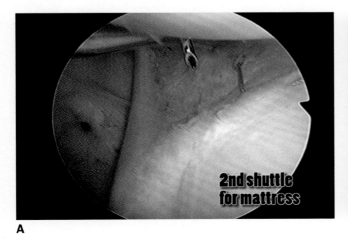

A

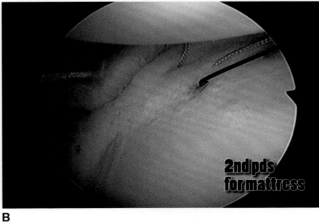

B

FIGURE 16-8

The suture hook is passed a second time through the inferior capsule **(A)** and labrum **(B)**.

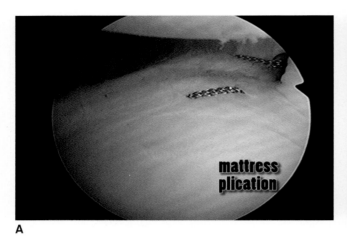
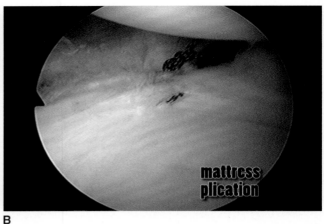

A   **B**

FIGURE 16-9

A: The second limb of nonabsorbable suture is shuttled and retrieved from the posterior portal. **B:** The mattress suture is tied, reducing capsular redundancy. The knot is away from the articular surface.

or they may be tied after passing multiple plication sutures. If the latter is chosen, some authors recommend using a Suture Saver (Linvatex, Inc., Largo, FL) to assist with suture management.

Next, attention is turned to the anteroinferior capsule. Anteriorly, we use a curve-to-the-left device for left shoulders and curve-to-the-right for right shoulders. Again, the capsule is excoriated with the shaver and an angled left Spectrum (left shoulder) is used to pass a 0-PDS as a shuttle, and then this maneuver is repeated for a mattress configuration at about the 6:30 position (Figs. 16-10 and 16-11). Subsequent knot tying rebolsters the labrum and allows capsular plication. The maneuver is repeated two additional times coming more cephalad to almost the 9 to 10 o'clock position (Fig. 16-12). The humeral head should be centered on the glenoid after accomplishing this part of the procedure.

Our decision on the use of suture anchors depends on the apparent quality of the labrum and its attachment to the glenoid. If the labrum is robust and has a secure attachment, we favor plication of the capsule to the labrum without suture anchors. However, we will use suture anchors if the labral tissue is deficient, detached, or degenerative with splitting. Anchor placement frequently requires the use of percutaneous portals. Posteriorly, an 18-gauge spinal needle is used to identify the appropriate trajectory of this portal (Fig. 16-13A and B). Our goal is to position this portal such that it allows an appropriate angle of insertion for more than one anchor (3-mm BioSutureTak, Arthrex, Inc., Naples, FL) if needed (Fig. 16-14). Anteriorly, a percutaneous

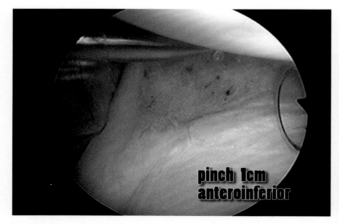
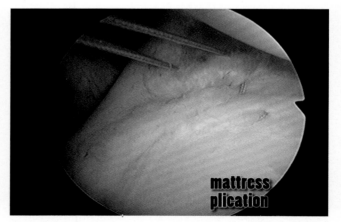

FIGURE 16-10

The plication steps are continued along the AIP glenoid. The suture hook (curve to the right for right shoulder) is inserted from the AIP portal.

FIGURE 16-11

Another mattress suture is prepared and tied from the AIP portal. Typically, we will place a total of two to three plication sutures posteriorly and three to four sutures anteriorly.

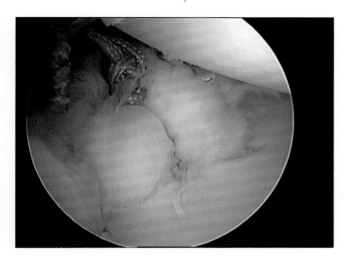

FIGURE 16-12

Sequential plication of the anterior capsule and labrum produces a robust anterior bumper.

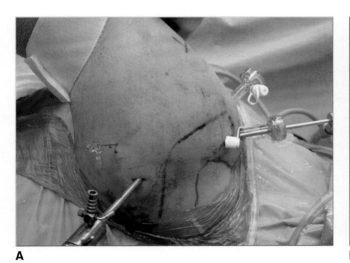

A

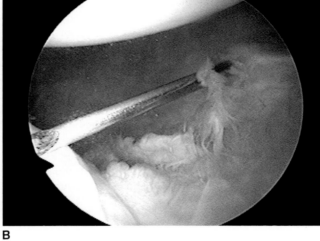

B

FIGURE 16-13

A: Percutaneous technique allows precise anchor placement for posterior and inferior glenoid. **B:** A spinal needle localizes the exact insertion directory for anchor placement.

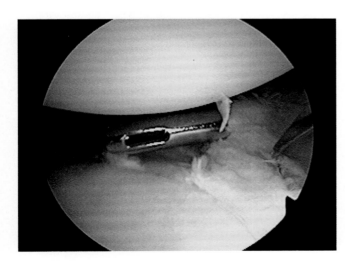

FIGURE 16-14

The drill guide for the 3-mm BioSutureTak (Arthrex, Inc., Naples, FL) is inserted percutaneously after localization with a spinal needle. It is possible to place two anchors through a well-positioned portal.

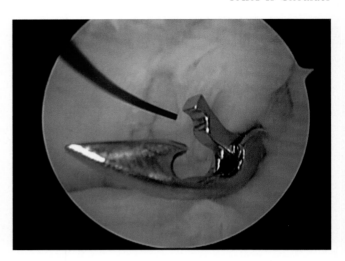

FIGURE 16-15

Rotator interval closure is performed by advancing an absorbable suture through the ASP. Next, the cannula in the AIP is backed out just superficial to the capsule in the rotator interval, and a penetrator is inserted through this cannula to retrieve the suture. The knot is tied extra-articularly, closing the rotator interval.

portal (5 o'clock portal) may be created from an outside-in technique, through the subscapularis tendon. The space available to view and work within the shoulder will diminish as the capsulorrhaphy continues. If suture anchors are used anteriorly, it is helpful to perform a pinch-tuck with the #0 PDS suture prior to anchor insertion. This creates a less obstructed view of the plication. Once the PDS is retrieved from the posterior portal, a suture anchor (3-mm BioSutureTak, Arthrex, Inc., Naples, FL) is inserted through a percutaneous "5 o'clock" portal. A limb of suture from this anchor can then be retrieved from the posterior portal and shuttled retrograde with the PDS out the AIP.

The arthroscope is then returned to the posterior viewing portal, and a #0 PDS suture is used to grasp the middle glenohumeral ligament from the AIP. The cannula is backed out of the capsule, and a BirdBeak (Arthrex, Inc., Naples, FL) penetrator is used, coming just anterior to the supraspinatus tendon edge to grasp the PDS (Fig. 16-15). A knot is tied outside the capsule to close the rotator interval. Figure 16-16 illustrates the finished repair. All weights are removed, and the portals are closed in a standard fashion.

FIGURE 16-16

Illustration demonstrates finished repair. Generally, two to three plication sutures are placed posterior to the 6 o'clock position (right shoulder) and three to four are placed anterior to this position. The rotator interval is closed in a medial to lateral direction, and the posterior portal has been closed as well.

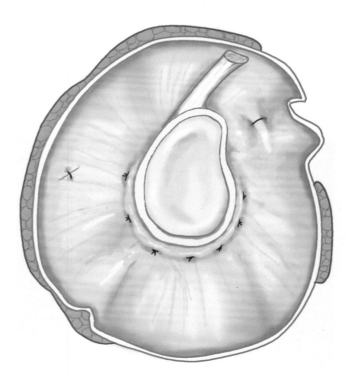

PEARLS AND PITFALLS

A precise diagnosis of MDI is critical when developing a treatment plan. Inaccurate diagnosis of inferior instability with subsequent inferior capsular shift with or without rotator interval closure can lead to significant loss of motion and poor clinical outcomes. The diagnosis of MDI must be made clinically and confirmed with examination under anesthesia and arthroscopically. The greatest pitfalls in the management of MDI occur either from "stabilizing" something that is not pathologic or failing to diagnose and treat all components of the pathology. For example, a large sulcus sign is not an independent indicator of inferior instability. The sulcus sign should only be considered pathologic if it does not diminish when the arm is externally rotated or if downward displacement of the arm reproduces the patient's symptoms. Either of these findings represents an indication for rotator interval closure. Routine rotator interval closure can diminish external rotation of the adducted arm without improving posterior stability.

It is possible to overtighten the anterior shoulder and insufficiently address the inferior pouch, which produces a shoulder with restricted external rotation and persistent inferior instability. The senior author (RAA) refers to this as the "Erlenmeyer flask phenomenon" where the humeral head translates inferiorly into the axillary pouch with range of motion. This can be avoided by starting the plication posteroinferiorly and then working systematically from AIP and to the anterior aspect of the glenoid and rotator interval.

Although most patients with MDI will report an insidious onset of symptoms, some will sustain a traumatic anteroinferior dislocation with a resultant Bankart lesion. The evaluation of patients with traumatic anterior dislocations requires the same clinical history and physical examination to establish whether the patient has underlying MDI. In this scenario, the posterior capsular plication is performed as described above. It is critical to mobilize the anterior labrum sufficiently prior to performing a capsulorrhaphy. The indication that the anteroinferior labrum has been mobilized sufficiently is that subscapularis muscle fibers are visualized in the window created between the labrum and the glenoid (Fig. 16-17). Special attention should be given to addressing the capsular redundancy as well as the labral repair in these instances.

POSTOPERATIVE MANAGEMENT

We immobilize our MDI patients in a sling with an abduction pillow for 4 to 6 weeks postoperatively. Active hand, wrist, and elbow motion is permitted immediately. Patients with MDI tend to have more generalized ligamentous laxity than do patients with unidirectional instability, and postoperative stiffness is less of a problem. Pendulum shoulder range of motion is initiated at 3 weeks. A formal range of motion program is initiated at 4 weeks. Sport-specific exercises are initiated at 3 to 4 months postoperative. Patients can return to noncontact sports at 6 months. Collision and contact athletics is permitted after 6 to 9 months provided the patient has full range of motion and full strength.

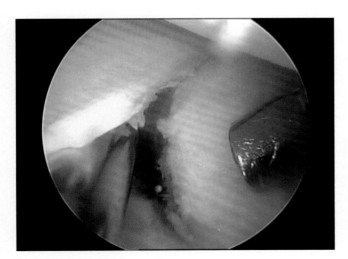

FIGURE 16-17

Anterior labrum of right shoulder viewed from ASP. The probe is directed toward the muscle fibers of the subscapularis. This indicates that the labrum has been elevated and mobilized from the glenoid sufficiently.

COMPLICATIONS

Risks of primary arthroscopic stabilization for MDI are generally rare. Loss of motion is infrequent in these patients. A meta-analysis of surgical management for MDI reported that open stabilization was associated with a 33.8% loss in range of motion, while arthroscopic stabilization was associated with a 5.5% range of motion loss (14). Furthermore, open and arthroscopic stabilization for MDI yielded similar redislocation rates in a systemic review comparing surgical treatment outcomes, with a rate of 7.5% for open stabilization and 7.8% for arthroscopic stabilization (15). Arthroscopic surgery minimizes the potential for subscapularis insufficiency that can occur after open anterior techniques. Residual postoperative pain can be seen after MDI operative management, reported in approximately 25% of patients. However, the pain is mostly mild to moderate, and the incidence of pain is not statistically different between the various operative treatment strategies (14). Infection is extremely rare with appropriate antibiotic prophylaxis. Neurologic injury has been reported to occur in up to 30% of shoulder arthroscopies, and these injuries are more common with lateral decubitus positioning. Although the vast majority of these injuries are neurapraxias that resolve over time, a number of steps should be taken to minimize direct or indirect neurologic trauma, which include careful attention to positioning and padding with neutral position of the cervical spine, use of an axillary roll, a pad under the proximal and distal fibula, avoiding excess traction, and edema control. When performing an inferior capsular plication, there is concern about iatrogenic injury to the axillary nerve as it traverses the quadrangular space inferior to the glenoid. Cadaveric studies have shown the nerve to pass between 2.5 and 3.2 mm from the inferior glenohumeral capsule, and this distance is smallest at the 6 o'clock position (16,17). Of the branches of the axillary nerve, the motor branch to the teres minor and the sensory branch to the lateral arm are closest to the inferior capsule. The authors are not aware of any reports documenting iatrogenic axillary nerve directly attributable to suture passing instruments. Nonetheless, care must be taken when penetrating the inferior capsule with curved suture hooks.

CONCLUSIONS

MDI patients are generally young and present with an insidious onset of symptoms, although trauma of variable severity is occasionally reported. To diagnose MDI, the patient must have symptoms attributable to glenohumeral laxity in more than one direction. Nonoperative treatment is initiated for all patients who present with signs and symptoms of MDI. If this fails, capsulorrhaphy for MDI requires symmetric tightening of the capsule so that the humeral head is concentrically reduced on the glenoid, yet normal range of motion is still permissible. Arthroscopic equipment continues to evolve, and this will facilitate capsular plication techniques. Multiple options are available to the surgeon performing arthroscopic shoulder stabilization. These include the type of suture (absorbable or nonabsorbable), the use of suture anchors, and the technique/instruments used to perform capsulorrhaphy. We are not aware of clinical outcomes in the literature that demonstrate superiority of one technique over another for MDI. Unfortunately, there are still no discrete guidelines to predict the amount of tightening that occurs following a particular degree of capsular shift. This may be defined through future biomechanical studies.

REFERENCES

1. Neer CS II, Foster CR. Inferior capsular shift for involuntary inferior and multidirectional instability of the shoulder. A preliminary report. *J Bone Joint Surg Am*. 1980;62:897–908.
2. McFarland EG, Kim TK, Neira CA, et al. Instability of the shoulder. The effect of variation in definition on the diagnosis of multidirectional instability of the shoulder. *J Bone Joint Surg Am*. 2003;85:2138–2144.
3. Richards RR. The diagnostic definition of multidirectional instability of the shoulder: searching for direction. *J Bone Joint Surg Am*. 2003;85:2145–2146.
4. Matsen FA III, Thomas SC, Rockwood CA Jr, et al. Glenohumeral instability. In: Rockwood CA Jr, Matsen FA III, eds. *The Shoulder*. 2nd Ed. Philadelphia, PA: WB Saunders; 1998:611–754.
5. Beighton P, Solomon L, Soskolne CL. Articular mobility in an African population. *Ann Rheum Dis*. 1973;32:413–418.
6. Lim CO, Park KJ, Cho BK, et al. A new screening method for multidirectional shoulder instability on magnetic resonance arthrography: labro-capsular distance. *Skeletal Radiol*. 2016;45:921–927.
7. Lee HJ, Kim NR, Moon SG, et al. Multidirectional instability of the shoulder: rotator interval dimension and capsular laxity evaluation using MR arthrography. *Skeletal Radiol*. 2013;42:231–238.
8. Caprise PA Jr, Sekiya JK. Open and arthroscopic treatment of multidirectional instability of the shoulder. *Arthroscopy*. 2006;22:1126–1131.

9. Flatow EL, Warner JJP. Instability of the shoulder: complex problems and failed repairs. *J Bone Joint Surg Am.* 1998;80:122–140.

10. Burkhead WZ Jr, Rockwood CA Jr. Treatment of instability of the shoulder with an exercise program. *J Bone Joint Surg Am.* 1992;74:890–896.

11. Warby SA, Watson L, Ford JJ, et al. Multidirectional instability of the glenohumeral joint: etiology, classification, assessment, and management. *J Hand Ther.* 2017;30:175–181.

12. Watson L, Warby S, Balster S, et al. The treatment of multidirectional instability of the shoulder with a rehabilitation program: Part 1. *Shoulder Elbow.* 2016;8(4):271–278.

13. Watson L, Warby S, Balster S, et al. The treatment of multidirectional instability of the shoulder with a rehabilitation program: Part 2. *Shoulder Elbow.* 2017;9(1):46–53.

14. Chen D, Goldberg J, Herald J, et al. Effects of a surgical management on multidirectional instability of the shoulder: a meta-analysis. *Knee Surg Sports Traumatol Arthrosc.* 2016;24:630–639.

15. Longo UG, Rizzello G, Loppini M, et al. Multidirectional instability of the shoulder: a systematic review. *Arthroscopy.* 2015;31(12):2431–2443.

16. Price MR, Tillett ED, Acland RD, et al. Determining the relationship of the axillary nerve to the shoulder joint capsule from an arthroscopic perspective. *J Bone Joint Surg Am.* 2004;86:2135–2142.

17. Bryan WJ, Schauder K, Tullos HS. The axillary nerve and its relationship to common sports medicine shoulder procedures. *Am J Sports Med.* 1986;14:113–116.

17 Subscapularis Repair

Jonas Pogorzelski, Erik M. Fritz, Zaamin B. Hussain, and Peter J. Millett

INDICATIONS

Several studies have reported the importance of the subscapularis (SSC) muscle for preservation of normal shoulder function, strength, and stability.

Nonoperative treatment often leads to a progression of tear size and fatty muscle infiltration over time.

Surgery is generally indicated for active patients of all ages.

Fox and Romeo reported a widely used classification. Lafosse et al. modified and expanded this classification by adding the results of MRI findings, more precisely the fatty degeneration of the muscle according to Goutallier et al. (Table 17-1).

Surgical options include an arthroscopic knotless single-anchor (Fig. 17-1) or double-row (Fig. 17-2) repair, mainly depending on the size of the SSC tear. While for Fox and Romeo Type I and II tears, a single-anchor repair is mostly sufficient, larger tears like Fox and Romeo III and IV often require a double-row repair.

CONTRAINDICATIONS

Possible contraindications are significant medical comorbidities including cardiac disease, pulmonary disease, and active infection. Other relative contraindications include massive glenohumeral osteoarthritis, fatty infiltration of the SSC muscle, and neuronal damage. In these patients, total shoulder arthroplasty is the preferred treatment.

PREOPERATIVE PREPARATION

Medical History and Clinical Examination

A thorough patient history and physical examination of the affected shoulder should be performed in each case. In general, patients with isolated SSC tears often present with a history of acute trauma.

TABLE 17-1 Classification Systems for Subscapularis Tendon Tears Proposed by Fox and Romeo (1) and Lafosse et al. (2)

CLASSIFICATION PER FOX AND ROMEO (1)	
Type I	Partial-thickness tear
Type II	Complete tear of the superior one-fourth of the tendon
Type III	Complete tear of the superior one-half of the tendon
Type IV	Complete rupture of the tendon
CLASSIFICATION PER LAFOSSE ET AL. (2)	
Type I	Partial lesion of the upper one-third of the tendon
Type II	Complete lesion of the upper one-third of the tendon
Type III	Complete lesion of the upper two-thirds of the tendon
Type IV	Complete lesion of the tendon but centered humeral head and fatty degeneration classified $\leq$ Goutallier et al. (3) stage III
Type V	Complete lesion of the tendon but eccentric humeral head and fatty degeneration classified $\geq$ Goutallier et al. (3) stage III

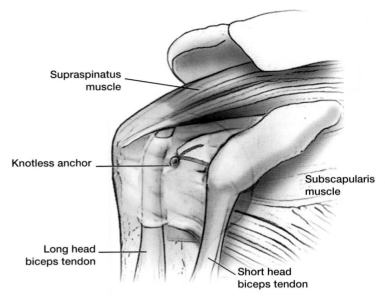

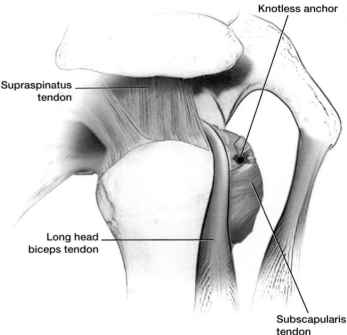

FIGURE 17-1

Illustration of a subscapularis tendon repair using a 1-anchor repair configuration.

Additionally, a history of anterior shoulder instability is not uncommon. On examination, patients will typically have weakness with internal rotation (IR) of the glenohumeral joint both at 0 and 90 degrees. At the same time, increased external rotation (ER) range of motion (ROM) may be present due to the lack of tension of the SSC tendon. With increasing size of the SSC tear, the patient shows a positive belly-press Test, in which, while pressing the hand into the abdomen, his or her elbow falls posteriorly relative to the coronal plane of the abdomen due to ancillary muscles compensating for the injured SSC. A positive lift-off test may also be present in which the patient is unable to hold his or her affected hand posterior to the lumbar spine. Finally, the bear-hug test may also be positive in which the patient is unable to hold the elbow of the affected arm in the horizontal plane while pushing down on his or her contralateral shoulder.

Imaging

Standardized radiographic evaluation is indicated preoperatively for all patients with a suspected SSC tendon tear. A true anteroposterior, axial, and y-view radiograph are each obtained to assess the articular surfaces for progressed osteoarthritis, joint incongruity, and to rule out any possible bony

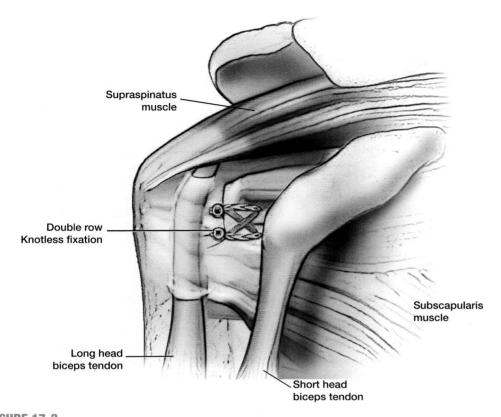

Supraspinatus
muscle

Double row
Knotless fixation

Subscapularis
muscle

Long head
biceps tendon

Short head
biceps tendon

FIGURE 17-2

Illustration of a subscapularis tendon repair using a knotless double-row knotless fixation configuration.

lesions or fractures. Magnetic resonance imaging (MRI) is also routinely performed for preoperative planning and to assess tendon and muscle quality. Additionally, the biceps reflection pulley should be carefully inspected, and the coracohumeral interval should be measured. Less than 10 mm in men and less than 8 mm in women is considered as a risk factor for coracoid impingement (4) and should be treated intraoperatively.

In the preoperative planning stage, it is important to distinguish between acute and chronic tears. Acute SSC tears may be repaired arthroscopically using a single-anchor repair or a double-row construct, depending on the size of the tear. However, with chronic tears, primary repair can be more challenging due to fatty infiltration, muscle atrophy, and tendon retraction. Thus, in cases where the repair is likely to fail and osteoarthritis of the shoulder is not present, the surgeon should consider instead performing a pectoralis major muscle transfer (5,6) or a replacement of the SSC tendon with a human acellular dermal allograft (7).

TECHNIQUE

Anesthesia and Patient Positioning

The surgery is performed with the patient under general anesthesia, and an interscalene block is routinely applied. Afterward, the patient is placed in the beach chair position with the operative extremity placed in a pneumatic arm holder to facilitate manipulation of the shoulder for optimal visualization. Another advantage of the beach chair position is the easy conversion to an open procedure if indicated. The bony landmarks are then marked on the skin indicating the acromion, clavicle, and coracoid process.

Diagnostic Arthroscopy and Portals

A standard posterior viewing portal is created approximately 2 cm inferior and 2 cm medial to the posterolateral acromion. Diagnostic arthroscopy is performed with a standard 30 degree arthroscope. To facilitate better visualization of the SSC and lesser tuberosity, the field of view may be manipulated with abduction, IR, or ER of the operative extremity. Following diagnostic arthroscopy, the anterior working portal is created under direct visualization with spinal needle localization through the rotator interval. This placement permits access to the lesser tuberosity at about a 45 degree angle and is particularly useful for anchor placement and suture management. In a similar fashion, the anterolateral portal is established next anterior and slightly medial to the anterolateral acromion. This portal approaches the tendon at a nearly parallel angle and facilitates preparation of the lesser tuberosity, mobilization of the SSC, and easy suture passage.

Biceps Tendon

During diagnostic arthroscopy, the long head of the biceps tendon should be thoroughly inspected as disruptions of the biceps reflection pulley are commonly associated with SSC tears. When a biceps pulley lesion or biceps tendon tear is present, the patient may experience persistent pain and even failure of the SSC repair postoperatively (8). Therefore, biceps tenotomy should be performed for later tenodesis, especially in chronic cases. We perform the tenodesis routinely at the end of the case using a mini-open subpectoral approach (9).

Coracohumeral Interval

Subcoracoid impingement is associated with SSC tears and may be implicated in its pathology. Therefore, intraoperative evaluation of the coracohumeral interval is imperative during this procedure. The surgeon may visualize intraoperative impingement of the coracoid process on the SSC with manipulation of the operative extremity through its ROM, particularly abduction, flexion, and IR. Moreover, when preoperative axial MRI demonstrates narrowing of the coracohumeral interval to <8 mm in women and 10 mm in men, coracoplasty is indicated. This provides the additional advantage of increasing the working space and making the subsequent SSC repair technically easier.

Coracoplasty and subcoracoid decompression begin with the creation of a window into the rotator interval using an arthroscopic shaver and radiofrequency device through the anterior working portal. The window is created just above the superior border of the SSC to expose the coracoid. The radiofrequency device can be used to remove the soft tissue from the tip and posterior aspect of the lateral coracoid. A 4-mm burr is then used through the anterior portal to remove approximately 3 to 5 mm of the lateroinferior side of the coracoid.

Subscapularis Tendon

Tendon mobility should be assessed using an arthroscopic grasper via the anterolateral portal. If the tendon mobilizes to the lesser tuberosity easily, such as in cases of acute tears, the repair may be performed right away. If the tendon does not mobilize, a three-sided release must be performed. A suture or grasper may be used at the superior border of the SSC tendon to provide traction during the release.

First, the anterior aspect of the tendon is released by dissecting the soft tissue between the anterior SSC and the coracoid process. Next, the superior aspect of the tendon is released by lysing the adhesions between the lateral arch of the coracoid process and the superior aspect of the SSC. Importantly, dissection should not extend medial to the base of the coracoid as this may put the musculocutaneous nerve, axillary nerve, and axillary artery at risk. Finally, the posterior release is performed dissecting the SSC from the glenoid neck; commonly, the capsulolabral interval needs to be divided to accomplish this final release, and complete release of the coracohumeral ligament (CHL) and medial glenohumeral ligament (MGHL) may also be necessary. Mobilization is completed when the tendon adequately reduces to the lesser tuberosity with appropriate tension.

For the SSC repair of tears of the upper one-third of the SSC, the arthroscope may completely remain in the posterior viewing portal; however, large tears may be obscured by the IGHL; therefore, the anterolateral portal or an open approach should be used for visualization.

Arthroscopic Transarticular Approach

In preparation for the repair, a 5-mm shaver through the anterior working portal is used to debride the edges of the torn SSC back to a stable margin of healthy tissue with healing capacity. A 4-mm burr is then used to prepare the SSC footprint on the lesser tuberosity, creating a bleeding bony surface to enhance and facilitate healing.

The more common type of SSC tendon tear is that of the upper one-third to one-half (Fig. 17-3), and these lesions can typically be repaired using a single anchor. Under direct visualization through the posterior viewing portal, an 18-gauge spinal needle is inserted percutaneously,

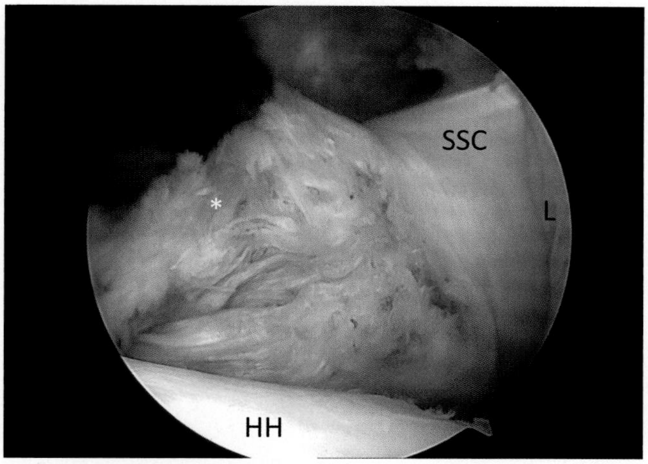

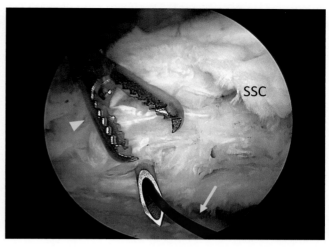

FIGURE 17-3

Arthroscopic view of a left shoulder through the standard posterior viewing portal demonstrating a delaminated full-thickness tear (*) of the upper one-half of the subscapularis tendon (SSC). HH, humeral head; L, labrum.

FIGURE 17-4

Arthroscopic view of a left shoulder through the standard posterior viewing portal demonstrating a subscapularis tendon tear. An 18-gauge spinal needle is inserted inferior to the anterior working portal and through the subscapularis tendon (SSC), a no. 1 PDS suture (*arrow*) is passed through the spinal needle, and an arthroscopic grasper (*arrowhead*) pulls the Ethibond suture through the anterior working portal.

inferior to the anterior working portal, and through the SSC tendon (Fig. 17-4). A no. 1 PDS suture is advanced through the spinal needle and pulled with an arthroscopic grasper out the anterior working portal.

A limb of suture tape is then secured to the limb of no. 1 PDS exiting the anterior working portal. The percutaneous limb is then gently pulled, shuttling the suture tape through the anterior portal, through the SSC, and out the skin percutaneously (Fig. 17-5). Through the anterior working portal, a grasper is then used to retrieve the percutaneous limb of the suture tape. Thus, both limbs of the tape exit the anterior working portal, creating a sling through the SSC (Fig. 17-6).

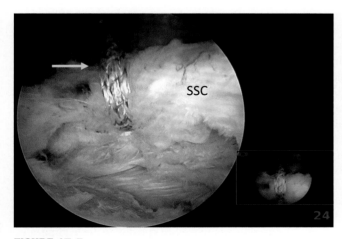

FIGURE 17-5

Arthroscopic view of a left shoulder through the standard posterior viewing portal demonstrating a subscapularis tendon tear. The suture tape (*arrow*) has been shuttled via the Ethibond suture through the anterior working portal, through the subscapularis tendon (SSC), and out the skin percutaneously (not seen here).

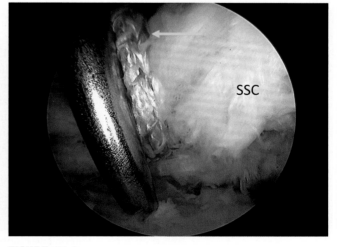

FIGURE 17-6

Arthroscopic view of a left shoulder through the standard posterior viewing portal demonstrating the subscapularis tendon (SSC). The suture tape (*arrow*) is passed though the tendon, and both limbs are exiting the anterior working portal. An arthroscopic punch is used to prepare the bone socket for subsequent suture anchor placement.

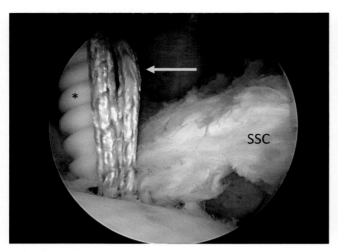

FIGURE 17-7

Arthroscopic view of a left shoulder through the standard posterior viewing portal demonstrating the subscapularis tendon (SSC). The suture tape (*arrow*) has been loaded through the eyelet of the 4.75-mm knotless suture anchor (*). Appropriate tension is applied to the SSC tendon via the suture tapes, and the anchor is loaded into the previously placed bone socket.

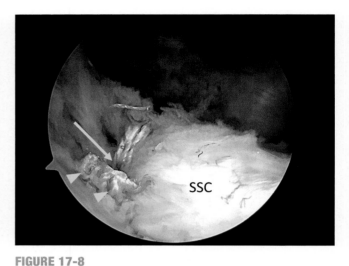

FIGURE 17-8

Arthroscopic view of a left shoulder through the standard posterior viewing portal demonstrating the completed knotless single-anchor repair of the subscapularis tendon (SSC). The suture anchor (*arrow*) has been placed and the free ends of the suture have been cut (*arrowhead*).

The SSC footprint on the lesser tuberosity is next prepared utilizing an arthroscopic shaver to creating a bleeding bony surface to enhance healing, and a radiofrequency device is used to mark the location for anchor placement. A punch is then used to create a bone socket for the suture anchor (Fig. 17-6). The limbs of suture tape are then threaded through the unloaded eyelet of a 4.75-mm knotless suture anchor, and the anchor is passed into the joint (Fig. 17-7). The suture limbs are pulled to generate the appropriate amount of tension on the SSC, and the anchor is finally placed (Fig. 17-8). The free ends of the suture tape are cut, completing the knotless single-anchor repair construct.

Arthroscopic Extra-articular Approach

High-grade full-thickness tears of the SSC tendon (Fox and Romeo Type III and IV) may be obscured by the IGHL; therefore, the anterolateral portal should be used for visualization. Thus, the arthroscope is placed in the aforementioned portal to get a better view down the SSC as this may facilitate the mobilization of a retracted tear. In general, a knotless double-row construct should be utilized for repair of larger tears (Fig. 17-2). This low-profile construct provides the benefit of even distribution of the compressive forces throughout the SSC tendon footprint. Unlike the tendon footprint of the supraspinatus, the SSC tendon footprint does not resemble a square but rather a trapezoidal shape. Thus, in order to optimize biomechanical load distribution, the superior-medial anchor is placed more medially than the inferior-medial anchor, resulting in a skewed double-row repair to fully cover the footprint. A superior-inferior bone bridge of about 10 mm in an inferior-lateral direction between each medial anchor is maintained.

For the medial row, double-loaded anchors are placed on the lesser tuberosity about 1 to 2 mm lateral to the articular margin through the anterior portal, and the sutures are then passed through the tensioned tendon using a tissue-penetrating device. One suture from each medial-row anchor is preloaded into the eyelet of the lateral row anchors, which are then placed approximately 15 mm lateral to their corresponding medial anchor. The suture tapes are pulled to achieve adequate tension, thus securing the tendon and completely covering the lesser tuberosity footprint and completing the repair. Additional side-to-side sutures may also be used to secure the SSC tendon to the leading edge of the supraspinatus tendon while being careful to leave the rotator interval open so as not to restrict postoperative ER.

Following completion of the SSC tendon repair, the arm is placed through ROM and tested for anterior instability. All arthroscopic instruments are then removed, and the portals are closed in standard fashion.

Open Approach for Massive and Contracted Subscapularis Tears

In more challenging cases, the surgeon may consider an open approach for complete repair of a full-thickness SSC tear involving the entire tendon as the arthroscopic view may be limited. Following a diagnostic arthroscopy, a standard deltopectoral incision of approximately 10 cm is made (Fig. 17-9). The subcutaneous tissue is carefully dissected down to the fascia in the deltopectoral groove, and the cephalic vein is exposed and retracted laterally, and if necessary, the vein may be ligated. Care is taken to dissect laterally to the conjoint tendon and retract it medially, thereby protecting the brachial plexus and the brachial vessels. In this way, the anterior glenohumeral joint is exposed revealing the SSC and anterior capsular deficiency.

For reparable tears, a knotless double-row construct is used, in an identical fashion as described above (Fig. 17-10). This construct can be extended to incorporate more anchors if required.

Anterior Capsule Reconstruction for Irreparable Subscapularis Tears

Patients with complete structural failure of the anterior capsule and the SSC muscle may experience weakness and chronic anterior shoulder instability. If retraction and poor tissue quality precludes primary repair, reconstruction with an allo- or autograft may be the only joint-preserving option. Even though pectoralis major tendon transfer surgeries have shown reliable results in the past, the procedure is technically challenging, invasive, and displays a relatively high failure rate. For that reason, the authors prefer an anterior capsule reconstruction with an acellular human dermal allograft for treatment of irreparable SSC tears (7).

To reconstruct the anterior shoulder capsule, the same open deltopectoral approach is taken that is described above (Fig. 17-11). The remaining cuff and capsular tissue is extensively debrided to create a bleeding bed for healing of the allograft tissue, and any residual anterior labrum is removed. The anterior glenoid is prepared with a motorized rasp to further enhance graft-to-bone healing. Three 3.0-mm knotted anchors preloaded with FiberWire are inserted into the anterior glenoid rim at the 1 o'clock, 3 o'clock, and 5 o'clock positions (Fig. 17-12).

Next, the tear size is measured in the coronal and axial planes with a ruler, and a 3.5-mm thick human acellular dermal patch is then prepared accordingly.

Two suture limbs from the middle glenoid suture anchor are then passed through the midpoint of medial edge of the graft. One limb from each of the inferior and superior anchors is then passed

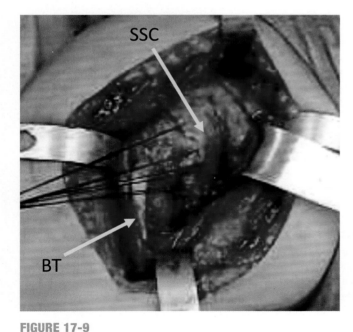

FIGURE 17-9
View of a right shoulder deltopectoral approach for open subscapularis repair. SSC, subscapularis; BT, long head of the biceps tendon.

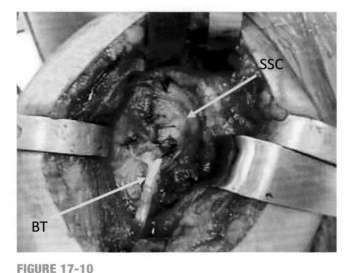

FIGURE 17-10
View of a right shoulder following open subscapularis repair. SSC, subscapularis; BT, long head of the biceps tendon.

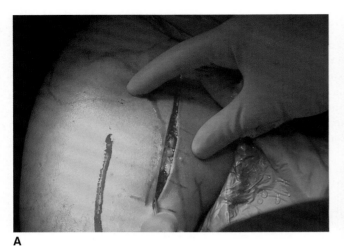
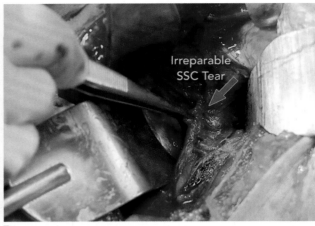

A   **B**

FIGURE 17-11

View of a right shoulder. **A:** A standard deltopectoral incision is made. **B:** The irreparable subscapularis (SSC) tear is exposed.

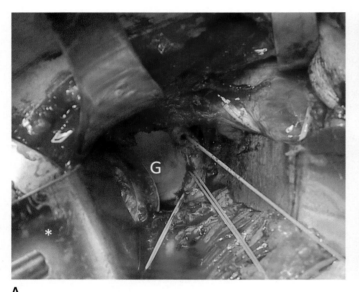
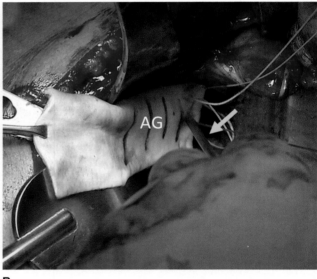

A   **B**

FIGURE 17-12

View of a right shoulder with the humeral head retracted using a Fukuda retractor (*) to expose the glenoid (G). **A:** Three suture anchors are placed along the anterior glenoid prior to allograft insertion. **B:** After the middle suture anchor limbs have been passed through the allograft (AG), it is inserted into the shoulder with the assistance of an arthroscopic knot pusher (*arrow*).

through the superior and inferior aspects of the graft, respectively. The graft is then shuttled down onto the glenoid (Fig. 17-12). Using an arthroscopic knot pusher, the middle suture limbs are tensioned and tied. The additional superior and inferior limbs that were not passed through the graft are now passed through the adjacent tissue and tied to their counterpart limb and tensioned, thus helping to prevent "dog-ear" formation on the glenoid side. This technique secures the graft along the anterior glenoid rim and surrounding structures.

The lesser tuberosity is then prepared with a motorized rasp (Fig. 17-13). Typically, a knotless double-row bridging repair with four anchors is performed for the lateral humeral-sided fixation. An arthroscopic punch is used to create a bone socket to accommodate the inferior-medial anchor approximately 1 to 2 mm lateral to the articular margin. A vented 4.75-mm knotless suture anchor

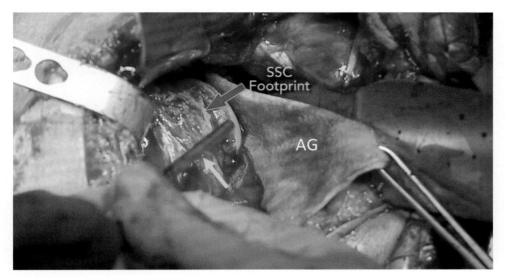

FIGURE 17-13

View of a right shoulder. The subscapularis (SSC) footprint on the lesser tuberosity is debrided with a motorized rasp (*arrow*) to prepare a bleeding bony surface prior to lateral fixation of the allograft (AG).

loaded with no. 2 suture tape and FiberWire sutures is placed in this inferior-medial socket. With an arthroscopic grasper and suture passer, each limb of the suture tape and one strand of FiberWire suture are passed through the inferior aspect of the graft, at a distance along the length of the graft that is determined by the size of the defect. One strand of FiberWire suture is not passed through the graft but is instead sutured to the surrounding rotator cuff tissue for additional stability. Next, preparation of the superior-medial anchor is performed in an identical fashion, taking care to maintain a 10-mm bone bridge relative to the first medial anchor.

The graft is then cut along its width, 1 cm lateral to the point where the graft has been sutured to the medial row, and the excess is discarded (Fig. 17-14).

An arthroscopic punch is then used to prepare the inferior-lateral bone socket approximately 15 mm lateral to the corresponding medial anchor. Limbs of suture tape from the two medial anchors are crossed and then loaded with the FiberWire sutures from the lateral corners of the

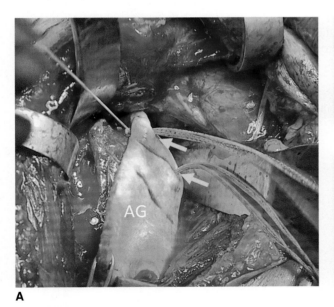
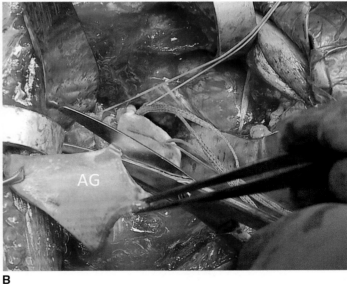

A   **B**

FIGURE 17-14

View of a right shoulder. **A:** The graft (AG) has been initially secured to the lesser tuberosity via two medial-row suture anchors (*arrows*). **B:** Prior to lateral-row fixation, the excess graft is removed.

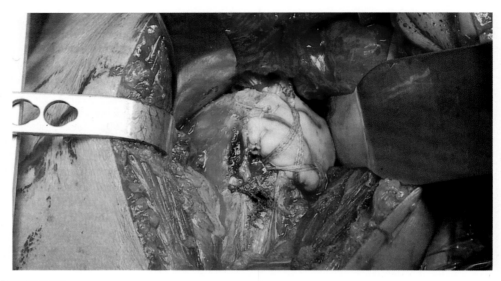

FIGURE 17-15

View of a right shoulder demonstrating the final knotless double-row lateral fixation construct for the anterior capsular reconstruction.

graft into the first lateral row anchor. The suture tapes are pulled to achieve adequate tension, thus securing the allograft patch laterally and completely covering the lesser tuberosity footprint. The suture tails are cut. This method is then repeated for the superolateral anchor to complete the repair (Fig. 17-15).

Two bone-to-tendon sutures are then placed at the lateral part of the superior aspect of the graft into the anterior edge of the supraspinatus tendon for further stability. However, care is taken to leave the rotator interval open. The wound is then thoroughly irrigated and closed in standard layers.

COMPLICATIONS

In general, arthroscopic repair of acute isolated SSC tendon tears is a safe, effective, and reliable procedure with positive outcomes and a low complication rate. Potential complications include infection, adhesive capsulitis, failure of the repair construct, and damage to the musculocutaneous nerve. Pearls and pitfalls for the procedure are outlined in Table 17-2.

TABLE 17-2 Pearls and Pitfalls of Arthroscopic Subscapularis Repair

Surgical Steps	Pitfalls	Pearls
Anterior working portal placement	Poor portal placement can make tendon repair technically difficult	Create portal lateral to coracoid and inferior to CA ligament permitting 45 degree access to the lesser tuberosity and helping anchor placement
Biceps tendon	A dislocated biceps tendon may injure the subscapularis tendon leading to rerupture	Perform biceps tenodesis to decrease risk of rerupture
Subcoracoid decompression and coracoplasty	A too far medial decompression may put neurovascular structures at risk. Too much resection of the coracoid process may lead to an iatrogenic fracture	Remain on the lateral side of the coracoid while dissecting and do not resect more than 5 mm of the lateroinferior side of the coracoid
Subscapularis tendon repair	Insufficient view	For SSC tears of the upper third, the posterior portal can be permanently used as camera portal. For bigger tears, the camera should be switched to an anterior portal
	Insufficient repair	For SSC tears Fox/Romeo Type I and II, a single-anchor repair is most commonly sufficient. For SSC tears Fox/Romeo Type III and IV, a knotless double-row construct should be used

TABLE 17-3 General Stages of Rehabilitation		
General Rehabilitation Stages		
Stage 1	Weeks 0–6	• Sling immobilization • External rotation ≤30 degree • PROM
Stage 2	Weeks 7–12	• Wean from sling • AAROM • AROM
Stage 3	Weeks 13–16	• Begin strengthening
Stage 4	Weeks 17–22	• Strengthen larger shoulder muscles • Full return to activities

Note that this is simply a general outline, and rehabilitation programs should be individualized to the patient. AAROM, active-assisted range of motion; AROM, active range of motion; PROM, passive range of motion.

POSTOPERATIVE MANAGEMENT

The rehabilitation program (Table 17-3) is individualized to each patient and varies based upon tear size, tissue quality, and security of the repair. In general, the arm is immobilized in a sling for 6 weeks with ER restricted to 30 degrees; during this time, the arm may come out of the sling for passive ROM beginning with pendulum exercises and advancing to low-load passive mid-ROM exercises. Patients with poor tissue quality or a less secure repair should have ER restricted to 0 degrees at this stage.

Between weeks 7 and 12, the patient is weaned from the sling and progresses to active-assisted and active ROM through the full range of the shoulder. At this stage, end-range stretching and joint mobilization techniques may be initiated.

Between 13 and 16 weeks, the patient begins strengthening exercises, provided sufficient gleno-humeral and scapulothoracic kinematics have been achieved in the previous stage; if patients experience persistent ROM limitations, they should be treated with prolonged passive and active-assisted ROM exercises, stretching, and manual therapy.

The final stage takes place approximately from 17 to 22 weeks and begins when the patient has achieved sufficient rotator cuff strength. This final stage involves strengthening the larger muscles of the shoulder, including the pectoralis major, latissimus dorsi, and deltoid muscles, and transitioning to full return to activities.

RESULTS

In general, arthroscopic repair of SSC tears is a safe and successful procedure. Saltzman and colleagues (10) recently performed a systematic review of arthroscopic SSC tendon repair. The authors identified eight studies, which demonstrated uniform improvements in patient-reported outcomes including the Constant score, strength, pain, and ROM with low complication rates.

Furthermore, Katthagen and colleagues (11) retrospectively reviewed the aforementioned technique of single-anchor repair of a partial- or full-thickness tear of the upper third of the SSC tendon in 31 patients with a minimum follow-up of 2 years. They showed high postoperative clinical outcome scores in combination with a high patient satisfaction, significantly improved clinical function, and significantly decreased pain postoperatively. Moreover, the authors found that full-thickness tears were associated with higher clinical outcomes and patient satisfaction compared to partial-thickness tears (ASES score 93.7 ± 10.8 and 86.7 ± 10.9, respectively) (11).

Comparable results were found by Lanz and colleagues (12) who retrospectively reviewed 46 patients who underwent arthroscopic repair of Lafosse type III and IV SSC tendon tears with a mean follow-up of 35 months. The mean Constant score improved from 46.5 to 79.9, UCLA score improved from 15.1 to 31.5, and subjective shoulder value improved from 51% to 88%; SSC strength was 92% compared to the contralateral shoulder at latest follow-up, and radiographic evaluation showed a rerupture rate of 11%. In total, 98% of patients were satisfied or very satisfied.

Also focusing on postoperative muscle strength, Bartl and colleagues (13) prospectively investigated outcomes of 21 patients with an average follow-up of 27 months after arthroscopic SSC repair. The average Constant score increased from 50 to 82 points, and 76% of patients went from positive to negative lift-off and belly-press tests following the surgery. Despite these excellent clinical results, SSC strength was still significantly lower compared to the contralateral extremity (65 vs. 87 N, respectively), and postoperative MRI demonstrated SSC muscle atrophy in about one-fourth of the patients (13).

Though outcomes for arthroscopic repair are positive, open repair may be another option, particularly in cases of difficult-to-access lesions. Achtnich and colleagues (14) investigated outcomes regarding isolated tears of the caudal SSC tendon, also known as the so-called "hidden lesion." Five patients underwent open repair of the caudal tear and demonstrated improved outcomes at an average follow-up of 12 months with a mean postoperative VAS score of one and ASES score of 93.3 (14).

In conclusion, arthroscopic repair of isolated SSC tendon tears is a rare but safe, effective, and reliable procedure with excellent clinical outcomes and high postoperative patient satisfaction.

REFERENCES

1. Fox J, Romeo A. Arthroscopic subscapularis repair. *Annual Meeting of AAOS*. New Orleans, Lousiana; 2003.
2. Lafosse L, Jost B, Reiland Y, et al. Structural integrity and clinical outcomes after arthroscopic repair of isolated subscapularis tears. *J Bone Joint Surg Am*. 2007;89(6):1184–1193.
3. Goutallier D, Postel JM, Bernageau J, et al. Fatty muscle degeneration in cuff ruptures. Pre- and postoperative evaluation by CT scan. *Clin Orthop Relat Res*. 1994;304:78–83.
4. Martetschlager F, Rios D, Boykin RE, et al. Coracoid impingement: current concepts. *Knee Surg Sports Traumatol Arthrosc*. 2012;20(11):2148–2155.
5. Gerber A, Clavert P, Millett PJ, et al. Split pectoralis major and teres major tendon transfers for reconstruction of irreparable tears of the subscapularis. *Tech Should Elbow Surg*. 2004;5(1):5–12.
6. Wirth MA, Rockwood CA Jr. Operative treatment of irreparable rupture of the subscapularis. *J Bone Joint Surg Am*. 1997;79(5):722–731.
7. Pogorzelski J, Hussain ZB, Fritz EM, et al. Open shoulder anterior capsular reconstruction with an acellular dermal graft for irreparable subscapularis tears. *Arthrosc Tech*. 2017;6(4):e951–e958.
8. Braun S, Millett PJ, Yongpravat C, et al. Biomechanical evaluation of shear force vectors leading to injury of the biceps reflection pulley: a biplane fluoroscopy study on cadaveric shoulders. *Am J Sports Med*. 2010;38(5):1015–1024.
9. Pogorzelski J, Beitzel K, Imhoff AB, et al. Surgical treatment of anterosuperior impingement of the shoulder. *Oper Orthop Traumatol*. 2016;28(6):418–429.
10. Saltzman BM, Collins MJ, Leroux T, et al. Arthroscopic repair of isolated subscapularis tears: a systematic review of technique-specific outcomes. *Arthroscopy*. 2017;33(4):849–860.
11. Katthagen JC, Vap AR, Tahal D, et al. Arthroscopic repair of isolated partial- and full-thickness upper third subscapularis tendon tears: minimum 2-year outcomes after single-anchor repair and biceps tenodesis. *Arthroscopy*. 2017;33(7):1286–1293.
12. Lanz U, Fullick R, Bongiorno V, et al. Arthroscopic repair of large subscapularis tendon tears: 2- to 4-year clinical and radiographic outcomes. *Arthroscopy*. 2013;29(9):1471–1478.
13. Bartl C, Salzmann GM, Seppel G, et al. Subscapularis function and structural integrity after arthroscopic repair of isolated subscapularis tears. *Am J Sports Med*. 2011;39(6):1255–1262.
14. Achtnich A, Braun S, Imhoff AB, et al. Isolated lesions of the lower subscapularis tendon: diagnosis and management. *Knee Surg Sports Traumatol Arthrosc*. 2015;25(7):2182–2188.

18 Superior Capsular Reconstruction

Jacob M. Kirsch, Neil Bakshi, Moin Khan, and Asheesh Bedi

INTRODUCTION

Massive rotator cuff tears pose significant challenges, particularly in the younger patient, despite advances in arthroscopic technique and equipment. Chronic attritional massive rotator cuff tears are a challenging clinical scenario due to a varying degree of tendon retraction, inelasticity, muscle atrophy, and fatty infiltration (1–6). Various treatment strategies have been proposed, including debridement, partial versus complete repair, repair with patch augmentation, tendon transfer and reverse total shoulder arthroplasty (7,8).

Many patients with massive, irreparable rotator cuff tears concomitantly have defects of the superior shoulder capsule (7,9,10). Biomechanically, it has been demonstrated that superior capsular defects can increase multidirectional glenohumeral translation, particularly with superior translation at 5 and 30 degrees of shoulder abduction (11). Mihata and colleagues (7) developed a technique for superior capsular reconstruction (SCR) using fascia lata autograft with the aim to recenter the humeral head, stabilize the shoulder, and restore the balanced force couples in patients with massive, irreparable rotator cuff tears (9,10).

INDICATIONS

The indications for SCR are largely directed by expert opinion, as limited clinical outcome data on the procedure are available in the literature. Our primary indication for performing an SCR is in the case of massive, irreparable supraspinatus and/or infraspinatus tears with minimal glenohumeral joint arthritis (Hamada stage 3 or less) in young patients (typically <65 years old) who have failed conservative management and have intolerable shoulder pain and subjectively unacceptable dysfunction (7,9,10). In these patients, reverse total shoulder arthroplasty is suboptimal due to the relatively high complication rate and limited longevity associated with this treatment in the young patient (12,13). Sershon and colleagues (14) demonstrated a 14% complication and 25% failure rate in young patients (mean age of 54 years old) undergoing reverse shoulder arthroplasty. Similarly, Ek and colleagues (15) reported a 37.5% complication rate and 25% rate of component exchange in a similar patient population. For these patient populations, SCR may be a viable alternative to reverse shoulder arthroplasty (7,9,10).

CONTRAINDICATIONS

Contraindications for SCR are evolving as more outcome data become available. In general, SCR should be avoided in patients with moderate to severe glenohumeral arthritis, as these patients would be better suited for reverse total shoulder arthroplasty to address pain generators from both the acromiohumeral and glenohumeral joint surfaces. In addition, patients with significant bone defects or stiffness at the glenohumeral joint may have poor results with SCR, and these conditions are contraindications to SCR as well. A lack of deltoid, latissimus dorsi, and pectoralis major function is another relative contraindication to SCR because of the importance of these dynamic stabilizers in providing the majority of the range of motion and function at the glenohumeral articulation (7,9,10). Subscapularis insufficiency is a relative contraindication also, as an inability to restore the force couple and contain the humeral head may compromise outcomes.

PREOPERATIVE PREPARATION

History and Physical Exam

Obtaining a comprehensive history is essential to evaluating patients with massive, irreparable rotator cuff tears. In addition to performing a general history and physical exam, critical questions during the evaluation of a patient with possible rotator cuff pathology include the age and activity level of the patient, chronicity of shoulder pain, presence of traumatic cause, radiation of pain, exacerbating activities/arm positions, relieving factors, and functional deficits.

Although there is no consistent presentation for patients with rotator cuff pathology (variable amounts of pain, unpredictable deficits in both active and passive range of motion, and inconsistent levels of disability), patients with symptomatic, massive rotator cuff tears often present with increased shoulder pain during activities of daily living (ADLs), overhead activities, and activities requiring reaching behind their back (1,16). Many patients also complain of increased pain at night that interrupts sleep. Some patients describe pain as radiating from the shoulder along the lateral aspect of the upper arm, sometimes to the elbow and proximally to the neck. Patients usually report either an insidious onset of symptoms or an acute traumatic event. They may report varying degrees of weakness and varying losses of the range of motion, depending on the tear size, location, and chronicity (1,16).

Performing a thorough physical exam is crucial to evaluating patients with massive rotator cuff tears, and the exam should begin with inspection, palpation, active/passive range of motion, and neurovascular testing of the affected and contralateral extremities. The physical examination includes inspection of the shoulder for supraspinatus and infraspinatus wasting/atrophy, as this is often present with chronic, massive rotator cuff tears. Pain with palpation of the acromioclavicular (AC) joint and crossbody adduction can point to the AC joint as a potential source of pathology. Passive motion is tested in all directions. Limitation of internal rotation can be common with any rotator cuff pathology and reflects a posterior capsular contracture. Inferior contracture can occur with large tears and superior migration of the humeral head. Significantly increased passive external rotation at the side compared to the opposite shoulder can indicate a very large subscapularis tear (1,16).

Active range of motion and rotator cuff strength testing can be performed using a variety of maneuvers. Functional deficits in shoulder strength and range of motion often correlate with the location of the tear. Posterosuperior cuff disruption typically causes decreases in abduction, flexion, and active external rotation. Patients often have weakness in external rotation, along with a positive external rotation lag sign, which is the inability to hold one's arm in a position of maximum external rotation. Patients with larger tears and significant decreases in external rotation strength compared to the contralateral shoulder may exhibit a positive hornblower sign. A positive hornblower sign—a patient's inability to externally rotate the shoulder in the motion required for a hornblower to raise the horn to the lips with the arm at the side—reflects significant teres minor dysfunction and has been found to be up to 100% sensitive and 93% specific for identifying irreparable tears of the teres minor (1,17–19).

With subscapularis involvement, the physical examination may reveal positive belly-press, lift-off, and bear-hug tests (1,17,20). The belly-press test is performed when the patient presses against his/her abdomen with the palm of the hand and the arm in an internally rotated position. The test is positive if the patient is unable to press the belly without the elbow moving posteriorly (behind the trunk of the body) and is indicative of deficiency of the upper portion of the subscapularis muscle. In the lift-off test, the patient is asked to bring his/her arm behind the back in an internally rotated position, with the palm facing outward. A positive lift-off test is indicated by an inability of the patient to push the examiner away from this internally rotated position and reflects lower subscapularis dysfunction (1,17). The bear-hug test for subscapularis tendon tears is performed by placing the palm of the affected side on the contralateral shoulder with the fingers extended and the elbow positioned anteriorly. The patient then holds this position while the physician tries to pull the patient's hand away from the shoulder with an external rotation force (1,20). While all tests had a specificity of >90%, Barth et al. found the bear-hug test to have greater sensitivity (60%) than the belly-press and lift-off tests for assessment of subscapularis tendon tears (1,20). Positive findings are a relative contraindication to SCR surgery.

Imaging

Imaging studies, including plain radiographs, computed tomography (CT) scans, ultrasound, and magnetic resonance imaging (MRI) scans, can help to guide both the diagnosis and the treatment of irreparable rotator cuff tears. Plain radiographs should evaluate for superior translation of the humeral head, evidence of degenerative arthritis of the glenohumeral joint, associated fractures, and disorders of the AC joint. A decreased acromiohumeral distance measured on radiographs may be evidence of a massive, irreparable rotator cuff tear that may benefit from SCR (1,16). However, evidence of degenerative arthritis of the glenohumeral joint may preclude the use of SCR and may favor reverse total shoulder or cuff tear arthropathy hemiarthroplasty. The stage of rotator cuff tear arthropathy as described by Hamada et al. (21) is an important part of preoperative assessment (Fig. 18-1). While clinical evidence regarding the indications for SCR continues to evolve, patients with Hamada stage ≤ 3 are best suited for SCR, whereas stage 4 and stage 5 disease should be considered relatively contraindicated.

Ultrasonography has also been used in the evaluation of irreparable rotator cuff tears. One of the main advantages of ultrasonography is the ability to evaluate the shoulder and the rotator cuff dynamically. Ultrasound allows for dynamic assessment of the rotator cuff during provocative

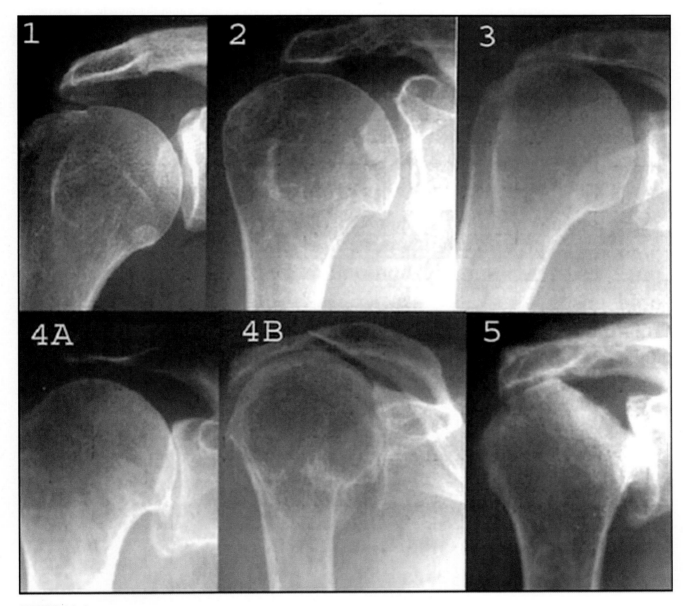

FIGURE 18-1

The Hamada classification of rotator cuff tear arthropathy. In stage 1, the head remains centered. Stage 2 has an acromiohumeral distance of <5 mm. Stage 3 has acetabularization of the acromion. Stage 4A is characterized by glenohumeral wear. Stage 4B has glenohumeral hear and acromial changes. Lastly, stage 5 has humeral head collapse. (From Ma CB, Feeley BT. *Basic Principles and Operative Management of the Rotator Cuff*. Thorofare, NJ: Slack Incorporated; 2012. Reprinted from SLACK Incorporated, with permission.)

maneuvers that reproduce symptoms and often can be useful in defining rotator cuff tendon tear size and morphology in the hands of a skilled ultrasonographer. In addition, unlike CT or MRI, ultrasonography is able to visualize the rotator cuff and nearby structures in the presence of metal implants without significant artifact. Furthermore, ultrasonography has no risk of exposure to radiation. However, there are multiple limitations of ultrasonography. First, the precision and accuracy of ultrasound can vary significantly with the skills of the technician. In addition, ultrasound cannot provide the osseous and soft tissue details of CT or MRI, respectively.

MRI has become the most common and most effective modality for the evaluation of rotator cuff pathology. MRI is a very sensitive and specific imaging test for the detection of rotator cuff tears. Iannotti et al. (22) demonstrated 100% sensitivity and 95% specificity for the diagnosis of complete rotator cuff tears. Goutallier et al. (2) initially classified the amount of rotator cuff degeneration by evaluating the amount of fat within the rotator cuff muscles using CT on a scale from 0 to 4. However, this is now most commonly evaluated using MRI. No fat within the rotator cuff muscles is classified as a 0. Minimal fatty degeneration within the muscle is classified as a 1. More muscle than fat within the rotator cuff is classified as a 2. Equivalent fat and muscle within the rotator cuff is classified as a 3. More fat than muscle in the rotator cuff is classified as a 4 (2). This can provide information regarding the ability to perform a rotator cuff repair, as the degree of fatty infiltration is correlated with healing rates, risk for retear, and functional outcomes postoperatively (1,16,23). Burkhart et al. (23) examined the functional results of 22 patients with stage 3 and stage 4 fatty degeneration of the rotator cuff and found significantly worse outcomes and decreased improvement in patients with stage-4 fatty degeneration. MRI can also provide exceptional soft tissue detail regarding the structures surrounding the rotator cuff to evaluate for concomitant pathology, including labral tears, paralabral cysts, cystic and degenerative bone changes, and articular cartilage damage. MRI also allows for evaluation of the biceps tendon and its location in the groove. In addition, accurate information can be obtained regarding the chronicity of the pathology, as acute tears often show edema and increased fluid in the affected tissue.

SURGICAL TECHNIQUE

An interscalene block is helpful and may be administered preoperatively for regional analgesia. In the operating room, and after induction of general anesthesia, the patient is placed in the beach chair position with a pneumatic arm holder (Fig. 18-2). Care is taken to pad all bony prominences. An examination under anesthesia of both shoulders is performed, which is part of our standard practice

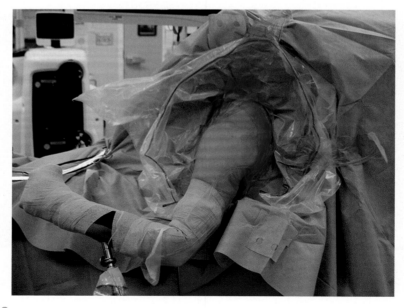

FIGURE 18-2

The patient is positioned in the beach chair position with the left arm in a pneumatic arm holder.

for all arthroscopic procedures. Intravenous antibiotics are administered preoperatively according to standard guidelines.

Standard diagnostic arthroscopy is initiated by making a posterior portal at the posterior soft spot, which is approximately 2 cm distal and 1 cm medial from the posterolateral aspect of the acromion (Fig. 18-3). This portal is deliberately maintained more lateral and superior in the setting of a known and massive posterosuperior cuff tear to facilitate visualization and instrumentation from the bursal side. After the arthroscope is introduced, an anterior portal is established under direct visualization using an outside-in technique with a spinal needle for localization above the leading edge of the subscapularis. Diagnostic arthroscopy is performed with attention to the integrity of the subscapularis, long head of the biceps tendon, and glenohumeral articular surface. The majority of patients in our experience have pathology of the long head of the biceps tendon, which can be managed either with tenotomy or tenodesis (Fig. 18-4).

The subacromial space is then entered through the posterior portal. An extensive lysis of adhesions and bursectomy is performed to fully define the rotator cuff defect and tear pattern. Capsular and soft tissue releases should be considered to mobilize retracted tissues, and primary or partial repair can be attempted if possible. In our patient, a massive irreparable posterosuperior tear involved the

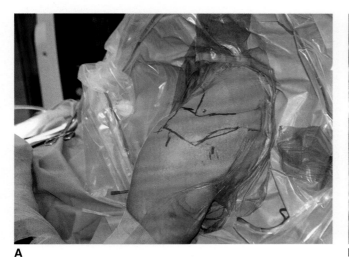
A

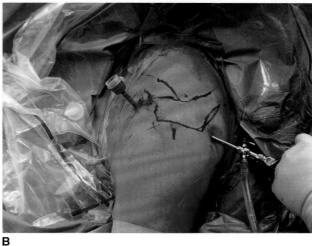
B

FIGURE 18-3

Standard arthroscopic landmarks are identified **(A)**, and diagnostic arthroscopy is initiated with posterior and anterior portals **(B)**.

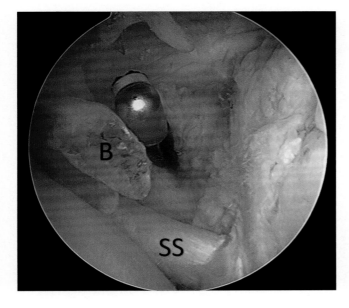

FIGURE 18-4

Biceps (B) tenotomy is performed with a radiofrequency ablation device adjacent to the superior labral anchor. The intact subscapularis (SS) is visible.

entire supraspinatus and nearly the entire infraspinatus. The superior glenoid could be visualized, and the rotator cuff native tissue was retracted well medial to the glenoid (Fig. 18-5). The subscapularis was intact, however if a tear was present, repair would be necessary prior to proceeding with SCR. If the remaining rotator cuff cannot be mobilized without undue tension despite lysis of adhesions on both the articular and bursal sides, SCR should be considered.

Glenoid preparation is approached from a lateral working portal. The superior margin of the glenoid neck is prepared by first removing all adherent soft tissue with a radiofrequency ablation device and then with a motorized shaver to expose healthy cancellous bone (Fig. 18-6). We aim to prepare at least 5 mm of bone medial to the articular border of the glenoid to ensure enough room for the suture anchors. The glenoid preparation is extended anteriorly to the level of the base of the coracoid and posteriorly to the posterior cuff remnant. In a left shoulder, as in the case presented here, this should be from approximately 10-o'clock anteriorly to the 2 to 3-o'clock position posteriorly. We attempt to maintain the integrity of the superior labrum whenever possible.

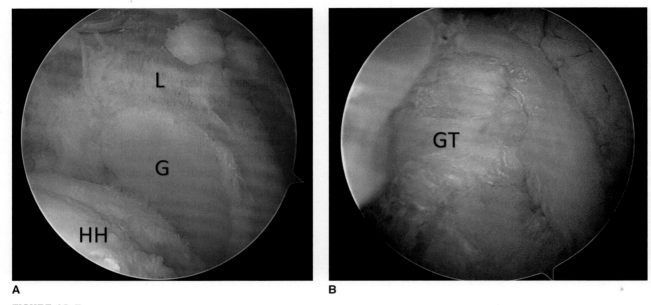

A   **B**

FIGURE 18-5

View from the subacromial space following bursectomy **(A)**. The massive cuff defect can be appreciated as the humeral head (HH), glenoid (G), and labrum (L) are all in view. **B:** Evaluation of the greater tuberosity (GT) footprint is devoid of rotator cuff attachment.

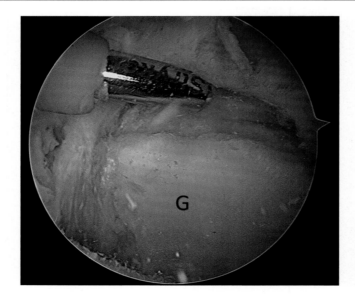

FIGURE 18-6

While viewing from the lateral portal, the superior margin of the glenoid (G) neck is biologically prepared with a burr.

Percutaneous anterior and posterior portals are used for placement of the glenoid suture anchors. We prefer to use a spinal needle to localize the anticipated location, and trajectory of the anchor can be optimized. A percutaneous anterior portal is made just anterior to the acromion for the placement of the anterior glenoid anchor (SutureTak BioComposite; Arthrex, Naples, FL) (Fig. 18-7). Ideally, the anterior glenoid suture anchor should be placed approximately at the level of the base of the cora-coid process, which is typically just anterior to the biceps tendon root, to help prevent anterosuperior escape. The bone quality at this location also tends to be favorable. After the anchor is drilled and placed, the suture tails are brought out the anterior portal. The ideal posterior portal can be variable and often depends on the anticipated trajectory at the glenoid face. It is essential to avoid being inclined toward the articular surface of the glenoid. We find that the posterior portal is often best established through the Neviaser portal (Fig. 18-8) or a percutaneous portal placed just posterior to the spine of the scapula (Fig. 18-9). Typically, two 2.9-mm anchors (SutureTak BioComposite; Arthrex, Naples, FL) are placed along the medial glenoid. If bone quality is suboptimal and there is

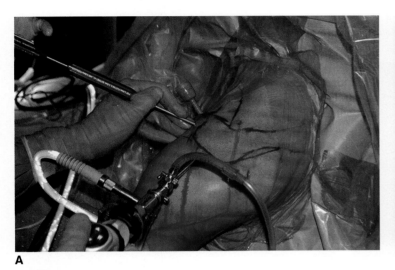
A

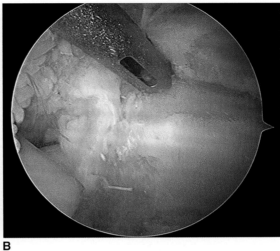
B

FIGURE 18-7

Viewing from the lateral portal **(A)**, the anterior glenoid suture anchor is placed on the medial glenoid neck **(B)** approximately just anterior to the biceps tendon root.

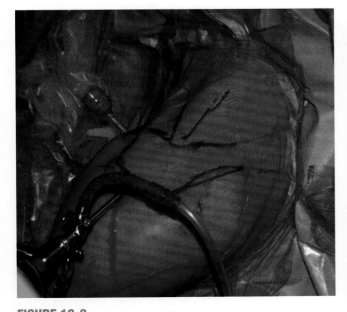

FIGURE 18-8

Using a spinal needle through the Neviaser portal to localize the posterior glenoid anchor trajectory.

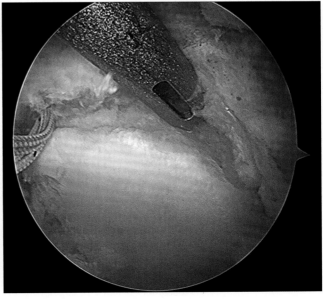

FIGURE 18-9

Placement of the posterior glenoid anchor.

poor pull-off strength, the anchors can be upsized to 4.75-mm anchors (SwiveLock BioComposite; Arthrex, Naples, FL). After placement of the posterior glenoid anchor, the suture tails are grasped and brought out the posterior portal, as having the suture tails exiting different portals is helpful for effective suture management.

The greater tuberosity footprint is prepared in a fashion similar to the preparation of the glenoid neck. The footprint is biologically prepared to create a vascular bed of healthy bleeding bone. Working from the anterolateral portal, two anchors (5.5-mm SwiveLock BioComposite; Arthrex, Naples, FL) are drilled and placed along the medial margin of the greater tuberosity footprint (Fig. 18-10). It is important to be cognizant that the overall shape of the dermal graft should be trapezoidal, and there should be more spread between the anchors on the greater tuberosity compared to the medial anchors on the glenoid. After placement of the greater tuberosity anchors, the suture tails from all the anchors are retrieved systematically starting with the anterior then posterior sutures of the glenoid followed by the sutures from the greater tuberosity. The suture tails are shuttled through a large cannula (12-mm Passport Cannula; Arthrex, Naples, FL) placed in the lateral portal. It is critical to perform this step in a controlled manner for effective suture management and to avoid entanglement (Fig. 18-11).

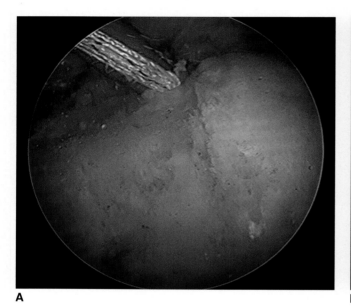 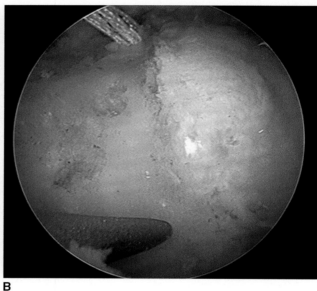

A   **B**

FIGURE 18-10

View from the anterolateral portal **(A,B)**, two anchors (5.5-mm SwiveLock BioComposite; Arthrex, Naples, FL) are drilled and placed along the medial margin of the greater tuberosity footprint.

FIGURE 18-11

All suture tails are brought through the lateral portal and placed in a different direction to avoid entanglement and confusion. AG, anterior glenoid; PG, posterior glenoid; AH, anterior humerus; PH, posterior humerus.

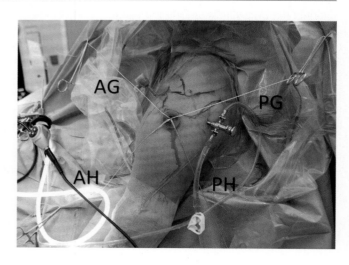

Measurements are made using a calibrated arthroscopic probe between the anchors in the anterior-posterior and medial-lateral planes to determine the size of the acellular dermal graft (Fig. 18-12). When preparing the graft, we typically allow 5 mm of circumferential overhang medially and 7 to 10 mm of overhang laterally to allow for double-row fixation over the greater tuberosity footprint. Ensuring adequate medial overhang is particularly important to help decrease the likelihood of suture cut out and increase graft to bone healing.

The graft (ArthroFlex; Arthrex, Naples, FL) is then prepared on the back table. A marking pen is used to mark the suture anchor locations and dimensions of the graft (Fig. 18-13). The graft can then be trimmed accordingly with scissors. A punch biopsy is then utilized to penetrate the thick ArthroFlex patch (Fig. 18-14). A suture passer (Micro Lasso; Arthrex, Naples, FL) is used to pass the sutures through the graft. While passing the sutures through the graft, we find that if the assistant pulls tension on the sutures, this decreases the likelihood of suture entanglement. The graft is marked on its superior surface to assure understanding of orientation once delivered into the joint space.

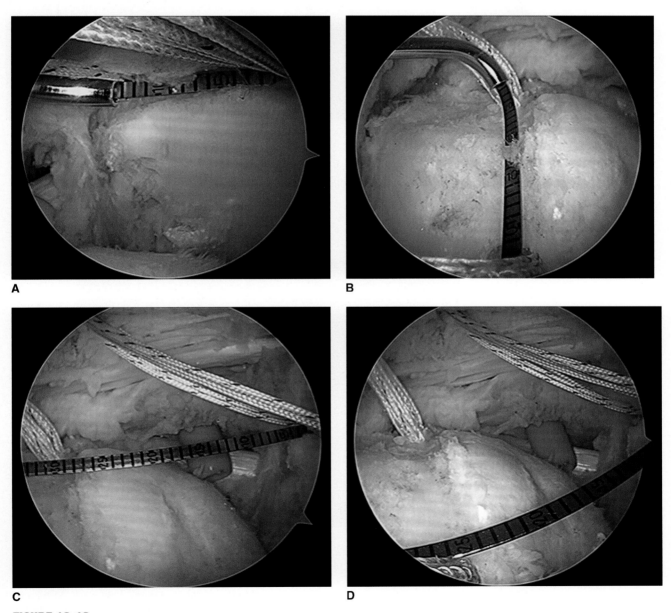

A   B

C   D

FIGURE 18-12

Measurement of the graft dimensions using a calibrated arthroscopic probe. The anteroposterior dimensions are measured on the glenoid **(A)** and the greater tuberosity **(B)**. The medial-lateral dimensions are measured both anteriorly **(C)** and posteriorly **(D)**.

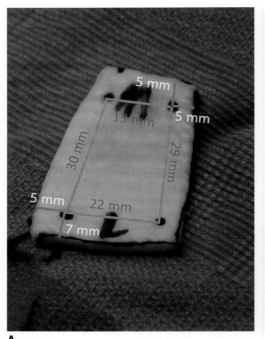
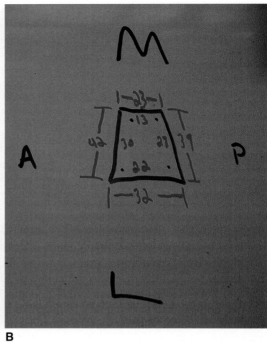

A   **B**

FIGURE 18-13

Actual **(A)** and schematic **(B)** representation of the graft (ArthroFlex; Arthrex, Naples, FL). We typically allow 5 mm of circumferential overhang medially (M), and 7 to 10 mm of overhang laterally (L) to allow for double-row fixation.

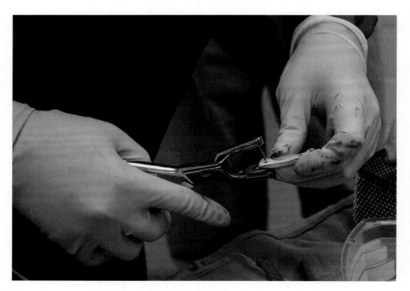

FIGURE 18-14

A punch biopsy is used to penetrate the graft at the marked sites.

While our preference is to use a commercially available decellularized dermal allograft, Mihata and colleagues (7,24) have demonstrated excellent results with fascia lata autograft. Recently, Mihata et al. (25) demonstrated that using a 8-mm-thick fascia lata graft provided better restoration of superior humeral head migration compared to a 4-mm graft. We prefer the decellularized dermal allograft due to the superior strength regarding load to failure and because it avoids the need for autograft procurement.

After all the sutures are placed through the graft, the graft is brought to the shoulder by the lateral portal. One suture from each glenoid anchor is tied over a finger to make a sliding construct, so a double pulley technique can be utilized as described by Koo and colleagues (26) (Fig. 18-15). The suture tails are cut and then the two remaining limbs from the glenoid anchors are tensioned in an alternating fashion to bring the graft into the passport cannula. A grasping instrument is used to aid in passing the graft through the cannula into the shoulder (Fig. 18-16). Tension should be maintained on the other suture limbs during graft passage to avoid entanglement. We find that this technique decreases the tension on the glenoid suture anchors and helps avoid anchor pull out. The two remaining limbs of the glenoid anchors are alternatingly tensioned to dock the graft medially on

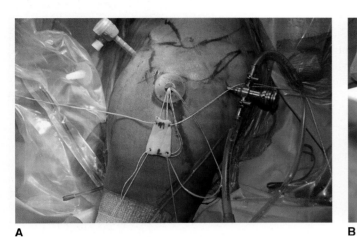
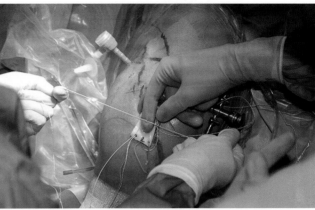

A   **B**

FIGURE 18-15

After the graft is brought to the shoulder **(A)**, one limb of each glenoid anchor is tied over a finger to make a sliding construct for the double pulley technique **(B)**.

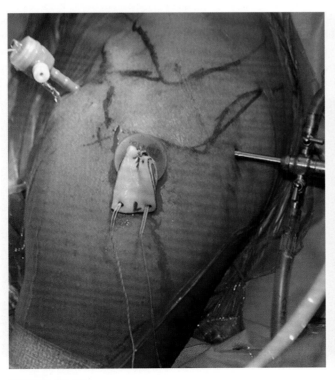
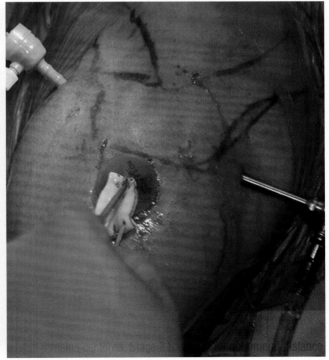

FIGURE 18-16

The graft is brought to the cannula **(A)**, and a grasping device is used to aid graft passage through the cannula **(B)**.

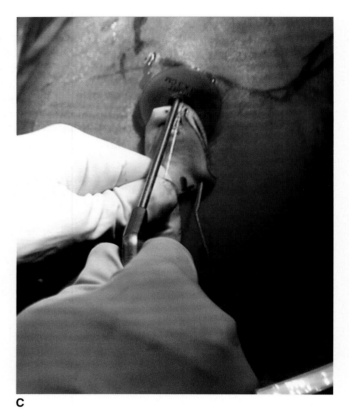

FIGURE 18-16 (*Continued*)

While doing this, it is imperative to maintain tension on the other suture limbs to avoid entanglement **(C)**.

C

the superior aspect of the glenoid. Once seated on the medial glenoid, the suture limbs are brought out the anterior portal to help avoid entanglement and then tied with a tension-slide construct along the medial glenoid (Fig. 18-17).

The lateral aspect of the graft to the greater tuberosity footprint is then secured. Prior to fixation, a grasper can be used to push down on the lateral aspect of the graft while pulling tension on the suture limb to take the tension out of the graft. A transosseous-equivalent double row SpeedBridge (Arthrex, Naples, FL) type construct is used to achieve lateral fixation, with the arm in 30 to 45 degrees of abduction to achieve adequate tensioning (7,27). Internal and external rotation

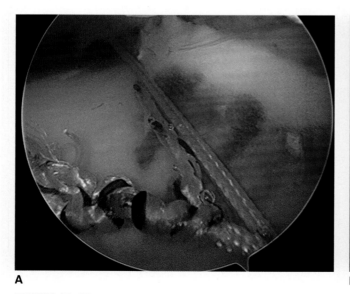

A

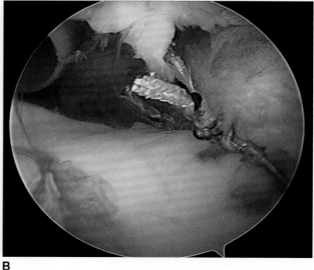

B

FIGURE 18-17

The graft is seated along the medial aspect of the glenoid **(A)** and tied with tension-slide construct **(B)**.

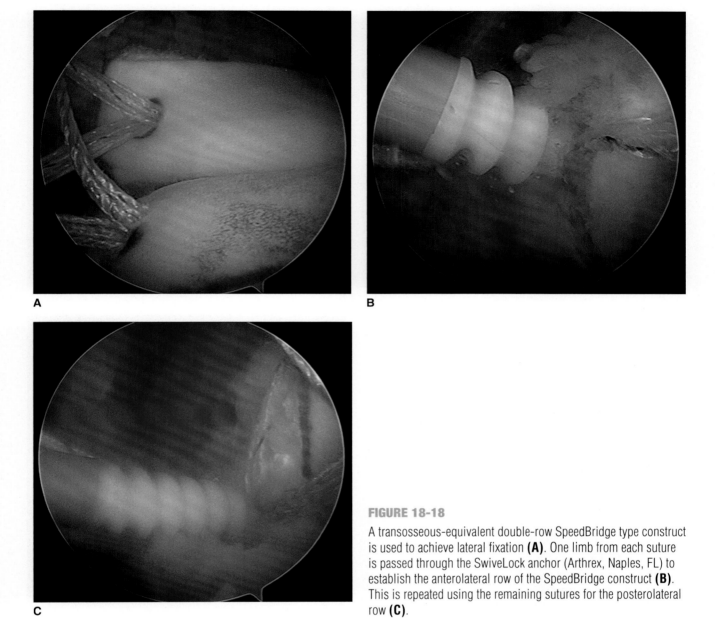

FIGURE 18-18

A transosseous-equivalent double-row SpeedBridge type construct is used to achieve lateral fixation **(A)**. One limb from each suture is passed through the SwiveLock anchor (Arthrex, Naples, FL) to establish the anterolateral row of the SpeedBridge construct **(B)**. This is repeated using the remaining sutures for the posterolateral row **(C)**.

of the arm can help aid in achieving the optimal position for anchor placement, which can be localized using a spinal needle. A pilot hole is made at the anterolateral aspect of the greater tuberosity footprint. One limb from each tuberosity footprint anchor is taken out and passed through the islet of a 4.75-mm SwiveLock anchor (Arthrex, Naples, FL) to establish the anterolateral row of the SpeedBridge construct. A similar procedure is performed to complete the SpeedBridge at the posterolateral aspect of the greater tuberosity footprint (Fig. 18-18).

If sufficient posterior rotator cuff remains, simple side-to-side margin convergence sutures can be placed between the posterior aspect of the graft and the most superior aspect of the remaining posterior superior rotator cuff. Caution should be used if deciding to place side-to-side sutures anteriorly as well as between the graft and the superior aspect of the subscapularis tendon, as this can over constrain the shoulder.

Once the graft is secured, a final inspection of the reconstruction is performed (Fig. 18-19). Gentle range of motion testing is performed to evaluate the tension on the graft. All portals are then irrigated and closed in a standard fashion.

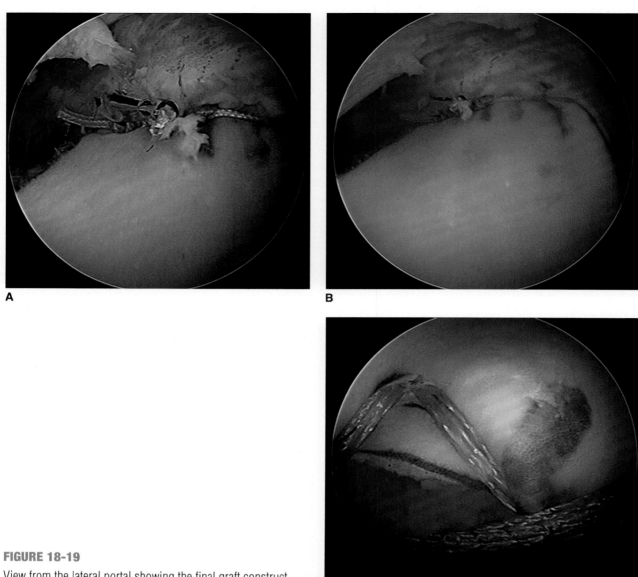

FIGURE 18-19

View from the lateral portal showing the final graft construct. The graft is secured medially on the superior glenoid neck **(A)**, and there is good superior **(B)** and lateral **(C)** coverage.

PEARLS AND PITFALLS

1. A thorough bursectomy and soft tissue release should be performed to assess rotator cuff mobility prior to opting for SCR.
2. Carefully evaluate for a tear of the subscapularis and repair if present.
3. A spinal needle is very helpful for localization of anchor placement and trajectory, especially on the glenoid. Often a Neviaser portal or a percutaneous portal just posterior to the spine of the scapula can be used to achieve proper anchor placement and trajectory.
4. The anterior glenoid suture anchor should be placed approximately at the level of the base of the coracoid process, which is typically just anterior to the biceps tendon root.
5. In the event that bone quality is suboptimal and the pull-off strength of the glenoid anchors is poor, anchor size can be increased.
6. Ensure an appropriate amount of overhang of the graft around the medial and lateral sutures to prevent cut out.
7. Meticulous suture management coupled with a large cannula through the lateral portal aids in successful graft passage.

8. A double-row transosseous equivalent construct provides excellent fixation and coverage of the graft to the humerus.
9. The graft should be tensioned with the arm in 30 to 45 degrees of abduction.

POSTOPERATIVE REHABILITATION

Postoperative rehabilitation typically follows a protocol similar to our massive rotator cuff repair protocol. The early phase focuses on limited and protected range of motion. Patients are in a sling immobilizer at all times except for exercises. We allow Codman pendulum exercises and active range of motion at the elbow and wrist. The next phase focuses on protected early motion. Patients work on flexion in scapular plane without restrictions while limiting external rotation to 45 degrees and internal rotation to 30 degrees. We encourage Codman pendulum exercises and rotator cuff isotonic exercises with the arm in 0 degree of abduction and neutral rotation. The next phases focus on progressive strengthening with a progressive scapular stabilization program.

COMPLICATIONS

Rates of complications following SCR are limited secondary to the paucity of clinical literature. In a study by Mihata and colleagues (7), 20 of 24 shoulders (83.3%) had an intact graft without subsequent rotator cuff tear during the follow-up period (mean follow-up 34.1 months). Three patients (12.5%) experienced a retear of the infraspinatus, all of which had preoperative Goutallier grade-4 fatty degeneration. One patient experienced a tear of the fascia lata graft after approximately 3 months. All patients who experienced either a retear of the infraspinatus or a graft tear had an acromiohumeral distance of 5 mm or less on postoperative radiographs (7). In a follow-up study of 48 additional patients, Mihata and Lee (24) reported only one graft tear at 12 months after surgery. In all, 67 of 72 patients (93%) had no graft tear or rotator cuff retear. No complication from the fascia lata graft harvest site had been reported.

RESULTS

Anatomical and biomechanical studies have recently begun to elucidate the importance of the superior shoulder capsule. The superior capsule attaches to approximately 30% to 60% of the greater tuberosity and plays an important role in passive glenohumeral stability (11,28). Mihata et al. (27) demonstrated that SCR completely restored superior translation of the humeral head to that of an intact rotator cuff in a cadaveric biomechanical study. Conversely, patch grafting to the supraspinatus tendon stump resulted in persistent superior translation of the humerus, which may explain the high retear rates associated with patch graft repairs (29–31).

Clinical outcomes following SCR are limited. Mihata and colleagues (7) were the first to report outcomes with this technique in 24 patients (mean age, 65.1 years) who underwent SCR for irreparable rotator cuff tears (11 large, 13 massive) at a mean follow-up of 34.1 months. Encouraging results were reported across a variety of parameters. Range of motion was significantly improved in forward flexion (84–148 degrees) and external rotation (26–40 degrees). Functional outcome scores were all significantly improved as measured by the American Shoulder and Elbow Surgeons (ASES) score (23.5–92.9 points), Japanese Orthopaedic Association (JOA) score (48.3–92.6 points), and the University of California, Los Angeles (UCLA) score (9.9–32.4 points). Additionally, the acromiohumeral distance increased from 4.6 ± 2.2 mm preoperatively to 8.7 ± 2.6 mm postoperatively.

Mihata and Lee (24) reported on 48 additional patients undergoing SCR for irreparable rotator cuff tears. Outcomes for the entire cohort of 72 patients were encouraging. Range of motion was significantly improved in forward flexion (97.1–152.7 degrees) and external rotation (28.2–43 degrees). Functional outcome scores were significantly improved for the ASES (31.3–92.8) and JOA (50.6–93.8). The acromiohumeral distance increased from 4.5 ± 2.1 mm preoperatively to 9.5 ± 2.7 mm at final follow-up.

Burkhart and colleagues have also demonstrated excellent success in their experience with SCR for massive irreparable rotator cuff tears (Burkhart SS, 2017, personal communication). Burkhart has reported excellent functional outcomes at 2 years in over 60 patients. According to global patient-reported surgical outcome registry data, more than 10,000 SCRs have been performed in the United States over a 5-year period with an adverse event reporting rate, monitored by the Food and Drug Administration, of <1% to date.

REFERENCES

1. Bedi A, Dines J, Warren RF, et al. Massive tears of the rotator cuff. *J Bone Joint Surg Am.* 2010;92:1894–1908. doi: 10.2106/JBJS.I.01531.
2. Goutallier D, Postel JM, Bernageau J, et al. Fatty muscle degeneration in cuff ruptures. Pre- and postoperative evaluation by CT scan. *Clin Orthop Relat Res.* 1994;78–83.
3. Melis B, Nemoz C, Walch G. Muscle fatty infiltration in rotator cuff tears: descriptive analysis of 1688 cases. *Orthop Traumatol Surg Res.* 2009;95:319–324. doi: 10.1016/j.otsr.2009.05.001.
4. Melis B, Wall B, Walch G. Natural history of infraspinatus fatty infiltration in rotator cuff tears. *J Shoulder Elbow Surg.* 2010;19:757–763. doi: 10.1016/j.jse.2009.12.002.
5. Oh JH, Kim SH, Choi JA, et al. Reliability of the grading system for fatty degeneration of rotator cuff muscles. *Clin Orthop Relat Res.* 2010;468:1558–1564. doi: 10.1007/s11999-009-0818-6.
6. Oh JH, Kim SH, Kang JY, et al. Effect of age on functional and structural outcome after rotator cuff repair. *Am J Sports Med.* 2010;38:672–678. doi: 10.1177/0363546509352460.
7. Mihata T, Lee TQ, Watanabe C, et al. Clinical results of arthroscopic superior capsule reconstruction for irreparable rotator cuff tears. *Arthroscopy.* 2013;29:459–470. doi: 10.1016/j.arthro.2012.10.022.
8. Rockwood CA Jr, Williams GR Jr, Burkhead WZ Jr. Debridement of degenerative, irreparable lesions of the rotator cuff. *J Bone Joint Surg Am.* 1995;77:857–866.
9. Adams CR, Denard PJ, Brady PC, et al. The arthroscopic superior capsular reconstruction. *Am J Orthop (Belle Mead NJ).* 2016;45:320–324.
10. Hirahara AM, Adams CR. Arthroscopic superior capsular reconstruction for treatment of massive irreparable rotator cuff tears. *Arthrosc Tech.* 2015;4:e637–e641. doi: 10.1016/j.eats.2015.07.006.
11. Ishihara Y, Mihata T, Tamboli M, et al. Role of the superior shoulder capsule in passive stability of the glenohumeral joint. *J Shoulder Elbow Surg.* 2014;23:642–648. doi: 10.1016/j.jse.2013.09.025.
12. Samuelsen BT, Wagner ER, Houdek MT, et al. Primary reverse shoulder arthroplasty in patients aged 65 years or younger. *J Shoulder Elbow Surg.* 2017;26:e13–e17. doi: 10.1016/j.jse.2016.05.026.
13. Villacis D, Sivasundaram L, Pannell WC, et al. Complication rate and implant survival for reverse shoulder arthroplasty versus total shoulder arthroplasty: results during the initial 2 years. *J Shoulder Elbow Surg.* 2016;25:927–935. doi: 10.1016/j.jse.2015.10.012.
14. Sershon RA, Van Thiel GS, Lin EC, et al. Clinical outcomes of reverse total shoulder arthroplasty in patients aged younger than 60 years. *J Shoulder Elbow Surg.* 2014;23:395–400. doi: 10.1016/j.jse.2013.07.047.
15. Ek ET, Neukom L, Catanzaro S, et al. Reverse total shoulder arthroplasty for massive irreparable rotator cuff tears in patients younger than 65 years old: results after five to fifteen years. *J Shoulder Elbow Surg.* 2013;22:1199–1208. doi: 10.1016/j.jse.2012.11.016.
16. Dines DM, Moynihan DP, Dines J, et al. Irreparable rotator cuff tears: what to do and when to do it; the surgeon's dilemma. *J Bone Joint Surg Am.* 2006;88:2294–2302.
17. Boes MT, McCann PD, Dines DM. Diagnosis and management of massive rotator cuff tears: the surgeon's dilemma. *Instr Course Lect.* 2006;55:45–57.
18. Gerber C, Fuchs B, Hodler J. The results of repair of massive tears of the rotator cuff. *J Bone Joint Surg Am.* 2000;82:505–515.
19. Zumstein MA, Jost B, Hempel J, et al. The clinical and structural long-term results of open repair of massive tears of the rotator cuff. *J Bone Joint Surg Am.* 2008;90:2423–2431. doi: 10.2106/JBJS.G.00677.
20. Barth JR, Burkhart SS, De Beer JF. The bear-hug test: a new and sensitive test for diagnosing a subscapularis tear. *Arthroscopy.* 2006;22:1076–1084. doi: 10.1016/j.arthro.2006.05.005.
21. Hamada K, Fukuda H, Mikasa M, et al. Roentgenographic findings in massive rotator cuff tears. A long-term observation. *Clin Orthop Relat Res.* 1990;92–96.
22. Iannotti JP, Zlatkin MB, Esterhai JL, et al. Magnetic resonance imaging of the shoulder. Sensitivity, specificity, and predictive value. *J Bone Joint Surg Am.* 1991;73:17–29.
23. Burkhart SS, Barth JR, Richards DP, et al. Arthroscopic repair of massive rotator cuff tears with stage 3 and 4 fatty degeneration. *Arthroscopy.* 2007;23:347–354. doi: 10.1016/j.arthro.2006.12.012.
24. Mihata T, Lee TQ. Clinical outcomes of superior capsule reconstruction for irreparable rotator cuff tears without osteoarthritis in the glenohumeral joint. *J Shoulder Elbow Surg.* 2015;24:e107–e109.
25. Mihata T, McGarry MH, Kahn T, et al. Biomechanical effect of thickness and tension of fascia lata graft on glenohumeral stability for superior capsule reconstruction in irreparable supraspinatus tears. *Arthroscopy.* 2016;32:418–426. doi: 10.1016/j.arthro.2015.08.024.
26. Koo SS, Burkhart SS, Ochoa E. Arthroscopic double-pulley remplissage technique for engaging Hill-Sachs lesions in anterior shoulder instability repairs. *Arthroscopy.* 2009;25:1343–1348. doi: 10.1016/j.arthro.2009.06.011.
27. Mihata T, McGarry MH, Pirolo JM, et al. Superior capsule reconstruction to restore superior stability in irreparable rotator cuff tears: a biomechanical cadaveric study. *Am J Sports Med.* 2012;40:2248–2255. doi: 10.1177/0363546512456195.
28. Nimura A, Kato A, Yamaguchi K, et al. The superior capsule of the shoulder joint complements the insertion of the rotator cuff. *J Shoulder Elbow Surg.* 2012;21:867–872. doi: 10.1016/j.jse.2011.04.034.
29. Moore DR, Cain EL, Schwartz ML, et al. Allograft reconstruction for massive, irreparable rotator cuff tears. *Am J Sports Med.* 2006;34:392–396. doi: 10.1177/0363546505281237.
30. Sclamberg SG, Tibone JE, Itamura JM, et al. Six-month magnetic resonance imaging follow-up of large and massive rotator cuff repairs reinforced with porcine small intestinal submucosa. *J Shoulder Elbow Surg.* 2004;13:538–541. doi: 10.1016/S1058274604001193.
31. Soler JA, Gidwani S, Curtis MJ. Early complications from the use of porcine dermal collagen implants (Permacol) as bridging constructs in the repair of massive rotator cuff tears. A report of 4 cases. *Acta Orthop Belg.* 2007;73:432–436.

19 Medial Patellofemoral Ligament Reconstruction

Miho J. Tanaka, Itai Gans, and Andrew J. Cosgarea

Medial patellofemoral ligament (MPFL) reconstruction is indicated for patients with recurrent lateral patellar instability; the goal of this procedure is to restore the primary medial restraint of the patella. However, patellofemoral instability is a complex entity. Although the MPFL is disrupted in 94% of patients after acute patellar dislocations (1), there are a multitude of factors that can contribute to patellofemoral instability, including bony deficiencies, malalignment, ligamentous laxity, and muscle imbalance. Successful outcomes after MPFL reconstruction require the recognition of both the function and limitations of this procedure in the setting of those other factors. An understanding of patellofemoral kinematics combined with thorough preoperative assessment and planning will allow one to provide the appropriate treatment for patients with lateral patellofemoral instability.

INDICATIONS/CONTRAINDICATIONS

Patients with recurrent episodes of lateral patellar instability typically present in adolescence, often after an acute inciting event. They may describe symptoms of anterior knee pain that accompany the episodes of instability. As with most conditions, the first line of treatment for patellar instability is nonoperative interventions, including activity modification, brace protection, and physical therapy. A brace with a lateral buttress, along with oral analgesics and icing, can help minimize the initial symptoms. Physical therapy is useful in helping the patient regain strength and function. The goals of rehabilitation are to minimize the lateral forces on the patellofemoral joint by strengthening the vastus medialis obliquus (the dynamic medial stabilizer of the patella) and by stretching the lateral extensor mechanism and retinaculum. Activity modification, which is generally not well accepted in a young, active patient, includes avoidance of activities involving planting and twisting motions.

If nonoperative treatment fails, choosing the appropriate operative intervention by correctly understanding the source of the patient's symptoms is the key in attaining successful outcomes. First, because MPFL reconstruction recreates the primary medial stabilizer of the patella, patellofemoral *pain* alone must be carefully differentiated from patellofemoral *instability* in the history and physical examination. MPFL reconstruction is reserved for lateral instability of the patella and should be regarded as a stabilization procedure. In contrast, symptoms of maltracking, arthrosis, and excessive lateral patellar pressure are better addressed by tuberosity osteotomy procedures that realign the extensor mechanism and unload the lateral patellofemoral cartilage.

Second, a thorough assessment of the factors contributing to the patient's patellofemoral instability must be considered before proceeding with MPFL reconstruction. Numerous factors can contribute to patellar instability, most of which involve a combination of hyperlaxity, malalignment, and bony abnormalities. Trochlear dysplasia and insufficiency of the medial retinaculum and MPFL can reduce the medial restraint of the patella and facilitate lateral instability. Such cases without concomitant malalignment can be treated with MPFL reconstruction. In contrast, instability secondary to substantial malalignment indicated by excessive lateralization of the tibial tuberosity (tibial tuberosity trochlear groove distance >15–20 mm), with or without patella alta, is better treated with tuberosity osteotomy procedures. MPFL reconstruction can be used to supplement these procedures in the event that adequate patellar stability is not attained after distal bony realignment.

Third, medial patellofemoral instability, although rare, should be distinguished from lateral instability because the former is a contraindication to MPFL reconstruction. Medial instability is usually an iatrogenic problem that occurs after an overly aggressive lateral retinacular release. MPFL reconstruction restores lateral patellar instability only and does not address medial instability. Other contraindications include active infection and inability to comply with postoperative instructions. Skeletal immaturity is not an absolute contraindication to MPFL reconstruction, but it necessitates an alternative procedure that avoids drilling a tunnel through the distal femoral physis (2).

PREOPERATIVE PLANNING

History

A thorough preoperative history and physical examination are required to evaluate each individual's causes of patellar instability. The obtained history should include the duration of symptoms and the number of episodes of instability. Patients may present after the first acute episode, describing it as a sense of giving way during a planting and twisting motion. Less commonly, direct trauma to the medial knee can also cause patellar instability. Patients may note an initial hemarthrosis and have tenderness along the course of the MPFL. Those with recurrent instability after the initial trauma may have associated anterior knee pain or mechanical symptoms from chondral injuries and loose bodies. Any previous treatment or procedure for their symptoms should be noted. Instability after a previous lateral retinacular release may indicate medial patellar instability, which should be noted in the examination.

Physical Examination

Physical examination begins with the patient in a standing position as the clinician notes any abnormalities in alignment, including genu varum or valgum, increased femoral anteversion, and excessive pronation of the foot. The examination continues with the patient sitting on the edge of the examination table: observation of patellar tracking in active extension may reveal a positive J sign, made apparent by lateral translation of the patella, as it exits the trochlear sulcus while the knee approaches full extension. Any hypoplasia of the vastus medialis obliquus or quadriceps should be noted. As always, a thorough ligamentous examination is obtained, with care taken to rule out concomitant injury. In particular, the knee should be assessed for injuries to the medial collateral and anterior cruciate ligaments because they may have a similar mechanism of injury.

Several tests are used specifically to assess patellar instability. With the knee in extension, the glide test is used to assess for incompetence of the medial soft tissue restraints. This test is performed by manually displacing the patella laterally (Fig. 19-1). Excursion is measured in patellar quadrants, which are described as one-quarter of the width of the patella. Normal lateral translation is quantified by comparing the test to the normal contralateral patella. In patients with bilateral patellar instability, it may be difficult to assess what degree of translation is pathologic or normal. The

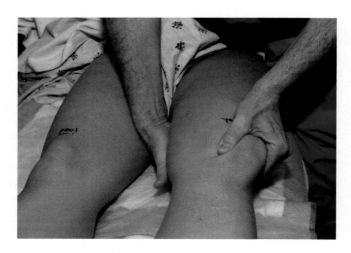

FIGURE 19-1

The glide test. In this patient, the patella can be easily dislocated laterally.

apprehension sign is assessed by displacing the patella laterally with the knee at 20 to 30 degrees of flexion. A sense of apprehension in the patient with this motion is often indicative of patellar instability. Finally, the tilt test is used to assess for tightness of the lateral structures. This examination involves lifting the lateral border of the patella. If the clinician is unable to elevate the lateral border of the patella above the horizontal plane, this test is considered positive and may be an indication for lateral retinacular release. Any medial patellar instability and associated medial apprehension should be ruled out during the physical examination.

Radiographic Imaging

Adequate imaging studies are critical in detecting anatomic abnormalities that may contribute to patellar instability. They may also help in identifying any associated injuries. Standard radiographs include anteroposterior, lateral, and axial views of the knee at 30 to 45 degrees of flexion. The lateral radiograph should be noted for any signs of patella alta or trochlear dysplasia. The crossing sign, seen on the lateral view of the knee, is present when the line of the anterior femoral condyles crosses that of the trochlear groove, indicating a dysplastic trochlea. Radiographs may also show the presence of loose bodies from chondral injury or calcifications along the medial border of the patella, indicative of MPFL injury.

Computed Tomographic Imaging

Computed tomography can also be used to assess the bony abnormalities associated with patellar instability. Precise measurements of the degree of patellar tilt, the height of the lateral trochlear ridge, and the degree of patellar subluxation are possible with computed tomographic imaging. The degree of subluxation is assessed by measuring the bisect offset index, which quantifies the ratio of the portion of the patellar width that is lateral relative to a line perpendicular to the posterior femoral condyles through the deepest point of the trochlear groove to the proportion of the patella that is medial to this line. Tibial tubercle malalignment can also be measured on superimposed axial views with the tibial tuberosity trochlear groove distance; measurements of more than 15 to 20 mm are considered abnormal and indicate an excessively lateralized tuberosity.

Magnetic Resonance Imaging

Magnetic resonance imaging can provide information regarding anatomic alignment, but it is most valuable in visualizing soft tissue and cartilage injuries. Magnetic resonance imaging can show the details of MPFL injury with regard to the type and location of the tear (3). It is also used to identify the presence of chondral lesions or concomitant ligamentous injury, which is particularly helpful in planning for concurrent procedures.

Potential Intraoperative Findings

When planning for MPFL reconstruction, the clinician should anticipate that additional or alternative intervention(s) may be required based on the intraoperative evaluation. For example, contractures of the lateral patellar soft tissues may require a lateral release, and the presence of chondral lesions found during diagnostic arthroscopy may necessitate debridement, microfracture, or other interventions. On the other hand, high-grade chondral lesions that require unloading may prompt the need for a distal realignment procedure instead of MPFL reconstruction. The potential need for these procedures should be adequately addressed in the preoperative consent and planning process.

TECHNIQUE

Preparation

The patient is placed in a supine position on the operating room table. Anesthesia is administered using general or regional techniques. Prophylactic intravenous antibiotics are given before the incision is made. A thorough physical examination of the operative and contralateral knees is performed. Standard evaluations include range of motion (ROM) testing and the Lachman test, posterior drawer test, and assessments of varus and valgus stability. The patellofemoral examination involves the assessment of patellar stability with the glide test, which demonstrates incompetence of the medial soft tissue restraints (Fig. 19-1), and tilt test to determine lateral retinacular tightness.

A thromboembolic deterrent stocking is applied to the nonoperative leg. A tourniquet is then applied to the operative proximal thigh, and a vertical post is placed distal to the tourniquet. The leg is next prepared and draped with sterile, impervious drapes.

Diagnostic Arthroscopy

Diagnostic arthroscopy is performed via the standard inferomedial and inferolateral portals. The suprapatellar pouch and medial and lateral parapatellar gutters are closely observed for loose bodies. Evaluation of the patellofemoral joint should include the visualization of patellar tracking during ROM of the knee, with special attention directed to observing the shape of the trochlea and condition of the patellar facets and trochlear ridges. Any chondral damage is noted, with appropriate cartilage procedures performed as needed. If a high-grade chondral lesion involving the inferior pole or lateral facet of the patella is found, the surgeon may, at this time, choose to proceed with a tibial tuberosity osteotomy instead. The complete diagnostic evaluation includes assessment of the anterior and posterior cruciate ligaments, medial and lateral compartments, and the posteromedial and posterolateral compartments through the femoral notch.

Landmarks and Graft Harvest

The leg is exsanguinated with an Esmarch bandage, and the tourniquet is inflated. The bony landmarks are identified and marked on the skin surface including the patella and patellar tendon, the medial femoral epicondyle, and adductor tubercle, as well as the site of the pes insertion. A short oblique incision is made over the pes anserine insertion, exposing the subcutaneous tissue to allow hamstring autograft harvest. Blunt dissection is used to expose and identify the sartorial fascia, and any vessels that cross the field are cauterized. The sartorial fascia is incised and everted, exposing the gracilis and semitendinosus tendons (Fig. 19-2). The semitendinosus tendon is released distally and tagged for harvesting. The fascial band from the semitendinosus to the medial head of the gastrocnemius (~7 cm proximal to the pes insertion) is released, and the graft is harvested using an open-ended pigtail tendon stripper. The gracilis tendon or allograft tendon may also be used in place of the semitendinosus tendon as an alternative graft for this procedure.

Graft Preparation

The semitendinosus tendon graft is prepared by removing the muscle and soft tissue debris from the graft. A No. 2 FiberLoop (Arthrex, Inc., Naples, Florida) is woven through the semitendinosus tendon graft (Fig. 19-3). The graft is sized in preparation for bone tunnel creation.

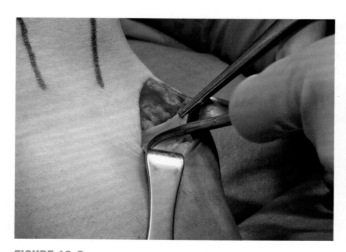

FIGURE 19-2

The sartorial fascia is incised and everted, exposing the gracilis and semitendinosus tendons.

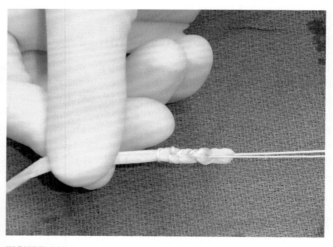

FIGURE 19-3

The semitendinosus tendon graft is prepared by removing the muscle and soft tissue debris from the graft. Next, a No. 2 Fiberloop (Arthrex, Inc., Naples, Florida) is woven through the semitendinosus tendon graft as depicted, starting at a point approximately 2 cm in from the end of the graft.

Patellar Tunnel

An incision is made along the medial border of the patella and along the MPFL remnant. The medial border of the patella is exposed at the level just proximal to the equator. A 2.5-mm drill bit is drilled through the medial cortex of the patella just proximal to the equator of the patella with extreme care taken to stay between the anterior cortex and articular surface (Fig. 19-4). A mini C-arm is used to confirm appropriate position. The drill bit is replaced with a 2.4-mm eyelet K-wire, which is drilled partially across the patella. The K-wire is overdrilled to a depth of 15 mm with a cannulated drill bit, 0.5 mm larger than the measured diameter of the graft. Diverging Keith needles (0.037 in. × 3.937 in.) are then drilled, exiting the skin on the lateral side of the patella (Fig. 19-5). One of the two suture strands from the graft is placed in the eyelet of each of the Keith needles, which are then pulled through their respective tunnels, thereby docking the graft in the blind patellar tunnel.

After confirmation that the graft is well docked in the blind tunnel, the sutures are captured through a small incision on the lateral edge of the patella, the soft tissue is cleared down to the lateral patella, and the sutures are tied securely over the bony patellar bridge. Fixation is confirmed by tugging on the graft.

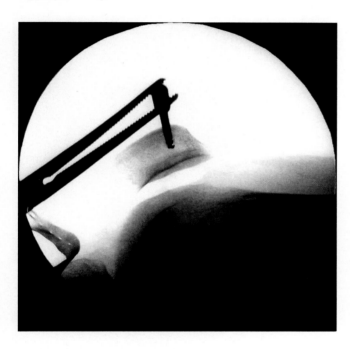

FIGURE 19-4

To prepare for placement of the medial patellofemoral ligament reconstruction graft, a 2.5-mm drill bit is drilled medial to lateral through patella, just proximal to the equator of the patella. Care is taken to maintain the drill bit between the anterior cortex of the patella and the articular surface. Position of the drill bit is confirmed using fluoroscopy. Depicted is a lateral view of the patella showing the position of the 2.5-mm drill bit.

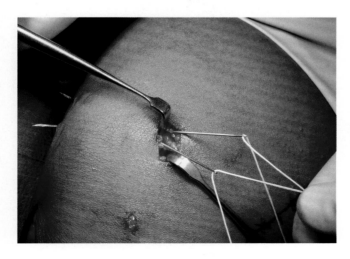

FIGURE 19-5

After the patella is prepared by overdrilling a K-wire to a depth of 15 mm with a cannulated drill bit 0.5 mm larger than the measured diameter of the graft, diverging Keith needles are drilled through the patella, exiting the skin on the lateral side of the patella. The suture tails from the prepared graft are passed through the eyelet of each of the Keith needles, which are then pulled through their respective tunnels to dock the graft into the blind patellar tunnel.

Femoral Tunnel

An incision is made centered over the saddle between the adductor tubercle and the medial epicondyle. Palpation and visualization are used to confirm tunnel position which should lie immediately adjacent to the medial epicondyle and distal to the adductor tubercle. A 2.5-mm drill bit is inserted at the MPFL attachment site. Position of the drill bit is confirmed using a mini C-arm, with minor position adjustments made as necessary (Fig. 19-6).

A soft tissue tunnel is created just deep to the medial retinaculum and MPFL remnant from the incision used for the femoral insertion to the medial incision at the patellar insertion of the graft, and the graft is passed through this tunnel (Fig. 19-7). The graft is wrapped around the drill bit and the knee is taken through full flexion and extension range of motion while tension is placed on the graft to determine tension manually. If the isometry of the graft remains appropriate throughout the full ROM of the knee, the femoral tunnel is in the appropriate position. Tension should decrease as

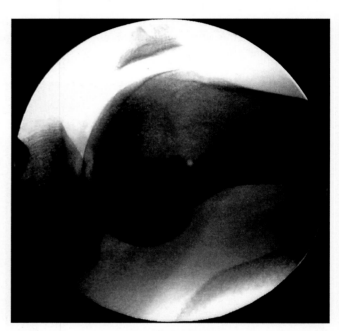

FIGURE 19-6

A fluoroscopic lateral view of the knee is obtained to confirm proper placement of the 2.5-mm drill bit at the MPFL attachment site. Seen in this image is a prior drill tract just proximal to the final position selected depicted by the radiographic shadow of the drill bit. The femoral tunnel was repositioned more distally because tension increased with flexion. After repositioning, the tension decreased as the knee was flexed to >60 degrees indicating an optimally positioned femoral tunnel.

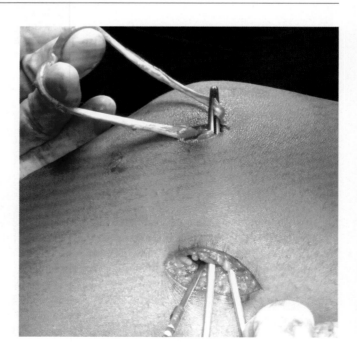

FIGURE 19-7

A soft tissue tunnel is created just deep to the medial retinaculum and medial patellofemoral ligament remnant between the incision used to create the femoral tunnel and the incision used to create the patellar insertion of the reconstruction graft. An instrument is used to pass the graft through this tunnel so that the knee can be cycled through range of motion while testing the tension of the graft manually.

the knee is flexed >60 degrees if the tunnel is optimally positioned. If tension increase with flexion, then the femoral tunnel is adjusted to a more distal position.

The graft is cut 20 mm longer than the distance between the tunnels (Fig. 19-8), and a No. 2 nonabsorbable suture (i.e., FiberWire [Arthrex, Inc., Naples, Florida]) is woven through the end of the graft. A No. 5 nonabsorbable pull-through suture is passed through a loop at the femoral end of the graft (Fig. 19-9). The drill bit is replaced with a 2.4-mm Beath needle, which is passed through the distal femur with a slightly anterior and proximal trajectory in order to protect the common peroneal nerve and popliteal artery and vein. The Beath needle is overdrilled with a 6.0-mm cannulated drill bit to a depth of 25 mm. The ends of the No. 5 pull-through suture are placed in the islet, and the Beath needle is pulled across the femur, docking the graft in the blind femoral tunnel (Fig. 19-10)

With tension placed manually on the pull-through suture, the knee is ranged again to determine the knee flexion angle with the greatest graft tension, attempting to recreate the normal lateral patellar translation equal to that of the contralateral patella. A 7.0-mm absorbable interference screw is placed in the femoral tunnel while holding the knee flexed at the angle that placed the greatest tension on the graft, typically between 70 and 90 degrees (Fig. 19-11). Once the screw is flush with the cortex, the knee is again extended and the lateral patellar translation is assessed. Care should be taken to avoid overtightening the graft. The patella should have lateral translation symmetric

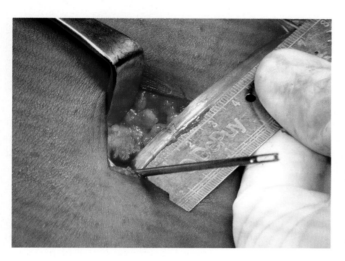

FIGURE 19-8

After the graft tension has been tested and is deemed appropriate, the graft is cut 20 mm longer than the distance between the patellar insertion and the femoral tunnel, indicated in this image by the position of the 2.4-mm Beath needle. The purple marking on the graft indicates the location at which the graft will be cut.

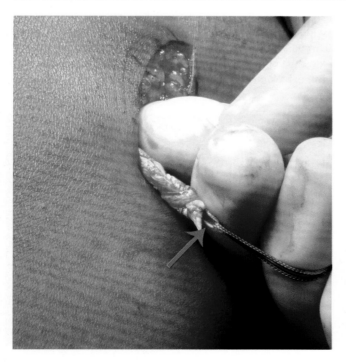

FIGURE 19-9

After the graft is cut at the appropriate length, a No. 2 nonabsorbable suture is woven through the end of the graft. A No. 5 nonabsorbable pull-through suture is passed through a loop at the femoral end of the graft (depicted by the *green arrow*). The No. 5 suture will be used to pass the graft into the femoral tunnel and hold tension while interference screw fixation of the femoral side of the medial patellofemoral ligament graft is obtained.

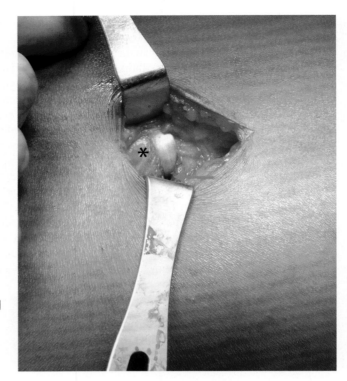

FIGURE 19-10

After the Beath needle is pulled across the femur, the medial patellofemoral ligament graft docks in the blind femoral tunnel demonstrated at the tip of the *green arrow*. The *asterisk* demonstrates the position of the medial femoral epicondyle.

to the normal contralateral knee or two to three quadrants of translation in patients with bilateral instability. The knee must flex fully without capture of the patella. If patellar translation is less than the normal contralateral side or the patella is felt to be overconstrained, the screw should be removed and the graft should be retensioned.

Closure

At the site of the graft harvest, the sartorial fascia and gracilis tendons are reattached to their insertion sites with 0 absorbable, braided sutures. The subcutaneous layer is closed with inverted 2-0 absorbable, braided sutures. The skin is closed with a running subcuticular 3-0 Prolene suture (Ethicon, Bridgewater, New Jersey) and covered with Steri-Strips (3M, St. Paul, Minnesota). The medial incision is closed in a similar fashion.

The portal sites are closed with 3-0 nylon sutures (Fig. 19-11). For pain control, a total of 10 mL of 0.25% bupivacaine is injected in and around the incisions. Sterile dressings are then applied, followed by a cryotherapy cooling unit, a loosely applied elastic bandage, a thromboembolic deterrent stocking, and a hinged brace locked in full extension. The tourniquet is then released.

FIGURE 19-11

Once the medial patellofemoral ligament reconstruction graft has been appropriately tensioned, a 7.0-mm absorbable interference screw is placed in the femoral tunnel while holding the knee flexed at the angle that places the greatest tension on the graft, typically between 70 and 90 degrees of knee flexion. Care should be taken not to overtighten the graft. The patella should have lateral translation symmetric to the normal contralateral knee or two to three quadrants of translation in patients with bilateral instability.

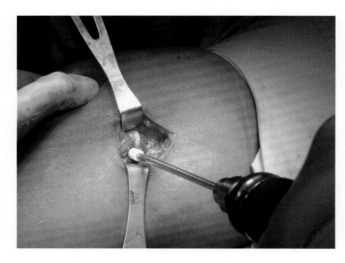

POSTOPERATIVE MANAGEMENT

- Postoperatively, the patients are kept in a brace for at least 4 weeks, with gradual progression of weight bearing and physical activities.
- Immediately after surgery, the patients are maintained in the brace, which is locked in full extension. Weight bearing is restricted to 5 lbs. The patients are instructed to do quadriceps sets and ankle pumps every hour and to ice and elevate as needed.
- Postoperative week 1: The portal sutures are removed, and the patients are advanced to 25% weight bearing in the brace (which is still locked in extension during ambulation). They begin flexion exercises with physical therapy, two to three times per week for 12 weeks.
- Postoperative week 2: The patients are reevaluated, and the incisional sutures are removed. The patients are progressed to full weight bearing in the brace and begin doing straight-leg raises with 1-lb weights. Activities are then increased as follows:
- Postoperative week 3: Patients are started on the stationary bike to increase ROM, and extension exercises are reemphasized.
- Postoperative week 4 to 6: Patients are encouraged to do 100 repetitions of straight-leg raises daily and are expected to have obtained 120 degrees of knee flexion. The brace is discontinued when patients exhibit adequate quadriceps control. ROM should be near normal. Recommendations at this point include single-leg stance, step-up exercises of several inches, and water exercises.
- Postoperative week 8: Treadmill walks, elliptical exercises, and isotonic exercises, including leg presses, toe presses, and leg curls, are allowed.
- Postoperative week 12: Patients are evaluated in the office and begun on a progressive treadmill jogging program, which is then transitioned to outdoor running.
- Postoperative week 16: Patients advance to cutting and sport-specific drills and may begin returning to regular sports if progress is satisfactory at this time.

COMPLICATIONS

Appropriate positioning and tensioning of the graft is critical to the success of this procedure. Overtightening or malpositioning of the graft can result in iatrogenic medial instability, medial facet arthropathy, and stiffness (4–9). Elias and Cosgarea (7) showed that malpositioning of the femoral tunnel proximally by 5 mm can cause significantly increased pressures on the medial patellar cartilage. Additionally, overtightening of the graft by as little as 3 mm can increase graft and patellofemoral joint reactive forces. The authors theorized that either scenario could lead to degeneration of the medial patellofemoral cartilage. As a result of overtightening, subsequent graft failure and recurrence of instability may also occur. Adequate tensioning of the graft is necessary to avoid continued instability. Similarly, Stephen et al. (10) described that overtightening an MPFL reconstruction graft or a femoral tunnel malpositioned proximally to the anatomic origin of the MPFL results in increases in mean medial joint contact pressure, medial patellar tilt, and medial patellar translation through range of motion.

Other potential complications after MPFL reconstruction are patellar fractures through the tunnel sites (9,11), recurrent lateral instability (12), hemarthrosis (13), minor wound complications (13), graft loosening after trauma (14), implant pain (12,14,15), arthrofibrosis (16), anterior knee pain, and injury to the saphenous vein or nerve.

RESULTS

Overall, MPFL reconstructions appear to provide long-term functional improvement with low rates of redislocation, improvement in Kujala scores, and decreases in apprehension and patellofemoral pain (14–20). A meta-analysis by Smith et al. (21) studying outcomes of MPFL reconstruction showed that there were "substantial methodologic limitations" in the current literature, including small samples sizes and limited follow-up times. The techniques for MPFL reconstructions are varied and evolving, and there are few studies that report similar techniques to allow for valid comparison. More recently, a systematic review by Mackay et al. (19) confirmed that while there is a paucity of high quality outcome-based research regarding MPFL reconstruction, the use of this technique improves validated subjective patient outcomes, has a low rate of redislocation, and low rate of complication. Despite the diversity of procedures, however, the results are generally favorable. Panagopoulos et al. (22) reviewed several techniques using hamstring autografts, which showed symptomatic improvement and low recurrence in 85% to 93% of the cases. Using a technique similar to that described in this chapter, Ahmad et al. (23) showed good postoperative stability after MPFL reconstruction in 20 consecutive patients, with statistical improvements in International Knee Documentation Committee (IKDC), Tegner, Kujala, and Lysholm questionnaire scores. There were no recurrent episodes of dislocation in any patients. Additionally, Christiansen et al. (15) showed good postoperative stability after MPFL reconstruction in 44 patients; they reported only one case of recurrent instability. Standardizing the technique and implementing an adequate sample size and follow-up will be necessary for future outcome studies.

PEARLS AND PITFALLS

- MPFL reconstruction is indicated for recurrent patellar instability and never for isolated patellofemoral pain.
- Patients with recurrent instability and substantial bony malalignment may be better treated with a distal realignment procedure.
- Concomitant injuries should be identified and addressed appropriately.
- When drilling the patellar tunnels, extreme care should be taken to avoid violating the articular surface.
- Placing the femoral attachment too proximally will cause the graft to be overly tight in flexion. The femoral attachment should not be proximal to the native origin of the MPFL, because it can cause excessive graft tension, with subsequent medial facet overload and arthrosis (4–7).
- In contrast, placing the femoral attachment too distally may cause the graft to be tight in extension, but it is less likely to cause patellofemoral degeneration. It is thus safer to err more distally if necessary (8).
- The graft should be tensioned so as to match the patellar excursion of the normal contralateral knee—usually two quadrants of lateral translation.

ALTERNATIVE PROCEDURES

There are numerous techniques described in the reconstruction of the MPFL. What we have described is one way to approach this procedure with a semitendinosus autograft, femoral interference fixation, and a patellar tunnel with modified docking technique (24). For the femoral attachment of the graft, we prefer fixation with an interference screw, although this procedure has been described using sutures (18), washers (25), and blind- and through-tunnel grafts. A variety of graft types have also been used in addition to the semitendinosus tendon, including the adductor muscle (14), gracilis tendon (15,26), quadriceps tendon (27), synthetic graft (28), and allograft. For patellar fixation, we use a modification of the docking technique, first described by Brown and Ahmad (24). Others recommend the use of single versus double patellar tunnels or the Endobutton (Smith and Nephew, Memphis, TN) (25). Multiple different methods have shown excellent results in reducing lateral patellar instability.

CONCLUSION

Patellofemoral instability is multifactorial and complex, and numerous procedures have been purported to address this issue. Although MPFL reconstruction is a relatively new procedure, the limited results thus far have been favorable when it is used for the appropriate indications. The key to MPFL reconstruction is understanding that its purpose is a stabilization procedure for medial soft tissue insufficiency, not a solution to arthropathy or marked malalignment. Understanding the indications and limitations of the procedure, as well as the importance of graft positioning and tensioning, will help the surgeon attain successful results in the treatment of patellofemoral instability.

REFERENCES

1. Sallay PI, Poggi J, Speer KP, et al. Acute dislocation of the patella. A correlative pathoanatomic study. *Am J Sports Med.* 1996;24:52–60.
2. Deie M, Ochi M, Sumen Y, et al. Reconstruction of the medial patellofemoral ligament for the treatment of habitual or recurrent dislocation of the patella in children. *J Bone Joint Surg Br.* 2003;85:887–890.
3. Nomura E, Horiuchi Y, Inoue M. Correlation of MR imaging findings and open exploration of medial patellofemoral ligament injuries in acute patellar dislocations. *Knee.* 2002;9:139–143.

4. Andrish JT. Surgical reconstruction of the medial patellofemoral ligament. *Tech Knee Surg.* 2006;5:121–127.
5. Bicos J, Carofino B, Andersen M, et al. Patellofemoral forces after medial patellofemoral ligament reconstruction. A biomechanical analysis. *J Knee Surg.* 2006;19:317–326.
6. Bollier M, Fulkerson J, Cosgarea A, et al. Technical failure of medial patellofemoral ligament reconstruction. *Arthroscopy.* 2011;27:1153–1159.
7. Elias JJ, Cosgarea AJ. Technical errors during medial patellofemoral ligament reconstruction could overload medial patellofemoral cartilage. A computational analysis. *Am J Sports Med.* 2006;34:1478–1485.
8. Thaunat M, Erasmus PJ. Management of overtight medial patellofemoral ligament reconstruction. *Knee Surg Sports Traumatol Arthrosc.* 2009;17:480–483.
9. Thaunat M, Erasmus PJ. Recurrent patellar dislocation after medial patellofemoral ligament reconstruction. *Knee Surg Sports Traumatol Arthrosc.* 2008;16:40–43.
10. Stephen JM, Kittl C, Williams A, et al. Effect of medial patellofemoral ligament reconstruction method on patellofemoral contact pressures and kinematics. *Am J Sports Med.* 2016;44:1186–1194.
11. Schiphouwer L, Rood A, Tigchelaar S, et al. Complications of medial patellofemoral ligament reconstruction using two transverse patellar tunnels. *Knee Surg Sports Traumatol Arthrosc.* 2017;25:245–250.
12. Hohn E, Pandya NK. Does the utilization of allograft tissue in medial patellofemoral ligament reconstruction in pediatric and adolescent patients restore patellar stability? *Clin Orthop Relat Res.* 2016;475(6):1563–1569. doi: 10.1007/s11999-016-5060-4.
13. Nomura E, Horiuchi Y, Kihara M. Medial patellofemoral ligament restraint in lateral patellar translation and reconstruction. *Knee.* 2000;7:121–127.
14. Steiner TM, Torga-Spak R, Teitge RA. Medial patellofemoral ligament reconstruction in patients with lateral patellar instability and trochlear dysplasia. *Am J Sports Med.* 2006;34:1254–1261.
15. Christiansen SE, Jacobsen BW, Lund B, et al. Reconstruction of the medial patellofemoral ligament with gracilis tendon autograft in transverse patellar drill holes. *Arthroscopy.* 2008;24:82–87.
16. Drez D Jr, Edwards TB, Williams CS. Results of medial patellofemoral ligament reconstruction in the treatment of patellar dislocation. *Arthroscopy.* 2001;17:298–306.
17. Deie M, Ochi M, Sumen Y, et al. A long-term follow-up study after medial patellofemoral ligament reconstruction using the transferred semitendinosus tendon for patellar dislocation. *Knee Surg Sports Traumatol Arthrosc.* 2005;13:522–528.
18. Ellera Gomes JL, Stigler Marczyk LR, Cesar de Cesar P, et al. Medial patellofemoral ligament reconstruction with semitendinosus autograft for chronic patellar instability: a follow-up study. *Arthroscopy.* 2004;20:147–151.
19. Mackay ND, Smith NA, Parsons N, et al. Medial patellofemoral ligament reconstruction for patellar dislocation: a systematic review. *Orthop J Sports Med.* 2014;2:2325967114544021.
20. Matsushita T, Oka S, Araki D, et al. Patient-based outcomes after medial patellofemoral ligament reconstruction. *Int Orthop.* 2017;41(6):1147–1153. doi: 10.1007/s00264-017-3433-2.
21. Smith TO, Walker J, Russell N. Outcomes of medial patellofemoral ligament reconstruction for patellar instability: a systematic review. *Knee Surg Sports Traumatol Arthrosc.* 2007;15:1301–1314.
22. Panagopoulos A, van Niekerk L, Triantafillopoulos IK. MPFL reconstruction for recurrent patella dislocation: a new surgical technique and review of the literature. *Int J Sports Med.* 2008;29:359–365.
23. Ahmad CS, Brown GD, Stein BS. The docking technique for medial patellofemoral ligament reconstruction: surgical technique and clinical outcome. *Am J Sports Med.* 2009;37:2021–2027.
24. Brown GD, Ahmad CS. The docking technique for medial patellofemoral ligament reconstruction. *Oper Tech Orthop.* 2007;17:216–222.
25. Schock EJ, Burks RT. Medial patellofemoral ligament reconstruction using a hamstring graft. *Oper Tech Sports Med.* 2001;9:169–175.
26. Schottle P, Schmeling A, Romero J, et al. Anatomical reconstruction of the medial patellofemoral ligament using a free gracilis autograft. *Arch Orthop Trauma Surg.* 2009;129:305–309.
27. Steensen RN, Dopirak RM, Maurus PB. A simple technique for reconstruction of the medial patellofemoral ligament using a quadriceps tendon graft. *Arthroscopy.* 2005;21:365–370.
28. Nomura E, Horiuchi Y, Kihara M. A mid-term follow-up of medial patellofemoral ligament reconstruction using an artificial ligament for recurrent patellar dislocation. *Knee.* 2000;7:211–215.

20 Tibial Tubercle Transfer

Robin Vereeke West

INTRODUCTION

This chapter addresses the surgical technique of a tibial tubercle transfer for the treatment of patellar instability and isolated patellofemoral arthritis.

Causes of patellofemoral joint instability and isolated patellofemoral arthritis are multifactorial and can be related to problems with limb alignment, the osseous architecture of the patella and trochlea, and the integrity of the surrounding soft tissues. The incidence of patellar dislocation is 5.8 per 100,000, and this increases to 29 per 100,000 in the 10- to 17-year-old age group. The recurrence rate averages 15% to 44% after nonoperative treatment of an acute injury. If there is a subsequent dislocation after the primary injury, the recurrence rate increases to 50%. Many patients continue to have mechanical symptoms and pain after a patellar dislocation. Atkin et al. reported that up to 55% of patients fail to return to sports activity after a primary patellar dislocation. He also showed that 58% of people have limitations with strenuous activity at 6 months after a primary dislocation.

The operative treatment of patellofemoral arthritis is variable depending on the degree and the location of the chondral damage, the age of the patient, and associated chondral injury to the tibiofemoral joint. Arthroscopic debridement can be used for isolated, superficial chondral flaps in the patellofemoral joint. Anteromedialization of the tibial tubercle can be used for the treatment of isolated lateral patellar facet arthritis. Patellofemoral replacement is used in patients with normal limb alignment and osseous anatomy who have diffuse patellofemoral arthritis. Total knee replacement offers the best clinical results in older patients or patients with associated tibiofemoral arthritis.

SIGNS AND SYMPTOMS

Patients with patellofemoral arthritis and recurrent patellar instability have similar symptoms. They may present with a sense of instability, pain, mechanical symptoms, and/or recurrent effusions. Most patients have tried a course of physical therapy to work on flexibility, proprioception, and strengthening around the knee and the hip. Bracing occasionally relieves some of the pain and instability. Hyaluronic acid injections can help relieve some of the swelling, pain, and mechanical symptoms.

PHYSICAL EXAM

A thorough examination of the entire lower limb should be performed and should be compared to the contralateral side. The following findings should be documented: limb rotation (femoral anteversion, external tibial torsion), muscle atrophy, core strength, crepitation, effusion, local or diffuse tenderness, patellar glide, patellar tracking throughout range of motion, patellar tilt, tuberosity position in relation to the center of the trochlea, apprehension (medial and lateral), and the Fulkerson medial instability test.

IMAGING

Radiographs (Both Knees)

Standard radiographs include 45-degree flexion weight-bearing posteroanterior and lateral view and Merchant view. The flexion weight-bearing radiographs show the degree of tibiofemoral joint space narrowing. The Merchant view is used to assess patellar tilt, subluxation, and trochlear dysplasia. The lateral view is used to evaluate the patellar height and trochlear dysplasia.

Magnetic Resonance Imaging

Magnetic resonance imaging (MRI) is useful in evaluating injury to the medial patellofemoral ligament (MPFL) and the articular cartilage, bone bruise patterns, and other associated ligamentous or meniscal injuries. When MRI findings were correlated with surgical findings, MRI was found to be 85% sensitive and 70% accurate in detecting disruption of the MPFL.

Computed Tomography

Cross-section imaging with computed tomography (CT) slices at different positions along the lower limb can provide a three-dimensional view of the patellofemoral joint. These CT cuts can be used to assess the lateral offset of the tibial tuberosity from the deepest point in the trochlear groove (TT-TG distance). A distance of >20 mm is nearly always associated with patellar instability and can be addressed with a tibial tubercle realignment.

INDICATIONS

Tibial tubercle transfer can be done for patellofemoral arthritis or instability. Indications for medialization of the tubercle include symptoms of patellofemoral instability along with an increased TT-TG distance (>20 mm). Indications for anteromedialization of the tibial tubercle include symptoms of patellofemoral instability and pain along with an increased TT-TG distance and/or distal/lateral patellar facet chondrosis or lateral trochlear chondrosis.

CONTRAINDICATIONS

Contraindications of tibial tubercle transfer include medial and/or proximal patellofemoral chondrosis that would be subjected to increased loading with a transfer of the tubercle. Standard contraindications to any osteotomy around the knee include osteoporosis, nicotine use, nonspecific pain, complex regional pain syndrome, inflammatory arthropathy, infection, patella baja, or arthrofibrosis.

ANESTHESIA

The type of anesthesia used for the case is decided by the surgeon, patient, and anesthesiologist. Options include general anesthesia, sedation along with local anesthesia, regional nerve blocks, or spinal anesthesia. The main concerns with regional nerve blocks are decreased motor function and slowed rehabilitation due to weakness. A narcotic prescription is sent home with all patients, and prophylactic antibiotics are given before the skin incision but not postoperatively.

POSITIONING

The patient is placed supine on the operating room table. All bony prominences are well padded. An eggcrate cushion is placed under the nonoperative leg. A tourniquet is applied and is insufflated to 250 mm Hg during the osteotomy portion of the case only.

SURGICAL LANDMARKS, INCISIONS, PORTAL PLACEMENT

Landmarks

- Patella
- Patellar tendon attachment on the tibial tubercle
- Gerdy tubercle
- Tibial crest

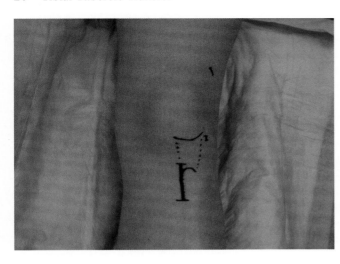

FIGURE 20-1

The landmarks of the inferior pole of the patella, the patellar tendon, the superolateral portal site, the inferolateral portal site, and the osteotomy site are marked on the skin.

Portals and Incisions

- The landmarks and arthroscopic portal sites and skin incisions are marked on the skin (Fig. 20-1).
- The best viewing portal for the patellofemoral joint is the superolateral portal. A 70-degree arthroscope is used to assess the articular cartilage in the patellofemoral joint and is used to evaluate patellofemoral tracking/glide/tilt.
- A 5- to 7-cm skin incision is made medial to the tibial tubercle, starting 1 cm proximal to the patellar tendon attachment and extending distally.

EXAMINATION UNDER ANESTHESIA

Under anesthesia, both knees are examined and compared. The range of motion, presence of effusion, generalized ligamentous exam, and patellar tracking/tilt/crepitation/glide are all documented. The patellar exam should be checked in full extension and then again at 20- to 30-degree knee flexion (when the patella is engaged in the trochlea).

DIAGNOSTIC ARTHROSCOPY

The diagnostic arthroscopy typically involves two portals. The standard anterolateral portal with the 30-degree arthroscope is used for the full diagnostic examination of the knee. The superolateral portal with the 70-degree arthroscope is used for evaluation of the patellofemoral joint (Fig. 20-2). This portal gives excellent visualization of the articular cartilage throughout the patellofemoral (PF) joint. Patellar tracking and glide can be examined from this portal.

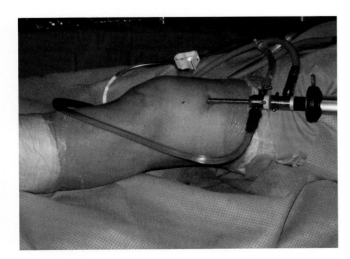

FIGURE 20-2

The superolateral portal site is used with a 70-degree arthroscope to assess the patellofemoral articular cartilage and patellar tracking.

PROCEDURE

Initially, the diagnostic arthroscopy is performed to assess the articular cartilage status and confirm that there is no contraindication to the realignment of the tubercle. An open lateral release is performed through a small 2- to 3-cm incision only if the retinaculum is exceptionally taut (negative patellar tilt). The release confirms that the retinaculum will not tether the patella after the tibial tubercle transfer. The release is not too extensive and only extends from the inferior pole to the superior pole, taking care not to injure the insertion of the vastus lateralis obliquus. A tourniquet set at 250 mm Hg is only used for the osteotomy portion of the case and released prior to wound closure.

The incision is made just medial to the tibial tubercle and is 5 to 7 cm in length, extending from just proximal to the patellar tendon insertion distally. The fascia is exposed and then elevated off of the tibia to expose the anterolateral tibial crest and Gerdy tubercle. The edges of the patellar tendon are identified. The osteotomy site is marked with a Bovie on the anteromedial tibial crest, starting at the medial edge of the patellar tendon insertion and extending distally about 5 cm.

The osteotomy is performed "free hand." With the tibial tubercle pointing directly at the ceiling (the foot is usually internally rotated), a Steinmann pin is placed from the medial tibial crest at the proximal portion of the osteotomy. The slope of the pin placement accounts for the slope of the osteotomy (Fig. 20-3). The slope is adjusted according to the amount of patellofemoral chondrosis. Once the slope of the osteotomy is determined, a microsagittal saw is used to perform the osteotomy (Fig. 20-4).

The osteotomy is completed with a ¼ in curved curette proximally at the patellar tendon insertion in a transverse fashion (Fig. 20-5). The osteotomy is hinged distally and is only completed if patella alta is identified on the preoperative radiographs, using the modified Insall-Salvati and Caton-Deschamps ratios. By completing the osteotomy, the patella can be easily distalized to correct patellar height.

The tibial tubercle is then shifted medially or anteromedially approximately 1 cm. Care is taken to make sure the tubercle has at least 50% contact with the underlying tibia to ensure good healing potential and minimize risk of nonunion. The tuberosity is temporarily fixed with Kirschner wires and

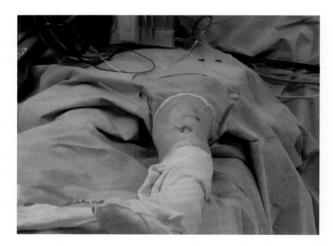

FIGURE 20-3

The Steinmann pin is placed from medial to lateral at the proximal portion of the tibial tubercle to mark the angle of the osteotomy slope. The slope is varied depending on the amount of medialization and anteriorization that is desired. This slope is determined by the amount of patellofemoral arthritis that is present.

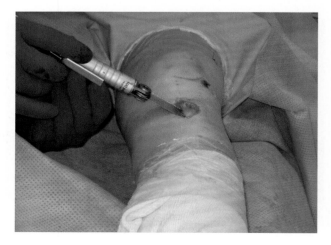

FIGURE 20-4

The osteotomy is performed with a microsagittal saw.

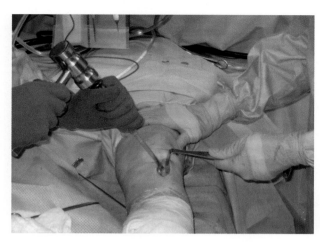

FIGURE 20-5
The osteotomy is completed proximally with a ¼ in curved osteotome. This cut is made transversally just proximal to the patellar tendon insertion.

then permanently fixed with two 4.5-mm fully threaded screws, using the AO compression technique. A mini C-arm is used to confirm good position and length of the two screws before wound closure.

The fascial layer is closed in an interrupted fashion, followed by a subcutaneous closure, then a subcuticular closure. Care is taken to provide hemostasis after releasing the tourniquet and prior to wound closure. A drain is not routinely used.

POSTOPERATIVE REHABILITATION AND RETURN TO PLAY

The patient is allowed immediate full weight bearing with crutches and a brace locked in full extension. The brace is unlocked at 6 weeks or when the osteotomy is radiographically healed and is discontinued when the patient has excellent quadriceps control. A CPM is started within a few days after surgery, and heel slides are allowed to 90 degrees of knee flexion until the osteotomy is healed. Physical therapy is started immediately to help regain quadriceps control and patellar mobility, control swelling, and begin a comprehensive core stabilization program.

Once the osteotomy is healed, activity is progressed from range of motion to strengthening, jogging, functional training, and then return to sports without restrictions by 5-6 months (Figs. 20-6 and 20-7).

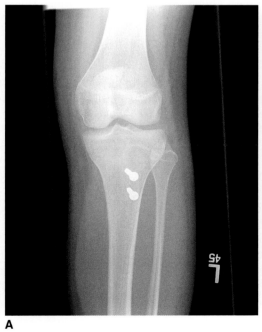
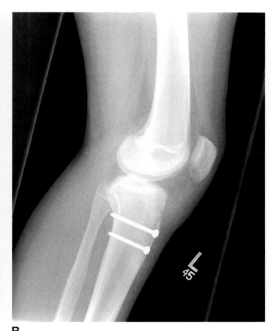

A   **B**

FIGURE 20-6

A,B: Preoperative and postoperative radiographs after a tibial tubercle realignment for patellar instability and a lateral patellar facet defect in a 15-year-old female.

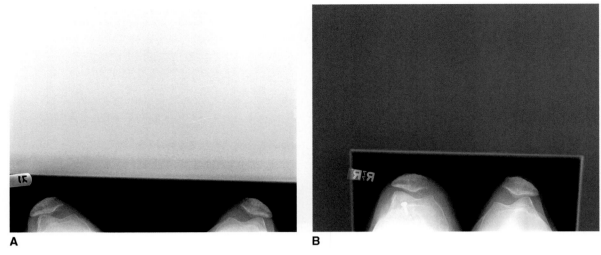

A   **B**

FIGURE 20-7

A,B: Preoperative and postoperative radiographs after a tibial tubercle realignment for severe bilateral patellofemoral arthritis in a 36-year-old woman.

COMPLICATIONS

Complications are similar to all bony procedures around the knee: infection, malunion, nonunion, compartment syndrome, arthrofibrosis, patella baja, worsening, or no improvement in symptoms. In Arthroscopy 2015, Payne et al. published a systematic review of 19 studies that included 787 tibial tubercle osteotomies. There was a 4.7% overall complication rate, with a 10.7% complication rate when there was complete detachment of the tubercle. Hardware removal was necessary in 36.7% of patients. In a retrospective review, Luhmann et al. performed a retrospective review of 101 tibial tubercle osteotomies. Of the patients included in the study, one third had a blunt cut, one third had a sloped or tapered cut, and one third had a greenstick cut with the periosteum left attached. In the blunt cut group, 11.8% of patients developed a tibial fracture. In the sloped group, 6.2% developed a nonunion that went onto a fracture. In the greenstick group, there was a 0% complication rate. This study showed that the fracture risk is much higher with a blunt cut and much lower with a shingle or greenstick technique.

PEARLS AND PITFALLS

- The lateral release is done in conjunction with tibial tubercle transfer to help "balance" the soft tissues. Overzealous lateral release can lead to poor quadriceps function, medial patellar instability, and increased lateral laxity. Be sure to preserve the vastus lateralis oblique (VLO) insertion.
- Avoid medializing the tubercle too much, which can lead to medial facet overload and posteriorization of the tubercle.
- Encourage smoking cessation.
- Hinge the shingle if distalization is not necessary to correct patella alta.
- Taper the shingle.
- Complete the osteotomy proximally with a ¼ in curved curette to avoid fracture extension into the lateral plateau.
- "Countersink" the screws to avoid prominent, painful hardware.
- Avoid early surgery on a swollen knee to decrease the risk of arthrofibrosis.
- Minimize tourniquet and nerve block use to decrease the quadriceps dysfunction postoperatively.
- Full weight bearing is allowed postoperatively only with the brace locked in full extension to avoid too much force across the osteotomy site.

SUGGESTED READINGS

Atkin DM, Fithian DC, Marangi KS, et al. Characteristics of patients with primary patellar acute lateral patellar dislocation and their recovery within the first 6 months of injury. *Am J Sports Med.* 2000;28:472–479.

Buuk DA, Fulkerson JP. Anteromedialization of the tibial tubercle: a 4 to 12 year follow-up. *Oper Tech Sports Med.* 2000;8:131–137.

Carofino BC, Fulkerson JP. Anteromedialization of the tibial tubercle for patellofemoral arthritis in patients >50 years. *J Knee Surg.* 2008;21:89–90.

Cofield RH, Bryan RS. Acute dislocation of the patella: results of conservative treatment. *J Trauma.* 1977;17:526–531.

Colvin AC, West RV. Current concepts review: patellar instability. *J Bone Joint Surg.* 2008;90A:2751–2762.

Cosgarea AJ, Schatzke MD, Seth AK, et al. Biomechanical analysis of flat and oblique tibial tubercle osteotomy for recurrent patellar instability. *Am J Sports Med.* 1999;27:507–512.

Dejour H, Walch G, Nove-Josserand L, et al. Factors of patellar instability: an anatomic radiographic study. *Knee Surg Sports Traumatol Arthrosc.* 1994;2:19–26.

Fithian DC, Paxton EW, Stone ML, et al. Epidemiology and natural history of acute patellar dislocation. *Am J Sports Med.* 2004;32:1114–1121.

Fulkerson JP, Becker GJ, Meaney JA, et al. Anteromedial tibial tubercle transfer without bone graft. *Am J Sports Med.* 1990;18:490–497.

Hawkins RJ, Bell RH, Anisette G. Acute patellar dislocations. The natural history. *Am J Sports Med.* 1986;14:117–120.

Kuroda R, Kambic H, Valdevit A, et al. Articular cartilage contact pressure after tibial tuberosity transfer. A cadaveric study. *Am J Sports Med.* 2001;29:403–409.

Luhmann SJ, et al. Tibial fractures after tibial tubercle osteotomies for patellar instability: a comparison of three osteotomy configurations. *J Child Orthop.* 2011;5(1):19–26.

Payne J, Rimmke N, Schmitt LC, et al. The incidence of complication of tibial tubercle osteotomy: a systematic review. *Arthroscopy.* 2015;31(9):1819–1825.

Pidoriano AJ, Weinstein RN, Buuck DA, et al. Correlation of patellar articular lesions with results from anteromedial tibial tubercle transfer. *Am J Sports Med.* 1997;25:533–537.

21 Patella Tendon and Quadriceps Tendon Ruptures

Stephen J. Rabuck and Conor I. Murphy

Ruptures of the extensor mechanism result in significant functional limitations. These injuries typically present after an acute injury. This commonly occurs with an eccentric contraction of the extensor mechanism as the knee is forced into flexion (1). These patients typically feel a pop accompanied by pain and an inability to perform straight leg raise. The proximal migration of the patella with patella tendon ruptures may be more apparent than the deformity present with quadriceps tendon ruptures.

Patella tendon ruptures are most common in patients < 40 years old, while the incidence of quadriceps tendon ruptures peaks in the sixth decade (2). In a healthy patient, rupture of these tendons requires major trauma (3). Systemic disease such as chronic renal insufficiency, diabetes mellitus, and rheumatoid arthritis can result in rupture with minor trauma or bilateral tendon ruptures. Local risk factors for rupture include corticosteroid injection and history of patella tendon graft harvest (4,5).

PREOPERATIVE PLANNING

A thorough history and physical exam are key components to the assessment of these injuries. Clinical findings include a palpable defect with swelling at the location of injury. Inability to perform straight leg raise and weakness with knee extension are common. Patients may also have limited knee flexion due to pain with distraction of the ruptured tendon. Patients may retain the ability to perform quadriceps contraction in cases with intact retinaculum, and the clinical and radiographic findings may not be appreciated resulting in a delay in diagnosis.

Radiographic examination includes AP and lateral views of the knee. Contralateral knee imaging may be necessary to appreciate subtle findings. The only radiographic finding may be a change in patella height. Several methods have been described to assess patella height including Caton-Deschamps ratio, Blumensaat line, the Insall-Salvati ratio, and Blackburne-Peel ratio.

Additional imaging modalities include ultrasound and MRI. Ultrasound is relatively inexpensive and can provide information of tear extent and location; however, MRI is commonly used to further characterize the injury and to visualize any associated pathology. These modalities can be beneficial in cases of atypical presentation. MRI is the most sensitive imaging modality and can be beneficial to characterize atypical cases including partial tears. Location of rupture can be characterized as myotendinous, intrasubstance, or tendinous avulsions. The distal quadriceps tendon contains a region of hypovascularity 1 to 2 cm from the proximal pole or the patella and is the most common location of quadriceps tendon rupture. Avulsion of the patella from the inferior pole of the patella is most common as strain is significantly elevated compared to the midsubstance of the patella.

INDICATIONS/CONTRAINDICATIONS

Surgical repair is the treatment of choice for complete rupture of the patella or quadriceps tendon. Timing of repair is an important factor in the management of these injuries as acute repair results in the best outcomes (6,7).

Contraindications to surgical repair include active infection, nonambulatory patients, or medical comorbidities that would preclude surgical intervention.

TECHNIQUE

The patient is positioned supine on the operative table. A tourniquet is placed on the proximal thigh. Regional anesthesia can be beneficial for pain control postoperatively as well as protecting the repair in the immediate postoperative period.

Quadriceps Tendon Repair

A longitudinal incision is centered over the patella extending to the retracted tendon and distal to the inferior pole of the patella. In acute cases, the hemarthrosis is entered after dissection through the subcutaneous tissue. Medial and lateral skin flaps are elevated to identify involvement of medial and lateral retinaculum (Fig. 21-1). All adhesions of the retracted tendon and soft tissue are released to mobilize the quadriceps tendon for a tension-free repair. A 1- to 2-cm stump of tendon is commonly present and the proximal pole of patella needs to be exposed. The proximal pole should be decorticated or create a trough to reapproximate the tendon edge to healing surfaces. All necrotic tissue must be removed from the distal tendon edge.

Orientation of the tendon fibers and the planned patella drill holes prior to suture passage (Fig. 21-2). Two No. 5 nonabsorbable sutures are passed as planned. Sutures are passed with a locking Krackow stitch.

A roll is placed under the knee to produce slight flexion of approximately 20 degrees. A 2-mm drill bit is utilized to pass three transosseous tunnels. The drill bit is left in place and a longitudinal incision through the overlying patella tendon is made with a No. 15 blade. A Hewson suture passer is advanced through the drill hole and identified through the split patella tendon. A passing suture is retrieved with the loop exiting the proximal pole of the patella. These steps are repeated for two more transosseous tunnels.

The roll is then moved distally to move the leg into extension. The tendon is reduced by pulling proximally with one set of sutures, while the other sutures are tied with a surgeon's knot followed by four half hitches (Fig. 21-3). The second set of sutures are tied in a similar fashion. The knee is slowly flexed with careful attention to the angle producing tension across the repair (Fig. 21-4). Medial and lateral retinaculum repairs are performed with No. 1 Vicryl. The patient is placed in a postop brace locked in extension or cylinder cast.

Suture anchor repair has been described as well. After exposure and preparation is completed, two 5.5-mm suture anchors are placed in the proximal pole of the patella. Careful attention to the articular and anterior surface is important in placing these anchors appropriately. One limb of each suture is passed proximally and then distally through the tendon stump. The remaining limb is utilized to remove tension and slide through the anchor, thus reducing the tendon back to the superior pole of the patella. This sliding limb can be passed once through the tendon in a nonlocking fashion to improve contact between tendon and bone. Sutures are then tied to complete repair.

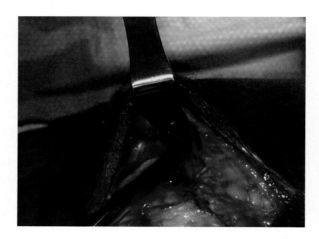

FIGURE 21-1

Retinaculum defect following extensor tendon rupture.

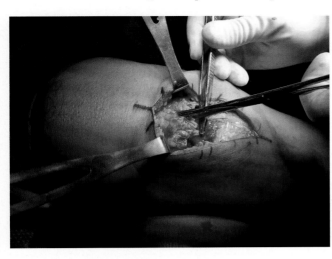

FIGURE 21-2

Planning suture and bone tunnel placement.

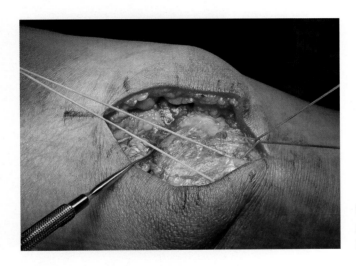

FIGURE 21-3

Sutures are tied while maintaining reduction.

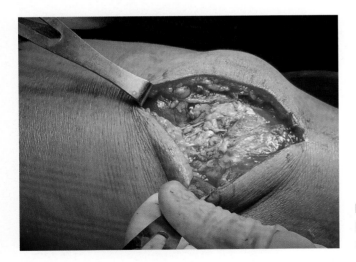

FIGURE 21-4

Final repair of quadriceps tendon rupture.

Patella Tendon Repair

A longitudinal midline incision is centered over the tendon rupture. In cases of proximal rupture, the incision is extended proximal to the superior pole patella. Exposure and evaluation of the retinaculum are performed as discussed with quadriceps tendon ruptures.

Proximal avulsions require careful attention to the orientation and alignment of the tendon stump to the inferior pole of the patella. Careful consideration is critical to perform an anatomic repair to restore patella alignment and patella height. This should be completed prior to suture passage so as not to distort the native anatomy. Two No. 2 nonabsorbable sutures are passed with a Krackow stitch (Fig. 21-5). A roll may be placed under the knee to allow slight knee flexion. Three transosseous tunnels are planned with a 1-cm bridge using a 2-mm drill bit (Fig. 21-6). The drill bit is left in place and a longitudinal incision is made with a No. 15 blade through the quadriceps tendon. A Hewson suture passer is advanced through the drill hole, and a passing suture is retrieved with the loop exiting the inferior pole of the patella. These steps are repeated for two more transosseous tunnels.

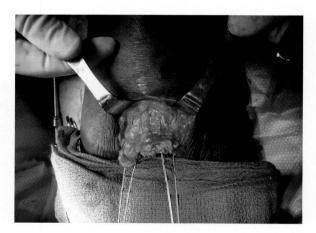

FIGURE 21-5

Sutures are passed with a Krackow stitch.

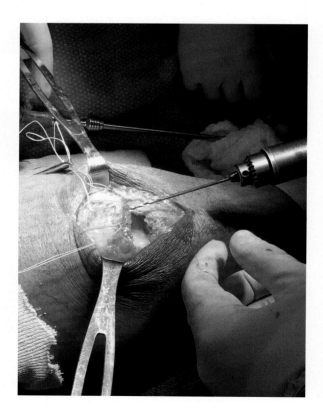

FIGURE 21-6

Parallel bone tunnels created with 2-mm drill bit.

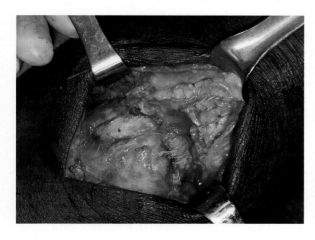

FIGURE 21-7

Final repair of inferior pole avulsion of the patella tendon.

One limb of each suture must be retrieved through the central tunnel, while the other sutures are retrieved through the medial and lateral bone tunnels, respectively. The tendon can be reduced by moving the knee into extension and pulling one set of sutures distally while tying the other set using a surgeon's knot followed by four half hitches (Fig. 21-7).

Ruptures from the tibial tubercle can be repaired with transosseous tunnels over a bone bridge. Careful attention to patella height is important in performing these repairs. Iatrogenic patella baja can result in poor outcomes by increasing contact pressures or resulting in a mechanical disadvantage. Alternatively, suture anchor repair can be completed with two 5.5-mm anchors at the proximal aspect of the insertion. Sutures are passed through the distal tendon and secured. This repair can be reinforced by bringing the tied sutures distally into a knotless suture anchor to restore the native footprint.

Intrasubstance repairs are performed in an end-to-end fashion. Similarly, the configuration of the tear must be evaluated and suture placement planned to prevent any significant change in patella height. Two No. 2 nonabsorbable sutures are passed in a locking fashion for each tendon stump, resulting in a total of four sutures utilized in this repair. The knee is kept in extension while sutures are tied.

Chronic Ruptures

Chronic quadriceps tendon ruptures can generally be mobilized adequately for a primary repair. In cases where lengthening is required, a V-Y advancement or turndown may be performed. The exposure and mobilization are performed as described for a primary repair. Within the proximal tendon, a full-thickness inverted V is created. The flap is turned down and repaired across the repair while a side-to-side repair is performed for the proximal tendon.

In cases of chronic patella tendon ruptures, there may not be adequate tissue to maintain appropriate patella height with primary repair. As a result, allograft reconstruction may be necessary. Achilles allograft allows for versatility in patella height while providing bone-to-bone fixation at the tibial tubercle. Both operative and nonoperative extremities may be prepped and draped to allow for comparison of patella height before final fixation. Exposure is performed as a primary repair. A rectangular bone trough is prepared for the calcaneal bone of the Achilles allograft. The bone plug is fixed with 4.5-mm bicortical screws. The tendon is then split and passed through two parallel longitudinal tunnels through the patella. The allograft Achilles tendon can then be secured and repaired across the intact quadriceps tendon. Alternatively, suture anchor repair can be performed after decorticating the inferior pole patella. This technique may be considered in cases where patella thickness increases concern for fracture. A relaxation suture can be placed through the tibial tubercle after graft fixation to the tibia and around the patella/quadriceps tendon to reinforce the graft.

PEARLS AND PITFALLS

Exposure is critical for planning tunnel position and trajectory. The articular surface should be visualized and medial/lateral aspect of patella clearly identified. An Awl can be utilized to plan the location of each transosseous tunnel and allows for the drill to maintain the desired starting position.

Positioning the tunnels closer to the articular surface allows for slight anterior angulation of the tunnels resulting in less dissection through the intact tendon.

Evaluation of the tear/injury pattern is important before preparing the ruptured tendon or passing sutures. The patella tapers to its inferior pole and may result in an irregular margin to the ruptured patella tendon. Care should be taken to not change patella height, and when uncertain, an intra-operative lateral radiograph can be beneficial. The extension of the tear to the medial and lateral retinaculum should be evaluated and repaired to minimize stress across the repair and restore patella tracking.

POSTOPERATIVE MANAGEMENT/REHABILITATION

Rehabilitation following repair of the extensor mechanism requires a balance between immobilization to allow for healing and mobilization/strengthening to minimize atrophy and restore function. The patient is locked in extension in a postop knee brace for the first 2 weeks with flat foot weight bearing. In rare circumstances, a cast is applied due to body habitus or compliance concerns. Weight bearing locked in extension is initiated at 2-week postoperative visit. Straight leg raise and isometric quadriceps contractions are initiated immediately. At 4 weeks, range of motion is initiated through the tension-free range of motion as determined intraoperatively. Each week, range of motion is advanced 20 to 30 degrees with a goal of 90 degrees of motion by 6 weeks from surgery. Strengthening is initiated at 6 weeks from surgery. Patients are released to sport participation once quadriceps strength is 80% of the contralateral side, usually at 6 months after surgery.

Relaxation or cerclage sutures techniques have been described to reinforce the repair site (8,9). A more aggressive rehab protocol is allowed due to relaxation suture reinforcing the repair. Aggressive range of motion is initiated with a goal to achieve 120-degree motion by 6 weeks, as most programs have a goal of 90 degrees by 6 weeks.

Complications/Outcomes

Repair of acute quadriceps and patella tendon ruptures results in favorable outcomes with patella tendon repairs having slightly better outcome scores than quadriceps tendon repairs (8,10). Most patients will regain strength within 90% and flexion within 5 degrees of the contralateral side (11). As many as 30% of patients will experience residual pain or patellofemoral symptoms (11).

Unlike acute tears, a prolonged delay in diagnosis can result in inferior outcomes. Chronic patella tendon ruptures can result in loss of tissue and necessitate reconstruction of the patella tendon to restore function of the extensor mechanism. Several methods have been described with allograft or autograft reconstruction. Discussions of these techniques are generally limited to case reports. Lamberti et al. compared extensor lag and functional scores following reconstruction for total knee arthroplasty patients (12). All methods resulted in excellent improvement from the prereconstruction state, and one technique was not concluded to be superior.

REFERENCES

 1. Nance E Jr, Kaye J. Injuries of the quadriceps mechanism. *Radiology.* 1982;142(2):301–307.
 2. O'Shea K, Kenny P, Donovan J, et al. Outcomes following quadriceps tendon ruptures. *Injury.* 2002;33(3):257–260.
 3. Kannus P, Josza L. Histopathological changes preceding spontaneous rupture of a tendon. *J Bone Joint Surg Am.* 1991;73(10):1507–1525.
 4. Busfield BT, Safran MR, Cannon WD. Extensor mechanism disruption after contralateral middle third patellar tendon harvest for anterior cruciate ligament revision reconstruction. *Arthroscopy.* 2005;21(10):1268.e1–1268.e6.
 5. Marumoto JM, Mitsunaga MM, Richardson AB, et al. Late patellar tendon ruptures after removal of the central third for anterior cruciate ligament reconstruction. A report of two cases. *Am J Sports Med.* 1996;24(5):698–701.
 6. Matava MJ. Patellar tendon ruptures. *J Am Assoc Orthop Surg.* 1996;4:287.
 7. Siwek CW, Rao JP. Ruptures of the extensor mechanism of the knee joint. *J Bone Joint Surg Am.* 1981;63A:932.
 8. West JL, Keene JS, Kaplan LD. Early motion after quadriceps and patellar tendon repairs: outcomes with single suture augmentation. *Am J Sports Med.* 2008;36:316–323.
 9. Kasten P, Schewe B, Maurer F, et al. Rupture of the patellar tendon: a review of 68 cases and a retrospective study of 29 ruptures comparing two methods of augmentation. *Arch Orthop Trauma Surg.* 2001;121(10):578–582.
10. Kelly DW, Carter VS, Jobe FW, et al. Patellar and quadriceps tendon rupture-jumpers knee. *Am J Sports Med.* 1984;12(5):375–380.
11. Marder RA, Timmerman LA. Primary repair of patella tendon rupture without augmentation. *Am J Sports Med.* 1999;27(3):304–307.
12. Lamberti A, Balato G, Summa PP, et al. Surgical options for chronic patella tendon rupture in total knee arthroplasty. *Knee Surg Sports Traumatol Arthrosc.* 2018;26(5):1429–1435.

22 Meniscal Débridement

Craig C. Akoh, Michael Shin, and Geoffrey S. Baer

INTRODUCTION

Much has been learned about the anatomy and function of the meniscus since 1897 when Bland-Sutton described the meniscus as "functionless remnants of intra-articular leg muscles" (1). Since that time, there has been a significantly better understanding of the meniscus's multiple important roles in load bearing, joint stability, shock absorption, proprioception, and lubrication (2,3).

Meniscal tears can occur both from acute injuries and from chronic degeneration. The exact incidence of meniscal tears is difficult to ascertain due to the high number of asymptomatic tears and the high rate of degenerative tears in patients with advanced degenerative joint disease. It is estimated that the incidence of acute meniscal tears in the United States is approximately 61/100,000 persons per year. An epidemiologic study from the United Kingdom estimated the incidence of acute meniscal tears to be about 23.8/100,000 persons (4). Meniscal tears are found up to a 4:1 male:female ratio, with two thirds of injuries occurring in the absence of sporting activities (5). Additionally, up to one third of tears are associated with anterior cruciate ligament (ACL) injuries (6).

The classification of meniscal tears can be based on tear location or blood supply or by tear pattern (Fig. 22-1). The classification of the tear, in addition to other patient and tear characteristics, assists in the process of deciding the appropriate treatment. Meniscal tears can also be found in meniscal variants, the most common of which is a lateral discoid meniscus. Arthroscopic studies have shown a prevalence of discoid menisci ranging from 0.4% to 16.6%, most of which are found incidentally (7–11). Discoid menisci are more common in patients of Japanese or Korean descent and can be bilateral in up to 20% of patients (12,13).

With an increased understanding of the importance of the meniscus and of preserving as much functional meniscal tissue as possible, meniscal repair has become an increasingly important option for the treatment of meniscal tears (14–19). The possibility of meniscal repair should be considered when evaluating meniscal injuries, especially in young, active patients with or without concomitant ACL reconstructions (19–22). However, some meniscal tears are not amendable to meniscal repair due to meniscal degeneration, tear location and pattern, limited vascular supply, or patient age (23–26). In these settings, meniscal repair can be impossible or unlikely to heal, and meniscal débridement is the treatment of choice for these patients with symptomatic meniscal tears. The American Academy of Orthopaedic Surgeons (AAOS) estimates that over 636,000 arthroscopic knee procedures are performed each year, with over 60% of cases composed of meniscal debridement (27,28).

PATIENT EVALUATION (HISTORY, PHYSICAL EXAMINATION, AND RADIOGRAPHIC EVALUATION)

A complete history and physical examination are essential when evaluating any patient with knee pain and possible meniscal pathology. Patients with meniscal tears typically complain of pain localizing to the joint line, swelling, locking, catching, giving way, and loss of motion. The mechanism of injury often is a twisting or hyperflexion injury that presents with acute pain and swelling. In a study of patients with normal radiographs and a meniscal tear at arthroscopy, Drosos and Pozo (5) reported that approximately 32% of the tears occurred during a sporting activity and 39% were sustained during nonsporting activities, the majority of which were during activities of daily living, most commonly squatting. Interestingly, 29% had no identifiable mechanism.

273

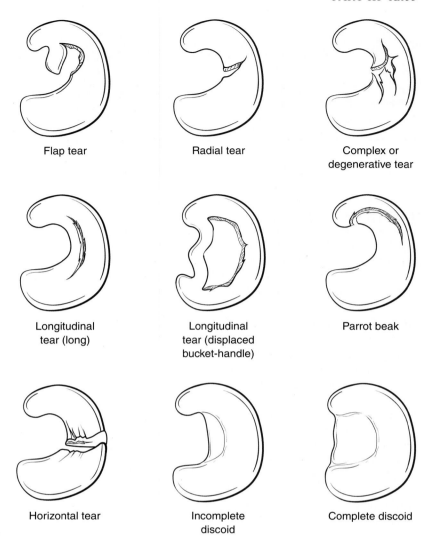

Flap tear

Radial tear

Complex or
degenerative tear

Longitudinal
tear (long)

Longitudinal
tear (displaced
bucket-handle)

Parrot beak

Horizontal tear

Incomplete
discoid

Complete discoid

FIGURE 22-1

Common types of meniscal tears and meniscal variants.

Physical examination usually demonstrates a patient with a joint effusion, pain in deep flexion, or pain with squatting. With a flipped bucket-handle meniscus tear, patients may have a mechanical block to motion, typically full extension. Specialized tests for meniscal tears include joint line tenderness, McMurray test (29), the Apley grind test (30), and the Thessaly test (31); however, these tests have been reported to have poor sensitivity, specificity, and positive predictive values and thus should be used in combination (32–36). Joint line tenderness with palpation is the most sensitive of the physical examination tests and has 92% and 86% sensitivity for lateral and medial meniscal tears, respectively (37). Joint line tenderness is less accurate in determining a meniscus tear in the setting of an ACL injury (38). The McMurray test is classically described as medial knee pain and clicking when the knee is slowly extended and externally rotated (29). Evans et al. demonstrated that a positive McMurray test with a palpable "clunk" at the joint line is very specific for a meniscal tear with 98% specificity but is only 16% sensitive (32), and pain alone with a McMurray test makes the test more sensitive but less specific (36). A positive Apley grind test has a sensitivity of 60% and a specificity of 70% (39–41). Patients with discoid menisci may present with the classic presentation of a "snapping knee," but this is the least common presentation. It usually presents as lateral-sided joint pain of insidious onset in a child or young adolescent (12). Kim et al. have described a paradoxical McMurray test for discoid meniscus pathology, in which lateral joint line pain or clicking occurs with the leg externally rotated (42,43). Physical examination should also include a ligamentous examination to assess for ligamentous damage and instability and an examination for degenerative joint disease.

Diagnostic studies are used to supplement and confirm diagnosis made through history and physical examination. Standing anteroposterior knee radiographs do not confirm a diagnosis of meniscal tears but are very important in evaluating the knee for knee alignment, joint space narrowing, and calcification of the meniscus (44). The 45-degree posteroanterior flexion is more sensitive than the standing weight-bearing radiograph for evaluating joint space narrowing (45). Radiographic findings suggestive of a discoid meniscus include widened lateral joint space, cupping of the lateral tibial plateau, or flattening/squaring of the lateral femoral condyle (12).

Magnetic resonance imaging (MRI) may be utilized to accurately evaluate tear location, tear pattern, and associated ligamentous and chondral pathology (Fig. 22-2). The limitations of MRI include its high cost and potential for misinterpretation, especially due to normal increased signal in the pediatric meniscus (46–49). Additionally, adults can have degenerative meniscus changes that are asymptomatic (50,51). Despite this potential for error, advances in technology and experience have increased the accuracy of MRI in diagnosing meniscal tears to 95% or better (52). Therefore, MRI should be used as a diagnostic tool to supplement the clinical diagnosis. Discoid menisci are often found incidentally on MRI (12,49). In the sagittal plane, three or greater contiguous 5-mm sections that show the classic "bow-tie" appearance representing continuity of the anterior and posterior horns are diagnostic for a discoid meniscus. In the coronal plane, when viewing an image from the midpoint from anterior to posterior, revealing the free edge of the lateral meniscus to extend past the midpoint of the femoral condyle or further toward the intercondylar notch is suggestive of a discoid meniscus.

INDICATIONS/CONTRAINDICATIONS

Indications for arthroscopic intervention for meniscal tears are typically reserved for patients who have failed nonoperative management such as activity modification, physical therapy, and pain medication. Patients indicated for surgery should have significant joint line pain and mechanical symptoms such as locking, catching, and giving way that affect activities of daily living, participation in sports, and work. Earlier surgical intervention may be warranted for radial tears and central meniscus tears that have a lower likelihood of spontaneous healing (53). Meniscal tears in young patients and tears associated with ACL reconstructions be repaired if possible. However, many tears found during surgery are not amendable to repair, in which case, a partial meniscectomy that removes unstable fragments and creates a smooth transition, while maintaining as much functional meniscus, should be undertaken (20).

Surgical intervention is contraindicated for asymptomatic patients with despite having tears on imaging studies. The incidence of meniscal tears, especially degenerative tears, increase with increasing age. A study evaluating 100 patients with an average age of 43 years with an MRI of asymptomatic knees showed a 37% prevalence of meniscal tears (54). Additionally, patients with degenerative meniscal tears in the setting of significant degenerative joint disease may obtain minimal benefit from arthroscopic meniscal débridement, and arthroscopic intervention should be undertaken only after exhausting nonoperative management. Degenerative changes and damage to the articular cartilage found at the time of arthroscopic partial meniscectomy had the greatest impact on long-term outcome and correlated with significantly worse functional outcomes at 12-year follow-up (16,55).

Modern treatment goals for meniscal tears include preserving as much functional meniscal tissue as possible without leaving unstable flaps or abrupt transitions. This evolution in treatment philosophy contrasts with historical treatment goals. In 1942, McMurray stated "a far too common error is shown in the incomplete removal of the injured meniscus" (29). The effects of total meniscectomy were described a short time later by Fairbank in 1948 (14). Fairbank described several radiographic changes in the knee joint after meniscectomy, including ridge formation, narrowing of the joint space, and flattening of the femoral condyle. Modern biomechanical studies have delineated the importance of preserving the meniscus. These studies have shown decreased contact areas and increased peak contact stresses after partial and total meniscectomies, leading to radiographic progression of osteoarthrosis. Baratz et al. showed that performing a partial meniscectomy at the central third and peripheral third of the meniscus increased peak local contact stress by 65% and 110%, respectively (15). Additionally, performing a total meniscectomy increased peak local contact stress by 235%. Another cadaveric study by Lee et al. demonstrated the importance of maintaining the peripheral circumferential meniscal fibers to preserve the ability of the meniscus to

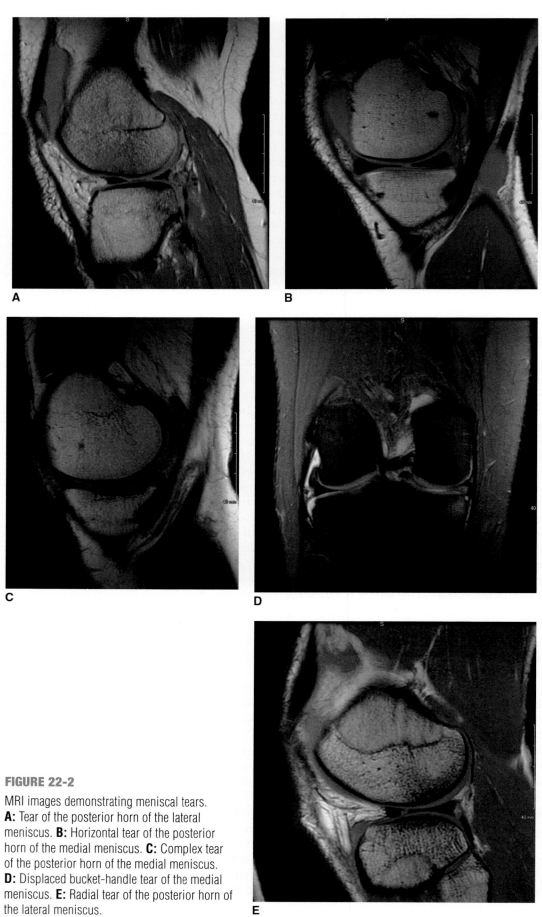

FIGURE 22-2

MRI images demonstrating meniscal tears.
A: Tear of the posterior horn of the lateral meniscus. **B:** Horizontal tear of the posterior horn of the medial meniscus. **C:** Complex tear of the posterior horn of the medial meniscus. **D:** Displaced bucket-handle tear of the medial meniscus. **E:** Radial tear of the posterior horn of the lateral meniscus.

resist hoop stresses (17). By retaining the periphery of the meniscus, there was a decrease in mean contact pressures. However, a loss of peripheral meniscus resulted in a segmental meniscectomy, which was functionally equivalent to a total meniscectomy. This cadaveric study demonstrated that this peripheral portion of the medial meniscus had a greater contribution to increasing contact area and decreasing mean contact stresses than did the central portions. Northmore-Ball studied 219 knees that underwent open total meniscectomy, open partial meniscectomy, or arthroscopic partial meniscectomy (18). Higuchi et al. retrospectively followed 67 patients who underwent partial meniscectomies. At 12-year follow-up, patients with >50% partial meniscectomies, cartilage injury, and medial meniscectomies had worse outcome (16).

SURGICAL TECHNIQUE (GENERAL, POSITIONING, TECHNIQUE)

Meniscal débridements have transitioned from total meniscectomies performed open to the current treatment of arthroscopic partial meniscectomies. Open total meniscectomies were originally thought to be benign procedures and were commonly performed for all types of meniscal pathology. However, as more has been learned about the long-term sequelae of open total meniscectomies and with the improvement of arthroscopic techniques, this procedure has fallen out of favor.

Arthroscopy can be performed under many forms of anesthesia including general, regional, and local based on multiple factors including length and type of procedure, patient's medical conditions, and the preferences of the patient, surgeon, and anesthesiologist (56–61). After adequate anesthesia has been achieved, the procedure begins with an examination under anesthesia (EUA). This examination utilizes the ability to perform a thorough examination with the patient relaxed and without causing the patient discomfort. The examination should evaluate for the presence of an effusion, passive range of motion (ROM), a Lachman test, anterior and posterior drawer tests, a pivot shift, varus and valgus testing at full extension and at 30 degrees of flexion, a Dial test, and patellar instability. Upon completion of the EUA, the patient is then positioned for the arthroscopic portion of the case. The patient is positioned supine on the operating room table, and care is taken to adequately pad the contralateral peroneal nerve and all bony prominences. A well-padded tourniquet is placed on the upper thigh of the operative leg but is typically not required unless necessary for visualization (62). Two common methods of setup include the use of a lateral post or leg holder, both of which assist the surgeon in positioning and manipulating the leg intraoperatively.

If the lateral post technique is used, the patient is positioned supine on the operating room table and the post is placed at the level of the tourniquet at approximately the level of the mid to upper thigh. A footrest can be secured to the bed and allows the leg to rest at 70 to 90 degrees of flexion and can be used with or without a bump under the ipsilateral hip. The lateral post assists in placing a valgus force through the knee, and advantages include better access to both posterior and superior accessory portals and the ability to rest the leg on the table when the knee is in full extension. A foot rest or hanging the leg off the side of the operative table assists with holding the leg when the knee is in flexion. The lateral post also has the advantages of not acting as a venous tourniquet and not fixing the thigh in place and therefore allowing more flexibility in positioning the leg, including in the figure-four position (Fig. 22-3).

When using the leg holder technique, the patient is positioned supine on the operating room table, and the patient's thigh is placed so that the knee is past the break of the table so that the bed does not block the ability of the knee to flex. The leg holder stabilizes the thigh while the foot of the table is dropped and the operative leg hangs free (Fig. 22-4). The nonoperative leg is then placed into a padded well-leg holder. The foot of the patient's operative leg can be placed on the surgeon's hip and then be manipulated into varus and valgus. Exsanguinating the leg by elevating the tourniquet prior to placement of the leg holder can help prevent venous bleeding. Proponents of the leg holder remark that it allows for greater valgus stress to be placed across the knee and therefore provides better visualization and access to the posteromedial joint. However, extra attention must be taken during patient positioning to assure that the leg holder is proximal on the thigh to not block access to accessory portals and to allow the knee to maximally flex. Proper positioning can be especially difficult in heavy patients with short thighs. The leg holder should also not be overtightened to avoid it acting as a venous tourniquet, which can be a significant concern during longer procedures.

Once the patient has been properly positioned, the leg is prepped and draped, and a diagnostic arthroscopy is performed to identify all areas of intra-articular pathology. Joint expansion with

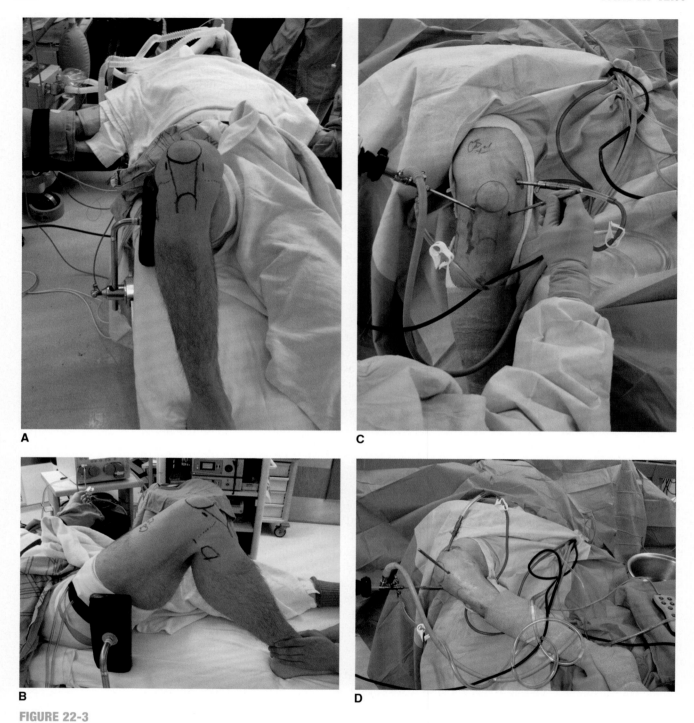

FIGURE 22-3

Lateral post technique. **A:** Anterior view. **B:** Lateral view with the post positioned at the upper thigh. **C:** Operating with knee in flexion.
D: Operative leg placed in figure four position.

arthroscopy fluid can be achieved through different methods, and the inflow and outflow can be brought into the joint in different locations. Some surgeons prefer water pressure through gravity flow while others choose a pump device. Also, both inflow and outflow can be placed on the arthroscope cannula or an accessory superolateral or superomedial portal can be utilized (63,64).

The standard portals for knee arthroscopy are utilized for meniscal débridement. The standard anterolateral viewing portal and anteromedial working portal are placed in the soft spots approximately 1 cm above the corresponding medial or lateral joint line and roughly 1 cm medial or lateral to the corresponding border of the patellar tendon. These portals are usually made as an approximately

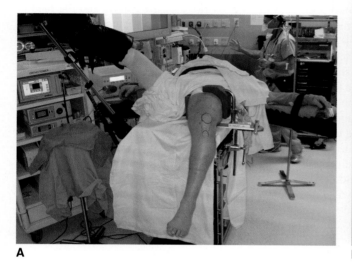
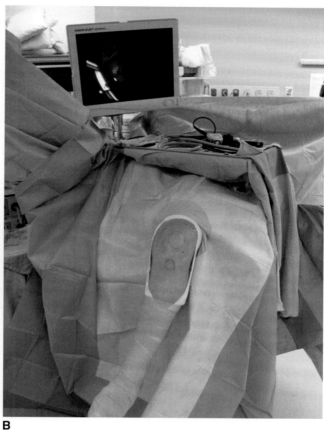

A   **B**

FIGURE 22-4

Leg holder technique. **A:** Patient positioned utilizing the leg holder. **B:** After draping, the operative leg is able to hang free.

1-cm vertical incision with the blade of the scalpel turned upward and away from the meniscus. Some surgeons prefer to utilize horizontal anterolateral and anteromedial portals. Horizontal portals should also be approximately 1 cm in length with the blade turned away from the patellar tendon to decrease the risk of iatrogenic injury. Proponents of horizontal anterior portal placement cite studies that suggest less iatrogenic nerve injury due to the anatomic route of the infrapatellar branches of the saphenous nerve as it traverses the knee (65,66). However, transverse portals have the disadvantage that they cannot be made extensile. Regardless of the type of incision, the portals should be made aiming toward the femoral notch to avoid iatrogenic articular cartilage damage. The anteromedial portal is made under direct visualization with the arthroscope in the anterolateral portal, and portal position should be localized using an 18-gauge spinal needle, observing the path of the needle such that optimal access to pathology may be achieved. Superomedial or superolateral portals placed with the knee in full extension approximately 25 mm above superior pole of patella and far enough from the midline to avoid injuring the quadriceps tendon. These portals can be used for inflow, outflow, or as a viewing or working portal. Both the posteromedial and the posterolateral accessory portals should be placed under direct visualization, again with a localizing 18-gauge spinal needle that allows optimal portal placement for accessing pathology. The posteromedial portal should be above the joint line and posterior to the medial collateral ligament, and the posterolateral should be posterior to the lateral collateral ligament, anterior to the biceps femoris tendon, and above the joint line. These posteromedial and posterolateral portals can be used during meniscal débridement as both viewing and working portals, and the posterior portals are especially useful for loose body removal as well as certain posterior horn and root tears. Risks from placing the posterior accessory portals include injury to the saphenous neurovascular bundle with the posteromedial portal and the peroneal nerve with the posterolateral portal (67).

Before any arthroscopic knee procedure, including meniscal débridement, a thorough diagnostic arthroscopy should be completed to identify all areas of pathology. The procedure begins by establishing the anterolateral portal and then inserting the cannula with a blunt introducer through the portal while the knee is at 90 degrees of flexion. After the cannula passes into the joint capsule, the knee is extended and the arthroscope is placed into the suprapatellar pouch. Some surgeons will utilize a superolateral or a superomedial accessory portal for inflow or outflow. The blunt trocar is then removed and a 30-degree arthroscope is placed, and a systematic evaluation is undertaken viewing the undersurface of the patella, the trochlea, and the patellofemoral articulation. The suprapatellar pouch is also thoroughly visualized looking for synovitis, adhesions, or loose bodies. The lateral trochlear ridge and lateral gutter should be examined starting from the patellofemoral joint to the lateral compartment by bringing the knee from full extension into flexion. The popliteal tendon and peripheral aspect of the lateral meniscus can be evaluated as well as examined for the presence of loose bodies, adhesions, and osteophytes. After viewing the lateral gutter, the arthroscope is brought back into the patellofemoral joint, and the medial ridge of the patella and the medial trochlear groove are evaluated. The medial gutter is evaluated from the suprapatellar pouch to the medial compartment while the knee is slowly brought from full extension to 90 degrees of flexion. The presence of pathologic plica, osteophytes, loose bodies, and synovitis should all be evaluated and noted. The anteromedial portal should now be established under direct visualization with the help of an 18-gauge localizing needle for optimal placement. The No. 11 blade is then used to make the anteromedial portal and should be visualized to assure that the joint capsule is incised and that the blade does not cause iatrogenic injury to the anterior horn of the meniscus or the articular cartilage. A straight hemostat can be used to help clear and expand the portal. The medial compartment is then examined from anterior horn to posterior horn and root. The knee can be placed into valgus and external rotation to improve visualization of the medial compartment and to allow space for the arthroscope. The meniscus should be probed for tears of the superior and inferior surface, for abnormal translation, and for root avulsions. If a meniscal tear is present, it should be thoroughly examined with the use of a probe to determine the type, location, size, and stability of the tear. The femoral and tibial articular surfaces should be evaluated and examined from full flexion to full extension to evaluate the entire chondral surface. If chondral defects are present, the probe should be used to test for flaps and stability and to determine the size of the defects.

The intercondylar notch is evaluated next, and the probe is used to examine the ACL, posterior cruciate ligament (PCL), intermeniscal ligament, and meniscofemoral ligaments. In some patients, an enlarged ligamentum mucosum may need to be débrided to allow access through the intercondylar notch and into the lateral compartment.

The lateral compartment is typically viewed with the arthroscope viewing through the anterolateral portal and the knee placed into flexion and a varus stress in the figure-four position. For greater varus stress, an assistant can lift the lateral aspect of the ankle off the table while the leg is in the figure-four position and/or place a hand on the medial aspect of the patient's operative knee or thigh and direct a force toward the lateral aspect of the patient's operative knee. After the knee has been positioned to optimally open the lateral compartment, the arthroscope is brought from the intercondylar notch into the compartment. It is sometimes necessary to débride parts of a hypertrophic fat pad or an enlarged ligamentous mucosum in order to visualize the lateral compartment. Once in the lateral compartment, the joint surfaces, meniscus, and popliteal tendon should be carefully examined. Any articular pathology or meniscal tears should be probed to characterize and define the extent of any tears in the same fashion as on the medial side. The articular surfaces should be examined through a full ROM to examine the entire surface for pathology (68).

If posterior compartment pathology is suspected, the posteromedial and posterolateral compartments should be examined. To visualize the posteromedial compartment for loose bodies and to view the posteromedial meniscus, the arthroscope can be passed through the intercondylar notch between the PCL and the medial wall of the intercondylar notch against the medial femoral condyle using the modified Gillquist maneuver (69). The arthroscope is replaced by the blunt trocar to facilitate passage of the cannula into the posteromedial compartment with the knee in 90 degrees of knee flexion and valgus stress to the knee. Once the cannula has been passed into the compartment, the blunt trocar is exchanged for the 30- or 70-degree scope for visualization. If needed, an accessory posteromedial portal can be established under direct visualization using a localizing 18-gauge needle. Once the localizing needle is in optimal position, an incision is made through just the skin to decrease the risk of injury to the saphenous nerve and vein, and the portal is completed with the use of a straight hemostat to penetrate the joint capsule and expand the portal. The established posteromedial portal can be used for both visualization and as a working portal.

The examination of the posterolateral compartment is through a similar maneuver where the arthroscope is brought into the knee through the anteromedial portal and directed into the intercondylar notch inferior to the ACL, and along the lateral wall of the notch. The arthroscope is replaced by a blunt trocar and with the knee in 90 degrees of flexion, and a varus stress onto the knee is advanced into the posterolateral compartment. The blunt trocar is then exchanged for a 30- or 70-degree scope. An accessory posterolateral portal can be created, if necessary, under direct visualization using a localizing 18-gauge needle for proper portal placement. The No. 11 blade is used for skin incision, and the straight hemostat is used to penetrate the joint capsule and expand the portal. This accessory portal can be used as both a working and a visualization portal.

Once the diagnostic arthroscopy has been completed and a tear has been identified, the tear should be more carefully evaluated to determine if the tear is repairable and if the meniscal tissue has a high probability to heal (Fig. 22-5). This evaluation should take into account not only the characteristics

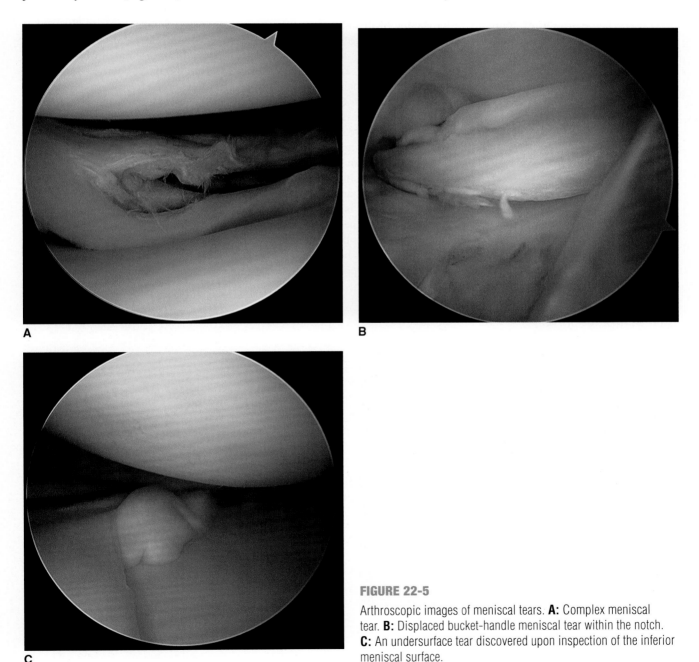

A

B

C

FIGURE 22-5

Arthroscopic images of meniscal tears. **A:** Complex meniscal tear. **B:** Displaced bucket-handle meniscal tear within the notch. **C:** An undersurface tear discovered upon inspection of the inferior meniscal surface.

of the tear (type, location, size, and stability) but also the patient's age, activity level of the patient, degeneration of the chondral surfaces or the meniscal tissue, the alignment and stability of the knee joint, and any concurrent procedures that may improve meniscal healing, such as an ACL reconstruction (70). The patient's desires regarding postoperative recovery and return to work should also be determined prior to surgery. Meniscal débridement should be undertaken if the determination is made that meniscal repair is not possible. For most tears, meniscal baskets and arthroscopic shavers should be used to resect all mobile fragments while preserving as much functional meniscus as possible (Fig. 22-6). A wide array of instruments are available for meniscal débridements that assist in accessing the various locations where tears of the meniscus can occur. The typical instruments used for meniscal tears are an up-angled basket for tears of the posterior horn of the medial meniscus and a straight basket for tears of the lateral meniscus. For tears of the midbody and anterior horn of the medial meniscus, one technique is to switch to the anteromedial portal as the viewing portal and use the straight basket through the anterolateral portal to access the tear. Other specialized baskets include back biters, narrow, 45-degree-angled, and right angle baskets, available in left and right (Fig. 22-7). The angled baskets and back-biting baskets may also be particularly useful for tears in the midbody of the medial meniscus and tears to the medial or lateral anterior horns. Shavers of various sizes are also available for meniscal débridements and should be selected based on the space available for the instrument (Fig. 22-8). Angled shavers may also be appropriate to optimize the ability to reach some meniscal tears. The remaining meniscal tissue should be contoured to leave a stable meniscal rim with smooth transitions to decrease the risk of retearing the meniscal remnants. The meniscal rim should be retained to maintain circumferential collagen fibers that preserve the meniscus's ability to absorb hoop stresses. After the partial meniscectomy is thought to be complete, the remaining meniscus should be reassessed and probed to confirm that the tear has been completely removed and that the remaining meniscus is stable (71–73).

For bucket-handle tears that cannot be repaired, a strategy frequently employed is to reduce the displaced tear back into normal position using a probe or blunt trocar. The posterior attachment is first resected to near completion, and then the anterior attachment is completely resected. The anterior tip of the meniscal fragment is then grasped, and the remaining posterior attachment is then avulsed free; a twisting or rolling maneuver may assist in completing the transection. The remaining meniscus is then evaluated and smoothed. This method for resecting bucket-handle tears prevents the fragment from becoming a loose body and decreases the chance that the tear will displace into the posterior aspect of the knee on a posterior hinge if the anterior attachment is transected first (73) (Fig. 22-9).

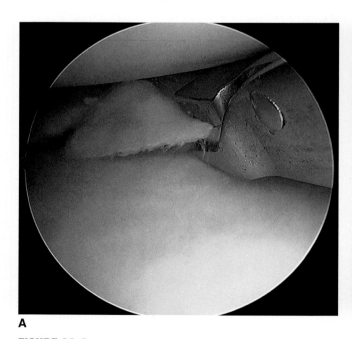
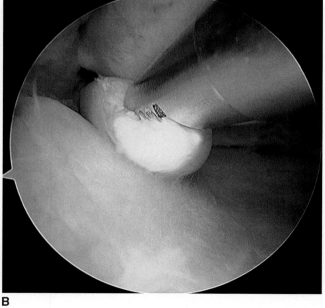

A   **B**

FIGURE 22-6

Arthroscopic instruments. **A:** Utilization of the biter during meniscal débridement. **B:** Use of a shaver during meniscal débridement.

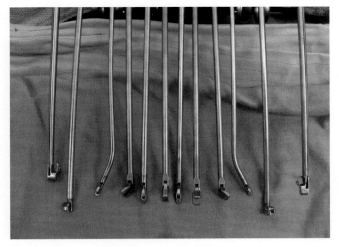

FIGURE 22-7

A variety of biters are available for resecting meniscal tears based upon tear location.

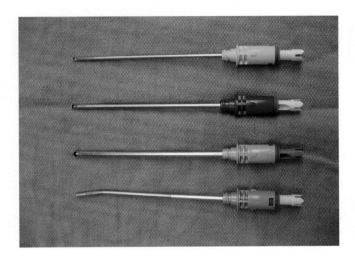

FIGURE 22-8

Shavers of various size and angle are available.

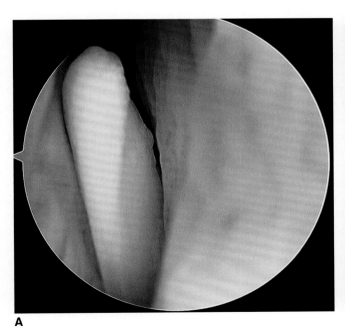

A

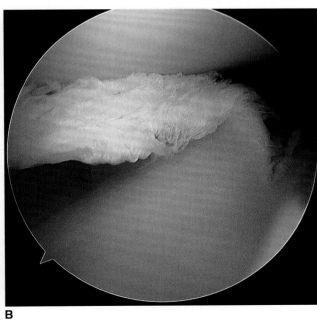

B

FIGURE 22-9

Partial meniscectomy of a displaced bucket-handle medial meniscus tear. **A:** Flipped fragment of meniscus in the medial gutter. **B:** Meniscal flap brought into medial joint.

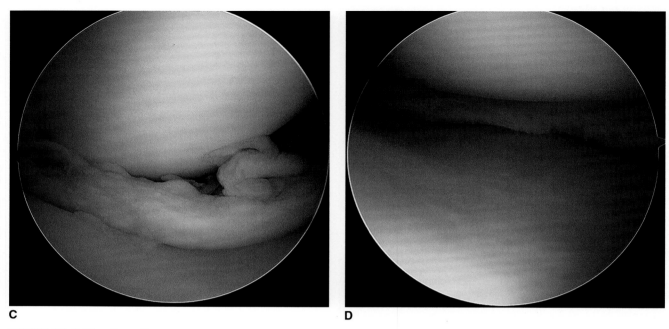

C   D

FIGURE 22-9 (*Continued*)
C: Posterior aspect of the complex tear. **D:** Post partial meniscectomy.

Horizontal meniscal tears may be treated in two ways, and its management is somewhat controversial as no good study was delineated which of the two methods is more advantageous. One method is a complete resection of both leaflets of the horizontal tear leaving a stable edge, which has a theoretic advantage of having a decreased risk of retearing. The other technique is to assess both the upper and the lower leaflets of the tear and then determining which leaf to preserve in order to retain as much meniscus as possible. Our preferred method is to attempt to preserve the more stable leaflet if possible, especially in younger patients.

The treatment for an asymptomatic discoid meniscus is observation. For a symptomatic tear in a patient with a discoid meniscus, the tear is resected and the meniscus is saucerized to a more "normal" shape (Fig. 22-10). For the patient with an unstable discoid meniscus, the unstable portion may need to be reattached, in addition to saucerization (30).

POST-OP MANAGEMENT

Postoperative management after arthroscopic meniscal débridement focuses on ROM, pain and effusion control, strengthening, and finally return to full activity. Weight bearing as tolerated can be started immediately postoperatively, and physical therapy with home exercise programs can be initiated within the first few days after surgery. Early therapy focuses on joint effusion control, ROM exercises especially achieving full extension, and quadriceps strengthening exercises. The judicious use of anti-inflammatory medications and use of icing can be very beneficial, especially in the early postoperative period. Excessive opioid prescriptions should be avoided unless concomitant surgeries such as ACL reconstructions are performed (74,75). Some surgeons will also provide crutches in the early postoperative period and/or cryotherapy, but both can be discontinued as soon as the patient is comfortable. Studies have shown mixed results with the use of cryotherapy and pain relief for non-ACL knee arthroscopy cases (76–78). The patient can advance therapy as the patient's symptoms and tolerance allow and with close monitoring of joint pain and effusions. The initiation of low-impact exercises and advancement to increasing impact and slow jogging can be accomplished with careful attention to the patient's symptoms and intra-articular effusions. The final step is to incorporate running, cutting, and sport-specific activities into the rehabilitation program. Once this final step is tolerated by the patient without pain or joint effusion, along with normal ROM and muscle strength, full return to sports and activity is permitted. The typical time frame for this return to full activity is typically 4 to 6 weeks but in our experience can frequently be expected to

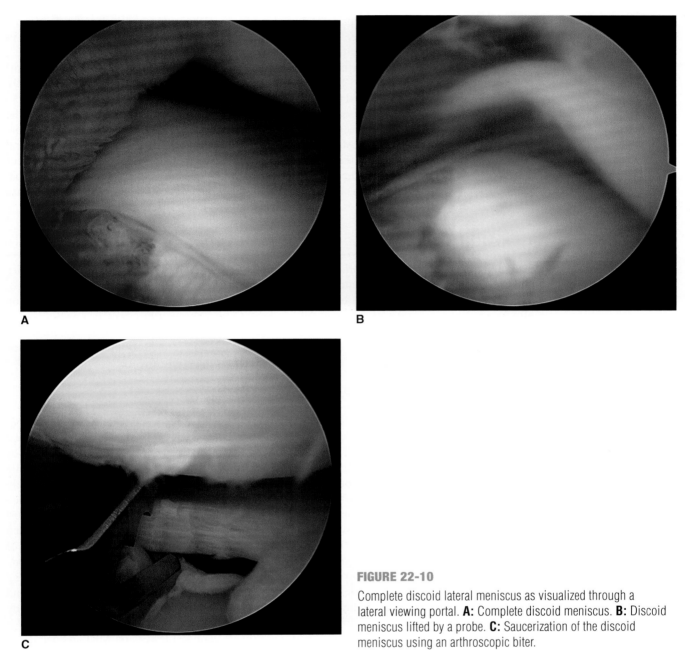

A

B

C

FIGURE 22-10
Complete discoid lateral meniscus as visualized through a lateral viewing portal. **A:** Complete discoid meniscus. **B:** Discoid meniscus lifted by a probe. **C:** Saucerization of the discoid meniscus using an arthroscopic biter.

take longer in patients with cartilage changes evident at time of arthroscopy (79,80) and in patients treated for lateral meniscal tears (81,82).

OUTCOMES

The results of arthroscopic partial meniscectomies are generally very favorable with reported satisfactory and good to excellent results in the 80% to 100% range with short-term follow-up (3,83,84). Northmore-Ball studied 219 knees that underwent open total meniscectomy, open partial meniscectomy, or arthroscopic partial meniscectomy (18). At a mean follow-up of 4.3 years, 90.5%, 85%, and 68% of patients had good or excellent outcomes for arthroscopic partial, open partial, and open total meniscectomies, respectively. Andersson-Molina et al. reported on 36 knees that underwent either partial or total meniscectomies. At 14-year follow-up, 33% of partial meniscectomy had radiographic arthritic changes compared to 72% for the total meniscectomy group (83). Some studies have demonstrated worse results and higher rates of radiographic degenerative changes with partial lateral meniscectomies when compared to partial medial meniscectomies with rates of radiographic degeneration as high as 84% at 12.3-year follow-up after partial lateral meniscectomy compared to 22.4% for partial medial meniscectomy at 11.5-year follow-up (85–88).

Long-term results following partial meniscectomies generally decline with time but are still favorable with reported satisfactory and good to excellent results in the 78% to 95% range (55,84,88,89). Paxton's systematic review showed that partial meniscectomies had a lower reoperation rate (1.4%) when compared to isolated meniscal repair (16.5%) (19). However, long-term outcomes may be improved with meniscal repair in acute traumatic tears in the young population (19,90). Two factors that have been shown to be prognostic for worse outcomes after partial meniscectomies are chondral injury evident at the time of meniscectomy and meniscectomies performed in ACL-deficient knees (3,16,55,89,91). Age and gender have not been proven to significantly alter outcomes after partial meniscectomies, especially when age was separated from age-related degenerative joint disease (16,89,92).

COMPLICATIONS

Complications from meniscal débridement are similar to those of other arthroscopic knee surgeries and include iatrogenic cartilage injury, anesthetic complication, infection, deep venous thrombosis, and neurovascular injury. Postoperative stiffness, joint effusions/hemarthrosis, and residual pain can also be adverse outcomes post meniscal débridement. Overall, knee arthroscopy is a well-tolerated procedure with very low complication rates. In one study, the overall complication rate following an arthroscopic meniscectomy was 2.8% (93). The most common complications were hemarthrosis, infection, deep venous thrombosis, and anesthetic complications (93–96).

SPECIAL CONSIDERATIONS

Special considerations should be given when evaluating meniscal tears and determining the proper surgical intervention in certain patient populations, particularly younger patients, athletic patients, and patients with concomitant ACL tears. In these younger, more active patients, we preserve as much meniscal tissue as possible by attempting to remove the least amount of meniscus, while still resecting the tear. Athletes represent a subgroup that until recently have not been extensively studied. In 1987, Jorgensen et al. published a longitudinal study on 147 athletes with isolated meniscal injuries that underwent total meniscectomies (97). At 4.5-year follow-up, 11% of the cohort underwent reoperation for additional injuries. Significantly worse results were in athletes compared to most other long-term results in the general population, with 36% of the cohort complaining of instability, 89% of the cohort demonstrating radiographic degeneration, and 34% cessation of sporting activity at the 14.5-year follow-up. A retrospective study on 72 NFL football players undergoing arthroscopic partial meniscectomies showed that the average return to play was 8.5 months and only 61% of players returned to play at their previous level of competition (82). Another NFL study that reported on 2,285 players who participated in the NFL combine showed that players with at least 10% of total meniscectomy volume had more severe chondral lesions on MRI and decreased performance (80).

The ACL-deficient knee represents another important subgroup of patients with meniscal pathology. Having an ACL-deficient knee is a poor prognostic factor for outcomes after a partial meniscectomy (23). Posterior horn tears of the medial meniscus leads to increased instability, even after ACL reconstruction (98-100). However, in acute ACL-deficient knees, there is an increased rate of healing for meniscus repairs at the time of concurrent ACL reconstruction, reportedly as high as 93%. Therefore, meniscal tears that would normally be débrided should be considered for repair (21,101,102).

Patients with certain tear morphologies including radial tears, flap tears, horizontal tears, and lateral meniscus tears also deserve extra attention (103). Flap tears were shown in one study to have a significantly longer time to return to sports, 20.1 weeks compared to 5.1 weeks, and a higher rate of repeat arthroscopy, 29% to 13%, when compared with bucket-handle tears (104). Radial tears disrupt the circumferential fibers of the meniscus, preventing the dissipation of hoop stresses during tibiofemoral loading. It can be more difficult in radial meniscal tears to assess tear depth and resect to the proper level to create a smooth transition. Radial tears that involve <90% may retain some protective properties and can be debrided (105–107). However, lateral meniscus radial tears >90% of the meniscus width that extend into the popliteal hiatus resemble forces experienced after a total meniscectomy (106). There is some controversy in the management of horizontal tears of the meniscus and whether a complete resection of the tear to a stable edge is preferable over assessing both the upper and the lower leaflets and retaining the larger or more normal appearing leaflet to retain meniscal tissue. One cadaveric study showed that resecting both horizontal leaflets leads to higher tibiofemoral peak contact pressures in the medial compartment when compared to removing only the inferior leaflet (108). Lateral meniscal tears have demonstrated in some studies to have slower return, higher rates of developing osteoarthrosis, and possibly worse clinical results (82,85–87). Finally, patients with degenerative articular changes are a special category due to worse outcomes in patients with articular changes at time of meniscectomy and slower recovery times and worse outcomes (109). One histologic study showed that patients over the age of 40 had fewer meniscus cells and may be more prone to degeneration and failure (110). Overall, worse outcomes following partial meniscectomies include obesity, female sex, and preexisting osteoarthritis (111).

REFERENCES

1. Bland-Sutton J. *Ligaments: Their Nature and Morphology*. 2nd Ed. London, UK: JK Lewis; 1897.
2. Greis PE, et al. Meniscal injury: I. Basic science and evaluation. *J Am Acad Orthop Surg*. 2002;10(3):168–176.
3. McDermott ID, Amis AA. The consequences of meniscectomy. *J Bone Joint Surg Br*. 2006;88(12):1549–1556.
4. Clayton RA, Court-Brown CM. The epidemiology of musculoskeletal tendinous and ligamentous injuries. *Injury*. 2008;39(12):1338–1344.
5. Drosos GI, Pozo JL. The causes and mechanisms of meniscal injuries in the sporting and non-sporting environment in an unselected population. *Knee*. 2004;11(2):143–149.
6. Poehling GG, Ruch DS, Chabon SJ. The landscape of meniscal injuries. *Clin Sports Med*. 1990;9(3):539–549.
7. Neuschwander DC, Drez D Jr, Finney TP. Lateral meniscal variant with absence of the posterior coronary ligament. *J Bone Joint Surg Am*. 1992;74(8):1186–1190.
8. Dickhaut SC, DeLee JC. The discoid lateral-meniscus syndrome. *J Bone Joint Surg Am*. 1982;64(7):1068–1073.
9. Fujikawa K, Iseki F, Mikura Y. Partial resection of the discoid meniscus in the child's knee. *J Bone Joint Surg Br*. 1981;63-b(3):391–395.
10. Ikeuchi H. Arthroscopic treatment of the discoid lateral meniscus. Technique and long-term results. *Clin Orthop Relat Res*. 1982;167:19–28.
11. Albertsson M, Gillquist J. Discoid lateral menisci: a report of 29 cases. *Arthroscopy*. 1988;4(3):211–214.
12. Jordan MR. Lateral meniscal variants: evaluation and treatment. *J Am Acad Orthop Surg*. 1996;4(4):191–200.
13. Bellier G, et al. Lateral discoid menisci in children. *Arthroscopy*. 1989;5(1):52–56.
14. Fairbank TJ. Knee joint changes after meniscectomy. *J Bone Joint Surg Br*. 1948;30b(4):664–670.
15. Baratz ME, Fu FH, Mengato R. Meniscal tears: the effect of meniscectomy and of repair on intraarticular contact areas and stress in the human knee. A preliminary report. *Am J Sports Med*. 1986;14(4):270–275.
16. Higuchi H, et al. Factors affecting long-term results after arthroscopic partial meniscectomy. *Clin Orthop Relat Res*. 2000;377:161–168.
17. Lee SJ, et al. Tibiofemoral contact mechanics after serial medial meniscectomies in the human cadaveric knee. *Am J Sports Med*. 2006;34(8):1334–1344.
18. Northmore-Ball MD, Dandy DJ, Jackson RW. Arthroscopic, open partial, and total meniscectomy. A comparative study. *J Bone Joint Surg Br*. 1983;65(4):400–404.
19. Paxton ES, Stock MV, Brophy RH. Meniscal repair versus partial meniscectomy: a systematic review comparing reoperation rates and clinical outcomes. *Arthroscopy*. 2011;27(9):1275–1288.
20. Metcalf R, Burks RT, Metcalf MS, et al. Arthroscopic meniscectomy. *Operative Arthroscopy*. Philadelphia, PA: Lippincott-Raven; 1996:263–297.
21. Cannon WD Jr, Vittori JM. The incidence of healing in arthroscopic meniscal repairs in anterior cruciate ligament-reconstructed knees versus stable knees. *Am J Sports Med*. 1992;20(2):176–181.
22. Noyes FR, Barber-Westin SD. Arthroscopic repair of meniscus tears extending into the avascular zone with or without anterior cruciate ligament reconstruction in patients 40 years of age and older. *Arthroscopy*. 2000;16(8):822–829.
23. Smith JP III, Barrett GR. Medial and lateral meniscal tear patterns in anterior cruciate ligament-deficient knees. A prospective analysis of 575 tears. *Am J Sports Med*. 2001;29(4):415–419.
24. Beaufils P, et al. Surgical management of degenerative meniscus lesions: the 2016 ESSKA meniscus consensus. *Joints*. 2017;5(2):59–69.
25. Arnoczky SP, Warren RF. Microvasculature of the human meniscus. *Am J Sports Med*. 1982;10(2):90–95.
26. Cipolla M, Cerullo G, Puddu G. Microvasculature of the human medial meniscus: operative findings. *Arthroscopy*. 1992;8(4):522–525.
27. Praemer A, Furner S, Rice DP. *Musculoskeletal Conditions in the United States*. Rosemont, IL: American Academy of Orthopaedic Surgeons; 1999.
28. Stahel PF, et al. Surgeon practice patterns of arthroscopic partial meniscectomy for degenerative disease in the United States: a measure of low-value care. *JAMA Surg*. 2018;153(5):494–496.
29. McMurray T. The semilunar cartilages. *Br J Surg*. 1942;29:407–414.
30. Apley AG. The diagnosis of meniscus injuries; some new clinical methods. *J Bone Joint Surg Am*. 1947;29(1):78–84.
31. Karachalios T, et al. Diagnostic accuracy of a new clinical test (the Thessaly test) for early detection of meniscal tears. *J Bone Joint Surg Am*. 2005;87(5):955–962.
32. Evans PJ, Bell GD, Frank C. Prospective evaluation of the McMurray test. *Am J Sports Med*. 1993;21(4):604–608.
33. Medlar RC, Mandiberg JJ, Lyne ED. Meniscectomies in children. Report of long-term results (mean, 8.3 years) of 26 children. *Am J Sports Med*. 1980;8(2):87–92.

34. Weinstabl R, et al. Economic considerations for the diagnosis and therapy of meniscal lesions: can magnetic resonance imaging help reduce the expense? *World J Surg.* 1997;21(4):363–368.

35. Goossens P, et al. Validity of the Thessaly test in evaluating meniscal tears compared with arthroscopy: a diagnostic accuracy study. *J Orthop Sports Phys Ther.* 2015;45(1):18–24, b1.

36. Fowler PJ, Lubliner JA. The predictive value of five clinical signs in the evaluation of meniscal pathology. *Arthroscopy.* 1989;5(3):184–186.

37. Eren OT. The accuracy of joint line tenderness by physical examination in the diagnosis of meniscal tears. *Arthroscopy.* 2003;19(8):850–854.

38. Shelbourne KD, et al. Correlation of joint line tenderness and meniscal lesions in patients with acute anterior cruciate ligament tears. *Am J Sports Med.* 1995;23(2):166–169.

39. Hegedus EJ, et al. Physical examination tests for assessing a torn meniscus in the knee: a systematic review with meta-analysis. *J Orthop Sports Phys Ther.* 2007;37(9):541–550.

40. Meserve BB, Cleland JA, Boucher TR. A meta-analysis examining clinical test utilities for assessing meniscal injury. *Clin Rehabil.* 2008;22(2):143–161.

41. Terry GC, Tagert BE, Young MJ. Reliability of the clinical assessment in predicting the cause of internal derangements of the knee. *Arthroscopy.* 1995;11(5):568–576.

42. Kim SJ, Min BH, Han DY. Paradoxical phenomena of the McMurray test. An arthroscopic investigation. *Am J Sports Med.* 1996;24(1):83–87.

43. Kim SJ, et al. The paradoxical McMurray test for the detection of meniscal tears: an arthroscopic study of mechanisms, types, and accuracy. *J Bone Joint Surg Am.* 2012;94(16):e1181–e1187.

44. Leach RE, Gregg T, Siber FJ. Weight-bearing radiography in osteoarthritis of the knee. *Radiology.* 1970;97(2):265–268.

45. Rosenberg TD, et al. The forty-five-degree posteroanterior flexion weight-bearing radiograph of the knee. *J Bone Joint Surg Am.* 1988;70(10):1479–1483.

46. Francavilla ML, et al. Meniscal pathology in children: differences and similarities with the adult meniscus. *Pediatr Radiol.* 2014;44(8):910–925; quiz 907–909.

47. McDermott MJ, et al. Correlation of MRI and arthroscopic diagnosis of knee pathology in children and adolescents. *J Pediatr Orthop.* 1998;18(5):675–678.

48. Takeda Y, et al. MRI high-signal intensity in the menisci of asymptomatic children. *J Bone Joint Surg Br.* 1998; 80(3):463–467.

49. Kramer DE, Micheli LJ. Meniscal tears and discoid meniscus in children: diagnosis and treatment. *J Am Acad Orthop Surg.* 2009;17(11):698–707.

50. Boden SD, et al. A prospective and blinded investigation of magnetic resonance imaging of the knee. Abnormal findings in asymptomatic subjects. *Clin Orthop Relat Res.* 1992;282:177–185.

51. LaPrade RF, et al. The prevalence of abnormal magnetic resonance imaging findings in asymptomatic knees. With correlation of magnetic resonance imaging to arthroscopic findings in symptomatic knees. *Am J Sports Med.* 1994;22(6): 739–745.

52. Muellner T, et al. The diagnosis of meniscal tears in athletes. A comparison of clinical and magnetic resonance imaging investigations. *Am J Sports Med.* 1997;25(1):7–12.

53. Weiss CB, et al. Non-operative treatment of meniscal tears. *J Bone Joint Surg Am.* 1989;71(6):811–822.

54. Zanetti M, et al. Patients with suspected meniscal tears: prevalence of abnormalities seen on MRI of 100 symptomatic and 100 contralateral asymptomatic knees. *AJR Am J Roentgenol.* 2003;181(3):635–641.

55. Schimmer RC, et al. Arthroscopic partial meniscectomy: a 12-year follow-up and two-step evaluation of the long-term course. *Arthroscopy.* 1998;14(2):136–142.

56. Cappellino A, Jokl P, Ruwe PA. Regional anesthesia in knee arthroscopy: a new technique involving femoral and sciatic nerve blocks in knee arthroscopy. *Arthroscopy.* 1996;12(1):120–123.

57. Casati A, et al. Regional anaesthesia for outpatient knee arthroscopy: a randomized clinical comparison of two different anaesthetic techniques. *Acta Anaesthesiol Scand.* 2000;44(5):543–547.

58. Shapiro MS, et al. Local anesthesia for knee arthroscopy. Efficacy and cost benefits. *Am J Sports Med.* 1995;23(1):50–53.

59. Yoshiya S, et al. Knee arthroscopy using local anesthetic. *Arthroscopy.* 1988;4(2):86–89.

60. Moura EC, et al. Minimum effective concentration of bupivacaine in ultrasound-guided femoral nerve block after arthroscopic knee meniscectomy: a randomized, double-blind, controlled trial. *Pain Physician.* 2016;19(1):E79–E86.

61. Charalambous CP, et al. Purely intra-articular versus general anesthesia for proposed arthroscopic partial meniscectomy of the knee: a randomized controlled trial. *Arthroscopy.* 2006;22(9):972–977.

62. Kirkley A, et al. Tourniquet versus no tourniquet use in routine knee arthroscopy: a prospective, double-blind, randomized clinical trial. *Arthroscopy.* 2000;16(2):121–126.

63. Ong BC, Musahl V, et al. Knee: patient positioning, portal placement, and normal arthroscopic anatomy. In: Miller MD, ed. *Textbook of Arthroscopy.* Philadelphia, PA: Saunders; 2004:463–469.

64. Baer GS, Knee arthroscopy-the basics. In: Miller MD, Cosgarea AJ, Sekiya JK, eds. *Operative Techniques: Sports Knee Surgery.* Philadelphia, PA: Saunders; 2008:24–39.

65. Mochida H, Kikuchi S. Injury to infrapatellar branch of saphenous nerve in arthroscopic knee surgery. *Clin Orthop Relat Res.* 1995;320:88–94.

66. Tifford CD, et al. The relationship of the infrapatellar branches of the saphenous nerve to arthroscopy portals and incisions for anterior cruciate ligament surgery. An anatomic study. *Am J Sports Med.* 2000;28(4):562–567.

67. Kim TK, et al. Neurovascular complications of knee arthroscopy. *Am J Sports Med.* 2002;30(4):619–629.

68. Diduch DR, Ong BC. Knee: diagnostic arthroscopy. In: Miller MD, ed. *Textbook of Arthroscopy.* Philadelphia, PA: Saunders, 2004:471–487.

69. Gillquist J, Hagberg G, Oretorp N. Arthroscopic visualization of the posteromedial compartment of the knee joint. *Orthop Clin North Am.* 1979;10(3):545–547.

70. Greis PE, et al. Meniscal injury: II. Management. *J Am Acad Orthop Surg.* 2002;10(3):177–187.

71. Baer GS. Arthroscopic meniscectomy. In: Miller MD, Cosgarea AJ, Sekiya JK, eds. *Operative Techniques: Sports Knee Surgery.* Philadelphia, PA: Saunders; 2008:69–85.

72. Safran MR. Meniscus: diagnosis and decision making. In: Miller MD, ed. *Textbook of Arthroscopy.* Philadelphia, PA: Saunders; 2004:497–506.

73. Soto G. Arthroscopic meniscectomy. In: Miller MD, ed. *Textbook of Arthroscopy.* Philadelphia, PA: Saunders; 2004:507–516.

74. Carrier CS, et al. Patient satisfaction with nonopioid pain management following knee arthroscopic partial meniscectomy and/or chondroplasty. *Orthopedics*. 2018;41(4):209–214.

75. Anthony CA, et al. Opioid demand before and after anterior cruciate ligament reconstruction. *Am J Sports Med*. 2017;45(13):3098–3103.

76. Lessard LA, et al. The efficacy of cryotherapy following arthroscopic knee surgery. *J Orthop Sports Phys Ther*. 1997;26(1):14–22.

77. Whitelaw GP, et al. The use of the Cryo/Cuff versus ice and elastic wrap in the postoperative care of knee arthroscopy patients. *Am J Knee Surg*. 1995;8(1):28–30; discussion 30–31.

78. Martin SS, et al. Cryotherapy: an effective modality for decreasing intraarticular temperature after knee arthroscopy. *Am J Sports Med*. 2001;29(3):288–291.

79. Lamplot JD, Brophy RH. The role for arthroscopic partial meniscectomy in knees with degenerative changes: a systematic review. *Bone Joint J*. 2016;98-b(7):934–938.

80. Chahla J, et al. Meniscectomy and resultant articular cartilage lesions of the knee among prospective national football league players: an imaging and performance analysis. *Am J Sports Med*. 2018;46(1):200–207.

81. Pena E, et al. Why lateral meniscectomy is more dangerous than medial meniscectomy. A finite element study. *J Orthop Res*. 2006;24(5):1001–1010.

82. Aune KT, et al. Return to play after partial lateral meniscectomy in national football league athletes. *Am J Sports Med*. 2014;42(8):1865–1872.

83. Andersson-Molina H, Karlsson H, Rockborn P. Arthroscopic partial and total meniscectomy: a long-term follow-up study with matched controls. *Arthroscopy*. 2002;18(2):183–189.

84. Hulet CH, et al. Arthroscopic medial meniscectomy on stable knees. *J Bone Joint Surg Br*. 2001;83(1):29–32.

85. Hoser C, et al. Long-term results of arthroscopic partial lateral meniscectomy in knees without associated damage. *J Bone Joint Surg Br*. 2001;83(4):513–516.

86. Jaureguito JW, et al. The effects of arthroscopic partial lateral meniscectomy in an otherwise normal knee: a retrospective review of functional, clinical, and radiographic results. *Arthroscopy*. 1995;11(1):29–36.

87. Scheller G, Sobau C, Bulow JU. Arthroscopic partial lateral meniscectomy in an otherwise normal knee: clinical, functional, and radiographic results of a long-term follow-up study. *Arthroscopy*. 2001;17(9):946–952.

88. Chatain F, et al. The natural history of the knee following arthroscopic medial meniscectomy. *Knee Surg Sports Traumatol Arthrosc*. 2001;9(1):15–18.

89. Burks RT, Metcalf MH, Metcalf RW. Fifteen-year follow-up of arthroscopic partial meniscectomy. *Arthroscopy*. 1997;13(6):673–679.

90. Stein T, et al. Long-term outcome after arthroscopic meniscal repair versus arthroscopic partial meniscectomy for traumatic meniscal tears. *Am J Sports Med*. 2010;38(8):1542–1548.

91. Neyret P, Donell ST, Dejour H. Results of partial meniscectomy related to the state of the anterior cruciate ligament. Review at 20 to 35 years. *J Bone Joint Surg Br*. 1993;75(1):36–40.

92. Fabricant PD, Jokl P. Surgical outcomes after arthroscopic partial meniscectomy. *J Am Acad Orthop Surg*. 2007;15(11):647–653.

93. Salzler MJ, et al. Complications after arthroscopic knee surgery. *Am J Sports Med*. 2014;42(2):292–296.

94. DeLee JC. Complications of arthroscopy and arthroscopic surgery: results of a national survey. Committee on Complications of Arthroscopy Association of North America. *Arthroscopy*. 1985;1(4):214–220.

95. Kieser C. A review of the complications of arthroscopic knee surgery. *Arthroscopy*. 1992;8(1):79–83.

96. Small NC. Complications in arthroscopic surgery performed by experienced arthroscopists. *Arthroscopy*. 1988;4(3):215–221.

97. Jorgensen U, et al. Long-term follow-up of meniscectomy in athletes. A prospective longitudinal study. *J Bone Joint Surg Br*. 1987;69(1):80–83.

98. Ahn JH, et al. Longitudinal tear of the medial meniscus posterior horn in the anterior cruciate ligament-deficient knee significantly influences anterior stability. *Am J Sports Med*. 2011;39(10):2187–2193.

99. Levy IM, Torzilli PA, Warren RF. The effect of medial meniscectomy on anterior-posterior motion of the knee. *J Bone Joint Surg Am*. 1982;64(6):883–888.

100. Seon JK, et al. The effect of anterior cruciate ligament reconstruction on kinematics of the knee with combined anterior cruciate ligament injury and subtotal medial meniscectomy: an in vitro robotic investigation. *Arthroscopy*. 2009;25(2):123–130.

101. Buseck MS, Noyes FR. Arthroscopic evaluation of meniscal repairs after anterior cruciate ligament reconstruction and immediate motion. *Am J Sports Med*. 1991;19(5):489–494.

102. Tenuta JJ, Arciero RA. Arthroscopic evaluation of meniscal repairs. Factors that effect healing. *Am J Sports Med*. 1994;22(6):797–802.

103. Feeley BT, Lau BC. Biomechanics and clinical outcomes of partial meniscectomy. *J Am Acad Orthop Surg*. 2018;26(24):853–863.

104. Fauno P, Nielsen AB. Arthroscopic partial meniscectomy: a long-term follow-up. *Arthroscopy*. 1992;8(3):345–349.

105. Ode GE, et al. Effects of serial sectioning and repair of radial tears in the lateral meniscus. *Am J Sports Med*. 2012;40(8):1863–1870.

106. Bedi A, et al. Dynamic contact mechanics of radial tears of the lateral meniscus: implications for treatment. *Arthroscopy*. 2012;28(3):372–381.

107. Bedi A, et al. Dynamic contact mechanics of the medial meniscus as a function of radial tear, repair, and partial meniscectomy. *J Bone Joint Surg Am*. 2010;92(6):1398–1408.

108. Brown MJ, et al. Biomechanical effects of a horizontal medial meniscal tear and subsequent leaflet resection. *Am J Sports Med*. 2016;44(4):850–854.

109. Englund M, et al. Patient-relevant outcomes fourteen years after meniscectomy: influence of type of meniscal tear and size of resection. *Rheumatology (Oxford)*. 2001;40(6):631–639.

110. Mesiha M, et al. Pathologic characteristics of the torn human meniscus. *Am J Sports Med*. 2007;35(1):103–112.

111. Englund M, Lohmander LS. Risk factors for symptomatic knee osteoarthritis fifteen to twenty-two years after meniscectomy. *Arthritis Rheum*. 2004;50(9):2811–2819.

23 Meniscal Repair Techniques

Zaira S. Chaudhry, Max R. Greenky, and Steven B. Cohen

INDICATIONS

Indications for meniscal repair are similar regardless of technique. It is generally agreed upon that factors that are favorable for repair include acute symptomatic tears, longitudinal orientation, peripheral zone (red-red/red-white tears), tears >7 to 10 mm in length, unstable tears with >3 mm excursion, concomitant reconstructive surgery (ACL or articular cartilage), and patients who prefer this procedure over continued nonoperative treatment.

Many find that tears of the anterior one-third of the meniscus are still most easily and predictably repaired with either outside-in or open techniques, with all-inside techniques being reserved for more posterior tears and those involving the body of the meniscus. Posterior one-third tears are more difficult to reach using an inside-out technique, and this technique also places the neurovascular structures, such as the saphenous nerve medially or peroneal nerve laterally, at greater risk for injury. Moreover, all-inside devices are designed to be inserted perpendicular to the tear. An anterior anatomic location may make this difficult despite switching portals or using an accessory portal. Some feel that traditional inside-out sutures placed in variable configurations are preferable for repairing bucket handle tears displaced into the notch because, traditionally, it had been thought that the inside-out technique allows more reliable tensioning of the suture into a meniscus that has been torn. However, with the advent of suture-based fixators, bucket handle tears may also be secured reliably using the all-inside devices. It is also important to note that some tears may be best addressed with hybrid repairs.

CONTRAINDICATIONS

Contraindications for meniscal repair may include degenerative tears in older patients, avascular tears in the white-white zone, complex tear patterns, stable/incomplete tears, associated infectious/rheumatologic/collagen vascular diseases, or patients unable to comply with weight bearing and motion restrictions. Some surgeons will allow immediate weight bearing in extension following repair, with the thought that hoop stresses placed through the meniscus will not harm and in fact may aid in healing. In spite of this, many still maintain the traditional protocol of nonweight or partial weight bearing for up to 6 weeks. This conversation with the patient and their ability to comply with these restrictions is necessary prior to every planned arthroscopy with the potential for meniscal repair. Moreover, the patient must understand that a tear may be found irreparable intraoperatively, and a final decision may be made at that time.

PREOPERATIVE PREPARATION

The patient is placed in the supine position and inducted with general anesthesia. A tourniquet is applied to the thigh, and a lateral post is utilized. The entire extremity is prepped and draped in a standard fashion to avoid contamination. Anterolateral and anteromedial portals are then established to perform an initial diagnostic arthroscopy to confirm that the meniscal tear is repairable and identify any concomitant pathology. The inferior and superior portions of the meniscus, meniscal root, and capsule attachment of the meniscus should be thoroughly evaluated. Depending on the location of the tear, additional portals may be required for adequate visualization.

TECHNIQUES

Meniscal Preparation

Once a meniscal tear is identified arthroscopically and indicated for repair, preparation of the site prior to repair is crucial. Meniscal preparation is performed in a standard fashion regardless of which repair technique is being utilized. Using a motorized shaver and/or rasp, both sides of the tear are debrided of fibrous tissue that may have formed during an attempt at healing. A peripheral tear near the meniscal/synovial junction may show signs of bleeding if the inflow is momentarily stopped and the intra-articular pressure is decreased. Also, a large bore needle may be used often "outside-in" to trephinate the meniscus and allow for vascular access channels.

FIBRIN CLOT TECHNIQUE

Use of exogenous fibrin clot has been shown in both animal and human studies to promote healing in what may be an avascular portion of the meniscus (1). The mechanism by which this technique improves the healing rate is not clear, but it coincides with the evidence that meniscal tears repaired during ACL reconstruction have a higher rate of healing presumably due to the hemarthrosis and its associated chemotactic and reparative properties. Moreover, it has been reported that isolated meniscal repairs without the addition of exogenous fibrin clots are associated with a 41% failure rate, whereas meniscal repairs with concomitant exogenous fibrin clots are associated with an 8% failure rate (1). This adjunct procedure can be used to promote meniscal healing regardless of the meniscal repair technique being utilized.

  Preparation of the clot is carried out on the back table while the surgeon is repairing the meniscus. The clot may or may not be secured with suture, and it is often placed on the undersurface of the tear between the meniscus and the tibia (1–3). An alternative to using fibrin clot is performing microfracture around the intercondylar notch to stimulate additional bleeding in the joint.

ALL-INSIDE TECHNIQUE

Regardless of the device chosen for implantation, several basic principles apply. Reduction of the meniscus is essential prior to fixation. Some recommend temporary K-wire or needle fixation to hold the reduction while the implant is placed. Fixators should be inserted perpendicular to the tear, and accessory or contralateral portals are often required to do so. When multiple devices are used, they are typically spaced in 3- to 5-mm intervals. Once the device is secured, the surgeon must be sure the fixator head or suture is not prominent in the joint to avoid articular damage. The repair site should then be probed for any gapping prior to and after the knee is taken through gentle range of motion. Any gapping or instability should be addressed with further fixation.

First-Generation All-Inside Repair Devices

Since their introduction over a decade ago, all-inside devices have undergone an evolution. The initial most commonly used "first-generation" fixators were:

  Meniscus Arrow (Bionx, Blue Bell, Pennsylvania, 1996)
  T-Fix (Acufex/Smith and Nephew, Andover, Massachusetts)
  SD Sorb Staple (Surgical Dynamics, Norwalk, Connecticut, 1997)
  Biostinger (Linvatec, Largo, Florida, 1998)
  Fastener (Mitek, Westwood, Massachusetts, 1998)
  Clearfix Screw (Mitek, Westwood, Massachusetts, 1998)
  Dart (Arthrex, Naples, Florida, 1999)

These devices were similar in that they were somewhat rigid devices made up of varying amounts of polymerized levorotatory polylactic acid (PLLA) and polyglactic acid (PGA). The manufacturers for two devices, the Arrow and the Dart, changed the composition of their implants in the early 2000s to include the polylactic acid dextrorotatory "D" stereoisomer configuration (PDLLA). This configuration is more amorphous and possesses different degradation properties (4).

Meniscus Arrow

The first popular fixation device, the Arrow, was "T" shaped with a 4-mm long cross bar and a shaft of varying lengths to be used at the surgeon's discretion. The shafts had reverse barbs projecting 90 degrees from each other. Each could be inserted manually or via a device known as the "crossbow" that held multiple arrows and facilitated multiple implant insertions. The disadvantages included chondral damage from retained PLLA fragments as well as suboptimal fixation strength. A systematic review showed that the Meniscus Arrow was by far the most studied device and had a failure rate between 5% and 43.5%, with higher rates occurring, as expected, in studies with longer follow-up (5). Siebold et al. reported on long-term outcomes of patients treated with all-inside arthroscopic Meniscus Arrow repair and noted a 28.4% failure rate at a mean follow-up of 6 years, with over 80% of these failures occurring during the first 3 postoperative years (6).

T-Fix

The T-Fix device was originally designed in 1984 but was made usable by the advent of the arthroscopic knot pusher by Joe Sklar, MD. The device consisted of a 17-gauge needle preloaded with blue nonabsorbable suture tied to a polyacetal absorbable bar or "T." A small obturator slid down the needle and pushed the "T" out and clear of the needle tip. A second T-Fix was then inserted 3 to 4 mm from the first, and arthroscopic knots were tied external to the knee and were tensioned using the knot pusher. Much research has been done on the T-Fix, mostly case series and retrospective reviews with failure rates ranging from 1.8% to 43% (5). Again, the studies with longer follow-up tended to reveal higher failure rates.

SD Sorb Staple

The SD Sorb Staple device consisted of two barbed 7-mm fixation posts linked by a 4-mm braided nonabsorbable suture providing two points of fixation. It could be inserted using a manual device or a multifire gun and reportedly resorbed in 15 months. Newer modifications of this device include a lower profile insertion system and longer fixation posts.

Biostinger

Linvatec's Biostinger was the first cannulated device with a lower profile head allowing insertion over a needle trocar. The violet-colored fixator was easily visualized in the joint, and the newly developed "Hornet" insertion device allowed for easy one-handed placement. The implant contained four rows of barbs that decreased pullout strength and came in three sizes each with its own disposable insertion device. Two studies by Barber et al. showed failure rates of 4.9% to 9.0% in 88 patients over a 2- to 3-year follow-up (7,8).

Fastener

Mitek's Fastener was part of their Meniscal Repair System introduced in 1998. The "T"- or "J"-shaped fixator device came in two sizes (6 and 8 mm) with two suture materials, nonabsorbable Prolene (Ethicon, Cincinnati, Ohio) and absorbable PDS (Ethicon). The insertion device also came in three angled tips. The reported advantage of the Fastener was that it was one of the few devices that could be used for a peripheral meniscus tear and that the cross-limb of the device could be placed beyond the capsule. In a study of 37 patients who underwent meniscal repair with this device, there were five retears at 1-year follow-up (9). The results were similar to other techniques at that time.

Clearfix Screw

The Clearfix Screw, a 2-mm-diameter by 10-mm long headless screw with a 0.3-mm variable pitch, was designed to allow for countersinking and compression across the tear site. Insertion was similar to other techniques via a cannulated needle-guided system. Multiple studies have reported a 10% to 25% failure rate for this device (5).

Dart

The meniscus repair Dart, released in 1999, was low profile and headless with a barb configuration of a double reverse design. This improved both pull-out strength as well as pull-through strength, thereby limiting migration of the implant. It could be inserted manually or using a spring-loaded delivery system and curved cannulae. Updates have included a preloaded insertion device called the "Dart Stick." Although lacking in clinical studies, the Dart showed inferior biomechanical properties of ultimate tensile load and stiffness as compared to other first-generation devices and traditional inside-out techniques (10).

Second-Generation All-Inside Repair Devices

There is no clear consensus as to which devices definitively belong to the first, second, or later generations. Many improvements and advances have been made on the original instrumentation described above making them second generation for that particular device. However, several newly designed devices have incorporated recent advancements and can truly be termed "second generation."

Disadvantages of first-generation devices included risk of injury to neurovascular structures, foreign body reaction, and chondral damage secondary to implant prominence. They were also less suitable for peripheral meniscus tears and continued to be inferior to more traditional techniques in biomechanical studies. New implants were designed to improve the surgeon's ability to repair a peripheral tear and increase the fixation strength using absorbable, permanent, or hybrid bioabsorbable fixator/anchor and suture constructs.

FasT-Fix

Designed in 2001 by Smith and Nephew, the FasT-Fix meniscal repair system uses the same 5-mm anchor bar as the T-Fix, but the new needle delivery system includes two anchors attached to a braided suture that can be deployed and tightened in series using a preloaded, pretied self-sliding knot. Advancements include the anchors that attach extracapsularly and the sequentially fired implants that allow for both a vertical or a horizontal mattress configuration and the ability to tension across the repair site (Fig. 23-1). The needle delivery system is supplied with three angles: 0, +22, and −22 degrees. The −22 degree needle can be used to place the implant on the undersurface of the meniscus. In a retrospective review of 81 patients who underwent meniscal repair using the FasT-Fix system, it was reported that 84% of patients continued to demonstrate intact repairs after a minimum follow-up of 5 years (11).

RapidLoc

Mitek released a similar device in 2001, which also utilizes a similar "backstop" anchor that crosses the tear site and attaches extracapsularly. Only one device is deployed and tensioned at a time using a sequentially loaded second anchor known as a "top hat," which then slides down the suture via an

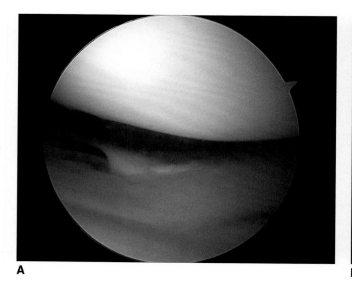
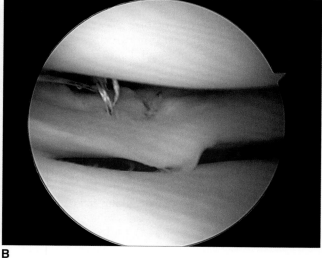

A   **B**

FIGURE 23-1

A: Arthroscopic view of a longitudinal tear of the lateral meniscus in a left knee from the lateral portal. **B:** Arthroscopic view of an all-inside meniscus repair of the lateral meniscus using two FasT-Fix devices.

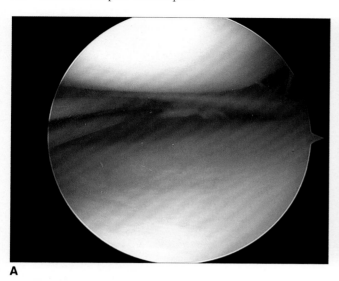

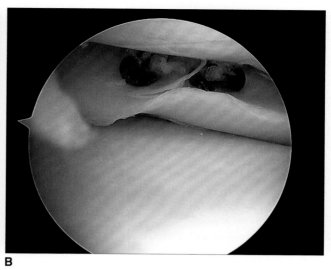

A   **B**

FIGURE 23-2

A: Arthroscopic view of an undersurface longitudinal medial meniscus tear in a left knee from the lateral portal. **B:** Arthroscopic view of an all-inside meniscus repair of the medial meniscus using two RapidLoc devices.

overlying preloaded, pretied, self-sliding knot and compresses the tear. An arthroscopic knot pusher may then be utilized to "cinch" the top hat down even further just until it "dimples" the meniscus (Fig. 23-2). The delivery needle systems are also available in multiple angles. A recent study with a median follow-up of 10 years reported a 48% failure rate among patients who underwent meniscal repair using the RapidLoc system, with approximately one-third of these failures occurring two or more years after the index meniscal repair (12).

The FasT-Fix and RapidLoc are currently two of the most widely used all-inside devices. Their techniques for use were well described in Chapter 9 of the 3rd edition of *Master Techniques in Orthopaedic Surgery: Reconstructive Knee Surgery.*

Third- and Fourth-Generation All-Inside Repair Devices

Over the past few years, several newer all-inside meniscal repair devices have emerged. Depending on the source, these devices may be regarded as third or fourth generation.

MaxFire

The Biomet MaxFire, introduced in March of 2007, is a suture-only system and utilizes "Ziploop" technology. "Ziploop" is a unique weave in which a single strand of braided polyethylene is woven through itself twice in opposing directions, thereby allowing the surgeon to customize the length and tension of the suture. It is a knotless system, yet has been found to be incredibly strong and resistant to slippage. Similar to other systems, the MaxFire has two sequentially loaded "anchors" that allow the surgeon to place either a horizontal or vertical mattress configuration (Figs. 23-3–23-5). The MarXmen gun, also provided by Biomet, is a one-handed trigger delivery system that uses a needle to insert the MaxFire device through the meniscus. Multiple biomechanical studies have demonstrated that the FasT-Fix and Meniscal Cinch devices can withstand significantly greater cyclic loads before failure than the MaxFire repair device (13,14).

Meniscal Cinch

The Arthrex Meniscal Cinch, approved in March 2008, uses a pistol grip handle and slotted curved cannula to deploy its double-loaded polyetheretherketone (PEEK) anchors. A pretied sliding knot of 2.0 Fiberwire can then be tensioned to compress across the repair site (Figs. 23-6–23-8). According to the manufacturer's studies, the ultimate load to failure is approximately 100 N, which exceeds that of comparable devices (15). Moreover, meniscal repairs using the Meniscal Cinch device have demonstrated equivalent biomechanical properties to the classic vertical mattress suture repair technique (13).

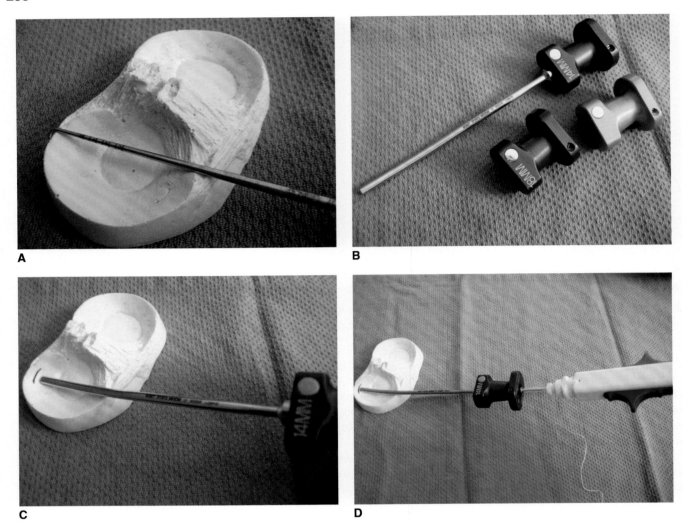

FIGURE 23-3

A: Once the location of the tear and optimal portal placement has been determined, measure the width of the tear using a meniscal depth gauge. **B:** After the correct measurement is determined, the appropriate color-coded barrel is attached to the cannula. **C:** An obturator is inserted into the cannula until desired position at the tear site is achieved at which point the obturator is removed. **D:** The MaxFire Meniscal Repair device is inserted into the cannula/barrel assembly by aligning the flats of the barrel with either flat on the tip of the MaxFire inserter handle.

SpeedCinch

The SpeedCinch (Arthrex, Naples, Florida) is a one-handed device with a low-profile needle that is designed to actively deploy small implants while limiting needle exposure. Low-profile 2-0 Fiberwire suture with a pretied knot allows for easy tensioning for either vertical or horizontal suture repairs. A recent biomechanical study by Milchteim et al. tested the mean maximum failure loads of meniscal repairs using two parallel vertical sutures created with the SpeedCinch, two crossed vertical sutures created with the SpeedCinch, two parallel vertical sutures created with the FasT-Fix 360, and two crossed vertical sutures created with the FasT-Fix 360; they noted that both devices had similar failure loads and stiffness regardless of the suture pattern (16).

Ultra FasT-Fix and FasT-Fix 360

Building upon the FasT-Fix device, Smith and Nephew designed the Ultra FasT-Fix system, an implant system with a pretied, self-sliding knot that does not require intra-articular knot tying. This system has an ultra-high molecular weight polyethylene suture (Ultrabraid) with the option of non-absorbable PEEK or bioabsorbable PLLA anchors. Standard straight and curved delivery needles are

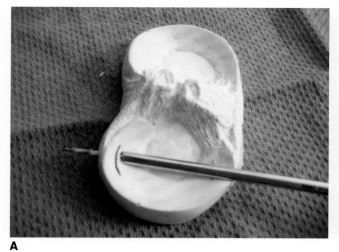

A

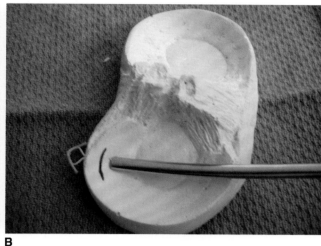

B

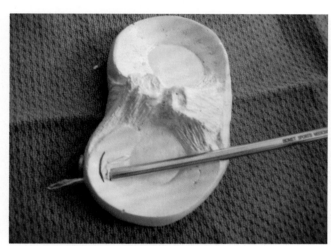

C

FIGURE 23-4

A: While maintaining gentle but firm pressure on the meniscus, the first all-suture anchor is passed by advancing the green trigger to its forward mechanical stop. **B:** Once the green lever has reached its forward mechanical stop, the green trigger is pulled back to its end point. **C:** The cannula is repositioned 5 to 10 mm away from the first anchor and toward the side corresponding with the red trigger of the inserter and the second anchor is fired.

available, and the device is deployed passively. Moreover, in an effort to minimize the risk of trauma to the ACL, this system contains no rigid structures. More recently, Smith and Nephew released the FasT-Fix 360 system. Advancements include an active deployment mechanism that enables deployment of implants in any hand position and built-in adjustable depth penetration (10–18 mm). Due to the smaller implants, the FasT-Fix 360 also allows for smaller insertion points, thereby allowing for minimal disruption to the meniscus.

Knee Scorpion

The Knee Scorpion suture passer and retriever (Arthrex, Naples, Florida) enables surgeons to pass 0 and 2-0 Fiberwire in tight recesses. It is a one-handed suture passer with an angled jaw that is designed for single step passage and retrieval of suture through a single portal, which eliminates the need for extra steps. However, considering that it is a relatively new device, there is currently a paucity of literature reporting the biomechanical results of repairs performed with the Knee Scorpion all-inside device.

Omnispan

The Omnispan (DuPuy Mitek, Raynham, Massachusetts) consists of a low-profile needle preloaded with two PEEK backstops connected by No. 2/0 Orthocord high strength orthopaedic suture, and it also has an active deployment applier. To avoid contact of rigid objects with the meniscal surface, the device was designed so that the backstops and suture knot are located at the periphery of the meniscus. An arthroscopic probe is used to tension the sutures, and each suture leg is then cut with the suture pusher/cutter.

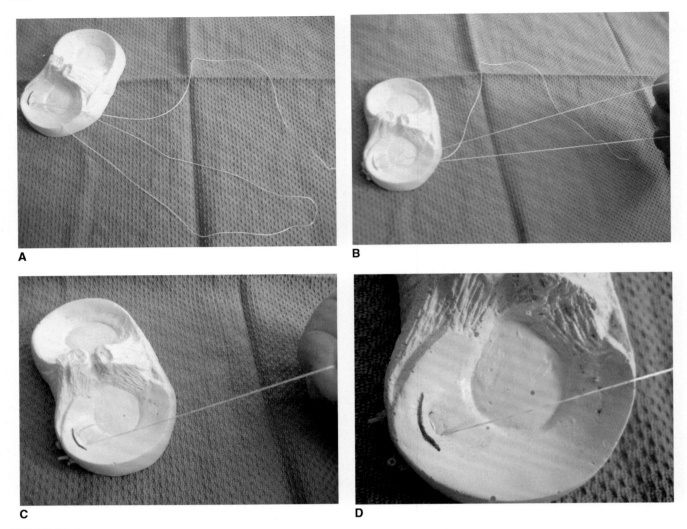

FIGURE 23-5
A: Once both suture anchors have been deployed across the tear, the MaxFire inserter/cannula/barrel assembly is removed from the joint. A large loop and a free strand of suture will remain outside the portal site. **B:** One finger is placed inside the large loop and pulled until the first stitch between the anchors slides down against the meniscus. **C:** The suture is pulled until the desired tension is achieved. The free strand is then pulled, which will reduce the large loop into the portal site and down to the meniscus. **D:** Next, using a MaxCutter device, the suture is passed through the bottom side (concave side) of the instrument. The MaxCutter device is inserted into the portal and advanced to cut the suture.

CrossFix

The CrossFix (Cayenne Medical, Scottsdale, Arizona) is an all-suture device with a pretied, sliding "Hot Knot" that creates an instantaneous 3-mm mattress stitch, replicating standard open suturing repair techniques. It allows for a single insertion with a dual needle design and is available with both straight and curved needles. In addition, the inserter has a built-in depth limiter that controls the degree of needle penetration. Barber et al. noted that repairs using an obliquely oriented stitch of No. 0 ultra high-molecular weight polyethylene suture inserted with the CrossFix device had a mean single-pull failure load of 77 N, whereas the Ultra FasT-Fix (121 N) and MaxFire (130 N) withstood greater loads (17).

Sequent

The Sequent (ConMed Linvatec, Largo, Florida) is composed of four or seven PEEK implants connected by Hi-FI braided suture. This device allows for a maximum of six sequential stitches that can be individually tensioned and fixed to create a knotless repair in any configuration. The implants are actively deployed, and the device can remain in the joint when making multiple suture

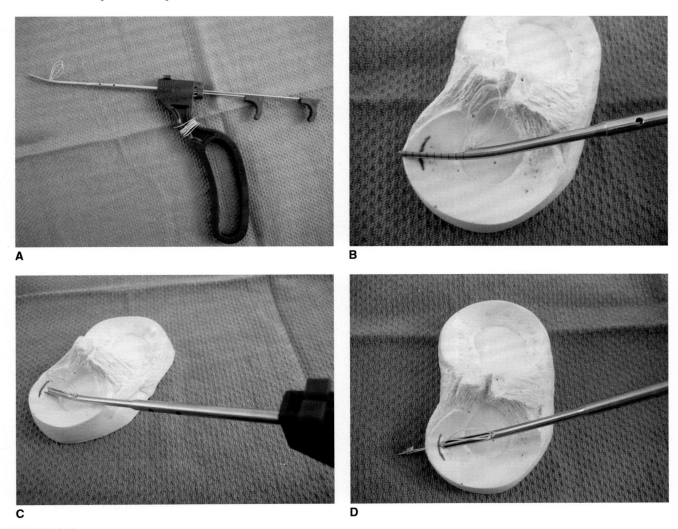

FIGURE 23-6

A: The Meniscal Cinch by Arthrex utilizes an ergonomic pistol grip handle, a slotted cannula, and external depth stop for the insertion of its implants. **B:** The measurement probe or the graduated tip of the Meniscal Cinch is used through a low arthroscopic portal, near the surface of the tibia, to measure the approximate distance from the entry point of the implant to capsule. **C:** The stop on the Meniscal Cinch handle is set based on the depth measurement. The tip of the cinch cannula is placed near the tear. The tip of the cannula may be used for manual reduction of the tear. **D:** The first implant is advanced through the meniscus by pushing trocar #1 until the trocar handle makes contact with the depth stop and the cannula rests on the surface of the meniscus.

placements. In a biomechanical study by Ramappa et al., the Sequent demonstrated significantly lower displacement in response to cyclic loading compared with both the Ultra FasT-Fix device and No. 0 Hi-FI inside-out repair, although the authors noted that this finding may not be clinically relevant (18).

NovoStitch Plus

The NovoStitch Plus (Ceterix Orthopaedics, Menlo Park, California), approved in 2015, allows for the placement of circumferential compression stitches, thereby providing anatomical reduction and uniform compression of the tear edges. This novel device enables surgeons to pass independent sutures to repair complex tear patterns as well as tears adjacent to the popliteal hiatus. The needle remains intra-articular without penetrating the capsule wall during sewing to minimize the risk of neurovascular injury. Although this is a relatively new device, according to a recent biomechanical study by Masoudi et al., the NovoStitch had comparable load to failure and displacement values during cyclic loading when compared with FasT-Fix 360 all-inside anchor-based repair and inside-out suture repair (19).

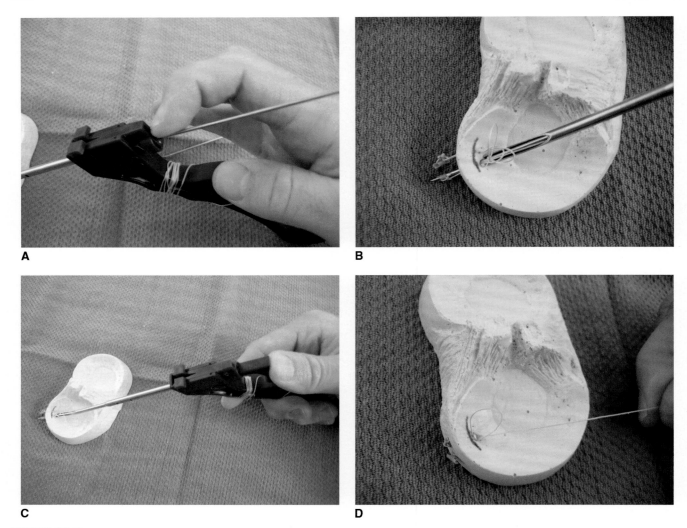

FIGURE 23-7

A: Trocar #1 is removed from the cannula completely and then trocar #2 is pushed down to release it from the holding position. The tip of the cannula is moved to the second insertion point over the meniscus. **B, C:** Trocar #2 is advanced forward by pushing the trocar handle forward and through the meniscus until the trocar handle makes contact with the depth stop and the cannula rests on the surface of the meniscus. **D:** Trocar #2 and the Meniscal Cinch are removed from the joint. The external suture is tensioned to advance the knot to the meniscus.

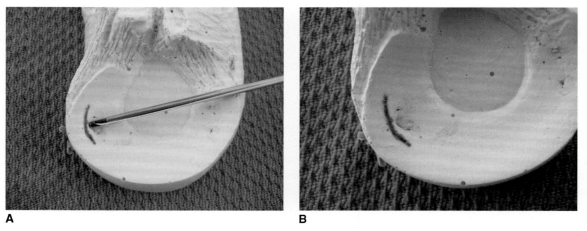

FIGURE 23-8

A: The suture is placed through the knot pusher/suture cutter. The knot is pushed while pulling on the free end of the suture until the knot is countersunk in the meniscal tissue. **B:** Using the knot pusher/suture cutter, the suture is cut.

INSIDE-OUT TECHNIQUE

Inside-out repair is the gold standard by which other meniscal repair techniques are judged (20). Prior to inside-out repair, tear debridement and perisynovial abrasion with a rasp or shaver are performed to promote healing as described earlier. The posterior border of the collateral ligaments is used as a landmark for the 3- to 4-cm skin incision, with two-thirds of the incision located distal to the joint line. When repairing the medial meniscus, the fascia is exposed, layer one is incised, and the medial gastrocnemius and hamstrings are retracted. To avoid iatrogenic injury to neurovascular structures and assist with needle passage, a popliteal or Henning retractor is placed between the posterior capsule of the joint and the medial head of the gastrocnemius (21). When repairing the lateral meniscus, the knee is positioned at 70 to 90 degrees of flexion in an effort to reduce tension on the peroneal nerve, and the lateral gastrocnemius is carefully reflected off of the posterior capsule.

Depending on the surgeon's preference, single or double lumen cannulas can be used. The suture cannula is placed through the contralateral portal and directed toward the meniscal tear under arthroscopic visualization. With the knee positioned at 10 to 20 degrees of flexion, a needle with a suture attached is advanced through the cannula and passed through the meniscus exiting laterally (21). Needle retrieval may be facilitated by further flexing the knee. The cannula is then repositioned to allow for passage and retrieval of a second needle. The second suture is placed adjacent to the first, creating a vertical, a horizontal, or an oblique suture pattern depending on tear morphology and surgeon preference. After suture placement, the sutures are cut free from the needles; the sutures are then tensioned and tied over the joint capsule. Tying is performed with the knee in 70 to 90 degrees of flexion when repairing lateral meniscus tears. When repairing medial meniscus tears, tying is performed with the knee in slight flexion or closer to full extension. Figures 23-9 and 23-10 illustrate arthroscopic inside-out repair of a bucket-handle tear.

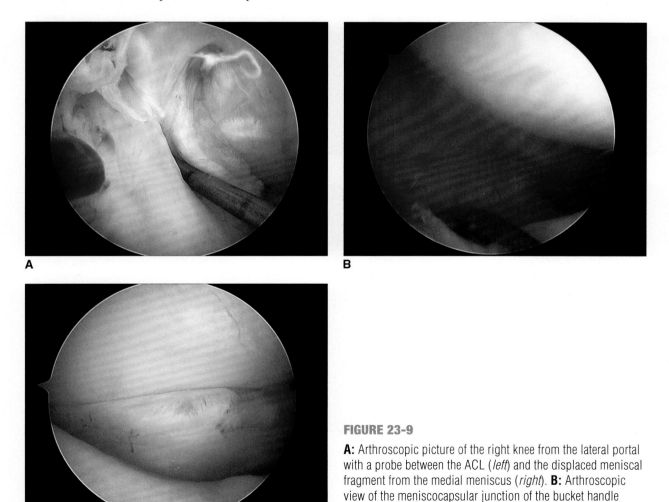

A

B

C

FIGURE 23-9

A: Arthroscopic picture of the right knee from the lateral portal with a probe between the ACL (*left*) and the displaced meniscal fragment from the medial meniscus (*right*). **B:** Arthroscopic view of the meniscocapsular junction of the bucket handle meniscus tear. **C:** Arthroscopic view of the displaced bucket handle tear in front of the medial femoral condyle.

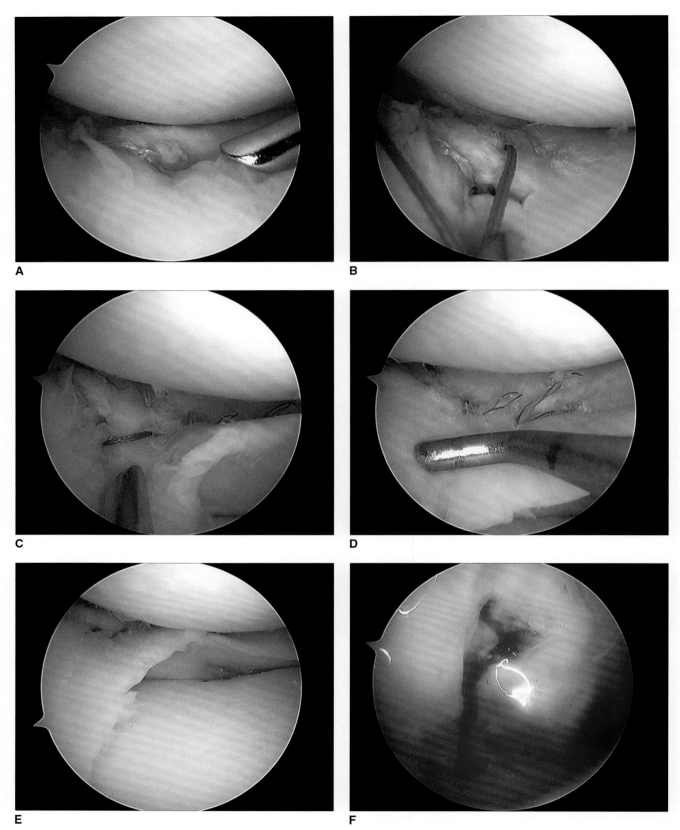

A

B

C

D

E

F

FIGURE 23-10

A–E: Arthroscopic view of the meniscal repair using inside-out repair technique. **F:** Arthroscopic view of the "crimson duvet" in the intercondylar notch after microfracture.

OUTSIDE-IN TECHNIQUE

The outside-in technique can be performed with 18-gauge spinal needles, an arthroscopic grasper, and rigid monofilament suture material (22). After preparing the tear and synovium as previously described, the knee is flexed appropriately depending on the location of the tear. A valgus or varus force can be placed on the knee to aid in needle passage. Under arthroscopic visualization, the needle is directed toward the superior or inferior meniscal surface. Care must be taken to avoid iatrogenic injury to the ACL surface during needle passage. After making a small incision around the initial needle puncture and spreading the subcutaneous tissue down to the capsule, a second needle is placed adjacent to the first to allow for proper suture orientation. A cannula may be used to assist in pulling the sutures out of the joint space. With a cannula placed in the appropriate portal, rigid monofilament suture is passed through each needle and pulled out anteriorly from the knee (23). Next, a 2-0 high strength suture is shuttled through the meniscus and passed through the capsule where the prior incision was made.

The orientation of the sutures (i.e., vertical, horizontal) is based on tear morphology and surgeon preference, although vertical mattress sutures have been found to be biomechanically superior (24,25). When placing a vertical mattress suture, the first needle is placed across the tear through the superior surface of the meniscus and the second needle is placed across the synovial junction (23). Under direct visualization, adjacent sutures are tied together over the joint capsule using a one-handed sliding locking knot technique.

PEARLS AND PITFALLS

All-Inside Repair

All-inside repair is an appropriate technique for meniscal tears involving the body and posterior horn region. However, it is generally not considered an optimal technique for tears involving the anterior horn or tears at the meniscocapsular junction because an intact meniscal rim is necessary for anchoring the repair device (26). All-inside repair offers the advantage of decreased operative time, less technical difficulty, and it eliminates the need for accessory incisions. However, extreme care must be taken to avoid chondral and neurovascular injury while manipulating the devices. The portal that allows for the most perpendicular approach to the tear should be utilized whenever possible (27).

All-inside repair can be used to treat meniscal root tears, with favorable outcomes reported in the literature (28). However, arthroscopic transtibial pullout repair is the more commonly used technique for meniscal root tears (29). Please note that repair of meniscal root tears is addressed extensively in Chapter 24 of the current text.

Inside-Out Repair

Inside-out repair is considered the gold standard for meniscal tears involving the body and posterior horn region. However, repair of meniscal tears involving the anterior horn may be challenging with this technique. With inside-out repair, an accessory incision is required in order to access the posterior joint capsule for suture retrieval; due to the anatomic proximity of key structures, this increases the risk of neurovascular injury. Placing suture cannulas from the contralateral portal of the repair may decrease the risk of injury (30). In addition, slight retraction of the suture cannula should allow the surgeon to visualize the precise placement of the needle prior to suture passage. When tying the sutures, it is important to ensure direct placement on the capsule to prevent nerve or soft tissue entrapment.

Outside-In Repair

Outside-in repair is most appropriate for meniscal tears involving the anterior horn region. In general, tears located in the posterior horn are less amendable to outside-in repair as orienting the needle and suture perpendicular to the tear can be particularly challenging. Considering that outside-in repair does not require the use of a rigid cannula, this technique decreases the risk of chondral injury (23). Moreover, because the spinal needle enters the joint under direct visualization during outside-in repair, the surgeon can avoid damage to articular cartilage and neurovascular structures. The use of a small cannula in the portal is critical for avoiding any soft tissue bridge when shuttling the suture back through the capsule.

Repair of Radial Tears

Radial tears transect the meniscus in a perpendicular fashion, which has more detrimental biomechanical consequences than longitudinal tears as disruption of the circumferential fibers impairs resistance to normal hoop stresses (31). This can result in increased joint contact stress, which has implications for the development of arthrosis. Radial tear patterns vary depending on which portion of the meniscus is involved, with differences noted in terms of whether the lateral meniscus or medial meniscus is affected. There is limited, albeit promising, literature indicating that repair of radial tears is feasible and can result in favorable outcomes (32). A recently published systematic review found six retrospective studies that evaluated outcomes in a total of 55 patients following repair of radial tears using various inside-out and all-inside techniques; their findings indicate that subjective outcome scores improve following repair of radial tears, and short-term clinical outcomes are favorable (32). However, there is a need for higher level evidence with larger data sets to evaluate the long-term outcomes of radial tear repair. In light of the paucity of higher-level evidence, recommendations regarding the optimal technique for repairing radial tears cannot be made.

POSTOPERATIVE MANAGEMENT

Differences exist from surgeon to surgeon regarding postoperative protocols for meniscal repair. However, several similar principles apply. The goal is to restore painless range of motion while ensuring that the repair site is not compromised during the rehabilitation course. In addition, adequate pain control is paramount in achieving early range of motion. This may begin in the operating room with intra-articular injections of long-acting analgesics and the application of a cryotherapy cuff to help control pain and inflammation.

Patients are allowed to partial weight bear in extension (locked in a range of motion hinged brace) immediately after surgery. We feel that after the repair of a longitudinal tear, weight bearing provides hoop stresses to further compress across the tear site. Active and passive range of motion is encouraged but limited to 90 degrees of flexion while the patient is not bearing weight for the first 4 weeks. Once protective quadriceps strength has returned, usually in 2 to 4 weeks, the patient is allowed to ambulate with the brace unlocked to 90 degrees. The brace is unlocked to fully open by 6 weeks with full unprotected weight bearing. The brace is then discontinued completely by 8 weeks. The patient is also instructed to avoid deep knee bends or loaded squats until closer to 10 to 12 weeks following surgery. These restrictions are often based on tear type, location, and the age of the patient.

To our knowledge, there are currently no multicenter prospective studies comparing rehabilitation protocols, although several small studies exist showing successful results with early accelerated rehabilitation including immediate unrestricted weight bearing and range of motion (33,34). A recent systematic review noted that both restricted weight bearing and early accelerated rehabilitation (immediate weight bearing) protocols produced similar results at a minimum follow-up of 2 years (35). However, it is important to note that the validity of direct comparisons between studies evaluating different rehabilitation protocols is limited by inconsistencies in objective criteria and surgical techniques used in different studies.

COMPLICATIONS

Complications associated with meniscal repair may arise due to preoperative, intraoperative, or postoperative factors. Complications related to errors in diagnosis include repair of chronic or degenerative tears as well as repair of tears located in the avascular zone, both of which have unfavorable healing potential (36). Complications related to technical error include failure to adequately prepare the tear for healing, iatrogenic chondral and meniscal injury, over-repair of tears, and improper suture tensioning. Moreover, failure to select the appropriate technique, suture type, or suture pattern may lead to a biomechanically inferior repair, tear recurrence, and the need for subsequent procedures (36). Neurovascular complications may arise due to injury to the saphenous nerve and vein, peroneal nerve, popliteal vessels, and lateral geniculate artery. All-inside device fracture or migration, particularly when using rigid devices, can lead to repair failure, chondral injury, and mechanical symptoms (36). The development of perimeniscal cysts, hemarthrosis or effusion, and arthrofibrosis may also complicate recovery from meniscal repair.

RESULTS

In a systematic review of all-inside meniscal repairs, failure rates of all techniques combined ranged from 0% to 43.5% (5). This included the most well-studied device, the Arrow, which had a failure rate of 5% to 43.5% (5). The majority of the studies were case series, and only a single prospective randomized study evaluating second- or third-generation devices had been published at the time of this systematic review (5). This was a study of Mitek's RapidLoc that showed a 35% failure rate in 20 patients with an average follow-up of 22 months (37). For devices that have been used for longer periods of time, such as the Arrow and T-Fix, there is a trend toward higher failure rates with longer follow-up (38). Overall, the systematic review noted that the success rate of all-inside repair is approximately 85% (5). Given the current literature and lack of prospective randomized trials, evidence-based recommendations regarding which type of all-inside meniscal repair device is associated with the best clinical outcomes cannot be made at this time. The theoretical benefit of suture-based fixators, which can apply compression across the tear site, seems to be a logical advantage over older devices. However, further studies are required to provide evidence that long-term success can be achieved using all-inside techniques.

A more recent systematic review compared outcomes of inside-out meniscal repair and modern all-inside devices in patients with isolated meniscal tears (39). Patients treated with inside-out repair were noted to have a clinical failure rate of 11%, an anatomic failure rate of 13%, and a complication rate of 5.1%, whereas patients who underwent repair with modern all-inside devices were noted to have a clinical failure rate of 10%, an anatomic failure rate of 16%, and a complication rate of 4.6% (39). However, these differences were not statistically significant. It is also important to note that most of the studies included in this systematic review were level IV evidence.

In contrast, a systematic review comparing outcomes of patients who underwent meniscal repair with concurrent anterior cruciate ligament reconstruction noted that the clinical failure rate of inside-out repair (10%) was significantly lower than the failure rate of all-inside repair (16%) in this setting (40). However, complication rates did not differ significantly between groups. While there is a paucity of literature on the outcomes of outside-in meniscal repair, a limited number of studies suggest that favorable outcomes can be achieved with this repair technique (41–43). In a study comparing arthroscopic all-inside, inside-out, and outside-in meniscal repair techniques in 57 patients, Hantes et al. noted a superior healing rate among patients treated with inside-out repair at a mean follow-up of 22 months, although complication rates did not differ significantly between groups (37).

A retrospective case series by Cohen et al. evaluated outcomes following arthroscopic repair of isolated meniscus tears using inside-out, outside-in, and all-inside techniques in 44 patients younger than 30 years of age (44). At a mean follow-up of 4.5 years, the overall clinical failure rate was 36.4%, and the patient satisfaction rate was 84.1% (44). Inability to return to preinjury function was reported by 10 patients (22.7%); for the remaining 34 patients (77.3%), the mean time to return to preinjury function following surgery was 5.0 months (44). More recently, a systematic review by Eberbach et al. noted that return to sports at the preinjury level of competition was achieved in 89% of 664 patients following isolated meniscal repair, with studies reporting a mean delay of return to sports between 4.3 and 6.5 months (45).

In summary, the existing literature indicates that the all-inside, inside-out, and outside-in repair techniques can all produce favorable results in patients with repairable meniscal tears. However, there is a need for additional prospective studies to evaluate the long-term outcomes of these repair techniques. Moreover, future studies should aim to elucidate the relationship between patient and tear characteristics (i.e., location, morphology) and technique-specific outcomes through direct, comparative clinical studies. Such information would be invaluable for surgical planning as it would enable surgeons to use empirical evidence to choose the most appropriate meniscal repair technique for their patients.

REFERENCES

1. Henning C, Lynch M, Yearout K, et al. Arthroscopic meniscal repair using an exogenous fibrin clot. *Clin Orthop.* 1990;252:64–72.
2. Arnoczky S, Warren R, Spivak J. Meniscal repair using an exogenous fibrin clot. An experimental study in dogs. *J Bone Joint Surg.* 1988;70:1209–1217.
3. Port J, Jackson DW, Lee TQ, et al. Meniscal repair supplemented with exogenous fibrin clot and autologous cultured marrow cells in the goat model. *Am J Sports Med.* 1996;24:547–555.
4. Ciccone W, Motz C, Bentley C, et al. Bioabsorbable implants in orthopaedics: new developments and clinical applications. *J Am Acad Orthop Surg.* 2001;9:280–288.
5. Lozano J, Ma C, Cannon W. All-inside meniscal repair: a systematic review. *Clin Orthop Relat Res.* 2006;455:134–141.
6. Siebold R, Dehler C, Boes L, et al. Arthroscopic all-inside repair using the Meniscus Arrow: long-term clinical follow-up of 113 patients. *Arthroscopy.* 2007;23(4):394–399.

7. Barber FA, Coons DA. Midterm results of meniscal repair using the Biostinger meniscal repair device. *Arthroscopy.* 2006;22:400–405.
8. Barber FA, Johnson DH, Halbrecht JL. Arthroscopic meniscal repair using the Biostinger. *Arthroscopy.* 2005;21:744–750.
9. Laprell H, Stein V, Peterson W. Arthroscopic all-inside meniscus repair using a new refixation device: a prospective study. *Arthroscopy.* 2002;18:387–393.
10. Becker R, Schroder M. Biomechanical investigations of different meniscal repair implants in comparison with horizontal sutures on human meniscus. *Arthroscopy.* 2001;17:439–444.
11. Bogunovic L, Kruse LM, Haas AK, et al. Outcome of all-inside second-generation meniscal repair: minimum five-year follow-up. *J Bone Joint Surg Am.* 2014;96(15):1303–1307.
12. Solheim E, Hegna J, Inderhaug E. Long-term outcome after all-inside meniscal repair using the RapidLoc system. *Knee Surg Sports Traumatol Arthrosc.* 2016;24(5):1495–1500.
13. Barber FA, Herbert MA, Bava ED, et al. Biomechanical testing of suture-based meniscal repair devices containing ultrahigh-molecular-weight polyethylene suture: update 2011. *Arthroscopy.* 2012;28(6):827–834.
14. Mehta VM, Terry MA. Cyclic testing of 3 all-inside meniscal repair devices: a biomechanical analysis. *Am J Sports Med.* 2009;37(12):2435–2439.
15. Arthrex, Inc. *The Meniscal Cinch All-Inside Repair.* Available at: https://www.arthrex.com/knee/meniscal-cinch-allin-side-repair. Accessed February 1, 2017.
16. Milchteim C, Branch EA, Maughon T, et al. Biomechanical comparison of parallel and crossed suture repair for longitudinal meniscus tears. *Orthop J Sports Med.* 2016;4(4):2325967116640263.
17. Barber FA, Herbert MA, Schroeder FA, et al. Biomechanical testing of new meniscal repair techniques containing ultra high-molecular weight polyethylene suture. *Arthroscopy.* 2009;25(9):959–967.
18. Ramappa AJ, Chen A, Hertz B, et al. A biomechanical evaluation of all-inside 2-stitch meniscal repair devices with matched inside-out suture repair. *Am J Sports Med.* 2014;42(1):194–199.
19. Masoudi A, Beamer BS, Harlow ER, et al. Biomechanical evaluation of an all-inside suture-based device for repairing longitudinal meniscal tears. *Arthroscopy.* 2015;31(3):428–434.
20. Henning CE. Arthroscopic repair of meniscus tears. *Orthopedics.* 1983;6(9):1130–1132.
21. Yoon KH, Park KH. Meniscal repair. *Knee Surg Relat Res.* 2014;26(2):68–76.
22. Rodeo SA. Arthroscopic meniscal repair with use of the outside-in technique. *Instr Course Lect.* 2000;49:195–206.
23. Vinyard TR, Wolf BR. Meniscal repair—outside-in repair. *Clin Sports Med.* 2012;31:33–48.
24. Asik M, Sener N. Failure strength of repair devices versus meniscus suturing techniques. *Knee Surg Sports Traumatol Arthrosc.* 2002;10:25–29.
25. Rimmer MG, Nawana NS, Keene GC, et al. Failure strengths of different meniscal suturing techniques. *Arthroscopy.* 1995;11(2):146–150.
26. Turman KA, Diduch DR, Miller MD. All-inside meniscal repair. *Sports Health.* 2009;1(5):438–444.
27. Tuman J, Haro MS, Foley S, et al. All-inside meniscal repair devices and techniques. *Expert Rev Med Devices.* 2012;9(2):147–157.
28. Jung YH, Choi NH, Oh JS, et al. All-inside repair for a root tear of the medial meniscus using a suture anchor. *Am J Sports Med.* 2012;40(6):1406–1411.
29. Chung KS, Ha JK, Ra HJ, et al. A meta-analysis of clinical and radiographic outcomes of posterior horn medial meniscus root repairs. *Knee Surg Sports Traumatol Arthrosc.* 2016;24(5):1455–1468.
30. Nelson CG, Bonner KF. Inside-out meniscus repair. *Arthrosc Tech.* 2013;2(4):e453–e460.
31. Newman AP, Anderson DR, Daniels AU, et al. Mechanics of the healed meniscus in a canine model. *Am J Sports Med.* 1989;17(2):164–175.
32. Moulton SG, Bhatia S, Civitarese DM, et al. Surgical techniques and outcomes of repairing meniscal radial tears: a systematic review. *Arthroscopy.* 2016;32(9):1919–1925.
33. Lind M, Nielsen T, Faune P, et al. Free rehabilitation is safe after isolated meniscus repair. *Am J Sports Med.* 2013;41:2753–2758.
34. Mariani PP, Santori N, Adriani E, et al. Accelerated rehabilitation after arthroscopic meniscal repair: a clinical and magnetic resonance imaging evaluation. *Arthroscopy.* 1996;12:680–686.
35. VanderHave KL, Perkins C, Le M. Weightbearing versus nonweightbearing after meniscus repair. *Sports Health.* 2015;7(5):399–402.
36. Gwathmey FW, Golish SR, Diduch DR. Complications in brief: meniscus repair. *Clin Orthop Relat Res.* 2012;470(7):2059–2066.
37. Hantes ME, Zachos VC, Varitimidis SE, et al. Arthroscopic meniscal repair: a comparative study between three different surgical techniques. *Knee Surg Sports Traumatol Arthrosc.* 2006;14(12):1232–1237.
38. Gill SS, Diduch DR. Outcomes after meniscal repair using the Meniscus Arrow in knees undergoing concurrent anterior cruciate ligament reconstruction. *Arthroscopy.* 2002;18:569–577.
39. Fillingham YA, Riboh JC, Erickson BJ, et al. Inside-out versus all-inside repair of isolated meniscal tears. *Am J Sports Med.* 2017;45(1):234–242.
40. Westermann RW, Duchman KR, Amendola A, et al. All-inside versus inside-out meniscal repair with concurrent anterior cruciate ligament reconstruction. *Am J Sports Med.* 2017;45(3):719–724.
41. Keyhani S, Abbasian MR, Siatiri N, et al. Arthroscopic meniscal repair: "modified outside-in technique." *Arch Bone Jt Surg.* 2015;3(2):104–108.
42. Morgan CD, Casscells SW. Arthroscopic meniscus repair: a safe approach to the posterior horns. *Arthroscopy.* 1986;2(1):3–12.
43. Morgan CD, Wojtys EM, Casscells CD, et al. Arthroscopic meniscal repair evaluated by second-look arthroscopy. *Am J Sports Med.* 1991;19(6):632–637.
44. Cohen SB, Hendy B, Khurana S, et al. The result of isolated arthroscopic meniscal repairs: evaluation of return to function and incidence of re-tear. *Arthroscopy.* 2009;25:e19–e20.
45. Eberbach H, Zwingmann J, Hohloch L, et al. Sport-specific outcomes after isolated meniscal repair: a systematic review. *Knee Surg Sports Traumatol Arthrosc.* 2018;26(3):762–771.

ADDITIONAL RECOMMENDED READING

Kurzweil PR. Meniscal repair with meniscal fixators. In: Jackson DW, ed. *Master Techniques: Reconstructive Knee Surgery.* 3rd Ed. Philadelphia, PA: Lippincott Williams & Wilkins; 2008:89–96.
Sgaglione N. Meniscus repair: update on new techniques. *Tech Knee Surg.* 2002;1:113–127.

24 Meniscal Root Repair

Patrick W. Kane, Kyle Muckenhirn, and Robert F. LaPrade

INDICATIONS

The menisci provide tibiofemoral joint stability and decrease contact pressures by converting 50% to 70% of axial loads (1) to hoop stresses, thereby preventing osteochondral damage (2,3). A meniscal root tear, described as a bony avulsion or a complete radial tear up to 9 mm from the posterior meniscal root attachment (4–6), has significant biomechanical consequences (7,8), compromising functionality to an extent comparable to complete meniscectomy (9). Improved understanding of the pathologic sequelae of meniscal root tears has led to increased recognition of the need for surgical management, but due to a lack of anatomic understanding, diagnoses are often missed on magnetic resonance imaging (MRI) and arthroscopy (10).

Meniscal root tears can classically be identified on sagittal MRI by the replacement of normal dark meniscus tissue signal with absent tissue or high signal, also known as the "ghost sign" (Fig. 24-1) (11–14). Axial and coronal views are also commonly used to visualize root tears, with the presence of ipsilateral tibiofemoral compartment bone marrow edema or insufficiency fractures indicating a possible tear (Fig. 24-2) (15). Further suspicion is warranted with anterior cruciate ligament (ACL) injuries, because lateral meniscal posterior root tears have been reported in up to 8% of cases (16). Conversely, a degenerative tear of the posterior medial meniscal root is more common and 5.8 times more likely to have chondral defects (17), but can also be seen acutely following multiple ligament knee injuries (16–18).

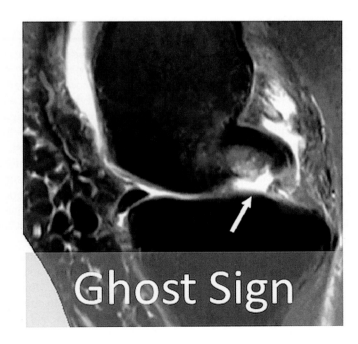

FIGURE 24-1

MRI sagittal section demonstrating the ghost sign in a right knee, which is the replacement of normal dark meniscus tissue signal with absent tissue or high signal.

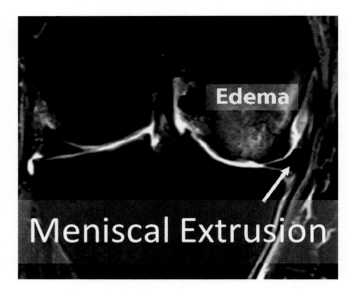

FIGURE 24-2

MRI coronal section demonstrating meniscal extrusion and medial femoral condylar bone marrow edema.

Another important indication of a meniscal root tear requiring surgical management is the presence of meniscal extrusion, defined by sagittal displacement on coronal sections at the level of the medial collateral ligament (Fig. 24-2) (10,14). Complex meniscal tear patterns, root tears, and degeneration of the meniscus and articular cartilage are all associated with 3 mm or more of meniscal extrusion (13,19), with greater extrusion associated with osteoarthritis severity (20). The rate of osteoarthritis development can significantly decelerate following a meniscal root repair compared to partial meniscectomy (14,21), but stringent surgical repair indications may restrict patient inclusion. Young or middle-aged patients who have yet to develop osteoarthritis and present acutely are ideal surgical candidates, but chronic symptomatic patients without significant osteoarthritis can also be successfully managed (3,12).

CONTRAINDICATIONS

Although repair is the preferred treatment option for posterior meniscal root tears to slow the progression of osteoarthritis, some patients may need to be treated nonoperatively or with partial meniscectomy. Chondral health and joint alignment are imperative to successful posterior meniscal root repair and can lead to better IKDC and Tegner scores. Comparatively, patients who have grade 3 cartilage changes or worse, or 5 degrees of malalignment or more, report no significant outcome difference to nonoperative treatment (22). The malalignment may be corrected before performing a meniscal root repair (11), but other general contraindications include patients with multiple comorbidities preventing surgery, high body mass index, asymptomatic chronic meniscal root tears, or advanced age (10,23). Controversially, advanced age alone should not exclude surgical candidacy, because there is no significant difference in reported outcomes following posterior meniscal root repair in patients older than 50 years compared to younger patients (24). Ultimately, the decision to attempt posterior meniscal root repair is multifactorial, and excluded patients should undergo a period of nonoperative treatment.

Patients who have posterior meniscal root tears who cannot be managed by surgical repair should first be offered nonoperative treatment with unloader bracing, anti-inflammatory medications, or intra-articular injections and modify activity to alleviate symptoms (10). However, poor clinical outcomes, osteoarthritis progression, and relative high rate of conversion to arthroplasty are associated with nonoperative treatment of medial meniscus posterior root tears, and expectations should be tempered (25). Similarly, advancement of radiographically evident osteoarthritis will continue if initial nonoperative treatment fails and partial meniscectomy is performed, though patients may find symptomatic relief (26).

PREOPERATIVE PREPARATION

If imaging fails to recognize the presence of a tear adjacent to the medial meniscus posterior root, which can happen in one third of cases (27), a history of acute injury or hyperflexion may provide other important cues to identify a meniscal root tear prior to operating (3,12,28). Another aspect of presurgical planning is classifying the tear into one of five broad tear types (Fig. 24-3): type 1 is a partial stable root tear; type 2 is a complete radial root tear located <3 mm (2A), 3 to <6 mm (2B), or 6 to 9 mm (2C) from the root attachment; type 3 is a bucket-handle tear with complete root detachment; type 4 is a complex oblique tear with a complete root detachments; and type 5 is a bony avulsion fracture of the root attachments (29). In one study evaluating the morphology of 71 meniscal root tears, they determined 67.6% were classified as type 2 with a complete radial tear up to 9 mm from the root, while 66 of the 71 injuries were to the posterior meniscal roots (29). Failure to diagnose and treat posterior medial meniscal root tears can lead to retraction, posteromedial extrusion, or scarring into the capsule (10,13,30), further emphasizing the need for prompt repair.

TECHNIQUE

The patient should be positioned on the operating room table in the supine position with the foot of the bed dropped for easy access to the knee throughout the procedure. The operative extremity should have a well-padded thigh high tourniquet applied and should be firmly secured in a leg holder; the nonoperative leg should be placed in an abduction stirrup.

After completing a thorough examination under anesthesia to assess for any concomitant pathology, standard anterolateral and anteromedial parapatellar arthroscopic portals are made. A thorough arthroscopic examination of the meniscal root is completed utilizing a probe to determine tear morphology and severity. An arthroscopic shaver should be utilized to help remove any adhesions that may be obscuring complete visualization of the tear pattern. Similarly, accessory arthroscopic portals can be made to enhance visualization and gain easier access to the posterior root. Clear visualization and a thorough understanding of meniscal root anatomy are key components to both achieving successful repair and also avoiding iatrogenic injury to local structures.

A surgical grasper is useful in positioning the torn meniscal root at the site of proposed repair on the tibial plateau, which is prepared and decorticated with a curved curette. Tension of the proposed repair and excursion of the posterior meniscus should be assessed at this time (Fig. 24-4). If excessive tension or adhesion formation to the posterior capsule is present, release of the meniscus, often with the aid of arthroscopic scissors, must be performed. Inadequate excursion of the meniscal root leading to malposition of the root repair can result in contact pressures equal to that of a meniscectomy (9).

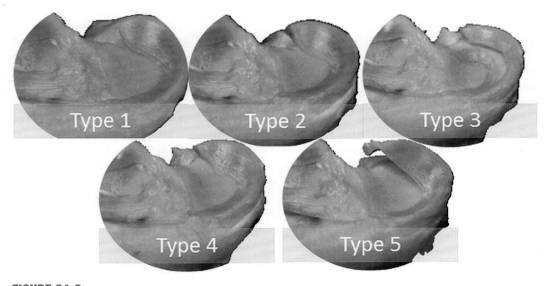

FIGURE 24-3

Cadaveric dissections of a right knee medial tibial plateau with the medial meniscus representing the five classifications of meniscal root tear.

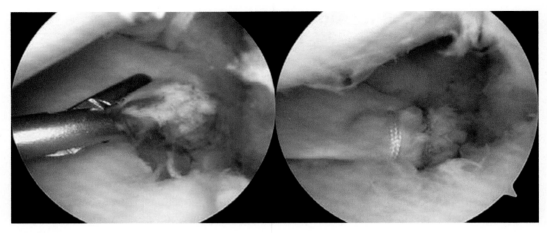

FIGURE 24-4

Arthroscopic view of a left knee medial meniscus root tear in an arthroscopic grasper (*left*) and after a medial meniscus root repair (*right*).

Two transtibial tunnels are drilled at the repair site to not only enhance biologic healing but also to better restore the footprint of the meniscal root. The incision and start point for the transtibial tunnels vary depending on the laterality of the root involved. For lateral meniscal root repairs, the incision is made slightly distal to the medial aspect of Gerdy tubercle on the anterolateral aspect of the tibia. For medial meniscal root repairs, the incision is made slightly medial to the tibial tubercle. After an approximately 2-cm incision is made at the respective location on the tibia, an ACL-aiming device is utilized to position a drill pin with a cannulated sleeve at the site of repair. The posterior tunnel is drilled first and the guide pin is removed, but the cannulated sleeve is left in place for later suture passage. Next, the anterior tunnel is created approximately 5 mm anterior to the first tunnel with the aid of an offset guide. The guide pin is similarly removed, but the cannulated sleeve is also left in place for later suture passage.

If not already present, accessory arthroscopic portals should be made at this time, because they are extremely useful in firmly grasping the meniscal root during suture passage. An accessory anteromedial portal should be made for medial meniscal root tears, and similarly, an accessory anterolateral portal should be made for lateral meniscal root tears. An accessory posteromedial or posterolateral portal can be made if access to the meniscal root is difficult through an accessory anterior portal. A suture-passing device is then used to pass a suture through the meniscal root from the tibial side to the femoral side at a distance approximately 5 mm from the edge of the meniscal root (5 mm medial to the lateral edge of the medial meniscal root and 5 mm lateral to the medial edge of the lateral meniscal root). Most suture-passing devices have a retrieving mechanism so the suture can be pulled out through a cannula with the device. It is important to use a cannula while shuttling the sutures through the anterior arthroscopic portals to ensure that there are no soft tissue bridges prior to passing the sutures down the tibial tunnels because this can lead to tearing of the sutures through the meniscal root during passage. In order to facilitate suture passage through the tibial tunnel, a looped passing wire is placed through the posterior cannulated sleeve and retrieved. The sutures are then placed inside the loop and shuttled down the posterior tibial tunnel. The same steps are repeated for suture passage and shuttling for the anterior tunnel. After both sutures are through their respective tibial tunnels, the sutures are secured to the tibia with a cortical fixation device, thereby completing the repair (Fig. 24-5).

PEARLS AND PITFALLS

- A thorough understanding of the relevant anatomy of the meniscal roots is essential prior to performing any repair. Repairs placed in nonanatomic locations have been shown to result in contact pressures equal to a meniscectomy.
- Any adhesions of the meniscal root to the posterior capsule that limit its excursion and ability to be placed at the anatomical site for repair should be thoroughly released, often with an arthroscopic scissors.

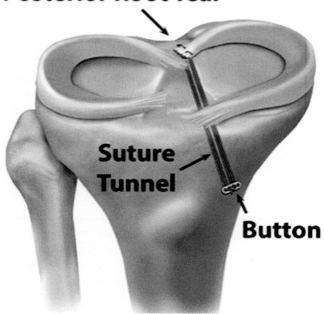

Posterior Root Tear

Suture Tunnel

Button

FIGURE 24-5

Diagram of the two-tunnel transtibial pullout technique for a posteromedial meniscal root repair on a right knee. (Reproduced from LaPrade CM, LaPrade MD, Turnbull TL, Wijdicks CA, LaPrade RF. Biomechanical evaluation of the transtibial pull-out technique for posterior medial meniscal root repairs using 1 and 2 transtibial bone tunnels. *Am J Sports Med.* 2015;43(4):899–904, with permission.)

- Accessory portals should be used to aid in suture passage and handling of the meniscal root.
- Ensure no soft tissue bridges are present prior to suture passage down the transtibial tunnels. The presence of a soft tissue bridge may lead to suture cutout and tearing through the meniscal root during passage through the tibial tunnels.
- Place passing sutures from the tibial side to the femoral side (bottom up).
- Retrieve and shuttle suture through the posterior tunnel prior to the passage of the second, anterior suture to facilitate suture management and help avoid intra-articular suture entanglement.

POSTOPERATIVE MANAGEMENT

Meniscal root repair patients are maintained on a non–weight-bearing protocol for 6 weeks following surgery. Weight-bearing activities increase circumferential or hoop stresses on the meniscal repair and are avoided in the initial postoperative period. After 6 weeks of non–weight bearing, patients are progressed to partial weight bearing from weeks 7 through 8 if the following conditions are met: no excessive joint effusion (>2-cm girth difference), no antalgic gait pattern, full active extension range of motion (ROM), and full quad sets demonstrated. Weight bearing as tolerated is allowed in postoperative week 9 if patients continue to demonstrate no evidence of an antalgic gait and there is no significant effusion or pain with partial weight-bearing outdoors for 20 minutes at a time.

A knee immobilizer locked in extension is used during the first 6 weeks following surgery to help reduce excessive tibiofemoral movement during the healing phase of the root repair.

The knee immobilizer is removed for physical therapy and ROM exercises, which are critical in reducing swelling and scar tissue formation following surgery. ROM is limited to passive ROM from 0 to 90 degrees in the first 2 postoperative weeks and progressed to ROM as tolerated thereafter. In order to reduce posterior tibial translation and sheer stress on the root repair, isolated hamstring contraction is limited for 6 weeks following surgery. Hyperextension is similarly avoided for 4 weeks following surgery.

COMPLICATIONS

Recreating the anatomic meniscal footprint is necessary for the restoration of tibiofemoral joint load conversion to circumferential tension, thereby reducing contact pressures and slowing the progression of osteoarthritis (2,3). However, meniscal root repairs are not without complications and technical difficulty. Failure, defined as a retear or loss of tension leading to extrusion, may be one of the most common complications. During a transtibial pullout repair, sutures may creep or become abraded in the tunnel prior to complete healing, and tunnel interference becomes an issue with concomitant ligament reconstruction (10). Conversely, fixation pullout is seen with the anchor repair technique. Other causes of nonanatomic repair include inadequate intraoperative tensioning or shortening of the root following debridement of the ruptured end. Furthermore, without proper exposure, iatrogenic damage to the ACL or neurovascular bundle may occur (31). Other common postoperative complications to be aware of include infection, arthrofibrosis, and deep vein thrombosis.

RESULTS

Preserving meniscal function through a posterior meniscal root repair should be attempted over partial meniscectomy or nonoperative treatment (32). One study evaluating 52 patients with meniscal root tears treated nonoperatively reported an 87% failure rate, with 31% undergoing conversion to a total knee arthroplasty (TKA) at a mean 30 ± 32 months (25). Similarly, 35% of meniscectomy patients were converted to TKA, compared to none in a repair group that also showed greater functional improvement scores, less joint space narrowing, and lower progression of arthritis (14,21).

The two most common repair techniques, suture anchor and pullout repair, have both demonstrated significant functional improvement, with no side-to-side difference in the latter (24). The all-inside suture anchor repair has had mixed results with one study reporting no change in meniscal extrusion (33), while another study resulted in significant improvement (34). Comparatively, 56% of patients demonstrated a significant reduction in meniscal extrusion following repair by transtibial pullout in a recent systematic review of posterior root tears of the medial meniscus (35). Furthermore, by restoring the native anatomy using a transtibial repair, contact areas and pressures return to near-normal values (7,8,10,36,37). This restoration of joint biomechanics is evident by lower progression of osteoarthritis and significant improvement in functional scores (38).

REFERENCES

1. Kidron A, Thein R. Radial tears associated with cleavage tears of the medial meniscus in athletes. *Arthroscopy.* 2002;18(3):254–256.
2. Fithian DC, Kelly MA, Mow VC. Material properties and structure-function relationships in the menisci. *Clin Orthop Relat Res.* 1990;(252):19–31.
3. Koenig JH, et al. Meniscal root tears: diagnosis and treatment. *Arthroscopy.* 2009;25(9):1025–1032.
4. Griffith CJ, et al. Posterior root avulsion fracture of the medial meniscus in an adolescent female patient with surgical reattachment. *Am J Sports Med.* 2008;36(4):789–792.
5. Johannsen AM, et al. Qualitative and quantitative anatomic analysis of the posterior root attachments of the medial and lateral menisci. *Am J Sports Med.* 2012;40(10):2342–2347.
6. Starke C, et al. The effect of a nonanatomic repair of the meniscal horn attachment on meniscal tension: a biomechanical study. *Arthroscopy.* 2010;26(3):358–365.
7. LaPrade CM, et al. Altered tibiofemoral contact mechanics due to lateral meniscus posterior horn root avulsions and radial tears can be restored with in situ pull-out suture repairs. *J Bone Joint Surg Am.* 2014;96(6):471–479.
8. Padalecki JR, et al. Biomechanical consequences of a complete radial tear adjacent to the medial meniscus posterior root attachment site: in situ pull-out repair restores derangement of joint mechanics. *Am J Sports Med.* 2014;42(3):699–707.
9. Allaire R, et al. Biomechanical consequences of a tear of the posterior root of the medial meniscus. Similar to total meniscectomy. *J Bone Joint Surg Am.* 2008;90(9):1922–1931.
10. Bhatia S, et al. Meniscal root tears: significance, diagnosis, and treatment. *Am J Sports Med.* 2014;42(12):3016–3030.
11. Chahla J, et al. Posterior meniscal root repair: the transtibial double tunnel pullout technique. *Arthrosc Tech.* 2016;5(2):e291–e296.
12. Papalia R, et al. Meniscal root tears: from basic science to ultimate surgery. *Br Med Bull.* 2013;106:91–115.
13. Lerer DB, et al. The role of meniscal root pathology and radial meniscal tear in medial meniscal extrusion. *Skeletal Radiol.* 2004;33(10):569–574.
14. Kim SB, et al. Medial meniscus root tear refixation: comparison of clinical, radiologic, and arthroscopic findings with medial meniscectomy. *Arthroscopy.* 2011;27(3):346–354.
15. Harner CD, et al. Biomechanical consequences of a tear of the posterior root of the medial meniscus. Surgical technique. *J Bone Joint Surg Am.* 2009. 91(suppl 2):257–270.
16. De Smet AA, Mukherjee R. Clinical, MRI, and arthroscopic findings associated with failure to diagnose a lateral meniscal tear on knee MRI. *AJR Am J Roentgenol.* 2008;190(1):22–26.
17. Matheny LM, et al. Posterior meniscus root tears: associated pathologies to assist as diagnostic tools. *Knee Surg Sports Traumatol Arthrosc.* 2015;23(10):3127–3131.

18. Feucht MJ, et al. Risk factors for posterior lateral meniscus root tears in anterior cruciate ligament injuries. *Knee Surg Sports Traumatol Arthrosc.* 2015;23(1):140–145.
19. Costa CR, Morrison WB, Carrino JA. Medial meniscus extrusion on knee MRI: is extent associated with severity of degeneration or type of tear? *AJR Am J Roentgenol.* 2004;183(1):17–23.
20. Lee DH, et al. Predictors of degenerative medial meniscus extrusion: radial component and knee osteoarthritis. *Knee Surg Sports Traumatol Arthrosc.* 2011;19(2):222–229.
21. Chung KS, et al. Comparison of clinical and radiologic results between partial meniscectomy and refixation of medial meniscus posterior root tears: a minimum 5-Year follow-up. *Arthroscopy.* 2015;31(10):1941–1950.
22. Ahn JH, et al. Comparison between conservative treatment and arthroscopic pull-out repair of the medial meniscus root tear and analysis of prognostic factors for the determination of repair indication. *Arch Orthop Trauma Surg.* 2015;135(9):1265–1276.
23. Moon HK, et al. Prognostic factors of arthroscopic pull-out repair for a posterior root tear of the medial meniscus. *Am J Sports Med.* 2012;40(5):1138–1143.
24. LaPrade RF, Matheny LM, Moulton SG, et al. Posterior meniscal root repairs: outcomes of an anatomic transtibial pull-out technique. *Am J Sports Med.* 2017;45(4):884–891.
25. Krych AJ, Reardon PJ, Johnson NR, et al. Non-operative management of medial meniscus posterior horn root tears is associated with worsening arthritis and poor clinical outcome at 5-year follow-up. *Knee Surg Sports Traumatol Arthrosc.* 2017;25(2):383–389.
26. Ozkoc G, et al. Radial tears in the root of the posterior horn of the medial meniscus. *Knee Surg Sports Traumatol Arthrosc.* 2008;16(9):849–854.
27. Bin SI, Kim JM, Shin SJ. Radial tears of the posterior horn of the medial meniscus. *Arthroscopy.* 2004;20(4):373–378.
28. Pagnani MJ, Cooper DE, Warren RF. Extrusion of the medial meniscus. *Arthroscopy.* 1991;7(3):297–300.
29. LaPrade CM, et al. Meniscal root tears: a classification system based on tear morphology. *Am J Sports Med.* 2015;43(2):363–369.
30. Magee T. MR findings of meniscal extrusion correlated with arthroscopy. *J Magn Reson Imaging.* 2008;28(2):466–470.
31. Vyas D, Harner CD, Meniscus root repair. *Sports Med Arthrosc Rev.* 2012;20(2):86–94.
32. Kim JH, et al. Arthroscopic suture anchor repair versus pullout suture repair in posterior root tear of the medial meniscus: a prospective comparison study. *Arthroscopy.* 2011;27(12):1644–1653.
33. Jung YH, et al. All-inside repair for a root tear of the medial meniscus using a suture anchor. *Am J Sports Med.* 2012;40(6):1406–1411.
34. Ahn JH, et al. Results of arthroscopic all-inside repair for lateral meniscus root tear in patients undergoing concomitant anterior cruciate ligament reconstruction. *Arthroscopy.* 2010;26(1):67–75.
35. Feucht MJ, et al. Arthroscopic transtibial pullout repair for posterior medial meniscus root tears: a systematic review of clinical, radiographic, and second-look arthroscopic results. *Arthroscopy.* 2015;31(9):1808–1816.
36. LaPrade CM, et al. Biomechanical consequences of a nonanatomic posterior medial meniscal root repair. *Am J Sports Med.* 2015;43(4):912–920.
37. LaPrade CM, et al. Biomechanical evaluation of the transtibial pull-out technique for posterior medial meniscal root repairs using 1 and 2 transtibial bone tunnels. *Am J Sports Med.* 2015;43(4):899–904.
38. Lee JH, et al. Arthroscopic pullout suture repair of posterior root tear of the medial meniscus: radiographic and clinical results with a 2-year follow-up. *Arthroscopy.* 2009;25(9):951–958.

25 Medial Meniscus Transplant

Justin W. Arner, Marcin Kowalczuk, Thierry Pauyo, and Volker Musahl

INDICATIONS

Although not initially appreciated as a vital structure, the medial meniscus' importance in force transmission and joint stability is now clear. Historically, treatment for knee pain and meniscal tears was total meniscectomy. Not surprisingly, patients developed arthritis and outcomes were found to be poor (1,2). One systematic review found that 53.5% of patients had arthritis at 7.4 years after meniscectomy (3). Even a partial meniscectomy has been shown in biomechanical studies to significantly increase cartilage contact pressures (4,5). Meniscal preservation is now recognized as critical with an emphasis on repair. However, many meniscal tears are often unable to be repaired or fail due to poor healing potential. Currently, many patients who fail repair or retear their meniscus end up with a subtotal meniscectomy.

Meniscal transplant is often the last resort, in particular in young patients, with the hope of preventing arthritic change. Long-term meniscal transplant outcomes are limited, but shorter-term studies have shown improvements in pain and function (6–9).

CONTRAINDICATIONS

Ideal patients for a meniscal transplant are young with isolated medial compartment pain with a history of a significant medial meniscectomy. Articular changes are also essential to evaluate. Meniscal transplants have been shown to be more successful in patients with no arthritic changes or low-grade (less than grade 2) unicompartmental changes only (10). Patients with arthritic changes in the compartment have been found to not have the same improvement in outcomes, and therefore, many do not recommend meniscal transplant for these patients (10,11).

Ligamentous stability is also essential for graft survival and improvement in symptoms. Patients with significant meniscal deficiency commonly have concurrent anterior cruciate ligament (ACL) injuries. With an ACL-deficient knee, the medial meniscus becomes an important knee stabilizer, and therefore if the ACL is not reconstructed appropriately, meniscal transplant failure is likely (12).

Appropriate mechanical alignment is also critical for success. A varus alignment must be corrected concomitantly or before a transplant is considered as medial meniscal transplantation has found to be better in those with a neutral mechanical axis (13,14).

Other relative contraindications include obesity, history of infection, inflammatory disorders, and inability to perform appropriate postoperative rehabilitation (10,15).

PREOPERATIVE PLANNING

A thorough preoperative evaluation is mandatory for a successful outcome of medial meniscus transplantation. During the physical examination, it is important to determine if any concomitant pathologies are present such as knee ligamentous instability or lower extremity malalignment. The treating surgeon should be prepared to treat any knee ligament instability or lower extremity malalignment at the time of medial meniscal transplant or prior to transplantation, in a staged fashion. Furthermore, operative reports of any previous procedures performed on the affected knee should be obtained to provide valuable insight on the general state of the joint.

The preoperative imaging evaluation should begin with radiographs, including a bilateral weight-bearing 45-degree posterior-anterior radiograph, a 30-degree flexion lateral radiograph, a sunrise or merchant radiograph, and bilateral full-length lower extremity weight-bearing radiograph for evaluation of the mechanical axis. In cases involving cruciate ligament revision, a computed tomography (CT) scan can be obtained to evaluate for tunnel enlargement. Next, a magnetic resonance imaging (MRI) scan of the affected knee is acquired to assess the state of the menisci, cruciates, collateral ligaments, and cartilage.

The last step in the preoperative planning is to appropriately size the medial meniscus allograft. There exists a myriad of methods to evaluate the dimension needed to obtain a sized-match medial meniscus allograft. We utilize a combination of radiograph and MRI to measure the anterior-posterior and medial-lateral dimension of the tibial plateau (16–18). It is important to note that any radiograph utilized should have a radiographic marker to obtain precise measurements (Figs. 25-1 and 25-2).

Before beginning the surgical procedure, the quality of the allograft is carefully examined on the back table. In the case of a degenerative or attenuated allograft medial meniscus, the surgeon should not hesitate to postpone the procedure to obtain an adequate graft for transplantation.

TECHNIQUE

Setup, Patient Positioning, and Exam under Anesthesia

The patient is positioned supine on the operating room table with all bony prominences well padded. Following the administration of a general anesthetic, a detailed physical examination is performed on both the operative and nonoperative lower extremities and the results recorded. Range of motion and ligamentous stability are assessed through Lachman, pivot shift, anterior/posterior drawer, and varus/valgus stress testing at 0 and 30 degrees. With the patient's heels even with the end of the

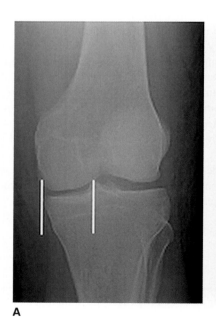 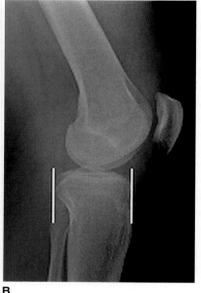

A   B

FIGURE 25-1

Meniscal allograft preoperative radiograph sizing. **A:** AP radiograph. The width of the meniscal allograft is the distance between the medial metaphyseal margin and peak of the tibial eminence. **B:** Lateral radiograph. The sagittal distance is measured between the anterior border of the tibial plateau and the posterior edge of the medial tibial. A 0.8 conversion factor is used.

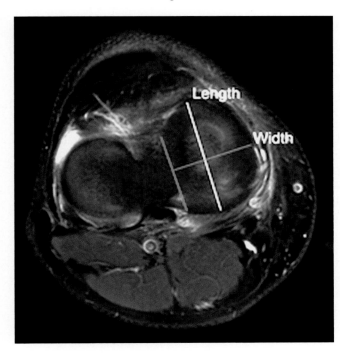

FIGURE 25-2

Medial meniscus MRI measurement for preoperative sizing: the length and width of the meniscus are measured from an axial T2 sequence. The length is measured from the most anterior point of the anterior horn and the most posterior point of the posterior horn of the meniscus (*white line*). The width is measured by first tracing a line joining the most lateral aspects of the anterior and posterior horns (*green line*). At the midpoint of this line, a perpendicular line is drawn to the most medial point on the body of the meniscus. The length of this line is the width (*blue line*).

operative table, the involved extremity is flexed to 80 degrees and a L-bar is secured to the operating room table to allow the heel to rest in this position during surgery. A lateral post is placed at the level of the greater trochanter to allow the extremity to balance in the flexed position and prevent it from falling into abduction (Fig. 25-3). A tourniquet is applied above the knee as high as possible to allow for a wide operative field.

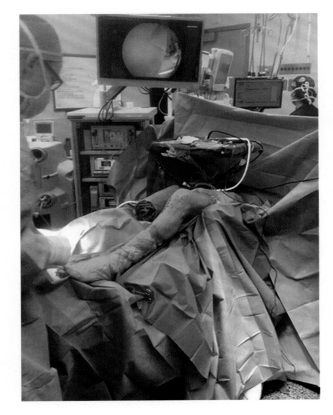

FIGURE 25-3

The patient is positioned with the knee flexed at 80 degrees with a bump at the foot and lateral post holding the thigh.

Anatomic Landmarks and Incisions

The identification of several anatomic landmarks is necessary, as multiple incisions are made for placement of the meniscal allograft. The inferior pole of the patella, patella tendon borders, tibial tubercle, and medial joint line are identified (Fig. 25-4). The patient is sterilely prepped and draped, and after exsanguinating the limb with an Esmarch bandage, the tourniquet is insufflated to 300 mm Hg for the duration of the procedure.

With the knee positioned in 80 degrees of flexion, standard anterolateral (ALP) and anteromedial (AMP) arthroscopy portals are utilized. The ALP is made on the lateral border of the patellar tendon at the level of the inferior pole of the patella and extended proximally approximately 1 cm. The AMP is also started at the same level, but approximately 1 cm medial to the medial border of the patellar tendon and extended distally. An accessory posteromedial portal (PMP) is also marked 1 to 1.5 cm above the posteromedial joint line and 1 cm lateral to the posteromedial aspect of the tibia. This portal should be high and lateral enough to provide good visualization of the posterior root of the medial meniscus.

An anterolateral 4-cm vertical incision is then marked halfway between the tibial tubercle and fibular head approximately two fingerbreadths below the joint line. This incision is used to secure the meniscal roots later on in the procedure.

Similar to inside-out meniscal repair techniques, a 5-cm vertical incision is marked one-third above and two-thirds below the joint line, just posterior to the medial collateral ligament (MCL) over the posteromedial aspect of the knee joint. This incision will be used to deliver the meniscal allograft into the knee joint via an eventual arthrotomy and may incorporate the PMP.

Diagnostic Arthroscopy

Prior to performing a meniscal transplant, it is necessary to perform a diagnostic arthroscopy. Although most patients have had a prior arthroscopy that resulted in a meniscectomy or as part of the evaluation for transplant suitability, there is often an extended interval as the allograft match process may take months to years. This delay may result in further arthritic changes that preclude

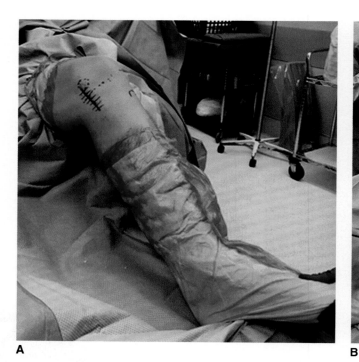
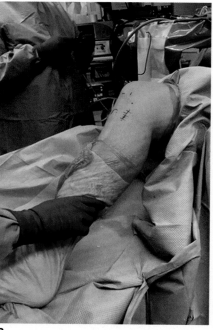

A   B

FIGURE 25-4

Anatomic landmarks and placement of surgical incisions. **A:** The posteromedial incision is made along the posterior border of the MCL. **B:** A lateral incision is made over the adductor tubercle. Standard anteromedial and anterolateral arthroscopic portals are also marked.

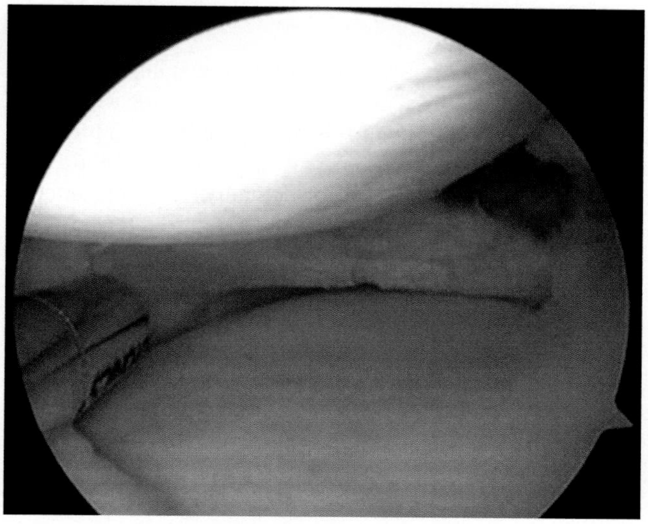

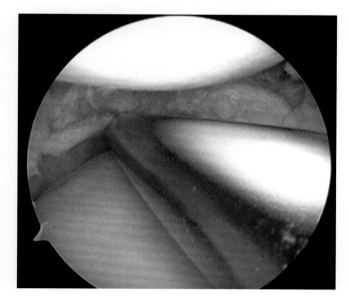

FIGURE 25-5

Arthroscopic view of medial compartment of the knee prior to debridement of remnant tissue. Note the near complete deficiency of the posterior horn and body.

transplantation. The standard anterolateral (AL) and AM portals are used. The medial, lateral, and patellofemoral compartments are assessed for pathologic changes involving the cartilage and menisci, and cruciate ligaments are also evaluated (Fig. 25-5). After evaluation of the medial compartment and determination that the patient is a suitable meniscal transplant candidate, the graft may be prepared. If the medial compartment is difficult to access arthroscopically, the MCL can be gently trephinated with an 18-gauge needle while a steady valgus stress is applied until visualization is adequate.

In the event that a concomitant ACL reconstruction is necessary, it is performed first. Both the femoral and tibial tunnels are created, and the graft may be passed but tibial fixation should be avoided until after the meniscal transplant is in place. Tibial fixation may create difficulty with visualization of the medial compartment.

MEDIAL COMPARTMENT PREPARATION

The degenerative medial meniscus is prepared for donor allograft. An arthroscopic 4.5-mm full radius shaver and arthroscopic basket forceps are used to debride the remaining meniscus to a stable rim in preparation for the allograft. The ideally outer one-third of the meniscus is preserved, as this provides hoop restraint and a well-vascularized foundation for the donor meniscal allograft to be sutured. A bleeding meniscal rim is critical to facilitate healing of the donor tissue (Fig. 25-6).

FIGURE 25-6

Preparation of the medial compartment. The medial compartment is prepared using an arthroscopic shaver to debride the remaining medial meniscus to a smooth rim.

Graft Selection and Preparation

Meniscal allografts are sourced from an AATB (American Association of Tissue Banks) approved tissue bank, and although specifications for sizing vary, they are usually based on measurements from imaging taken from the affected knee preoperatively. The graft is often supplied as a proximal tibia with both menisci present. After a 20-minute thaw in 0.9% normal saline and antibiotic bath (cefazolin), the specimen is inspected for any defects. Using a No. 15 blade scalpel, both the anterior and posterior root insertions are released via subperiosteal dissection, as our preferred technique is to perform the transplant without bone blocks.

The superior surface of the allograft is marked "T.O.P." to maintain orientation during arthroscopy and also marks the anterior, middle, and posterior thirds of the graft. A No. 5 Ethibond (Ethicon Incorporated, Somerville, New Jersey) is passed first in a modified Bunnell fashion through the anterior root followed by the posterior root of the allograft meniscus. Four to five No. 2 Ethibond (Ethicon Incorporated, Somerville, New Jersey) sutures are then passed sequentially in a simple vertical fashion from posterior to anterior into the posterior third of allograft meniscus. Once the graft is prepared, it is set aside in a moist sponge until the recipient site is ready (Fig. 25-7).

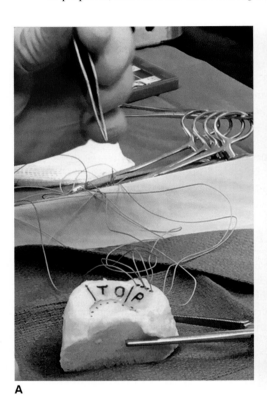

A

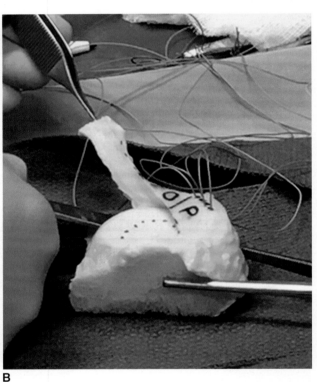

B

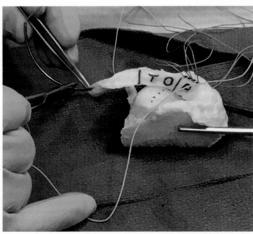

C

FIGURE 25-7

Graft preparation. **A:** Proximal tibial allograft with menisci intact with top labeled and a line marking the anterior, middle, and posterior one-third. Marks are made for four sutures beginning at the middle and posterior one-third junction. Sutures are placed in this region, while the meniscus is still attached to the allograft bone. **B:** The anterior root is elevated from its bony attachment. **C:** Suture is then passed through the anterior root insertion.

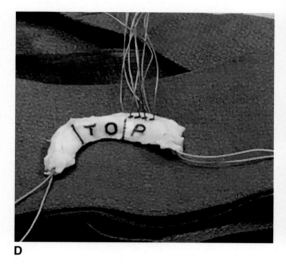

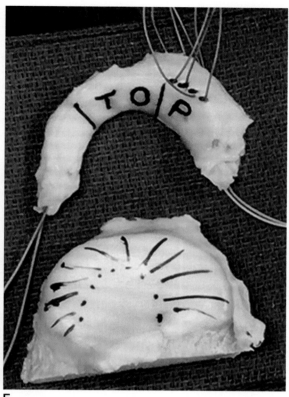

D   **E**

FIGURE 25-7 (*Continued*)

D: The suture ends are then brought through a loop to make a luggage tag. After the posterior root is elevated and sutured in the same fashion, the loops are tensioned around the roots. **E:** The meniscal allograft is seen with its original bony portion.

POSTERIOR ROOT TUNNEL PREPARATION

The posterior root insertion is prepared first. With the arthroscope in the AM portal, an arthroscopic shaver is inserted through the AL portal and the posterior root insertion is debrided. A standard arthroscopic curette or ring curette is used to denude the area immediately next to the posterior root attachment of articular cartilage creating a bleeding surface to further facilitate healing.

If visualization of the posterior root of the medial meniscus is poor, the PMP previously mentioned can now be made. An 18-gauge spinal needle is used to establish the trajectory of the portal, and the Gillquist interval with the arthroscope in the ALP is utilized to observe the needle and switching stick entering the posterior joint. Arthroscopic visualization may then switch between the AM and PM portals as needed.

With the knee in 80 degrees of flexion, an ACL tip guide set at 45 degrees is placed in the ALP portal and via the Gillquist is carefully centered in the posterior root footprint. If the native root is not obvious, the position is immediately posterior to the medial tibial spine.

The guide pin sleeve of the ACL tibial drill guide is placed directly on cortical bone within the anterior tibial compartment approximately 1 cm off the tibial crest. This is approached via the previously marked incision on the anterolateral tibial aspect of the proximal tibia. The skin and subcutaneous tissue are sharply incised and then the tibialis anterior muscle is reflected off the anterolateral tibia in turn protecting underlying neurovascular structures. A second tunnel anchoring the anterior meniscal allograft root will be placed in the area; therefore, the initial tunnel needs to be slightly proximal and posterior, allowing for a 1-cm bone bridge. With the ACL guide locked, a 3.2-mm drill bit is inserted under arthroscopic visualization. If necessary, the drill bit may be left just under the cortical bone of the plateau, and a mallet is used to complete the advancement as not to over penetrate or deflect. The ACL drill guide is now removed and the drill bit is left in situ for the time being (Fig. 25-8).

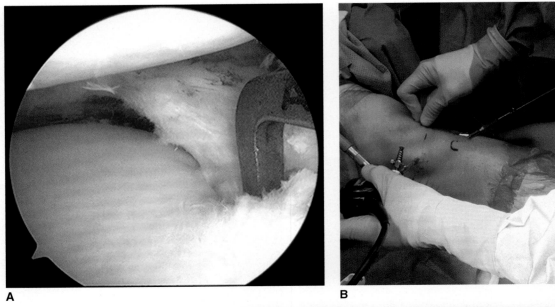

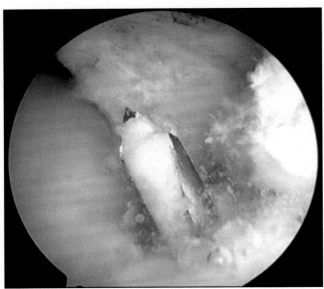

FIGURE 25-8

A: Preparation of the posterior root tibial tunnel. The tip of the drill guide is placed in the center of the footprint of the posterior meniscal root with the camera in the anteromedial portal. **B:** External view showing the drill guide through the anterolateral incision. **C:** The drill bit is left in situ while the anterior root tibial tunnel is drilled. The anterior root tibial tunnel should start 1 cm away from the posterior root tunnel.

Anterior Root Tunnel Preparation

Attention is then turned to preparation of the anterior horn and root of the medial meniscus. With the arthroscope in the AL portal, the anterior root insertion is identified. Analogous to preparation of the posterior root attachment following debridement with an arthroscopic shaver, a standard arthroscopic curette or ring curette is once again used to denude the area immediately next to the anterior root attachment of articular cartilage creating a bleeding surface to further facilitate healing.

With the knee in 80 degrees of flexion, an ACL tip drill guide set at 55 degrees is placed in the AMP portal and is centered in the anterior root footprint. The guide boom is placed within the same anterolateral proximal tibial incision and locked onto the bone 1 cm anterior and distal to the posterior root tunnel. A second 3.2-mm drill bit is used to create the tunnel and the drill bit is once again left in situ upon removal of the ACL tip drill guide (Fig. 25-9).

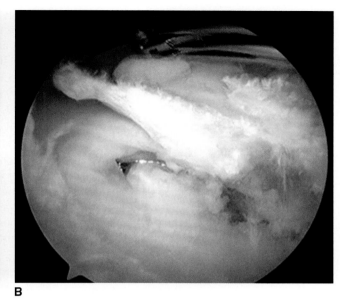

A   **B**

FIGURE 25-9

Preparation of the anterior root tibial tunnel. **A:** The tip of the drill guide is placed in the center of the footprint of the anterior meniscal root. **B:** The drill guide is removed and the drill bit is left in situ until graft passage.

POSTEROMEDIAL PREPARATION

A 5-cm medial-based vertical incision is planned just posterior to the MCL with the knee at 80 degrees of flexion. The vertical incision should be placed one-third superior and two-thirds inferior to the joint line Fig. 25-4A. The skin is incised and carefully dissected to the level of the sartorial fascia. Taking care to preserve the infrapatellar branch of the saphenous nerve, the sartorial fascia is sharply divided in line with the skin incision down to the level of the joint capsule. A 1.5-cm arthrotomy is performed just posterior to the MCL. The arthrotomy should be large enough to accommodate one finger and therefore allow safe passage of the meniscus allograft into the joint (Fig. 25-10).

Graft Passage

The entry sites of the drill bit left in situ for the anterior and posterior roots are then visualized. With the knee at 80 degrees of flexion, the anterior and posterior drill bits are removed and replaced by loop suture passers, which are advanced into the medial compartment. A clamp is then inserted through the medial arthrotomy, and the posterior root suture passer is retrieved and delivered out

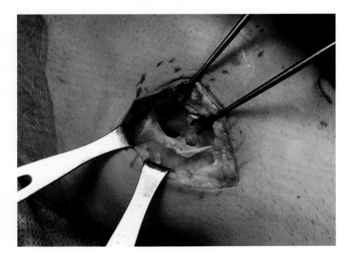

FIGURE 25-10

The posteromedial incision posterior to the MCL is made and dissection is carried down to the capsule, which is then incised longitudinally large enough for passage of the meniscal allograft.

of the joint. The allograft posterior root sutures are then loaded in the posterior root suture passer and brought through the posterior root tibial tunnel. The process is repeated for the anterior root sutures, which are brought out of the anterior root tibial tunnel with the loop suture passer. The meniscus allograft is then pushed into the joint taking care for the multiple sutures not to tangle. The anterior and posterior root sutures are then pulled and held with constant tension throughout the entire remainder of the procedure to provisionally reduce the allograft into its final position and facilitate securing the graft (Fig. 25-11).

Securing the Graft

The four No. 2 Ethibond sutures (Ethicon Incorporated, Somerville, New Jersey) placed in the posterior horn are passed through the capsule with a free needle starting closest to the posterior root insertion and proceeding toward the arthrotomy (Fig. 25-12A). The body of the meniscus is then secured to the capsule using 8 to 12 inside-out vertical mattress suture no. 2-0 Ticron (Covidien, Mansfield, Massachusetts), which is passed in a posterior to anterior fashion (Fig. 25-12D). The vertical mattress sutures should be placed three-fourth superior and one-fourth inferior to the meniscus in order

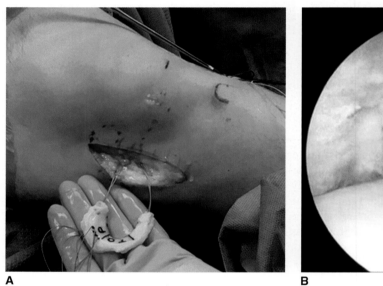

A

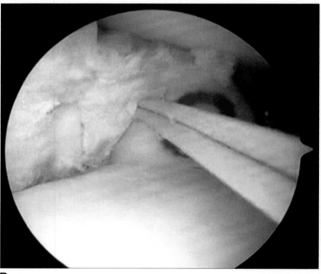

B

FIGURE 25-11

The meniscal graft is now ready to be passed. **A:** The arthroscope is reinserted and a suture grasper is inserted through the anterolateral bone tunnel, and the posterior sutures are passed through the medial arthrotomy and grasped and passed through the bone tunnel. **B:** Allograft is seen after the sutures are passed through the bone tunnels and the allograft is being passed through the medial arthrotomy. **C:** The roots are reduced and sutures held with constant tension.

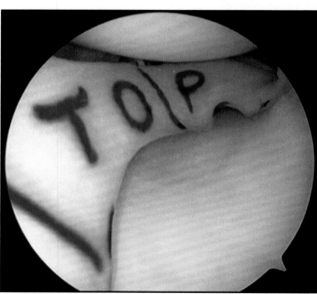

C

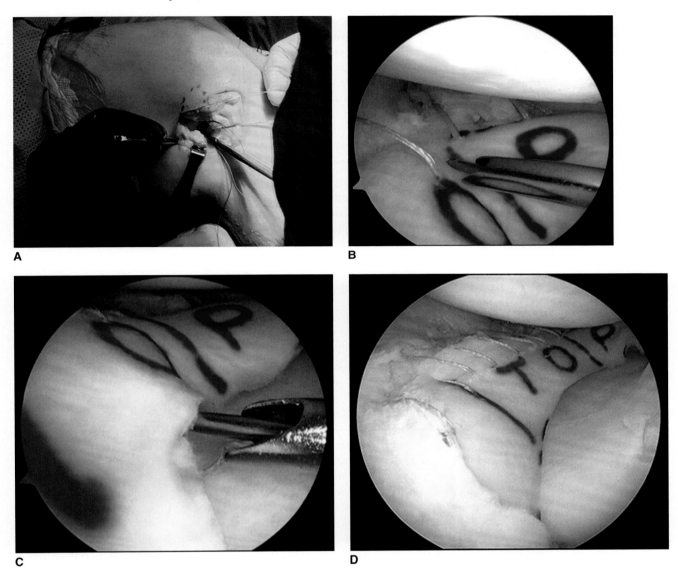

FIGURE 25-12

Placement of meniscal sutures. **A:** The four sutures placed in the allograft before dissection from the allograft bone are then passed through the medial capsule with a free needle. The capsule is then closed. **B, C:** The arthroscope is then inserted, and inside-out sutures are placed in the remaining regions in a vertical mattress fashion from posterior to anterior on top and bottom of the meniscus. **D:** Arthroscopic view of the meniscal allograft with sutures in place which are then tied from posterior to anterior. The meniscal roots are then tied over a bone bridge with the knee flexed at 60 degrees. If ACL reconstruction is done, the tibial side is then tied and the wounds are closed.

to balance the position of the meniscus. The anterior horn of the allograft is secured to the capsule with an outside-in Prolene suture (Fig. 25-12). The capsule is sutured closed with a No. 0 absorbable suture. With the knee at 60 degrees of flexion, the allograft meniscal sutures are then tied from posterior to anterior. Finally, the anterior and posterior root sutures are then tied together over the bony 1-cm tibial bridge, and the knot is tucked under the soft tissue of the anterior muscle compartment.

CLOSURE

Once the medial meniscal allograft is appropriately secured, the medial and lateral incisions are closed in layers. For the medial incision, the sartorial fascia is closed with a 0 absorbable braided suture. The subcutaneous layer is then closed with interrupted 2-0 absorbable braided sutures and the skin is approximated with a 3-0 absorbable monofilament suture in a running subcuticular fashion. For the lateral incision, the anterior compartment is closed over the meniscal root suture with an interrupted 0 absorbable braided suture. The subcutaneous layer is closed with interrupted 2-0 absorbable braided suture and the skin is approximated with a 3-0 absorbable monofilament suture in a running subcuticular fashion. The arthroscopic portals are closed with 3-0 nonabsorbable monofilament sutures. A sterile dressing is applied on the incisions and the leg is placed in a hinged knee brace locked in extension.

PEARLS AND PITFALLS

- The ideal patient for meniscal transplant is young with isolated medial compartment pain with a history of a significant medial meniscectomy.
- Concomitant knee instability or lower extremity malalignment needs to be addressed prior or at the time of medial meniscus transplant.
- The surgeon should carefully examine the quality and sidedness of the meniscus allograft prior to beginning the procedure and should not hesitate to postpone the surgery if the graft is not adequate (e.g., too small, hypoplastic, etc.).
- A solid posterior horn-based meniscocapsular fixation is primordial to the successful outcome of the medial meniscus transplant.
- During the fixation of the allograft, the suture should be tied from posterior to anterior with the knee at 60 degrees of flexion.
- The patient's expectations and the importance of patient compliance to the postoperative physical therapy regimen should be thoroughly discussed prior to performing the medial meniscus transplant.

POSTOPERATIVE MANAGEMENT

A supervised and regimented physical therapy protocol is essential after meniscal transplant (Tables 25-1 and 25-2). Patients are initially restricted to toe-touch weight bearing for 6 weeks, with their knee locked in extension for 2 weeks, then unlocked and progressively increased for another 4 weeks. After 6 weeks in a hinged knee brace, a medial unloader brace is recommended at all times besides sleep for 6 months. Isometric quad sets, straight leg raises (SLRs), and therapy supervised range of motion are begun immediately. At 6 weeks, patients begin using an exercise bike and doing closed kinetic chain exercises. Patients remain on crutches for 10 weeks total with their weight bearing slowly increased from week 6 to 10. Running is allowed at week 16 and return to full activity at around 6 to 9 months postoperative.

COMPLICATIONS

Complications after meniscal transplant are similar to those seen in meniscal repairs with repeat operation for meniscal debridement being the most common and failure being rare. One recent study found 5-year survival to be 93.8% in patients with ideal indications, 90.9% in those with relative indications, and 62.2% in patients with preexisting arthritis (6). Another study found a complication rate of 21% in patients who returned to active duty military at a mean of 2 years, 4.4% requiring a meniscal debridement (9). However, another study of adolescents found a 6% complication rate at 7 years while one meta-analysis found a 10.6% failure rate and 13.9% complication rate at 4.7 years (7,19).

Other complications include neurovascular injury and infection. Although low risk, any allograft transplantation has a risk of disease transmission; the most concerning being HIV and hepatitis C.

TABLE 25-1 Rehabilitation Protocol	
Phase I (0–12 wk)	
Goals	Protect graft
	Develop quadriceps
	Regain motion
	Normal gait
Weight bearing	touchdown weight bearing 0-6 wk
	partial weight bearing 6-10 wk
	weight bearing as tolerate after wk 10
	d/c crutches wk 10–12
ROM	Wk 0–4: 0–70 degrees
	Wk 4–8: 0–90 degrees
	Wk 8: Full ROM
Brace	Locked for 2 wk
	d/c brace after wk 6
	Medial unloader at wk 8
	d/c medial unloader brace at 6 mo
Physical therapy	Immediate isometric quad sets, SLR
	Knee ROM as above
	6 wk: exercise bike and closed kinetic chain
	Normal gait mechanics
Phase II (8–12 wk)	
Goals	Protect graft
	Develop quadriceps
	Normal gait
Weight bearing	As tolerated
ROM	Full
Brace	Medial unloader
Physical therapy	Exercise bike
	Closed kinetic chain (0–60 degrees)
	Open kinetic chain (45–90 degrees)
	Balance
	ROM
Phase III (3–9 mo)	
Goals	Develop hamstrings
	Full ROM
	Strengthening
Physical therapy	Hamstring curls
	Aquatic therapy
	Pool jogging
	Stationary bike, elliptical, stair machine
	More ROM
Phase IV (9 mo)	
Goals	Maintenance of strength, ROM
	Gradual return to activity
Physical therapy	Home regimen with activity-specific exercises

RESULTS

Meniscus transplant is an effective operation for salvage of the postmeniscetomized and painful knee. Concomitant procedures to correct malalignment, ligamentous instability, or focal articular cartilage loss can be successfully done. Many techniques for medial meniscus transplantation exist. Medial meniscus transplantation with posterior peripheral suture technique is the author's preferred technique. When chondral changes in the ipsilateral compartment are minimal, clinical outcome studies show successful long-term outcomes for patients.

TABLE 25-2 Surgical Steps

1 Diagnostic arthroscopy using AL and AM portals
2 Prepare medial compartment, leave outer 1/3 of meniscal rim if possible
3 Prepare allograft
4 Reconstruct ACL if necessary without fixation on tibial side
5 Make anterolateral incision
6 Prepare posterior root footprint and tunnel
7 Prepare anterior root footprint and tunnel
8 Make PM incision and develop plane between layers I and II, make arthrotomy
9 Load posterior and anterior root allograft sutures into respective tunnels through PM arthrotomy
10 Insert allograft into PM arthrotomy with assistant keeping tension in root sutures
11 Posterior horn horizontal mattress sutures passed
12 Capsulotomy closed
13 Inside-out vertical mattress sutures passed on upper surface of meniscus from posterior to anterior
14 Inside-out vertical mattress sutures passed on under surface of meniscus from posterior to anterior
15 Maintain tension on root sutures and all sutures are tied over capsule from posterior to anterior
16 Place knee in 60 degrees of flexion and tie root sutures
17 Secure tibial side of ACL reconstruction if necessary
18 Close wounds

REFERENCES

1. Cox JS, Nye CE, Schaefer WW, et al. The degenerative effects of partial and total resection of the medial meniscus in dogs' knees. *Clin Orthop Relat Res.* 1975;178–183.
2. Johnson RJ, Kettelkamp DB, Clark W, et al. Factors effecting late results after meniscectomy. *J Bone Joint Surg Am.* 1974;56:719–729.
3. Papalia R, Del Buono A, Osti L, et al. Meniscectomy as a risk factor for knee osteoarthritis: a systematic review. *Br Med Bull.* 2011;99:89–106.
4. Edd SN, Netravali NA, Favre J, et al. Alterations in knee kinematics after partial medial meniscectomy are activity dependent. *Am J Sports Med.* 2015;43:1399–1407.
5. Koh JL, Yi SJ, Ren Y, et al. Tibiofemoral contact mechanics with horizontal cleavage tear and resection of the medial meniscus in the human knee. *J Bone Joint Surg Am.* 2016;98:1829–1836.
6. Lee BS, Bin SI, Kim JM, et al. Survivorship after meniscal allograft transplantation according to articular cartilage status. *Am J Sports Med.* 2017;45:1095–1101.
7. Riboh JC, Tilton AK, Cvetanovich GL, et al. Meniscal allograft transplantation in the adolescent population. *Arthroscopy.* 2016;32:1133.e1131–1140.e1131.
8. Saltzman BM, Bajaj S, Salata M, et al. Prospective long-term evaluation of meniscal allograft transplantation procedure: a minimum of 7-year follow-up. *J Knee Surg.* 2012;25:165–175.
9. Waterman BR, Rensing N, Cameron KL, et al. Survivorship of meniscal allograft transplantation in an athletic patient population. *Am J Sports Med.* 2016;44:1237–1242.
10. Cole BJ, Carter TR, Rodeo SA. Allograft meniscal transplantation: background, techniques, and results. *Instr Course Lect.* 2003;52:383–396.
11. Noyes FR, Barber-Westin SD. Long-term survivorship and function of meniscus transplantation. *Am J Sports Med.* 2016;44:2330–2338.
12. Walker PS, Arno S, Bell C, et al. Function of the medial meniscus in force transmission and stability. *J Biomech.* 2015;48:1383–1388.
13. Amendola A. Knee osteotomy and meniscal transplantation: indications, technical considerations, and results. *Sports Med Arthrosc.* 2007;15:32–38.
14. LaPrade RF, Wills NJ, Spiridonov SI, et al. A prospective outcomes study of meniscal allograft transplantation. *Am J Sports Med.* 2010;38:1804–1812.
15. Rosso F, Bisicchia S, Bonasia DE, et al. Meniscal allograft transplantation: a systematic review. *Am J Sports Med.* 2015;43:998–1007.
16. Jang SH, Kim JG, Ha JG, et al. Reducing the size of the meniscal allograft decreases the percentage of extrusion after meniscal allograft transplantation. *Arthroscopy.* 2011;27:914–922.
17. Netto AD, Kaleka CC, Toma MK, et al. Should the meniscal height be considered for preoperative sizing in meniscal transplantation? *Knee Surg Sports Traumatol Arthrosc.* 2018;26(3):772–780.
18. Samitier G, Alentorn-Geli E, Taylor DC, et al. Meniscal allograft transplantation. Part 1: systematic review of graft biology, graft shrinkage, graft extrusion, graft sizing, and graft fixation. *Knee Surg Sports Traumatol Arthrosc.* 2015;23:310–322.
19. Smith NA, MacKay N, Costa M, et al. Meniscal allograft transplantation in a symptomatic meniscal deficient knee: a systematic review. *Knee Surg Sports Traumatol Arthrosc.* 2015;23:270–279.

26 Lateral Meniscus Transplant

Matthew H. Blake, M. Christopher Yonz, and Darren L. Johnson

INTRODUCTION

The menisci serve several important roles in knee function, including load distribution, shock absorption, joint lubrication, enhancing joint congruity, and serving as secondary stabilizers (1). At one time, the meniscus was thought to be a vestigial remnant with little consequence to removal. Thus, subtotal or complete meniscectomies were performed for meniscal pathology. In 1948, Fairbank published on a series of patients who developed osteoarthritis after meniscectomy. He noted that arthritic changes were more common after lateral meniscectomy. He postulated that the menisci may play a role in load bearing (1). Several studies have demonstrated the importance of the meniscus in knee mechanics (2,3).

Now, meniscal preservation using modern repair techniques is advocated whenever possible (2). However, not all meniscus tears are repairable. For these tears, partial meniscectomy to remove only torn portions of the meniscus is recommended. Unfortunately, some circumstances still require subtotal or total meniscectomy. While some patients can tolerate subtotal or total meniscectomies, others develop persistent pain in the deficient compartment with degenerative changes (1,4).

During gait, the articular surface of the knee bears up to six times the body weight, with over 70% of that load borne by the medial tibial plateau (5). The menisci serve to increase the contact area and dissipate the compressive forces at the articular cartilage. The lateral meniscus carries 70% of the lateral compartment load, compared to just 40% by the medial meniscus. By converting joint loading forces to radial hoop stresses on circumferential collagen fibers, the menisci transmit 50% of the joint load when the knee is extended and 90% when the knee is in flexion (7). Loss of just 20% of a meniscus can lead to a 350% increase in contact forces (6). Radial meniscus tears extending to the periphery, and thus disrupting all hoop stresses, results in tibiofemoral contact forces equivalent to a completely meniscectomized knee.

Patients tend to have poorer clinical outcomes after lateral meniscectomy compared to medial meniscectomy. In addition, degenerative changes occur more rapidly after lateral meniscectomy (1,3,7,8). This may be especially concerning to patients with genu valgum after a subtotal or total lateral meniscectomy.

Meniscal allograft transplantation was developed in the 1980s as a potential solution for patients with symptomatic meniscal deficient compartments (7). With several decades of published evidence, it is now considered a viable option for symptomatic meniscus-deficient patients. In this chapter, we discuss the indications, evaluation of these patients, basic science considerations, technical points for sizing, surgical procedure, and rehabilitation. We also review the complications and outcomes of this procedure.

INDICATIONS

The ideal patient for a lateral meniscal allograft is one who presents with lateral-sided knee pain in a meniscus-deficient knee who is skeletally mature and not obese. The knee should be ligamentously stable, in neutral alignment with minimal chondrosis or max International Cartilage Repair Society (ICRS) grade IIIa changes (9,10). Although there is no upper chronologic age limit, patients who have a meniscus-deficient knee and are over the age of 50 often have significant arthritis. Skeletal maturity is necessary to avoid causing asymmetric physeal arrest and progressive angular deformity with the use of current meniscal allograft techniques.

If needed, concomitant procedures should be performed to address malalignment, knee stability, or cartilage deficiency. There is little evidence that, in an asymptomatic knee, performing a meniscal transplant delays the radiographic advancement of arthritis (11). Clinical symptoms, however, rarely correlate with radiographic progression. As such, lateral meniscal allograft transplantation should not be performed in an asymptomatic patient. These patients should be educated and closely monitored for signs of postmeniscectomy syndrome (12).

Contraindications include inflammatory arthritis, synovial disease, history of septic arthritis, immunodeficiency, obesity, and skeletal immaturity. The most common contraindication is advanced arthritis (Outerbridge grade III or IV) on the tibia, flattening of the femoral condyle, or marked osteophyte formation (13).

The surgeon must identify the specific motivation for a patient seeking transplantation and adjust expectations for partial short-term pain relief. Meniscal allograft transplantation may potentially delay osteoarthritis, but it is primarily a pain-relieving operation. The patient should seek treatment for pain in the meniscal deficient compartment and understand that, at best, meniscal transplantation does not prevent the need for future total knee arthroplasty.

PATIENT EVALUATION

Postmeniscectomy patients present with unicompartment joint line pain, effusions, and knee pain induced by changes in barometric pressure. They may also present with occasional giving way and crepitus. After a detailed history, the physical examination should assess ligament stability, alignment, and evaluation of the articular cartilage. If available, previous operative pictures and video are beneficial to see. Evaluation of the location and reason for previous incisions is also critical as many of these patients have undergone prior surgical procedures, including ligament reconstructions and attempted meniscal repair. Patients generally will have tenderness in the involved joint line, full range of motion, and potentially a slight effusion.

Routine radiographs include weight-bearing anteroposterior (AP) views of both knees in full extension and a Rosenberg view to identify joint space narrowing that may not be appreciated on the full extension view (14). A non–weight-bearing 45-degree flexion lateral view and a Merchant view of the patellofemoral joint should also be obtained. Long-leg alignment films must be taken to evaluate any malalignment (10).

A recent magnetic resonance imaging (MRI) is mandatory prior to meniscal transplant. MRI, in conjunction with intraoperative pictures, is useful in determining how much meniscus remains (Fig. 26-1A and B). MRI also allows for evaluation of any cartilage defects. If the status of the cartilage and the

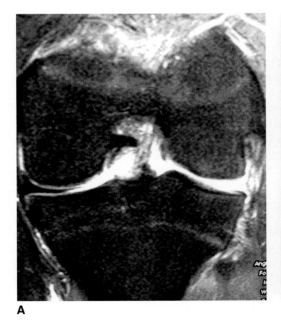
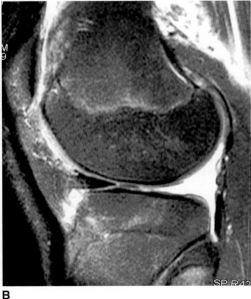

A   **B**

FIGURE 26-1

A and B: Coronal and sagittal MRI views demonstrating a significant amount of lateral meniscus missing.

amount of meniscus that was previously resected are unclear, it is strongly encouraged to perform a diagnostic arthroscopy in order to evaluate the knee for meniscal allograft. This is especially true if the patient has not had any surgical intervention for over a year as it is not uncommon for articular cartilage degeneration to occur over this time frame. This is particularly true on the lateral side where once articular cartilage begins to break down and degeneration rapidly progresses. MRI is also beneficial in evaluating ligamentous structures of the knee that may also need to be addressed at time of surgery (15).

ALLOGRAFT SIZING

Inappropriate sizing of the meniscus can lead to inferior outcomes (15). The appropriate size of an absent meniscus cannot be determined by measuring the meniscus in the contralateral knee as meniscal allografts are side and compartment specific.

The International Meniscus Reconstruction Experts Forum (IMREF) recommends use of a quantitative method for sizing the patient for meniscus allograft transplant (MAT) (10). Pollard's technique is commonly used. This is done by measuring the distance between the peak of the involved compartment's tibial eminence and the compartment's tibial metaphyseal margin as seen on AP radiographs. The length is measured on the lateral radiographic view from the anterior aspect of the tibia above the tibial tuberosity to the posterior plateau margin on the lateral radiographs (Fig. 26-2A and B). After correction for magnification, meniscal length measurements are multiplied by 0.8 for the medial meniscus and by 0.7 for the lateral meniscus (16). This technique has been shown to lead to a size match in at least 95% of cases, which is crucial to optimizing graft survival and protection of the articular surfaces as undersizing will lead to meniscal tears once activities are resumed. This is especially true when using a bone bridge technique as the distance between the anterior and posterior horns of the lateral meniscus is a fixed distance and attached to the bone block.

Pollard's method has been shown to be less accurate when sizing the lateral meniscus. Yoon et al. modified Pollard's method based on a mathematical model to increase accuracy (0.52 × length of the tibia plateau established by the Pollard method) + 5.2 (17).

MRI of the contralateral knee has been described to potentially more accurately size the allograft. This is based on specific meniscus measurements (10). Many have also suggested adding correlation between donor's and recipient's gender, weight, and height (18,19). Other authors have advocated that meniscal allograft tissue should be from a donor <45 years of age (20).

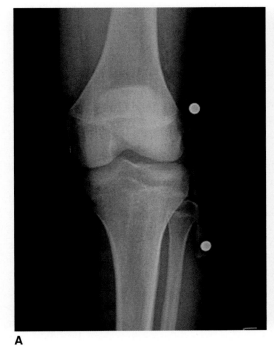
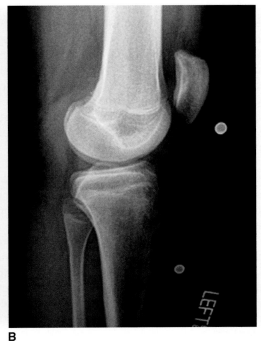

A   **B**

FIGURE 26-2

A and B: AP and lateral views of the left knee with magnification markers in place.

GRAFT PROCUREMENT AND PRESERVATION

Meniscal allografts are harvested within 12 hours of death or within 24 hours of death if the body has been stored at 4°C. Allograft tissue can be obtained either in a sterile environment or in a nonsterile environment and secondarily sterilized. In order to reduce the risk of disease transmission, donor screening should be performed before and after harvest. The American Association of Tissue Banks has defined a stringent protocol to increase the likelihood of obtaining disease-free grafts (21). Serologic screening is performed for HIV p24 antigen, HIV-1/HIV-2 antibody, human T-lymphocyte virus 1 and human T-lymphocyte virus 2, hepatitis B core antibody, antibodies to hepatitis C virus, and syphilis. Most banks also perform polymerase chain reaction testing, which can detect one HIV-infected cell in over 1 million cells. The current window of time for development of detectable antibodies to HIV is approximately 20 to 25 days. The current risk for HIV transmission from frozen connective tissue allografts is estimated to be 1 in 8 million (22). Blood cultures for aerobic and anaerobic bacteria are conducted as well, and lymph node sampling may be performed.

After harvesting, meniscal allografts can be kept as a fresh, viable graft or preserved. Fresh grafts should be ideally harvested within 12 hours of death and are stored in a culture medium at 4°C or 39°F (23). Fresh grafts should be implanted no later than 14 days after procurement (24). The advantages of fresh graft are that it provides the highest number of viable cells and the least alteration to the structure of the meniscus. Its disadvantages are that it is expensive, is logistically demanding for the surgeon and tissue bank, and has the highest risk of disease transmission (due to having less time to test grafts) (25,26). In addition, studies have shown that meniscal allografts become repopulated with host cells, which calls into question the importance of viable cells (27). Because of these limitations, most meniscal allografts are now preserved grafts.

Meniscal allografts can be preserved in several ways: fresh frozen, cryopreserved, or lyophilization (freeze-drying). Fresh frozen grafts are rapidly frozen in a saline and antibiotic solution at −80°C. The freezing process may destroy viable cells as well as result in some collagen disruption. In addition, multiple freeze-thaw cycles may reduce a graft's resistance to compression (28). Advantages of fresh frozen grafts are ease of processing and storage, lower immunogenicity (which may result from denaturing of histocompatibility antigens during the freezing process), and the ability to use secondary stabilization techniques to reduce disease transmission (24). Nonirradiated, fresh frozen grafts are the most common meniscal allografts reported in the literature (9).

Cryopreservation involves placing harvested grafts in a cryoprotective solution with an antiseptic agent. The graft is then slowly frozen to −196°C. The cryoprotective agent is usually glycerol or dimethyl sulfoxide and works by preventing the formation of intracellular ice crystals during the freezing process. The advantages of cryopreservation are that it provides more viable cells compared to fresh frozen and does not alter the ultrastructure of the meniscus. However, cryopreservation is a technically difficult and expensive process. Also, studies have shown that cryopreservation has variable success with preserving viable cells. As studies have shown that host cells repopulate allograft tissue, the importance of viable cells is also questionable. Finally, cryopreserved allografts are not able to be secondarily sterilized, which may increase the risk of disease transmission (29).

Lyophilization involves drying tissue under freezing and vacuum conditions. Cryoprotective solutions are used during this process to preserve cell viability (29). This process allows tissue to be stored for prolonged periods of time at room temperature. However, lyophilization is expensive and reduces the mechanical properties and tissue properties of grafts. This is especially true if the tissue is also sterilized by irradiation.

Graft tissue can be secondarily stabilized to reduce the risk of disease transmission. This is not performed on fresh or cryopreserved grafts in order to preserve cell viability. The most common methods are gamma irradiation or ethylene oxide. Gamma irradiation is bactericidal and viricidal through direct alteration of genetic material and the generation of free radicals. Higher doses are required for frozen compared to fresh or thawed grafts (30). Also, irradiation can reduce the biomechanical properties of soft tissue grafts. Ethylene oxide acts as a chemical sterilizer with bactericidal and viricidal properties. However, it is seldom used in soft tissue grafts because it produces ethylene chlorohydrin as a by-product. This by-product can lead to a significant cell response and synovial inflammation (29). Newer sterilization methods such as supercritical CO_2 sterilization are also being explored. Bui et al. found supercritical CO_2 to cause fewer biomechanical and histologic changes compared to gamma irradiation (31). Despite its disadvantages, gamma irradiation remains the most common method of secondary sterilization.

IMMUNOGENICITY

Animal studies have not demonstrated a predictable humeral or cellular-based immunologic rejection response from bone allografts in rabbits or implanted meniscal allografts in goats or mice (32,33). The most immunogenic portions of the meniscal allograft are the cellular elements of the cancellous bone anchors or trough (29). However, studies of even massive bone allograft implantation demonstrated a low rate of clinically meaningful immunogenic reactions (25). Although meniscal allograft rejection has been reported, most series have not reported significant sequelae related to immunologic reaction. De Boer and Koudstaal (26) implanted a non–tissue antigen-matched cryopreserved meniscal allograft in the lateral compartment of a patient's knee that remained metabolically active with excellent clinical results. Several other studies have reported antibodies against the HLA complex using non–tissue antigen-matched cryopreserved meniscal allografts without accompanying graft failure (27). Rodeo et al. biopsied in vivo meniscal allografts at a mean of 16 months after human transplant. They found evidence of a subtle immune response but noted this had no effect on outcomes (34).

SURGICAL TECHNIQUES

Lateral meniscus transplantation can be performed either open or with an arthroscopically assisted technique. The two methods have similar outcomes, but arthroscopic techniques are now routinely used because of the reduced surgical morbidity.

Multiple techniques, such as the bone bridge, bone plug, and suture fixation, have been described. Seventy-four percent of the surgeons of the International Meniscal Reconstruction Experts Forum (IMREF) prefer bone fixation compared to soft tissue techniques with preference for the bone bridge technique for the lateral side (10). Bone plugs are not recommended for lateral meniscal allografts because the distance between the meniscal horns is only 1 cm or less and, as such, presents a risk of tibial tunnel communication with compromised fixation (35). The suture-only technique has a higher extrusion rate, complication rate, and allograft failure rate; however, both suture-only and bone bridge technique provide similar functional and radiographic results at midterm follow-up (36,37). Fixation of soft tissue with bone is preferred because of its superior load transmission properties (28).

The two most common bone bridge techniques are the bridge-in-slot technique and the dovetail technique. We prefer the bridge-in-slot technique because of its simplicity, its secure bone fixation, the ability to more easily perform concomitant procedures such as osteotomy and ligament reconstruction, and the advantages of maintaining the relationship of the native anterior and posterior horns of the meniscus.

The graft must also be securely sutured to the capsule using standard meniscal repair techniques. Peripheral capsular fixation is a prerequisite for healing and vascularization of the graft. A peripheral meniscal remnant is considered to be important in establishing and maintaining vascular supply to allow ingrowth of the meniscal allograft. The absence of peripheral healing and revascularization induces cell death and matrix disorganization, leading to failed meniscal transplantation. Vertical mattress stitches using nonabsorbable suture material in an inside-out fashion is the gold standard and our preferred technique. All-inside bioabsorbable devices are a reasonable alternative to sutures, but their pullout strength is less than that of vertical sutures and they provide only single-point fixation.

Initial Preparation

The patient is placed under general anesthesia with regional block and intravenous prophylactic antibiotics are administered. An examination under anesthesia is performed on the affected knee to assess for range of motion and ligament stability. A tourniquet is placed high on the thigh and the leg placed in an arthroscopic leg holder. The leg holder should be placed proximally on the thigh

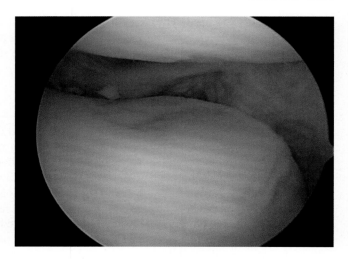

FIGURE 26-3

Arthroscopic view of the lateral compartment after debriding back to a 1- to 2-mm rim of lateral meniscus.

to allow access to perform a safe inside-out meniscal repair. The contralateral leg is placed in the lithotomy position in a well-padded leg holder.

Standard arthroscopic portals are made, and a diagnostic arthroscopy is performed in order to assess for chondral injuries, particularly in the operative compartment. Debridement of the residual meniscus should be performed without inflation of the tourniquet to verify a vascularized recipient meniscocapsular interface. An arthroscopic rasp or 18-gauge spinal needle can be used to generate a vascular rim with punctate bleeding for vascular ingrowth.

A remnant of the posterior and anterior horns should be left for identification later when sliding in the bone bridge (Fig. 26-3). A low modified notchplasty of the lateral femoral condyle, protecting the ACL femoral insertion site, should be performed with an electrocautery unit and a 5.5 shaver. This allows increased visualization of the posterior horn of the lateral meniscus and is also helpful when passing the graft.

A posterolateral incision is also necessary for suture passage during the meniscal repair portion of the procedure. The incision should extend approximately one third above and two thirds below the lateral joint line, posterior to the lateral collateral ligament, and allow adequate exposure to protect neurovascular structures during passage of the inside-out sutures. The short head of the biceps musculature is stripped from the posterior capsule, and a spoon is placed to protect the peroneal nerve. By staying above the tendon of the long head of the biceps, the peroneal nerve is always safe. An additional incision is made through the iliotibial band in line with its fibers and spread with a self-retainer. This is in order to ensure that the sutures are tied beneath these structures to minimize the chances of capturing the knee due to soft tissue tethering.

Bridge-in-Slot Technique

The allograft arrives from the tissue bank as a hemiplateau with the meniscus attached. All non-meniscal tissue is removed, and the exact locations of the anterior and posterior horn anchors are identified. Using a cutting guide, the bridge is then cut to a width of 7 or 8 mm and a depth of 10 mm (Fig. 26-4). The bone bridge should intentionally be undersized by 1 mm to facilitate graft passage and to reduce the risk of inadvertent bridge fracture during insertion. The prepared bridge is then tested for ease of passage through calibrated troughs on the back table. The posterior wall of the bridge should be flush or slanted slightly anterior to the fibers of the posterior horn attachment to allow for insertion at the most posterior edge of the prepared slot. Bone anterior to the anterior horn should be left in place to allow for safer graft manipulation during insertion. A vertical mattress traction suture of 0 polydioxanone (PDS) is placed at the junction of the posterior and middle thirds of the meniscus to assist with graft insertion (Fig. 26-5).

On occasion, the anterior horn attachment can be larger, up to 9 mm wide. If the anterior horn attachment site is wider than the intended width of the bone bridge, the attachment should be left intact, and the width of the bone bridge should be increased accordingly in the area of the anterior horn insertion only. The remainder of the bone bridge should be trimmed to 7 mm as intended.

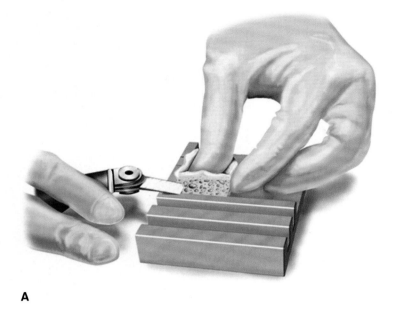

A

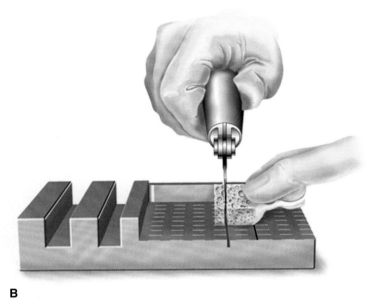

B

FIGURE 26-4

A and B: A diagram showing the allograft bone block being cut to appropriate size. (Courtesy of Stryker Endoscopy, San Jose, CA.)

To accommodate the increased width, the corresponding area of the recipient slot should be widened accordingly.

A 2- to 3-cm mini-arthrotomy is performed in line with the anterior and posterior horn insertion sites of the lateral meniscus. This allows correct orientation of the slot and introduction of the graft. This arthrotomy should be performed directly adjacent to the patellar tendon. An electrocautery device is used to demarcate a straight line from the anterior to posterior root attachments. A 4-mm burr is then used to make a reference slot in the tibial plateau. Its height and width will equal the dimensions of the burr, and its alignment in the sagittal plane should parallel the slope of the tibial plateau (Fig. 26-6). Slot dimensions should be confirmed by placement of a depth gauge in the reference slot, which also measures the AP length of the tibial plateau (Fig. 26-7).

With use of a drill guide, a guide pin is placed just distal and parallel to the reference slot and advanced to but not through the posterior cortex (Fig. 26-8). This is a critical step in ensuring that

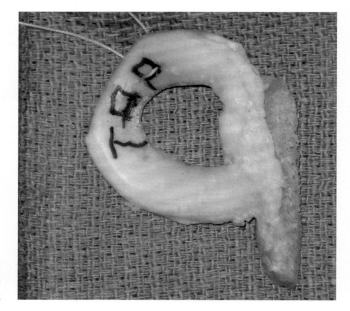

FIGURE 26-5

Lateral meniscal allograft with bone bridge cut to size and traction suture placed at the junction of the posterior and middle thirds.

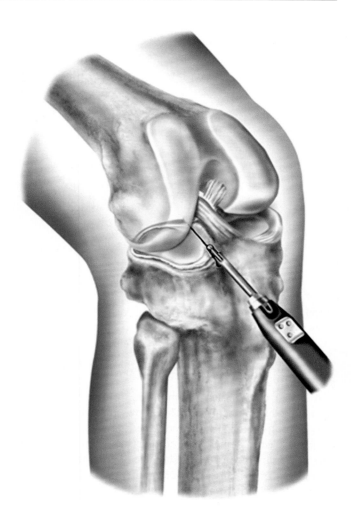

FIGURE 26-6

A 4-mm burr is used to make a reference slot in line with the anterior and posterior horns, parallel to the sagittal slope of the tibial plateau and a width no greater than the burr. (Courtesy of Stryker Endoscopy, San Jose, CA.)

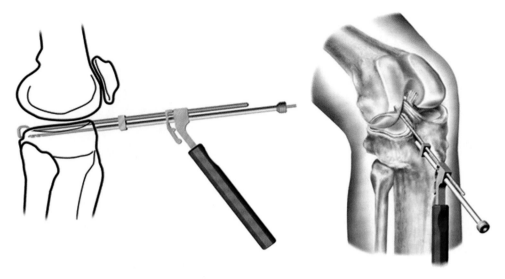

FIGURE 26-7

Stryker guide placed within the reference slot and hooked onto the posterior tibial plateau. The drill guide is in place to measure length of the tibial slot. (Courtesy of Stryker Endoscopy, San Jose, CA.)

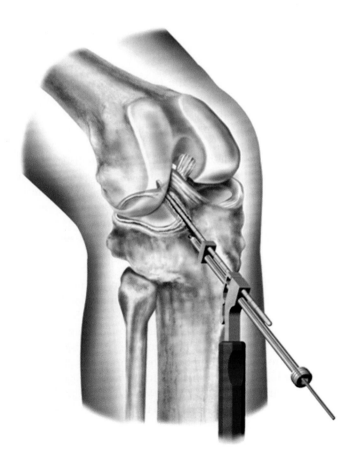

FIGURE 26-8

Guide pin placed through the guide handle, care taken to drill to the posterior tibial cortex but not through it. (Courtesy of Stryker Endoscopy, San Jose, CA.)

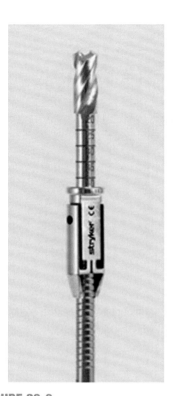
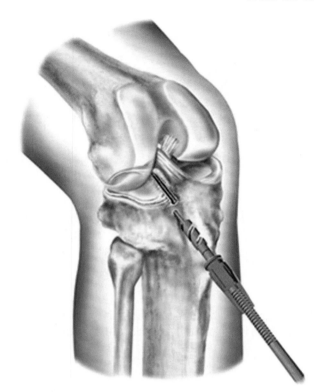

FIGURE 26-9

An 8-mm cannulated reamer is advanced over the guide to the measure depth. (Courtesy of Stryker Endoscopy, San Jose, CA.)

the graft is placed in an anatomic location. The pin is subsequently overreamed with an 8-mm cannulated drill bit, again with care not to breach the posterior cortex (Fig. 26-9). The trough can then be unroofed with the aid of a pituitary. A box cutter is then used to make a slot 8 mm wide by 10 mm deep, which is smoothed and refined with an 8-mm rasp to ensure that the bone bridge will slide smoothly into the slot (Fig. 26-10).

With the arthroscope in the anterolateral portal, a single-barrel zone-specific meniscal repair cannula is placed through the anteromedial portal and is directed toward the capsular attachment of the posterior and middle thirds of the meniscus. A long, flexible nitinol suture passing-pin is placed through the capsule, just anterior to the popliteus tendon, to exit the accessory posterolateral incision. The proximal end of the nitinol pin is then withdrawn from the anterior arthrotomy site, the allograft traction sutures are passed through the loop of the nitinol pin, and the pin and sutures are withdrawn through the posterolateral incision.

Varus stress is placed on the knee to open the lateral compartment. With the aid of traction sutures, the meniscal allograft is pulled into the joint through the anterior arthrotomy while the bone bridge is advanced into the tibial slot, and the meniscus is manually reduced under the condyle with a finger placed through the arthrotomy (Fig. 26-11).

Once the meniscus is reduced, the knee is cycled to ensure proper anatomic placement and capturing by the tibiofemoral articulation. Once again, it is critical that the trough is posterior enough. If there is any question, x-ray may be brought in to confirm trough and bone bridge position. The graft is then attached to the capsule with standard inside-out vertical mattress sutures placed from posterior to anterior, equally on the dorsal and ventral meniscal surfaces (Fig. 26-12). This fixation can be supplemented with appropriate all-inside fixation devices placed in the most posterior aspect of the meniscus to minimize the risk of neurovascular injury.

In regard to the bone bridge fixation, there are a variety of ways to ensure fixation. Some advocate leaving the bone bridge without supplemental fixation. Others use an interference screw to add additional compression of the bone bridge within the slot. Still others supplement fixation with sutures tied over a distal tibial bone bridge. Standard closure of the arthrotomies and accessory incisions is then performed.

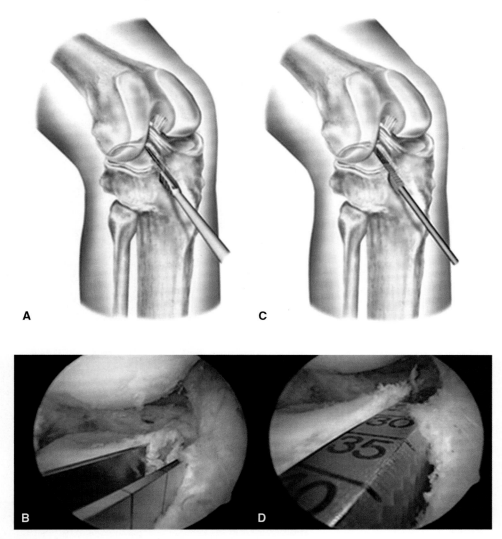

FIGURE 26-10

A: Box cutter is used to convert the rounded slot to a box shape. **B:** Arthroscopic view of the box cutter in place. **C:** Rasp is used to smooth the edges of the slot. **D:** Arthroscopic view of 8-mm rasps in the bone trough. (Courtesy of Stryker Endoscopy, San Jose, CA.)

REHABILITATION

There are no standardized rehabilitation protocols that exist for patients undergoing meniscal allograft transplantation. However, the goal of rehabilitation is to regain motion and function of the knee while protecting the healing allograft tissue.

In our postoperative protocol, patients begin quadriceps sets, straight leg raises, and calf pumps immediately after surgery. Many authors recommend the use of a continuous passive motion machine. We recommend active and passive range of motion from 0 to 90 degrees with protected weight bearing using a hinged knee brace locked in extension during weight bearing for the initial 4 weeks. Goals for range of motion are to achieve full knee extension symmetrical to the noninvolved side within 1 week and 90 degrees of flexion within 4 weeks. Weight bearing, at week 4, is then gradually increased, and full weight bearing is allowed by week 8. During this time period, activities such as cycling, swimming, and closed chain kinetic exercises are begun. It is important that during the first 3 months, no impact loading of the knee flexed past 90 degrees occurs. Forced flexion and pivoting activities should also be avoided during this time period. Running is started at 16 weeks. Return to sporting activities begins at 6 to 9 months following surgery provided that the strength of the leg is at least 85% of normal. It appears most authors limit athletic activity to light sports in the first year (15,38).

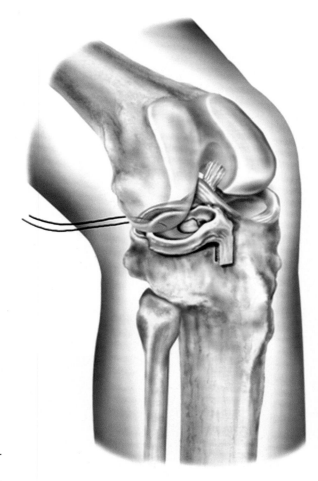

FIGURE 26-11

Diagrammatic representation of meniscus insertion.
(Courtesy of Stryker Endoscopy, San Jose, CA.)

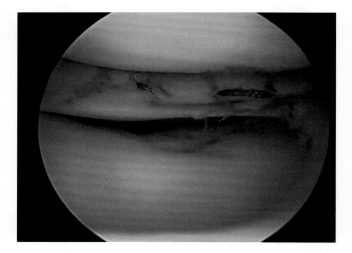

FIGURE 26-12

View of the meniscal allograft in place,
secured with inside/out sutures.

COMPLICATIONS

Meniscal allograft transplant has a complication rate between 10% and 35% (9,39,40). Fortunately, most complications are minor. The most common complication is a graft tear requiring debridement or partial or subtotal meniscectomy. This has been reported in 5% to 30% of patients (9,30,39,40). Meniscal repair has been reported in 2% of cases (9). A review by Myers and Tudor found that graft removal was required in 1.95% of patients (9). Case series have reported on the need for manipulation under anesthesia for stiffness (34). Myers and Tudor found a 1.9% rate of manipulation (9). The bacterial infection rate has been reported to be between 0.7% and 4.5% (9,34). Most have been managed with arthroscopic irrigation and debridement. There have been no reports of viral infection, namely HIV or hepatitis transmission, in the literature. Three studies (34,41,42) reported postoperative immunologic responses but no follow-up. No reports of neurovascular injury are in the literature. Meniscus transplantation performed with concomitant procedures (i.e., ligament reconstruction, cartilage repair/transplantation, osteotomy) is also subject to potential complications from those other procedures including nonunion, ligament failure, and hardware failure.

The criterion for graft failure has been inconsistent across the literature. Some define failure as removal of the graft or conversion to arthroplasty, while others also include patient-reported outcomes below a certain score as graft failures. Others also include structural failure of the graft as a failure. Given these inconsistencies, the failure rate has been reported to be between 8% and 35% (9,39,43). There is still considerable debate regarding what constitutes a failure (9,10). Finally, while meniscus transplant can provide good outcomes and survival rates, it is important for patients to know the rate of reoperation can be over 30%. In case series by Stollsteimer et al. (42) and Graf et al. (31), reoperation was required in 26% and 25% of patients with tears, respectively. These were mostly meniscal trimming or repairs. A case series by McCormick et al. had a 32% reoperation rate (44). Most were debridements and occurred within the first 2 years. Saltzman et al. reported a 36% reoperation rate (40).

OUTCOMES

Favorable clinical outcomes have been reported after meniscal allograft transplant. A systematic review by Rosso et al. determined that Lysholm scores increase from 55.5 ± 2.1 to 82.7 ± 2.7. Visual analog scale (VAS) pain scores decreased from 6.4 ± 0.4 to 2.4 ± 0.4. Overall patient satisfaction rate was 81% ± 3.8% (39). De Bruycker et al. conducted a meta-analysis and found a mean 25% improvement in Lysholm scores, 24 point gain in International Knee Documentation Committee (IKDC) scores, 40 point improvement (on a scale of 100) for VAS pain scores, and 23 point improvement in Knee injury and Osteoarthritis Outcome Score (KOOS) scores (45).

Graft survival rates have varied across the literature. Verdonk et al. reported a 69.8% survival rate for lateral allografts at 10 years (23). Parkinson et al. report an 89% 5-year survival rate for lateral allografts (46). Noyes and Barber-Westin conducted a survivorship analysis in patients <50 years and found survivor rates to be 88% at 5 years, 63% at 10 years, and 40% at 15 years (47). A second survivorship analysis of consecutive meniscus transplants demonstrated 77% survivorship at 5 years with rates falling sharply after 7 years (48). De Bruycker et al. found a mean survivorship around 80% at 5 years. However, they noted that by 10 to 15 years, almost half of the allografts had failed (45).

In addition to patient-reported outcomes and survivorship, graft extrusion is frequently studied. Rosso et al. found a weighted mean graft extrusion of 3.8% (39). A systematic review by Smith et al. found reported mean extrusions between 1.7 and 5.8 mm (11). The anterior horn and mid body of the meniscus are the most likely to extrude (49). Most cases of extrusion occur within the first 6 weeks (50). Studies have been inconsistent regarding whether medial or lateral grafts are more likely to extrude. Some have shown greater extrusion with medial grafts, some greater extrusion with lateral grafts, and some no difference between medial or lateral meniscus allografts (11). Suture-only fixation has been found to have a higher percentage of extrusion compared to bone plug or trough fixation (51). However, multiple studies have demonstrated that graft extrusion does not affect patient-reported outcomes and no significant differences have been found in outcomes when comparing extruded versus nonextruded grafts (9). Meniscal extrusion has also not been found to impact radiologic degeneration (11).

Graft shrinkage is a complication of meniscal allograft transplant related to preservation techniques. Lee et al. found 36% of grafts had mild to moderate shrinkage based on MRI at 1-year postop. However, graft shrinkage did not correlate with clinical outcomes (50). Milachowski et al. (34) found that graft shrinkage does not affect outcomes. Moreover, Stollsteimer et al. (42) described significant pain relief in all 23 patients despite graft shrinkage of 37% on average.

Meniscus allograft horns can be secured with suture-only or with bone plug or trough fixation. Biomechanical studies show that bony fixation more accurately restores contact mechanics in the knee (52,53). As mentioned above, suture-only fixation is associated with a higher rate of graft extrusion compared to bone fixation. Suture-only fixation may also have a higher complication rate (37). Despite possible biomechanical superiority, studies have demonstrated that both techniques produce similar clinical improvement. There is not sufficient evidence to proclaim one technique clinically superior (9,10).

Meniscus transplant is often performed with other concomitant procedures, such as ligament reconstruction, mechanical realignment, and/or cartilage restoration. No significant clinical differences have been found for isolated transplants when compared to transplants performed with concomitant procedures (39,43). As mentioned below, concomitant procedures probably improved survivorship and outcomes by correcting factors associated with failure.

A number of factors have been found to correlate to poorer outcome after meniscus transplant. Meniscus survivorship decreases when performed in compartment with more advanced cartilage lesions (46). A study by Stone et al. demonstrated a survivorship of 12 years with transplant in knees with Outerbridge III and IV lesions (54); however, multiple studies demonstrate poorer outcomes in patients with more advanced cartilage degeneration and osteoarthritis (9). Additionally, mechanical malalignment is associated with poorer results. Thus, realignment procedures are often recommended in patients with a nonneutral mechanical axis to decrease mechanical stress on the graft and compartment (10). Other factors associated with poor results may be increased BMI and patients desiring return to high-impact activity (43).

Traditionally, meniscus transplant is considered a procedure to help young patients return to low-impact activities of daily living. A recent systematic review concluded that many patients return to low-impact recreational sports (55). Several studies have also been published demonstrating a 75% to 85% return to high-level sports (56). However, these results should be interpreted with caution as it is unclear how return to high-level, high-impact activities may affect graft longevity.

In addition to improving pain and function, a goal of meniscus transplant is to protect remaining cartilage. A systematic review of several studies shows no significant joint space narrowing after meniscus transplant (11). Most patients either have no change in Kelligren-Lawrence grade or 1 grade worsening. Up to 78% have no degradation of cartilage signal on MRI at 2.6 years, though this decreases to 40% with longer-term follow-up of 12 years.

CONCLUSION

Allograft meniscus transplantation is a reasonable treatment alternative for patients who have a meniscus-deficient knee. While some studies show promising results in more advanced arthrosis, outcomes are best for patients with no more than grade II or early grade III arthrosis. Clinical studies support the procedure's effectiveness in alleviating pain, swelling, and improving functional outcomes. The procedure can provide reliable pain relief for low-impact activity. While some studies report good outcomes with high-impact activity, the long-term impacts of high-impact activity are not known. Finally, mechanical alignment, ligament stability, and healthy cartilage are required to optimize outcomes. These should be evaluated prior to surgery, and the surgeon should be prepared to perform concomitant procedures if needed to optimize outcome and survival.

REFERENCES

1. Fairbank TJ. Knee joint changes after meniscectomy. *J Bone Joint Surg Br.* 1948;30B(4):664–670.
2. Baratz ME, Fu FH, Mengato R. Meniscal tears: the effect of meniscectomy and of repair on intraarticular contact areas and stress in the human knee. A preliminary report. *Am J Sports Med.* 1986;14(4):270–275.
3. Walker PS, Erkman MJ. The role of the menisci in force transmission across the knee. *Clin Orthop Relat Res.* 1975;(109):184–192.
4. Tapper EM, Hoover NW. Late results after meniscectomy. *J Bone Joint Surg Am.* 1969;51(3):517–526 passim.
5. Rohrle H, Scholten R, Sigolotto C, et al. Joint forces in the human pelvis-leg skeleton during walking. *J Biomech.* 1984;17(6):409–424.
6. Seedhom BB, Hargreaves DJ. Transmission of load in the knee joint with special reference to the role of the menisci, part II: experimental results, discussions, and conclusions. *Eng Med.* 1979;8:220–228.
7. Paletta GA Jr, Manning T, Snell E, et al. The effect of allograft meniscal replacement on intraarticular contact area and pressures in the human knee. A biomechanical study. *Am J Sports Med.* 1997;25(5):692–698.
8. Levy IM, Torzilli PA, Gould JD, et al. The effect of lateral meniscectomy on motion of the knee. *J Bone Joint Surg Am.* 1989;71(3):401–406.
9. Myers P, Tudor F. Meniscal allograft transplantation: how should we be doing it? A systematic review. *Arthroscopy.* 2015;31(5):911–925.
10. Getgood A, LaPrade RF, Verdonk P, et al. International Meniscus Reconstruction Experts Forum (IMREF) 2015 consensus statement on the practice of meniscal allograft transplantation. *Am J Sports Med.* 2017;45(5):1195–1205.
11. Smith NA, Parkinson B, Hutchinson CE, et al. Is meniscal allograft transplantation chondroprotective? A systematic review of radiological outcomes. *Knee Surg Sports Traumatol Arthrosc.* 2016;24(9):2923–2935.
12. Sherman SL, Thomas DM, Gulbrandsen TR, et al. Meniscus allograft transplantation. *Oper Tech Sports Med.* 2018;26(3):189–204.
13. Veltri DM, Warren RF, Wickiewicz TL, et al. Current status of allograft meniscal transplantation. *Clin Orthop Relat Res.* 1994;(303):44–55.
14. Rosenberg TD, Paulos LE, Parker RD, et al. The forty-five-degree posteroanterior flexion weight-bearing radiograph of the knee. *J Bone Joint Surg Am.* 1988;70(10):1479–1483.
15. Frank RM, Cole BJ. Meniscus transplantation. *Curr Rev Musculoskelet Med.* 2015;8(4):443–450.
16. Pollard ME, Kang Q, Berg EE. Radiographic sizing for meniscal transplantation. *Arthroscopy.* 1995;11(6):684–687.

17. Yoon JR, Kim TS, Lim HC, et al. Is radiographic measurement of bony landmarks reliable for lateral meniscal sizing? *Am J Sports Med*. 2011;39(3):582–589.

18. Stone KR, Walgenbach AW, Turek TJ, et al. Meniscus allograft survival in patients with moderate to severe unicompartmental arthritis: a 2- to 7-year follow-up. *Arthroscopy*. 2006;22(5):469–478.

19. Van Thiel GS, Verma N, Yanke A, et al. Meniscal allograft size can be predicted by height, weight, and gender. *Arthroscopy*. 2009;25(7):722–727.

20. Bursac P, York A, Kuznia P, et al. Influence of donor age on the biomechanical and biochemical properties of human meniscal allografts. *Am J Sports Med*. 2009;37(5):884–889.

21. Osborne JC, Norman KG, Maye T, et al. *Standards for Tissue Banking*. McLean, VA: American Association of Tissue Banks; 2016.

22. Buck BE, Resnick L, Shah SM, et al. Human immunodeficiency virus cultured from bone. Implications for transplantation. *Clin Orthop Relat Res*. 1990;(251):249–253.

23. Verdonk R, Van Daele P, Claus B, et al. [Viable meniscus transplantation]. *Orthopade*. 1994;23(2):153–159.

24. Mickiewicz P, Binkowski M, Bursig H, et al. Preservation and sterilization methods of the meniscal allografts: literature review. *Cell Tissue Bank*. 2014;15(3):307–317.

25. Friedlaender GE, Strong DM, Sell KW. Studies on the antigenicity of bone. II. Donor-specific anti-HLA antibodies in human recipients of freeze-dried allografts. *J Bone Joint Surg Am*. 1984;66(1):107–112.

26. De Boer HH, Koudstaal J. The fate of meniscus cartilage after transplantation of cryopreserved nontissue-antigen-matched allograft. A case report. *Clin Orthop Relat Res*. 1991;(266):145–151.

27. Khoury MA, Goldberg VM, Stevenson S. Demonstration of HLA and ABH antigens in fresh and frozen human menisci by immunohistochemistry. *J Orthop Res*. 1994;12(6):751–757.

28. Chen MI, Branch TP, Hutton WC. Is it important to secure the horns during lateral meniscal transplantation? A cadaveric study. *Arthroscopy*. 1996;12(2):174–181.

29. Goble EM, Kohn D, Verdonk R, et al. Meniscal substitutes—human experience. *Scand J Med Sci Sports*. 1999;9(3):146–157.

30. Matava MJ. Meniscal allograft transplantation: a systematic review. *Clin Orthop Relat Res*. 2007;455:142–157.

31. Bui D, Lovric V, Oliver R, et al. Meniscal allograft sterilisation: effect on biomechanical and histological properties. *Cell Tissue Bank*. 2015;16(3):467–475.

32. Jackson DW, McDevitt CA, Simon TM, et al. Meniscal transplantation using fresh and cryopreserved allografts. An experimental study in goats. *Am J Sports Med*. 1992;20(6):644–656.

33. Ochi M, Ishida O, Daisaku H, et al. Immune response to fresh meniscal allografts in mice. *J Surg Res*. 1995;58(5):478–484.

34. Rodeo SA, Seneviratne A, Suzuki K, et al. Histological analysis of human meniscal allografts. A preliminary report. *J Bone Joint Surg Am*. 2000;82-a(8):1071–1082.

35. Johnson DL, Swenson TM, Livesay GA, et al. Insertion-site anatomy of the human menisci: gross, arthroscopic, and topographical anatomy as a basis for meniscal transplantation. *Arthroscopy*. 1995;11(4):386–394.

36. De Coninck T, Huysse W, Verdonk R, et al. Open versus arthroscopic meniscus allograft transplantation: magnetic resonance imaging study of meniscal radial displacement. *Arthroscopy*. 2013;29(3):514–521.

37. Abat F, Gelber PE, Erquicia JI, et al. Prospective comparative study between two different fixation techniques in meniscal allograft transplantation. *Knee Surg Sports Traumatol Arthrosc*. 2013;21(7):1516–1522.

38. Chalmers PN, Karas V, Sherman SL, et al. Return to high-level sport after meniscal allograft transplantation. *Arthroscopy*. 2013;29(3):539–544.

39. Rosso F, Bisicchia S, Bonasia DE, et al. Meniscal allograft transplantation: a systematic review. *Am J Sports Med*. 2015;43(4):998–1007.

40. Saltzman BM, Meyer MA, Weber AE, et al. Prospective clinical and radiographic outcomes after concomitant anterior cruciate ligament reconstruction and meniscal allograft transplantation at a mean 5-year follow-up. *Am J Sports Med*. 2017;45(3):550–562.

41. Noyes FR, Barber-Westin SD. Irradiated meniscal allografts in the human knee: a two to five year follow-up study. *Orthop Trans*. 1995;19:417.

42. Stollsteimer GT, Shelton WR, Dukes A, et al. Meniscal allograft transplantation: a 1- to 5-year follow-up of 22 patients. *Arthroscopy*. 2000;16(4):343–347.

43. Hergan D, Thut D, Sherman O, et al. Meniscal allograft transplantation. *Arthroscopy*. 2011;27(1):101–112.

44. McCormick F, Harris JD, Abrams GD, et al. Survival and reoperation rates after meniscal allograft transplantation: analysis of failures for 172 consecutive transplants at a minimum 2-year follow-up. *Am J Sports Med*. 2014;42(4):892–897.

45. De Bruycker M, Verdonk PCM, Verdonk RC. Meniscal allograft transplantation: a meta-analysis. *SICOT J*. 2017;3:33.

46. Parkinson B, Smith N, Asplin L, et al. Factors predicting meniscal allograft transplantation failure. *Orthop J Sports Med*. 2016;4(8):2325967116663185.

47. Noyes FR, Barber-Westin SD. Meniscal transplantation in symptomatic patients under fifty years of age: survivorship analysis. *J Bone Joint Surg Am*. 2015;97(15):1209–1219.

48. Noyes FR, Barber-Westin SD. Long-term survivorship and function of meniscus transplantation. *Am J Sports Med*. 2016;44(9):2330–2338.

49. Samitier G, Alentorn-Geli E, Taylor DC, et al. Meniscal allograft transplantation. Part 1: systematic review of graft biology, graft shrinkage, graft extrusion, graft sizing, and graft fixation. *Knee Surg Sports Traumatol Arthrosc*. 2015;23(1):310–322.

50. Lee DH, Kim TH, Lee SH, et al. Evaluation of meniscus allograft transplantation with serial magnetic resonance imaging during the first postoperative year: focus on graft extrusion. *Arthroscopy*. 2008;24(10):1115–1121.

51. Abat F, Gelber PE, Erquicia JI, et al. Suture-only fixation technique leads to a higher degree of extrusion than bony fixation in meniscal allograft transplantation. *Am J Sports Med*. 2012;40(7):1591–1596.

52. Alhalki MM, Howell SM, Hull ML. How three methods for fixing a medial meniscal autograft affect tibial contact mechanics. *Am J Sports Med*. 1999;27(3):320–328.

53. McDermott ID, Lie DT, Edwards A, et al. The effects of lateral meniscal allograft transplantation techniques on tibio-femoral contact pressures. *Knee Surg Sports Traumatol Arthrosc*. 2008;16(6):553–560.

54. Stone KR, Pelsis JR, Surrette ST, et al. Meniscus transplantation in an active population with moderate to severe cartilage damage. *Knee Surg Sports Traumatol Arthrosc*. 2015;23(1):251–257.

55. Barber-Westin SD, Noyes FR. Low-impact sports activities are feasible after meniscus transplantation: a systematic review. *Knee Surg Sports Traumatol Arthrosc*. 2018;26(7):1950–1958.

56. Trentacosta N, Graham WC, Gersoff WK. Meniscal allograft transplantation: state of the art. *Sports Med Arthrosc Rev*. 2016;24(2):e23–e33.

27 Bone-Patellar Tendon-Bone ACL Reconstruction

Matthew J. Deasey, MaCalus V. Hogan, and Mark D. Miller

INTRODUCTION

The anterior cruciate ligament (ACL) has an important stabilizing and biomechanical function for the knee. Reconstruction of the ACL is one of the most commonly performed procedures in the field of sports medicine. With an incidence of 68 tears per 100,000 person years, over 200,000 ACL tears occur each year with 100,000 ACL reconstructive surgeries done each year in the United States (1,2). The rate of tear recognition and reconstruction has increased by over 20% in the first two decades of the 21st century (3). Restoration of normal knee function, protection from further intra-articular injury, and return to play are the goals of treatment and have led to research for the development of new operative techniques. Preparation for ACL surgery should include consultation with the patient regarding functional expectations and postoperative activity. Reconstruction of the ACL with the bone-patella tendon-bone (BPTB) autograft secured with an interference screw has been described as a successful method of ACL reconstruction, in particular for young men with no antecedent knee pain.

Reconstruction of the ACL with BPTB autograft secured with interference screws was first described by Jones in 1963 and later popularized by Clancy in 1982 (4,5). The BPTB autograft reconstruction accomplishes some of the fundamental goals of ACL reconstruction: ease of graft harvest, minimal harvest-site morbidity, and biomechanical properties that are similar to those of the native ligament. It also possesses high initial strength and stiffness and can be secured predictably with rapid incorporation into host tissue that allows for early, aggressive rehabilitation while recreating the anatomy and function of the native knee (6–8). Arthroscopically assisted BPTB autograft also has the advantage of a single incision, leading to shorter operating times, reduced postoperative morbidity, improved cosmesis, and quicker rehabilitation. The disadvantages of BPTB ACL reconstruction include graft site morbidity, disruption of the extensor mechanism, patella fracture, patella baja, and patellofemoral pain (9–11). It is important for the orthopedic surgeon to be aware of the advantages and disadvantages of using BPTB autograft and compare those to factors related to other graft choices and apply pertinent information to each individual patient who is a candidate for reconstruction. Regardless of graft choice, a clear understanding of the critical stages of arthroscopic ACL reconstruction and knowledge of the potential pitfalls can help avoid complications and produce consistent results. This chapter seeks to provide a reproducible technique for arthroscopic ACL reconstruction using BPTB autograft.

HISTORY AND PHYSICAL EXAMINATION

ACL injuries can occur in numerous ways, but there are a few mechanisms that predominate. Up to one third of the time the patient is unable to give clarity to the mechanism of injury; however, when an account is given, patients often report a noncontact pivoting injury with a deceleration and rotational component during running, cutting, or jumping (12,13). The injury is often associated with an audible "pop" heard by the patient at the time of injury. The patient usually falls to the ground and is not able to resume activity. An effusion ensues within a few hours in contrast to a meniscus tear where swelling usually occurs within 24 hours (1,14). Contact injuries can also lead to ACL disruption and usually involve a hyperextension and/or valgus force to the knee by a direct blow.

The physical examination and preoperative assessment of the knee joint is critical to successful outcomes from ACL surgery. With an adequate history and physical examination, an ACL injury can often be diagnosed proficiently without additional studies. Most sports medicine physicians agree that the examination is most accurately performed immediately after the injury, before swelling, pain, and muscle spasms occur. Collateral ligament and meniscal injuries can be identified through the history and physical examination; therefore, a complete examination of the knee should be performed in order for improved interpretation of diagnostic studies, recognition of concomitant injuries, surgical planning, and optimal physician-patient communication about expected outcomes. Poor outcomes are associated with poor range of motion, weak quadriceps function, and excessive swelling. Therefore, it is reasonable to delay surgery until full extension is achieved, optimal skin and soft tissue factors have resolved (minimal swelling), and quadriceps function is in the activated state (15).

The physical examination should begin with examination of the uninjured knee. This helps to familiarize the patient with the knee examination and helps the examiner determine patient-specific normal parameters. Examination of the injured knee begins with visual inspection for evidence of swelling and lacerations. After inspection, palpation ensues for qualitative assessment of patella position and potential knee effusions. Next, quantitative measures of the patient's active and passive range of motion are obtained and recorded. After taking the patient through a range of motion, the patient's knee can be brought to 90 degrees and inspection of meniscal pathology may proceed with palpation of the medial and lateral joint line. While at 90 degrees of flexion, the anterior drawer test is performed to evaluate anterior tibial translation. This is performed by stabilizing the foot of the affected knee while placing an anterior force on the tibia. Next, the patient is brought out into 20 to 30 degrees of flexion, and the Lachman test is performed (Fig. 27-1). This test has become the hallmark of anterior laxity testing in the knee and involves stabilization of the femur with one hand while an anterior force is applied to the tibia with the other hand (16). The degree of translation of the tibia as well as the characterization of the endpoint is recorded. The laxity is based on comparison of the contralateral knee and not as the degree of absolute translation. Grade 1 laxity is 1 to 5 mm of translation. Grade 2 laxity is 6 to 10 mm of translation. Grade 3 laxity is more than 10 mm of translation. This test is most specific for the anteromedial bundle of the ACL (17). Varus and valgus stressing can also be applied to the knee at 20 to 30 degrees to assess lateral collateral ligament and the medical collateral ligament (MCL) competency, respectively. The knee can then be brought out into extension with varus and valgus stressing applied once again to determine if there are other associated injuries (14). The pivot shift test is a special maneuver to assess the rotational component of ACL competency, requires an intact MCL, and begins with the patient in extension (1). The examiner places a valgus-directed force, axial load, and internal rotation on the extended knee and proceeds to slowly flex the knee. At approximately 30 degrees of flexion, a reduction of the subluxation can be felt or heard. The test is based on the lateral tibial plateau subluxing anteriorly with extension and reducing with flexion

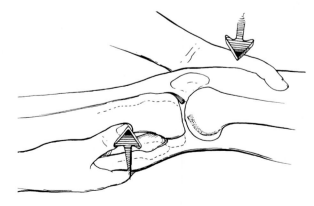

FIGURE 27-1
Lachman test.

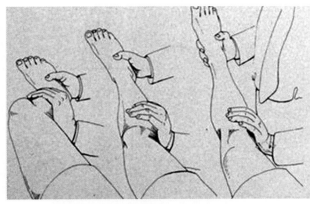

FIGURE 27-2
Pivot shift test.

and is pathognomonic of ACL deficiency (18,19) (Fig. 27-2). This maneuver is often poorly tolerated by awake patients and should be performed toward the end of the physical examination secondary to subsequent patient apprehension and guarding. If equivocal on awake exam, the pivot shift can and should be tested and documented under anesthesia both before and after reconstruction.

DIAGNOSTIC STUDIES

Plain radiographs of the knee should be obtained during the initial evaluation to rule out fractures about the femorotibial joint. The Segond fracture is an avulsion of the anterolateral capsule of the tibia and is thought to be a pathognomonic radiographic finding of ACL injury (20). If the patient is immature skeletally or skeletally mature with osteopenia, an avulsion of the tibial insertion of the ACL, which results in a nonfunctioning ACL, can also be seen on plain radiographs. Plain radiographs also can reveal osteochondral lesions, loose bodies, degenerative joint disease, and overall alignment of the knee. Specific to planning for BPTB autograft reconstruction, appropriate preoperative radiographic assessment of the patellar tendon with a true lateral radiograph is important to ensure adequate graft length (7,21). Radiographs also help to note the presence of any ossicles within the tendon. These ossicles can be associated with Sinding-Larsen-Johansson (proximal ossicles) or Osgood-Schlatter syndrome (distal ossicles) and can compromise graft competency or length if improperly addressed (22).

Following radiographs, an MRI is the most useful diagnostic study for detecting ACL tears with a reported accuracy of 70% to 100% (1,23). The normal ACL is seen as a defined band through the intercondylar notch. With disruption, the ligament is ill defined, with a mixed signal intensity representing local edema and hemorrhage (24). MRI can also reveal any associated meniscal tears, chondral injuries, or bone bruises. The typical bone bruise pattern is increased signal intensity on T2-weighted images on the posterolateral tibial plateau and anterolateral femoral condyle. This "kissing contusion" pattern is present in up to 80% of patients with ACL injuries (25–27). Patients who cannot undergo MRI imaging may be candidates of stress radiographs; however, these are primarily used to diagnose posterior cruciate ligament (PCL) injuries.

ANESTHESIA AND POSITIONING

Reconstruction of the ACL can be performed under regional (spinal or epidural) or general anesthesia supplemented by a femoral and/or sciatic nerve block to assist with postoperative analgesia (7,28). Once the appropriate anesthesia has been chosen and induced, preoperative antibiotics should be given to the patient. An examination under anesthesia can then be performed. The previously mentioned tests specific for ACL function are performed bilaterally. The surgeon should also test the extent of combined injuries by assessing external rotation stability in 30 and 90 degrees of flexion indicating a posterolateral corner (PLC) or combined PCL/PLC injury, respectively. This exam is essential to avoid missing PLC injuries, which, if missed, can lead to failure of the ACL reconstruction.

After performing the examination under anesthesia, a nonsterile tourniquet is placed on the operative extremity high on the thigh. A reliable technique for placement of the tourniquet is to bend the knee of the operative leg and place the foot on the edge of the bed with the hip in about 40 to 45 degrees of abduction. The person applying the tourniquet uses their chest against the anterior portion of the patient's knee for stabilization. Padding is applied to the upper thigh, and the tourniquet is

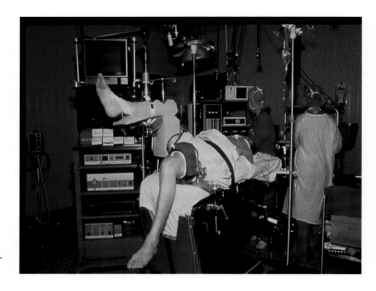

FIGURE 27-3

Positioning for BPTB ACL reconstruction.

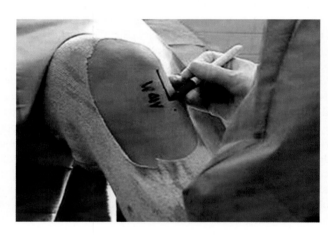

FIGURE 27-4

Marking from anterior patella to tibial tubercle for graft harvest.

applied as far proximal as possible. After application, the skin just distal to the tourniquet is tugged slightly to prevent slippage. The contralateral leg can rest in extension on the OR table. A well-padded post should be attached to the operating table just distal to the tourniquet. Proper positioning of this post will allow the leg to be abducted for the diagnostic arthroscopy and will should provide support for the operative knee during ACL reconstruction. The operative leg is then prepped and draped using standard sterile technique. An Alvarado boot and plate are attached to the patient and to the table, respectively (Fig. 27-3). Once draped, markings are made on the patient's skin for the tibial tubercle, the borders of the patella, and portal sites. A marking is then made for the proposed incision for graft harvest (Fig. 27-4). The operative leg is exsanguinated with a commercially available Esmarch bandage. The tourniquet is inflated to 275 to 300 mm Hg, and the procedure begins.

PREFERRED OPERATIVE TECHNIQUE

A diagnostic arthroscopy is performed to verify injury to the ACL and to assess for associated injuries that may be present. The standard anterolateral and anteromedial portals are made, and the suprapatellar pouch is entered. A limited fat pad debridement is performed to enhance visualization. After debridement of the fat pad, the patellofemoral joint is visualized, the lateral gutter is inspected, and then the medial gutter is inspected. The gutters are cleared of any loose bodies and then the scope is introduced into the medial compartment. Associated cartilage damage and meniscal pathology is identified and noted and then the scope is introduced into the lateral compartment, and the cartilage and meniscus is evaluated in the lateral compartment as well. Injuries seen during the diagnostic arthroscopy are addressed during graft preparation. During assessment of the intercondylar notch, the PCL is identified and examined with a probe and the probe is then used to confirm the incompetency of the ACL. Arthroscopic photographs of the torn ACL are taken for both office and patient records. To confirm the ACL tear, the arthroscope is used to inspect the lateral wall of the intercondylar notch and an anterior drawer test can be performed to assess ligament failure (Fig. 27-5).

Once the diagnostic arthroscopy is complete and the ACL tear has been confirmed, the patellar tendon autograft harvest begins. A 4- to 6-cm incision is made along the previously made skin markings from the midpatella to the tibial tubercle. The incision is made slightly medial to midline to avoid scarring over the prominent parts of the patella and tibial tubercle. The skin incision is taken down through the skin and subcutaneous fat and full-thickness flaps are made down to the paratenon. The paratenon is then divided and dissected off of the tendon both medially and laterally. Care is taken to preserve the paratenon for later reapproximation and closure. This layer has been shown to be important in tendon regeneration (7,29).

The patellar tendon width is measured, and the central third of the patellar tendon is chosen. For patellar tendons that measure <30 or >38 mm, the harvested graft width should be 9 and 11 mm, respectively. Once the proper graft size is determined, a no. 15 blade is used for graft harvest. The surgeon should aim to harvest a distal bone plug of 23 mm and a proximal bone plug of 20 mm length. The graft is harvested with the knee in flexion in order to keep the tendon under tension. A rectangular bone block is then harvested from the tibial tubercle cutting through the cortex to a depth of approximately 10 mm. A curved ¼ in osteotome is used to make sure that the corners of the bone block are free from the remaining tubercle. The osteotome is then inserted into the distal aspect of the tibial tubercle cut horizontally and used as a lever to release the bone block from the tibial tubercle (Fig. 27-6).

The patella graft harvesting retractor is placed under the skin, and the patella is levered distally for better exposure of the patella bone block harvest site. The oscillating saw is angled toward the midline, in a convergent manner, for the longitudinal cuts to create a trapezoidal or triangular bone block (Fig. 27-7). Care should be taken to avoid diving too deep into the patella in order to prevent patella fracture and chondral damage. The ¼ inch osteotome used for the tibial tubercle osteotomy can be used in the patella to complete the osteotomy at the corners and periphery. The osteotome is also used to lever the bone block from the surrounding patella. The patella tendon graft is then carefully dissected free from the remaining patella tendon and brought to the back table for preparation.

Once the graft is brought to the back table, the bone blocks are sculpted using a small rongeur and an ACL graft-shaper clamp so that they fit through the appropriately sized hole of a sizing block (usually 10-mm sizing block). The tibial bone block should be rounded at the leading end to assist in graft passage from the tibial tunnel into the femoral tunnel. Excess bone removed from the bone blocks should be saved to fill harvest defect sites prior to closure at the end of the case. A single hole is drilled using a 2-mm drill bit 5 to 8 mm from the end of the tibial bone block in an anterior-to-posterior direction and a number 5 nonabsorbable suture is threaded through the hole (Fig. 27-8). Two evenly spaced holes are made in the patella bone block perpendicular to each other (90–90 holes), and 5 nonabsorbable sutures are threaded through each hole (Fig. 27-8). The bone-tendon junction at each end of the BTPB graft is marked with a surgical pen, and measurements of the entire

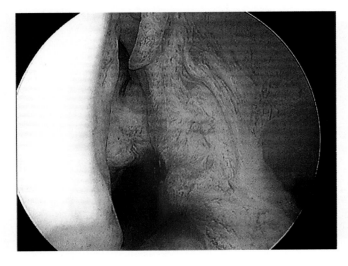

FIGURE 27-5

Empty lateral wall seen on arthroscopy.

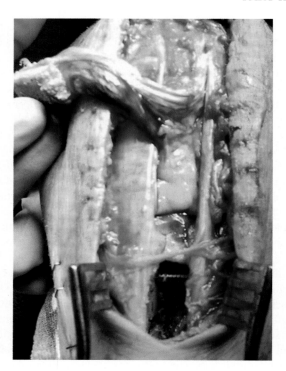

FIGURE 27-6

BPTB graft harvest seen from lateral side.

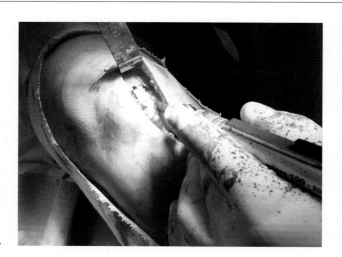

FIGURE 27-7

BPTB graft harvest patellar cuts.

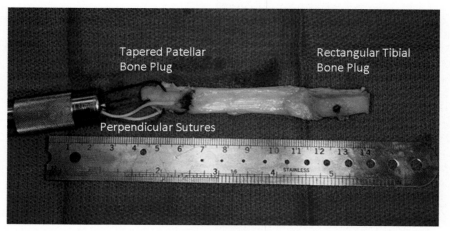

FIGURE 27-8

BPTB graft with bone plugs.

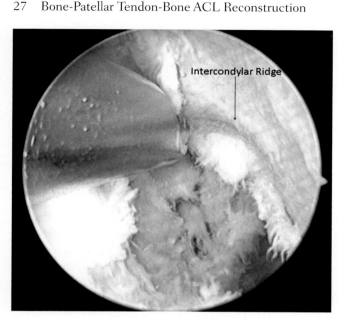

FIGURE 27-9
Intercondylar ridge.

graft including the bone blocks are made for tunnel angulation. The graft is then placed in a moist lap and is stored in a safe place to prevent inadvertent contamination on the back table.

While the graft is being prepared on the back table, any meniscal work can be addressed. Chondral repair procedures such as osteochondral transplantation or microfracture should be performed prior to ACL reconstruction to improve arthroscopic visualization. The remnant ACL is excised using a shaver and biters to allow full access to the lateral wall of the intercondylar notch and to prevent impingement of the graft on soft tissue. The tibial footprint of the ACL insertion site is cleared allowing for visualization of an outline for proper tibial tunnel placement. The roof and lateral wall of the intercondylar notch is then cleared of soft tissue as well with special attention paid to protection of the PCL while débridement of the wall ensues. After the soft tissue is débrided, a large burr and a rasp are used to complete the notchplasty if needed.

The notchplasty can be performed to ensure the creation of a smooth tunnel-shaped notch that allows for easy visualization and access to the posterior notch and avoids impingement of the ACL graft on the lateral wall and roof. The over-the-top position is then identified with care to avoid mistaking the intercondylar ridge (resident's ridge) for the over-the-top position (Fig. 27-9) (30). However, this intercondylar ridge has become a recent area of interest for double-bundle reconstruction. A fringe of white periosteal tissue, denoting the junction of the femur and the posterior joint capsule, usually can be seen posteriorly when the over-the-top position has been identified (Fig. 27-10).

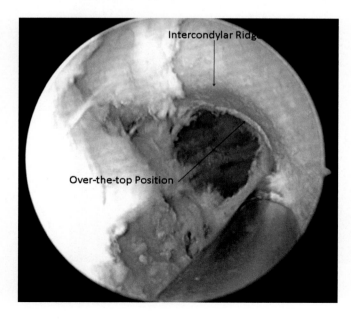

FIGURE 27-10
Femoral tunnel position.

An arthroscopic probe is then used to verify this position. An accessory medial portal is created 1.5 cm medial and 5 mm inferior to the standard anteromedial portal. The knee is hyperflexed, and a Beath pin (a long guidewire with an eyelet at one end) with a heavy FiberWire or TiCron suture through the eyelet is placed into the femoral footprint.

Attention is then turned to tunnel placement. The femoral tunnel should be located near the 10 o'clock position on the femur for the right knee and the 2 o'clock position on the left knee for optimal results and to resist rotatory loads more effectively (6,29). The starting point on the tibia should be the midpoint from inferior to superior with respect to the tibial tubercle harvest site and midpoint between and the tibial tubercle and the posteromedial edge of the tibia. Too medial or too central a starting point results in compromise of the medial collateral ligament or vertical tunnel placement, respectively. A commercially available guide is used to ensure property entry of the tibial tunnel into the joint. Landmarks for placement of the tibial tunnel include a position 7 mm anterior to the fibers of the PCL, the upslope of the lateral face of the medial tibial intercondylar eminence, the posterior aspect of the anterior horn of the lateral meniscus, and center of the native ACL footprint (7,31,32). In the sagittal plane, the tunnel should be angled posteriorly to prevent graft impingement, and in the coronal plane, the tibial tunnel should be angled 70 degrees to the medial tibial plateau (7,33). The elbow or tip aimer of the ACL tibial guide is placed through the anteromedial portal, and the tip of the guide is visualized arthroscopically and placed at the landmarks mentioned above. The angle of the guide is set to 50 to 55 degrees. The guide pin is inserted using the commercially available guide and placing the starting point along the medial aspect of the anterior surface of the tibia between the tibial tubercle and the posteromedial edge of the tibia. The guide pin is inserted and proper positioning can be confirmed with a lateral radiograph showing the guide pin at 40% of the anterior to posterior width of the tibia. The position of the proposed femoral tunnel should be at the junction of the third and fourth quadrants and below Blumensaat line (Fig. 27-11). Soft tissues are resected using an arthroscopic shaver if necessary (Fig. 27-12). The commercially available guide is then removed. A reamer based on graft size (usually 10 or 11 mm) is used to ream the tunnel until the reamer is seen arthroscopically just past the tibial articular surface (Fig. 27-13). The inflow pump is turned off just before penetration of the joint by the reamer; determined by resistance to advancement of the reamer during tibial drilling. Once the articular surface is reached, the reamer is removed and excess bone from reaming of the tibial tunnel is saved for incorporation into the graft harvest sites. The arthroscopic shaver is then used to débride all soft tissue surrounding the tibial tunnel to allow easier graft passage and to smooth the posterior edge of the tunnel to prevent graft abrasion.

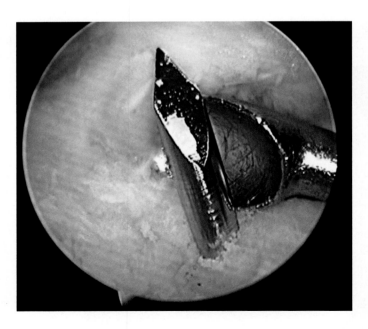

FIGURE 27-11
Tibial guide pin insertion.

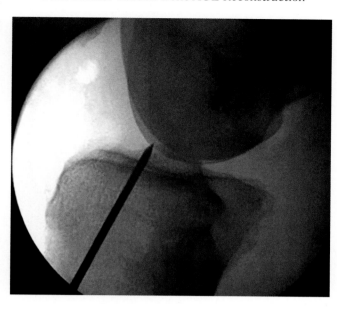

FIGURE 27-12
Proper tibial and femoral position on
fluoroscopy lateral.

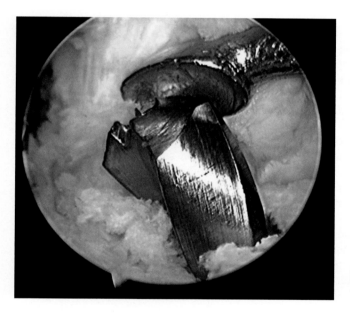

FIGURE 27-13
Tibial tunnel reamer.

The knee is hyperflexed. After inserting a soft tissue protector through the accessory medial portal, the femoral tunnel is drilled using a cannulated reamer (usually 8–10 mm) placed over the Beath pin inserted previously. Care is taken to protect the medial femoral condyle. This tunnel is drilled to a depth of 25 to 35 mm. The shaver is used to clear all excess bone debris out of the tunnel and posterior notch. Heavy suture, such as FiberWire or no. 5 TiCron, is threaded through the pin's eyelet. The Beath pin is then pushed deep into the femoral tunnel under arthroscopic visualization to ensure that a loop of suture remains in the joint. This suture is grasped and pulled out through the tibial tunnel (Fig. 27-14).

The graft is then obtained from the back table, and the sutures from the patella bone block are clamped to the drape close to the knee to ensure that the graft will not fall to the ground. The suture limbs from the proximal bone block are threaded through the eyelet of the Beath needle, and the needle is pulled through the anterolateral thigh. The knee is then brought out into a neutral position, and the remainder of the graft is pulled carefully into the knee. Markings previously placed on the

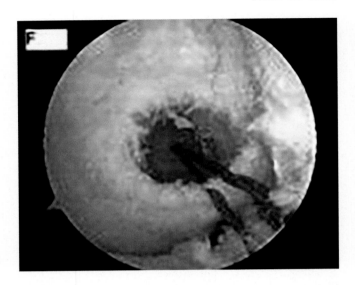

FIGURE 27-14

Femoral tunnel with suture visualized in joint.

graft measuring 5 mm less than the depth drilled for the femoral tunnel are used to ensure full incorporation of the graft into the femoral tunnel.

FIXATION

Now that the graft has been passed, we turn our attention to fixation. A well-agreed upon advantage of BPTB graft use is the ability to obtain early rigid fixation and stability in the setting of bone-to-bone healing (34). Both aperture (i.e., interference screws), nonaperture (i.e., extracortical suspensory) systems, as well as screw and washer constructs are available. Both femoral and tibia fixation can be achieved through the use of such devices. Our preference is to use interference screws for both femoral and tibia fixation. Interference screws have been shown to provide initial strength in excess of that needed for early range of motion and rehabilitation (35). Both metal and bioresorbable screw options are available, with controversy regarding which material provides the ultimate advantage over the other. However, to date several studies have shown there is no difference in initial strength of fixation or bone-to-bone healing between the two materials (36,37).

We first determine our interference screw diameter. We take into consideration both bone block quality and size. In the setting of good bone quality and size (i.e., a 10-mm bone block), we use a 7-mm diameter screw. When bone quality is in question or there is a loose fit, we recommend a 9-mm screw. Our practice is to match the screw length to that of the graft plug while maintaining 10 mm of bone plug-interference screw contact.

Once we have selected a screw, we hyperflex the knee to facilitate parallel screw placement in relation to our bone plug. Using either the anteromedial portal, accessory medial, or the patella tendon defect, we put in place an offset femoral guide (tunnel notcher), which is used to ensure optimal guidewire placement. The interference screw is then introduced over the guidewire while equal tension is applied to the sutures that were previously placed at the ends of the graft. The screw is placed against the cancellous surface of the bone and inserted until flush with the bone block (Fig. 27-15). Tension is then applied to the sutures at the end of the tibial block to check fixation strength. Simultaneously, the knee is brought through full range of motion and into full extension a dozen or more time to remove crimp. During this step, we address any signs of impingement and/or graft motion. Any motion >2 mm signifies poor placement and should be corrected.

We then turn our attention to tensioning and fixation of the tibial end of our graft. We prefer to tension and secure the tibial graft in full knee extension. An interference screw is then introduced over a guidewire anterior to the bone block (Fig. 27-16). If needed, additional fixation can be obtained through the use of a staple or screw and washer construct. Any excess bone is removed and used as bone graft for our patella and tibial harvest sites during closure.

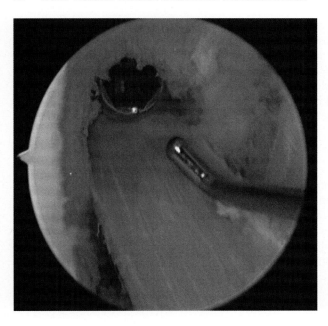

FIGURE 27-15
Femoral interference screw.

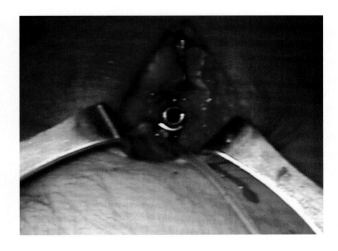

FIGURE 27-16
Tibial interference screw.

CLOSURE

The wounds are well irrigated, and 0-Vicryl (Ethicon, Summerville, NJ) is used to close the patella defect by close approximation of the paratenon. The remainder of the incision is closed in layers using Vicryl suture, and the skin is closed using a running subcuticular Prolene (Ethicon, Summerville, NJ). The portal sites are closed using a 2-0 nylon suture. A sterile dressing is applied followed by an elastic bandage from the toes proximally past the knee.

POSTOPERATIVE REHABILITATION

The top priority and goal of rehabilitation during the early phase is reducing knee stiffness. Range of motion should be assessed during the patient initial presentation, particularly the ability to reach full extension. If preoperative range of motion is a concern, we refer patients for physical therapy prior to undertaking surgery. After surgery, ice and cryotherapy are used to minimize effusion and pain. A protocol-driven rehab program is initiated 2 to 3 days after surgery. Both the patient and the physical therapist are given a copy of the rehab protocol. We allow patients to weight bear as tolerated without a brace, provided no meniscal repair was performed. In the event of meniscal repair, a hinged knee brace is used with range of motion set at 0 to 90 degrees of flexion and the patient is allowed only partial weight bearing for 6 weeks.

Early rehab goals include proprioceptive training and closed chain exercises with focus on proper quadriceps recruitment. During the later phase of rehabilitation, the primary goal is strengthening. A stationary bicycle, treadmill walking, and aquatic therapy are used to maximize knee motion and strength. Crutches are used until the patient is able to weight bear without a limp. Weight machines are used at 5 to 6 weeks, with plyometrics at 8 weeks. By 12 weeks, patients are usually allowed to return to jogging and progress toward return to sport. Return to sport is usually allowed between 4 and 6 months. Our return goals include strength at least 85% that of the nonoperative side.

COMPLICATIONS

The most common complication following BPTB ACL reconstruction is postoperative patellofemoral pain. Anterior knee pain has also been accredited to graft harvest during autogenous BPTB procedures (38,39). Others have associated this complication with postoperative flexion and extension, as well as quadriceps strength (40,41). In one of the largest series to date, Shelbourne and Trumper showed that there was no difference in the incidence of patellofemoral pain between patients who underwent ACL reconstruction and control patients who had not undergone surgical intervention (42). They concluded that anterior knee was not an intrinsic complication to BPTB harvest, and that the incidence of such pain could be prevented with a rehabilitation program focused on restoration of full hyperextension. Decreased sensitivity as a result of disturbance to the infrapatellar branch of the saphenous nerve and patella tendonitis may also contribute to postoperative anterior knee pain; however, these findings usually resolve within a year (7).

Patella fractures have also been reported following BPTB ACL reconstruction and have been associated with both direct and indirect forces (43,44). This complication can be avoided with careful technique during graft harvest and not creating additional stress risers during the bone block cut. In the event of intraoperative patella fracture, rigid fixation should be done immediately as to allow early postoperative range of motion. Extensor mechanism disruption is also rare but has been reported during the postoperative period (45,46).

Proper tunnel placement and adequate fixation are imperative to ACL reconstruction. Careful technique during reaming, guide pin placement, notchplasty, and fixation can help minimize these complications. One must make sure not to violate the posterior cortex of the femur during reaming. This can be prevented by maintaining the knee in flexion and not reaming more than 35 mm in depth. A poorly done notchplasty can lead to impingement and therefore loss of extension. Impingement can also occur if the tibial tunnel is placed too anteriorly and ultimately can lead to pathologic laxity. Care also must be taken not to lacerate the suture or cause graft fracture during interference screw placement. Each of the above-mentioned complications can be prevented with careful technique and direct visualization during each step. In the unfortunate event of any of these complications, they should be addressed immediately.

The importance of postoperative early range of motion cannot be overstated. The incidence of arthrofibrosis has decreased over the years as a result of advances in rehabilitation protocols. If motion is not restored by 6 weeks postoperatively, the senior author performs a manipulation under anesthesia followed by aggressive physical therapy. If this approach fails, then an arthroscopic debridement or revision procedure may be needed. Any subsequent procedures must be followed by aggressive physical therapy.

REFERENCES

1. Miller RH, Azar FM. Sports medicine: knee injuries. In: Canale ST, Beaty JH, eds. *Campbell's Operative Orthopaedics*. Philadelphia, PA: Mosby Elsevier; 2008.
2. Sanders TL, Maradit Kremers H, Bryan AJ, et al. Incidence of anterior cruciate ligament tears and reconstruction: a 21-year population-based study. *Am J Sports Med*. 2016;44(6):1502–1507.
3. Herzog MM, Marshall SW, Lund JL, et al. Incidence of anterior cruciate ligament reconstruction among adolescent females in the United States, 2002 through 2014. *JAMA Pediatr*. 2017;171(8):808–810. doi:10.1001/jamapediatrics.2017.0740.
4. Clancy WG Jr, Nelson DA, Reider B, et al. Anterior cruciate ligament reconstruction using one-third of the patellar ligament, augmented by extra-articular tendon transfers. *J Bone Joint Surg Am*. 1982;64(3):352–359.
5. Jones KG. Reconstruction of the anterior cruciate ligament. A technique using the central one-third of the patellar ligament. *J Bone Joint Surg Am*. 1963;45:925–932.
6. Cain EL Jr, Clancy WG Jr. Anatomic endoscopic anterior cruciate ligament reconstruction with patella tendon autograft. *Orthop Clin North Am*. 2002;33(4):717–725.
7. Gladstone JN, Andrews JR. Endoscopic anterior cruciate ligament reconstruction with patella tendon autograft. *Orthop Clin North Am*. 2002;33(4):701–715, vii.
8. Miller SL, Gladstone JN. Graft selection in anterior cruciate ligament reconstruction. *Orthop Clin North Am*. 2002;33(4):675–683.
9. Ejerhed L, Kartus J, Sernert N, et al. Patellar tendon or semitendinosus tendon autografts for anterior cruciate ligament reconstruction? A prospective randomized study with a two-year follow-up. *Am J Sports Med*. 2003;31(1):19–25.

10. Laxdal G, Kartus J, Hansson L, et al. A prospective randomized comparison of bone-patellar tendon-bone and hamstring grafts for anterior cruciate ligament reconstruction. *Arthroscopy*. 2005;21(1):34–42.

11. Laxdal G, Sernert N, Ejerhed L, et al. A prospective comparison of bone-patellar tendon-bone and hamstring tendon grafts for anterior cruciate ligament reconstruction in male patients. *Knee Surg Sports Traumatol Arthrosc*. 2007;15(2):115–125.

12. Hardaker WT Jr, Garrett WE Jr, Bassett FH III. Evaluation of acute traumatic hemarthrosis of the knee joint. *South Med J*. 1990;83(6):640–644.

13. Noyes FR, Bassett RW, Grood ES, et al. Arthroscopy in acute traumatic hemarthrosis of the knee. Incidence of anterior cruciate tears and other injuries. *J Bone Joint Surg Am*. 1980;62(5):687–695, 757.

14. Skinner HB. Knee injuries. In: *Current Diagnosis and Treatment in Orthopedics*. New York: Lange Medical Books/McGraw-Hill; 2003.

15. Schoderbek RJ Jr, Treme GP, Miller MD. Bone-patella tendon-bone autograft anterior cruciate ligament reconstruction. *Clin Sports Med*. 2007;26(4):525–547.

16. Torg JS, Conrad W, Kalen V. Clinical diagnosis of anterior cruciate ligament instability in the athlete. *Am J Sports Med*. 1976;4(2):84–93.

17. Christel PS, Akgun U, Yasar T, et al. The contribution of each anterior cruciate ligament bundle to the Lachman test: a cadaver investigation. *J Bone Joint Surg Br*. 2012;94:68–74.

18. Galway H, Beaupre A, MacIntosh D. Pivot shift: a clinical sign of symptomatic ACL insufficiency. *J Bone Joint Surg Br*. 1972;54:763–776.

19. Galway HR, MacIntosh DL. The lateral pivot shift: a symptom and sign of anterior cruciate ligament insufficiency. *Clin Orthop Relat Res*. 1980;147:45–50.

20. Woods GW, Stanley RF, Tullos HS. Lateral capsular sign: x-ray clue to a significant knee instability. *Am J Sports Med*. 1979;7(1):27–33.

21. McAllister DR, Bergfeld JA, Parker RD, et al. A comparison of preoperative imaging techniques for predicting patellar tendon graft length before cruciate ligament reconstruction. *Am J Sports Med*. 2001;29(4):461–465.

22. McCarroll JR, Shelbourne KD, Patel DV. Anterior cruciate ligament reconstruction in athletes with an ossicle associated with Osgood-Schlatter's disease. *Arthroscopy*. 1996;12(5):556–560.

23. Nogalski M, Bach B Jr. Acute anterior cruciate ligament injuries. In: Fu F, Harner C, Vince K, eds. *Knee Surgery*. Baltimore, MD: Williams & Wilkins; 1994.

24. Turner DA, Prodromos CC, Petasnick JP, et al. Acute injury of the ligaments of the knee: magnetic resonance evaluation. *Radiology*. 1985;154(3):717–722.

25. Johnson DL, Bealle DP, Brand JC Jr, et al. The effect of a geographic lateral bone bruise on knee inflammation after acute anterior cruciate ligament rupture. *Am J Sports Med*. 2000;28(2):152–155.

26. Rosen MA, Jackson DW, Berger PE, Occult osseous lesions documented by magnetic resonance imaging associated with anterior cruciate ligament ruptures. *Arthroscopy*. 1991;7(1):45–51.

27. Speer KP, Spritzer CE, Bassett FH III, et al. Osseous injury associated with acute tears of the anterior cruciate ligament. *Am J Sports Med*. 1992;20(4):382–389.

28. Mulroy MF, Larkin KL, Batra MS, et al. Femoral nerve block with 0.25% or 0.5% bupivacaine improves postoperative analgesia following outpatient arthroscopic anterior cruciate ligament repair. *Reg Anesth Pain Med*. 2001;26(1):24–29.

29. Sanchis-Alfonso V, Subias-Lopez A, Monteagudo-Castro C, et al. Healing of the patellar tendon donor defect created after central-third patellar tendon autograft harvest. A long-term histological evaluation in the lamb model. *Knee Surg Sports Traumatol Arthrosc*. 1999;7(6):340–348.

30. Almekinders LC, Chiavetta JB, Clarke JP. Radiographic evaluation of anterior cruciate ligament graft failure with special reference to tibial tunnel placement. *Arthroscopy*. 1998;14(2):206–211.

31. McGuire DA, Wolchok JW. The footprint: a method for checking femoral tunnel placement. *Arthroscopy*. 1998;14(7):777–778.

32. Morgan CD, Kalman VR, Grawl DM. Definitive landmarks for reproducible tibial tunnel placement in anterior cruciate ligament reconstruction. *Arthroscopy*. 1995;11(3):275–288.

33. O'Neill DB. Arthroscopically assisted reconstruction of the anterior cruciate ligament. A follow-up report. *J Bone Joint Surg Am*. 2001;83-A(9):1329–1332.

34. Noyes FR, Butler DL, Grood ES, et al. Biomechanical analysis of human ligament grafts used in knee-ligament repairs and reconstructions. *J Bone Joint Surg Am*. 1984;66(3):344–352.

35. Steiner ME, Hecker AT, Brown CH Jr, et al. Anterior cruciate ligament graft fixation. Comparison of hamstring and patellar tendon grafts. *Am J Sports Med*. 1994;22(2):240–246; discussion 246–247.

36. Barber FA, Elrod BF, McGuire DA. et al. Preliminary results of an absorbable interference screw. *Arthroscopy*. 1995;11(5):537–548.

37. Marti C, Imhoff AB, Bahrs C, et al. Metallic versus bioabsorbable interference screw for fixation of bone-patellar tendon-bone autograft in arthroscopic anterior cruciate ligament reconstruction. A preliminary report. *Knee Surg Sports Traumatol Arthrosc*. 1997;5(4):217–221.

38. Freedman KB, D'Amato MJ, Nedeff DD, et al. Arthroscopic anterior cruciate ligament reconstruction: a metaanalysis comparing patellar tendon and hamstring tendon autografts. *Am J Sports Med*. 2003;31(1):2–11.

39. Prodromos CC, Joyce BT, Shi K, et al. A meta-analysis of stability after anterior cruciate ligament reconstruction as a function of hamstring versus patellar tendon graft and fixation type. *Arthroscopy*. 2005;21(10):1202.

40. Aglietti P, Buzzi R, D'Andria S, et al. Arthroscopic anterior cruciate ligament reconstruction with patellar tendon. *Arthroscopy*. 1992;8(4):510–516.

41. Sachs RA, Daniel DM, Stone ML, et al. Patellofemoral problems after anterior cruciate ligament reconstruction. *Am J Sports Med*. 1989;17(6):760–765.

42. Shelbourne KD, Trumper RV. Preventing anterior knee pain after anterior cruciate ligament reconstruction. *Am J Sports Med*. 1997;25(1):41–47.

43. Simonian PT, Mann FA, Mandt PR. Indirect forces and patella fracture after anterior cruciate ligament reconstruction with the patellar ligament. Case report. *Am J Knee Surg*. 1995;8(2):60–64; discussion 64–65.

44. Stein DA, Hunt SA, Rosen JE, et al. The incidence and outcome of patella fractures after anterior cruciate ligament reconstruction. *Arthroscopy*. 2002;18(6):578–583.

45. Marumoto JM, Mitsunaga MM, Richardson AB, et al. Late patellar tendon ruptures after removal of the central third for anterior cruciate ligament reconstruction. A report of two cases. *Am J Sports Med*. 1996;24(5):698–701.

46. Mickelsen PL, Morgan SJ, Johnson WA, et al. Patellar tendon rupture 3 years after anterior cruciate ligament reconstruction with a central one third bone-patellar tendon-bone graft. *Arthroscopy*. 2001;17(6):648–652.

28 Anatomical Single-Bundle ACL Reconstruction: Hamstring Autograft

Michael G. Baraga and Hayley E. Ennis

INTRODUCTION

The anterior cruciate ligament (ACL) is an important stabilizer of the knee that primarily prevents anterior translation of the tibia on the femur. ACL injury most commonly occurs due to a non-contact mechanism—typically "cutting" which involves a sudden deceleration followed by change in direction (1). ACL injuries are estimated to represent one quarter of all knee injuries with the annual incidence of ACL tear in the general population found to be approximately 70 per 100,000 population (2,3). Furthermore, the incidence of ACL injury is higher in competitive athletes, and ACL injury rates are continuing to rise in both men's and women's sports (4). Although difficult to estimate, data suggest that this equates to more than 246,000 ACL injuries and upwards of 175,000 reconstructions in the United States annually (2). Extensive research efforts on the topic of ACL reconstruction and evolution of operative techniques have developed over the years due to the high volume of this injury, need for restoration of knee stability, interest in quick return to sport, and prevention of graft failure.

In preparation for ACL reconstruction, graft selection should be discussed with the patient and is dependent on multiple factors such as concomitant ligament injuries, donor site morbidity, age and activity level, and surgeon's preference. Benefits of using autograft include decreased cost, no risk of disease transmission, and quicker graft incorporation time compared to allografts (5,6). Age and activity level of the patient plays a role in the decision, as some studies have demonstrated increased failure rate of allografts in younger and more active populations (7–10). The exact reason for this is unclear; however, it may be related to increased incorporation time of allograft alongside timing of return to full activity.

Hamstring (HS) autograft typically consists of the semitendinosus (ST) tendon and gracilis tendon, which are doubled over to create a four-stranded graft. Additionally, more recent graft preparation techniques involving tripling or quadrupling the semitendinosus or both semitendinosus and gracilis tendons have been described. The benefits of the HS autograft when compared to bone patellar tendon bone (BTB) autograft are a less morbid harvest procedure, decreased anterior knee pain, and a decreased risk of knee extension deficit (11,12). The potential drawbacks of the HS autograft are decreased knee flexion strength, potential of higher retear rate compared to BTB in young athletes participating in pivoting sports, and potential for small graft size that necessitates augmentation (13,14). However, need for augmentation may be anticipated prior to surgery and is further described in the next section. Lastly, studies examining overall graft survival comparing HS to BTB have shown mixed results making it difficult to truly determine superiority (15–17).

PREOPERATIVE PLANNING

Consideration for Graft Augmentation

The ideal size for HS autograft remains undefined in the literature, though it appears to be around 8 mm, with recent studies demonstrating that HS grafts 8 mm or greater have decreased failure rates compared to those that are smaller (18). The diameter of HS autograft obtained from the patient is variable, and the size has been shown to correlate with anthropometric factors such as patient height, BMI, thigh circumference, and gender (19–21). Furthermore, preoperative MRI and/or ultrasound using cross-sectional area of the HS tendons has been shown to be useful in predicting graft diameter and thus allows planning for likelihood of graft augmentation prior to surgery (22,23).

ANESTHESIA AND POSITIONING

ACL reconstruction is most commonly performed under general anesthesia with addition of a regional block to aid with postoperative analgesia. The patient is placed in the supine position, and a full ligamentous exam of both knees is then performed under anesthesia. Attention is then turned to positioning the patient. We prefer performing arthroscopy with a side post with the leg free, though a circumferential leg holder may be used as well. The nonoperative leg is well padded and secured to the bed in the extended position. A sand bag is placed on the side of the operative extremity and fixed down so that the patient's knee can be flexed to about 90 degrees with the foot resting on the sand bag to keep the knee in a flexed position. A lateral post is then placed roughly a hand's width above the superior pole of the patella while the leg is in an extended position. A nonsterile tourniquet is then placed as proximal as possible on the thigh of the operative extremity followed by a nonsterile adhesive drape. We inject the planned incisions with 1% lidocaine with epinephrine. The skin is then prepped and draped in sterile fashion. After timeout, the limb is exsanguinated with an Esmarch bandage, tourniquet is inflated, and the initial incision is made.

SEMITENDINOSUS/GRACILIS GRAFT HARVEST

We typically begin the procedure with the graft harvest. If any doubt remains regarding the diagnosis of complete ACL tear, then the diagnostic arthroscopy would be performed first. We begin the harvest by making a longitudinal 3-cm incision centered over the palpable pes tendons, 2 cm medial to the medial edge of the tibial tubercle (Fig. 28-1). Sharp dissection is carried through the skin and hemostasis achieved. Branches of the saphenous nerve may be encountered during the dissection (Fig. 28-2). An incision through the sartorial fascia along the superior edge of the gracilis is made (Fig. 28-3). Care is taken to avoid cutting sharply to bone, as this may lead to iatrogenic injury to the underlying medial collateral ligament (Fig. 28-4). This incision is then extended anterolaterally toward the lateral most aspect of the hamstring insertion on the tibia. The sartorial fascia is then carefully dissected free from the underlying gracilis and ST tendons. A right-angled clamp is then used to secure the tendons, and these are resected off of the lateral-most insertion on the tibia. Reflecting the deep aspect of the tendons reveals the natural split between the gracilis and ST, and a second right-angled clamp is added to secure the ST (Fig. 28-5). This interval is then sharply developed with Metzenbaum scissors. The free ends of the tendons are then whipstitched with No. 2 nonabsorbable braided suture (Fig. 28-6). Care is taken to ensure that tendons are adequately mobilized, as fascial bands between the ST and medial gastrocnemius may cause premature graft truncation if not incised off of the hamstring tendons (Fig. 28-7). These are released, and circumferential palpation around the tendons is performed to confirm full release (Fig. 28-8). Closed-loop harvesters are then used to harvest each individual tendon (Fig. 28-9), taking care to harvest in line with the tendon's origin (Fig. 28-10). These are then prepared on the back table (Fig. 28-11).

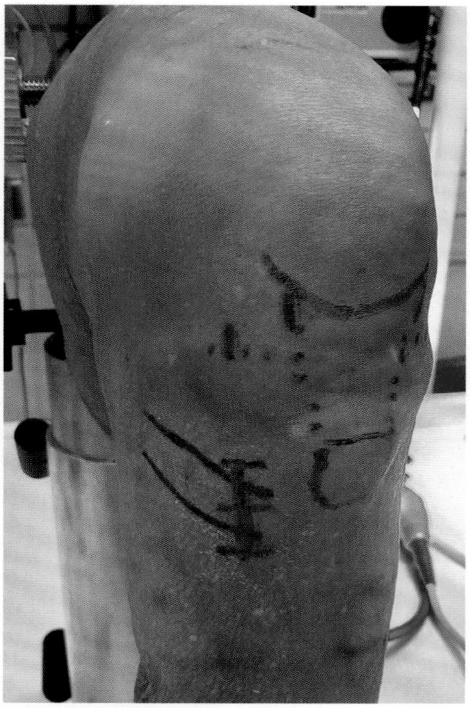

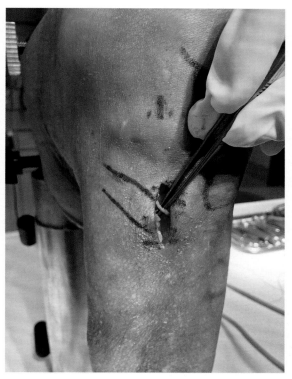

FIGURE 28-1

Harvest incision centered over the palpable pes tendons, roughly 2 cm medial to the medial edge of the tibial tubercle.

FIGURE 28-2

Branches of the saphenous nerve may be encountered during the dissection.

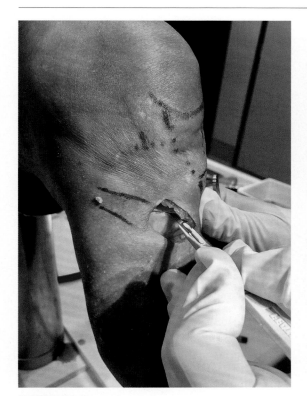

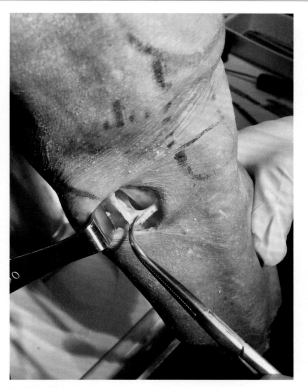

FIGURE 28-3

An incision along the superior edge of the gracilis is made, this being into sartorial fascia. Care must be taken to avoid cutting sharply to bone, as this may lead to iatrogenic injury to the MCL.

FIGURE 28-4

ST and gracilis tendons reflected. The *green dot* denotes the MCL, which lies just deep to the hamstrings. Care must be taken during dissection to avoid iatrogenic injury.

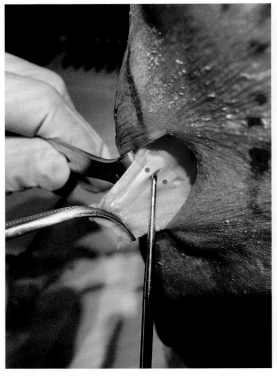

FIGURE 28-5

After releasing the hamstrings off the tibia and reflecting them, the ST tendon (*red dot*) and gracilis tendon (*green dot*) can be visualized.

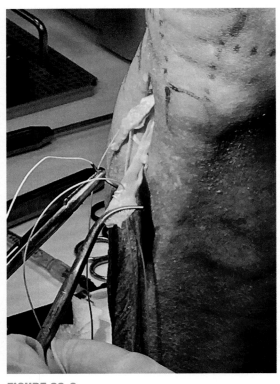

FIGURE 28-6

The free ends of the tendons are then whipstitched with No. 2 nonabsorbable braided suture.

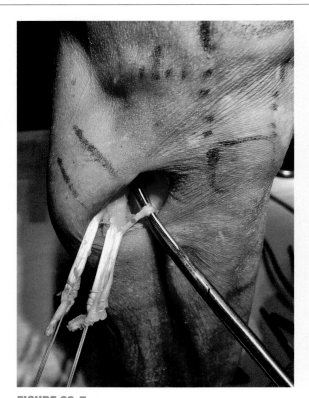

FIGURE 28-7

Care is taken to ensure that tendons are adequately mobilized, as fascial bands between the ST and medial gastrocnemius (*green dot*) may lead to premature graft truncation.

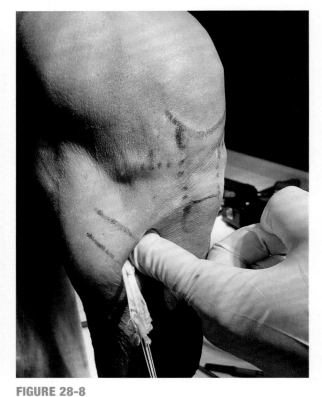

FIGURE 28-8

Palpation should be performed to ensure that all fascial bands have been released circumferentially around each tendon.

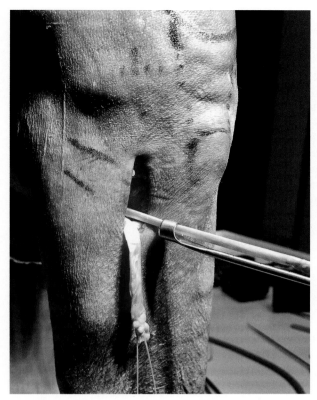

FIGURE 28-9
Closed-loop harvesters are then used to harvest each tendon—here shown harvesting the gracilis tendon.

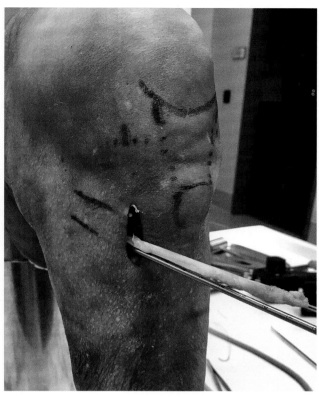

FIGURE 28-10
Closed-loop harvester being used to harvest ST tendon with care taken to harvest in line with the tendon's origin.

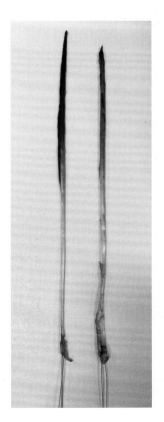

FIGURE 28-11
Gracilis (*left*) and ST (*right*) after harvest, prior to graft preparation.

GRAFT PREPARATION

Once all muscle tissue is removed from the tendons, the tendons are measured to length and cut. We prefer between 90 and 95 mm for a doubled graft length. The free ends are whipstitched with No. 2 nonabsorbable braided suture. The graft is then pulled through sizing tubes and measured (Fig. 28-12). With the doubled ST-gracilis graft, we augment any graft smaller than 8 mm in diameter with allograft, unless one of the tendons harvested is long enough to triple (requires 27 cm length of harvested tendon). The tissue is then doubled over a cortical suspensory device loop and placed under tension until ready for graft passage (Fig. 28-13). Length from the insertion site to the lateral femoral cortex is marked from the trailing end of the cortical suspensory button to identify the amount of suture that should be pulled prior to the button engaging the femoral cortex. Conversely, if the button is resting perpendicular to the sutures in a proprietary button holder, we simply add 6 mm to our measurement to avoid the need to remove from the button holder. More recently, techniques describing quadrupling of the ST, such as Lubowitz et al., to yield a larger diameter graft have been described. These can be used in a setting of femoral and tibial suspensory fixation but also allow for femoral suspensory and tibial interference fixation.

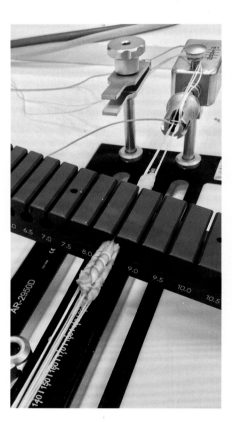

FIGURE 28-12

Whipstitched doubled graft being pulled through sizing block for measurement of diameter.

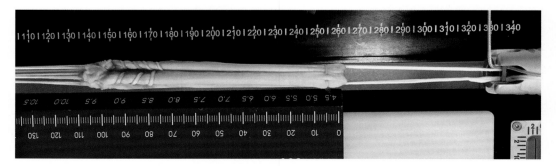

FIGURE 28-13

Final graft construct with cortical suspensory fixation device on femoral side, placed under tension.

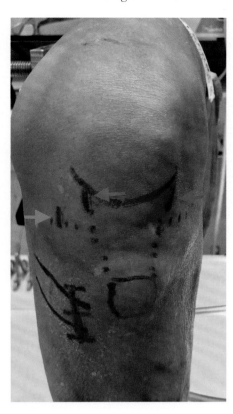

FIGURE 28-14

Arthroscopic portal placement: anterolateral portal (*blue arrow*), high anteromedial (*red*), and low anteromedial (*green*).

ARTHROSCOPIC PORTAL PLACEMENT AND DIAGNOSTIC ARTHROSCOPY

We prefer a three portal techniques for all of our ACL reconstructions. These are an anterolateral, high anteromedial, and low anteromedial portals (Fig. 28-14). Both the anterolateral portal, which is the primary viewing portal, and anteromedial portals are made at the start. Both are placed high above the level of the joint line and tight to the lateral and medial edges of the patellar tendon, respectively. A diagnostic arthroscopy is then carried out. This is done in a systematic fashion, ensuring complete visualization of the knee joint to address any meniscal or chondral pathology.

FEMORAL SOCKET PREPARATION

We prefer a separate low anteromedial reaming portal for preparation of the femoral socket. Once the fat pad and femoral notch have been debrided to optimize visualization, a spinal needle is used to localize the optimal angle that allows for safe portal placement just above the medial meniscus and as perpendicular as possible to the ACL femoral insertion, while ensuring protection of the medial femoral condyle cartilage (Fig. 28-15). We find this technique achieves avoidance of posterior cortical breach and allows for reproducible bone socket length. We prefer leaving some ACL remnant to use as guides for anatomic reconstruction (Fig. 28-16). An offset guide is used to help place a spade-tipped guide pin into the center of the femoral anatomic footprint. The knee is then flexed to approximately 120 degrees and adjusted to fit the pin in the center of the footprint. The pin is then advanced and engaged on the lateral femoral cortex, and the length from the insertion site to the lateral femoral cortex is measured. The appropriate size acorn reamer is then used to create the femoral socket to the desired depth, while a cannula is placed in the high anteromedial portal to help remove bone debris while reaming (Fig. 28-17). A small stab incision is made with a No. 11 blade along the path of the guide pin exiting the distal lateral thigh, thus allowing us to retension the femoral suspensory device after tibial fixation and secure with alternating half hitches. After all debris is removed, a shuttling suture is passed and the knee is brought back to 90 degrees of flexion (Fig. 28-18).

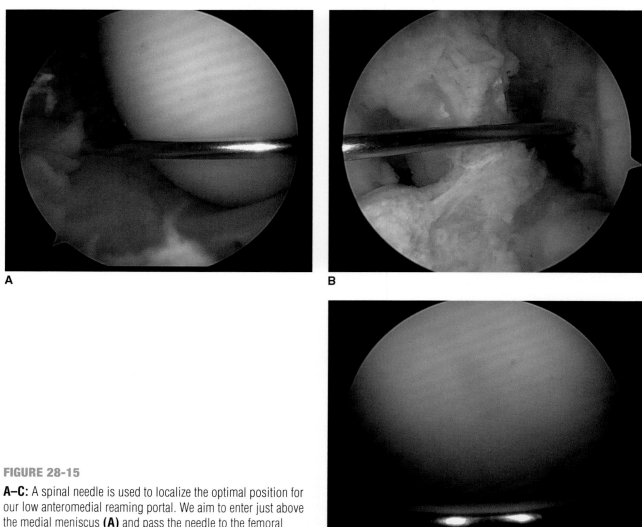

FIGURE 28-15

A–C: A spinal needle is used to localize the optimal position for our low anteromedial reaming portal. We aim to enter just above the medial meniscus **(A)** and pass the needle to the femoral footprint **(B)**. Once set on the footprint, we verify the space between the needle and the medial femoral condyle to ensure safe entry of the reamer to avoid iatrogenic injury to the cartilage **(C)**.

FIGURE 28-16

After debridement, some remnant is left to identify the anatomic insertion sites as landmarks for reconstruction. Femoral footprint is pictured here.

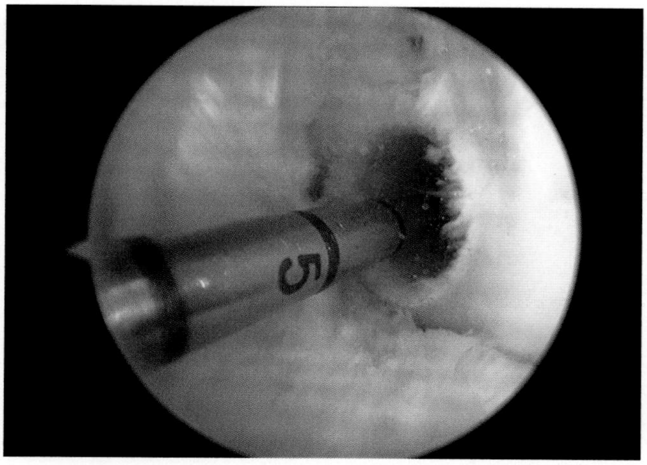

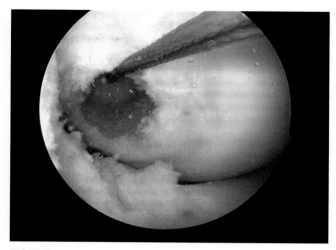

FIGURE 28-17

Femoral tunnel after reaming, view from high anteromedial portal.

FIGURE 28-18

Shuttling suture in femoral socket, view from low anteromedial portal.

TIBIAL TUNNEL PREPARATION

Although landmarks of the posterior aspect of the anterior horn of the lateral meniscus as well as medial and lateral tibial spines have been described for tibial tunnel placement, we prefer to leave some tibial ACL remnant to use as a guide for proper anatomic restoration of the ACL (Fig. 28-19). A tibial ACL guide is inserted through the low anteromedial reaming portal, and the guide is set on the tibia through the hamstring harvest incision (Fig. 28-20). We typically set our guide at 50 degrees. A 2.4-mm guide pin is advanced into the center of the tibial ACL insertion. This is removed once reaming is completed with the appropriate size reamer (Fig. 28-21). Soft tissue is debrided from the tunnel aperture at the anteromedial tibia to decrease the risk of soft tissue impingement during graft passage.

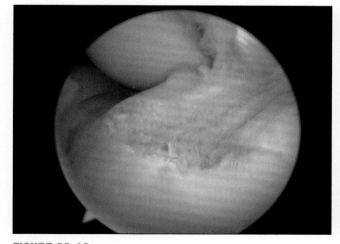

FIGURE 28-19

Tibial ACL remnant footprint, which is used as a guide for proper anatomic restoration of the ACL.

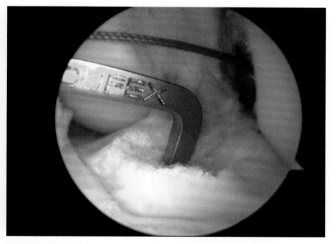

FIGURE 28-20

Tibial ACL guide, typically set to 50 degrees, placed on the tibial ACL remnant footprint.

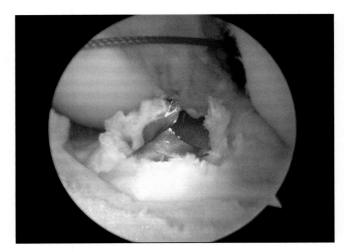

FIGURE 28-21
Reaming of the tibial tunnel.

PASSING THE GRAFT

The shuttling suture is then pulled out through the tibial tunnel, and the hamstring graft is brought to the field. The sutures from the cortical suspensory device are shuttled through the tibial and femoral tunnels and out the anterolateral thigh. While visualizing from the low anteromedial portal, we observe that the cortical button penetrates the lateral aspect of the femoral socket and confirms deployment on the lateral femoral cortex. The graft is then delivered into the femoral socket until it has bottomed out (Fig. 28-22). It is then cycled 25 times and tibial fixation performed with interference screw sized to the same diameter of the drilled tunnel. The femoral suspensory fixation is then retensioned with the knee in full extension, and a knot pusher is used to back this up with alternating half hitches. Care is taken to ensure that the knots are tied deep to the iliotibial band. The tibial fixation is then backed up with a knotless suture anchor incorporating the excess sutures from the tibial aspect of the graft.

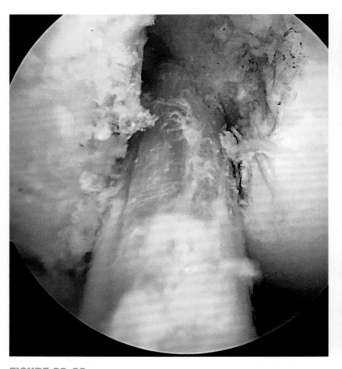
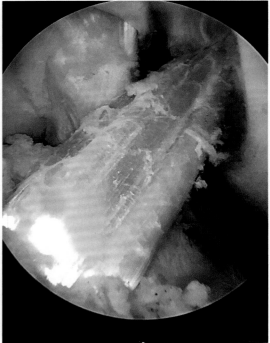

FIGURE 28-22
View through medial portal **(left)** and lateral portal **(right)** of the ACL graft after fixation.

FIXATION

Fixation of the HS graft can be achieved via either suspensory fixation, which includes cortical button, washer, or post screw methods, or aperture fixation, which is accomplished by fixation within the confines of the bone tunnel. The best fixation method of HS autograft is still debatable; however, recent articles have suggested possible superiority of suspensory methods due to significant improved overall arthrometric stability and fewer graft ruptures when compared to aperture fixation (24).

CLOSURE OF SKIN

After irrigation, the sartorial fascia is closed with No. 0 braided absorbable suture. A layered closure is performed, and 4-0 absorbable monofilament suture is used for skin.

POSTOPERATIVE BRACING AND REHABILITATION

Rehabilitation guidelines are surgeon-specific. We utilize postoperative range of motion bracing for protection during ambulation in the early postoperative period and utilize axillary crutches for assistance. These are discontinued once gait has normalized. Emphasis is placed on controlling effusion and establishing full extension as quickly as possible. Physical therapy is initiated 2 to 3 days after surgery.

REFERENCES

1. Sutton KM, Bullock JM. Anterior cruciate ligament rupture: differences between males and females. *J Am Acad Orthop Surg.* 2013;21(1):41–50.
2. Frobell RB, Roos HP, Roos EM, et al. The acutely ACL injured knee assessed by MRI: are large volume traumatic bone marrow lesions a sign of severe compression injury? *Osteoarthritis Cartilage.* 2008;16:829–836.
3. Sanders TL, Kremers HM, Bryan AJ, et al. Incidence of anterior cruciate ligament tears and reconstruction. *Am J Sports Med.* 2016;44(6):1502–1507.
4. Agel J, Rockwood T, Klossner D. Collegiate ACL injury rates across 15 sports: National Collegiate Athletic Association injury surveillance system update (2004/2005 through 2012/2013). *Clin J Sport Med.* 2016;26:518–523.
5. Bhatia S, Bell R, Frank RM, et al. Bony incorporation of soft tissue anterior ligament grafts in an animal model: autograft versus allograft with low-dose gamma irradiation. *Am J Sports Med.* 2012;40(8):1789–1798.
6. Muramatsu K, Hachiya Y, Izawa H. Serial evaluation of human anterior cruciate ligament grafts by contrast-enhanced magnetic resonance imaging: comparison of allografts and autografts. *Arthroscopy.* 2008;24(9):1038–1044.
7. Engelman GH, Carry PM, Hitt KG, et al. Comparison of allograft versus autograft anterior cruciate ligament reconstruction graft survival in an active adolescent cohort. *Am J Sports Med.* 2014;42(10):2311–2318.
8. Ellis HB, Matheny LM, Briggs KK, et al. Outcomes and revision rate after bone-patellar tendon-bone allograft versus autograft anterior cruciate ligament reconstruction in patients aged 18 years or younger with closed physes. *Arthroscopy.* 2012;28(12):1819–1825.
9. Pallis M, Svoboda SJ, Cameron KL, et al. Survival comparison of allograft and autograft anterior cruciate ligament reconstruction at the United States Military Academy. *Am J Sports Med.* 2012;40(6):1242–1246.
10. Barrett AM, Craft JA, Replogle WH, et al. Anterior cruciate ligament graft failure: a comparison of graft type based on age and Tegner activity level. *Am J Sports Med.* 2011;39(10):2194–2198.
11. Kartus J, Movin T, Karlsson J. Donor-site morbidity and anterior knee problems after anterior cruciate ligament reconstruction using autografts. *Arthroscopy.* 2001;17(9):971–980.
12. Xie, X, Liu X, Chen Z, et al. A meta-analysis of bone-patellar tendon-bone autograft versus four-strand hamstring tendon autograft for anterior cruciate ligament reconstruction. *Knee.* 2015;22(2):100–110.
13. Gifstad T, Foss OA, Engebretsen L, et al. Lower risk of revision with patellar tendon autografts compared with hamstring autografts: a registry study based on 45,998 primary ACL reconstructions in Scandinavia. *Am J Sports Med.* 2014;42(10):2319–2328.
14. Rahr-Wagner L, Thillemann TM, Pedersen AB, et al. Comparison of hamstring tendon and patellar tendon grafts in anterior cruciate ligament reconstruction in a nationwide population-based cohort study: results from the Danish registry of knee ligament reconstruction. *Am J Sports Med.* 2014;42(2):278–284.
15. Mohtadi NG, Chan DS, Dainty KN, et al. Patellar tendon versus hamstring tendon autograft for anterior cruciate ligament rupture in adults. *Cochrane Database Syst Rev.* 2011;9:CD005960.
16. Persson A, Fjeldsgaard K, Gjertsen JE, et al. Increased risk of revision with hamstring tendon grafts compared with patellar tendon grafts after anterior cruciate ligament reconstruction: a study of 12,643 patients from the Norwegian Cruciate Ligament Registry, 2004–2012. *Am J Sports Med.* 2014;42(2):285–291.
17. Thompson SM, Salmon LJ, Waller A, et al. Twenty-year outcome of a longitudinal prospective evaluation of isolated endoscopic anterior cruciate ligament reconstruction with patellar tendon or hamstring autograft. *Am J Sports Med.* 2016;44(12):3083–3094.
18. Conte EJ, Hyatt AE, Gatt CJ, et al. Hamstring autograft size can be predicted and is a potential risk factor for anterior cruciate ligament reconstruction failure. *Arthroscopy.* 2014;30(7):882–890.
19. Schwartzberg R, Burkhart B, Lariviere C. Prediction of hamstring autograft diameter and length for anterior cruciate reconstruction. *Am J Orthop.* 2008;37:157–159.
20. Treme G, Diduch DR, Billante MJ, et al. Hamstring graft size prediction: a prospective clinical evaluation. *Am J Sports Med.* 2008;36:2204–2209.

21. Tuman JM, Diduch DR, Rubino LJ, et al. Predictors for hamstring graft diameter in anterior cruciate ligament reconstruction. *Am J Sports Med.* 2007;35:1945–1949.

22. Wernecke G, Harris IA, Houang MTW, et al. Using magnetic resonance imaging to predict adequate graft diameter for autologous hamstring double-bundle anterior cruciate ligament reconstruction. *Arthroscopy.* 2011;27(8):1055–1059.

23. Erquicia JI, Gelber PE, Doreste JL, et al. How to improve the prediction of quadrupled semitendinosus and gracilis autograft sizes with magnetic resonance imaging and ultrasonography. *Am J Sports Med.* 2013;41(8):1857–1863.

24. Browning WM, Kluczynski MA, Curatolo C. Suspensory versus aperture fixation of a quadrupled hamstring tendon autograft in anterior cruciate ligament reconstruction: a meta-analysis. *Am J Sports Med.* 2017;45(10):2418–2427. doi: 10.1177/0363546516680995.

29 ACL Reconstruction: Quadriceps Tendon Autograft

Andrew Schwartz, Harris Slone, and John Xerogeanes

INDICATIONS

Optimal graft choice for anterior cruciate ligament (ACL) reconstruction remains a controversial and contested topic. There is an increasing body of evidence supporting the use of quadriceps tendon autograft for ACL reconstruction. The quadriceps tendon can be used for primary or revision reconstruction and can be used in various reconstruction and drilling techniques. The quadriceps tendon is unique in that the surgeon can harvest as much or as little graft as needed, leaving normal anatomy behind. This is especially useful for an all-epiphyseal reconstruction where shorter grafts are required. The graft can be harvested with or without a bone block according to surgeon preference, although we currently utilize all soft tissue grafts exclusively for our quadriceps tendon autograft ACL reconstructions.

The quadriceps tendon is used relatively infrequently compared to hamstring and bone-tendon-bone autografts despite favorable clinical outcomes, biomechanical properties, and low donor site morbidity. This may be related to lack of surgeon familiarity with harvest techniques and relevant anatomy. Historically, quadriceps tendon harvests have been performed through larger, less-cosmetic incisions. Recently developed minimally invasive harvest techniques and specialized commercially available instrumentation have facilitated an easy and reproducible graft harvest through small incisions.

We currently employ an "individualized ACL reconstruction" philosophy and prefer quadriceps tendon autograft reconstruction for nearly all patients where a soft tissue autograft reconstruction is indicated. We have found quadriceps tendon autografts to be especially useful in patients where kneeling pain is unacceptable due to professional or recreational demands. Contrary to hamstring autografts, there is little variability with regard to quadriceps tendon graft diameter, and the thickness of the tendon can be measured easily on magnetic resonance imaging.

CONTRAINDICATIONS

Few contraindications for quadriceps tendon ACL reconstruction exist. Specific relative contraindications specific to quad tendon autografts include: prior quadriceps tendon injury or preexisting quadriceps tendinopathy, prior quadriceps tendon surgery or parapatellar approach to the knee, and large cystic or cavitary bony lesions in the revision setting.

PREOPERATIVE PLANNING

When evaluating a patient for suspected ACL tear, one should always start with a detailed history and physical examination. Assessing patients' functional demands, activity level, and expectations following surgery allows the surgeon to choose the most appropriate graft after a diagnosis has been established.

Restoration of preoperative knee motion, especially extension, is essential prior to any ACL reconstruction, unless a bucket-handle meniscus tear or comparable injury limits motion. Comparison to the contralateral side should serve as reference for normal motion.

Once the decision has been made to perform a quadriceps tendon autograft ACL reconstruction, the MRI can be evaluated to assess quadriceps tendon thickness. The quadriceps tendon is measured

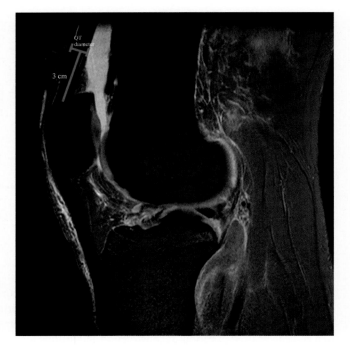

FIGURE 29-1

Sagittal MRI demonstrating measurement of quadriceps tendon thickness 3 cm proximal from the superior pole of the patella.

midsagittal from anterior to posterior, 3 cm above the proximal pole of the patella (Fig. 29-1). In general, we prefer partial-thickness quadriceps tendon harvest; however, full-thickness grafts can be harvested in patients with thinner tendons (≤6 mm). We have found no increased morbidity when harvesting full-thickness grafts, as long as the capsular rent is closed or approximated.

TECHNIQUE

In this chapter, we describe our minimally invasive harvest technique, which has evolved with newer instrumentation. Some surgeons prefer a larger incision and more "open" technique, but we have found our minimally invasive technique to be reproducible, easy, and more cosmetic. Patients tend to dislike larger incisions over the quadriceps tendon, as the scar is readily visible when they are sitting.

Positioning

After successful general anesthetic, examination under anesthesia is performed and findings are recorded. A tourniquet is applied to the operative thigh. We prefer positioning the operative leg in a circumferential leg holder with the foot of the bed dropped, and the contralateral side in a lithotomy positioner with bony prominences well padded. Alternatively, the bed can be left flat with an arthroscopic post, and the knee can be flexed over the side of the bed. The operative extremity is then prepped and draped. An Esmarch bandage is used to exsanguinate the leg, and the tourniquet is inflated.

Graft Harvest

We generally start with graft harvest, although it can be performed before or after diagnostic arthroscopy. If diagnostic arthroscopy is performed first, it is helpful to completely drain the knee of fluid prior to graft harvest. This limits capsular distention and pressure on the deep surface of the quadriceps tendon, making capsular violation less likely.

With the knee flexed to 90 degrees, the proximal pole of the patella, medial patellar border, lateral patellar border, and vastus medialis obliquus (VMO) are marked. It is important to distinguish the lateral trochlear ridge from the superior pole of the patella, which can be difficult at 90 degrees of flexion. Gentle flexion and extension of the knee helps to distinguish between the mobile patella and the immobile lateral trochlear ridge.

When this technique was initially developed, we utilized a longitudinal incision over the distal quad tendon, extending proximally from the superior pole of the patella by 1.5 to 2 cm. We have now transitioned to a transverse incision, again about 1.5 to 2 cm in length, running perpendicular to the distal quadriceps tendon about 0.5 cm proximal to the superior pole of the patella. We have

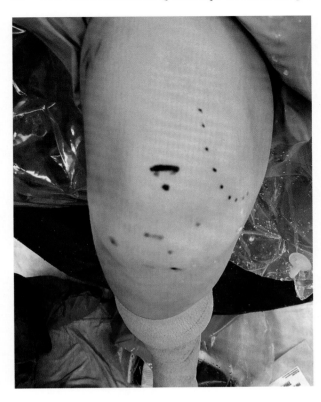

FIGURE 29-2

Preoperative marking of quadriceps tendon autograft harvest incision and vastus medialis obliquus.

found the transverse incision to be more cosmetically appealing and requires less retraction by the assistant. A second mark is made at 7 cm from the proximal pole of the patella (Fig. 29-2).

A 15-blade scalpel is used to make the incision. It is critical to widely ellipse the subcutaneous fat and paratenon to allow for visualization (Fig. 29-3). A Ray-Tech sponge over a key elevator is used to sweep away tissue on the anterior surface of the quadriceps tendon and patella. Soft tissue should be removed at least 7 cm proximal to the incision. An Army-Navy retractor is placed into the proximal apex of the incision, and the arthroscope (fluid off, looking down toward the tendon) is placed in the wound. The VMO, proximal aspect of the rectus, and vastus lateralis are identified (Fig. 29-4). When the proximal rectus tendon is identified, the arthroscope is turned so the light is shining through the skin on the anterior thigh, and this point is marked (Fig. 29-5). If any crossing vessels are seen, they should be coagulated with the radiofrequency or electrocautery device.

The Arthrex (Naples, FL) minimally invasive double blade harvest knife is designed to cut a predetermined width and depth based on surgeon preference. We generally use a 10-mm-wide by 7-mm-

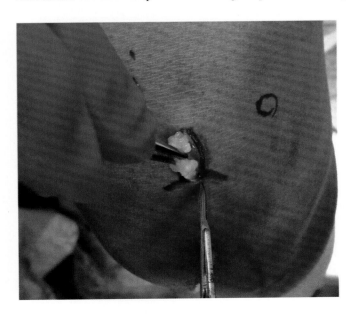

FIGURE 29-3

Pretendinous fat pad must be widely excised to gain access to the tendon.

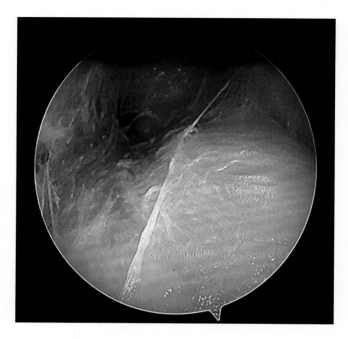

FIGURE 29-4

The musculotendinous junction of the quadriceps, viewed arthroscopically.

deep blade for most adult patients, but a 9-mm-wide blade can used for smaller or skeletally immature patients. The design of the blade allows for a "push" or "pull" cutting technique; we recommend using a push technique as cutting seems to be easier in this direction. The knife handle has markings that allow for appropriate length incision based off the superior pole of the patella. The knife carefully is placed into the wound incising in line with the proximal pole of the patella and the previously placed mark of transillumination, indicating the direction of the rectus femoris (Fig. 29-6). The longitudinal incisions are extended down to the patella with a 15-blade. The tendon is then dissected off its insertion on the proximal pole of the patella, connecting the two longitudinal incisions. The depth of the

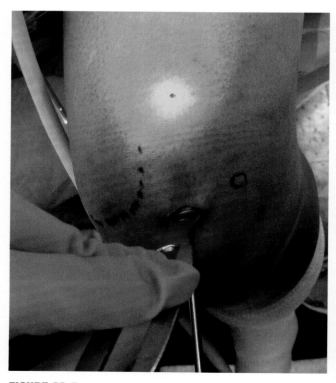

FIGURE 29-5

Transillumination of the skin above the musculotendinous junction of the quadriceps.

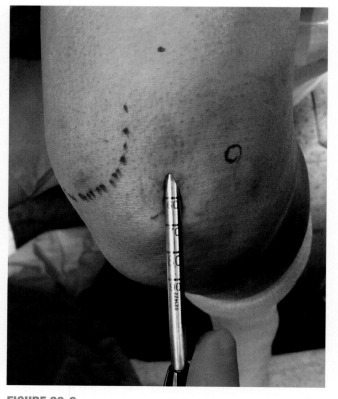

FIGURE 29-6

Insertion of quadriceps tendon double blade.

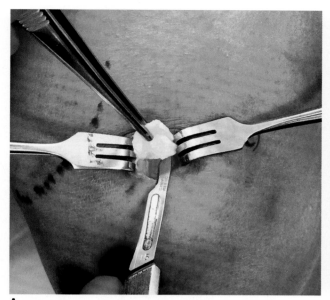 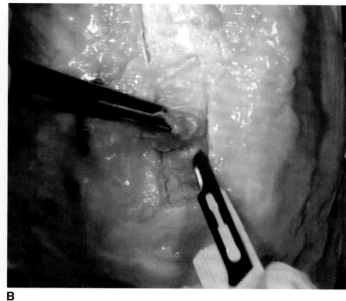

A **B**

FIGURE 29-7

A: Fat encountered deep to the quadriceps tendon. **B:** Cadaver demonstration of fat behind quadriceps tendon.

dissection can be determined based on the depth of the longitudinal incisions from the double blade knife. If fat is encountered, avoid deeper dissection or risk capsular violation (Fig. 29-7A and B). An Allis clamp is used to lift the central soft tissue quadriceps graft anteriorly, and Metzenbaum scissors are used to continue proximal dissection. It is important to taper the distal end of the graft slightly, as additional 1 mm of girth will be added with suture. Once 3 cm of graft has been elevated, an Arthrex (Naples, FL) Fiber Loop suture is placed about 2 cm proximal from the end of the graft (Fig. 29-8). Four suture throws are placed from proximal to distal, and the last suture is "locked" by entering the tendon proximal to the last throw and exiting the central portion of the tendon (Fig. 29-9). The needle is left attached to the suture for later graft preparation. With tension on the sutures, proximal dissection is carried bluntly with a key elevator or, if needed, sharply with Metzenbaum scissors. When taking a partial thickness graft, blunt dissection with key elevator is usually sufficient to developed a plane and to dissect the graft proximally. Once 5 to 6 cm of graft has been elevated, the Arthrex (Naples, FL) Quadriceps Tendon Stripper/Cutter is used to strip the tendon proximally, with firm

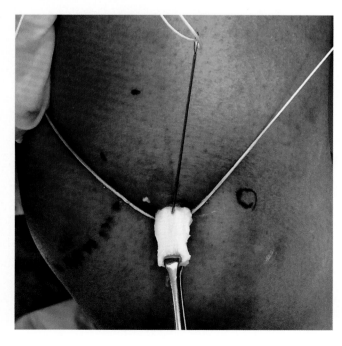

FIGURE 29-8

Initiating whipstitch of distal quadriceps tendon, in situ.

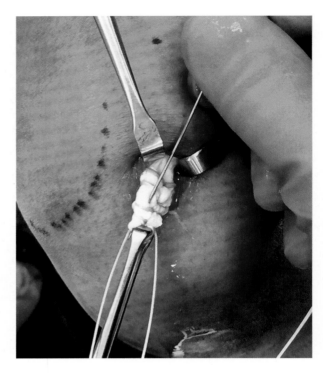

FIGURE 29-9
Locking of distal whipstitch of quadriceps tendon.

tension on the placed sutures. It is important to note that this tendon stripper is used differently than a hamstring tendon stripper, since only a portion of the tendon is being harvested. Markings on the shaft of the Stripper/Cutter allow the surgeon to identify graft length. We generally cut the graft at 7 cm for skeletally mature patients, which allows for 2 cm or more of graft in both the femoral and tibial tunnels. Harvesting grafts >8 cm can lead to an increased incidence of both bleeding and cosmetic deformity. Once the desired graft length has been obtained, the handle of the Stripper/Cutter is squeezed while tension is applied to the sutures, cutting the graft proximally (Fig. 29-10A and B). The graft is then removed from the wound and taken to the back table for preparation.

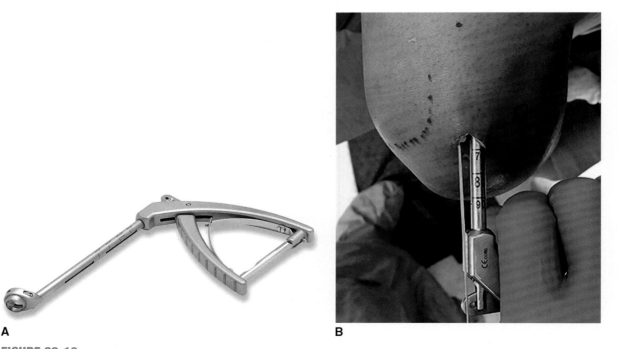

A   B

FIGURE 29-10

A: Graphic representation of quadriceps tendon stripper/cutter (Arthrex, Naples, FL). **B:** Advancement of quadriceps tendon stripper/cutter.

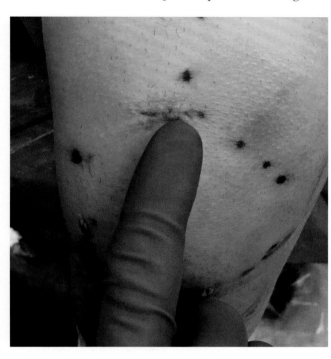

FIGURE 29-11

Closure of quadriceps tendon autograft harvest site.

The arthroscope (fluid off, looking down toward the tendon) is placed back into the wound and partial thickness harvest can be confirmed. If full-thickness rents or capsular violation is identified, they are closed with #0 Vicryl. A rotator cuff type suture passer can be used to close more proximal defects. Subcutaneous layer is closed with 2-0 Vicryl, and the skin is closed with 3-0 Monocryl (Fig. 29-11). While there is no functional difference seen with closing the defect, it limits fluid extravasation and eliminates a palpable defect postoperatively. Remember when using an arthroscopy pump, check the tenseness of the thigh periodically during the case to ensure no significant fluid extravasation is occurring.

Graft Preparation

The previously sutured end of the graft is secured to the graft preparation stand. An Allis clamp is placed on the free multilaminar end of the graft, which is controlled by an assistant to facilitate graft preparation. It is critical to trim the free side of the graft slightly, as the end diameter of the graft will increase between 0.5 and 1 mm following suture addition. A looped suture is used to whip stitch the graft in the same manner as was done during graft harvest, starting 2 cm away from the end of the graft (i.e., toward the middle of the graft) progressing toward the end (Fig. 29-12). The last suture is also locked in the same manner, passing behind the previously placed stitch, and exiting the central portion of the graft. After both ends of the graft are prepared, their respective diameters are measured. Depending on the size of each end of the graft, a decision can be made as to which end will be used for the femoral or tibial tunnels. One must keep in mind that the side selected for the femoral tunnel will have its diameter increased 0.5 mm after the attachment of the femoral fixation device.

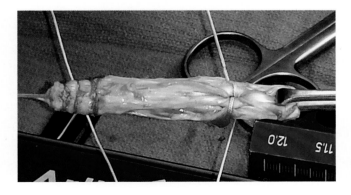

FIGURE 29-12

Quadriceps tendon autograft, being prepared on back table with proximal whipstitch.

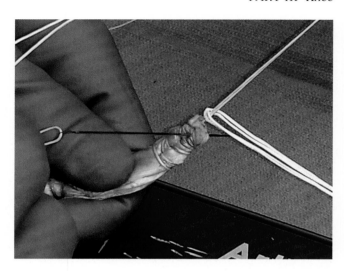

FIGURE 29-13

Locking or proximal whipstitch of quadriceps tendon.

We prefer adjustable loop suspensory fixation for the femoral side, which provides the opportunity for graft adjustment on the femoral side after the graft is passed. The previously placed fiber-loop (with attached needle) is passed through the loop of the Arthrex Tightrope RT (Naples, FL). The needle is then passed through the central portion of the graft exiting the surface of the graft 5 mm away from the graft end (Fig. 29-13). Three or four subsequent whipstitches are placed in the graft proceeding centrally. The needle is then cut from the suture, and the two limbs of suture are wrapped around the graft in opposite directions from each other and tied. The ends of sutures can be passed through the needle, and the knot can be shuttled into the midsubstance of the tendon, before suture tails are cut on the opposite side of the tendon.

The tibial side can be fixed with a variety of methods, including suspensory fixation with a button, or tie-over-post screw. If a suspensory button is used for the tibial side, it is attached to the graft in the same manner as the femoral side. The final diameter of each graft ends are then measured.

ACL Reconstruction

We use three arthroscopic portals: the standard anterior lateral (AL) portal, a low anterior medial (AM) portal placed just medial to the patellar tendon, and an accessory far medial (FM) portal. When identifying the correct placement of the femoral tunnel, we look through the AM portal with the arthroscope. In the acute setting, there is often sufficient soft tissue left on the wall, which can help identify the center of the footprint. We drill anatomic tunnels centered on the bifurcate ridge in the center of the ACL femoral origin. No matter which femoral drilling technique a surgeon utilizes, it is vital to accurately measure the distance from the ACL footprint to the lateral femoral cortex or "potential femoral tunnel length." We prefer to do this with a spade-tipped eyelet pin with measurement marking. The potential tunnel length is normally between 30 and 40 mm with an AM portal technique. In general, no more than a 25-mm tunnel is needed with a 7-cm graft (Fig. 29-14). A looped suture is placed in the femoral tunnel for later graft passage. The adjustable loop button is shortened to the length of the potential femoral tunnel +5 mm (Fig. 29-15).

The arthroscope is then switched to the AL portal, and the tibial side is marked in the center of the tibial footprint. When present, we leave a small stump of tibial footprint to aid in anatomic graft placement. The mark is approximately 2 mm anterior to the posterior aspect anterior horn of the lateral meniscus. Either a full length or blind socket tibial tunnel can be drilled, based on surgeon preference. If a blind socket is preferred, we generally prepare 25 mm of tunnel with the Arthrex Flip Cutter (Naples, FL) to allow for adequate graft tensioning. A looped suture is placed in the tibial tunnel for later graft passage.

Graft Passage

We prefer graft passage through the FM portal. Passing the graft through the FM is not only easier but also provides flexibility to place the larger diameter end on the femoral side without enlarging the tibial tunnel, which may be helpful in revision settings.

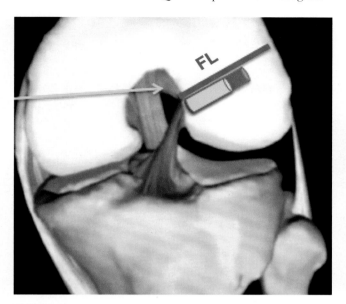

FIGURE 29-14

Femoral tunnel length, graphic representation. FL, femoral length, the length of the femoral tunnel.

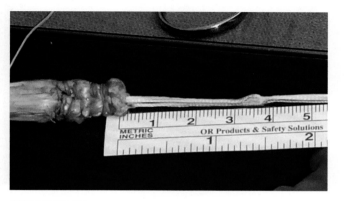

FIGURE 29-15

The adjustable loop is shortened to the length of the femoral tunnel, +5 mm.

Opening the FM portal with a large hemostat facilitates easy suture and graft passage. A grasper is used to retrieve passing sutures from both the femoral and tibial side out the FM portal. Care must be taken to ensure no soft tissue suture bridge is created. A hemostat is used to clamp the tibial passing suture out of the way (Fig. 29-16).

The passing suture is used to shuttle the sutures from the femoral Tight Rope RT (Arthrex, Naples, FL) out through the lateral thigh. The graft is then pulled through the FM portal until the proximal end of the graft reaches the aperture of the femoral tunnel (Fig. 29-17). If the potential femoral tunnel measurement and the loop shortening were done correctly, the button should be deployed on the lateral aspect of femoral cortex, and not outside of the IT band. Deployment can be confirmed by performing the "tight rope bounce" maneuver. To perform this maneuver, the femoral sutures are grasped in one hand, and the tibial in the other hand. The button is pulled a 1 to 2 mm off of the femoral cortex and then tension is quickly placed on the tibial sutures (Fig. 29-18). The

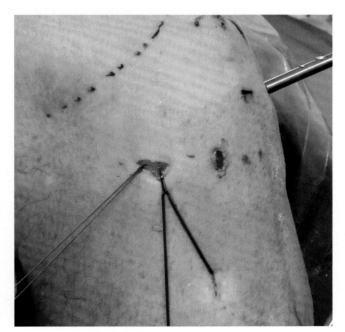

FIGURE 29-16

The femoral- and tibial-tunnel passing sutures are passed through the far medial portal. The tibial tunnel suture is held in place by passing the other end through the loop.

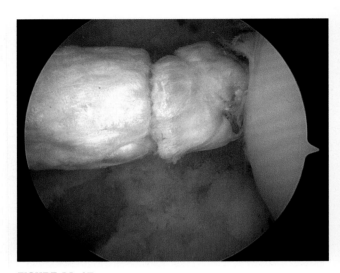

FIGURE 29-17

The proximal end of the graft at the notch orifice of the femoral tunnel.

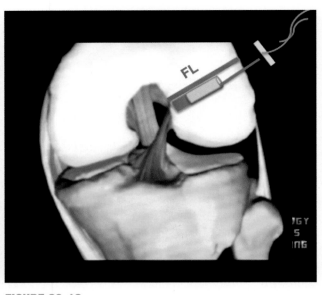

FIGURE 29-18

Graphical representation of the graft being passed through the femoral tunnel. FL, femoral length.

surgeon should feel a firm end point as the button reaches the femoral cortical bone (Fig. 29-19). Once the femoral button is successfully deployed, the adjustable loop is shortened until 20 mm of graft enters the femoral tunnel (i.e., when no suture is seen on the femoral side) (Fig. 29-20). Approximately 5 mm of space is left in the femoral socket for final tightening after tibial-sided fixation.

The sutures from the distal end of the graft are then placed through the loop of the tibial passing suture. The passing suture is then pulled out of the tibia bringing the tibial end of the graft into the tibial tunnel. Again the suture from graft preparation should be in the tibial tunnel, ensuring at least 20 mm of graft in the tunnel.

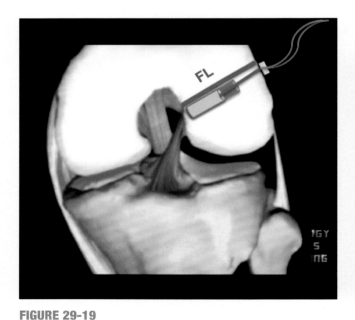

FIGURE 29-19

Graphic representation of the graft being tightened on the femoral side. FL, femoral length.

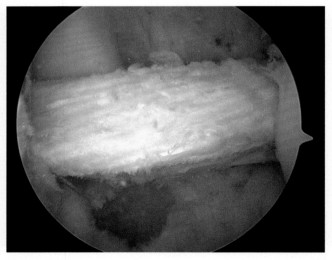

FIGURE 29-20

There is no visible suture on the femoral side of the graft once it is tightened into place in the femoral tunnel.

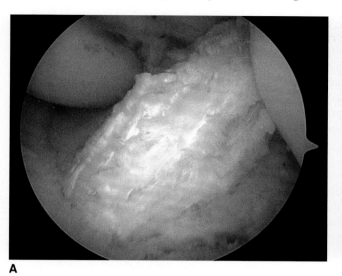

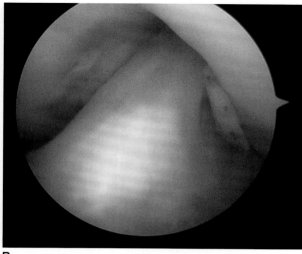

A   **B**

FIGURE 29-21

A: Tibial side of the graft is passed. **B:** Arthroscopic evaluation to ensure that there is no graft-bone impingement.

Graft Tensioning

With firm tension applied to the tibial fixation sutures, the knee is cycled approximately 20 times. Prior to fixing the distal end of the graft, we again look intraarticularly to ensure that the proper amount of graft is in the femoral tunnel, which can be adjusted by shortening the Tightrope (Arthrex, Naples, FL) construct. With the knee in full extension (but not hyperextension), the graft is tensioned, and the tibial side secured. If a screw is used, we prefer the Arthrex (Naples, FL) low profile flat-headed screw, which does not require a washer. Alternatively, the tibial side can be fixed with an adjustable loop cortical button as previously noted. The adjustable loop(s) is then maximally shortened while maintaining the knee in extension. A Lachman's maneuver and final arthroscopic evaluation are then performed to confirm appropriate graft tension (Fig. 29-21A and B).

PEARLS AND PITFALLS

- If arthroscopy is performed prior to graft harvest, ensure all fluid is drained from the knee to minimize capsular distention on the deep surface of the quadriceps tendon.
- It is critical to adequately excise the subcutaneous fat and overlying paratenon following skin incision to allow for adequate visualization following incision for graft harvest.
- Any crossing vessels identified with the arthroscope prior to graft harvest should be coagulated.
- A layer of fat lies deep to the quadriceps tendon as it attaches to the patella; if fat is encountered, avoid deeper dissection or risk capsular violation.
- The ends of the graft should be trimmed prior to suture addition, as the graft diameter will increase by 0.5 to 1 mm following suture addition.
- Passing the graft from the far medial portal allows the surgeon to customize tunnel diameter on both the femoral and tibial sides.
- Ensure that FM portal is large enough to ensure easy graft passage and cleared of fat and soft tissue so that passing sutures do not get tangled or caught.
- Shorten femoral tight rope so it is just 5 mm longer than femoral length measurement so that it is not pulled through the IT band.
- Cycle knee 20 times and look at graft position in femoral tunnel to ensure the proper amount of graft remains in the tunnel.
- Evaluate harvest site at the conclusion of the case to ensure that there is no excessive fluid extravasation.

POSTOPERATIVE MANAGEMENT

Postoperatively, we treat our quadriceps tendon autograft ACL reconstructions similar to alternative graft options. We do not routinely use a brace, except with meniscal repair or coexisting extra-articular ligamentous injury. Extension (prone hangs, forced extension) is emphasized in the immediate postoperative period. Patients are instructed to use crutches with minimal weight bearing for their first 3 to 4 days, which coincides with their first postoperative visit. At that point they began full weight bearing with crutches for 2 weeks. They are then transitioned off crutches when they can walk without a limp.

COMPLICATIONS

One complication specific to quadriceps tendon graft harvest includes harvest site hematoma. This condition presents with swelling directly under the harvest site wound and must be differentiated from intra-articular hematoma. Wound hematomas can either be from damage to a crossing vessel overlying the quadriceps tendon, inadvertent muscle damage, or intra-articular bleeding, which may escape through a full-thickness rent. Although uncommon, this can be a source of pain within 2 to 3 days of surgery. Once identified, this should be evacuated, or closely monitored if small in size and the wound is healing well. We have seen no long-term sequelae of harvest site hematoma following evacuation. Most of these complications happened early in the development of this technique, although they can still occur. Since we have started to identify and coagulate any crossing vessels and limited graft harvest length to <8 cm, we have observed fewer problems with postoperative hematoma.

Although extremely rare, we have diagnosed one impending thigh compartment syndrome following quadriceps tendon harvest in the post-anesthesia care unit. This was immediately evacuated, explored, and found to emanate from a proximal muscle arteriole. This complication occurred early in our quadriceps harvest experience and was secondary to harvesting a graft >8 cm in length going into the rectus femoris muscle. It is part of our standard postoperative protocol to check the thigh for atypical swelling prior to discharge.

We have seen two postoperative deformity with proximal retraction of the rectus femoris muscle belly. Despite the deformity, the patient reported no functional deficit and had an otherwise normal recovery. Rates of other complications such as reruptures and arthrofibrosis are similar to alternative autografts and will be discussed in more detail below.

RESULTS

Over the past 4 years, the senior author has performed over 1,000 primary ACL and revision reconstructions using the quadriceps tendon with mean follow-up of over 2 years. This is the senior author's primary graft choice for all patients under 25 years old and all elite collegiate and professional athletes. All of the patients have been prospectively followed. Our overall failure rate of all reconstructions by the primary author stands at 4.6% with 2- to 5-year follow-up. The percentage of patients with ≤3 mm side-to-side difference on KT-1000 arthrometer testing at 6-weeks, 3-months, and 6-months was found to be 97%, 96%, and 93%, respectively. No significant increase ($p > 0.05$) in side-to-side measurements was found between the 6-week to 3-month or the 3-month to 6-month intervals, suggesting our preferred method of fixation is sufficient.

Overall rate of arthrofibrosis (loss of extension) was 8.2% with the majority being in patients under 20 years old. Initially, we did not recognize the importance of tensioning the graft in full extension and emphasizing early postoperative full extension and believe this may have contributed to higher early rates of extension loss. If the patient does not achieve full extension within 6 weeks of surgery, the odds of them having a Cyclops type lesion are very high. Patients who did not achieve full extension by 3 months underwent an arthroscopy, all were found to have a Cyclops lesion and all achieved full or near full extension after the procedure.

SUGGESTED READINGS

Lund B, Nielsen T, Fauno P, et al. Is quadriceps tendon a better graft choice than patellar tendon? A prospective randomized study. *Arthroscopy*. 2014;30(5):593–598.

Slone HS, Ashford WB, Xerogeanes JW. Minimally invasive quadriceps tendon harvest and graft preparation for all-inside anterior cruciate ligament reconstruction. *Arthrosc Tech*. 2016;5(5):e1049–e1056.

Slone HS, Romine SE, Premkumar A, et al. Quadriceps tendon autograft for anterior cruciate ligament reconstruction: a comprehensive review of current literature and systematic review of clinical results. *Arthroscopy*. 2015;31(3):541–554.

30 Augmentation of Single-Bundle ACL Tears

Ryan T. Li, Benjamin B. Rothrauff, and Freddie H. Fu

INTRODUCTION

As the goal of anatomic anterior cruciate ligament (ACL) reconstruction is functional restoration of the ACL to its native dimensions, collagen orientation, and insertion sites, consideration should be given to characteristics of the individual patient's injury (1). Partial ACL tears, including isolated tears of either the anteromedial (AM) bundle or the posterolateral (PL) bundle, constitute 5% to 25% of all ACL ruptures (2–4). In such cases, it may be possible to reconstruct the torn bundle while preserving the intact bundle, termed single-bundle ACL augmentation. Retention of the intact bundle provides several advantages, as reported in preclinical and emerging clinical studies, including maintenance of the vascular supply, preservation of proprioceptive receptors, and provision of mechanical support to the healing graft, theoretically permitting earlier rehabilitation (5). Furthermore, remnant preservation can facilitate appropriate drilling of tunnels in the correct anatomical positions. Recent literature suggests that anatomic single-bundle augmentation yields equivalent or superior clinical outcomes compared to standard techniques for patients undergoing primary ACL reconstruction (6). However, the decision regarding when to perform single-bundle augmentation, as opposed to anatomic single-bundle or double-bundle ACL reconstruction, should be informed by findings on clinical examination, preoperative imaging, and intraoperative evaluation.

INDICATIONS

Indications for single-bundle ACL augmentation are the same as those more broadly considered for individualized anatomic ACL reconstruction, as the former is a technique utilized appropriately to achieve the latter. Notably, the principal indication for individualized anatomic ACL reconstruction is ACL incompetence that prevents the patient from performing at his or her desired activity level. Although a subset of patients, commonly termed "copers," can return to a preinjury level of activity following rehabilitation, the majority of patients with a complete ACL rupture will experience persistent instability (7,8). In young, active patients seeking to resume activities that require pivoting or cutting, or for those that will otherwise place high functional demand on the knee, ACL reconstruction should be strongly considered. While the indications for treatment are the same for complete and partial ACL tears, the preservation of intact fibers may mitigate preoperative measurements of objective laxity and subjective instability, obscuring the clinical picture. Careful preoperative workup and intraoperative corroboration are needed to identify patients in whom partial tears are most likely and thereby most amenable to single-bundle augmentation.

CONTRAINDICATIONS

Contraindications to single-bundle augmentation are the same as those for single-bundle or double-bundle ACL reconstruction, as described in Chapter 31, and include the following:

1. Older or more sedentary individuals who can successfully return to their preinjury level of activity without pain or knee instability

2. The presence of medical comorbidities that preclude safe surgical intervention (e.g., active infection)
3. Open tibial or femoral physes or a Tanner stage < 3 (relative contraindication, if planning transphyseal drilling)
4. Decreased range of motion in the injured knee when compared to the contralateral normal side
5. Significant osteoarthritis (Kellgren-Lawrence grade > 2)
6. Unwillingness or inability to comply with the required postoperative rehabilitation protocol

Additionally, if complete rupture of a suspected partial ACL tear is discovered during intraoperative examination, or if the preserved remnant/bundle is so tenuous as to be mechanically incompetent, single-bundle or double-bundle ACL reconstruction should instead be performed. Concomitant pathology, such as tears of the menisci or ligaments, malalignment, and PL corners injuries, should be addressed concurrent with ACL reconstruction or appropriately addressed in staged procedures if necessary.

PREOPERATIVE PREPARATION

Clinical Examination

Diagnosis of an isolated bundle ACL tear is often suggested by injury mechanism and physical examination findings but necessitates sufficient knowledge of ACL anatomy and biomechanical function (9). The AM bundle is nearly isometric from 0 to 90 degrees of knee flexion and possesses relatively constant levels of in situ forces, as it principally resists anterior translation of the tibia relative to the femur (10). On the other hand, the PL bundle is tight in extension and experiences high in situ forces from 0 to 30 degrees of flexion, which rapidly decrease with increasing flexion. While both the AM and PL bundles contribute to anterior stability, especially when the knee is flexed between 0 and 30 degrees, the PL bundle more strongly contributes to rotational stability (5,10,11).

With preservation of some continuous fibers, patients with isolated AM or PL bundle tears often deny the frank instability associated with complete ACL rupture but may complain of nonspecific symptoms such as recurrent swelling and pain. When subjective instability is noted, patients with isolated AM bundle tears describe anterior instability with activities of daily living (ADLs) and/or sports, similar to a complete ACL rupture. Conversely, patients with symptomatic PL bundle tears complain of rotational instability, most pronounced with pivoting or cutting movements, rather than anterior instability. Nonpivoting sports can often be performed without instability, while pivoting sports, such as soccer or football, induce incidents of instability that ultimately prevent continued participation (3,5). As the AM bundle principally resists anterior translation, anterior drawer test at 90 degrees of flexion is commonly positive (≥1+) with a KT side-to-side difference of 2 to 4 mm. Anterior translation with the Lachman test at 30 degrees of knee flexion is relatively small (0 to 1+), with an absent or small pivot shift (0 to 1+). In contrast, patients with PL bundle tears often possess a positive pivot shift (≥1+) while the anterior drawer and Lachman tests often measure 0 to 1+. KT side-to-side differences of 1 to 3 mm may be seen (3). These differential patterns on physical examination are summarized in Table 30-1.

TABLE 30-1 Distinguishing Isolated AM versus PL Bundle Tears		
Exam Finding	**AM Bundle Tear**	**PL Bundle Tear**
Preoperative		
Injury mechanism	Explosive, anterior direction	Pivoting, rotational
Anterior drawer test	≥1+	0 to 1+
Lachman test	0 to 1+	0 to 1+
Pivot shift test	0 to 1+	≥1+
KT-1000 side-to-side difference	2–4 mm	1–3 mm
Intraoperative		
Anterior drawer (90-degree flexion)	**No tension (torn)**	No tension (physiologic)
Lachman (20–30-degree flexion)	Some tension (if PL intact)	Some tension (if AM intact)
Internal tibial rotation (90-degree flexion)	No tension (physiologic)	**No tension (torn)**

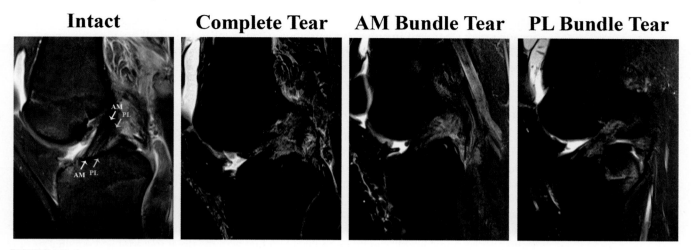

FIGURE 30-1

T2 fat-suppressed MR images in sagittal plane showing intact ACL, complete tear of ACL, isolated AM bundle tear, and isolated PL bundle tear. ACL fibers often appear continuous from the femoral to tibial insertions in partial tears; wavy fibers or increased signal in a particular bundle should increase suspicion for isolated bundle tear.

Preoperative Imaging

Suspicion for isolated ACL bundle tears can be further clarified by preoperative MRI imaging (Fig. 30-1). In a retrospective evaluation of 51 patients with arthroscopy-confirmed partial ACL tears, partial ACL tears were accurately diagnosed by two experienced, blinded radiologists using a 1.5-T scanner in 25% to 53% of cases with moderate interobserver agreement and good intraobserver agreement (12). In another retrospective study in which preoperative MRIs of 156 patients who underwent ACL reconstruction were evaluated by blinded radiologists, 83% of the 11 partial tears were accurately diagnosed (4). Diagnostic accuracy for isolated AM bundle tears was better than was that for PL bundle tears, as the latter were further obscured in MRIs obtained acutely after injury (i.e., <6 weeks of injury) (4). Identification of partial ACL tears can be further challenged by intrasubstance mucoid degeneration, which can mirror the increased MRI signal seen in isolated bundle tears. However, determination of partial tears has recently improved due to implementation of higher magnetic field strengths (e.g., 3 T) and more common use of oblique views of coronal, sagittal, and axial planes (12,13).

Determination of Tibial Insertion Site Area and Potential Graft Diameter

As is our approach with all patients undergoing individualized anatomic ACL reconstruction, the area of the tibial ACL footprint is estimated by measuring the footprint length and width on several cuts of the sagittal oblique and coronal views, respectively, of T2 fat-suppressed MR images (14). Concurrently, the graft diameter of potential autografts harvested from the quadriceps, patellar, and hamstring tendons are determined by both MRI and ultrasound (15,16). Based on clinical experience and with the knowledge that the tibial footprint area is on average 200% larger than the midsubstance cross-sectional area, it is the senior author's preference to use a graft diameter that restores 50% to 80% of the tibial insertion site area (17). However, as it is not currently possible to accurately determine the area preserved by the ACL remnant bundle, the choice of graft diameter for single-bundle augmentation may be made in consideration of anatomical studies showing that the ratio of areas of the AM:PL bundles on the tibial insertion site ranges from 50:50 to 60:40 (18). Hamstring autografts and soft tissue allografts are most commonly used in single-bundle augmentation, but both quadriceps and patellar tendons (with bone blocks) have also been employed with success.

TECHNIQUE

Positioning

Following examination under anesthesia, the patient is positioned in the hemilithotomy position with the contralateral extremity placed in a well-leg holder. A tourniquet is placed on the operative extremity, which is secured in an arthroscopic leg holder and allowed to hang at 90-degree flexion for joint distraction and improved visualization. Care is taken to pad all bony prominences with special attention paid to padding the fibular head to protect the peroneal nerve. Following standard prepping and draping, the operative extremity is exsanguinated using an Esmarch bandage, and the tourniquet is inflated to 300 mm Hg for the duration of the procedure.

Portals

The procedure is performed with a three-portal technique. Arthroscopy is initiated using a high anterolateral portal (ALP). This portal is made with the knee in 45 degrees of flexion. The position of the portal should be just lateral to the lateral border of the patella and approximately 3 to 4 mm proximal to the inferior pole of the patella. A No. 11 blade should be angled 45 degrees distal and posterior. The high position of this portal allows for a clear view of the joint unobstructed by the infrapatellar fat pad. The central portal (CP) should be made under spinal needle localization and is located just medial to the medial border of the patellar tendon just proximal to the joint line. The trajectory of the spinal needle should be cephalad, in line with the tibial footprint and directed toward the femoral origin of the ACL. The accessory anteromedial portal (AAMP) should be made under spinal needle localization and is located approximately 1 cm medial to the patellar tendon. This portal should be located above the medial meniscus and allow for easy access to the ACL femoral origin as it will be used to drill the femoral tunnel. The trajectory of the spinal needle should avoid the medial femoral condyle. Portals should be made using a No. 11 blade with the bevel of the blade pointed cephalad to avoid iatrogenic meniscal injury.

Intraoperative Examination

Prior to preparing the ACL footprints, a diagnostic arthroscopy should be performed to assess the status of the menisci and cartilage. An intraoperative examination should also be performed to confirm the integrity of the bundles. The two bundles may be visualized based on their origin and insertion on the femur and tibia, respectively. The AM bundle may be directly visualized in the notch and should have tensioned fibers from full extension to 90 degrees of knee flexion. The integrity of the AM bundle may be tested by observing appropriate tension in the bundle while applying an anterior drawer force under arthroscopic visualization. The PL bundle is often obstructed by the AM bundle and may be visualized by using a probe to retract the AM bundle medially. The integrity of the PL bundle may be tested by observing appropriate tension in the bundle while internally rotating the tibia with the knee at 90-degree flexion under arthroscopic visualization. The fibers of both bundles are probed to gauge tension. If both AM and PL bundles are incompetent on intraoperative examination, the decision should be made to perform an anatomic single- or double-bundle ACL reconstruction rather than an augmentation procedure.

Preparation of Femoral and Tibial ACL Footprints

Following thorough diagnostic arthroscopy, the remnant fibers of the injured bundle are gently debrided with the use of an arthroscopic shaver. Special care is taken to preserve the fibers of the intact bundle as well as the tibial and femoral remnant fibers of the injured bundle. In the absence of ACL remnant tissue, bony landmarks should be preserved, as they can be used to dictate the position of the bone tunnels. An arthroscopic ruler is then inserted through the CP. The tibial footprint is measured in the midcoronal and midsagittal planes confirming preoperative MRI measurements. However, accuracy of the measurement maybe compromised by the presence of the remnant bundle. Measurement of the femoral PL insertion site is possible, while measurement of the AM femoral insertion site is often blocked by an intact PL bundle. The choice of graft is finalized, and an appropriately sized graft to match the tibial insertion site is harvested and prepared using standard technique.

Placement of Bone Tunnels

Correct placement of bone tunnels is critical to the success of single-bundle ACL augmentation. Anatomic tunnel position places appropriate force vectors on the reconstructed graft, leading to knee kinematics that more closely approximate that of the preinjury state. Femoral and tibial remnant tissue represents the most reliable landmark to identify the site of the origin and insertions of the AM and PL bundles. Prior to drilling tunnels, the femoral origin and tibial insertion sites of the injured bundle are marked with electrocautery.

In instances where the remnant tissue is unable to be preserved, the location of the femoral origin and tibial insertion may be identified based on the relationship to bony landmarks and the intact bundle. On the femoral side, the PL bundle is bordered by the intercondylar ridge superiorly and the bifurcate ridge posteriorly. The AM bundle is bordered by the intercondylar ridge superiorly and the bifurcate ridge anteriorly. The femoral tunnel is reamed through the AAMP with the knee in 120 degrees of flexion using a flexible reaming system (Fig. 30-2A and B). Optimal visualization during femoral tunnel preparation is achieved with the arthroscope in the CP.

On the tibial side, the center of the PL bundle is located just medial and anterior to the posterior horn of the lateral meniscus. The center of the AM bundle is located just medial and posterior to the anterior horn of the lateral meniscus. The tibial tunnel is drilled using a standard tibial aiming guide set at 55 degrees, which is inserted through the AAMP. The tibial tunnel is initially reamed 1 mm smaller than its desired diameter and then dilated in 0.5 mm increments up to the final size (Fig. 30-2C and D).

AM Tunnels   PL Tunnels

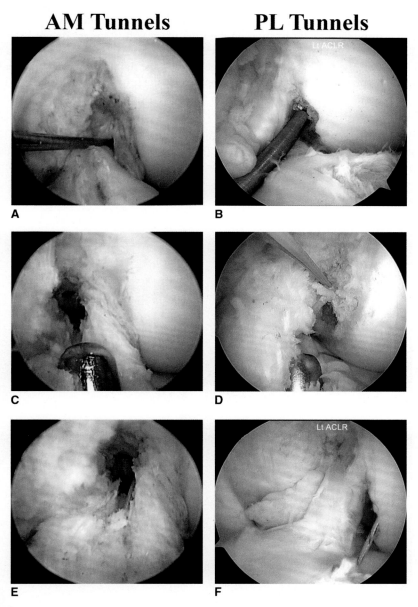

FIGURE 30-2

Bone tunnels for isolated AM or PL bundle augmentation in left knees. **A and B:** Femoral tunnels at the center of the **(A)** AM or **(B)** PL footprint are drilled with a flexible reamer system. **C and D:** Tibial tunnels with dilator positioned in center of AM or PL footprint, respectively, with femoral tunnels visualized in background. **E and F:** Suture loop spanning femoral to tibial tunnels will be used to pull graft (not shown) from distal to proximal before fixation.

Prior to reaming, the position of the guide pin for each tunnel should be viewed through all three portals to ensure appropriate position. This is especially helpful in visualizing the posterior aspect of lateral wall of the intercondylar notch, which is not always possible when viewing through the ALP alone. The guide pin should be located at the center of the origin or insertion site of the injured bundle (Fig. 30-2E and F). Care should be taken to avoid iatrogenic injury to the intact bundle during placement of the guide pin and tunnel reaming. This is particularly important when reaming the tibial tunnel during isolated PL bundle reconstruction. A curette placed over the tip of the guide pin is especially helpful to avoid iatrogenic injury. Prior to drilling the tibial tunnels, the knee can be brought into extension, and the position of the guide pins can be checked relative to the roof of the intercondylar notch to ensure there is no impingement.

Graft Tensioning and Fixation

A variety of graft fixation options are available to the surgeon. It is the senior author's preference to use suspensory fixation (15-mm EndoButton: Smith & Nephew Endoscopy, Andover, MA) on the femur and interference screw fixation on the tibia when soft tissue grafts are used. Following femoral-sided fixation, the knee is placed in neutral rotation and 20 degrees of flexion to fix the AM bundle and full extension to fix the PL bundle. The graft on the tibial side is manually tensioned and secured while a gentle posterior drawer force is applied to the proximal tibia (Fig. 30-3).

Postoperative Management

Following the procedure, the knee is placed in a long-leg hinged knee brace. The patient is permitted crutch-assisted weight bearing as tolerated, with the brace locked in full extension. In the immediate postoperative period, the brace is unlocked for range of motion exercises such as heel slides and

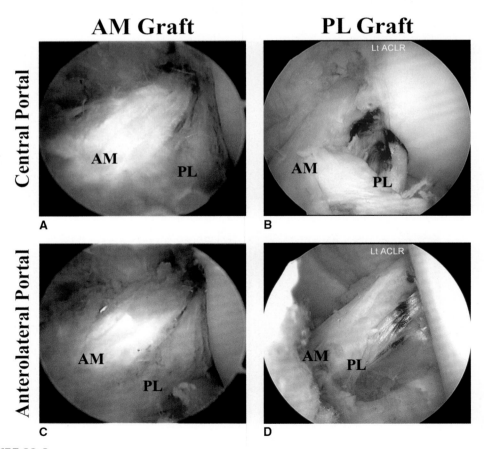

FIGURE 30-3

AM and PL grafts in place, as viewed from **(A and B)** central portal and **(C and D)** anterolateral portal.

the use of a continuous passive motion device. A customized rehabilitation protocol tailored to the procedure performed (e.g., AM vs. PL bundle augmentation with or without concomitant meniscal repair) is instituted 7 to 10 days after surgery following the first postoperative visit.

PEARLS AND PITFALLS

- Preoperative planning is critical, including a thorough history and physical examination and close scrutiny of preoperative imaging to determine the injury pattern, as well as the size of the tibial ACL footprint, patellar tendon, quadriceps tendon, and hamstring tendons.
- Confirm intact fibers of the uninjured bundle by performing a thorough intraoperative examination. The uninjured bundle may be probed and assessed for appropriate tension with either anterior drawer (intact AM bundle) or internal rotation of the tibia (intact PL bundle).
- Carefully and meticulously debride the fibers of the injured bundle while preserving the origin and insertion sites of the uninjured bundle on the femur and tibia.
- When placing the guide pins and reaming the tibial tunnel, place a curette over the guide pin to avoid iatrogenic injury to the AM bundle when performing isolated PL bundle reconstruction.
- Mark the center of the footprint on the femur and tibia prior to placing the guide pin. Failure to do so may result in nonanatomic placement of the graft or iatrogenic injury to the intact bundle.

COMPLICATIONS

Potential complications following single-bundle ACL augmentation are the same as those for ACL reconstruction and include arthrofibrosis, graft retear, infection, deep vein thrombosis, injury to neurovascular structures, and an increased risk for future degenerative joint disease. The use of allograft is further associated with increased risk for disease transmission and, though not yet demonstrated for single-bundle augmentation, increased risk for failure in young patients. Remnant-preserving ACL reconstruction has been anecdotally associated with an increased risk of cyclops lesion formation, yet numerous clinical studies have failed to find an increased risk of this particular complication as compared to traditional ACL reconstruction (19–21). Furthermore, the overall complication rate, including graft retear, appears equivalent between single-bundle augmentation and traditional ACL reconstruction techniques as recently described in two meta-analyses (6,22).

RESULTS

Although partial tears of the ACL may account for up to 25% of cases of symptomatic ACL insufficiency, single-bundle augmentation remains less commonly employed than complete ACL reconstruction in treating isolated AM or PL bundle tears (2). Despite the demonstrated short-term benefits of retaining the intact remnant with regard to accelerated revascularization and improved proprioception, it remains uncertain if these advantages persist or if they improve clinical outcomes (3,5,21). In a retrospective cohort study comparing outcomes following one of three interventions—single-bundle ACL augmentation, single-bundle ACL reconstruction, and double-bundle ACL reconstruction—Nakamae et al. found that single-bundle augmentation induced better synovial coverage than the other two groups and restored anterior tibial translation (KT-2000 side-to-side mean difference, 0.4 mm) significantly better than single-bundle ACL reconstruction (mean 1.3 mm) (21). However, there were no differences in Lysholm scores or pivot-shift grades among groups (21). In a similar study comparing single-bundle augmentation with double-bundle ACL reconstruction, the former produced superior improvements in the anterior drawer test but no added benefit in objective measures of knee stability nor subjective measures including visual analog scale score, Lysholm score, Tegner score, or International Knee Documentation Committee (IKDC) knee evaluation (20). In a systematic review of studies comparing remnant-preserving augmentation against traditional ACL reconstruction, the clinical outcomes at up to 3-year follow-up were found to be equivalent between techniques (22). In a more recent meta-analysis that included only randomized controlled studies, the remnant preservation technique showed better clinical outcome than standard ACL reconstruction technique with regard to Lysholm score and side-to-side difference in tibial translation (6). However, the durability of these effects, and their clinical meaningfulness, is still unclear.

REFERENCES

1. van Eck CF, Lesniak BP, Schreiber VM, et al. Anatomic single- and double-bundle anterior cruciate ligament reconstruction flowchart. *Arthroscopy.* 2010;26(2):258–268.
2. Zantop T, Brucker PU, Vidal A, et al. Intraarticular rupture pattern of the ACL. *Clin Orthop Relat Res.* 2007;454:48–53.
3. Siebold R, Fu FH. Assessment and augmentation of symptomatic anteromedial or posterolateral bundle tears of the anterior cruciate ligament. *Arthroscopy.* 2008;24(11):1289–1298.
4. Chang MJ, Chang CB, Choi J-Y, et al. How useful is MRI in diagnosing isolated bundle ACL injuries? *Clin Orthop Relat Res.* 2013;471(10):3283–3290.
5. Borbon CA, Mouzopoulos G, Siebold R. Why perform an ACL augmentation? *Knee Surg Sports Traumatol Arthrosc.* 2012;20(2):245–251.
6. Wang H-D, Wang F-S, Gao S-J, et al. Remnant preservation technique versus standard technique for anterior cruciate ligament reconstruction: a meta-analysis of randomized controlled trials. *J Orthop Surg Res.* 2018;13(1):231.
7. Chalmers PN, Mall NA, Moric M, et al. Does ACL reconstruction alter natural history? A systematic literature review of long-term outcomes. *J Bone Joint Surg Am.* 2014;96(4):292–300.
8. Beynnon BD, Johnson RJ, Abate JA, et al. Treatment of anterior cruciate ligament injuries. Part I. *Am J Sports Med.* 2005;33(10):1579–1602.
9. Woo SL-Y, Debski RE, Withrow JD, et al. Biomechanics of knee ligaments. *Am J Sports Med.* 1999;27(4):533–543.
10. Sakane M, Fox RJ, Woo SL, et al. In situ forces in the anterior cruciate ligament and its bundles in response to anterior tibial loads. *J Orthop Res.* 1997;15(2):285–293.
11. Gabriel MT, Wong EK, Woo SL-Y, et al. Distribution of in situ forces in the anterior cruciate ligament in response to rotatory loads. *J Orthop Res.* 2004;22(1):85–89.
12. Van Dyck P, De Smet E, Veryser J, et al. Partial tear of the anterior cruciate ligament of the knee: injury patterns on MR imaging. *Knee Surg Sports Traumatol Arthrosc.* 2012;20(2):256–261.
13. Park HJ, Kim SS, Lee SY, et al. Comparison between arthroscopic findings and 1.5-T and 3-T MRI of oblique coronal and sagittal planes of the knee for evaluation of selective bundle injury of the anterior cruciate ligament. *Am J Roentgenol.* 2014;203(2):W199–W206.
14. Guenther D, Irarrázaval S, Albers M, et al. Area of the tibial insertion site of the anterior cruciate ligament as a predictor for graft size. *Knee Surg Sports Traumatol Arthrosc.* 2017;25(5):1576–1582.
15. Zakko P, van Eck CF, Guenther D, et al. Can we predict the size of frequently used autografts in ACL reconstruction? *Knee Surg Sports Traumatol Arthrosc.* 2017;25(12):3704–3710.
16. Takenaga T, Yoshida M, Albers M, et al. Preoperative sonographic measurement can accurately predict quadrupled hamstring tendon graft diameter for ACL reconstruction. *Knee Surg Sports Traumatol Arthrosc.* 2018.
17. Fujimaki Y, Thorhauer E, Sasaki Y, et al. Quantitative in situ analysis of the anterior cruciate ligament. *Am J Sports Med.* 2016;44(1):118–125.
18. Siebold R, Ellert T, Metz S, et al. Tibial insertions of the anteromedial and posterolateral bundles of the anterior cruciate ligament: morphometry, arthroscopic landmarks, and orientation model for bone tunnel placement. *Arthroscopy.* 2008;24(2):154–161.
19. Ochi M, Adachi N, Uchio Y, et al. A minimum 2-year follow-up after selective anteromedial or posterolateral bundle anterior cruciate ligament reconstruction. *Arthroscopy.* 2009;25(2):117–122.
20. Park SY, Oh H, Park SW, et al. Clinical outcomes of remnant-preserving augmentation versus double-bundle reconstruction in the anterior cruciate ligament reconstruction. *Arthroscopy.* 2012;28(12):1833–1841.
21. Nakamae A, Ochi M, Deie M, et al. Clinical outcomes of second-look arthroscopic evaluation after anterior cruciate ligament augmentation. *Bone Joint J.* 2014;96B(10):1325–1332.
22. Hu J, Qu J, Xu D, et al. Clinical outcomes of remnant preserving augmentation in anterior cruciate ligament reconstruction: a systematic review. *Knee Surg Sports Traumatol Arthrosc.* 2014;22(9):1976–1985.

31 Individualized Anatomic Approach to ACL Reconstruction

Marcin Kowalczuk, Jeremy M. Burnham, Marcio B. V. Albers, and Freddie H. Fu

INTRODUCTION

The anteromedial (AM) and posterolateral (PL) bundles of the anterior cruciate ligament (ACL) work synergistically to impart knee stability. Surgical treatment of ACL injuries has progressed from extra-articular tenodeses to traditional nonanatomic transtibial reconstruction and more recently to tibial tunnel–independent drilling of the femoral tunnel. With modern femoral tunnel reaming methods, remnant ACL soft tissue and identifiable bony landmarks are used to achieve a more anatomic reconstruction (1,2). A natural evolution of this concept is individualized anatomic ACL reconstruction, which can be summarized by the following four concepts (3):

1. Restore both functional bundles of the ACL, the AM and PL, whether it be through a single- (SB) or double-bundle (DB) type of reconstruction.
2. The graft or grafts need to be placed anatomically, with the tibial and femoral tunnel apertures placed within the native ACL insertion sites.
3. To ensure functional properties similar to that of the native ACL bundles, each bundle should be tensioned in accordance with native tensioning patterns from full knee extension through flexion.
4. Each surgical procedure should be customized for each patient taking into account variation in anatomic characteristics, activity level, lifestyle, and personal preferences.

INDICATIONS

The indications for individualized anatomic ACL reconstruction are similar to that for standard ACL reconstruction. The chief indication is knee instability due to ACL incompetence that precludes a patient's desired level of activity (4). Although a certain subset of patients, known as "copers," are able to function at a high level despite ACL deficiency, ACL reconstruction should be strongly considered in young active individuals who participate in activities that require cutting and/or pivoting-type motions and in other patients with high functional demands and/or excessive knee instability (5).

CONTRAINDICATIONS

Contraindications to anatomic individualized ACL reconstruction include the following:

1. Older or more sedentary individuals who can successfully return to their preinjury level of activity without pain or knee instability
2. The presence of medical comorbidities that preclude safe surgical intervention (e.g., active infection)
3. Open tibial or femoral physes or a Tanner Stage <3
4. Decreased range of motion in the injured knee when compared to the contralateral normal side
5. Significant osteoarthritis (Kellgren-Lawrence Grade >2)
6. Unwillingness or inability to comply with the required postoperative rehabilitation protocol

Caution should also be exercised in the setting of chronic ACL deficiency or recurrent ACL rupture. The surgeon should maintain a high index of suspicion for concomitant pathology such as sagittal and coronal malalignment or PL corner injury, which should be addressed in conjunction with the ACL deficiency.

PREOPERATIVE PREPARATION

The cornerstone of preoperative planning is a thorough history and physical examination. Information regarding injury mechanism, history of previous knee injury or surgery, level of activity, and future patient goals should be noted. The physical exam should carefully examine both knees and document alignment, knee range of motion (including native hyperextension or ligamentous laxity), and any other concomitant ligamentous or meniscal injury.

Preoperative imaging including standard radiographs and magnetic resonance image (MRI) of the injured knee are obtained. The radiographs are used to assess bony anatomy and alignment, rule out fracture, and assess skeletal maturity.

On the preoperative MRI, the pattern of injury is closely scrutinized. Close attention is paid to whether the ACL rupture involves both the AM and PL bundles or if a partial tear involving only a single bundle is present. The dimensions of the tibial footprint of the ACL in the midcoronal and midsagittal planes are recorded (Fig. 31-1). The thickness of the patellar and quadriceps tendons is also recorded (Fig. 31-2). The prospect of single versus DB reconstruction or potential SB augmentation as well as graft choice can now be considered. The indications, contraindications, and surgical technique for SB augmentation are discussed in Chapter 30.

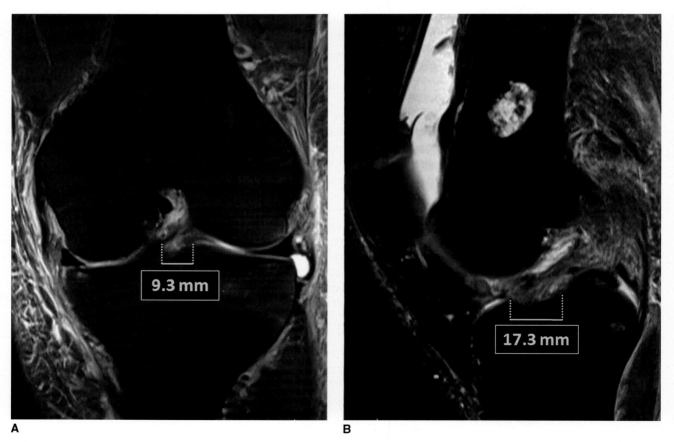

A   **B**

FIGURE 31-1

A: T2-weighted MRI demonstrating the tibial ACL footprint in the midcoronal plane. The mediolateral dimensions of the tibial ACL footprint are measured. **B:** T2-weighted MRI image of the tibial ACL footprint in the midsagittal plane. The anterior-posterior dimensions of the tibial ACL footprint are measured. An incidental benign enchondroma is also seen within the femur.

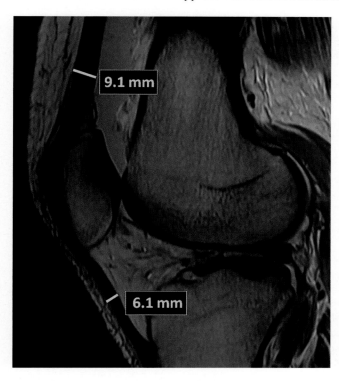

FIGURE 31-2

A proton density–weighted sagittal MRI image is used to measure the thickness of both the quadriceps tendon and patellar tendon. This aids the surgeon in determining the optimal graft choice.

SINGLE- VERSUS DOUBLE-BUNDLE RECONSTRUCTION

The dimensions of the anatomic tibial insertion have been show to vary in size considerably (6). Based on previous anatomic studies, the target graft size for ACL reconstruction should restore 50% to 80% of the estimated native tibial insertional area in order to adequately restore knee stability (7,8). A graft that is too small increases the risk of residual instability and rerupture postoperatively, while a graft that is too large can lead to graft impingement in the notch and decreased range of motion (7–9).

The percentage area reconstructed (PRA) can be calculated using the following formula (9):

PRA = tibial tunnel aperture area / native tibial insertion site area

The tibial tunnel aperture area, which is elliptical in shape, can be calculated with the following formula where α is the drill angle and d is instrument (drill or dilator) diameter:

$$A_{ellipse} = \pi(d^2/(4 \times \sin \alpha))$$

The area of the active tibial insertion can be calculated using the formula for area of an ellipse:

Area of Native Tibial Insertion: $\left[(\text{mid sagittal plane length} \times \text{mid coronal plane width})/4 \right]$

Based on the above, a formula to determine the required graft size can be created (8):

Single-bundle reconstruction: (tunnel aperture area) = (aimed percentage of reconstructed area) $\times$ (native tibial insertion site area).

Double-bundle reconstruction: (tunnel aperture area of anteromedial bundle) + (tunnel aperture area of posterolateral bundle) = (aimed percentage of reconstructed area) $\times$ (native tibial insertion site area).

For an SB reconstruction, the drilling angle for the tibial tunnel is 55 degrees by convention. For a DB reconstruction, the tibial AM and PL tunnels are drilled with the tibial guide set at 55 and 45 degrees, respectively (10,11). The AM and PL bundles are of equal size or the AM bundle can be made 1 to 2 mm larger in diameter than the PL bundle.

Table 31-1 illustrates an example of how to match potential graft size and tibial insertion site size for single- and double-bundle reconstructions.

TABLE 31-1 Percentage Reconstructed Area of the Tibial ACL Footprint-Based Graft Size				
Single-Bundle Reconstruction		**Double-Bundle Reconstruction**		
		Graft Diameter (mm)		
Graft Diameter (mm)	**Percentage Reconstructed Area (%)**	**AM Bundle**	**PM Bundle**	**Percentage Reconstructed Area (%)**
8	36	7	6	48
8.5	40	7	7	55
9	45	8	6	56
9.5	51	8	7	63
10	56			
10.5	62			

Midcoronal and midsagittal insertion site dimensions are based on MRI images seen in Figure 31-1.
AM, anteromedial; PL, posterolateral.

In most cases, a large SB graft reconstruction or DB reconstruction with two smaller grafts can be utilized to restore 50% to 80% of the tibial foot print. Using the mid–anteroposterior dimension as a guide, the senior author will perform an SB technique for insertion sites <14 mm and prefers a DB reconstruction in those with a tibial insertion site >18 mm (3,4,12). In patients with a tibial insertion site 14 to 18 mm in size, an SB or DB reconstruction may be performed although most frequently an SB reconstruction is chosen, as it is more technically straightforward and less likely to result in complications.

Although these preoperative measurements act as a guide, the final decision whether to perform an SB versus DB reconstruction is made intraoperatively after remeasuring the tibial insertion size with an arthroscopic ruler and also considering the dimensions of the femoral intercondylar notch. If considering a DB reconstruction, particularly in patients with a tibial insertion site in the 14 to 18 mm range, a notch width of <12 mm may not allow for placement and drilling of the tunnels at the native insertion site without damaging the medial femoral condyle, while a shallow notch (<12 mm) may potentially lead to graft impingement (3,11,12). In such cases, an SB reconstruction is performed.

GRAFT CHOICE IN ANATOMIC INDIVIDUALIZED ACL RECONSTRUCTION

A multitude of graft options are available to the surgeon, and all must be considered. The advantages and disadvantages of each graft choice can be seen in Table 31-2. The thickness of the quadriceps and patellar tendon can be evaluated on preoperative MRI. The patellar tendon should not be the primary option if the anteroposterior maximum thickness is <5 mm on the sagittal cuts of the MRI. The quadriceps tendon is considered to be of adequate size if the anteroposterior thickness is >7 mm.

If a DB reconstruction is being considered, the graft of choice is either quadriceps or hamstring autograft. If the use of an autograft hamstring graft is being considered, the patient is made aware that augmentation with allograft, which should always be available, may be necessary. Whether hamstring autograft diameter can be reliably predicted preoperatively remains controversial (13–16).

SURGICAL TECHNIQUE

Positioning

Following a thorough examination under anesthesia, the patient is positioned in the hemilithotomy position with the uninjured leg secured in a well-leg holder. The tourniquet is applied to the thigh of the operative leg, which is then also secured into an arthroscopic leg holder allowing the leg to hang freely at 90 degrees of flexion (Fig. 31-3). Care is taken to pad all bony prominences, particularly the

TABLE 31-2 Graft Options for Anatomic ACL Reconstruction

Graft	Advantages	Disadvantages
Quadriceps tendon	• Large graft • Option of a one-sided bone block	• Invasive, large incision • Risk of patellar fracture with bone block harvest
Hamstring	• Ease of harvest • Cosmesis • Minimal donor site morbidity	• Soft tissue healing • Graft size can be unpredictable • Not suitable for certain athletes who rely heavily on their hamstring muscles • Less stiffness than native ACL
Patellar tendon	• Bone to bone healing • Large graft	• Single bundle only • Residual kneeling pain • Graft-tunnel mismatch • Risk of patellar fracture
Allograft	• No donor site morbidity • Available in various types and sizes • Shortens operative time	• Risk of disease transmission • Healing time • Increased risk of rerupture with irradiated allografts, especially in younger patients • Costly

From Rahnemai-Azar AA, Sabzevari S, Irarrazaval S, et al. Anatomical individualized ACL reconstruction. *Arch Bone Jt Surg.* 2016;4(4):291–297.

fibular head of the nonoperative leg. Following standard draping, the operative leg is exsanguinated with the aid of an Esmarch bandage, and the tourniquet is inflated to 300 mm Hg for the duration of the procedure.

Arthroscopic Portals

The arthroscopic portion of the procedure is commenced using a three-portal technique. An initial high anterolateral portal (ALP) is created to allow good visualization of the ACL tibial footprint. It is made with the knee in 45 degrees of flexion and placed just off the lateral border of the patella approximately 3 to 4 mm superior to a transverse line drawn at the inferior pole of the patella. The "high" position of the ALP helps avoid visual obstruction by the infrapatellar fat pad and provides a "bird's-eye" view of the tibial insertion site. The central portal (CP) is then created just off the medial border of the patellar tendon just above the joint line. It should first be localized with a spinal needle whose trajectory should be slightly cephalad, in line with the tibial ACL footprint and heading toward the femoral ACL origin. The accessory anteromedial portal (AAMP) is created approximately 10 mm medial to the patellar tendon and just above the medial meniscus. This portal will be used to drill the femoral tunnel; therefore, the trajectory is checked with a spinal needle. The spinal needle should avoid the medial femoral condyle to prevent later cartilage damage during femoral tunnel preparation while also easily reaching the femoral insertion of the ACL.

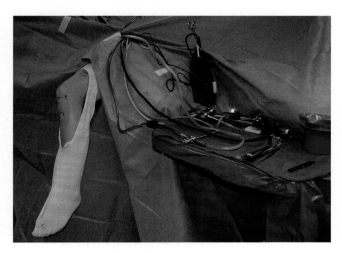

FIGURE 31-3

The operative limb is secured with an arthroscopic leg holder and allowed to hang freely at 90 degrees of knee flexion. Under the surgical drapes, a tourniquet is placed around the thigh and is inflated for the duration of the operative procedure. Note how the operative limb can be easily flexed more than 90 degrees to facilitate drilling of the femoral tunnel.

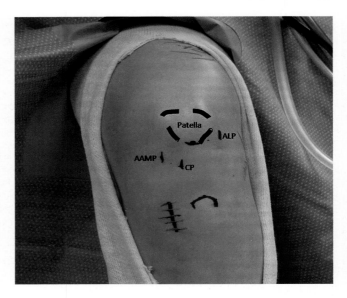

FIGURE 31-4

The anatomic landmarks including the patella and tibial tubercle are marked on the skin. A vertical skin incision 1 cm medial and 3 to 5 cm distal to the joint line is also marked for drilling the tibial tunnel or harvesting the hamstring tendons if required. Following palpation of the medial and lateral margins of the patellar tendon, the *ALP, CP,* and *AAMP* are marked. ALP, anterolateral portal; CP, central portal; AAMP, accessory anteromedial portal.

All portals are created with a No. 11 blade, taking care to point the beveled edge away from the meniscus (Fig. 31-4).

Preparation of the Tibial and Femoral ACL Footprints

Following a thorough diagnostic arthroscopy, the remnant ACL fibers are gently debrided with the use of an arthroscopic shaver. Care is taken to preserve the tibial and femoral remnant ACL fibers if possible. With the arthroscope in the ALP, a No. 11 scalpel blade is inserted via the CP, and the tibial ACL stump is transected sharply to reveal the insertions of the AM and PL bundles (Fig. 31-5). In the absence of the ACL remnant tissue, which occurs in a small proportion of the chronic cases, bony landmarks should be preserved by subtle dissection, as they can be used to dictate the position of the bone tunnels.

The scalpel blade is then exchanged for a malleable arthroscopic ruler (Smith & Nephew Endoscopy, Andover, MA), and via the CP, the tibial footprint is measured in the midcoronal and midsagittal planes confirming preoperative MRI measurements (Fig. 31-6). The intercondylar notch height (medially and laterally) and width along with the length and width of the femoral ACL footprint are also measured (Fig. 31-7). At this juncture, the decision to perform a DB or SB reconstruction is made. The choice of graft is also finalized, which is subsequently harvested and prepared according to standard technique.

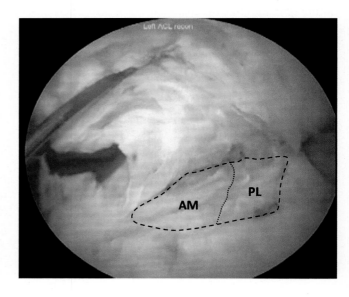

FIGURE 31-5

Viewing from the ALP, a No. 11 scalpel blade is inserted through the CP, and the remnant ACL stump is sharply transected revealing the tibial insertions of the *AM* and *PL* bundles. CP, central portal; ALP, anterolateral portal.

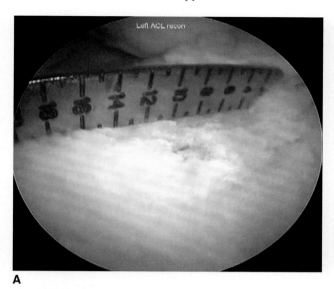
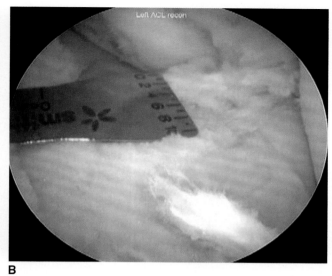

FIGURE 31-6

Viewing from the ALP, the scalpel blade is exchanged for a malleable arthroscopic ruler, and the tibial footprint is measured and compared to preoperative MRI measurements. **A:** The tibial ACL footprint is measured in its midportion in the sagittal plane. **B:** The tibial ACL footprint is also measured at its midportion in the coronal plain. ALP, anterolateral portal.

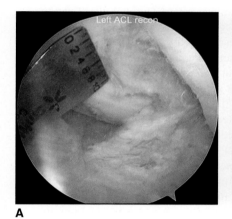
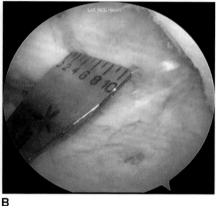
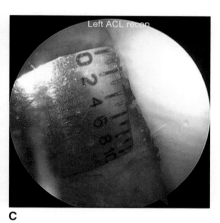

FIGURE 31-7

The dimensions of the intercondylar notch are assessed with a malleable arthroscopic ruler. **A:** The height is measured medially. **B:** The width of the intercondylar notch is recorded. **C:** The height is also measured laterally.

Placement of Bone Tunnels

The placement of bone tunnels in the anatomic position is critical to successful anatomic ACL reconstruction. Proper tunnel placement ensures that the reconstructed ligament experiences appropriate force vectors leading to knee kinematics that most closely resemble the preinjury state. The most reliable landmark for femoral and tibial tunnel placement is the remnant ACL tissue, which is usually seen in acute cases (1,11). The importance of meticulous arthroscopic dissection of the AM and PL bundle footprints cannot be overstated (Fig. 31-8). In more chronic cases, the lateral intercondylar and bifurcate ridges can be used on the femoral side, while the tibial spines and the intermeniscal ligament are suggested landmarks for placement of the tibial tunnel (17,18). Fluoroscopy can also be used as an adjunct in difficult cases and has been shown to be reproducible, reliable, and accurate (19–21).

In the case of SB reconstruction, the femoral tunnel should be centered halfway between the origin of the AM and PL bundles. When a DB reconstruction is being performed, the femoral tunnels are centered directly over the anatomic origin of the AM and PL bundles. All femoral tunnels

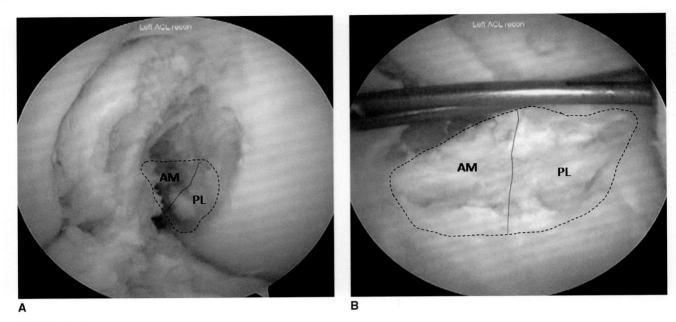

FIGURE 31-8

To optimize anatomic tunnel placement, meticulous dissection of the femoral and tibial ACL footprints is critical. **A:** The femoral ACL footprint is visualized. **B:** The tibial ACL footprint is visualized.

irrespective of SB or DB technique are drilled with the knee in 120 degrees of flexion via the AAMP, and it is the senior author's preference to use a flexible reaming system. Optimal visualization during femoral tunnel preparation is achieved with the arthroscope in the CP.

Analogous to the femoral tunnel in the setting of SB reconstruction, the tibial tunnel is located midway between the tibial insertions of the AM and PL bundles and drilled with the aid of a standard tibial aiming guide inserted through the AAMP set at 55 degrees. For a DB reconstruction, the AM and PL tibial tunnels are drilled with the guide set at 55 and 45 degrees, respectively, and centered over the anatomic insertions of each bundle (10). The drill guide is inserted via the CP in both instances, and the guide pins for both tunnels are inserted first, and the tunnel positions are confirmed before reaming is commenced. The tunnels are positioned to allow for a 2-cm boney bridge between tunnels on the AM tibial cortex, with the AM tunnel just medial to the tibial tubercle and the PL tunnel located more posteriorly (10,11). The tibial tunnels are reamed 1 mm smaller than their desired diameter and then dilated to their final size in 0.5-mm increments.

Adequate direct arthroscopic visualization is critical to appropriate tunnel placement. The position of the guide pin for each tunnel is visualized through the ALP, CP, and AAMP (if possible) to ensure it is in the appropriate anatomic position before final tunnel reaming is performed (Fig. 31-9). This is especially helpful in visualizing the posterior aspect of the inner wall of the lateral intercondylar notch, which is not always possible via the ALP. The PL femoral tunnel is drilled first followed sequentially by the AM and PL tibial tunnels and finally the AM femoral tunnel (10,11). Prior to drilling the tibial tunnels, the knee can also be brought into extension, and the position of the guide pins can be checked relative to the roof of the intercondylar notch to ensure there is no impingement.

Graft Tensioning and Fixation

A variety of graft fixation options are available to the surgeon. It is the senior author's preference to use suspensory fixation (15-mm EndoButton: Smith & Nephew Endoscopy, Andover, MA) on the femur and interference screw fixation on the tibia when soft tissue grafts are used. Metal or bioabsorbable interference screws can be used. If bone plugs are present, then interference screw fixation is used most frequently to secure the tibial and femoral aspects of the graft although suspensory fixation (EndoButton CL BTB: & Nephew Endoscopy, Andover, MA) is also occasionally used on the femoral side.

There is no standard protocol for preconditioning the graft nor is there a consensus with regard to graft tensioning (11). Following femoral-sided fixation for SB reconstructions, the knee is placed in

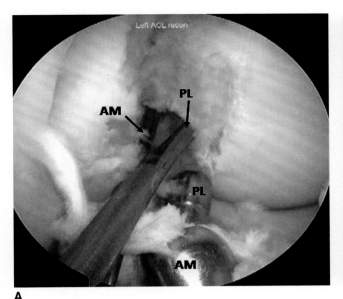
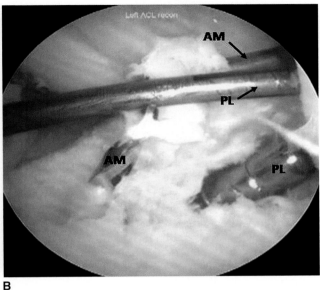

FIGURE 31-9

Tunnel position should be checked from various perspectives. In the case of this double-bundle reconstruction, visualization through the AAMP could not be achieved due to the presence of hardware. **A:** The position of the femoral and tibial *AM* and *PL* tunnels as visualized from the CP. Note that during femoral tunnel drilling, the posterior aspect of the inner wall of the lateral intercondylar notch can be easily visualized. **B:** The position of the femoral and tibial *AM* and *PL* tunnels as visualized from the ALP. Note the suboptimal visualization of the femoral tunnels highlighting the importance of using a three-portal technique. ALP, anterolateral portal; CP, central portal.

neutral rotation and 20 degrees of flexion, and while a gentle posterior drawer is applied, the graft on the tibial side is manually tensioned and secured. The same protocol is used for DB reconstruction except that after both the PL and AM bundles are secured sequentially on the femoral side using suspensory fixation (15-mm EndoButton: Smith & Nephew Endoscopy, Andover, MA), PL bundle fixation on the tibia is performed first in full extension followed by AM bundle fixation in 20 to 40 degrees of flexion (Fig. 31-10) (10).

PEARLS AND PITFALLS

- Preoperative planning is critical, including a thorough history and physical exam and close scrutiny of preoperative imaging to determine the injury pattern, as well as the size of the tibial ACL footprint, patellar tendon, and quadriceps tendon.
- The goal should be to recreate 50% to 80% the native tibial ACL insertion area with the ACL reconstruction.
- Use of all three portals, including a "high" ALP that is above the infrapatellar fat pad, is critical for visualization and allows for anatomic tunnel placement.
- An appropriately positioned SB reconstruction functionally restores both the AM and PL bundles.
- The final decision regarding the type of reconstruction and graft choice is made intraoperatively.
- If hamstring autograft is used, all patients should be made aware that augmentation with allograft maybe necessary.
- Postoperative rehabilitation protocols should be tailored to the procedure that was performed.

POSTOPERATIVE MANAGEMENT

Following the procedure, the knee is placed in a long leg hinged knee brace postoperatively, and crutch-assisted weight bearing as tolerated, with the brace locked in full extension, is permitted. In the immediate postoperative period, the brace is unlocked for range of motion exercises such as heel slides and the use of a continuous passive motion device. A customized rehabilitation protocol tailored to the procedure performed (e.g., SB vs. DB reconstruction with or without concomitant meniscal repair) is instituted 7 to 10 days after surgery following the first postoperative visit.

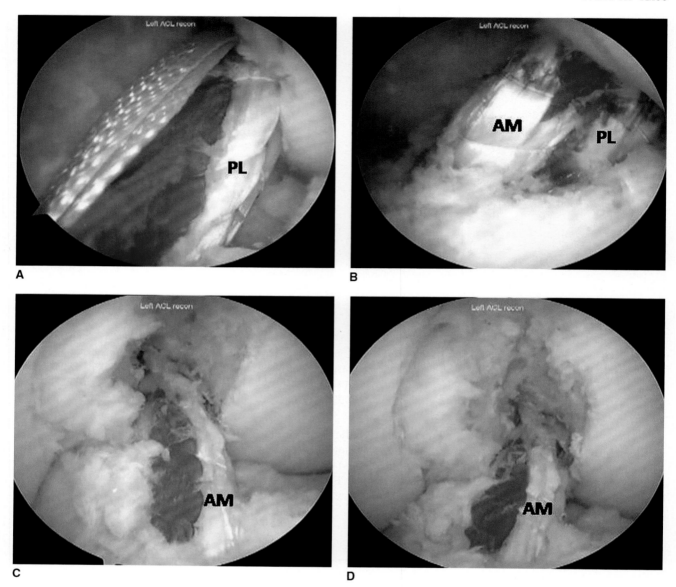

FIGURE 31-10

A: The PL bundle is passed first with the shuttling sutures for the *AM* bundle also visible. Note the fibrin clot sutured to the PL bundle graft with an undyed absorbable 3-0 or 4-0 suture (Caprosyn: Medtronic, Minneapolis, MN) to facilitate healing between the *AM* and *PL* bundles. **B:** The position of both the *AM* and *PL* bundles in an anatomic double-bundle ACL reconstruction as seen from the ALP. **C:** The position of both the *AM* and *PL* bundles as seen from the CP. **D:** The position of both the *AM* and *PL* bundles as seen from the AAMP.

COMPLICATIONS

The complications following anatomic individualized ACL reconstruction do not differ from those of traditional ACL reconstruction procedures. The potential for arthrofibrosis, graft rerupture, deep vein thrombosis, infection, and damage to neurovascular structures and the risk for future degenerative joint disease are discussed with every patient. The risks of allograft use, particularly disease transmission and higher failure rates in young patients, are also discussed.

Importantly, if <50% of the tibial foot print area is restored, the risk of residual instability and rerupture increases (22,23). If >80% of the tibial footprint area is restored, the risk of graft impingement increases (8). Tunnel position is critical, and inappropriate positioning can result in failure to restore rotatory stability (vertical graft placement), reduced range of motion, and potentially increased rates of rerupture (2,24).

RESULTS

A recent level I prospective randomized control trial of 281 patients with 3- to 5-year follow-up compared conventional SB ACL reconstruction to anatomic SB or DB reconstructions (25). Decreased anteroposterior translation and improved rotatory stability were noted with the use of DB and SB techniques when compared to conventional SB ACL reconstruction. In a subsequent level II cohort study, the concept of individualized ACL surgery was examined, and patients received either SB or DB reconstruction based on the size of the tibial ACL footprint. No differences in terms of anteroposterior laxity, rotatory laxity, or patient-reported outcomes were seen at a mean of 2.5 years' follow-up (26). This confirms that in the appropriately selected patient, SB reconstruction functionally confers the stability afforded by a DB reconstruction and leads to comparable outcomes.

REFERENCES

1. Fu FH, van Eck CF, Tashman S, et al. Anatomic anterior cruciate ligament reconstruction: a changing paradigm. *Knee Surg Sports Traumatol Arthrosc.* 2015;23(3):640–648. doi:10.1007/s00167-014-3209-9.
2. Salzler MJ, Harner CD. Tunnel placement for the ACL during reconstructive surgery of the knee: a critical analysis review. *JBJS Rev.* 2014;2(4). doi:10.2106/jbjs.rvw.m.00054.
3. Hofbauer M, Muller B, Murawski CD, et al. The concept of individualized anatomic anterior cruciate ligament (ACL) reconstruction. *Knee Surg Sports Traumatol Arthrosc.* 2014;22(5):979–986. doi:10.1007/s00167-013-2562-4.
4. Murawski CD, van Eck CF, Irrgang JJ, et al. Operative treatment of primary anterior cruciate ligament rupture in adults. *J Bone Joint Surg Am.* 2014;96(8):685–694. doi:10.2106/jbjs.m.00196.
5. Johnson D. *ACL Made Simple.* New York: Springer-Verlag; 2004.
6. Kopf S, Pombo MW, Szczodry M, et al. Size variability of the human anterior cruciate ligament insertion sites. *Am J Sports Med.* 2011;39(1):108–113. doi:10.1177/0363546510377399.
7. Fujimaki Y, Thorhauer E, Sasaki Y, et al. Quantitative in situ analysis of the anterior cruciate ligament: length, midsubstance cross-sectional area, and insertion site areas. *Am J Sports Med.* 2016;44(1):118–125. doi:10.1177/0363546515611641.
8. Guenther D, Irarrazaval S, Albers M, et al. Area of the tibial insertion site of the anterior cruciate ligament as a predictor for graft size. *Knee Surg Sports Traumatol Arthrosc.* 2017;25(5):1576–1582. doi:10.1007/s00167-016-4295-7.
9. Middleton KK, Muller B, Araujo PH, et al. Is the native ACL insertion site "completely restored" using an individualized approach to single-bundle ACL-R? *Knee Surg Sports Traumatol Arthrosc.* 2015;23(8):2145–2150. doi:10.1007/s00167-014-3043-0.
10. Karlsson J, Irrgang JJ, van Eck CF, et al. Anatomic single- and double-bundle anterior cruciate ligament reconstruction, part 2: clinical application of surgical technique. *Am J Sports Med.* 2011;39(9):2016–2026. doi:10.1177/0363546511402660.
11. Rahnemai-Azar AA, Sabzevari S, Irarrazaval S, et al. Reconstruction. *Arch Bone Jt Surg.* 2016;4(4):291–297.
12. van Eck CF, Lesniak BP, Schreiber VM, et al. Anatomic single- and double-bundle anterior cruciate ligament reconstruction flowchart. *Arthroscopy.* 2010;26(2):258–268. doi:10.1016/j.arthro.2009.07.027.
13. Conte EJ, Hyatt AE, Gatt CJ Jr., et al. Hamstring autograft size can be predicted and is a potential risk factor for anterior cruciate ligament reconstruction failure. *Arthroscopy.* 2014;30(7):882–890. doi:10.1016/j.arthro.2014.03.028.
14. Mardani-Kivi M, Karimi-Mobarakeh M, Mirbolook A, et al. Predicting the Hamstring tendon diameter using anthropometric parameters. *Arch Bone Jt Surg.* 2016;4(4):314–317.
15. Treme G, Diduch DR, Billante MJ, et al. Hamstring graft size prediction: a prospective clinical evaluation. *Am J Sports Med.* 2008;36(11):2204–2209. doi:10.1177/0363546508319901.
16. Zakko P, van Eck CF, Guenther D, et al. Can we predict the size of frequently used autografts in ACL reconstruction? *Knee Surg Sports Traumatol Arthrosc.* 2017;25(12):3704–3710. doi:10.1007/s00167-015-3695-4.
17. Ferretti M, Doca D, Ingham SM, et al. Bony and soft tissue landmarks of the ACL tibial insertion site: an anatomical study. *Knee Surg Sports Traumatol Arthrosc.* 2012;20(1):62–68. doi:10.1007/s00167-011-1592-z.
18. Ferretti M, Ekdahl M, Shen W, et al. Osseous landmarks of the femoral attachment of the anterior cruciate ligament: an anatomic study. *Arthroscopy.* 2007;23(11):1218–1225. doi:10.1016/j.arthro.2007.09.008.
19. Bernard M, Hertel P, Hornung H, et al. Femoral insertion of the ACL. Radiographic quadrant method. *Am J Knee Surg.* 1997;10(1):14–21; discussion 21–22.
20. Dhawan A, Gallo RA, Lynch SA. Anatomic tunnel placement in anterior cruciate ligament reconstruction. *J Am Acad Orthop Surg.* 2016;24(7):443–454. doi:10.5435/jaaos-d-14-00465.
21. Staubli HU, Rauschning W. Tibial attachment area of the anterior cruciate ligament in the extended knee position. Anatomy and cryosections in vitro complemented by magnetic resonance arthrography in vivo. *Knee Surg Sports Traumatol Arthrosc.* 1994;2(3):138–146.
22. Magnussen RA, Lawrence JT, West RL, et al. Graft size and patient age are predictors of early revision after anterior cruciate ligament reconstruction with hamstring autograft. *Arthroscopy.* 2012;28(4):526–531. doi:10.1016/j.arthro.2011.11.024.
23. Mariscalco MW, Flanigan DC, Mitchell J, et al. The influence of hamstring autograft size on patient-reported outcomes and risk of revision after anterior cruciate ligament reconstruction: a Multicenter Orthopaedic Outcomes Network (MOON) Cohort Study. *Arthroscopy.* 2013;29(12):1948–1953. doi:10.1016/j.arthro.2013.08.025.
24. Bedi A, Maak T, Musahl V, et al. Effect of tibial tunnel position on stability of the knee after anterior cruciate ligament reconstruction: is the tibial tunnel position most important? *Am J Sports Med.* 2011;39(2):366–373. doi:10.1177/0363546510388157.
25. Hussein M, van Eck CF, Cretnik A, et al. Prospective randomized clinical evaluation of conventional single-bundle, anatomic single-bundle, and anatomic double-bundle anterior cruciate ligament reconstruction: 281 cases with 3- to 5-year follow-up. *Am J Sports Med.* 2012;40(3):512–520. doi:10.1177/0363546511426416.
26. Hussein M, van Eck CF, Cretnik A, et al. Individualized anterior cruciate ligament surgery: a prospective study comparing anatomic single- and double-bundle reconstruction. *Am J Sports Med.* 2012;40(8):1781–1788. doi:10.1177/0363546512446928.

32 ACL Reconstruction in Children and Adolescents

Peter D. Fabricant and Mininder S. Kocher

INDICATIONS

Tears of the anterior cruciate ligament (ACL) were once considered rare in skeletally immature athletes; however, they are now observed with increasing frequency. Adolescents and teenagers in fact represent the largest per capita demographic of ACL reconstructions (1). Nonoperative management has been shown to lead to high rates of sport dropout, with up to 94% unable to participate at preinjury level of activity and up to 50% unable to participate at all due to recurrent knee instability (2–4). Furthermore, continued instability can result in progressive meniscal and cartilage damage, as well as arthritic changes in 61% of knees (3,5,6). This is particularly true in children and adolescents, as they are not frequently compliant in modifying their postinjury activity levels. Therefore, with few exceptions, young athletes with ACL tears are frequently indicated for surgical reconstruction.

Although skeletal maturity occurs around age 14 in girls and age 16 in boys, negligible (<1 cm in each limb segment) growth remains around the knee after age 12 to 13 years in girls and 14 to 15 years in boys (7). Therefore in children prior to skeletal maturity but with little growth remaining (Tanner stage ≥3; skeletal age ≥12 years in females and ≥13 years in males), anatomic soft tissue autograft ACL reconstruction without transphyseal fixation hardware (e.g., suspensory cortical fixation button on the femur and nonmetal tibial metaphyseal interference screw) is preferred. Hamstring autograft ACL reconstruction technique is covered in Chapter 28 and will therefore not be repeated here; in this chapter, we will focus on considerations and technique of ACL reconstruction in prepubescent children (Tanner stage 1 to 2; skeletal age ≤11 years in females and ≤12 years in males) using the iliotibial (IT) band combined extra- and intra-articular ACL reconstruction (Fig. 32-1).

CONTRAINDICATIONS

Contraindications for ACL reconstruction in children and adolescents are rare, given recent understanding of the risks of nonoperative treatment and surgical delay (8–13). While skeletal immaturity has been considered a historical relative contraindication to ACL reconstruction, surgical methods and instrumentation have evolved, in order to accommodate the unique anatomy of skeletally immature patients. In current practice, contraindications to ACL reconstruction in young athletes include incompletely addressed polytrauma, active infection, and arthrofibrosis. Relative contraindications also include morbidly obese and sedentary patients and those with developmental delay and/or behavioral disturbances that preclude the child's ability to participate in safe, structured postoperative rehabilitation.

Children with a skeletal age of 14 years or younger with tears less than half of the thickness of the ACL, tears of the anteromedial bundle only, and a grade A pivot shift examination have been shown in one study to have a higher rate of success with bracing and structured rehabilitation (14). Therefore, it may be reasonable to consider a trial of nonoperative treatment in patients who meet all

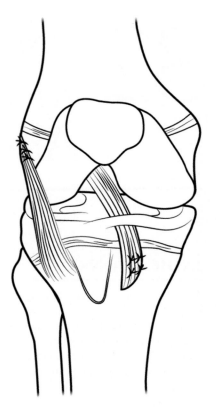

FIGURE 32-1

Illustration of the iliotibial band combined extra- and intra-articular ACL reconstruction (modified MacIntosh procedure). (Reprinted from Fabricant PD, Jones K, Delos D, et al. Reconstruction of the anterior cruciate ligament in the skeletally immature athlete: a review of current concepts. *J Bone Joint Surg Am.* 2013;95(5):e28, with permission.)

these criteria, with the understanding that recurrent instability requiring delayed ACL reconstruction may inevitably persist.

PREOPERATIVE PREPARATION

In addition to standard ACL reconstruction, preoperative evaluation, and workup covered elsewhere in this text (e.g., history, physical examination, plain radiographs, MRI, and ruling out concomitant meniscal, cartilage, or ligamentous injury), there are additional steps in the pediatric athlete that warrant special mention. First, skeletal age should be determined for children and adolescents with open physes and is most frequently assessed using a posteroanterior left hand radiograph (15–17); however, alternative methods based on pelvis, elbow, and calcaneal radiographs have also been described (18–21). Timing of peak growth velocity may be derived from Tanner staging, as well as time since menarche (22). Second, surgeons can quantify baseline leg length discrepancy and angular deformity using standing AP hip-to-ankle radiography (23–25). By characterizing preexisting length and angular deformities as well as calculating remaining growth, the surgeon is able to both document preexisting deformity and consider realignment using minimally invasive implant-mediated guided growth in extreme cases. Because children often have more physiologic laxity than adults, examination of the contralateral uninjured knee is important to determine normal findings, including a physiologic pivot shift/glide (26). Finally, psychological assessment of the child's ability to actively participate in rehabilitation after surgery should be determined.

A course of prereconstruction physical therapy is prescribed focusing on reducing pain, swelling, and effusion; regaining normal gait mechanics; and maximizing quadriceps and hamstring strength preoperatively. This delay of approximately 4 weeks helps to minimize postoperative arthrofibrosis (27). In the event of an urgent meniscal (e.g., locked bucket-handle tear) or osteochondral injury with loose body, the reconstructive surgery can either be staged or performed earlier after appropriate counseling of the risks, benefits, and requirements involved in either approach.

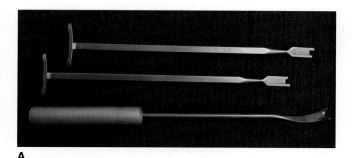

A

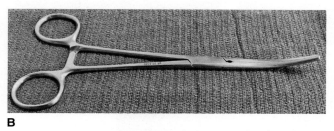

B

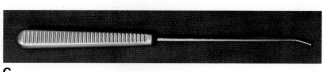

C

FIGURE 32-2

Surgical equipment used for the modified MacIntosh procedure. Meniscotomes **(A)**, large curved hemostat/clamp **(B)**, and rat-tail rasp **(C)** are used for graft harvest, passing, and tibial footprint preparation, respectively.

TECHNIQUE

In addition to standard knee arthroscopy equipment and a nonsterile thigh tourniquet, the modified MacIntosh combined extra- and intra-articular IT band ACL reconstruction is performed with minimal additional equipment, including:

- Cobb elevator
- Burr
- Periosteal elevator
- Meniscotomes (left, right, end cutting) (Fig. 32-2A)
- Large curved hemostat/clamp (Fig. 32-2B)
- "Rat-tail" rasp (Fig. 32-2C)
- Heavy nonabsorbable suture

The patient is positioned supine, and bumps can be placed under the hip and at the foot of the table to help with knee flexion if the surgeon prefers. The nonsterile pneumatic tourniquet is placed as proximal as possible on the thigh, in order to prevent compression on the IT band during graft harvest. A lateral knee arthroscopy post is used based on surgeon preference; however, we prefer a fold-down "breakaway" post that allows knee arthroscopy with the operative leg flexed to 90 degrees over the side of the table.

IT band graft harvest is performed through a 6- to 8-cm longitudinal/oblique incision, which is centered over the midportion of the iliotibial band just proximal to the lateral joint line. A Cobb elevator is utilized to elevate the subcutaneous tissue off the superficial surface of the IT band a minimum of 15 cm up the thigh. The IT band is incised first with a No. 15 scalpel near the border of the fascia of the vastus lateralis anteriorly and the posterior intermuscular septum posteriorly, leaving a few millimeters of IT band intact on both sides. Then, left- and right-angled meniscotomes are used to carry this IT band dissection proximally in line with its fibers (Fig. 32-3A). A curved end-cutting meniscotome or an open-ended tendon harvester with a mechanical end-cutting device is used to truncate the graft proximally. The graft is further freed from the lateral joint capsule using a knife or dissecting scissors but left attached to Gerdy tubercle distally (Fig. 32-3B). Finally, the

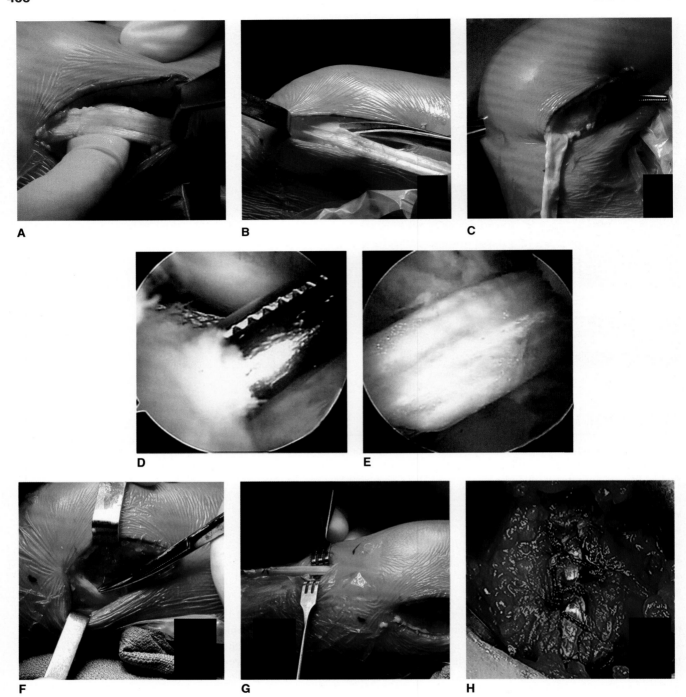

A   **B**   **C**

D   **E**

F   **G**   **H**

FIGURE 32-3

Modified MacIntosh procedure: combined extra- and intra-articular ACL reconstruction using iliotibial band autograft. Meniscotomes are used to carry this IT band dissection proximally in line with its fibers **(A)**. The graft is freed from the lateral joint capsule using a knife or dissecting scissors but left attached to Gerdy tubercle distally **(B)**. The graft is passed with the assistance of a large curved clamp **(C)**, and after tibial epiphyseal preparation with a rat-tail rasp, it is retrieved under the intermeniscal ligament **(D, E)**. In 90 degrees of relaxed flexion with neutral foot rotation, the extra-articular limb is sewn into the periosteum of the lateral femoral condyle and the intermuscular septum **(F)**. With longitudinal tension on the graft with the knee in 30 degrees of flexion with a posterior drawer force applied **(G)**, the graft is fixed to the tibia using a Mason-Allen (self-locking) stitch with three to four heavy nonreabsorbable sutures **(H)**. (Parts **A–G**, Reprinted from Kocher MS, Garg S, Micheli LJ. Physeal sparing reconstruction of the anterior cruciate ligament in skeletally immature prepubescent children and adolescents. *J Bone Joint Surg Am*. 2005;87(11):2371–2379, with permission; Part **H**, Reprinted from Fabricant PD, Kocher MS. Management of ACL injuries in children and adolescents. *J Bone Joint Surg Am*. 2017;99(7):600–612, with permission.)

graft is tubularized and whipstitched for 2 cm using a heavy nonabsorbable suture and placed back in the lateral thigh wound to prevent desiccation during the arthroscopic portion of the procedure.

A diagnostic knee arthroscopy is then performed using standard anterolateral and anteromedial portals to address any concurrent intra-articular pathology (e.g., meniscus tears). The ACL remnant is gently debrided. The intermeniscal ligament should be visualized. Intact posterolateral bundle fibers may be left in place to increase collagen mass. In order to ease graft passage, the medial portal is widened for easier clamp spreading and a minimized chance of traumatic and irregular enlargement of the portal. A small hemostat (e.g., Schnidt tonsil) is used to create a path in the over-the-top position between bone and soft tissue, leaving a sling of soft tissue to prevent graft subluxation. This tract is widened with a large curved hemostat and directed proximal to the lateral femoral condyle with bimanual palpation through the lateral graft harvest incision (Fig. 32-3C). The graft sutures are passed via the large clamp and retrieved through the joint and out the anteromedial portal, docking the graft in the over-the-top position. A longitudinal 3- to 4-cm incision is made medial to the tibial tubercle and dissected down to the level of the periosteum. This is followed by blunt dissection with a curved clamp (e.g., Schnidt tonsil) proximally along the tibia and into the knee joint (under the intermeniscal ligament) (Fig. 32-3D). The passageway is dilated by spreading the clamp in order to aid with tibial footprint preparation and graft passage. A groove in the tibial ACL footprint is created using a "rat-tail" rasp, which facilitates intra-articular healing of the graft and posteriorizes the tibial footprint to a more anatomic position that minimizes the chance of impingement in extension. Once an adequate groove is created, the clamp is reintroduced in the knee and the intra-articular sutures are brought out through the tibial incision to their final position (Fig. 32-3E).

Attention is then turned to graft fixation. The arthroscope is removed and the knee is allowed to hang in 90 degrees of relaxed flexion with neutral foot rotation, which prevents overconstraining the knee. With tension on the graft distally, the extra-articular component of the reconstruction is sewn into the periosteum of the lateral femoral condyle and the intermuscular septum (Fig. 32-3F) with at least three figure-of-8 passes of heavy nonabsorbable suture. Tibial fixation is performed in a footprint just medial to the tibial tubercle, distal to the proximal tibial physis, and proximal to the pes anserinus. The periosteum in this area is incised longitudinally and elevated medially and laterally using a periosteal elevator and then lightly decorticated using a burr. With firm tension on the graft distally (Fig. 32-3G) and with the knee in 30 degrees of flexion with a posterior drawer force applied, the graft is fixed to the tibia using a Mason-Allen (self-locking) stitch with three to four heavy non-reabsorbable sutures (Fig. 32-3H). Advancing 1 cm with each pass through graft and periosteum assists in further tensioning the graft. Portals and wounds are closed per the surgeon's preference.

PEARLS AND PITFALLS

- When placing the thigh tourniquet, it is important to apply it as proximal on the thigh as possible, so it does not interfere with graft harvest.
- During graft harvest, if end-cutting meniscotomes or an open-ended tendon harvester with a mechanical end-cutting device are not available, a small counter incision may be made proximally to detach the graft proximally.
- Radiofrequency ablation is avoided in the intercondylar notch due to the close proximity of the distal femoral physis to the over-the-top position.
- When performing tibial graft fixation, advancing 1 cm proximally in the graft from each periosteal pass assists with further graft tensioning.

POSTOPERATIVE MANAGEMENT

Postoperatively, children are typically kept overnight for a 23-hour observation period in order to ensure adequate analgesia and compliance with weight-bearing and range of motion restrictions. Patients who undergo this procedure are maintained with touchdown weight bearing (20% body weight) for 4 to 6 weeks postoperatively with range of motion limited to 0 to 30 degrees for 2 weeks followed by 0 to 90 degrees through week 6. This allows for adequate protection of the implant-free periosteal graft fixation. After 6 weeks, rehabilitation is similar to other protocols and consists of regaining full range of motion, working on closed-chain strengthening, with straight line jogging initiated 10 weeks postoperatively. Running and agility training are started at 12 weeks and progressed toward sport-specific training and jump landing. Patients are evaluated with an ACL return to play (RTP) assessment at 6 months including range of motion, strength, thigh girth, balance, and functional testing. Any identified deficits are targeted for improvement. RTP is gradual and initiated at 6 to 9 months depending on RTP assessment. Patients wear a hinged knee brace postoperatively until week 6 when quadriceps control returns, at which point they are converted to functional ACL brace for use during exercise and sports out to 2 years postoperatively. Two years after surgery, bracing becomes optional but is encouraged for these younger prepubescent patients, particularly those who compete in high-risk sports.

COMPLICATIONS

To date, there have been no reports to our knowledge of clinical or radiographic growth disturbances using this technique. The two largest series of this technique reported revision rates of 4.5% in 44 patients of mean age 10.3 years at a mean follow-up of 5.3 years (28) and 6.6% in 237 patients of mean age 11.2 years at a mean follow-up of 6.2 years (29). The latter series also reported 2.1% rate of arthrofibrosis, 0.4% rate of septic arthritis, and no limb length or angular deformities (29). Two additional smaller series reported revision rates of 14% in 21 patients of mean age 11.8 years at 3 years postoperatively (30) and 0% in 13 patients of mean age 12.2 years at 2 years of follow-up (31).

RESULTS

The iliotibial band combined extra- and intra-articular reconstruction has several advantages, including complete avoidance of the physes, improving the ease of revision surgery (no previous tunnels and all other autograft sources remain intact), and providing an additional extra-articular reconstruction limb analogous to the anterolateral ligament (28,32–34). Currently, the technique is indicated as a primary or revision ACL reconstruction for prepubescent children (Tanner stage 1–2; skeletal age ≤11 years in females and ≤12 years in males). While some opponents of this technique cite its nonanatomic configuration, biomechanics studies have shown restoration of kinematic constraint (35) and good clinical outcomes with low revision rates at a mean of 5.3 years postoperatively (28).

Outcomes after ACL reconstruction using this technique have been excellent. In a cohort of 44 patients (mean age of 10.3 years, mean follow-up of 5.3 years), the mean International Knee Documentation Committee (IKDC) subjective knee score was 96.7 ± 6.0 and the Lysholm knee score was 95.7 ± 6.7 (28). All patients except three with congenital limb anomalies returned to cutting and pivoting sports. There were no clinical or radiographic growth disturbances. These results have been maintained in the longer term as well with a subsequent study of 237 patients at an average of 6.2 years postoperatively showing Pedi-IKDC and Lysholm scores averaging 93 points each (29). Clinical success has been replicated in other series as well (30,31). Twenty-two knees at average 3-year follow-up had mean Pedi-IKDC and Lysholm scores of 96.5 and 95, respectively, with high patient satisfaction and no limb length or angular deformities (30).

REFERENCES

1. Dodwell ER, Lamont LE, Green DW, et al. 20 years of pediatric anterior cruciate ligament reconstruction in New York state. *Am J Sports Med.* 2014;42:675–680.
2. McCarroll JR, Rettig AC, Shelbourne KD. Anterior cruciate ligament injuries in the young athlete with open physes. *Am J Sports Med.* 1988;16:44–47.
3. Mizuta H, Kubota K, Shiraishi M, et al. The conservative treatment of complete tears of the anterior cruciate ligament in skeletally immature patients. *J Bone Joint Surg Br.* 1995;77:890–894.
4. Moksnes H, Engebretsen L, Risberg MA. Prevalence and incidence of new meniscus and cartilage injuries after a nonoperative treatment algorithm for ACL tears in skeletally immature children: a prospective MRI study. *Am J Sports Med.* 2013;41:1771–1779.
5. Graf BK, Lange RH, Fujisaki CK, et al. Anterior cruciate ligament tears in skeletally immature patients: Meniscal pathology at presentation and after attempted conservative treatment. *Arthroscopy.* 1992;8:229–233.
6. Aichroth PM, Patel DV, Zorrilla P. The natural history and treatment of rupture of the anterior cruciate ligament in children and adolescents. A prospective review. *J Bone Joint Surg Br.* 2002;84:38–41.
7. Kelly PM, Dimeglio A. Lower-limb growth: how predictable are predictions? *J Child Orthop.* 2008;2:407–415.
8. Fabricant PD, Lakomkin N, Cruz AI, et al. ACL reconstruction in youth athletes results in an improved rate of return to athletic activity when compared with non-operative treatment: a systematic review of the literature. *J ISAKOS.* 2016;1:62–69.
9. Fabricant PD, Lakomkin N, Cruz AI, et al. Early ACL reconstruction in children leads to less meniscal and articular cartilage damage when compared with conservative or delayed treatment. *J ISAKOS.* 2016;1:10–15.

10. Newman JT, Carry PM, Terhune EB, et al. Factors predictive of concomitant injuries among children and adolescents undergoing anterior cruciate ligament surgery. *Am J Sports Med.* 2015;43:282–288.
11. Anderson AF, Anderson CN. Correlation of meniscal and articular cartilage injuries in children and adolescents with timing of anterior cruciate ligament reconstruction. *Am J Sports Med.* 2015;43:275–281.
12. Lawrence JT, Argawal N, Ganley TJ. Degeneration of the knee joint in skeletally immature patients with a diagnosis of an anterior cruciate ligament tear: is there harm in delay of treatment? *Am J Sports Med.* 2011;39:2582–2587.
13. Dumont GD, Hogue GD, Padalecki JR, et al. Meniscal and chondral injuries associated with pediatric anterior cruciate ligament tears: relationship of treatment time and patient-specific factors. *Am J Sports Med.* 2012;40:2128–2133.
14. Kocher MS, Micheli LJ, Zurakowski D, et al. Partial tears of the anterior cruciate ligament in children and adolescents. *Am J Sports Med.* 2002;30:697–703.
15. Zerin JM, Hernandez RJ. Approach to skeletal maturation. *Hand Clin.* 1991;7:53–62.
16. Acheson RM, Fowler G, Fry EI, et al. Studies in the reliability of assessing skeletal maturity from X-rays. I. Greulich-Pyle atlas. *Hum Biol.* 1963;35:317–349.
17. Heyworth BE, Osei DA, Fabricant PD, et al. The shorthand bone age assessment: a simpler alternative to current methods. *J Pediatr Orthop.* 2013;33:569–574.
18. Dimeglio A, Charles YP, Daures JP, et al. Accuracy of the Sauvegrain method in determining skeletal age during puberty. *J Bone Joint Surg Am.* 2005;87:1689–1696.
19. Hans SD, Sanders JO, Cooperman DR. Using the Sauvegrain method to predict peak height velocity in boys and girls. *J Pediatr Orthop.* 2008;28:836–839.
20. Nicholson AD, Liu RW, Sanders JO, et al. Relationship of calcaneal and iliac apophyseal ossification to peak height velocity timing in children. *J Bone Joint Surg Am.* 2015;97:147–154.
21. Sitoula P, Verma K, Holmes L Jr, et al. Prediction of curve progression in idiopathic scoliosis: validation of the sanders skeletal maturity staging system. *Spine (Phila Pa 1976).* 2015;40:1006–1013.
22. Granados A, Gebremariam A, Lee JM. Relationship between timing of peak height velocity and pubertal staging in boys and girls. *J Clin Res Pediatr Endocrinol.* 2015;7:235–237.
23. Shifflett GD, Green DW, Widmann RF, et al. Growth arrest following ACL reconstruction with hamstring autograft in skeletally immature patients: a review of 4 cases. *J Pediatr Orthop.* 2016;36(4):355–361.
24. Fabricant PD, Jones KJ, Delos D, et al. Reconstruction of the anterior cruciate ligament in the skeletally immature athlete: a review of current concepts: AAOS exhibit selection. *J Bone Joint Surg Am.* 2013;95:e281–e313.
25. Fabricant PD, Kocher MS. Management of ACL injuries in children and adolescents. *J Bone Joint Surg Am.* 2017;99:600–612.
26. Baxter MP. Assessment of normal pediatric knee ligament laxity using the Genucom. *J Pediatr Orthop.* 1988;8:546–550.
27. Nwachukwu BU, McFeely ED, Nasreddine A, et al. Arthrofibrosis after anterior cruciate ligament reconstruction in children and adolescents. *J Pediatr Orthop.* 2011;31:811–817.
28. Kocher MS, Garg S, Micheli LJ. Physeal sparing reconstruction of the anterior cruciate ligament in skeletally immature prepubescent children and adolescents. *J Bone Joint Surg Am.* 2005;87:2371–2379.
29. Kocher MS, Heyworth BE, Fabricant PD, et al. Outcomes of physeal-sparing ACL reconstruction with iliotibial band in skeletally immature children. J Bone Joint Surg. 2018. [In Press].
30. Willimon SC, Jones CR, Herzog MM, et al. Micheli anterior cruciate ligament reconstruction in skeletally immature youths: a retrospective case series with a mean 3-year follow-up. *Am J Sports Med.* 2015;43:2974–2981.
31. Fanelli D, Hennrikus W. Pediatric ACL reconstruction with iliotibial band autograft. *J Knee Surg.* [In Press].
32. Vincent JP, Magnussen RA, Gezmez F, et al. The anterolateral ligament of the human knee: an anatomic and histologic study. *Knee Surg Sports Traumatol Arthrosc.* 2012;20:147–152.
33. Parsons EM, Gee AO, Spiekerman C, et al. The biomechanical function of the anterolateral ligament of the knee. *Am J Sports Med.* 2015;43:669–674.
34. Claes S, Vereecke E, Maes M, et al. Anatomy of the anterolateral ligament of the knee. *J Anat.* 2013;223:321–328.
35. Kennedy A, Coughlin DG, Metzger MF, et al. Biomechanical evaluation of pediatric anterior cruciate ligament reconstruction techniques. *Am J Sports Med.* 2011;39:964–971.

33 Revision ACL Reconstruction

Matthew H. Blake and Darren L. Johnson

INTRODUCTION

At the turn of the century, it was estimated that 100,000 anterior cruciate ligament reconstructions (ACLRs) were being performed in the United States every year (1). It has recently been documented that over 200,000 anterior cruciate ligament (ACL) ruptures occur each year and over 175,000 ACLRs are being performed in the same time period (2). The increased incidence of ACLRs has been theorized to be associated with the increase of female athletes participating in ACL-dependent sports, high-velocity sports, year-round sports participation without a break, as well as a larger population participating in competitive and recreational sporting activities.

Despite improved surgical techniques and rehabilitation protocols, ACLR failure rates range from 5% to 35% (3–5). Half of these failures occur within 12 months after the index procedure (6). Younger patients have a higher re-tear rate than do older individuals with patients <21 years of age having an eightfold increase in re-tear in comparison with individuals >40 years of age (7). Return to play is lower after revision ACL surgery, and studies have shown similar or higher rate of ACL tear on the contralateral side (6,8).

INDICATIONS

As with primary ACLR, indications for revision ACLR include patients with symptomatic instability or those wishing to return to ACL-dependent activities. Revision ACLR has a low probability for helping patients who have a functional ACL with continued pain. The principal purpose to perform a revision ACLR is to restore knee stability, not to relieve pain.

FACTORS

There are numerous reasons why ACLRs fail. The primary cause of failure of primary ACLR must be determined to devise a plan for revision surgery. Failures within the first 6 months of index operation are typically associated with technical error, unrecognized associated ligamentous injury, malalignment, too early return to play or biologic failure, or failure of the graft to incorporate.

Malposition of the femoral and/or tibial tunnel is the most common technical error why ACLRs fail (Fig. 33-1A and B) (9). Nonanatomic tunnel placement can result in loss of knee motion, graft impingement, and graft attenuation. A vertical femoral tunnel, as may be seen with the transtibial technique, often results in anteroposterior (AP) stability but continued rotational instability or a residual pivot shift. Hyperflexion ACL technique with an accessory medial portal can result in an anteriorly placed femoral tunnel that results in a graft that is tight in flexion and lax in extension. This will lead to either stretching of the graft or loss of knee flexion. A posteriorly placed femoral tunnel results in excessive graft tension in full extension with laxity in flexion. Anterior placement of the tibial tunnel will result in graft-notch impingement and possible loss of terminal extension while posterior placement will cause impingement on the PCL in knee flexion as well as no elimination of the pivot shift. Medial or lateral placement of the tibial tunnel may result in notch impingement and iatrogenic injury to the chondral surfaces (10).

Inadequate operative tension may contribute to graft failure. The optimal graft tension and knee position remain controversial; however, tensioning in a nonanatomic position or in flexion

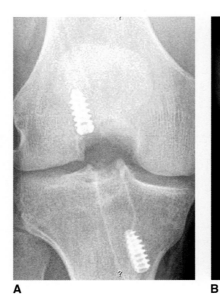
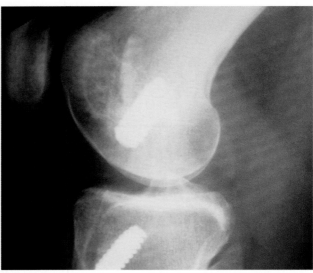

A   **B**

FIGURE 33-1

A: Vertical tunnel malposition. **B:** Anterior femoral tunnel malposition.

may constrain the knee and increase articular contact pressures. Inadequate tensioning results in a ligamentously lax knee at time zero. Loss of graft fixation prior to graft incorporation will also result in a rotational unstable knee.

Varus malalignment, increased posterior tibial slope, collateral ligament injury, and loss of menisci can place nonanatomic loads on a reconstructed ACL that can lead to premature graft failure.

Late failure with appropriately placed tunnels is often due to return to competitive activity prior to achieving adequate proprioception and strength.

PREOPERATIVE EVALUATION

History

A detailed history regarding the initial injury, associated injuries (cartilage, meniscus, and ligamentous), graft type, fixation method, and other concomitant procedures performed is necessary to evaluate the failed ACL. Prior clinical notes, imaging studies, operative report, and arthroscopic images provide information regarding changes to the knee and techniques that were implemented at the primary surgery. The patient's postoperative course, rehabilitation, return to sport, knee function, and time and mode of failure are imperative to obtain. Instability prior to return to preinjury level of function points toward a technical error at the index procedure, postoperative complication, or inadequate rehabilitation. One must ask the patients if they were ever able to return to Level 1 sports with complete confidence in their knee.

At the time of revision surgery, a surgeon must be cognizant of a variety of factors, such as the prior surgical technique performed, prior graft used, previous tunnel placement, limb alignment, tibial slope, tunnel osteolysis, and any fixation devices that may be implanted. Any of these factors can make revision ACLR more technically demanding than the index procedure. Surgical planning for revision ACLR is often guided by these factors.

Physical Examination

The patient should be initially evaluated in the standing position. In this position, the condition of the skin can be evaluated, location of prior incisions documented, and the presence of any muscle atrophy evaluated. Limb alignment with any asymmetry to the contralateral extremity is noted. The patient is allowed to ambulate to assess gait mechanics for possible varus or valgus thrust or a bent-knee gait in your office hallway.

With the patient supine on a table, the knee is evaluated for an effusion. If an effusion is present, an arthrocentesis may be performed. A hemarthrosis will indicate if a new structural injury has occurred. If there is concomitant loss of extension with instability, one must be concerned about the presence of a bucket-handle meniscal injury. An urgent MRI is required in this situation. Synovial fluid without hemarthrosis should be submitted for cell count, crystals, and culture.

We find it helpful to evaluate knee range of motion with the patient lying prone. In this position, both passive extension and active and passive knee flexion can be assessed and compared to the contralateral knee. Loss of motion may be secondary to pain and swelling from a recent traumatic event or may be chronic in nature. When diminished range of motion related to a recent traumatic event and a bucket-handle meniscal tear has been ruled out a period of physical therapy followed by a repeat physical examination is warranted before a more definitive assessment of the knee and treat plan can be formulated.

Chronic motion loss can stem from swelling in or around the joint, chronic region pain syndrome, infection, arthrofibrosis, a mechanical block (i.e., cyclops lesion, graft impingement, meniscal tear) or capturing of the knee related to nonanatomic tunnel positions. With decreased motion resulting from a prior operative procedure, particularly lack of full extension, a treatment protocol (nonsurgical and/or surgery) aimed at restoring knee motion takes precedence over performing a revision ACLR. The revision procedure can be entertained only after functional range of motion has been reestablished, particularly extension.

To evaluate the instability pattern found as a result of an incompetent ACL, the amount of anterior translation (Lachman test) and anterolateral rotatory instability (pivot-shift test) is documented. The ability to elicit a pivot shift in the office and grade its magnitude is inconsistent and variable, depending upon a multitude of factors.

Assessment for combined instabilities is critical. The PCL is examined with posterior drawer at 90 degrees; evaluation of Godfrey sign, quadriceps active test, and reverse pivot shift is performed. The collateral ligaments are evaluated with varus and valgus stress at full extension and 30 degrees of flexion. The posterior lateral and posteromedial structures are likewise evaluated with the dial test at 30 and 90 degrees of flexion, PL drawer test, PL external rotation test, and Slocum test. If there is a combined instability pattern, this should be corrected at the time of revision ACLR.

Imaging

Standing full-length AP, Rosenburg, lateral, and patellar (Merchant, sunrise, or infrapatellar) roentgenograms should be obtained. Important information can be gleaned from these films including limb and patellar alignment, degree of tibial slope, the notch sign, the size and location of prior bone tunnels, nature and location of graft fixation devices, geometry of the intercondylar notch, and the presence or absence of degenerative changes. Stress x-rays may be used to pick up subtle laxity patterns of the medial or lateral side (Fig. 33-2) (11). This is particularly important in the multiple failed ACL-deficient knee or in a chronic case.

If limb malalignment and/or increased posterior tibial slope exists, correctional osteotomy may be necessary, particularly in the twice failed ACLR. The combination of osteotomy and ACLR may be carried out as a two-stage procedure, with the osteotomy being done prior to the ligament reconstruction (12). Correction of the posterior slope to neutral will often eliminate the excessive anterior translation from ACL deficiency. If they are accomplished simultaneously, the osteotomy with fixation should be completed initially followed by creation of bone tunnels, graft passage, and finally, graft tensioning and fixation. If an osteotomy is performed due to malalignment, the normal posterior tibial slope should be decreased to aid in decreasing anterior translation (12).

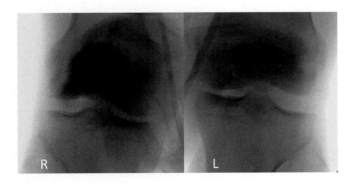

FIGURE 33-2

Positive varus stress x-ray of the left knee.

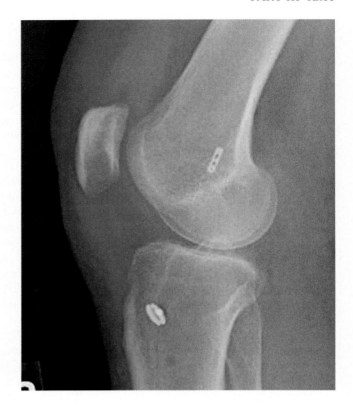

FIGURE 33-3

Appropriate tibial tunnel placement with the tibial tunnel entering the knee in the posterior third of quadrant 2.

Gross tunnel malposition can be seen on standard preoperative radiographs. The tibial tunnel should penetrate the articular surface at the midpoint of the tibial plateau on the AP view. The tunnel should also be parallel and just behind Blumensaat line with the knee in full extension entering the knee in the posterior third of quadrant 2 if the plateau is divided into four equal parts (Fig. 33-3) (13,14). AP radiographs with femoral fixation that is fixed along the anterior rather than the lateral cortex is indicative of a vertical graft. Lateral radiographs should reveal that a femoral tunnel should be seen just inferior to Blumensaat line at a position on the posterior aspect of the notch.

Graft fixation types can be visualized on x-ray, and sites of fixation must be determined. We elect to leave prior hardware in place if the fixation device does not interfere with anatomic revision tunnel placement as removal may create residual bony defects that may be problematic to fill (Fig. 33-4). If removal is necessary, many devices require specialized instruments for removal. Bone overgrowth, scar tissue, and implant migration can make hardware removal more difficult and should be assessed with an appropriate plan established prior to the day of surgery.

Computed tomography (CT) or three-dimensional CT scans can be helpful in assessing prior bone tunnel locations, tunnel expansion, or tunnel osteolysis. Tunnel osteolysis or expansion >15 mm require bone grafting followed by revision ACLR 4 to 6 months later.

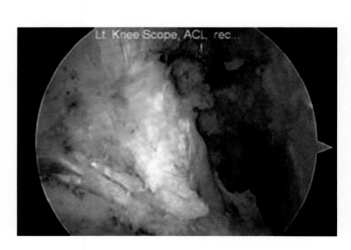

FIGURE 33-4

Retained femoral interference screw high in the notch (anterior, vertical position) after removal of residual graft tissue and minimal notch debridement. The PCL is seen in the foreground to the left.

MRI will reveal the integrity of the prior ACL graft, injury to the secondary supporting structures, the status of the menisci, and the status of the articular cartilage. Absence or near absence of the medial or lateral menisci will lead the surgeon to the consideration of a concomitant meniscal allograft reconstruction as well as revision ACL surgery. This information is critical to allow appropriate counseling of the patient to create honest objective goals of the operation. This information assists the surgeon in planning for any concomitant procedures that may be performed in conjunction with the revision ACLR. Assessment of bone bruise patterns may also provide insight into injury mechanisms. Metal implants may cause artifact and decreases the sensitivity and specificity of MRI to identify these structures.

Staging

Revision ACLR may need to be staged. Motion loss, tunnel lysis, malalignment, increased tibial slope, and other concomitant knee pathology may be best treated by a staged procedure.

Range of motion of the operative knee should be similar to that of the contralateral knee prior to revision ACLR. Motion loss, particularly in extension, will cause functional limitations after revision ACLR (15). When physical therapy, splinting, and pharmacotherapy fail to regain flexion or extension, a staged manipulation under anesthesia and arthroscopic lysis of adhesions, combined with an arthroscopic posteromedial capsular release, may be performed to regain motion (16). Postoperatively an aggressive rehabilitation program must be implemented to prevent motion loss (17).

Bone grafting of the femoral and tibial tunnels should be performed when prior tunnel placement prohibits anatomic new tunnel placement and/or when tunnel osteolysis (>15 mm) prevents secure fixation and biologic healing of the revision ACL (Fig. 33-5) (18). Initially, all prior hardware is removed. A guidewire is placed into the prior femoral and tibial tunnels. Sequential drilling is performed to remove all prior soft tissue graft. An arthroscope and shaver can also be used to remove soft tissue from the tunnels. Visual confirmation of cleaned tunnels is performed using the arthroscope (Fig. 33-6). A femoral head allograft can be used to create appropriately sized bone graft plugs. Likewise, Cloward plugs can also be utilized (Fig. 33-7). The bone graft is press fit and impacted into the cleaned tunnels (Fig. 33-8). X-rays should be performed at 4 months to verify that bone integration has occurred prior to the revision surgery (19).

Coronal and sagittal plane alignment should be evaluated prior to performing revision ACLR. A normal posterior tibial slope is 7 to 9 degrees (20). When compared to uninjured controls, females and males both had increased lateral tibial slope (21). Normalizing the posterior tibial slope decreases anterior tibial translation and thus decreases the stresses to the reconstructed ACL (Fig. 33-9) (22). Similarly, Noyes et al. advocated high tibial osteotomy to correct coronal malalignment prior to performing revision ACLR to help preserve the ACL and articular surface (23).

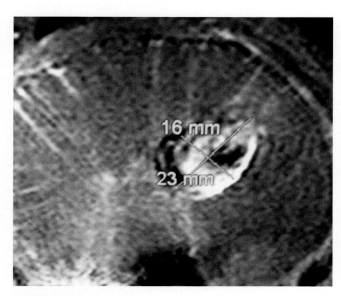

FIGURE 33-5
Tibial tunnel osteolysis measuring 23 mm x 16 mm.

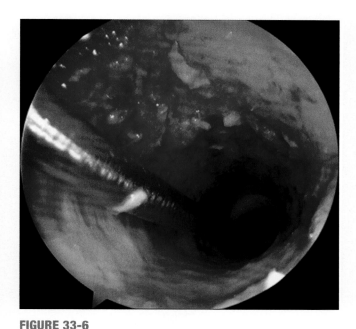

FIGURE 33-6
Arthroscopic visualization of the tibial tunnel that has been reamed and all soft tissue excised.

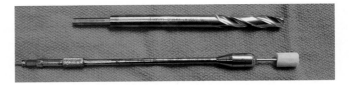

FIGURE 33-7

Cloward bone plug that is sized equal to last reamer used. The Cloward bone plug is placed on K-wire, and a cannulated impactor is used for placement and impaction of the bone graft.

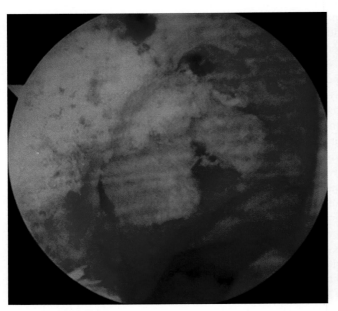
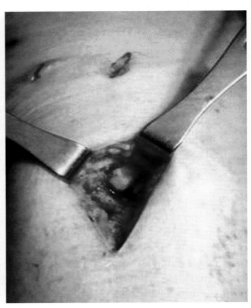

FIGURE 33-8

Press-fit bone in the femoral and tibial tunnels, respectively.

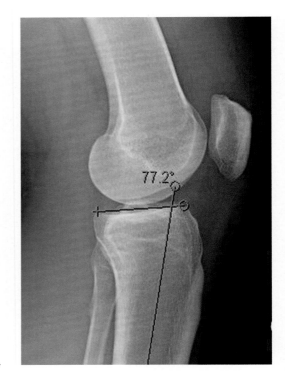

FIGURE 33-9

Posterior tibial slope is the angle formed at the intersection of a line parallel to the posterior tibial inclination and a line that bisects the shaft of the tibia.

Depending on the skill set of the surgeon and available intraoperative assistance, a surgeon may wish to treat concomitant knee pathology such as combined ligament reconstruction, cartilage restoration, and meniscus transplantation in a staged manner.

Surgery

A surgeon must be able to employ a variety of techniques to obtain appropriate tunnel placement, deal with tunnel expansion and prior placed hardware, treat meniscal injury, chondral damage, and malalignment, as well as handle concomitant ligament injuries so that a stable functional knee can be obtained.

A general anesthesia with block is used for all procedures. Preoperative IV antibiotics are administered. A padded pneumatic tourniquet is applied at the proximal thigh. A detailed examination under anesthesia is performed and compared to the contralateral "normal" knee. Range of motion and laxity patterns are assessed. In the anesthetized state, knee guarding does not occur, and the quality of endpoints with degree of translation is often increased than what was found during examination in the office setting. If there is concomitant ligamentous laxity that was not recognized prior to surgery, this should also be addressed as repeat failure of the reconstructed ACL will likely result. When there is a combined pattern of ligamentous laxity options for reconstruction include stating the surgical procedures with the secondary restrains addressed initially followed by lateral ACLR or reconstruction of all pathologic laxity through simultaneous surgical correction.

Patient Positioning

The patient is placed supine on the operating table in a hemi-lithotomy position. A tourniquet is placed high on the operative thigh and then placed into an arthroscopic leg holder which is secured to the surgical table at the break point of the bed. The nonoperative extremity is placed in a lithotomy position with the leg resting upon a well-padded support in approximately 90 degrees of hip and knee flexion with hip abduction and external rotation. The foot of the bed is then removed or maximally flexed. This position allows the surgeon and assistant an unobstructed access to the whole knee should any accessory procedures (PCL, PLC, MCL, or inside-out meniscal repair) be necessary. We angle the bed so that the femur is perpendicular to the floor with the knee flexed to 90 degrees (Fig. 33-10).

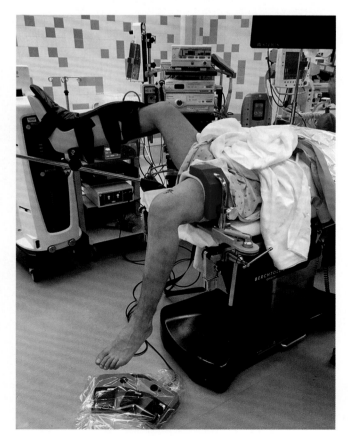

FIGURE 33-10

Patient positioning for a revision ACL reconstruction.

Arthroscopy

After sterile preparation and draping of the operative extremity, prior incisions are marked. The leg is exsanguinated and the tourniquet inflated.

The importance of appropriately placed arthroscopic portals cannot be overemphasized. We create new portals if the previous portals are not in the correct location. Poorly positioned portals block adequate visualization and compromise the use of instrumentation during the procedure. We utilize three anterior portals for visualization and instrumentation during all revision and primary ACLRs. The portals are created with an 11-blade with the knee in a 90-degree flexed position after spinal needle localization (Fig. 33-11).

The anterior lateral portal is established 5 mm proximal to the distal pole of the patella and adjacent to the patella. This position will typically avoid the fat pad, allow access to all three compartments of the knee, and allow for a bird's-eye view of the anterior horn of the lateral meniscus and the tibial ACL footprint.

The anterior medial portal is localized with a spinal needle and established directly adjacent to the medial border of the patellar tendon in line with the ACL and superior to the medial meniscus. This is used as both a working portal and a viewing portal. When visualizing through this portal (femoral tunnel work), the surgeon is provided an unobstructed view of the entire lateral intercondylar wall, posterior aspect of the notch, and ACL attachment on the femur.

The accessory medial portal is then established 2 cm medial to the anteromedial portal just above the anterior horn of the medial meniscus. This portal is utilized as a working portal (Fig. 33-12).

An additional superomedial or superolateral portal for inflow or outflow may be employed based upon surgeon preference.

Following creation of the standard arthroscopic portals, a systematic diagnostic assessment of the knee is performed. Any chondral or meniscal abnormalities are identified and addressed. Attention

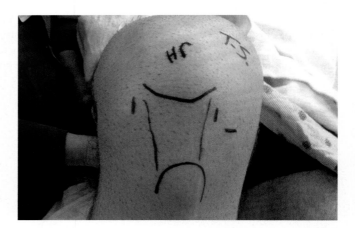

FIGURE 33-11

From left to right: the anterolateral, central medial, and accessory medial portals are drawn on the skin of this right knee. A prior ACL reconstruction scar is visible along the medial border of the patellar tendon.

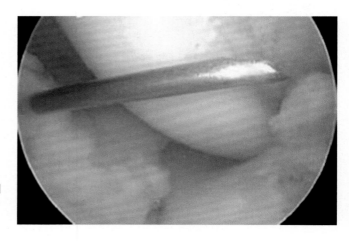

FIGURE 33-12

Arthroscopic view from anterolateral portal looking medially, showing a spinal needle localizing the position of the accessory AM portal.

is then focused upon the revision ACLR. All remaining ACL graft material is resected. Identifying and visualizing the over-the-top position in the posterior aspect of the notch is critical. To appropriately identify this region, we visualize through the anteromedial portal and use the shaver in the accessory medial portal. The intra-articular locations of the prior bone tunnels and the fixation hardware are sought. A methodical debridement is performed so as to minimize bone removal or distortion of anatomy.

A notchplasty may be performed for improved visualization from the anterolateral portal; this is not necessary when viewing from the anteromedial portal. Osteophytes or notch overgrowth should be resected. These occur at the anterior aspect of the notch. The surgeon should avoid removal of bone posterior to the aperture of the intercondylar notch so as not to lateralize the position of the femoral tunnel, changing the normal length of the ACL.

Tunnel Placement

The most important technical aspect of revision ACL surgery is the location and creation of anatomic bone tunnels. In revision ACL surgery, the patient's native anatomy has often been distorted or removed. By clarifying the positions of the previously placed bone tunnels and having knowledge of ACL insertion site anatomy the surgeon is able to begin the process of establishing new tunnels for the revision reconstruction. Our approach to a revision surgery applies the same anatomic concepts that are employed during a primary ACLR. The characteristics and positions of the prior tunnels will dictate the specifics of our surgical technique.

We initially address the femoral tunnel and subsequently proceed with creation of the tibial tunnel. The femoral tunnel size will dictate the dimension of the tibia tunnel. Prior to creating new bone tunnels, a thorough assessment of the patient's intercondylar anatomy as well as prior tunnel locations and characteristics is performed. Evaluating the tibial anatomy prior to drilling the femoral tunnel is necessary to assure that there are no specific findings present that may prohibit or impact the ability to perform anatomic reconstruction.

Comfort and familiarity with multiple techniques for creation of the femoral tunnel is recommended. Possessing these skills will arm the surgeon with the means by which to address the planned as well as unplanned details that may arise during the procedure. We have found that using an outside-in technique or two-incision technique for creation of the femoral tunnel allows for increased precision and accuracy at obtaining the appropriate tunnel placement as well as greater freedom in selecting a starting point. The revision ACL surgeon, however, must be comfortable with transtibial, medial portal, two-incision outside-in, and over-the-top femoral-sided techniques.

Our current experience has found that the vast majority of revisions are done with the index procedure having been accomplished via a transtibial drilling technique with a vertical graft or utilizing an accessory medial portal with an anterior graft. When this situation is encountered, we proceed with creation of the femoral tunnel in a manner identical to that used for a primary anatomic ACLR.

The knee is held at 90 degrees of flexion, and the outside-in drill guide is brought through the anterolateral portal and placed on the anatomic location of the ACL femoral footprint on the lateral intercondylar wall with 2 mm of posterior wall remaining (Fig. 33-13). Visualization of the lateral condylar wall is performed through the anteromedial portal. A guide pin is advanced into the knee. If the pin is not in appropriate location then a second pin is advanced utilizing a parallel pin guide. Once the pin is in appropriate position, the pin is grasped with a pituitary rongeur through the accessory medial portal. Sequential reaming from outside-in commences to the desired tunnel diameter while adjustments of the tunnel position is performed utilizing the pituitary rongeur.

If concern exist that creation of the new femoral tunnel will extend into a portion of the previous tunnel and thereby compromise the integrity of the new tunnel, the surgeon has several options. The first option would be to utilize the anatomic starting point but drill the new tunnel divergent from the old tunnel. The two tunnels may have a small area of coalescence at their origin but diverge from one another more proximally, thereby maintaining integrity of the new tunnel over the majority of its length. When this situation arises, use of suspensory fixation or fixation distant from the tunnel entrance into the knee would be recommended. A second option would be to place the graft in the over-the-top position. This is also an excellent option when during the course of drilling the posterior cortical integrity is compromised. The final option would be to bone graft the prior femoral tunnels and stage the reconstruction.

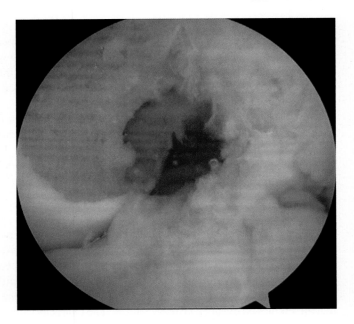

FIGURE 33-13

Notch view from the medial portal of the femoral tunnel with 2 mm of posterior wall remaining.

The size, characteristics (prior soft tissue graft vs. bone plug, type of previous fixation device), and location of the previous tibial tunnel will dictate the options available for creation of the revision tibial tunnel. Options include creation of a new tunnel, use of the prior tunnel, or bone grafting the prior tunnel and stage the reconstruction. The preoperative assessment will often alert the surgeon the presence of this latter possibility. However, it may arise expectantly based upon intraoperative findings, and this potential option should be discussed with the patient prior to surgery.

The knee is held at 90 degrees of flexion, and the arthroscope is placed in the anterolateral portal with the viewfinder looking down at the anterior horn of the lateral meniscus and the ACL footprint on the tibia. To initiate establishment of the tibial tunnel, a commercially available guide is employed for placement of the guide wire (Fig. 33-14). The proximal arm of the guide is positioned through the accessory medial portal and the guide set at 55 to 60 degrees. The guide tip is placed within the center of the ACL footprint on the tibia medial to the anterior horn of the lateral meniscus and just lateral to the medial tibial eminence. If desired, a lateral fluoroscopic image with the knee in full extension can be obtained to confirm anatomic tunnel placement. The guide pin is advanced and docked into the femoral notch. Sequential reaming commences to the desired tunnel diameter while adjustments of the tunnel position can be performed in-between reaming by moving the guide pin.

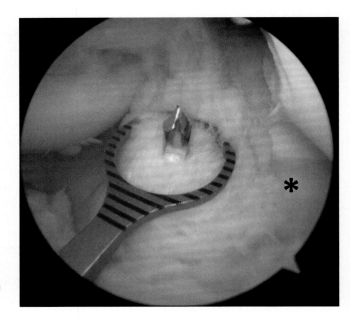

FIGURE 33-14

The posterior edge of the anterior horn of the lateral meniscus (*) is utilized to determine the position of the guide wire for the tibial tunnel.

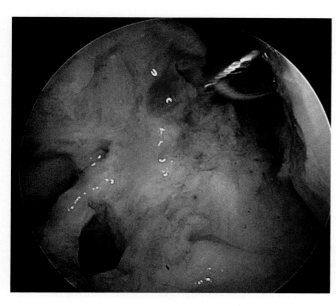

FIGURE 33-15

A passing suture entering the knee from the femoral tunnel. This will be grasped through the tibial tunnel for passing the graft through the tibial tunnel and into the femoral tunnel.

If the previous tibial tunnel is utilized then the prior graft should be reamed out to assure exposed bone throughout the circumference of the tunnel.

After the tunnels have been created, a passing suture is placed from outside-in through the femoral tunnel and into the notch. The suture is then grasped through the anteromedial portal and brought to the tibial tunnel and then pulled through the tibial tunnel (Fig. 33-15).

Graft Selection/Graft Preparation

The choice of potential graft material for a revision ACLR includes autograft of allograft tissue. A variety of factors play a role in selecting the specific type of graft to be utilized for a particular revision ACLR. These include, but are not limited to, the type of prior graft, amount and size of the revision graft needed, patient and surgeon preference, as well as cost. Autograft tissue can be obtained from either the ipsilateral or the contralateral knee. Graft options include bone-patellar tendon bone, hamstring tendon, and quadriceps tendon with or without attached patellar bone plug. The advantages of autograft tissue include lack of potential disease transmission, lack of additional cost, lower failure rate, and improved healing potential within bone tunnels. Disadvantages consist of increased operative time, potential graft harvest site morbidity, limitation of graft size, in addition to the possibility of limited graft choice based upon prior graft harvest.

The advantages and disadvantages surrounding the use of allograft tissue are reciprocal to those involving use of an autograft. Allograft tissue may have prolonged incorporation time in bone tunnels and higher failure rate; does carry the possibility of disease transmission; and has an associated cost. At the same time, use of allograft tissue has no associated harvest site morbidity, does not have a limited supply, and can be customized with respect to graft size and type. Achilles tendon–calcaneus and bone-patellar-tendon bone are the most common allograft tissues that are utilized; semitendinosus and anterior tibialis all soft tissue grafts are also frequently employed but not recommended.

When available and appropriate based upon preoperative preparation, we prefer the use of autograft tissue. We recommend at least an 8-mm-diameter graft size. If anatomy permits, a bone–patellar tendon–bone autograft is utilized; this is particularly true if the failed primary reconstruction was done with allograft or hamstring autograft. Bone plugs can be created to accommodate tunnel lysis of 12 mm.

Hamstring tendon size is quite unpredictable prior to its harvest. Graft thickness can be achieved by creating a three-stranded semitendinosus and double gracilis graft, quad-stranded semitendinosus graft with or without gracilis augmentation, or a double-stranded semitendinosus and gracilis graft with an additional hamstring allograft.

Even when the presurgical plan is for use of only autogenous tissue, the surgeon must discuss with the patient the possibility of allograft utilization. The need for allograft tissue may occur because of intraoperative anatomic findings or unforeseen circumstances that arise during the procedure precluding the graft tissue comprised solely of autogenous origin. When such a scenario is encountered, a hybrid reconstruction should be considered (autograft + allograft) if at all possible. The hybrid graft is created by first folding the allograft over an EndoButton (Smith & Nephew Endoscopy, Andover, MA), and then the other hamstring tendons are folded over the EndoButton and sutured together so that the allograft tissue is covered by and central to the autograft hamstrings.

Each case is inherently unique and requires thoughtful discussion between surgeon and patient regarding the multitude of possible graft options and why plans may need to be altered in order to optimize outcome.

Graft Fixation

The graft is placed in mineral oil for easier passage of the graft. The sutures from the graft are pulled up the tibial tunnel and out the femoral tunnel using the passing suture. With the knee stabilized, the graft is pulled into the notch. A hemostat or probe can be used as a pulley to guide the graft into the femoral tunnel. The hemostat can also aid in turning the femoral bone block to enter the femoral tunnel.

We typically employ suspensory fixation with the use of a 10-mm EndoButton with ExtendoButton for fixation of hamstring grafts. This is a soft tissue graft, and fixation outside of the tunnel will allow maximal tendon-to-bone contact through the entire circumference of the tunnel, an important variable for optimizing graft incorporation. If bone-patellar tendon-bone graft is used, then the bone plug is pulled flush with the lateral femoral cortex; a nitinol wire and an interference screw are placed. If there is any concern regarding the integrity of the posterior wall, the femoral graft sutures can be tied around a bicortical screw and washer placed across the distal femur through the lateral incision.

The graft is then pretensioned by taking the knee through 25 repetitions of full motion while holding the tibial sutures taut. This maneuver will also permit a relative check of femoral fixation stability. The arthroscope is introduced into the knee, and the graft is assessed while taking the knee through a full arc of motion. If there is graft impingement in the notch, a careful notchplasty can be performed. Any adjustments deemed necessary can be made at this time, prior to committing to final graft fixation. There should be minimal graft length changes when taking the knee through a complete range of motion. Graft length changes >5 mm should alert you that one of your tunnels may not be anatomic.

Tibial fixation is the final step in the procedure. The knee is held in 30 degrees of flexion, external rotation, with a posterior drawer force placed. If performing a bone patellar tendon bone graft another interference metal screw is placed. Because early fixation compromise or graft slippage usually occurs on the tibial side, we routinely utilize both primary and back up tibia fixation. If a hamstring graft is placed a bioabsorbable screw is placed and the graft is backed up with a screw and washer.

Following completion of the fixation process, knee range of motion is assessed to assure that no impediment to either full flexion or extension is present. The arthroscope is reintroduced into the knee and a final inspection of the graft is undertaken. The graft is probed to assure stability and appropriate tension in varying degrees of knee flexion.

Closure

If BPTB graft has been harvested, the excess bone reamings and bone from the harvested graft is replaced in the patellar defect first then the tibial defect. The periosteum is closed over the grafted sites. All portal incisions are closed with skin sutures. Incisions utilized for graft harvest or tunnel placement are closed in layers. A well-padded sterile dressing and a cold therapy unit are applied to the operative extremity. The leg is wrapped from the groin to the toes with an ACE bandage followed by application of a postoperative double upright brace, locked in full extension.

Pearls and Pitfalls

- Expect the unexpected; challenges will frequently arise. The ability to accept and compensate for the unforeseen is often necessary, even in the face of optimal presurgical preparation.
- Identify the likely contributing cause(s) of prior graft failure and use that information to avoid the same errors during the revision procedure.
- Patient positioning is the initial prerequisite component to a technically successful revision ACLR.
- Assure necessary equipment availability for both planned and unplanned intraoperative findings and occurrences.

- Proper arthroscopic portal placement cannot be overemphasized.
- Knowledge and comfort with several techniques for creation of femoral tunnels (i.e., accessory medial portal with hyperflexion; the use of a rear-entry guide; the use of the over-the-top graft position) can be invaluable and will allow the revision surgeon an array of means by which to deal with patient-specific anatomy and obstacles presented as a result of the prior surgical procedure(s).
- Bone grafting a tunnel from the previous surgery and staging the revision reconstruction is preferable to accepting less than optimal anatomic tunnel positioning as a consequence of the anatomic alterations created from prior bone tunnel positions and/or osteolysis. Anatomic tunnel placement is critically important to overall outcome.
- Primary and supplemental tibial-sided graft fixation is recommended for soft tissue grafts or other situations where impaired graft fixation is present.
- Intraoperative fluoroscopic images can be beneficial for confirming positions of bone tunnels whether or not uncertainty exists.
- An overly accelerated and aggressive rehabilitation protocol is not appropriate following a revision ACLR.
- Failure to identify and address laxity of the static secondary restraints will commonly lead to suboptimal restoration of knee stability and probable compromise or failure of the revision ACL graft.

Postoperative Management

The historical development and promotion of an accelerated rehabilitation program following primary ACLR allowed for improved functional outcomes while diminishing associated complications resulting from prolonged immobilization and a delay in initiation of strengthening exercises. Until biologic incorporation of the graft into host bone occurs, graft fixation must be capable of withstanding normal cyclical forces during rehabilitation without graft slippage or pullout occurring (24). Animal studies have provided timelines with respect to graft incorporation, healing, and remodeling following an ACLR (25–27) and have served as guidelines for structuring the early phases of postsurgical rehabilitation protocols; knowledge of the native ACL strain behavior during various exercises has been of additional benefit in guiding development of these protocols (28).

Two concerns have led to our use of a less aggressive, more prolonged rehabilitation protocol following a revision ACLR. First, we believe the revision patient may provide a "compromised" host environment, and as such, the biology of graft healing/incorporation could be impaired and lengthier relative to a primary ACLR. In addition, although graft revascularization may be complete at 6 months, further remodeling and development of increased tensile strength continues up until 12 months following placement of an intra-articular graft (26,27). It is our belief that an overly accelerated rehabilitation protocol, even in its latter phases, may have as a consequence, a negative impact upon graft maturation; the functional implications could be detrimental, particularly to the patient who strives to return to participation in ACL-dependent sporting activities. Principles outlined in a postsurgical rehabilitation protocol developed for patients recovering from a primary ACLR serve as a template to which we adhere following a revision procedure (29). In our revision patients, the timeline of progression through the protocol is, however, slower. When concomitant secondary procedures have been performed, adapting certain aspects of the rehabilitation protocol accordingly may be necessary.

Following an isolated revision ACLR, the surgical extremity is protected with a postoperative long leg hinged brace for 8 weeks. The patient is permitted crutch-assisted weight bearing as tolerated with the brace locked in full extension for the initial 4 weeks and unlocked during ambulation for an additional 4 weeks. The patient is encouraged to remove the brace whenever in a non–weight-bearing position and highly encouraged to move the knee as well as perform manual patellar mobility exercises.

The brace may be unlocked for range of motion exercises (i.e., continuous passive motion [CPM], seated knee flexion, heel slides) immediately following surgery. Early restoration of symmetric knee extension is of primary importance. This must occur within the first 2 weeks. Swelling is controlled through cold therapy, use of a compression stocking, and limitation of prolonged weight-bearing activity. During the period of protected weight bearing, physical therapy exercises are focused on achieving full range of motion, improving patellar mobilization while also initiating quadriceps isometric and closed kinetic chain strengthening. If available, aquatherapy can be utilized after the surgical incisions have healed. When in a pool, brace-free gait mechanics can be employed. As gait mechanics normalize and quadriceps strength improves, proprioception training and resistive exercises of increased intensity are begun. Initiation of plyometric exercises, introduction of running, and progression to functional training exercises are all delayed relative to a primary ACLR. The patient is fit with a functional knee brace prior to beginning his or her functional training regimen. A return to unrestricted activity, including sports, is typically delayed until 9 to 12 months following surgery.

Complications

Complications and untoward outcomes do not differ inherently from those that may be seen following a primary ACLR. There is nothing intrinsic to the revision procedure itself, which creates or exposes the patient to specific defined risks or potential complications not seen in the setting of a primary reconstruction. Infection, deep vein thrombosis, neurovascular compromise, risks associated with the use of allograft tissue, loss of motion, persistent effusion, failure of graft incorporation, loss of graft fixation, recurrent development of graft laxity or instability, progressive degenerative changes, etc., all may occur following a revision ACLR and warrant appropriate discussion with the patient as part of the standard preoperative dialogue and consent process.

Results

While results of revision ACLR are generally inferior to those of primary ACLR, results can provide for a gratifying outcome to both patient and surgeon. It has been reported that anywhere between 57% and 90% of patients undergoing revision ACL reconstructive surgery return to their preinjury level of function (30–32). The failure rate of revision ACLR has been documented to be between 4% and 13% at 2-year follow-up (3,33).

The necessary elements to achieve a positive result include the implementation of proper preoperative planning followed by critical attention to technical details during performance of the surgery. Specific presurgical consultation with the patient regarding motivation, expectations, and compliance with rehabilitation is another critical component of the presurgical preparation serving to maximize potential outcomes.

REFERENCES

1. Brown CH Jr, Carson EW, Revision anterior cruciate ligament surgery. *Clin Sports Med.* 1999;18(1):109–171.
2. Bogunovic L, Yang JS, Wright RW. Anterior cruciate ligament reconstruction: contemporary revision options. *Oper Tech Sports Med.* 2013;21(1):64–71.
3. Spindler KP, et al. Anterior cruciate ligament reconstruction autograft choice: bone-tendon-bone versus hamstring: does it really matter? A systematic review. *Am J Sports Med.* 2004;32(8):1986–1995.
4. Wright RW, et al. Risk of tearing the intact anterior cruciate ligament in the contralateral knee and rupturing the anterior cruciate ligament graft during the first 2 years after anterior cruciate ligament reconstruction: a prospective MOON cohort study. *Am J Sports Med.* 2007;35(7):1131–1134.
5. Azar FM. Revision anterior cruciate ligament reconstruction. *Instr Course Lect.* 2002;51:335–342.
6. Webster KE, et al. Younger patients are at increased risk for graft rupture and contralateral injury after anterior cruciate ligament reconstruction. *Am J Sports Med.* 2014;42(3):641–647.
7. Maletis GB, et al. Age-related risk factors for revision anterior cruciate ligament reconstruction: a cohort study of 21,304 patients from the Kaiser Permanente Anterior Cruciate Ligament Registry. *Am J Sports Med.* 2016;44(2):331–336.
8. Wright RW, et al. Ipsilateral graft and contralateral ACL rupture at five years or more following ACL reconstruction: a systematic review. *J Bone Joint Surg Am.* 2011;93(12):1159–1165.
9. Greis PE, Johnson DL, Fu FH. Revision anterior cruciate ligament surgery: causes of graft failure and technical considerations of revision surgery. *Clin Sports Med.* 1993;12(4):839–852.
10. Liechti DJ, et al. Outcomes and risk factors of rerevision anterior cruciate ligament reconstruction: a systematic review. *Arthroscopy.* 2016;32(10):2151–2159.
11. James EW, Williams BT, LaPrade RF. Stress radiography for the diagnosis of knee ligament injuries: a systematic review. *Clin Orthop Relat Res.* 2014;472(9):2644–2657.
12. Dejour D, et al. Tibial slope correction combined with second revision ACL produces good knee stability and prevents graft rupture. *Knee Surg Sports Traumatol Arthrosc.* 2015;23(10):2846–2852.
13. Howell SM, Clark JA. Tibial tunnel placement in anterior cruciate ligament reconstructions and graft impingement. *Clin Orthop Relat Res.* 1992;(283):187–195.
14. Harner CD, et al. Anterior cruciate ligament reconstruction: endoscopic versus two-incision technique. *Arthroscopy.* 1994;10(5):502–512.
15. Shelbourne KD, et al. Arthrofibrosis in acute anterior cruciate ligament reconstruction. The effect of timing of reconstruction and rehabilitation. *Am J Sports Med.* 1991;19(4):332–336.
16. LaPrade RF, Pedtke AC, Roethle ST. Arthroscopic posteromedial capsular release for knee flexion contractures. *Knee Surg Sports Traumatol Arthrosc.* 2008;16(5):469–475.
17. Shelbourne KD, Klootwyk TE, Decarlo MS. Update on accelerated rehabilitation after anterior cruciate ligament reconstruction. *J Orthop Sports Phys Ther.* 1992;15(6):303–308.
18. Thomas NP, et al. Revision anterior cruciate ligament reconstruction using a 2-stage technique with bone grafting of the tibial tunnel. *Am J Sports Med.* 2005;33(11):1701–1709.

19. Franceschi F, et al. Two-stage procedure in anterior cruciate ligament revision surgery: a five-year follow-up prospective study. *Int Orthop.* 2013;37(7):1369–1374.
20. Giffin JR, et al. Importance of tibial slope for stability of the posterior cruciate ligament deficient knee. *Am J Sports Med.* 2007;35(9):1443–1449.
21. Todd MS, et al. The relationship between posterior tibial slope and anterior cruciate ligament injuries. *Am J Sports Med.* 2010;38(1):63–67.
22. Marouane H, et al. Steeper posterior tibial slope markedly increases ACL force in both active gait and passive knee joint under compression. *J Biomech.* 2014;47(6):1353–1359.
23. Noyes FR, Barber-Westin SD, Hewett TE. High tibial osteotomy and ligament reconstruction for varus angulated anterior cruciate ligament-deficient knees. *Am J Sports Med.* 2000;28(3):282–296.
24. Kurosaka M, Yoshiya S, Andrish JT. A biomechanical comparison of different surgical techniques of graft fixation in anterior cruciate ligament reconstruction. *Am J Sports Med.* 1987;15(3):225–229.
25. Rodeo SA, et al. Tendon-healing in a bone tunnel. A biomechanical and histological study in the dog. *J Bone Joint Surg Am.* 1993;75(12):1795–1803.
26. Arnoczky SP. Biology of ACL reconstructions: what happens to the graft? *Instr Course Lect.* 1996;45:229–233.
27. Clancy WG Jr, Smith L. Arthroscopic anterior and posterior cruciate ligament reconstruction technique. *Ann Chir Gynaecol.* 1991;80(2):141–148.
28. Beynnon BD, et al. Anterior cruciate ligament strain behavior during rehabilitation exercises in vivo. *Am J Sports Med.* 1995;23(1):24–34.
29. Irrgang JJ. Follow-up to the clinical and cost-effectiveness of two different programs for rehabilitation following ACL reconstruction. *J Orthop Sports Phys Ther.* 1997;26(1):39–40; author reply 40-6.
30. Garofalo R, Djahangiri A, Siegrist O. Revision anterior cruciate ligament reconstruction with quadriceps tendon-patellar bone autograft. *Arthroscopy.* 2006;22(2):205–214.
31. Battaglia MJ II, et al. Results of revision anterior cruciate ligament surgery. *Am J Sports Med.* 2007;35(12):2057–2066.
32. Noyes FR, Barber-Westin SD. Revision anterior cruciate ligament reconstruction using a 2-stage technique with bone grafting of the tibial tunnel. *Am J Sports Med.* 2006;34(4):678–679; author reply 679-80.
33. Wright RW, et al. Outcome of revision anterior cruciate ligament reconstruction: a systematic review. *J Bone Joint Surg Am.* 2012;94(6):531–536.

SUGGESTED READINGS

George MS, Dunn WR, Spindler KP. Current concepts review: revision anterior cruciate ligament reconstruction. *Am J Sports Med.* 2006;34:2026–2037.
Johnson DL, Fu FH. Anterior cruciate ligament reconstruction: why do failures occur? In: Jackson DW, ed. *Instructional Course Lectures,* vol. 44. Rosemont, IL: American Academy of Orthopaedic Surgeons; 1995:391–406.
Lubowitz JH, Bernardini BJ, Reid JB. Current concepts review: comprehensive physical examination for instability of the knee. *Am J Sports Med.* 2008;36:577–594.
Shen W, Forsythe B, Ingham SM, et al. Application of the anatomic double-bundle reconstruction concept to revision and augmentation anterior cruciate ligament surgeries. *J Bone Joint Surg.* 2008;90:20–34.
Steiner ME, Murray MM, Rodeo SA. Strategies to improve anterior cruciate ligament healing and graft placement. *Am J Sports Med.* 2008;36:176–189.

34 The Anterolateral Ligament

Thierry Pauyo, Marcio B. V. Albers, Jeremy M. Burnham, and Freddie H. Fu

INTRODUCTION

In the recent literature, there is a renewed interest in the anatomy of the anterolateral structures of the knee (1,2). More precisely, there exists a debate regarding the existence of the anterolateral ligament (ALL) and its role in knee rotational and dynamic stability. The controversy regarding the anatomy and function of the ALL has been well studied in anatomic, biomechanical, histologic, and radiologic studies (3,4). Anatomic studies have not consistently found a distinct ALL in the lateral capsule sheet of the knee. In an anatomical study of fetuses 18 to 22 weeks, Sabzevari et al. could not distinguish any ALL in the capsule (5,6). Furthermore, histologic and radiologic evaluation performed by Dombrowski et al. demonstrated that only 30 % of specimen had a capsular thickening with histology not consistent with ligament properties (7).

Biomechanical and robotic studies of the anterolateral complex of the knee found that the iliotibial band was three times stiffer than the anterolateral capsule and that the ALL had five times less load to failure compared to other ligaments (4,5). Furthermore, Spencer et al. demonstrated that reconstruction of the ALL did not restore pathologic rotational laxity (8). While at the current time isolated reconstruction of the ALL is not recommended, there are some instances where it could potentially provide supplemental knee stability. There are cases of anterior cruciate ligament (ACL) reconstruction with residual pathologic laxity and increased pivot shift that can be attributed to the damage of the lateral extra-articular soft tissue structures (9,10).

INDICATIONS/CONTRAINDICATIONS

Currently, there are no high evidence studies in the literature supporting the reconstruction of the ALL or the anterolateral structures of the knee. There are still, however, some situations where the reconstruction of the anterolateral complex of the knee can be performed with an extra-articular tenodesis. We believe that extra-articular tenodesis of the anterolateral structures of the knee can be warranted in cases of ACL reconstruction failures where all other causes of pathologic laxity have been excluded. For instance, ACL revision in a patient with Grade 3 pivot shift with no other etiologies of failure poses an adequate indication for extra-articular tenodesis.

It is important to stress that while the extra-articular tenodesis of the anterolateral capsule of the knee can, in theory, provide increased rotational stability, some studies have found that it may over-constrain the knee (11).

A thorough evaluation of the cause of instability of the knee must be completed prior to performing an anterolateral complex stabilizing procedure. Patient with lower extremity malalignment or increased tibial slope must have their bone morphology corrected with osteotomies prior to considering ALL surgery. Furthermore, patients with advance arthritis and impaired lower extremity neurologic function are not appropriate candidates for ALL surgery.

PREOPERATIVE PREPARATION

A thorough preoperative evaluation of the knee is paramount in determining the necessity to perform an ALL reconstruction. There is often a concomitant ipsilateral knee ACL intra-articular pathology that should be identified during the preoperative evaluation. The treating surgeon should obtain a detailed history of the knee injury, including prior physical therapy and surgical treatment. If surgical treatment was previously performed, the operative records should be acquired to fully comprehend the overall state of the knee, the surgical technique, as well as the specifics of the retained hardware. An extensive physical examination should be performed with the goal to correlate the patient's symptoms to the clinical picture. The rotational stability of the affected knee should be carefully examined using specialized tests such as the pivot shift.

The diagnostic imaging series of the affected knee includes weight-bearing 45-degree posterior-anterior radiographs, lateral view in 30 degrees of knee flexion (Fig. 34-1). In cases of instability, we routinely performed ultrasound imaging of the anterolateral structure of the knee. The ultrasound enables a dynamic evaluation of the lateral structures of the knee (Fig. 34-2). Since the extra-articular tenodesis is done in the case of an ACL revision, we also obtain weight-bearing entire lower extremity radiograph to assess the coronal alignment of the lower extremities, along with a computed tomography (CT) to further evaluate tunnel positioning.

Magnetic resonance imaging is obtained to investigate the overall state of the knee. All soft tissues, ligaments, bone, and cartilage surface are carefully examined in order to diagnose concomitant pathology. The surgeon must have an adequate conversation with the patient regarding his or her expectations and goals concerning the ACL revision surgery with extra-articular tenodesis given that this surgery is not as successful as the isolated primary ACL reconstruction.

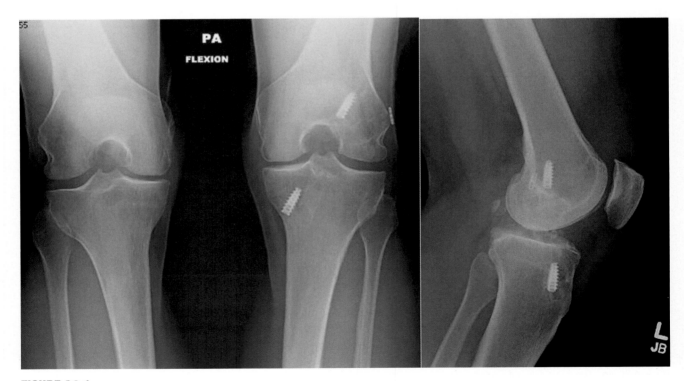

FIGURE 34-1

Weight-bearing 45-degree posterior-anterior radiographs and lateral view in 30 degrees of knee flexion. Previous tunnel placements are evaluated during the preoperative evaluation.

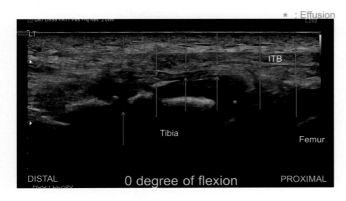

FIGURE 34-2

Ultrasound of the lateral soft tissue of the knee of a failed ACL reconstruction. An increased opacity is noted in the posterior capsule (*blue arrows*) of the knee. An intra-articular effusion is noted (*red star*).

SURGICAL TECHNIQUE

The surgical technique for the extra-articular tenodesis in complement to the ACL reconstruction is based on a modified Marcacci technique (12).

Patient Positioning and Exam under Anesthesia

Once the patient is properly anesthetized and time-out had been completed, the patient is placed supine with the affected leg in a leg holder, which allows application of varus and valgus stress to the knee during the procedure. A tourniquet is placed as proximal as possible on the affected thigh. The examination under anesthesia of both lower extremities is then performed including range of motion, Lachman test, anterior and posterior drawer, valgus and varus stress at 0 degree and 30 degrees of flexion, a pivot shit, and a dial test. The leg is then prepped and draped, and an Esmarch wrap is used to exsanguinate the leg before the tourniquet is inflated. A three-portal ACL reconstruction technique is utilized (see Chapter 31: Individualized Anatomic Approach to ACL Reconstruction).

Arthroscopy

The arthroscopic portion of the ACL reconstruction is undertaken with standard diagnostic arthroscopy. The surgeon then processes with the proper identification and preparation of the tibial and femoral footprint according to the individualized ACL reconstruction principles (Chapter 31). It is important to address all other necessary procedures including those relating to concomitant meniscal injury or chondral damage. Furthermore, it is important to adequately identify and prepare the over-the-top (OTT) position on the posterior-superior aspect of the femoral ACL footprint (Fig. 34-3).

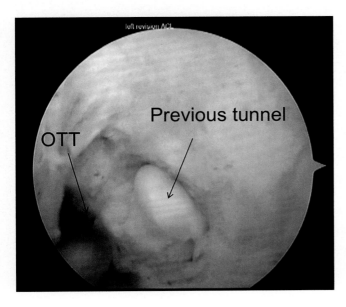

FIGURE 34-3

The over-the-top (OTT) position is identified in the posterior-superior aspect of the femoral footprint.

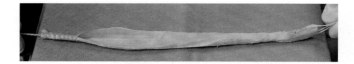

FIGURE 34-4

Achilles tendon allograft with bone block. The soft tissue end of the graft is whipstitched using a Krackow technique, and two No. 2 fiber wire sutures are passed through the bone block 10 mm apart from each other.

Graft Preparation

An Achilles tendon allograft is utilized for the ACL with extra-articular tenodesis of the lateral soft tissue complex of the knee. In cases where allografts are not available, autologous semitendinosus and gracilis grafts can be harvested according to Marcacci's surgical technique (12). It is important to prepare a graft of sufficient length, 15 to 20 cm, to enable the reconstruction of both the ACL and the extra-articular tenodesis with the same graft. The soft tissue end of the Achilles tendon allograft is whipstitched using a Krackow technique, and two No. 2 fiber wire sutures are passed through the bone block 10 mm apart from each other (Fig. 34-4). The soft tissue end of the graft can be bulleted to allow easy passage of the graft through the tibial tunnel and the OTT position.

Extra-articular Tenodesis

Once the tibial tunnel has been appropriately positioned and sized according to the graft dimension, the attention is turned toward the extra-articular portion of the procedure. With the knee at 90 degrees of flexion, a 5-cm superior-lateral incision is made starting at Gerdy tubercle to just proximal to the posterior aspect of the femoral condyle (Fig. 34-5). The iliotibial (IT) band is then incised in line with the incision at the posterior one third of the IT band. The IT band is then retracted anteriorly, and the dissection is carried down to the intermuscular septum, separating the vastus lateralis and the lateral head of the gastrocnemius. A retractor is placed over the lateral intermuscular capsule to expose the posterior joint capsule. With finger dissection, the OTT position is identified by palpating the posterior tubercle of the lateral femoral condyle and creating a potential place.

The arthroscope is then placed back into the knee, and a curved Kelly clamp is placed in the posterior-superior notch, and the tip is pushed superiorly and posteriorly while maintaining contact with the posterior aspect of the lateral femoral condyle. The tip of the curved Kelly clamp is then felt with a finger posterior to the lateral intermuscular septum, in the OTT position previously identified

FIGURE 34-5

Superior-lateral incision. During arthroscopic transillumination of lateral soft tissue, no thickening of the anterolateral capsule was seen, and we could not identify an anterolateral ligament.

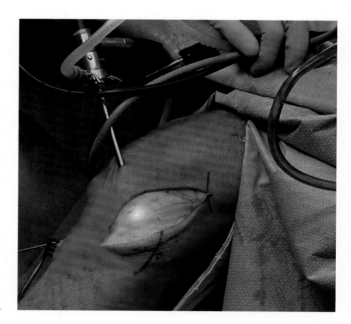

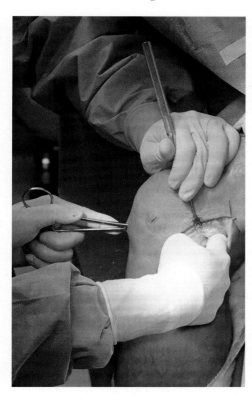

FIGURE 34-6

A curved Kelly clamp is placed from the accessory portal into the posterior-superior aspect of the notch, and the tip is felt posterior to the lateral intermuscular septum in the over-the-top position.

(Fig. 34-6). Once the tip of the curved Kelly clamp is clearly palpated, it is pushed through the posterior capsule into the OTT potential place previously created. The lateral aspect of the femur at the OTT position is then decorticated with a curette to provide bleeding surface. Next, a malleable wire loop is gripped by the tip of the curved Kelly clamp and pulled into the knee joint. A grasper is then placed into the tibial tunnel, and the wire loop is then pulled from the joint out through the tibia (Fig. 34-7).

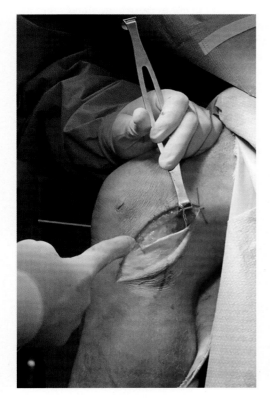

FIGURE 34-7

The wire loop is gripped by the tip of the curved Kelly clamp and pulled from the over-the-top position through the joint. A grasper is then placed into the tibial tunnel and the wire loop is pulled out through the tibial tunnel.

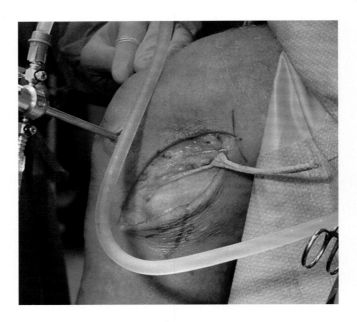

FIGURE 34-8

The fiber wire sutures at the bony end of the Achilles tendon allograft are then loaded in the wire loop, and the graft is pulled from the over-the-top position through the joint into the tibial tunnel.

Graft Passage and Fixation

The fiber wire sutures at the bony end of the Achilles tendon allograft are then loaded in the wire loop, and the graft is pulled from the OTT position through the joint into the tibial tunnel (Fig. 34-8). A bioabsorbable interference screw (Smith & Nephew, Richards Inc., Memphis, USA) is used to secure the tibial portion of the graft (Fig. 34-9). The graft is then tensioned coming out of the lateral incision, and the knee is cycled 15 times through a full range of motion (Fig. 34-10). While maintaining tension on the graft, it is fixed with two staples with the knee at 20 degrees of flexion with a posterior drawer applied to the tibia (Fig. 34-11). It is important to not overdrive the staples into the femur to prevent graft rupture. Next, the graft is tensioned and placed onto the Gerdy tubercle with the knee at 90 degrees of flexion and cycled through a full range of motion to evaluate graft isometry and to ensure that the knee is not captured. The graft is fixed in placed with two staples at the center of the Gerdy tubercle (Fig. 34-12). Intraoperative fluoroscopy is obtained to evaluate position of the staples and to ensure that they do not encroach on the cartilage surface (see Fig. 34-13).

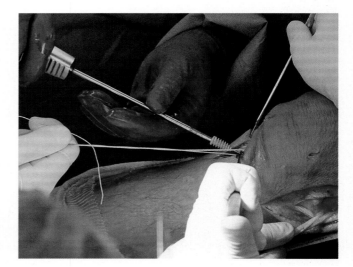

FIGURE 34-9

The tibial portion of the Achilles tendon allograft is fixed with a bioabsorbable screw (Smith & Nephews, Richards Inc., Q5 Memphis, USA).

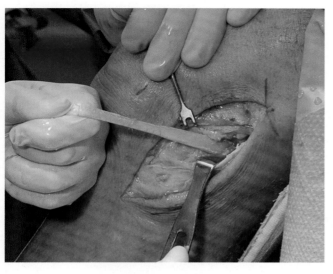

FIGURE 34-10
The graft is then tensioned coming out of the lateral incision.

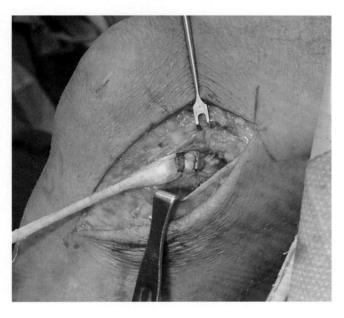

FIGURE 34-11
The Achilles tendon allograft is fixed to the lateral femoral condyle in the over-the-top position with two staples.

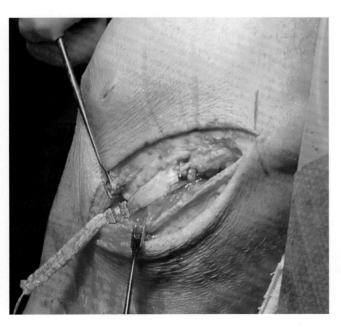

FIGURE 34-12
The extra-articular lateral tenodesis is completed by securing the graft to the Gerdy tubercle with two staples.

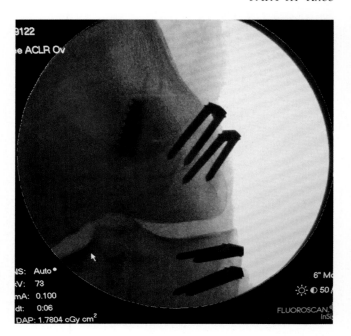

FIGURE 34-13

Intraoperative fluoroscopy is obtained to ensure the staples are well positioned and do not encroach on cartilage surface.

Closure

The incisions are then thoroughly irrigated, and the arthroscopic portals are closed with a 3-0 non-absorbable monofilament suture. For the lateral incision, the IT band is closed with a 0 absorbable braided suture in an interrupted figure-of-eight fashion. The subcutaneous layer is then approximated with interrupted 2-0 absorbable braided suture, and the skin is closed with a 3-0 absorbable monofilament suture in a running subcuticular fashion. For the medial incision, the subcutaneous layer is closed with interrupted 2-0 absorbable braided suture, and the skin is approximated with a 3-0 absorbable monofilament suture in a running subcuticular fashion. A sterile dressing is then applied, and the knee is placed in a braced locked in extension.

PEARLS AND PITFALLS

- Appropriate preoperative evaluation is necessary to assess for any concomitant injury using a thorough physical examination and proper diagnostic imaging.
- In the absence of other etiology, the presence of a high-grade pivot shift in cases of ACL revision failure should prompt the treating physician to consider lateral soft tissue extra-articular tenodesis.
- An ultrasound can be invaluable in obtaining a dynamic exam of the lateral structure of the knee.
- An isolated lateral extra-articular tenodesis is not recommended.
- Anterolateral extra-articular tenodesis is contraindicated in patients with advanced arthritis and impaired lower extremity neurologic function.
- Proper identification and preparation of the OTT position are paramount to the success of this procedure.
- During the fixation of the graft with staples, care must be taken not to rupture the graft by over-driving the staples into the cortical surface.
- Intraoperative fluoroscopy should be obtained to verify correct placement of the staples and ensure that they do not encroach on the cartilage surface.

POSTOPERATIVE MANAGEMENT

The patient should be followed closely during the postoperative course. The patient is seen at postoperative day 7 to remove the nonabsorbable suture and evaluate the incision for signs of infection or for signs of deep venous thrombosis. Straight leg raises and supervised range of motion are initiated at the first postoperative visit (Fig. 34-14). Furthermore, during this visit,

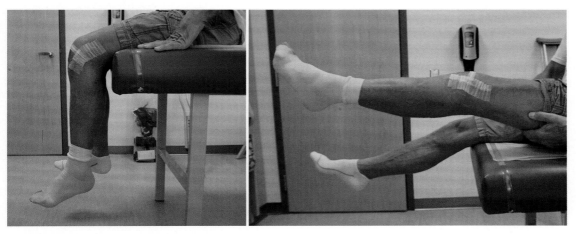

FIGURE 34-14

Straight leg raises and supervised range of motion are initiated at the first postoperative visit.

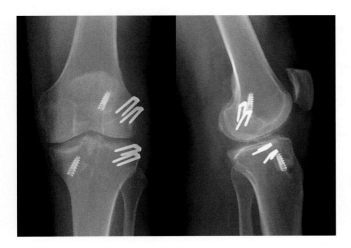

FIGURE 34-15

45-degree flexion posterior-anterior and 30-degree flexion lateral radiograph on postoperative day 7.

the patient should be evaluated with a 45-degree knee flexion posterior-anterior radiograph and a 30-degree flexion lateral view of the knee to evaluate the tunnel and hardware positioning (Fig. 34-15).

The patients are restricted to toe-touch weight bearing in brace for the first 2 weeks and then progressed to full weight bearing. The brace is discontinued at 6 weeks, once quadriceps control is judged to be adequate. At 6 weeks postoperative, closed chain exercises are begun. Running is permitted at 3 to 4 months, and return to sports is considered between 6 and 9 months postoperative.

COMPLICATIONS

The perioperative complications following extra-articular tenodesis of the anterolateral structures of the knee parallel the complications of ACL reconstruction. The patient should be evaluated for post-operative infection, deep vein thrombosis, and neurologic injury. Furthermore, it should be noted that the allograft tendon carries inherently the potential for disease transmission. The extra-articular tenodesis can potentially overconstrain the knee and provoke stiffness and may precipitate arthritis. While taking these into consideration, the patient expectation is primordial to maximize the potential for success of this procedure that is often done in a revision setting.

RESULTS

Currently, there are no level 1 studies evaluating the proper indications for extra-articular tenodesis of the anterolateral structures of the knee. The extra-articular tenodesis has a theoretical application in revision ACL surgery when there is significant persistent rotational instability. Until such high-level evidence is brought forward by the research community, the extra-articular tenodesis of the lateral structures of the knee should only be performed in specific revision settings.

REFERENCES

1. Claes S, Vereecke E, Maes M, et al. Anatomy of the anterolateral ligament of the knee. *J Anat.* 2013;223(4):321–328.
2. Dodds AL, Halewood C, Gupte CM, et al. The anterolateral ligament: anatomy, length changes and association with the Segond fracture. *Bone Joint J.* 2014;96-b(3):325–331.
3. Thein R, Boorman-Padgett J, Stone K, et al. Biomechanical assessment of the anterolateral ligament of the knee: a secondary restraint in simulated tests of the pivot shift and of anterior stability. *J Bone Joint Surg Am.* 2016;98(11):937–943.
4. Rahnemai-Azar AA, Miller RM, Guenther D, et al. Structural properties of the anterolateral capsule and iliotibial band of the knee. *Am J Sports Med.* 2016;44(4):892–897.
5. Musahl V, Rahnemai-Azar AA, van Eck CF, et al. Anterolateral ligament of the knee, fact or fiction? *Knee Surg Sports Traumatol Arthrosc.* 2016;24(1):2–3.
6. Sabzevari S, Rahnemai-Azar AA, Albers M, et al. Anatomic and histological investigation of the anterolateral capsular complex in the fetal knee. *Am J Sports Med.* 2017;45(6):1383–1387.
7. Dombrowski ME, Costello JM, Ohashi B, et al. Macroscopic anatomical, histological and magnetic resonance imaging correlation of the lateral capsule of the knee. *Knee Surg Sports Traumatol Arthrosc.* 2016;24(9):2854–2860.
8. Spencer L, Burkhart TA, Tran MN, et al. Biomechanical analysis of simulated clinical testing and reconstruction of the anterolateral ligament of the knee. *Am J Sports Med.* 2015;43(9):2189–2197.
9. Williams A, Ball S, Stephen J, et al. The scientific rationale for lateral tenodesis augmentation of intra-articular ACL reconstruction using a modified 'Lemaire' procedure. *Knee Surg Sports Traumatol Arthrosc.* 2017;25(4):1339–1344.
10. Lewis PB, Parameswaran AD, Rue JP, et al. Systematic review of single-bundle anterior cruciate ligament reconstruction outcomes: a baseline assessment for consideration of double-bundle techniques. *Am J Sports Med.* 2008;36(10):2028–2036.
11. Branch T, Lavoie F, Guier C, et al. Single-bundle ACL reconstruction with and without extra-articular reconstruction: evaluation with robotic lower leg rotation testing and patient satisfaction scores. *Knee Surg Sports Traumatol Arthrosc.* 2015;23(10):2882–2891.
12. Marcacci M, Zaffagnini S, Iacono F, et al. Arthroscopic intra- and extra-articular anterior cruciate ligament reconstruction with gracilis and semitendinosus tendons. *Knee Surg Sports Traumatol Arthrosc.* 1998;6(2):68–75.

35 Extra-articular Tenodesis of the Knee

W. Scott McGuffin and Alan Getgood

BACKGROUND

The goals of surgical reconstruction of the anterior cruciate ligament (ACL)-deficient knee include restoration of both anteroposterior (AP) and rotational knee stability. Conventional intra-articular ACL reconstruction is widely accepted as a means of achieving satisfactory AP stability, but it does not reliably restore rotational control in all patients (1–3). Reestablishing rotational stability correlates with return to sport, functional scores, overall knee function, and patient satisfaction (4,5). Newer intra-articular reconstruction techniques including anatomic femoral tunnel positioning have demonstrated improvements in rotational stability (6–8), but significant rates of rerupture and revision surgery persist (9–12). This has propelled investigation into further techniques to improve rotational stability after ACL reconstruction.

Several structures in addition to the ACL have been identified as important contributors to rotational knee stability including the lateral meniscus (13), the medial meniscotibial ligament (14), and the iliotibial band (ITB) (15). Moreover, the anterolateral ligamentous structures have long been known to provide restraint to anterolateral rotation of the tibia (16), and injuries in this region have been reported to occur at the time of ACL injury (17,18). Recent anatomic descriptions of the anterolateral ligament (ALL) (19,20) have revived interest in the biomechanical properties of the ALL (21–24) and its importance in stabilizing the ACL-deficient knee (25). Concerns over residual rotational laxity following ACL reconstruction have generated interest in surgical options, specifically ALL reconstruction (26) and lateral extra-articular tenodesis (LET), for augmenting anterolateral stability at the time of ACL reconstruction.

Descriptions of LET procedures are numerous (27–29). Their use in isolation is largely historical due to concerns of overconstraint of the knee and poor clinical outcomes (30,31); however a recent systematic review reported significant reduction in anterolateral rotational laxity when LET was performed in combination with intra-articular ACL reconstruction (32). When performing intra-articular ACL reconstruction, our preference has been to augment rotational control where indicated with LET rather than reconstruction of the ALL because an extra-articular tenodesis based on a distal attachment to the Gerdy tubercle results in graft orientation that is more optimal for resisting tibial internal rotation (33). Recent biomechanical findings support this and have demonstrated improved restoration of rotational stability with LET when compared to ALL reconstruction (34,35). The modified Lemaire extra-articular tenodesis procedure has been shown to restore native rotational kinematics to the knee without overconstraining tibial internal rotation (35).

INDICATIONS/CONTRAINDICATIONS

We advocate performing LET only on patients most likely to benefit from the additional procedure given that a majority of patients undergoing intra-articular ACL reconstruction experience satisfactory results. As yet, there exists no high-level prospective evidence to guide the use of LET during primary ACL reconstruction. Based on expert opinion, the patient most likely to benefit from primary LET may have one or more of young age (<25 years), high-grade rotational laxity (Grade 2 to Grade 3 pivot shift or >5 mm lateral compartment translation), generalized ligamentous laxity (knee hyperextension >10 degrees), elevated tibial posterior slope, meniscal deficiency, magnetic resonance imaging (MRI) evidence of anterolateral capsule injury, or

437

participation in pivoting sport (36). At our center, we strongly consider performing LET during primary ACL procedures on patients with a Grade 3 pivot shift and generalized ligamentous laxity, with additional consideration given to patients wishing to return to pivoting sport. We routinely perform LET during revision ACL reconstruction when the knee displays no other rotational (i.e., posterolateral) laxity.

PREOPERATIVE PREPARATION

Preoperative clinical evaluation includes a history of the patient's age, medical history, mechanism of injury, preferred sport(s) and level of participation, as well as presence of any prior ipsilateral or contralateral ACL injury. Physical examination of both lower limbs mandates assessment of the ACL including AP laxity with the Lachman test and anterolateral rotational laxity with the pivot shift maneuver. Grading is done according to International Knee Documentation Committee (IKDC) standards. Collateral ligament stability should be assessed with varus and valgus stress testing at 0 and 30 degrees of knee flexion. The posterior cruciate ligament is examined by inspection for posterior tibial sag and the posterior drawer test. Integrity of the posterolateral corner should be confirmed with the posterolateral drawer test, the external rotation recurvatum test, and the dial test for external rotation asymmetry. Knees with meniscal pathology may display joint line tenderness to palpation, and provocative tests may reproduce pain or mechanical symptoms. Knee range of motion is documented and signs of generalized ligamentous laxity are considered.

Preoperative investigations include AP, lateral, skyline, and 45-degree knee flexed (Rosenberg view) radiographs of the knee to assess for presence of bony injury, degenerative change, and tibial posterior slope. We do not routinely obtain preoperative MRI for isolated ACL tears. In revision ACL situations, plain radiographs and often computerized tomography (CT) of the knee with three-dimensional reconstructions are obtained to determine previous tunnel size and position.

TECHNIQUE

Patients are positioned supine with a tourniquet on the upper thigh and a side arthroscopy post and two foot rests for limb positioning. After completion of passage, tensioning, and fixation of the ACL graft, we perform extra-articular tenodesis using the modified Lemaire procedure (Fig. 35-1A–F). The knee is placed at 90 degrees of flexion and a 6-cm longitudinal incision is made approximately 1 cm posterior to the lateral femoral epicondyle. Subcutaneous tissue is divided sharply down to the level of the ITB, and fat is swept off the ITB posteriorly with a gauze sponge to identify its posterior margin. Ensuring the posterior fibers of the ITB are undisturbed, we harvest an 8-cm-long by 1-cm-wide strip of ITB that is released proximally and freed of any deep attachments leaving it attached distally at the Gerdy tubercle. The proximal 2 cm of ITB are then whip stitched with no. 1 Vicryl suture.

We then identify the fibular collateral ligament (FCL) using palpation. With a no. 15 scalpel, small capsular incisions are made just anterior and posterior to the proximal aspect of the FCL, and Metzenbaum scissors are passed deep to the FCL taking care to remain extracapsular and prevent damage to the popliteus tendon. A Fraser clamp is then passed deep to the FCL, and the ITB graft is brought under FCL from distal to proximal using the Fraser clamp.

The femoral attachment site of the tenodesis is just posterior and proximal to the origin of the fibula collateral ligament, just anterior to the attachment site of the distal Kaplan fibers of the ITB. The periosteum is removed by using a Cobb elevator on the metaphyseal flare of the lateral femoral condyle. The knee is then placed in 60 degrees of flexion with the tibia and foot in neutral rotation to avoid overconstraining the lateral joint compartment and restricting rotational freedom. The graft is held taut with minimal tension and secured to the femur with a Richards staple (Smith and Nephew Inc, Andover, MA), and excess graft length is then folded and sutured back onto itself using a free needle on the No. 1 Vicryl whip stitch.

The wound is irrigated after ensuring hemostasis and closure is performed. At the level of the vastus lateralis, the defect in the ITB is gently reopposed using interrupted figure-of-8 No. 1 Vicryl sutures. To avoid overconstraint of the lateral patellofemoral joint, we refrain from closing the ITB defect distally at the level of the transverse ligament. Standard subcutaneous and skin closure is performed.

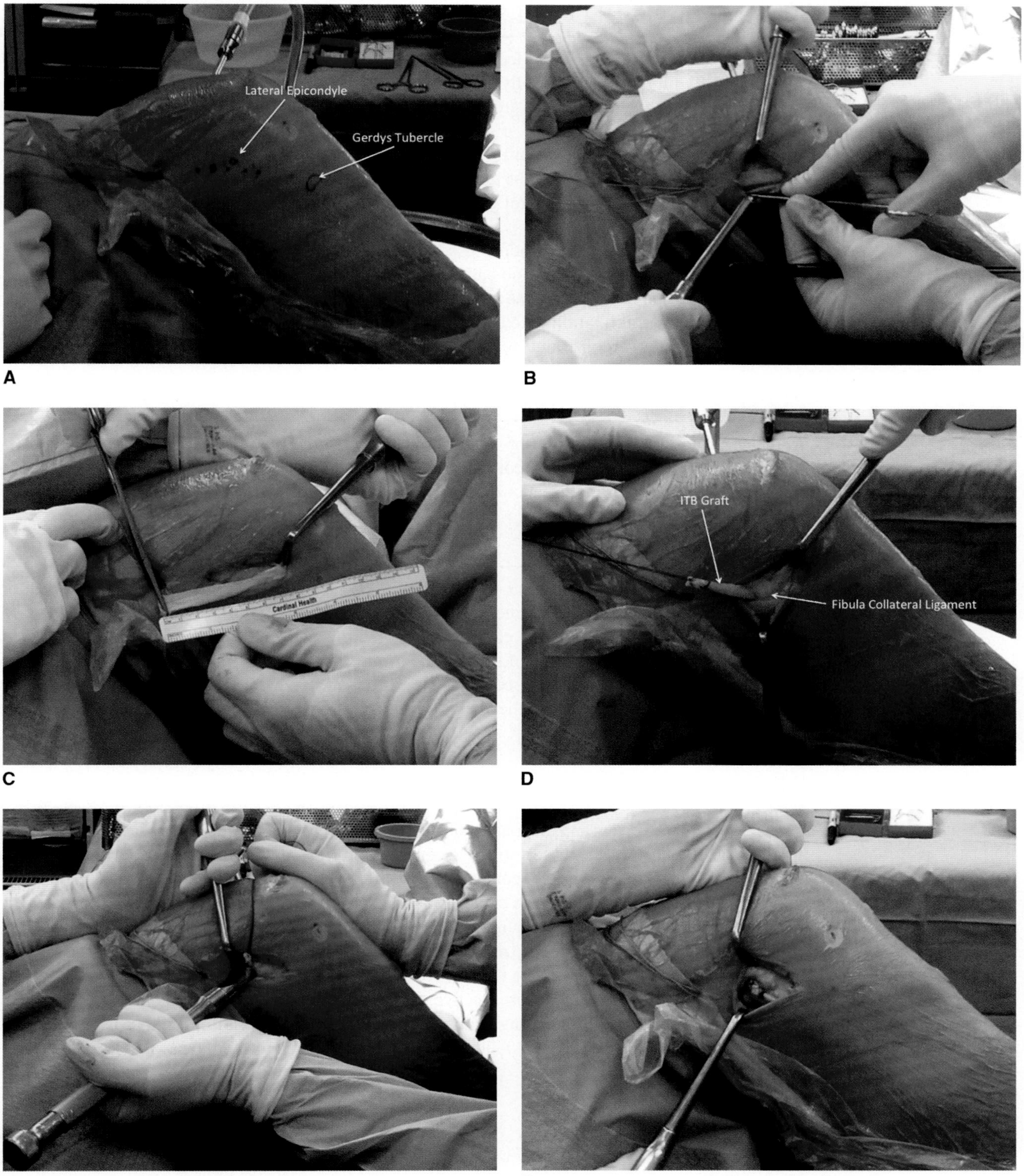

FIGURE 35-1

Surgical technique of the modified Lemaire LET. **A:** A 6-cm curvilinear incision (dotted line) is placed just posterior to the lateral femoral epicondyle. **B,C:** An 8-cm-long × 1-cm-wide strip of ITB is harvested from the posterior half of the ITB, ensuring that the most posterior fibers of the capsulo-osseous layer remain intact. **D:** The FCL is identified and the ITB graft is then passed beneath the FCL from distal to proximal. **E:** The attachment site should be identified just anterior and proximal to the lateral gastrocnemius tendon. The graft is fixed with a small Richards staple, held taut but not overtensioned, with the knee at 60 degrees of flexion and the foot in neutral rotation to avoid lateral compartment overconstraint. **F:** The graft is sutured back on itself, and the ITB is left open at the transverse ligament to avoid overtightening the lateral retinaculum and increasing patellofemoral pressure.

PEARLS AND PITFALLS

- Use Metzenbaum scissors to dissect the deep plane of the ITB graft proximally first as this plane is more difficult to identify distally.
- The knee can be placed into figure-of-four position to place the FCL on stretch and aid its identification by palpation.
- At the femoral attachment site of the tenodesis, there is a small fat pad in the area proximal and lateral to the lateral gastrocnemius tendon. This fat pad should be cleared down to the femur with electrocautery as the superolateral geniculate artery is in close proximity as well as small veins are usually present within it.
- If suspensory loop femoral fixation is used for the ACL graft, the button is typically in the area of femoral LET graft attachment, and care should be taken to avoid damaging the button.
- The tenodesis can be thought of as a checkrein, and as such, minimal tension is placed on the LET graft during femoral fixation with the knee placed at 60 degrees of flexion and the foot in neutral rotation to avoid overconstraint.

POSTOPERATIVE MANAGEMENT

Weight-bearing status and range of motion can be performed as tolerated as part of a standard rehabilitation protocol for ACL reconstruction. Modifications to rehabilitation parameters may be made for any concurrent meniscal or cartilage treatment performed.

COMPLICATIONS

The modified Lemaire procedure as described above is a safe procedure with few complications noted. We have infrequently encountered postoperative hematoma of the lateral aspect of the knee, which we feel can be prevented by careful use of electrocautery during identification and preparation of the femoral attachment site of the IT band graft. Both overconstraint of tibial internal rotation and increased lateral compartment compressive stress can be avoided by fixating the graft on the femur under minimal tension with the knee positioned at 60 degrees of flexion and the tibia and foot in neutral rotation.

RESULTS

A recent systematic review and meta-analysis of 29 articles revealed a statistically significant reduction in the pivot shift when LET was performed in combination with ACLR when compared to ACLR alone (32); however, there was no improvement seen in IKDC scores with the addition of LET. Similarly, a meta-analysis published by Rezende et al. reported improvements in pivot shift testing with the combined procedure, yet no difference in functional outcomes was noted (37). The quality of included studies in both meta-analyses was poor to moderate. At present, there is no high-quality published evidence comparing ACLR with and without LET. At our center, we have recently completed enrollment of approximately 630 patients into a prospective, randomized controlled trial (Stability Study: Clinical Trials.gov NCT02018354) comparing primary ACL reconstruction with or without LET in patients considered to be at high risk of graft failure, and 2-year clinical results will be available in 2019.

REFERENCES

1. Woo SLY, Kanamori A, Zeminski J, et al. The effectiveness of reconstruction of the anterior cruciate ligament with hamstrings and patellar tendon. A cadaveric study comparing anterior tibial and rotational loads. *J Bone Joint Surg Am.* 2002;84-A(6):907–914.
2. Ristanis S, Stergiou N, Patras K, et al. Excessive tibial rotation during high-demand activities is not restored by anterior cruciate ligament reconstruction. *Arthroscopy.* 2005;21(11):1323–1329. doi:10.1016/j.arthro.2005.08.032.
3. Georgoulis AD, Ristanis S, Chouliaras V, et al. Tibial rotation is not restored after ACL reconstruction with a hamstring graft. *Clin Orthop Relat Res.* 2007;454:89–94. doi:10.1097/BLO.0b013e31802b4a0a.
4. Ayeni OR, Chahal M, Tran MN, et al. Pivot shift as an outcome measure for ACL reconstruction: a systematic review. *Knee Surg Sports Traumatol Arthrosc.* 2012;20(4):767–777. doi:10.1007/s00167-011-1860-y.
5. Kocher MS. Relationships between objective assessment of ligament stability and subjective assessment of symptoms and function after anterior cruciate ligament reconstruction. *Am J Sports Med.* 2004;32(3):629–634. doi:10.1177/0363546503261722.

6. Zampeli F, Ntoulia A, Giotis D, et al. Correlation between anterior cruciate ligament graft obliquity and tibial rotation during dynamic pivoting activities in patients with anatomic anterior cruciate ligament reconstruction: an in vivo examination. *Arthroscopy.* 2012;28(2):234–246. doi:10.1016/j.arthro.2011.08.285.

7. Webster KE, Wotherspoon S, Feller JA, et al. The effect of anterior cruciate ligament graft orientation on rotational knee kinematics. *Knee Surg Sports Traumatol Arthrosc.* 2012;21(9):2113–2120. doi:10.1007/s00167-012-2310-1.

8. Porter MD, Shadbolt B. "Anatomic" single-bundle anterior cruciate ligament reconstruction reduces both anterior translation and internal rotation during the pivot shift. *Am J Sports Med.* 2014;42(12):2948–2954. doi:10.1177/0363546514549938.

9. Hettrich CM, Dunn WR, Reinke EK, et al. The rate of subsequent surgery and predictors after anterior cruciate ligament reconstruction: two- and 6-year follow-up results from a multicenter cohort. *Am J Sports Med.* 2013;41(7):1534–1540. doi:10.1177/0363546513490277.

10. Mariscalco MW, Flanigan DC, Mitchell J, et al. The influence of hamstring autograft size on patient-reported outcomes and risk of revision after anterior cruciate ligament reconstruction: a Multicenter Orthopaedic Outcomes Network (MOON) Cohort Study. *Arthroscopy.* 2013;29(12):1948–1953. doi:10.1016/j.arthro.2013.08.025.

11. Shelbourne KD, Gray T, Haro M. Incidence of subsequent injury to either knee within 5 years after anterior cruciate ligament reconstruction with patellar tendon autograft. *Am J Sports Med.* 2009;37(2):246–251. doi:10.1177/0363546508325665.

12. Wright RW, Magnussen RA, Dunn WR, et al. Ipsilateral graft and contralateral ACL rupture at five years or more following ACL reconstruction. *J Bone Joint Surg Am.* 2011;93(12):1159–1165. doi:10.2106/JBJS.J.00898.

13. Musahl V, Citak M, O'Loughlin PF, et al. The effect of medial versus lateral meniscectomy on the stability of the anterior cruciate ligament-deficient knee. *Am J Sports Med.* 2010;38(8):1591–1597. doi:10.1177/0363546510364402.

14. Peltier A, Lording T, Maubisson L, et al. The role of the meniscotibial ligament in posteromedial rotational knee stability. *Knee Surg Sports Traumatol Arthrosc.* 2015;23(10):2967–2973. doi:10.1007/s00167-015-3751-0.

15. Vieira ELC, Vieira EÁ, da Silva RT, et al. An anatomic study of the iliotibial tract. *Arthroscopy.* 2007;23(3):269–274. doi:10.1016/j.arthro.2006.11.019.

16. Hughston JC, Andrews JR, Cross MJ, et al. Classification of knee ligament instabilities. Part II. The lateral compartment. *J Bone Joint Surg Am.* 1976;58(2):173–179.

17. Claes S, Luyckx T, Vereecke E, et al. The Segond fracture: a bony injury of the anterolateral ligament of the knee. *Arthroscopy.* 2014;30(11):1475–1482. doi:10.1016/j.arthro.2014.05.039.

18. Dyck P, Clockaerts S, Vanhoenacker FM, et al. Anterolateral ligament abnormalities in patients with acute anterior cruciate ligament rupture are associated with lateral meniscal and osseous injuries. *Eur Radiol.* 2016:1–9. doi:10.1007/s00330-015-4171-8.

19. Claes S, Vereecke E, Maes M, et al. Anatomy of the anterolateral ligament of the knee. *J Anat.* 2013;223(4):321–328. doi:10.1111/joa.12087.

20. Caterine S, Litchfield R, Johnson M, et al. A cadaveric study of the anterolateral ligament: re-introducing the lateral capsular ligament. *Knee Surg Sports Traumatol Arthrosc.* 2015;23(11):3186–3195. doi:10.1007/s00167-014-3117-z.

21. Parsons BO, Parsons BO, Boileau P, et al. Surgical management of traumatic anterior glenohumeral instability: an international perspective. *Instr Course Lect.* 2010;59:245–253.

22. Corbo G, Norris M, Getgood A, et al. The infra-meniscal fibers of the anterolateral ligament are stronger and stiffer than the supra-meniscal fibers despite similar histological characteristics. *Knee Surg Sports Traumatol Arthrosc.* 2017. doi:10.1007/s00167-017-4424-y.

23. Kennedy MI, Claes S, Fuso FAF, et al. The anterolateral ligament. *Am J Sports Med.* 2015;43(7):1606–1615. doi:10.1016/S0021-9290(01)00222-6.

24. Van der Watt L, Khan M, Rothrauff BB, et al. The structure and function of the anterolateral ligament of the knee: a systematic review. *Arthroscopy.* 2015;31(3):569.e3–582.e3. doi:10.1016/j.arthro.2014.12.015.

25. Monaco E, Ferretti A, Labianca L, et al. Navigated knee kinematics after cutting of the ACL and its secondary restraint. *Knee Surg Sports Traumatol Arthrosc.* 2011;20(5):870–877. doi:10.1007/s00167-011-1640-8.

26. Sonnery-Cottet B, Thaunat M, Freychet B, et al. Outcome of a combined anterior cruciate ligament and anterolateral ligament reconstruction technique with a minimum 2-year follow-up. *Am J Sports Med.* 2015;43(7):1598–1605. doi:10.1007/s00167-011-1589-7.

27. Lemaire M. Instabilité chronique du genou. Techniques et résultats des plasties ligamentaires en traumatologie sportive. *J Chir.* 1975;110(4):281–294.

28. Ireland J, Trickey EL. Macintosh tenodesis for anterolateral instability of the knee. *J Bone Joint Surg Br.* 1980;62(3):340–345.

29. Ellison AE. Distal iliotibial-band transfer for anterolateral rotatory instability of the knee. *J Bone Joint Surg Am.* 1979;61(3):330–337.

30. Fox JM, Blazina ME, Del Pizzo W, et al. Extra-articular stabilization of the knee joint for anterior instability. *Clin Orthop Relat Res.* 1980;(147):56–61.

31. Engebretsen L, Lew WD, Lewis JL, et al. The effect of an iliotibial tenodesis on intraarticular graft forces and knee joint motion. *Am J Sports Med.* 1990;18(2):169–176. doi:10.1177/036354659001800210.

32. Hewison CE, Tran MN, Kaniki N, et al. Lateral extra-articular tenodesis reduces rotational laxity when combined with anterior cruciate ligament reconstruction: a systematic review of the literature. *Arthroscopy.* 2015;31(10):2022–2034. doi:10.1016/j.arthro.2015.04.089.

33. Amis AA. Anterolateral knee biomechanics. *Knee Surg Sports Traumatol Arthrosc.* 2017;25(4):1015–1023. doi:10.1007/s00167-017-4494-x.

34. Spencer L, Burkhart TA, Tran MN, et al. Biomechanical analysis of simulated clinical testing and reconstruction of the anterolateral ligament of the knee. *Am J Sports Med.* 2015;43(9):2189–2197. doi:10.1097/BLO.0b013e31802ba45c.

35. Inderhaug E, Stephen JM, Williams A, et al. Biomechanical comparison of anterolateral procedures combined with anterior cruciate ligament reconstruction. *Am J Sports Med.* 2017;45(2):347–354. doi:10.1177/0363546516681555.

36. Musahl V, Getgood A, Neyret P, et al. Contributions of the anterolateral complex and the anterolateral ligament to rotatory knee stability in the setting of ACL Injury: a roundtable discussion. *Knee Surg Sports Traumatol Arthrosc.* 2017;25(4):997–1008. doi:10.1007/s00167-017-4436-7.

37. Rezende FC, Moraes VY, Martimbianco ALC, et al. Does combined intra- and extraarticular ACL reconstruction improve function and stability? A meta-analysis. *Clin Orthop Relat Res.* 2015:1–10. doi:10.1007/s11999-015-4285-y.

36 Single-Bundle Posterior Cruciate Ligament Reconstruction: Transtibial Technique

S. Joseph de Groot Jr, William Schulz, and Dharmesh Vyas

Posterior cruciate ligament (PCL) injuries remain relatively uncommon injuries especially as compared to anterior cruciate ligament (ACL) injuries. As such, research in the fixation of PCL injuries historically has lagged behind the ACL literature. However, over the past several decades, there has been an increase in both basic science research detailing the anatomy and biomechanics of the native PCL and outcome studies evaluating management of the ruptured PCL.

INDICATIONS AND CONTRAINDICATIONS

The goal of PCL reconstruction regardless of technique is to restore normal knee biomechanics (1) by addressing the various components of the complex anatomy of the PCL. Typical single-bundle reconstruction aims to reproduce the anterolateral bundle of the PCL. In the isolated PCL injury, which occurs much less frequently, absolute indications for surgical treatment include persistent symptoms of knee instability following a grade III (complete) PCL rupture or a bony PCL avulsion. Contraindications include traumatic knee arthrotomy, active infection, or significant knee stiffness.

In acute isolated symptomatic PCL injuries in which the posteromedial bundle and the meniscofemoral ligament remain intact, a single-bundle augmentation procedure may be the preferred surgical technique. In more complex PCL ruptures with associated injuries involving the posterolateral structures (PLS) or medial collateral ligament, more benefit may be derived from double-bundle reconstruction. Again, cadaveric testing of double-bundle PCL reconstruction has not consistently outperformed single-bundle techniques in combined PCL/PLS injury (2). Multiligamentous injuries are commonly associated with PCL rupture (3), and their management should be considered carefully in the decision to reconstruct one or both of the functionally distinct PCL bundles. However, the technical complexity of double-bundle reconstruction, the longer surgical time required, as well as the inconclusive clinical outcome are all factors that must be weighed carefully.

PREOPERATIVE PREPARATION

A complete PCL rupture can be accurately diagnosed by means of a thorough history and physical examination. In light of the known association between PCL rupture and multiligament knee injuries, the neurovascular status of the leg must be carefully assessed and documented. Furthermore, careful evaluation of the integrity of the PLS is of paramount importance given the high incidence of associated injury to these structures. Failure to recognize and treat associated PLS instability and/or injury to other secondary restraints will compromise the success of a PCL reconstruction.

Preoperative imaging includes bilateral standing AP radiographs with the knees in both full extension and in 30 degrees of flexion (tunnel view), a lateral radiograph with the knee in 30 degrees of flexion, and a skyline view of the patellofemoral joint. If any clinical or radiographic concerns exist regarding varus or valgus alignment of the lower extremity, long leg standing views from pelvis to the ankles are obtained to determine if a concurrent or staged tibial osteotomy may be required.

Magnetic resonance imaging (MRI) can be helpful prior to PCL reconstruction to identify additional ligamentous injuries. One must keep in mind, however, that while the sensitivity and specificity of MRI in detecting acute PCL rupture have been reported to be 99% and 100%, respectively (4,5), the accuracy in the chronic setting is significantly reduced (6). Associated meniscal injuries occur much less frequently than in ACL rupture (3) and should be managed at the time of arthroscopic PCL reconstruction.

TECHNIQUE

Surgery

Patients routinely receive 1 g of cefazolin intravenously 30 minutes prior to surgery. Those with allergies to cefazolin are given vancomycin or clindamycin.

Patient Positioning

A nonsterile tourniquet is placed on the patient's upper thigh. A comprehensive bilateral knee exam is performed under anesthesia to confirm the diagnosis, while identifying other potential undetected ligamentous injuries (7). The patient is placed in the supine position, and a lateral post is placed at the level of the tourniquet with a footrest or beanbag placed on the table near the foot. This is done to allow the knee to be flexed and maintained at 90-degree flexion when needed (Fig. 36-1). This is the working position for notch preparation, tibial tunnel drilling, and autologous graft harvest. The knee is shaved with electric clippers 5 cm above the proximal pole of the patella to 5 cm distal to the tibial tubercle. Care is taken to incorporate areas of incisions for potential meniscal repairs. Arthroscopy portals are marked, as well as the incision planned for graft harvest and tibial tunnel drilling. The leg is washed, and the incision sites are preinjected with 20 mL of 0.25% Sensorcaine with 1:200,000 (5 μg/mL) epinephrine. Intra-articular injection is avoided. The leg is prepped with a chlorhexidine solution and allowed to dry before sterile drapes and an iodophor impregnated adhesive drape are applied.

Arthroscopy

Inferomedial and inferolateral parapatellar working portals and a superomedial outflow portal are created vertically with a no. 11 blade. The inferolateral portal is placed slightly more lateral than in routine knee arthroscopy to improve the visualization of the medial femoral condyle when drilling the femoral tunnel. The inferomedial portal is placed medial to the medial border of the patellar tendon and proximal to the medial meniscus. A diagnostic arthroscopy is performed and any meniscal pathology addressed. The medial and lateral compartments are assessed for meniscal or chondral injuries. The ACL and PCL are also visualized, while arthroscopically visualizing the degree of ligament laxity via posterior drawer stress (7).

Two additional posteromedial portals are created for visualization and preparation of the tibial insertion of the PCL. The safety of posteromedial portals and the value of utilizing dual portals to

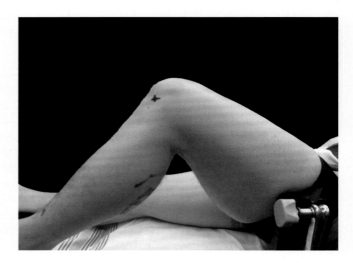

FIGURE 36-1

Knee is placed in a self-supported position of 70 to 80 degrees of flexion with a lateral side post. A tourniquet is applied.

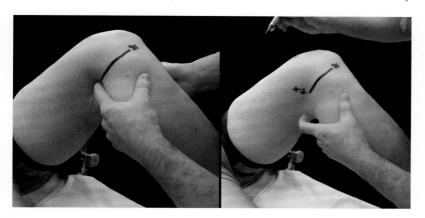

FIGURE 36-2

Arthroscopic portals are marked. Two posteromedial are positioned proximal and posterior to the medial femoral condyle, approximately a two-finger breadth proximal to the medial joint line.

assist with medial meniscal repair have been well documented (8,9). A 30-degree arthroscope is inserted into the inferolateral portal and directed posteriorly through the femoral notch just lateral to the medial femoral condyle. This allows the surgeon to directly visualize the placement of portals in the posteromedial joint capsule. An 18-gauge spinal needle is inserted through the skin into the knee joint at the location of the first posteromedial portal. Portals should be positioned proximal and posterior to the medial femoral condyle, approximately two-finger breadths proximal to the medial joint line (Fig. 36-2). The second posteromedial portal is placed just proximal to the first (Fig. 36-3). Two small separate or one common larger skin incision may be used for the placement of the two posteromedial portals. A frequent error is to place the portals too anterior and distal causing the medial femoral condyle to become an obstacle to instrument maneuverability.

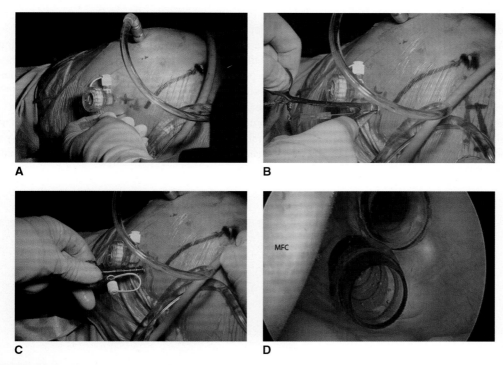

FIGURE 36-3

Posteromedial portal placement is demonstrated. **A:** Under arthroscopic guidance, a spinal needle is introduced into the knee to ensure accurate portal placement. **B:** Once a portal has been created with a no. 11 blade, it is dilated with a hemostat. **C:** Insertion of the 5-mm arthroscopic cannula. **D:** Arthroscopic view of the 5- and 8-mm cannula placement.

A no. 11 blade is advanced into the knee joint directly in line with the previously placed spinal needle. This path is subsequently dilated with a hemostat. An arthroscopic cannula is placed through each of the posteromedial portals to accommodate the mechanical shaver through a 5-mm cannula and the arthroscope through an 8-mm cannula. The large cannulas minimize fluid extravasation during preparation of the tibia.

The order of tunnel preparation depends on the chronicity of the injury. In the chronic PCL injury, either the tibial or femoral tunnel can be prepared first. In more acute cases, extravasation of arthroscopic fluid from the knee can quickly distort surrounding soft tissue planes, complicate ligament repair or reconstruction of collateral restraints, and increase the risk of compartment syndrome. Because it is more difficult to convert arthroscopic tibial tunnel preparation to an open technique, than it is to convert femoral tunnel preparation, we prioritize tibial tunnel preparation in acute (<3 weeks from injury) PCL reconstruction, especially if additional ligamentous or capsular compromise is present.

Tunnel Location and Preparation

Tibial Tunnel

The PCL tibial insertion site is prepared using the 30-degree arthroscope and mechanical shaver through the superior and inferior posteromedial portals, respectively (Figs. 36-4–36-8). Often the tibial insertion of the PCL is intact and can serve as a reference point. Debridement of the inferior aspect of the posterior septum of the knee (below the level of the middle geniculate artery) is carried out posterior to the PCL insertion utilizing a shaver and/or radiofrequency ablation (7). This technique preserves the native tibial insertion and any remaining intact fibers, which is very important for PCL injuries where the posteromedial bundle and meniscofemoral ligament remain intact. The debridement is continued until the most distal and lateral borders of the PCL insertion are visualized. A small amount is left on the femoral condyle, making footprint visualization possible.

The calibrated tibial PCL guide is set at a 55-degree angle and inserted through the inferomedial portal and the notch medial to any preserved PCL fibers. Under direct visualization and with the arthroscope in the posteromedial portal, the tip of the guide is placed 1.5 to 2 cm distal to the top of the tibial plateau in the lateral most aspect of the PCL footprint. A small incision is made along the anteromedial border of the tibia, and the guide sleeve is seated against bone.

A nonthreaded guidewire on power is advanced to the posterior tibial cortex through the guide parallel to the orientation of the proximal tibiofibular joint, as viewed on lateral fluoroscopy. Under direct visualization with the arthroscope in the posteromedial portal, the guidewire is advanced by hand through the posterior tibial cortex to exit posteriorly in the lower one third of the PCL insertion. The same process is repeated with a reamer that corresponds to the graft in diameter. A curette can be placed through the second posteromedial portal over the guidewire to ensure it is not inadvertently advanced during reaming. The tunnel is cleared of any debris with a shaver and rasped superiorly at the posterior cortex to smooth any sharp edges to protect the graft where it will make its abrupt turn.

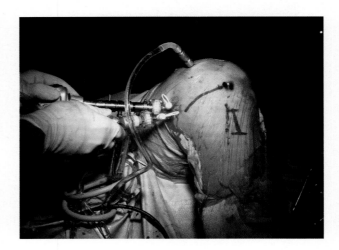

FIGURE 36-4

During preparation of the tibial insertion site, the surgeon works from the opposite side of the operating table through the two posteromedial portals.

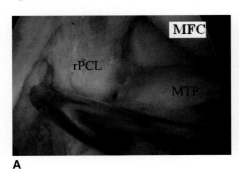
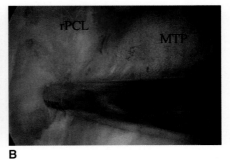

FIGURE 36-5

Preparation of the tibial insertion site is demonstrated. **A, B:** Debridement of the inferior aspect of the posterior septum of the knee, posterior to the PCL insertion. This technique preserves the remaining intact PCL fibers (*rPCL*). The medial femoral condyle (*MFC*) and medial tibial plateau (*MTP*) are shown.

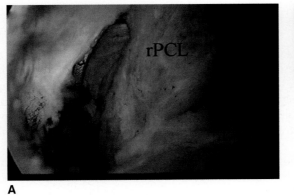
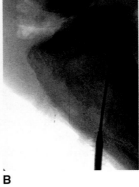

FIGURE 36-6

The tibial tunnel is created. **A:** Under direct visualization, the tip of the guide is placed 1.5 to 2 cm distal to the top of the tibial plateau. **B:** Fluoroscopy is used to confirm the position of the wire.

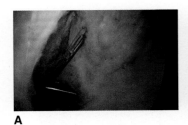
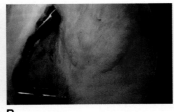
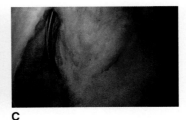

FIGURE 36-7

A: A pediatric feeding tube is inserted retrograde into the tibial tunnel. **B, C:** It curves superiorly and can be easily retrieved using a grasper through the inferolateral portal. The tube is used to pull the traction sutures anterograde into the tibial tunnel.

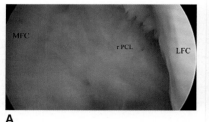
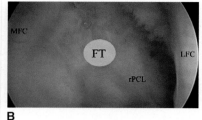

A   **B**

FIGURE 36-8

The femoral tunnel is prepared. **A:** The PCL femoral footprint that often remains intact is shown. **B:** The center of the proposed femoral tunnel (*FT*) is shown within the footprint of the anterolateral bundle on the medial femoral condyle. The remaining PCL (*rPCL*), medial femoral condyle (*MFC*), and lateral femoral condyle (*LFC*) are indicated.

A pediatric feeding tube is inserted retrograde into the tibial tunnel and its exit from the posterior cortex of the tibia visualized arthroscopically. A grasper through the inferolateral portal is used to retrieve the feeding tube medial to any preserved PCL fibers. A polydioxanone monofilament 0 suture is shuttled through the tibial tunnel with the feeding tube. A looped nonabsorbable no. 5 suture is tied to the polydioxanone strand at its tibial end and retrieved through the inferolateral portal.

Femoral Tunnel

The femoral isometric point of the PCL is suggested to be in the far posterior region of the intercondylar region (10). Studies suggest that the majority of the anterior and middle portions of the PCL are likely nonisometric with respect to length (11) (Fig. 36-9). Isometric single-bundle PCL reconstruction may therefore not only prove challenging but also be less effective than anatomical PCL reconstruction in restoring posterior tibial translation (12). Furthermore, studies have shown over constraint of isometric reconstructions during extension accompanied by under constraint at greater degrees of flexion (13).

A 30-degree arthroscope is placed through the inferolateral portal. A hooked cautery tip in the inferomedial portal is used to mark the center of the proposed femoral tunnel within the footprint of the anterolateral bundle on the medial femoral condyle. Fortunately, the PCL footprint on the femur often remains intact. Using cautery to remove any synovium from the insertion site of the PCL, care is taken to leave any underlying fibers undisturbed. If no intact PCL fibers remain, a Steadman awl is used to mark the starting point on the medial femoral condyle.

A Beath pin loaded through the appropriate diameter cannulated reamer (sized for graft) is inserted through the inferolateral portal. The tip of the Beath pin is gently impacted into the medial femoral condyle at the center of the proposed femoral tunnel drilling site. The cannulated reamer is advanced by hand over the Beath pin to a depth of approximately 1 to 2 mm into the medial

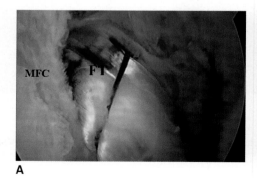
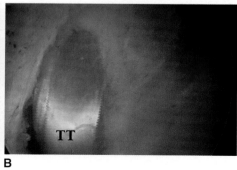

A   **B**

FIGURE 36-9

Final graft position is shown. **A:** Demonstrates the femoral tunnel (*FT*) insertion. **B:** The tibial tunnel (*TT*) insertion is shown. The medial femoral condyle (*MFC*) is indicated as well.

femoral condyle and then removed. The location of the reamer etching is viewed with either a 30- or 70-degree scope through the inferomedial portal to ensure it is acceptable and does not compromise the articular cartilage of the medial femoral condyle. Occasionally, an accessory inferolateral portal is required to bring the angle of the Beath pin as close to the face of the lateral femoral condyle as possible. This serves to reduce the acuity of the angle the graft encounters at its insertion into the femur.

With the knee positioned in 110 to 120 degrees of flexion, the Beath pin is reinserted and advanced through the medial femoral cortex. The 4.5-mm cannulated EndoButton drill is advanced over the Beath pin and through the medial femoral cortex. Care must be taken to ensure that the anterior aspect of the lateral femoral condyle is not damaged during reaming. The femoral tunnel length is measured, and an EndoButton of a size that will allow placement of a minimum of 20 mm of graft within the femoral tunnel is selected. A cannulated reamer is used by hand to create the femoral tunnel. The Beath pin is pulled through the medial femoral cortex shuttling an absorbable polydioxanone monofilament suture size 0 through the femoral tunnel from the inferolateral portal. The femoral tunnel can alternatively be drilled with an outside-in technique and interference screw fixation utilized.

Graft Passage

The inferolateral portal is enlarged sufficiently to allow unimpeded insertion of the PCL graft into the knee. It is critical to have both the tibial and femoral shuttling sutures free of any interposed soft tissue when exiting the inferolateral portal. The sutures attached to the EndoButton are shuttled through the medial femoral condyle. The EndoButton and attached graft are inserted through the inferolateral portal and pulled out of the femoral tunnel. The EndoButton is flipped. The sutures on the remaining end of the PCL graft are shuttled antegrade through the tibial tunnel using the previously placed nonabsorbable shuttling suture. The free end of the PCL graft is inserted into the inferolateral portal and retrieved from the tibial tunnel distally.

Graft Fixation

As described, EndoButton fixation is used on the femoral side. Tibial fixation is accomplished with either staples or interference screws. The graft is secured with the knee in 90 degrees of flexion while applying a strong anterior drawer force on the proximal aspect of the tibia (7). According to studies, the optimal tension of the PCL graft allowing for full range of knee motion is 15 lb (68 N) (14). An anterior load is placed on the tibia in order to recreate both normal knee kinematics and in situ forces previously described in the PCL reconstruction utilizing a single anterolateral bundle technique (15) (Fig. 36-10).

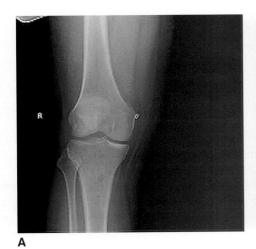
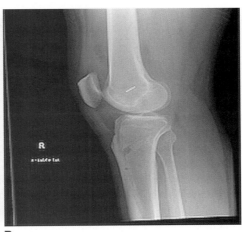

A   B

FIGURE 36-10

Immediate postoperative x-rays demonstrating the final position of the graft after PCL reconstruction.

Pearls and Pitfalls

Arthroscopic Fluid Extravasation

Fluid extravasation has an incidence of 0.8% to 1.3% during knee arthroscopy. Fluid extravasation is associated with increased intra-articular pressure, capsular tears, as well as extended operation time. Increases in flexion angles in addition to obstructed outflow may increase intra-articular pressure and capsular ruptures. The capsular volume of the knee decreases with increasing angles of flexion, making flow rates with low distension pressures recommended (16). In arthroscopic reconstruction, care must be taken to avoid excess arthroscopic fluid extravasation from the knee when associated ligamentous and capsular damage exist. Using a large diameter shaver for tibial and femoral tunnel preparation will save time and as well facilitate the evacuation of a greater quantity of arthroscopic fluid from the knee than a smaller diameter shaver. The outflow cannula must be constantly monitored to ensure that it does not become blocked.

Graft Contamination

Recent studies have shown that the best agent for sterilizing a dropped graft is chlorhexidine. Implanting a contaminated graft can have serious consequences, including septic arthritis (17). The ways to manage an intraoperative graft contamination range from sterilization and implantation of the graft, discarding the graft and procuring another from the ipsilateral or contralateral knee, or using an allograft while discarding the contaminated graft. Studies have shown the most effective sterilization protocols to be a combination of 7 to 8 minutes of irrigation with 3 L of 2% chlorhexidine, serial dilution with a polymyxin B-bacitracin solution, and mechanical agitation (17).

Medial Femoral Cortex Breach

The exit point for the femoral tunnel in PCL reconstruction is often situated in the softer metaphyseal cortex of the femur. If the medial femoral cortex is breached, fixation may be accomplished with the Xtendobutton (Smith and Nephew, Corp., Andover, MA), a femoral interference screw or by securing the sutures around a femoral post using a two incision technique.

Short Graft

There is no current consensus on potential harvest site morbidity. Certain grafts, such as bone–patellar tendon–bone grafts, raise the concern of being too short for use as a substitute for the PCL if the patient has a short patellar tendon. To avoid premature amputation of the graft during harvest, an extra 2 to 2.5 cm of graft can be obtained by releasing the common insertion site of the two tendons on the anterior tibia with a large sleeve of periosteum attached. This may provide enough length to proceed with the reconstruction as planned. However, if staple fixation cannot be utilized due to insufficient graft, an interference screw may be used.

POSTOPERATIVE MANAGEMENT

The rehabilitation and postoperative management for PCL injuries tends to vary from surgeon to surgeon, but all postoperative protocols have one thing in common: avoiding excess stress on the graft until it has been incorporated. It is difficult to measure stress on the ligaments during weight bearing and passive and active range of motion in vivo so most of the research has been derived from cadaveric specimens (18).

For range of motion, studies have shown that PCL tension is increased with increasing passive flexion of the knee (19). Further, stabilizing the tibia with constant anterior pressure on the posterior aspect of the leg decreases the force on the PCL (20).

Concerning weight-bearing status, experimental models have demonstrated that weight bearing causes the tibia to move anterior to the femur and thus decreases the stress on the PCL (21). Further, axial compression, that is, weight bearing, actually decreases femorotibial shearing and subsequently leads to less stress on the PCL (22).

Finally, timing for beginning muscle strengthening is very surgeon dependent and the status of the patient also plays a large role in determining when he or she is capable of initiating strengthening exercises. However, multiple studies have shown that when the hamstrings are contracted, the force on the tibia increases the stress on the PCL and that is why most surgeons wait 6 to 10 weeks before beginning any hamstring strengthening (21–23). Open chain quad strengthening exercises are usually started earlier as they are less likely to place stress on the PCL.

The protocol of this senior author which is adopted from Edson et al. is as follows (24):

Post-op weeks 0 to 6:

- Nonweight bearing for all ambulatory activities, and patient must use a long leg brace locked in full extension at all times.
- Cryotherapy, quad sets, patella mobilization, ankle pumps are all encouraged.

Post-op weeks 6 to 10:

- Patient able to begin partial weight bearing of approximately 20% of body weight and increase incrementally by 20% each week.
- Long leg brace opened to full flexion and patient encouraged to begin passive- or active-assisted flexion without active hamstring activity. Stationary cycling is permitted.
- Continue with quad strengthening and patella mobilization. Patient able to begin short-arc and long-arc quad strengthening.

Post-op weeks 10 to 16:

- Long leg brace is discontinued and fitted for functional brace for ADLs.
- Closed chain exercises are initiated in 0- to 60-degree range.
- Proprioception is emphasized in addition to proper gait mechanics.

Post-op months 4 to 6:

- Patient may begin straight-line jogging if adequate strength and proprioception achieved.
- Isolated hamstring strengthening against gravity without weight initiated at the end of post-op month 5 and resisted exercises may begin at post-op month 6.
- Aggressive quadriceps strengthening implemented, and patient can begin low-intensity plyometric and low-intensity sport-specific activities at the end of post-op month 5.

Post-op months 6 to 12:

- Patient must have symmetric strength and proprioception before returning to unrestricted activity.
- Functional bracing is used for sports or work activities for the first 18 months after surgery.

COMPLICATIONS

Complications in PCL surgery are thought to be more common than complications in ACL surgery not only because surgeons generally have less experience performing PCL reconstructions but the fact that it is a technically demanding surgery (25).

The most feared complication in PCL transtibial surgery is neurovascular injury particularly to the popliteal artery and tibial nerve. These are particularly vulnerable when the surgeon is drilling the tibial tunnel. This is an even more demanding situation in revision surgery as scarring may affect the positioning of the nerve and artery and make dissection more difficult (25). The distance between the tibial insertion and the popliteal artery is only 7 to 9 mm. However, that distance increases as the knee is flexed up to 100 degrees. At 100 degrees, the distance between the PCL insertion site and the artery increases to 9 to 10 mm (26).

Another complication of PCL surgery is fracturing of the tibia or femur. Fractures have been reportedly more common when hammering in staples for fixation so interference screws or ligament washers are preferred for fixation (25).

Postoperatively, patients undergoing PCL reconstruction run the risk of motion loss particularly in flexion. The reason for this loss of motion are multifactorial and can include poor tunnel placement, noncompliance with postoperative therapy, and the development of adhesions and arthrofibrosis (25,27,28). On the other hand, PCL reconstructions can also have residual posterior laxity. This can be the result of unrecognized concomitant ligamentous injuries, poor graft tensioning, poor graft placement, overly aggressive rehabilitation, or choosing an improper graft size (25).

RESULTS

Early biomechanical studies examining the transtibial approach raised concern about graft abrasion and damage to the integrity of the graft due to the acute angle of the graft (7). Despite studies showing transtibial grafts with signs of fraying and thinning at this acute angle (29), clinical studies have shown no significant short-term difference in posterior drawer test, knee laxity, subjective knee scores, or functional test scores when compared to tibial inlay (30). Further, long-term follow-up has also shown no difference between tibial inlay and transtibial techniques when comparing knee laxity, development of arthritic changes, and subjective knee scores (31).

The focus of many recent studies has been on double-bundle versus single-bundle reconstruction techniques. Multiple biomechanical studies have shown that the double-bundle technique provides more AP stability, but the results appear to be more due to positioning of the graft than the technique (12,15). The majority of clinical studies comparing the two techniques, however, have shown no significant clinical difference in double- versus single-bundle reconstruction (32–35).

In a meta-analysis looking at outcomes of transtibial single-bundle PCL reconstructions, patients undergoing a transtibial single-bundle PCL reconstruction reported preoperative Lysholm Knee Scores ranging from 55.5 to 67. Follow-up Lysholm Knee Scores in this study were shown to range from 81 to 100. Transtibial single-bundle PCL reconstructions have also been shown to improve posterior laxity by one grade as compared to the preoperative condition. Although posterior laxity shows improvement with this procedure, normal stability is not fully restored (13).

REFERENCES

1. Amis AA, Bull AM, Gupte CM, et al. Biomechanics of the PCL and related structures: posterolateral, posteromedial and meniscofemoral ligaments. *Knee Surg Sports Traumatol Arthrosc.* 2003;11(5):271–281.
2. Apsingi S, Nguyen T, Bull AM, et al. Control of laxity in knees with combined posterior cruciate ligament and posterolateral corner deficiency: comparison of single-bundle versus double-bundle posterior cruciate ligament reconstruction combined with modified Larson posterolateral corner reconstruction. *Am J Sports Med.* 2008;36(3):487–494.
3. Shelburne KB, Pandy MG. Determinants of cruciate-ligament loading during rehabilitation exercise. *Clin Biomech (Bristol, Avon).* 1998;13(6):403–413.
4. Fischer SP, Fox JM, Del Pizzo W, et al. Accuracy of diagnoses from magnetic resonance imaging of the knee. A multicenter analysis of one thousand and fourteen patients. *J Bone Joint Surg Am.* 1991;73(1):2–10.
5. Ogilvie-Harris DJ, Biggs DJ, Mackay M, et al. Posterior portals for arthroscopic surgery of the knee. *Arthroscopy.* 1994;10(6):608–613.
6. Shelbourne KD, Davis TJ, Patel DV. The natural history of acute, isolated, nonoperatively treated posterior cruciate ligament injuries. A prospective study. *Am J Sports Med.* 1999;27(3):276–283.
7. Shelbourne KD, Jennings RW, Vahey TN. Magnetic resonance imaging of posterior cruciate ligament injuries: assessment of healing. *Am J Knee Surg.* 1999;12(4):209–213.
8. Ahn JH, Kim SH, Yoo JC, et al. All-inside suture technique using two posteromedial portals in a medial meniscus posterior horn tear. *Arthroscopy.* 2004;20(1):101–108.
9. Markolf KL, O'Neill G, Jackson SR, et al. Effects of applied quadriceps and hamstrings muscle loads on forces in the anterior and posterior cruciate ligaments. *Am J Sports Med.* 2004;32(5):1144–1149.
10. Jeong Woon-Seob, et al. An analysis of the posterior cruciate ligament isometric position using an in vivo 3-dimensional computed tomography–based knee joint model. *Arthroscopy.* 2010;26(10):1333–1339.
11. Covey DC, Sapega AA, Sherman GM. Testing for isometry during reconstruction of the posterior cruciate ligament. Anatomic and biomechanical considerations. *Am J Sports Med.* 1996;24(6):740–746.
12. Qi Y-S, et al. A systematic review of double-bundle versus single bundle cruciate ligament reconstruction. *BMC Musculoskelet Disord.* 2016;17:45.
13. Kim Y-M, et al. Clinical results of arthroscopic single-bundle transtibial posterior cruciate ligament reconstruction: a systematic review. *Am J Sports Med.* 2011;39(2):425–434.
14. Toutoungi DE, Lu TW, Leardini A, et al. Cruciate ligament forces in the human knee during rehabilitation exercises. *Clin Biomech (Bristol, Avon).* 2000;15(3):176–187.
15. Harner CD, Janaushek MA, Ma CB, et al. The effect of knee flexion angle and application of an anterior tibial load at the time of graft fixation on the biomechanics of a posterior cruciate ligament-reconstructed knee. *Am J Sports Med.* 2000;28(4):460–465.
16. Race A, Amis AA. PCL reconstruction. In vitro biomechanical comparison of 'isometric' versus single and double-bundled 'anatomic' grafts. *J Bone Joint Surg Br.* 1998;80(1):173–179.
17. Khan M, et al. Management of the contaminated anterior cruciate ligament graft. *Arthroscopy.* 2014. Available at: www.sciencedirect.com/science/article/pii/S0749806313011973
18. de Paula Leite Cury R, Kiyomoto HD, Rosal GF, et al. Rehabilitation protocol after isolated posterior cruciate ligament reconstruction. *Rev Bras Ortop.* 2015;47(4):421–427. doi:10.1016/S2255-4971(15)30122-1.
19. Dürselen L, Claes L, Kiefer H. The influence of muscle forces and external loads on cruciate ligament strain. *Am J Sports Med.* 1995;23(1):129–136.
20. MacGillivray JD, Stein BE, Park M, et al. Comparison of tibial inlay versus transtibial techniques for isolated posterior cruciate ligament reconstruction: minimum 2-year follow-up. *Arthroscopy.* 2006;22(3):320–328.

21. Romero, J, et al. Massive intraperitoneal and extraperitoneal accumulation of irrigation fluid as a complication during knee arthroscopy. *Arthroscopy*. 1998;14(4):401–404.
22. Song EK, Park HW, Ahn YS, et al. Transtibial versus tibial inlay techniques for posterior cruciate ligament reconstruction: long-term follow-up study. *Am J Sports Med*. 2014;42(12):2964–2971.
23. Wijdicks CA, Kennedy NI, Goldsmith MT, et al. Kinematic analysis of the posterior cruciate ligament, part 2: a comparison of anatomic single- versus double-bundle reconstruction. *Am J Sports Med*. 2013;41(12):2839–2848.
24. Edson CJ, Fanelli GC, Beck JD. Postoperative rehabilitation of the posterior cruciate ligament. *Sports Med Arthrosc Rev*. 2010;18(4):275–279.
25. Zawodny SR, Miller MD. Complications of posterior cruciate ligament surgery. *Sports Med Arthrosc Rev*. 2010;18(4):269–274.
26. Matava MJ, Sethi NS, Totty WG. Proximity of the posterior cruciate ligament insertion to the popliteal artery as a function of the knee flexion angle: implications for posterior cruciate ligament reconstruction. *Arthroscopy*. 2000;16: 796–804.
27. Fanelli GC, Monahan T. Complications in posterior cruciate ligament and posterolateral corner surgery. *Oper Tech Sports Med*. 2001;9:96–99.
28. Irrgang JJ, Harner CD. Loss of motion following knee ligament reconstruction. *Sports Med*. 1995;19:150–159.
29. Bergfeld JA, Graham SM, Parker RD, et al. A bio-mechanical comparison of posterior cruciate ligament reconstructions using single- and double-bundle tibial inlay techniques. *Am J Sports Med*. 2005;33(7):976–981.
30. Li Y, Li J, Wang J, et al. Comparison of single-bundle and double-bundle isolated posterior cruciate ligament reconstruction with allograft: a prospective, randomized study. *Arthroscopy*. 2014;30(6):695–700.
31. Shin J, Maak TG. Arthroscopic transtibial PCL reconstruction: surgical technique and clinical outcomes. *Curr Rev Musculoskelet Med*. 2018;11:307. https://doi.org/10.1007/s12178-018-9489-9
32. Wang C-J, et al. Effects of knee position, graft tension, and mode of fixation in posterior cruciate ligament reconstruction. *Arthroscopy*. 2002;18(5):496–501.
33. Kim SJ, Kim TE, Jo SB, et al. Comparison of the clinical results of three posterior cruciate ligament reconstruction techniques. *J Bone Joint Surg Am*. 2009;91(11):2543–2549.
34. Lee D-Y, et al. Posterior cruciate ligament reconstruction with transtibial or tibial inlay techniques: a meta-analysis of biomechanical and clinical outcomes. *Am J Sports Med*. 2018;46(11).
35. Polly DW Jr, Callaghan JJ, Sikes RA, et al. The accuracy of selective magnetic resonance imaging compared with the findings of arthroscopy of the knee. *J Bone Joint Surg Am*. 1988;70(2):192–198.

37 Single-Bundle PCL Reconstruction: Inlay Technique

Matthew J. Deasey and Mark D. Miller

HISTORY OF THE TECHNIQUE

The posterior cruciate ligament (PCL) is infrequently injured with an estimated incidence of 3% to 16% of all knee injuries (1). In recent years, a better understanding of the short- and long-term consequences of PCL deficiency has spurred research to find the optimal method for reconstructing this ligament. There have been several techniques of PCL reconstruction developed; however, no single operation has emerged as the gold standard to predictably restore posterior stability and PCL function. We believe that, as with other procedures in orthopedic surgery, the best results stem from procedures that recreate normal anatomy.

The PCL originates at the posterolateral aspect of the medial femoral condyle, inserting extra-synovial in a central sulcus located 1 cm distal to the posterior edge of the tibial plateau. The ligament consists of a large anterolateral portion and a smaller posteromedial portion, each of which has distinct and consistent insertions, in addition to variable meniscofemoral ligaments. These ligaments originate from the lateral meniscus and insert anterior and posterior to the PCL on the medial femoral condyle. The meniscofemoral ligaments (ligaments of Humphrey and Wrisberg) commonly remain intact following PCL rupture and provide some posterior stability to the knee. The smaller posteromedial portion of the PCL consists of shorter fibers that are taut in knee extension. The anterolateral bundle is thicker in diameter, contains the longest fibers, and is taut with knee flexion. This anterolateral bundle of the PCL provides the greatest tensile strength and resists posterior tibial translation beginning at 30 degrees of flexion (2,3).

Historically, most PCL reconstructions have emphasized an anterior-to-posterior approach to recreate the anterolateral bundle. This has been performed through a long oblique interosseous tunnel that creates difficulty with graft passage. These reconstructions require the graft to bend around a large angle at the back of the tibia, which has been dubbed the "killer turn," and has been implicated as a cause of graft failure (4).

The tibial inlay technique was originally developed in Europe and introduced to the United States by Berg (5) in 1995. This method processes a more anatomic reconstruction of the PCL by placing the distal portion of the graft directly in the PCL sulcus, in the posterior aspect of the tibia. Thus, the tibial inlay method avoids creating the "killer turn" of the graft associated with other reconstruction techniques.

This chapter describes a combination of the original concept of the tibial inlay with a posterior approach to the tibia as described by Burks and Schaffer (6). Additional refinements have been added, leading to the technique discussed herein.

INDICATIONS AND CONTRAINDICATIONS

Diagnosis

A thorough history of the events of the injury is needed to make the diagnosis of a PCL injury. Common mechanisms of PCL injury include "dashboard injuries" during motor vehicle accidents or overloading of the knee and quadriceps in hyperflexion during athletic events. Isolated PCL injuries are more likely to be associated with athletic injury than any other mechanism. Acute, isolated PCL rupture is often associated with a smaller hemarthrosis than with anterior cruciate ligament (ACL) injury. Problems with knee instability with cutting or rapid deceleration movements are less common than with ACL-injured patients, although they may give a history recounting a sensation of instability with deceleration, especially when on uneven ground. Many athletes will continue to play on a PCL-injured knee and will not seek medical attention until they develop pain or aching in the days or weeks after the initial injury. Patients with PCL injuries may complain that the knee is just "not right" or have other subjective complaints such as a generalized "aching." Chronic PCL-injured patients will report pain (medial and patellofemoral) with ambulation or descending stairs.

PCL tears frequently occur with concomitant ligamentous, bony, or capsular injuries to the knee. In the trauma setting, these associated injuries can occur up to 60% of the time (7). Following medial or lateral collateral ligament damage, varus or valgus stress to the tibia may result in PCL injury. A hyperextension mechanism of PCL rupture can occur after the ACL is torn and is also associated with a posterior capsular injury. The most common combination is the combined PCL and postero-lateral corner injury, which accounts for up to 60% of combined injuries involving the PCL.

The physical examination is critical to making the correct diagnosis of PCL injury. The posterior drawer test is 90% sensitive and 99% specific for PCL pathology and should be considered the gold standard for diagnosis (8). The posterior sag test, the Godfrey test, the prone drawer, the quadriceps active test, and the dynamic posterior shift test may all be used to confirm a PCL injury. Knee dislocation must be ruled out any time when there is a possibility of a multiligamentous injury. A careful hip and ankle examination as well as a neurovascular examination should be performed, especially if associated with high-energy trauma or a potential knee dislocation. Posterolateral instability is commonly associated with PCL injury and may be diagnosed with external rotation asymmetry, the external rotation recurvatum test, posterolateral and posteromedial drawer test, or the reverse pivot shift test. External rotation asymmetry has been proven to be the most reliable indicator of postero-lateral instability.

Radiographic studies, including plain films, stress radiography, and magnetic resonance imaging (MRI), are used to confirm clinical suspicion for a PCL injury. Plain films can be used to assess for any bony avulsion, tibial plateau fracture, or fibular head fracture ("arcuate fracture") suggesting possible posterolateral corner injury. Stress films are used to quantify posterior instability and can confirm clinical suspicions. Stress radiography is a noninvasive, reproducible, and reliable method for determining the amount of posterior tibial translation (Fig. 37-1).

Historically, the management of PCL injuries has been nonoperative. Conservative management usually involves early brace treatment with progressive range of motion (ROM) exercise, followed by a quadriceps strengthening program early in the post–injury period. Protecting the knee from posterior tibial translation is crucial. Patients are typically restricted from full participation in athletics until 90% of contralateral quadriceps and hamstring strength is obtained. Recently, the accepted management of complete PCL tears has become more aggressive, with a lower threshold for operative treatment. This is the result of long-term follow-up studies that demonstrate worse results with nonoperative treatment. These studies also show radiographic deterioration with time, especially in the medial and patellofemoral compartments (9). The rate of arthrosis severity and progression depends upon the degree of posterior instability, quadriceps weakness, and the presence of additional ligamentous or meniscal damage. Nonoperative treatment is now reserved for asymptomatic, acute isolated PCL tears with mild posteriorly laxity (grades I and II), or chronic isolated PCL injuries that are asymptomatic.

The development of pain and degenerative arthritis is more common in patients with combined PCL injuries. Thus, patients who suffer from PCL injuries in combination with bony avulsion injuries, posterolateral corner injuries, or concomitant ligamentous injuries (grade III medial collateral ligament [MCL] or ACL rupture) require operative reconstruction of the PCL. Combined MCL-PCL and posterolateral corner injuries necessitate operative treatment, as both the primary (PCL) and secondary (PLC) stabilizers to posterior displacement of the tibia relative to the femur are injured. Posterolateral corner injuries should be reconstructed within 2 weeks of injury. Isolated PCL injuries with grade III posterior laxity/instability are also an indication for operative management. Finally, active, young patients who demonstrate <10 mm of posterior laxity on displacement testing (grade II) but with symptomatic complaints of instability or pain should also have the PCL reconstructed.

Another relative indication for the use of the tibial inlay technique involves the revision setting. The tibial inlay technique is useful when a previous nonanatomic reconstruction has been

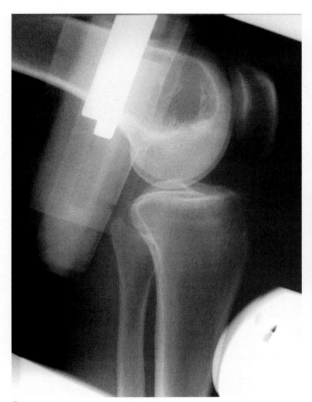
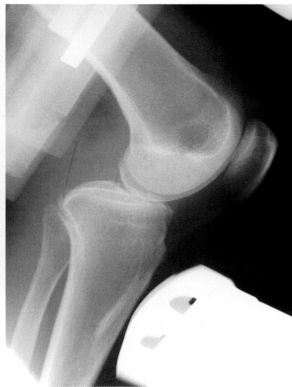

A   B

FIGURE 37-1

Stress radiography. **A:** Normal stress radiograph. Note that there is no posterior displacement of the tibia as the drawer test is applied. **B:** Abnormal stress radiograph. Note the posterior displacement of the tibia suggesting PCL injury.

performed. This avoids complications associated with previous tibial tunnels that are too wide in diameter or too proximal on the tibia. Patients with tibial osteopenia, previous fracture, or previous osteotomy may benefit from the tibial inlay technique to prevent proximal graft migration (10).

When operative management is indicated, the type and site of injury is critical in choosing the correct surgical procedure. Bony avulsion injuries involving the PCL insertion at the posterior tibia are treated with primary repair using lag screws or suture fixation. Mid-substance tears of the PCL require ligament reconstruction, which attempts to reproduce normal anatomy. We believe that the tibial inlay technique procedures have the most anatomic PCL reconstruction.

The tibial inlay technique is contraindicated in patients who have had prior vascular surgical procedures, especially those who have had remote vascular repairs.

SURGICAL TECHNIQUE

Preoperative Planning

Prior to surgery, it is necessary to diagnose concomitant knee pathology and to quantify the degree of posterior instability. With the assistance of stress radiography (Fig. 37-1A and B) or instrumented ligament testing using the KT-1000/2000 (MedMetric, San Diego, CA), PCL instability may be quantified (11,12) (Fig. 37-2). Plain radiographs are used to exclude associated bony injury and to assess radiographic signs of arthrosis. MRI is also used as an adjunct in diagnosis and development of treatment plan. MRI is nearly 100% sensitive and specific for diagnosing PCL tears (13). In addition, MRI may be used to diagnose meniscal injuries, which should be addressed at the time of surgery. The arthroscopic examination is used as the final confirmation of intracapsular pathology (14). At the time of surgery, arthroscopy provides direct visualization in the knee's internal structures, allowing the surgeon to assess for the presence of complete versus partial PCL tears, bony avulsions, ACL pseudolaxity, and degenerative changes.

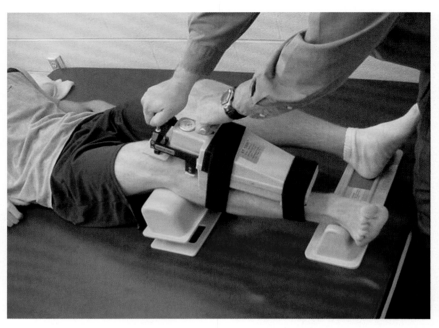

FIGURE 37-2

KT-1000. KT-1000-developed to provide objective measurements of sagittal plane motions of the tibia relative to the femur.

Anesthesia, Positioning, and Setup

For anesthesia, we prefer the use of a general anesthetic to allow for proper positioning and control during the procedure. Often, we will employ the use of a femoral or sciatic nerve block that is placed prior to surgery for use in postoperative pain control. Epidural catheter placement is also an option for use in postoperative pain control.

Once adequate anesthesia is obtained, an examination under anesthesia is performed prior to final positioning and preparation of the patient. This is useful for confirmation of ligamentous laxity associated with PCL rupture and for ruling out previously unrecognized combined knee injuries. A broad-spectrum cephalosporin antibiotic or a suitable alternative is given preoperatively. Following examination, the patient is placed in the lateral decubitus position with the injured leg up. The contralateral leg remains extended, with padding placed around the fibular head in order to protect the common peroneal nerve (Fig. 37-3). The injured leg is abducted and externally rotated at the hip, flexed at the knee, and locked in place with a commercially available leg holder. From this position, graft harvest, arthroscopy, and drilling of the femoral tunnel are easily accomplished (Fig. 37-4). The posterior approach and the tibial inlay are performed

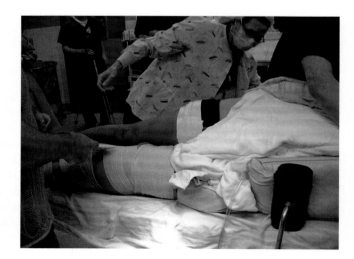

FIGURE 37-3

Preoperative positioning. The patient is placed in the lateral decubitus position with the contralateral leg padded.

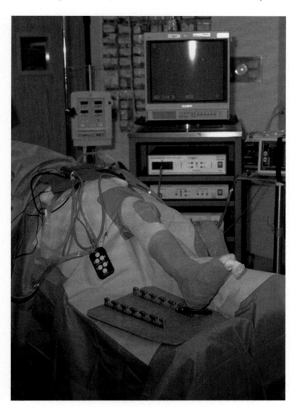

FIGURE 37-4

External rotation and abduction of the leg allow for graft harvest and arthroscopy.

with leg positioned in extension, neutral rotation, and resting on a Mayo stand. Finally, a tourniquet is placed on the proximal thigh, and the patient is prepped and draped in the usual sterile fashion.

Patellar Graft Harvest

Following preparation and draping, an 8-cm longitudinal incision is extended from the inferior pole of the patella to the tibial tubercle centered on the medial aspect of the patellar tendon. Care is taken to preserve saphenous nerve branches. The dissection is taken down to the paratenon, and skin flaps are raised. The paratenon is carefully dissected off the patellar tendon both proximally and distally for use in later closure. A central third 11- to 12-mm patellar tendon graft with 20-mm bone-patellar tendon-bone blocks is harvested, taking special care to make parallel incisions. A graft of this size can be readily obtained from most patients and is of suit length to negotiate the angle needed for entry into the femoral tunnel.

The tibial bone plug is trimmed to achieve a trapezoidal shape with a flattened surface, and a 3.2-mm hole is drilled centrally. This hole is then tapped in preparation for tibial inlay fixation using a 4.5-mm bicortical screw (Fig. 37-5). The patellar bone plug is sized to fit through a 10- to 12-mm

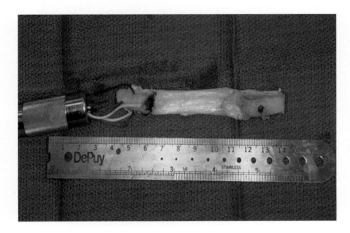

FIGURE 37-5

PCL patellar tendon graft. Note the preparation of the tibial plug for passage of a 4.5-mm bicortical screw. Patellar side with tapered bone plug and perpendicular sutures for femoral graft passage.

tunnel. The patellar bone plug is cylindrically contoured, tapering the leading edge such that it is bullet shaped for ease of insertion. Two perpendicularly oriented drill holes are placed approximately 5 and 10 mm from the distal tip of the patellar end of the graft. Two no. 5 nonabsorbable sutures are placed through the leading edge of the bone plug at the drill hole sites. These sutures will later be used to manipulate the patellar bone plug into the femoral tunnel. A no. 2 Ethibond or TiCron suture is also placed at the patella-bone-tendon junction and will be used laterally to toggle the graft, permitting easier entry into the femoral tunnel. Finally, all bone plug trimmings should be saved for use as bone graft.

Given that the native PCL is comprised of two distinct bundles, a novel technique for double-bundle reconstruction has been described (15). These authors recommend the use of Achilles tendon allograft for the anterolateral bundle and tibialis anterior or semitendinosus allograft for the posteromedial bundle. The surgical technique described in this chapter could be modified to pass these two grafts. Despite modest advantages in rotational stability in biomechanical testing, no evidence of clinical improvement with double-bundle reconstruction has yet been found (16).

Arthroscopy and Femoral Tunnel Placement

The affected limb is held in abduction, external rotation, and flexion by the leg holder. Standard anterolateral and medial arthroscopic portals are created. A thorough diagnostic arthroscopy is performed to confirm PCL deficiency, to identify comorbid intra-articular pathology, and to landmarks for reconstruction. Special attention should be directed to the lateral joint space of patients who have excessive opening with varus stress. These patients should be evaluated with a high index of suspicion for posterolateral corner injuries (17). Following PCL débridement, all meniscal and cartilage work should be performed, and uninjured meniscofemoral ligaments should be left intact. After débridement of the PCL femoral footprint, a standard PCL femoral guide is placed into the knee via the anteromedial portal. This guide will be used to place the guide pin for the femoral tunnel. The drill guide is placed in the anterior portion of the PCL femoral insertion site, located 8 to 10 mm behind the medial femoral condyle articular surface at the 1 o'clock position in the notch for a right knee and 11 o'clock for a left knee. A small 2- to 3-cm incision is made at the superior and the medial borders of the patella. The vastus medialis oblique muscle fibers are split or retracted, and the external tunnel guide is positioned on the cortical surface of the femur away from the articular surface of the medial femoral condyle (Fig. 37-6A). A guide pin is inserted from outside in and identified on the intra-articular medial femoral condyle (Fig. 37-6B). After confirming the guide pin to be in the anterolateral PCL bundle footprint, the tunnel is overdrilled from outside in

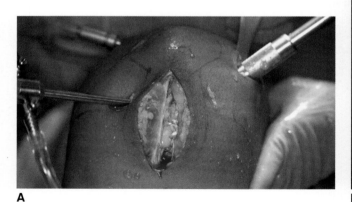
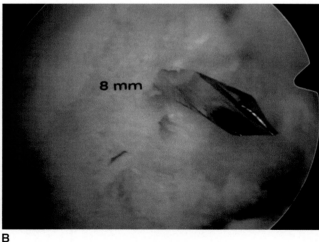

A   **B**

FIGURE 37-6

Femoral tunnel placement. **A:** The vastus medialis oblique muscle fibers are split and the external tunnel guide is positioned on the cortical surface of the femur away from the articular surface of the medial femoral condyle. **B:** A guide pin is inserted from outside in and identified on the intra-articular medial femoral condyle. Note that the guide pin is to be in the anterolateral PCL bundle footprint approximately 8 mm behind the medial femoral condyle articular surface.

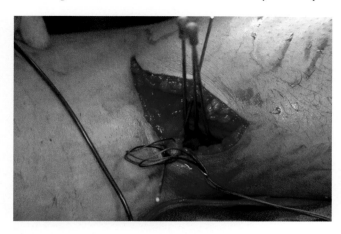

FIGURE 37-7

Positioning for the posterior approach to the knee.

with a cannulated reamer-sized appropriately for the graft. A small curette is placed into the joint to prevent the guide pin from injuring any intra-articular structures. Bone graft should be saved from the flutes of the reamer. Following drilling, the posterior aspect of the tunnel is rasped, or smoothed, with a reverse cutting reamer to decrease abrasive forces on the graft. Once the femoral tunnel is fully prepared for graft placement, a looped 18-gauge wire is introduced in the tunnel from outside to inside. The guide wire is passed into the posterior aspect of the knee joint and will be used later to initiate and facilitate graft passage (Fig. 37-7). At this time, the pump/inflow is turned off, and the arthroscope and the equipment are removed from the knee. Attention is directed to the inlay portion of the case.

Posterior Approach and Inlay

The patient is repositioned, placing the injured leg on the padded Mayo stand in full extension and neutral rotation (Fig. 37-8). A transverse incision is made in the flexion crease. The medial head of the gastrocnemius muscle is exposed by incising the medial aspect of the gastrocnemius fascia both transversely and distally on the medial side. Blunt dissection is used to develop an interval between the gastrocnemius and the semimembranosus muscles. The medial sural cutaneous nerve must be kept in mind at this point, although it usually perforates the deep fascia distal to the incision. Once the interval is developed, the medial head of the gastrocnemius muscle is retracted laterally, exposing the posterior knee capsule. The middle and the medial geniculate arteries may be encountered near the mid-posterior capsule and can be ligated if necessary. The medial head of the gastrocnemius is surprisingly mobile, but it is occasionally necessary to release a portion of its tedious origin medially in order to gain adequate exposure. Slight knee flexion will also allow for greater lateral retraction of the medial head of the gastrocnemius and increase exposure. A cadaveric study previously demonstrated that the gastrocnemius muscle protects the popliteal artery during lateral retraction,

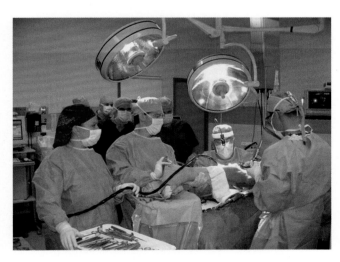

FIGURE 37-8

Looped 18-gauge wire used for passage of patella end through arthrotomy.

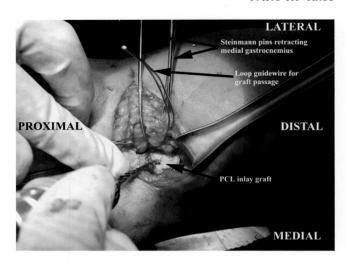

FIGURE 37-9

Tibial inlay. Note the Steinmann pins used for lateral retraction of the gastrocnemius and the looped guide wire for passage of the graft into the femoral tunnel. The tibial portion of the patellar tendon graft is placed into the unicortical window and drilled from posterior to anterior.

and this exposure is safe, although one must be aware of anatomic variations (18). Steinmann pins can be placed posteriorly into the tibia and bent laterally in order to assist with retraction of the medial head of the gastrocnemius.

Next, the PCL sulcus is palpated through the fibers of the popliteus muscle. The sulcus is defined by a large medial and a smaller lateral bump. Electrocautery and an elevator are used to dissect the popliteus muscle from its origin, exposing the posterior tibial cortex. The position of the PCL sulcus is reconfirmed at the central aspect of the posterior tibial. A generous capsular incision is made vertically, contiguous with the PCL sulcus. Any remaining scar tissue or PCL remnant is débrided at this time. At this point, the preplaced 18-gauge passing wire may be retrieved through the new posterior arthrotomy site (Fig. 37-7). The 18-gauge wire will later be used to pass the no. 5 nonabsorbable sutures and graft through the femoral notch and into the femoral tunnel. A trough is developed at the PCL insertion site using an osteotome, burr, and tamp. The inlay site is fashioned such that it matches the size and the shape of the tibial portion of the PCL graft. The graft is inlaid into the unicortical window. The graft/bone plug is carefully adjusted such that it fits snugly within the trough, flush with the posterior tibia. Before securing the graft, a second 18-gauge looped guide wire is passed from the anteromedial arthroscopic portal and out of the posterior arthrotomy (Fig. 37-9). This looped guide wire is used to pull the no. 2 Ethibond suture out of the anteromedial portal. The patellar end of the graft is then passed into the knee joint and the femoral tunnel using the 18-gauge wire and no. 5 sutures.

After all necessary sutures and the patellar end of the bone-patellar tendon-bone graft are passed into the knee joint, the tibial bone plug is secured by lagging 4.5-mm bicortical screw and washer through the predrilled tibial bone plug hole and into the anterior cortex of the tibia (Fig. 37-10). Additional fixation with a second screw or a staple is sometimes beneficial.

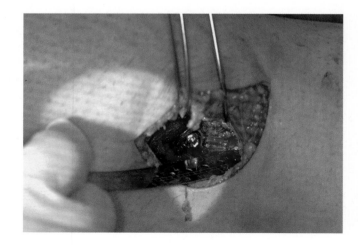

FIGURE 37-10

Inlay fixation. Tibial inlay following placement of a 4.5-mm posterior to anterior bicortical screw.

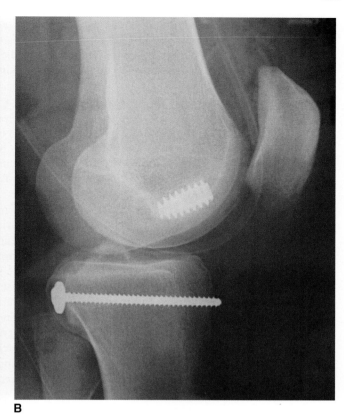

A   **B**

FIGURE 37-11

Postoperative films **(A)** AP and **(B)** lateral radiograph of a patient's knee after PCL tibial inlay technique.

Graft Passage and Fixation

Using the original looped 18-gauge wire as a graft passer, the patellar end of the graft is passed through the posterior arthrotomy, into the notch, and then into the femoral tunnel. The knee is then passively taken through a full ROM cycles while palpating the tibial inlay site in order to ensure that there are no hang-ups at the posterior arthrotomy. The leg is then repositioned for arthroscopy and final graft placement. The no. 5 and no. 2 sutures should be pulled through the femoral tunnel and anteromedial arthroscopic portal, respectively, if this has not been already performed. The no. 5 suture is used to pull the patellar bone plug into the femoral tunnel, while the no. 2 suture is used to toggle the graft for easier passage. The graft is optimally positioned with the patellar-bone plug-tendon junction located at the articular margin of the femoral tunnel. This graft/tunnel angle is sometimes referred to as the "critical corner" because poor positioning can contribute to excessive sheer stress and early graft failure (19). While keeping moderate tension on the no. 5 suture, the knee is again passively cycled through full ROM cycles in order to rule out kinks in the graft and reconfirm a lack of impedance at the posterior arthrotomy site.

The graft is tensioned by placing an anterior drawer on a knee flexed to 70 to 80 degrees while maintaining the desired intra-articular position of the patellar-bone plug-tendon junction. Proximal fixation is achieved with a 9-mm by 20-mm interference screw. Additional fixation with a plastic button tied with the no. 5 nonabsorbable sutures over the cortex at the tunnel entrance is also utilized. Intraoperative radiographs should be obtained to ensure proper graft and hardware placement (Fig. 37-11A and B).

Wound Closure

Prior to wound closure, all bone graft from femoral tunnel drilling and graft preparation should be packed into the patella and tibial tubercle harvest sites. Anteriorly, the paratenon is closed in an interrupted fashion using 0 Vicryl sutures over the patellar tendon and previous bone harvest sites. All subcutaneous tissue and skin layers are closed in standard fashion, and a sterile dressing is applied.

At the end of the procedure, the posterior capsule is closed and sutured with no. 0 absorbable suture. A one-eighth inch closed drain is placed deep to the medial head of the gastrocnemius muscle for hematoma prevention. The medial gastrocnemius is allowed to fall into place, the subcutaneous layers are approximated, and the skin is closed in a routine fashion.

TECHNICAL ALTERNATIVES AND PITFALLS

The surgeon should be particularly vigilant during certain periods of the PCL reconstruction in order to prevent operative complications. One potential pitfall is the failure to recognize an associated injury. Isolated PCL injury is uncommon; thus, most injuries will involve other knee structures. This can lead to residual laxity on the posterior drawer test and present as recurrent symptomatic laxity following reconstruction.

Avascular necrosis (AVN) of the medial femoral condyle has been reported after PCL reconstruction. Patients will usually present with medial knee pain and tenderness to palpation of the medial femoral condyle. To avoid this potential problem, care must be taken to start the femoral tunnel 8 to 10 mm posterior to the articular margin as the etiology secondary to femoral drilling is too close to the articular surface or the extensive soft tissue dissection over the medial femoral condyle. AVN of the medial femoral condyle can present months to years after surgery and is thought to be caused by local trauma to the subchondral bone blood supply causing increased pressure in the area. By using a more proximal entry site, maximal subchondral bone is preserved, thereby reducing the risks of AVN. It is also critical to ensure that the graft does not kink or hang up during passage from the posterior arthrotomy, through the femoral notch, and into the femoral tunnel. This complication decreases the stability of the reconstruction, causing persistent posterior laxity, but can be easily avoided by palpating the PCL inlay site and using direct arthroscopic visualization of the graft while the knee is taken through passive full ROM cycles. Persistent laxity can also be caused by overly aggressive rehabilitation, poor graft fixation or placement, and a previously stated failure to recognize any associated injuries. In addition, particular care should be taken to ensure that the patellar bone tendon junction is located at the intra-articular margin of the femoral tunnel in order to decrease graft degradation at this "critical corner." Finally, we previously used a hockey stick–shaped incision for the posterior approach to the knee. This approach was associated with an increased incidence of wound breakdown superiorly. By using a transverse incision on the flexion crease of the posterior knee, we nearly eliminated the problem of wound breakdown, while providing a better cosmetic result (Fig. 37-12).

The most feared potential complication with any posterior exposure to the knee is vascular injury. Injury to the vascular structures is always a risk during posterior knee exposure, especially in the revision setting where normal anatomy can be altered secondary to previous scar formation. The surgeon should be aware of potential vascular anomalies during the exposure as even the superficial dissection in the semimembranosus-gastrocnemius interval can lead to inadvertent injury.

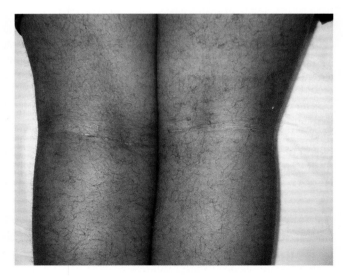

FIGURE 37-12

Using a transverse incision at the flexion crease of the posterior knee decreases problem of wound breakdown while providing a better cosmetic result.

Subperiosteal dissection of the popliteus provides additional soft tissue protection against any anatomic variants. The use of k-wires or Steinman pins allows for continuous retraction during posterior dissection, thus avoiding repetitive repositioning of retractors and further potential for injury.

REHABILITATION

In the immediate postoperative period, the extended leg is placed in a hinged knee brace. Special care is taken to support the tibia and prevent posterior translation. On postoperative day 1, the patient is permitted to bear weight as tolerated and ambulate with crutches. When bearing weight, the patient is always in the brace locked at 0 degrees. Continuous passive motion, isometric quadriceps training, and straight leg raises should be implemented into the rehabilitation program as soon as the patient can tolerate such activity. Partner-assisted ROM exercises are also useful in the immediate postoperative period. These exercises are performed with the patient in the prone position in order to prevent posterior translation of the tibia. In the early postoperative period, weeks 0 to 4, gravity-assisted flexion exercises to 90 degrees and closed-chain exercises for quadriceps strengthening are important. At 1 month postop, the patient is allowed to transition to unlocking the brace for ambulation and activities under supervision of the therapist. The patient may start to wean off crutches as tolerated. When the patient exhibits independent quadriceps control, he or she may progress to open-chain extension exercise, mini squats, and isometric exercises. At 2 months, the patient may add in stationary bike or stairmaster activities as well as leg presses within available ROM. From months 3 to 9, the patient may progress within his or her level of function and symptoms. The patient should ideally be allowed to return to normal activities 9 to 12 months postoperatively if the knee is stable, with full ROM and quadriceps strength equal to the contralateral leg.

OUTCOMES AND FUTURE DIRECTIONS

Even among experts, PCL reconstruction is a relatively uncommon procedure, and there are a limited number of published reports in the literature. A growing body of data suggests that the tibial inlay technique is effective at decreasing posterior knee instability with good long-term results. A 2-year follow-up study performed by Jung et al. (20) in Korea demonstrated that the average posterior displacement on stress radiography decreased from 10.8 to 3.4 m, with 90% of patients reporting a satisfactory outcome. Likewise, Cooper (21,22) has presented two reports showing good results using the tibial inlay. The standard transtibial tunnel technique of PCL reconstruction has been popular, but biomechanical studies raise concern about the long-term outcomes of this method. A cadaveric, matched pair comparison of the tibial inlay versus tibial tunnel techniques found that the tibial tunnel group had greater anterior-posterior laxity postoperatively. Upon evaluation of the grafts, the tibial tunnel group revealed greater evidence of mechanical degradation at the acute angle (23). These findings were confirmed by a second matched pair biomechanical comparison that demonstrated the tibial inlay method to be superior to the tibial tunnel technique with respect to graft failure, permanent graft lengthening, and graft thinning (24).

REFERENCES

1. Miyasaka KC, Daniel DM, Stone ML, et al. The incidence of knee ligament injuries in the general population. *Am J Knee Surg.* 1991;4:3–8.
2. Butler DL, Noyes FR, Grood ES. Ligamentous restraints to anterior-posterior drawer in the human knee: a biomechanical study. *J Bone Joint Surg Am.* 1980;63:259–270.
3. Gollehon DL, Torzili PA, Warren RF. The role of the posterolateral and cruciate ligaments in the stability of the human knee; a biomechanical study. *J Bone Joint Surg Am.* 1987;69:233–242.
4. Miller MD, Bergeld JA, Folwer PJ, et al. The posterior ligament injured knee: principles of evaluation and treatment. *Instr Course Lect.* 1999;48:199–207.
5. Berg EE. Posterior cruciate ligament tibial inlay reconstruction. *Arthroscopy.* 1995;11:69–76.
6. Burks RT, Schaffer JJ. A simplified approach to the tibial attachment of the posterior cruciate ligament. *Clin Orthop.* 1990;254:216–219.
7. Fanelli GC, Edson CJ. Posterior cruciate ligament injuries in trauma patients; part II. *Arthroscopy.* 1995;11:526–529.
8. Miller MD, Johnson DL, Harner CD, et al. Posterior cruciate ligament injuries. *Orthop Rev.* 1993;22:1201–1210.
9. Dejour H, Walch G, Peyrot J, et al. The natural history of rupture of the posterior cruciate ligament. *Rev Chir Orthop Reparatrice Appar Mot.* 1988;2:112–120.
10. Noyes FR, Medvecky MJ, Bhargava M. Arthroscopically assisted quadriceps double-bundle tibial inlay posterior cruciate ligament construction: an analysis of techniques and a safe operative approach to the popliteal fossa. *Arthroscopy.* 2003;10:894–905.

11. Puddu G. Radiographic view for PCL injuries: instructional course lecture. Paper presented at: Western Pacific Orthopaedic Association meeting, Taipei, Taiwan, November 1997.

12. Hewett TE, Noyes FR, Lee MD. Diagnosis of complete and partial posterior cruciate ligament ruptures: stress radiography compared with KT-1000 arthrometer and posterior drawer testing. *Am J Sports Med*. 1997;25:648–655.

13. Gross ML, Grover JS, Bassett LW, et al. Magnetic resonance imaging of the posterior cruciate ligament: clinical use to improve diagnostic accuracy. *Am J Sports Med*. 1992;20:732–737.

14. Fanelli GC, Giannotti BG, Edson CJ. The posterior cruciate ligament arthroscopic evaluation and treatment: current concepts review. *Arthroscopy*. 1994;10:673–688.

15. Chahla J, Nitri M, Civitarese D, et al. Anatomic double-bundle posterior cruciate ligament reconstruction. *Arthrosc Tech*. 2016;5(1):e149–56. doi:10.1016/j.eats.2015.10.014.

16. Tucker CJ, Joyner PW, Endres NK. Single versus double-bundle PCL reconstruction: scientific rationale and clinical evidence. *Curr Rev Musculoskelet Med*. 2018;11(2):285–289.

17. LaPrade RF. Arthroscopic evaluation of the lateral compartment of knees with grade 3 posterolateral knee complex injuries. *Am J Sports Med*. 1997;25:596–602.

18. Miller MD, Line AJ, Gonzales J, et al. Vascular risk associated with a posterior approach for posterior cruciate ligament reconstruction using the tibial inlay technique. *J Knee Surg*. 2002;15:137–140.

19. Mariani PP, Adriani E, Bellelii A, et al. Magnetic resonance imaging of tunnel placement in posterior cruciate ligament reconstruction. *Arthroscopy*. 1999;15:733–740.

20. Jung Y-B, Tae S-K, Jin W-J, et al. Reconstruction of posterior cruciate ligament by the modified tibial inlay method. In: *Proceedings of the 20002 Annual Meeting of the American Academy of Orthopaedic Surgery*. Vol. 3. Dallas, TX: AAOS; 2002:602.

21. Cooper DE. Revision PCL reconstruction with the tibial inlay technique. In: *AOSSM Proceedings*. Keystone, CO: AOSSM; 2001.

22. Cooper DE, Stewart D. Posterior cruciate ligament reconstruction using single-bundle patella tendon graft with tibial fixation. 2- to 10-year follow-up. *Am J Sports Med*. 2004;32:346–360.

23. Bergfeld JA, McAllister DK, Parker RD, et al. A biomechanical comparison of posterior cruciate ligament reconstruction techniques. *Am J Sports Med*. 2001;29:129–136.

24. Markolf KLK, Zemanovic JR, McAllister DR. Cyclic loading of posterior cruciate ligament replacements fixed with tibial tunnel and tibial inlay methods. *J Bone Joint Surg Am*. 2002;84:518–524.

38 Double-Bundle PCL Reconstruction

Christopher Kim and Scott G. Kaar

HISTORY OF THE TECHNIQUE

Posterior cruciate ligament (PCL) reconstruction techniques continue to evolve. The PCL is the primary restraint to posterior tibial translation and is composed of the anterolateral (ALB) and posteromedial (PMB) bundles. Recent biomechanical studies have also suggested that the PCL resists internal rotation, particularly between 90 and 120 degrees of flexion (1). Traditional single-bundle reconstruction has focused on reconstructing the ALB to restore anteroposterior stability. Similar to anterior cruciate ligament (ACL) reconstructions, PCL surgery has evolved from isometric to anatomic reconstructions. These techniques have ranged from the transtibial technique, with the reported concern of the "killer turn," (2) to the tibial inlay technique requiring a posterior knee incision. Despite the increased understanding of PCL anatomy and surgical techniques, there have been reports suggesting residual laxity after a single-bundle procedure (3). Although the ALB and PMB were traditionally thought to have provided stability in flexion and extension, respectively, studies have found them to act codominantly (4,5). Therefore, some have suggested reconstructing both the ALB and PMB to best simulate stability of the native PCL. The significance of the technique is still unknown; however, some studies have suggested improved stability and outcomes with double-bundle techniques (6–9). In both single- and double-bundle procedures, no single operation has emerged as the gold standard. The variation in double-bundle reconstruction techniques mirrors that of single-bundle procedures. Namely, there are variations in transtibial versus inlay techniques, graft options, fixation methods, and tunnel positioning. This chapter describes an anatomic double-bundle reconstruction through the traditional transtibial drilling technique using an Achilles allograft.

INDICATIONS AND CONTRAINDICATIONS

Diagnosis and Physical Examination

A PCL injury may occur in isolation or combined with other ligamentous, meniscal, capsular, or bony injuries. Isolated injuries typically occur in the athlete during sports, while combined injuries are usually traumatic such as "dash-board" injuries in motor vehicle accidents. Acutely, patients with isolated injuries will present with pain and a small hemarthrosis. They describe injury during either hyperflexion or extension of the knee. They may also describe a sense of instability, particularly with a flexed knee. Symptoms such as pain and instability may not be as pronounced as with an ACL rupture however, and a thorough history and physical examination are important. It is important to recognize concomitant injuries, which can occur 60% of the time (10). The most commonly injured structure is the posterolateral corner (up to 60%), although associated medial collateral, lateral collateral, and ACL injuries also occur frequently.

The physical examination should begin with a general inspection, and this should always be compared to the contralateral knee. The amount of swelling, deformity, and any bruising should be noted. A thorough neurovascular examination should be performed, particularly when suspecting a multiligamentous knee injury. A hip and ankle exam should be done to rule out other injuries. The gold standard for diagnosing a PCL rupture is the posterior drawer test, which is 90% sensitive and 99% specific (Fig. 38-1) (11). Other tests for PCL injury include the quadriceps activation test, posterior sag test, and the dynamic posterior shift test. It is important to rule out other ligamentous injuries, including to the posterolateral corner. Prone dial testing can be done to check for asymmetry in external rotation to evaluate the posterolateral corner.

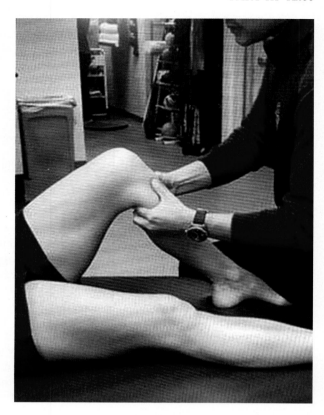

FIGURE 38-1

The posterior drawer test—The knee is placed in 90 degrees of flexion and then a posteriorly directed force is applied to the proximal tibia.

Radiographic studies may show posterior subluxation of the tibia, particularly if stress radiographs are performed. Plain films can also show bony avulsions or tibial plateau fractures. Ultimately, MRI is highly specific and sensitive for diagnosing PCL injury.

Traditionally, most PCL injuries have been treated nonoperatively. Reconstruction was typically reserved for patients with symptomatic instability despite conservative treatment, in the setting of a multiligament knee injury, or sometimes in elite athletes. As our understanding of PCL anatomy and function increases and as surgical techniques improve, the indications for PCL reconstruction have expanded. Indeed, there have been reports of poor clinical and radiographic outcomes with conservative treatment as well (12). The PCL should be reconstructed when the injury is associated with other ligamentous injuries, as these patients treated nonoperatively will often develop pain, arthritis, and symptomatic instability. Isolated ruptures have traditionally been treated nonoperatively. However, given some reports of poor outcomes, many have lowered their threshold for recommending surgery. Likewise, athletes with grade II injuries (<10 mm laxity) can also be recommended for surgery if there are symptoms of chronic pain and instability. Isolated PCL ruptures can be treated nonoperatively if the patient is asymptomatic, only has mild laxity (grades I and II), or if the injury is chronic.

SURGICAL TECHNIQUE

Preoperative Planning

In almost all situations, an MRI is performed in addition to radiographs to confirm PCL injury and evaluate for other ligamentous involvements. It is important to note associated pathology that should be addressed at the time of surgery, such as chondral or meniscal injuries. Examination under anesthesia is the optimal time to carefully assess the patient's level of instability with care to compare the examination with the contralateral uninjured knee. Arthroscopic examination ultimately serves as final confirmation of PCL rupture and allows direct visual diagnosis of other intra-articular pathology.

When planning for the transtibial drilling technique, one should plan tunnel locations carefully, particularly when creating multiple tunnels such as in a multiligamentous reconstruction. The placement of hardware, such as screws and suspensory devices, should also be planned, so there is adequate bone for fixation. Any bony deformities from previous fractures or coronal plane malalignment should be noted as well.

Anesthesia, Positioning, and Setup

The type of anesthesia should be discussed with the anesthesiologist prior to surgery. Options include general anesthetic or a spinal anesthetic. Regional nerve blocks are often applied either before or after surgery to assist with postoperative pain control. We prefer use of general anesthesia in addition to a femoral and/or sciatic nerve block prior to surgery.

After general anesthesia is administered, the patient is positioned supine on the operating table. Examination under anesthesia of both lower extremities is performed, confirming the grade of PCL laxity, checking for other ligamentous injuries, and noting range of motion. A well-padded tourniquet is applied on the upper thigh, and a small bump is placed under the ipsilateral hip to prevent excessive external rotation of the operative extremity. We place a sand bag distally on the bed on which to rest the foot when flexing the knee to 90 degrees during arthroscopy (Fig. 38-2). Particularly for PCL reconstructions, we prefer this positioning, as it allows the posterior knee structures to fall back while working in the posterior compartment. A post is placed laterally to help valgus stressing during arthroscopy and to prevent the knee from falling laterally while positioned in flexion. We use a sterile bump and place this between the knee and post while the knee is flexed. It is important to position the post proximal enough to allow external rotation and figure-4 positioning during arthroscopy. The arthroscopy monitor and towers are positioned near the head of the patient on the side ipsilateral to the operative extremity. This allows easy visualization while working on the medial side of the knee.

Graft Preparation

An Achilles tendon-bone allograft is used (Fig. 38-3). We place the single calcaneal bone plug within the tibial tunnel and the prepared soft tissue ends of the Achilles in the two femoral tunnels. A 12 × 25 mm bone plug is prepared, and we pass two No. 5 nonabsorbable sutures in perpendicular orientations to act as grasping sutures and for later backup fixation. The Achilles tendon is then cut from the distal end in line with the fibers using scissors to create two tendon ends. The cut is stopped approximately 3 to 5 cm from the bone plug. The medial tendon is tubularized and prepared to pass

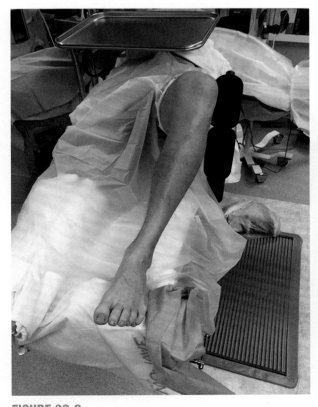

FIGURE 38-2

Patient positioning.

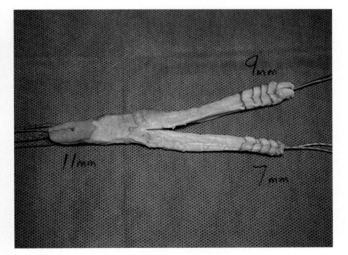

FIGURE 38-3

Prepared Achilles tendon allograft—Sutures from the two tendon ends are different colors for easy identification within the intercondylar notch. The 9-mm tendon will serve as the anterolateral bundle, and the 7-mm tendon is for the posteromedial bundle.

through a 7-mm femoral tunnel. This is to act as the PMB. The lateral tendon is prepared for a 9-mm femoral tunnel and will be used for the ALB. At least 25 mm of tendon length are whip-stitched at the ends of each tendon, and these will later be used as passing/grasping sutures and for backup fixation. We ensure that the sutures from each tendon are of different colors for later identification within the notch. We like to ensure that the tendon lengths are at least 180 mm from the bone plug. The allograft is then placed under tension, and a moist gauze is placed over the tendon to ensure tissue quality during tunnel preparation.

Arthroscopy and Tunnel Preparation

The procedure always begins with a diagnostic arthroscopy to confirm PCL rupture and identify associated intra-articular pathology. The injured PCL is debrided and we make note of the femoral and tibial footprints. Other meniscal or cartilage pathologies are then addressed.

We prefer to begin with tibial tunnel creation, as this can be the most challenging. The knee is flexed to approximately 90 degrees on the bed with the foot resting on the distal sand bag. This allows the popliteal tissues to fall posteriorly creating a larger safe zone from the posterior neurovascular structures. We then switch to a 70-degree arthroscope to help visualize the posteromedial compartment and the PCL tibial footprint. A posteromedial portal is created using a spinal needle to confirm accurate trajectory. We use both an arthroscopic shaver and radiofrequency device, introduced through the posteromedial portal, to clear the tibial footprint (Fig. 38-4). A tibial PCL guide set at 55 degrees is introduced through the anteromedial portal and positioned for the guide pin to exit at the center of the PCL footprint, typically 13 to 15 mm distal to the articular surface. An approximately 3- to 4-cm longitudinal incision is made over the proximal medial tibia to introduce the guide pin. Intraoperative fluoroscopy may be used to confirm guide pin placement, which should be about 6 to 7 mm proximal to the champagne glass drop-off on the lateral view and just at the medial aspect of the lateral tibial eminence on the anteroposterior view. A reamer is used to create a 12-mm tibial tunnel. Both tunnel apertures are then cleared of debris using a shaver and curette. The tunnel is temporarily plugged at its anterior tibial entry to prevent fluid extravasation.

The femoral tunnels are subsequently drilled. A PCL femoral guide is used to place a guide pin from outside-in. We make an approximately 3- to 4-cm longitudinal incision on the medial thigh to introduce the pins (Fig. 38-5). The guide pin for the ALB tunnel is positioned at the 11 o'clock position (for the left knee) and 6 mm proximal to the articular edge. The guide pin for the PMB is placed in the 9 o'clock position and 6 mm proximal to the articular edge (Fig. 38-6). We recommend placing both pins prior to reaming to ensure good tunnel position. A 9-mm acorn reamer is used to create the ALB tunnel from outside-in. Then, a 7-mm tunnel is created in the same manner for the PMB. We try to have at least 2 mm of bone bridging the two femoral tunnels (Fig. 38-7). An

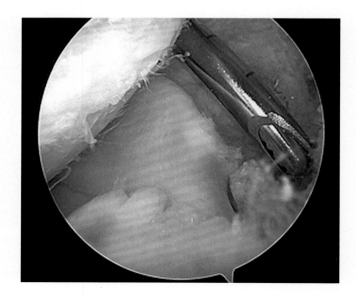

FIGURE 38-4

An arthroscopic shaver and radiofrequency device can be placed through the posteromedial portal to clear the PCL footprint.

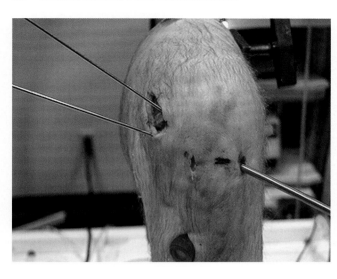

FIGURE 38-5

Guide pins for the two femoral tunnels are placed from outside-in through a medial incision.

arthroscopic shaver, curette, and radiofrequency device are then used to clear the tunnel apertures to facilitate smooth graft passage.

Graft Passage and Fixation

We use a heavy suture for passing the graft placed into the tibial tunnel in a retrograde direction. The suture is grasped intra-articularly and pulled out through the anteromedial portal. We then place all the sutures from the two tendon ends into the looped end of the passing suture, which are then pulled up into the tibial tunnel, into the joint, and out the anteromedial portal. The sutures of the two tendon ends are now exiting the anteromedial portal. We then pull on these sutures to deliver both tendons up the tibial tunnel and into the intercondylar notch (Fig. 38-8). This is stopped when the tendon ends reach the apertures of the two femoral tunnels. Then, an arthroscopic ring grasper is introduced from outside-in through each femoral tunnel (Fig. 38-9). The suture ends from the ALB are grasped and pulled out the ALB femoral tunnel. This is repeated for the sutures of the PMB. These sutures are then individually pulled to deliver each prepared tendon up through their respective femoral

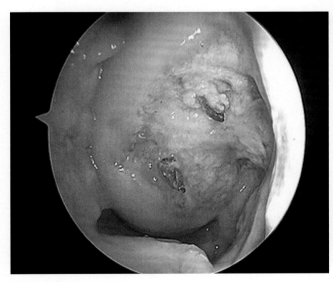

FIGURE 38-6

Guide pin placement is checked arthroscopically.

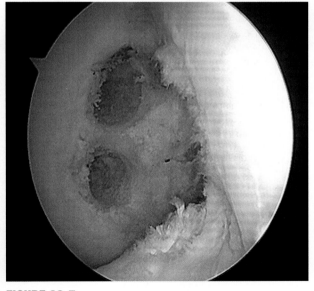

FIGURE 38-7

Two femoral tunnels are created, with at least 2 mm of bone remaining between the tunnels.

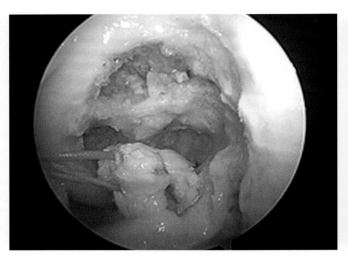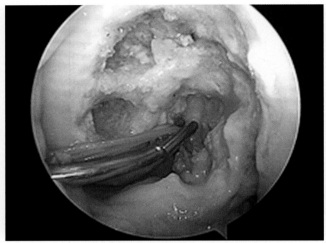

FIGURE 38-8

The sutures from both tendons are pulled into the intercondylar notch and stopped when they reach the femoral tunnel apertures.

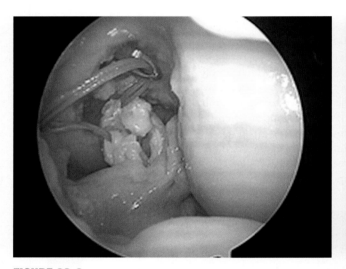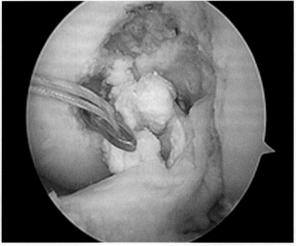

FIGURE 38-9

A grasper can be introduced from outside-in through the femoral tunnels. The sutures from each bundle are retrieved out their respective femoral tunnels.

tunnels and out the medial cortex (Fig. 38-10). Each tendon end is pulled out the medial femoral cortex until the calcaneal bone plug lies flush against the proximal medial tibial cortex. This is then fixed using a 10 × 25 mm bioabsorbable interference screw. The tibial fixation is backed up with a knotless lateral row rotator cuff anchor more distal in the tibia. The tendon ends on the femoral side are then individually tensioned. The knee is placed in 90 degrees of flexion and neutral rotation, an anterior drawer force is applied. The ALB is fixed using a 9 × 25 mm bioabsorbable interference screw from outside-in. The knee is then placed in full extension, and the PMB is fixed in the same manner using a 7 × 25 mm bioabsorbable screw. We then apply backup fixation on the femur using the sutures from the tendon ends and two additional knotless lateral row anchors.

Wound Closure

The tourniquet is released prior to wound closure to check for unexpected bleeding. All open incisions and portals are thoroughly irrigated and then closed in routine fashion. Sterile dressings are applied, and a hinged knee brace is applied locked in extension. A cryotherapy device is placed over the knee.

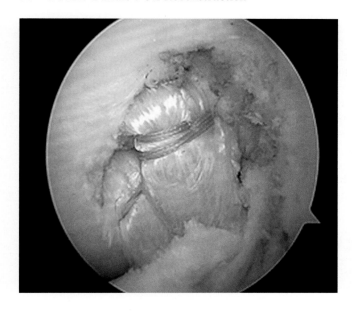

FIGURE 38-10

The sutures from each bundle are used to pull the tendons into their respective femoral tunnels.

TECHNICAL ALTERNATIVES AND PITFALLS

Preoperatively, it is important to evaluate for associate knee injuries (2,7). Isolated PCL tears of sufficient grade to warrant reconstruction are uncommon. Posteromedial and posterolateral instability should be carefully evaluated in the clinic prior to planning surgery. Alternatively, if the patient's knee is too swollen or they are guarding due to the acute nature of their injury, a systematic knee examination under anesthesia should be performed prior to starting surgery. In this case, any necessary surgical equipment and grafts should also be available for use. The patient and their family should be counselled on the possibility that more than an isolated PCL reconstruction may be necessary. Whether in the clinic or operating room, both knees should be carefully assessed for comparison as a unilateral exam is unreliable. Failure to diagnose an associated collateral or corner injury can lead to chronic attritional failure of the PCL graft and recurrence of their instability (1,13).

Intraoperatively, there are certain technical pitfalls to be aware of. By far, the most serious concern would be of neurovascular injury (2,7,10,11). The popliteal vessels in particular are in close proximity to the posterior knee capsule. They are protected by the popliteus muscle belly, though aggressive pin drilling or reaming can lead to vascular injury. Protective instruments are available in most PCL trays that can be used to catch the pin and reamer thereby protecting against plunging. If not available, a curette placed through a posteromedial portal can accomplish the same level of protection. Furthermore, some surgeons prefer to drill until they reach the posterior tibial cortex and then complete the drilling/reaming by hand to afford better control.

Another intraoperative technical pitfall is to place the exit point for the tibial tunnel too proximal. The native PCL footprint is between the mammillary bodies of the proximal tibia and roughly 1 cm distal to the posterior tibial plateau chondral surface. Too proximal tunnel placement can lead to graft attrition in part attributable to there being too acute a graft angle (14). A more anatomic distal placement lessens the acuity of the "killer curve" (15,16).

In our double-bundle PCL reconstruction technique, there are two distinct femoral tunnels. It is important to carefully place these tunnels at an appropriate distance from each other (Figs. 38-6 and 38-7). If the tunnels are too close, then can converge in a "figure-of-8" pattern and turn a double-bundle graft into a single-bundle reconstruction. Alternatively, if the tunnels are too far apart, they will not represent the locations of the anatomic footprint of the femoral insertions sites of the PCL. While not proven, it is likely that nonanatomic femoral tunnel placement can lead to suboptimal long-term surgical outcomes.

Lastly, as is in the case for all ligament reconstruction procedures, though perhaps more so for a three-tunnel reconstruction, difficulties with graft passage can arise. Some techniques can be done to ensure smooth graft passage. First, it is important to be sure that the graft is whipstitched in a way that is secure and easily fits through the appropriate tunnel size with tunnel sizers. The soft tissue ends should be bulleted so that the graft fits easier entering the tunnels. There are commercially available graft smoothers that can be used to smooth the tunnels. The edges of the tunnels can be smoothed with a curette, bur, or other devices to eliminate sharp corners. The graft can be precompressed to a size smaller than the drilled tunnels. During passage itself, there are v-shaped instruments designed to align the vector of pull of the passing suture with the tibial tunnel. The graft sutures can be pulled towards or out the anterior knee portal to improve the vector of pull into the femoral tunnels as well.

A rare though debilitating postoperative complication is AVN of the medial femoral condyle. There have been case reports of osteonecrosis occurring after cruciate ligament reconstruction, and it can present with delayed pain and disability months to years after surgery. It is felt to be typically due to the femoral tunnel being drilled relatively distal within the condyle. This coupled with devascularization from soft tissue dissection over the medial femoral condyle can impair the vascularity of the underlying bone. Of note, the blood supply to the medial femoral condyle is more tenuous and less redundant than that of the lateral femoral condyle perhaps adding to its susceptibility of injury (17–19).

POSTOPERATIVE MANAGEMENT AND REHABILITATION

Immediately after surgery is complete, the patient's leg is placed in a hinged knee brace locked in full extension. Overall, PCL reconstruction postoperative rehab is a slower process than after other ligament reconstruction surgeries. The goal is minimizing graft forces that are seen with weight-bearing and deep knee flexion. The patient is maintained toe-touch weight bearing on the operative extremity for the initial 8 weeks after surgery. Early on ROM is limited to the prone position avoiding posterior directly tibial forces. Later in the first month, patients are allowed to unlock their brace to allow 90-degree knee flexion. Hamstring active contractions are avoided for the first 6 weeks to limit posterior directed forces on the proximal tibia (20).

By 2 months after surgery, full knee range of motion is allowed, in particular deep knee flexion. Additionally, the patient is transitioned to full weight bearing. Quadriceps strengthening followed by more functional strengthening exercises can begin by 3 months post-op. At this point, the patient can stop wearing their brace. Rehab continues with a sports- or job-specific functional progression in mind. Supervised physical therapy typically continues for 4 to 5 months postoperatively at which point patients are transitioned to a home program. Ideally, the patient is released to full activities without restrictions sometime after 6 months once their affected quadriceps strength is >90% of the contralateral side as measured by a leg press or functional hop test (20).

SURGICAL OUTCOMES

Comparing studies on double-bundle PCL reconstruction is challenging due to a variety of techniques that are reported. Furthermore, there is no standardization of graft tension angle at fixation for the two different bundles. This leads to significant heterogeneity in the literature. Some biomechanical data have found no difference between single and double-bundle reconstructions. At the same time, other studies support double-bundle PCL reconstruction as mechanically superior and better able to restore near normal knee laxity. Some research notes that it is possible to overconstrain the knee with double-bundle reconstruction, possibly due to fixing the posteromedial bundle in too much flexion (7,21–23).

Similarly, reported clinical outcomes of double-bundle PCL reconstruction are also mixed with regard to its benefits when compared to single-bundle anterolateral reconstruction. The surgical case numbers reported, while limited, do show good results in terms of postoperative knee stability. Some studies show improved biomechanical benefit, namely in anteroposterior stability with double-bundle reconstruction, while others do not. No studies show higher patient-reported outcomes or functional outcomes with double-bundle reconstruction. The majority of clinical outcome studies are short-term reviews. It is possible that longer-term follow-up would be necessary to find a superior outcome for double-bundle reconstruction. A 10-year comparison of single- vs double-bundle reconstruction using hamstring autografts failed to find a clinical difference. However, to date, there is no level 1 comparison study published to definitively determine a difference (7,21–23).

REFERENCES

1. Sekiya JK, Whiddon DR, Zehms CT, et al. A clinically relevant assessment of posterior cruciate ligament and postero-lateral corner injuries. Evaluation of isolated and combined deficiency. *J Bone Joint Surg Am.* 2008;90:1621–1627.
2. Miller MD, Bergfeld JA, Fowler PJ, et al. The posterior cruciate ligament injured knee: principles of evaluation and treatment. *Instr Course Lect.* 1999;48:199–207.
3. Kennedy NI, LaPrade RF, Goldsmith MT, et al. Posterior cruciate ligament graft fixation angles, part 2: biomechanical evaluation for anatomic double-bundle reconstruction. *Am J Sports Med.* 2014;42:2346–2355.
4. Harner CD, Janaushek MA, Kanamori A, et al. Biomechanical analysis of a double-bundle posterior cruciate ligament reconstruction. *Am J Sports Med.* 2000;28:144–151.
5. Papannagari R, DeFrate LE, Nha KW, et al. Function of posterior cruciate ligament bundles during in vivo knee flexion. *Am J Sports Med.* 2007;35:1507–1512.
6. Kim SJ, Kim SH, Kim SG, et al. Comparison of the clinical results of three posterior cruciate ligament reconstruction techniques: surgical technique. *J Bone Joint Surg Am.* 2010;92(suppl 1 Pt 2):145–157.
7. LaPrade CM, Civitarese DM, Rasmussen MT, et al. Emerging updates on the posterior cruciate ligament: a review of the current literature. *Am J Sports Med.* 2015;43:3077–3092.
8. Li Y, Li J, Wang J, et al. Comparison of single-bundle and double-bundle isolated posterior cruciate ligament reconstruction with allograft: a prospective, randomized study. *Arthroscopy.* 2014;30:695–700.
9. Yoon KH, Bae DK, Song SJ, et al. A prospective randomized study comparing arthroscopic single-bundle and double-bundle posterior cruciate ligament reconstructions preserving remnant fibers. *Am J Sports Med.* 2011;39:474–480.
10. Fanelli GC, Edson CJ. Posterior cruciate ligament injuries in trauma patients: part II. *Arthroscopy.* 1995;11:526–529.
11. Miller MD, Johnson DL, Harner CD, et al. Posterior cruciate ligament injuries. *Orthop Rev.* 1993;22:1201–1210.
12. Dejour H, Walch G, Peyrot J, et al. The natural history of rupture of the posterior cruciate ligament. *Rev Chir Orthop Reparatrice Appar Mot.* 1988;74:35–43.
13. Mauro CS, Sekiya JK, Stabile KJ, et al. Double-bundle PCL and posterolateral corner reconstruction components are codominant. *Clin Orthop Relat Res.* 2008;466:2247–2254.
14. Okoroafor UC, Saint-Preux F, Gill SW, et al. Nonanatomic tibial tunnel placement for single-bundle posterior cruciate ligament reconstruction leads to greater posterior tibial translation in a biomechanical model. *Arthroscopy.* 2016;32:1354–1358.
15. Anderson CJ, Ziegler CG, Wijdicks CA, et al. Arthroscopically pertinent anatomy of the anterolateral and posteromedial bundles of the posterior cruciate ligament. *J Bone Joint Surg Am.* 2012;94:1936–1945.
16. Chahla J, Nitri M, Civitarese D, et al. Anatomic double-bundle posterior cruciate ligament reconstruction. *Arthrosc Tech.* 2016;5:e149–e156.
17. Athanasian EA, Wickiewicz TL, Warren RF. Osteonecrosis of the femoral condyle after arthroscopic reconstruction of a cruciate ligament. Report of two cases. *J Bone Joint Surg Am.* 1995;77:1418–1422.
18. Lerebours F, ElAttrache NS, Mandelbaum B. Diseases of subchondral bone 2. *Sports Med Arthrosc Rev.* 2016;24:50–55.
19. Reddy AS, Frederick RW. Evaluation of the intraosseous and extraosseous blood supply to the distal femoral condyles. *Am J Sports Med.* 1998;26:415–419.
20. Kim JG, Lee YS, Yang BS, et al. Rehabilitation after posterior cruciate ligament reconstruction: a review of the literature and theoretical support. *Arch Orthop Trauma Surg.* 2013;133:1687–1695.
21. Deie M, Adachi N, Nakamae A, et al. Evaluation of single-bundle versus double-bundle PCL reconstructions with more than 10-year follow-up. *ScientificWorldJournal.* 2015;2015:751465.
22. Qi YS, Wang HJ, Wang SJ, et al. A systematic review of double-bundle versus single-bundle posterior cruciate ligament reconstruction. *BMC Musculoskelet Disord.* 2016;17:45.
23. Montgomery SR, Johnson JS, McAllister DR, et al. Surgical management of PCL injuries: indications, techniques, and outcomes. *Curr Rev Musculoskelet Med.* 2013;6:115–123.

39 Surgical Management of Medial Collateral Ligament Injuries

Mitchell B. Meghpara and Bryson P. Lesniak

INTRODUCTION

The medial collateral ligament (MCL) is the most commonly injured ligament in the knee (1–5). Injury generally results from trauma to the knee following a valgus load with or without a rotational force applied. MCL injuries present as an isolated injury or commonly in combination with injury to the anterior cruciate ligament (ACL), posterior cruciate ligament (PCL), or both. The MCL has a relative increased ability to heal primarily without surgical intervention compared to the other ligaments of the knee. There are certain MCL injuries, mostly in combination with concomitant ligamentous injuries, that do not reliably heal nonoperatively and leave patients with significant joint instability that require an operation. The purpose of this chapter is to delineate which patients are indicated for surgery and how they are treated.

INDICATIONS

Relative indications for acute primary repair should be considered in isolated injuries if the MCL is entrapped within the joint in the medial compartment. In addition, a grade III MCL injury in a valgus aligned knee is not well tolerated and potentially less likely to heal nonoperatively given the increased stress on the injured ligament when compared to a varus aligned patient. Also, a displaced distal avulsion injury off of the tibia as well as ruptures in combination with tibial plateau fractures can be treated with primary repair (6).

The treatment of MCL injuries with combined ACL or PCL injuries is more controversial than that of isolated MCL injuries. There have been studies completed that support nonoperative treatment of the MCL with both acute (7) and delayed (8) treatment of the ACL after the MCL is healed. There is also support in the literature for acute operative treatment of both the ACL and the MCL (9). It is our opinion that each injury should be thoroughly evaluated on an individual basis to determine the most optimal treatment plan.

In a grade I or II MCL injury, ACL reconstruction should be completed between 4 and 6 weeks after injury. This permits nonoperative healing of the MCL and reduces the risk of arthrofibrosis that often occurs with immediate surgery. Determination of the location of the grade III MCL injury may have prognostic value as femoral avulsion injuries tend to heal more reliably than do tibial avulsion injuries. In our opinion, tibial-sided MCL injuries need to be followed closely to assess healing and the need for operative repair. Operative repair should be considered if there is medial laxity still present after a trial of rehabilitation. Our current approach is to allow 4 weeks of rehabilitation to allow the MCL to heal and allow the patient to regain knee motion and reduce swelling. Our final determination of the operative procedure is not complete until after the examination under anesthesia. If valgus laxity with gentle stress persists after 4 weeks of nonoperative management, we will proceed with both the cruciate reconstruction and an MCL repair versus reconstruction.

Relative indications for operative reconstruction should be considered in a patient who presents with a chronic MCL injury and remains symptomatic and unstable after nonoperative treatment has failed.

CONTRAINDICATIONS

Relative contraindications for surgical management of MCL injuries include grade I or II injuries that have not undergone conservative treatment, degenerative changes within the medial and/or lateral compartment of the knee, an ongoing infection, suboptimal wound healing potential, or a patient with multiple comorbidities who is medically unfit for surgery.

PREOPERATIVE PREPARATION

History

A proper history and physical with appropriate imaging must be undertaken prior to any intervention. Typically, the mechanism for an MCL injury involves an isolated valgus force to the knee, or a valgus force combined with a rotational force. It is usually the result of a sports-related impact injury or a twisting noncontact injury. When rotational injury is suspected, concomitant injury to the postero-medial corner structures and/or the ACL should be considered. The patient will present with varying degrees of swelling, pain, instability, and loss of motion. Location of swelling can be variable. An isolated MCL tear may only have swelling at the medial aspect of the knee. A hemarthrosis may be present if there is injury to the deep MCL and capsule, or if there is other associated intra-articular pathology. Studies have found up to 80% of MCL injuries to have additional ligamentous injury (1).

Physical Examination

The injured knee should be examined completely and compared with the contralateral knee. This includes a thorough neurovascular examination. Although potentially difficult, the patient should be relaxed to achieve a useful physical examination. Tenderness along the MCL should be assessed by palpation and note made of whether pain can be localized to a specific region of the MCL. In order to isolate the MCL on examination, a valgus force in the coronal plane should be applied while avoiding any rotational component. The endpoint of varus and valgus stress to the knee should be noted. A complete tear of the MCL may or may not have an endpoint detected with valgus stress. If there is any uncertainty, comparison to the contralateral knee can provide further confirmation of the injury. The MCL should also be tested at 0 and 30 degrees of flexion (Figs. 39-1 and 39-2).

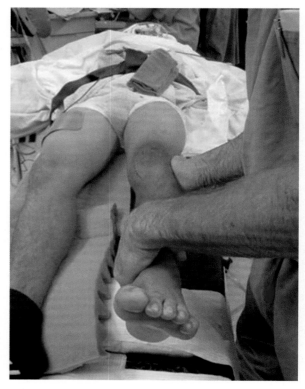

FIGURE 39-1
Valgus stress testing of the patient in full extension.

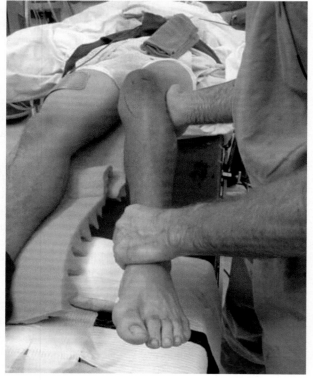

FIGURE 39-2
Valgus stress testing of the knee at 30 degrees of flexion.

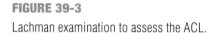

FIGURE 39-3

Lachman examination to assess the ACL.

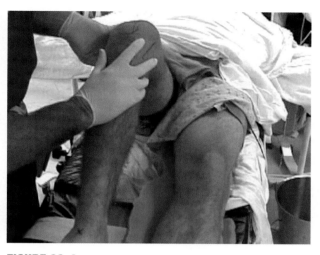

FIGURE 39-4

Posterior drawer examination to assess the PCL.

Increased laxity to valgus stress in full extension is an ominous sign as it implies possible injury to a cruciate ligament and/or posteromedial capsular structures. Flexion of the knee reduces the second-ary restraint of the posterior capsule and better isolates the MCL. The ACL and the PCL provide secondary restraint to varus and valgus stress, so the knee should remain stable with stress in full extension if the cruciate ligaments are intact, even in the setting of MCL injury. The ACL, PCL, LCL, and posterolateral corner should all be examined to determine the severity and pattern of the injury (Figs. 39-3 and 39-4).

Imaging

When an MCL injury is suspected, radiographic evaluation begins with a standard knee series. This should include a 45 degree–flexion weight-bearing AP, lateral and merchant views. Plain radiographs usually provide limited information, but may show evidence of a bony avulsion or an osteochondral fragment that could alter the treatment plan. In skeletally immature patients, stress radiographs should be obtained to evaluate for physeal injury as the cause of valgus laxity as this is more common than an MCL tear. Stress radiographs may also be used to better confirm the extent of laxity of the medial knee. LaPrade et al. demonstrated that grade III MCL injuries should be suspected with >3.2 mm of medial compartment gapping compared to the contralateral knee at 20 degrees of flexion with valgus stress (10). This valgus stress view is very useful in objectively identifying medial knee injuries (11).

Magnetic resonance image (MRI) can provide significant data that can assist in treatment of an MCL injury. First and foremost, an MRI can assist in determining the severity of the MCL injury as well as any associated cruciate ligament, meniscal, or capsular damage. MRI can also determine the location of the MCL tear that, as stated previously, can have therapeutic implications. Occasionally, a displaced MCL tear that becomes incarcerated in the knee joint is seen on MRI, thus obligating operative intervention (Fig. 39-5). Information from the MRI combined with physical examination findings allows for formulation of the appropriate treatment plan.

TECHNIQUE

Patient Positioning

The patient is placed in supine position after general or spinal anesthesia is administered. In our practice, we do not use a tourniquet, especially in the setting of a knee dislocation where an undi-agnosed arterial injury may be exacerbated by tourniquet use. A complete examination under anes-thesia is performed to confirm or refine the diagnosis made by the examination in the office and the imaging studies. All bony prominences are well padded, and all relevant anatomic landmarks and incisions are drawn on the skin. The planned incisions are then prepped with Betadine and injected with epinephrine (1:100,000). Prophylactic intravenous antibiotics are given preoperatively.

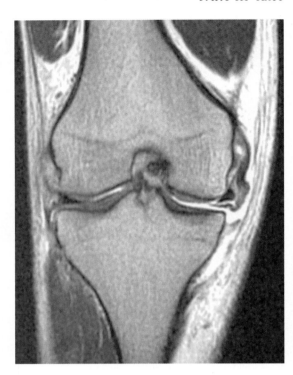

FIGURE 39-5

MRI demonstrating incarceration of the MCL into the medial compartment, mandating operative reduction of the MCL.

A 5-lb sand bag is taped to the operative table to allow the knee to rest in 90 degrees flexion and a side post is placed at the midthigh level to serve as an abduction block when the knee is in flexion and provide an abduction post when performing arthroscopy (Fig. 39-6). The entire limb is then prepped with alcohol and Betadine and draped free. A sterile bolster is then made and placed between the thigh and the side post.

Arthroscopic examination of the knee can be performed before or after the medial dissection. We recommend performing the approach prior to the arthroscopic examination because the tissue planes are more readily identified making the dissection more straightforward. However, the difficulty of performing arthroscopy after an arthrotomy must be considered as well.

Approach

Most commonly when approaching the medial structures of the knee, a medial "hockey stick"–type incision is used (Fig. 39-7). The landmarks for the medial incision are the adductor tubercle, the medial epicondyle, the joint line, and the medial facet of the patella. Often, the incision

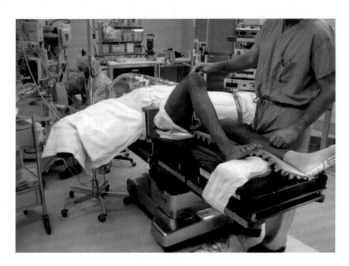

FIGURE 39-6

Operative setup: All boney prominences are well padded and a sandbag is placed to maintain 90 degrees of flexion for the operative leg. A post is placed at the midthigh level to allow for abduction during arthroscopy.

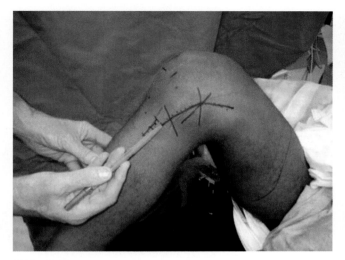

FIGURE 39-7

Planned surgical incision: the MCL and planned curvilinear incision are drawn on the medial knee.

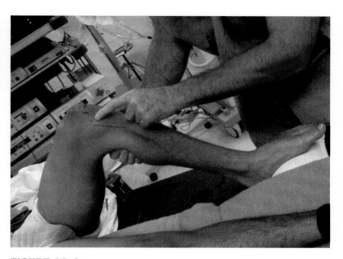

FIGURE 39-8

A minimized incision planned for a tibial-sided MCL repair.

size can be adjusted and minimized by centralizing the incision over the specific location of the MCL injury (Fig. 39-8).

Skin and subcutaneous tissue is incised with a scalpel to the sartorial fascia (Fig. 39-9). Care must be taken to identify and protect the infrapatellar branch of the saphenous nerve as it emerges from under the sartorius 1 cm above the joint line and travels anteriorly on the fascia. The nerve should be identified and retracted gently with a vessel loop. Skin flaps are then made at the fascial layer using a lap sponge and finger dissection.

Sartorial fascia is then incised in line with the skin incision proximally from the medial epicondyle to the gracilis tendon distally. The hamstring tendons as well as the sartorius are retracted posteriorly. The pes bursa is removed thereby exposing the superficial MCL and the posterior oblique ligament (POL). Access to the joint is made by creating an arthrotomy between the posterior edge of the superficial MCL and the anterior border of the POL (Fig. 39-10). An important note is to perform this arthrotomy with caution as transecting the medial meniscus is possible. With the medial structures of the knee now exposed, all structures should be identified and evaluated for any injury.

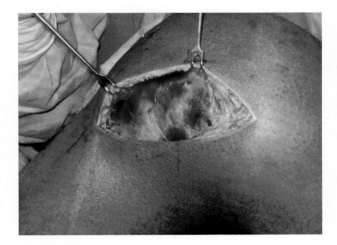

FIGURE 39-9

Dissection through subcutaneous tissue with the underlying exposed layer 1.

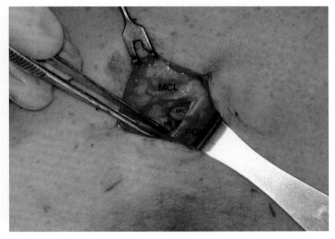

FIGURE 39-10

The capsule is incised between the MCL and the POL, exposing the medial joint and meniscus.

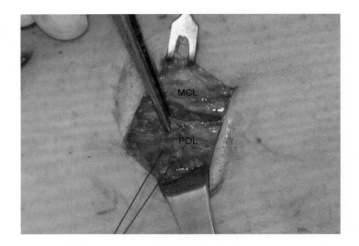

FIGURE 39-11

The medial meniscus is tagged (*black suture*) for eventual incorporation into the final repair.

Primary MCL Repair

The sequence of repair should proceed from deep to superficial. First, any meniscal injuries that are accessible are addressed. Any peripheral meniscal injuries should be repaired using nonabsorbable suture. Care must be taken to reduce the capsule that the meniscus is being sewn to prior to passing any sutures to ensure proper reduction of the meniscal injury. We routinely place the knee in extension to avoid restricting motion by overconstraining the knee. When all sutures are passed, these are tagged until the remaining structures are repaired and are then tied at the end of the case (Fig. 39-11).

The MCL is then addressed. For the repair, the knee is kept in approximately 30 degrees of flexion by placing a soft bolster under the distal thigh. If the tibial insertion of the deep MCL is avulsed, this should be sutured to the tibial periosteum deep to the superficial MCL. If the superficial MCL is avulsed off of the tibia (most common MCL pattern requiring operative repair), this should be repaired with multiple suture anchors with mattress sutures or a screw with a soft tissue washer (Fig. 39-12A–D). To ensure appropriate placement of the anchors or screw, we use intraoperative fluoroscopy to ensure all anchors are adequately distal from the joint line (Fig. 39-13). The goal is to reapproximate the MCL anatomically and prevent synovial fluid from being able to disrupt bone-ligament contact.

If the MCL is avulsed from its femoral insertion, the deep and superficial portions must be repaired directly just posterior to the medial epicondyle (Fig. 39-14). The MCL can be sutured to periosteum either directly with a No. 0 or No. 1 nonabsorbable suture or with suture anchors. In cases of midsubstance tear patterns, the MCL is repaired anatomically with direct suturing. With

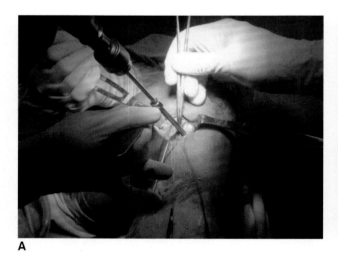

A

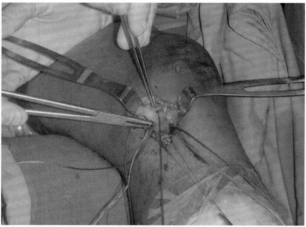

B

FIGURE 39-12

A: After preparation of the MCL and tibial surface, the suture anchors are drilled sequentially. **B,C:** Mattress sutures are then thrown to secure the MCL to the tibial surface. **D:** All mattress sutures tied sequentially.

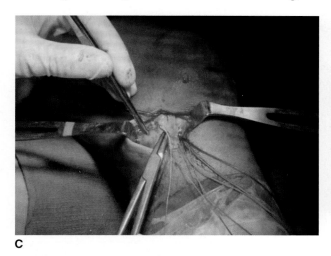

C

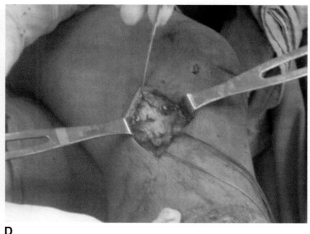

D

FIGURE 39-12 (*Continued*)

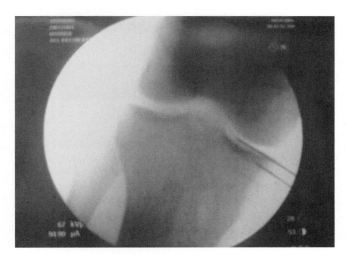

FIGURE 39-13

Fluoroscopic confirmation of anchor placement can be a helpful technique to ensure proper location (note one improper needle location in the medial joint space and one proper location in the medial tibia).

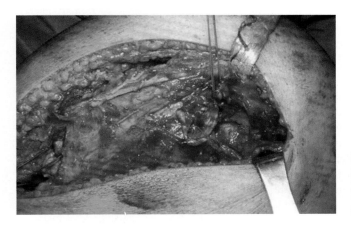

FIGURE 39-14

Direct fixation of a femoral-sided MCL tear with suture anchors in the medial epicondyle.

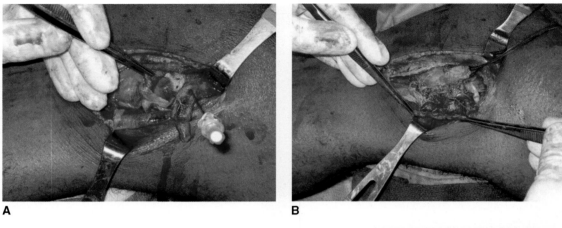

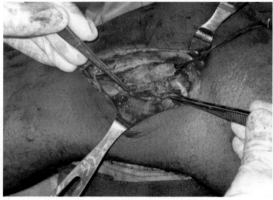

FIGURE 39-15

A: Dissection through layer 1 exposing the torn ends of the MCL. Note the 18-gauge needle in the medial epicondyle and the distal portion of the MCL in the forceps. **B:** MCL repaired with direct suturing. Note the POL held in the forceps posterior to the repaired MCL. **C:** Advancement of the POL to the posterior edge of the MCL.

femoral-sided or midsubstance tears, the anterior edge of the POL is advanced to the level of the repair and used to reinforce the repair. This provides increased strength to the repair and assists with medial stability (Fig. 39-15A–C).

Recently, there have been newer techniques described in the literature (12) to augment the primary repair with suture augmentation for added stability. For femoral-sided pathology, interlocking repair sutures placed through the proximal stump of the MCL can be shuttled into the eyelet of a suture anchor also loaded with FiberTape (Arthrex, Naples, FL) that will act as an internal brace. Once the femoral attachment of the ligament is secured with a suture anchor in the femur, a guide pin can be drilled into the tibial footprint of the MCL. The FiberTape is then passed from the femoral attachment distally to the tibial footprint and can then be wrapped around the guide pin to check for isometry. With the knee in approximately 30 degrees of flexion, neutral rotation, and a slight varus reduction, an anchor with the FiberTape loaded can be placed into an appropriately drilled tibial socket achieving final fixation and an augmented repair (Fig. 39-16). For tibial-sided pathology, the technique is similar, except that the primary anchor and repair are done at the tibial insertion and the internal brace is tensioned at the femoral insertion point.

Posterior Oblique Ligament Repair

If the patient has anteromedial rotary instability or valgus instability in full extension, an injury to the POL should be suspected and a repair should be attempted. The medial joint line is identified, and an incision is marked along the posterior one third of the medial femoral condyle that is approximately 5 cm long with two thirds of the incision distal to the joint line and one third proximal. Again, layer 1 is identified and incised in similar manner to that described in the above paragraph describing MCL repair. Once layer 2 is identified, the anterior edge of the POL and posterior edge of the superficial MCL is found. If there is difficulty identifying the plane between these two structures, a valgus stress maneuver can be utilized. With a valgus stress, the MCL will become taught whereas the POL will remain relatively lax. The interval is then divided, and the medial capsule deep to these structures is identified (Fig. 39-17). The MCL and the POL are dissected off of the capsule with an elevator. For imbrications, we use four horizontal mattress sutures (braided No. 2 nonabsorbable sutures) to advance the POL anteriorly and restore posteromedial tension (Fig. 39-18). The POL is advanced

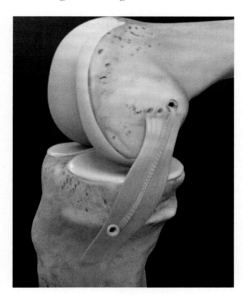

FIGURE 39-16

Illustration of augmentation of primary MCL repair with internal bracing. (This image provided courtesy of Arthrex, Inc.)

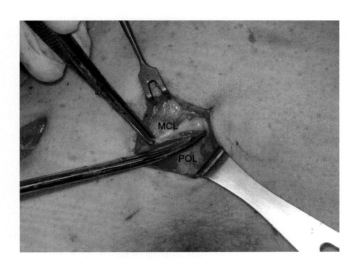

FIGURE 39-17

The demarcation between the MCL and the POL is split to allow for the imbrication.

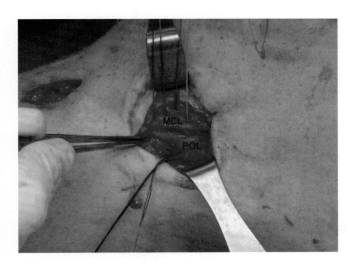

FIGURE 39-18

Sutures are passed through the POL and advanced through the MCL, thereby completing the imbrications.

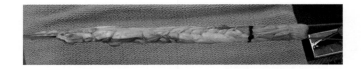

FIGURE 39-19

Tibialis anterior allograft whipped stitched prior to MCL reconstruction.

underneath the MCL at the level of the MCL tear (midstance or femoral sided), thus reinforcing the area of injury. In addition to the proximal-distal level of advancement, the depth of advancement of the POL under the superficial MCL is determined by the severity of the MCL injury and subsequent laxity. Once the appropriate imbrication is determined, the sutures are all tied in 15 degrees of knee flexion. Any meniscal repair sutures are included into the repair at this time as well. It is important to take the knee through a full range of motion after this repair to ensure no flexion contracture.

MCL Reconstruction

If surgery is indicated in a chronic situation, primary repair is attempted initially. It is important to note that in chronic conditions, the medial structures can be poorly defined and poorly identi-fied making primary repair more difficult. Because of this, augmentation of primary repair with an anatomic reconstruction is often necessary.

Numerous graft choices for reconstruction are available including hamstring autograft or multiple allografts. Our preference is tibialis anterior allograft (Fig. 39-19); however, given its proximity and ease of harvest, semitendinosus autograft is also reasonable.

For anatomic reconstruction, the femoral and tibial insertion sites of the superficial MCL should be identified as reported by LaPrade et al. (13). Tibial fixation can be achieved by using a screw with a soft tissue washer through the graft. The proximal end of the graft is then held (manually or with temporary K-wire fixation) at the location of the medial epicondyle. The knee should be taken through a full range of motion to ensure the MCL reconstruction is isometric. A pilot hole is drilled at the isometric point, and the graft is fixed proximally with a screw and soft tissue washer with the knee in full extension. If needed, the POL is advanced in a similar fashion that was previously described for acute repairs. It is our opinion that chronic repairs tend to require POL advancement more often than do acute repairs. Again, horizontal mattress sutures should be passed through the superficial MCL (and graft) and into the tibial periosteum (Fig. 39-20).

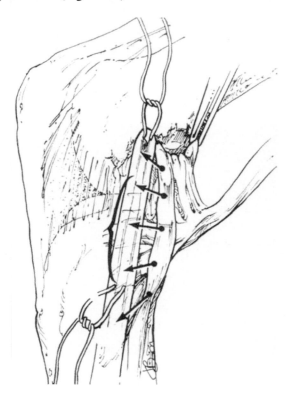

FIGURE 39-20

The graft is placed from the medial epicondyle to the anteromedial tibial surface. The POL can be advanced similar to the MCL repair to reinforce the reconstruction.

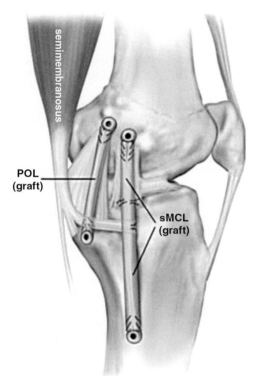

FIGURE 39-21

Illustration of the POL and MCL reconstruction grafts. (Reprinted from Coobs BR, Wijdicks CA, Armitage BM, et al. An in vitro analysis of an anatomical medial knee reconstruction. *Am J Sports Med.* 2010;38(2):339–347. Copyright © 2010 SAGE Publications, with permission.)

POL and MCL Reconstruction

If the POL is unable to be advanced or repaired, POL reconstruction along with MCL reconstruction can be attempted. LaPrade and Wijdicks have developed an anatomical medial knee reconstruction technique using two grafts that has shown to improve patient function and restore valgus instability (14). A 16-cm allograft is used for the MCL, and a 12-cm allograft is used for the POL (Fig. 39-21). This technique first involves properly identifying the femoral and tibial anatomic attachment sites for the POL and MCL. Tunnels are then reamed at each site over a guidewire, and the two grafts are first secured into the femur using interference screws. Then, the grafts are passed distally within the substance of their native tissue. The POL screw is tightened first in full extension, and then the MCL is tightened in 20 degrees of flexion, neutral rotation, and a varus reduction. The proximal tibial attachment of the MCL is also secured approximately 12.2 mm distal to the joint line directly medial to the anterior portion of the semimembranosus with a suture anchor (14).

PEARLS AND PITFALLS

Pearls

- Valgus stress radiographs are very useful to objectively identify medial knee injuries.
- Use MRI to correctly identify MCL tear location as this may help guide treatment method.
- A thorough understanding of the anatomic landmarks for MCL and POL insertion is critical for proper anchor or screw placement.
- Identify and repair any meniscal tears that may be present; tie down meniscal repair sutures once the repair or reconstruction is completed at the end of the case.
- Ensure isometry of the ligament is obtained prior to fixation.
- Anterior edge of the POL or an internal brace can be used for augmentation of primary repair.
- Keep knee in 30 degrees of flexion and neutral rotation, and hold a varus reduction when final tensioning is performed.

Pitfalls

- Primary repair may not be feasible for a chronically injured MCL.
- In a combined ACL/MCL injured knee, perform examination under anesthesia and make surgical decision to repair or reconstruct the MCL prior to reconstruction of ACL as the knee will become artificially tight after ACL fixation.
- Avoid overtensioning with the knee in extension to avoid overconstraining the medial knee.
- Failure to address POL pathology may result in residual side-to-side laxity and poor outcomes.

POSTOPERATIVE MANAGEMENT

If a medial-sided repair/reconstruction is performed in isolation, our postoperative protocol is to maintain the leg in full extension in a locked hinged brace for 2 to 4 weeks. A continuous passive range of motion machine is used twice daily. At 4 weeks, the brace is unlocked and motion exercises are begun. The patients are non–weight bearing with crutches for 2 weeks and then progressive weight bearing is allowed. Crutches are only discontinued when ambulation without a limp is achieved. Strengthening is initiated at 6 weeks post-op with closed-chain exercises. The brace is discontinued at 8 weeks from the date of surgery.

With combined injuries, the postoperative protocol follows cruciate reconstruction rehabilitation regimen. Achieving full extension is the initial goal, in particular with combined ligamentous injury. Any decrease in range of motion or failure to progress in range of motion should be treated aggressively.

COMPLICATIONS

The primary complication of operative treatment of the MCL is arthrofibrosis. While this complication may occur with any knee ligament surgery, it is accepted that surgical treatment of the MCL is a risk factor for loss of motion. This risk can be minimized by careful dissection and an appropriate repair with care taken not to overtension the POL or MCL. As we stated earlier, after repairing the MCL the knee should be taken through a full range of motion prior to skin closure. If full range of motion is possible in the operating room, then motion should be able to be restored with aggressive physical therapy. Another important consideration is the preoperative range of motion. We routinely allow 1 to 2 weeks after injury to pass to allow reduction of swelling and restoration of motion prior to operative management.

RESULTS

In isolated MCL injuries indicated for primary repair as mentioned herein, surgical management has yielded favorable outcomes. DeLong and Waterman conducted a systematic review that demonstrated that repair of the MCL and posteromedial corner of the knee may be an effective and reliable treatment for medial-sided knee injuries. The results show improved valgus stability and patient-reported function scores with low rates of secondary failure (15). An anatomical medial knee reconstruction has been shown to restore near-normal stability for MCL injuries that are not amenable to repair (14,16).

Many fixation methods have been presented in the literature for MCL repair. Although No. 2 braided sutures and suture anchors are our preferred method of fixation, Omar et al. showed in a biomechanical study that spiked polyether ether ketone (PEEK) washers secured with polyester sutures is the most appropriate fixation technique for MCL anatomical augmented repair (6).

Internal bracing is a more recent technique that has grown in popularity for augmentation of MCL repair. This bridging concept has shown positive results for Achilles tendon repair (17) and may justify broadening its indications for MCL injuries (18). MCL internal bracing for grade II and III injuries at the time of ACL reconstruction has shown good clinical results with restoration of knee stability without any complications of stiffness (9). Also, biomechanical analysis has demonstrated internal bracing to be superior for femoral-sided avulsions to repair alone and similar to allograft reconstruction (19).

Much controversy still exists regarding the optimal surgical procedure and timing when associated with other cruciate injuries. Successful repairs and reconstructions of the MCL both acutely and in a delayed fashion have been reported in the literature; thus, it is our belief that each injury should be comprehensively evaluated to determine the most optimal treatment plan.

REFERENCES

1. Fetto JF, Marshall JL. Medial collateral ligament injuries of the knee: a rational for treatment. *Clin Orthop.* 1978;132:206–218.
2. Grood ES, Noyes FR, Butler DL, et al. Ligamentous and capsular restraints preventing straight medial and lateral laxity in intact human cadaver knees. *J Bone Joint Surg Am.* 1981;63:1257–1269.
3. Hughston JC. The importance of the posterior oblique ligament in repairs of acute tears of the medial ligaments in knees with and without an associated rupture of the anterior cruciate ligament. *J Bone Joint Surg Am.* 1994;76:1328–1344.
4. Kannus P. Long-term results of conservatively treated medial collateral ligament injuries of the knee joint. *Clin Orthop Relat Res.* 1988;226:103–112.
5. LaPrade RF. The medial collateral ligament complex and the posterolateral aspect of the knee. In: Arendt EA, ed. *Orthopaedic Knowledge Update. Sports Medicine 2.* Rosemont, IL: American Academy of Orthopaedic Surgeons; 1999:327–340.
6. Omar M, Petri M, Dratzidis A, et al. Biomechanical comparison of fixation techniques for medial collateral ligament anatomical augmented repair. *Knee Surg Sports Traumatol Arthrosc.* 2016;24(12):3982–3987.
7. Millett PJ, Pennock AT, Sterett WI, et al. Early ACL reconstruction in combined ACL-MCL injuries. *J Knee Surg.* 2004;17(2):94–98.
8. Grant JA, Tannenbaum E, Miller BS, et al. Treatment of combined complete tears of the anterior cruciate and medial collateral ligaments. *Arthroscopy.* 2012;28(1):110–122.
9. Ateschrang A, Döbele S, Freude T, et al. Acute MCL and ACL injuries: first results of minimal-invasive MCL ligament bracing with combined ACL single-bundle reconstruction. *Arch Orthop Trauma Surg.* 2016;136(9):1265–1272.
10. Laprade RF, Bernhardson AS, Griffith CJ, et al. Correlation of valgus stress radiographs with medial knee ligament injuries: an in vitro biomechanical study. *Am J Sports Med.* 2010;38(2):330–338.
11. Laprade RF, Wijdicks CA. The management of injuries to the medial side of the knee. *J Orthop Sports Phys Ther.* 2012;42(3):221–233.
12. Van der list JP, Difelice GS. Primary repair of the medial collateral ligament with internal bracing. *Arthrosc Tech.* 2017;6(4):e933–e937.
13. LaPrade RF, Engebretsen AH, Ly TV, et al. The anatomy of the medial part of the knee. *J Bone Joint Surg Am.* 2007;89(9):2000–2010.
14. Laprade RF, Wijdicks CA. Surgical technique: development of an anatomic medial knee reconstruction. *Clin Orthop Relat Res.* 2012;470(3):806–814.
15. Delong JM, Waterman BR. Surgical repair of medial collateral ligament and posteromedial corner injuries of the knee: a systematic review. *Arthroscopy.* 2015;31(11):2249.e5–2255.e5.
16. Coobs BR, Wijdicks CA, Armitage BM, et al. An in vitro analysis of an anatomical medial knee reconstruction. *Am J Sports Med.* 2010;38(2):339–347.
17. Witt BL, Hyer CF. Achilles tendon reattachment after surgical treatment of insertional tendinosis using the suture bridge technique: a case series. *J Foot Ankle Surg.* 2012;51(4):487–493.
18. Lubowitz JH, Mackay G, Gilmer B. Knee medial collateral ligament and posteromedial corner anatomic repair with internal bracing. *Arthrosc Tech.* 2014;3(4):e505–e508.
19. Gilmer BB, Crall T, Delong J, et al. Biomechanical analysis of internal bracing for treatment of medial knee injuries. *Orthopedics.* 2016;39(3):e532–e537.

40 LCL/PLC Reconstruction

George F. LeBus, Bradley Kruckeberg, and Robert F. LaPrade

INDICATIONS

Treatment of posterolateral corner (PLC) injuries is dependent upon the degree and chronicity of the pathology and the presence of associated injury. In general, surgery is recommended for isolated grade III PLC injuries, PLC injury with concomitant anterior cruciate ligament (ACL) or posterior cruciate ligament (PCL) injuries, or grade II PLC injuries that have failed nonoperative treatment. With regard to the degree of injury, some studies have reported good results following nonsurgical treatment with an early mobilization protocol for grade I and II injuries (1,2). On the contrary, grade III injuries treated nonoperatively have demonstrated poor functional outcomes, persistent instability, and degenerative changes (3). Adequate surgical treatment of chronic PLC injuries in patients with varus alignment may mandate an osteotomy for limb alignment correction in the same setting or in a staged fashion (4). PLC injuries occurring in conjunction with ACL or PCL tears can lead to increased force on ACL or PCL grafts if the PLC is not appropriately stabilized along with the deficient cruciate ligaments (5). While repair of PLC structures may be an option in some settings, such as an acute injury (<2–3 weeks) or fibular collateral ligament (FCL) or popliteus tendon (PLT) avulsions without midsubstance injury, reconstruction is necessary in more chronic cases and for midsubstance injuries. Attempted repair in these latter situations has consistently demonstrated significantly higher failure rates than reconstruction (6,7).

CONTRAINDICATIONS

In patients with acute injuries, surgery is contraindicated when there is an extensive injury to the subcutaneous tissues or skin that could compromise wound healing, associated abrasions or open lacerations over the area of surgical incision, or active infection. Patients with chronic injuries should not undergo reconstructive surgery if they have severe knee osteoarthritis or uncorrected varus alignment of the ipsilateral extremity.

PREOPERATIVE PREPARATION

A thorough understanding of the complex anatomy and biomechanics of the PLC is essential to performing a comprehensive physical exam, interpreting diagnostic imaging, and executing the appropriate surgical techniques for PLC injuries.

Anatomy

Three main structures act as the primary static stabilizers of the PLC: FCL, the PLT, and the popliteofibular ligament (PFL) (8). Additional structures act as secondary stabilizers of the knee in both a static and dynamic fashion including the lateral capsular thickening of the mid-third lateral capsular ligament, the coronary ligament, the fabellofibular ligament, the long head of the biceps femoris, and the iliotibial band (ITB) (9).

Fibular Collateral Ligament

The femoral and fibular attachments of the FCL have been well described in the literature by LaPrade et al. (8). The femoral attachment of the FCL is in a small bony depression that lies 1.4 mm proximal and 3.1 mm posterior to the lateral epicondyle (8). The distal insertion of the FCL on the fibular head is located 8.2 mm posterior to the anterior margin of the fibular head and 28.4 mm distal to the tip of the fibular styloid. Most of the distal attachment is in a bony depression that extends to about the distal one third of the lateral fibular head. This attachment occupies approximately 38% of the fibular head. The FCL averages 7 cm in length and travels beneath the superficial layer of the ITB (8).

Popliteus Tendon

The PLT runs obliquely from the posteromedial aspect of the tibia. Its femoral insertion is 18.5 mm anterior to the FCL attachment with the knee at 70 degrees of flexion (8). From its insertion on the anterior fifth of the popliteal sulcus, the PLT runs deep to the FCL and travels posteriorly and distally to insert onto the posteromedial tibia. The average total length of the PLT to its musculotendinous junction is 54.5 mm (8).

Popliteofibular Ligament

The PFL originates from the popliteus musculotendinous junction and inserts on the posteromedial aspect of the fibular head with an anterior and a posterior division. The anterior division attaches distally on the anterior downslope of the fibular styloid process. The attachment of the posterior division inserts on the tip and posteromedial aspect of the fibular styloid process (8).

Secondary Stabilizers

In addition to the three main static stabilizers of the PLC, other structures contribute to the stability of the lateral knee including the lateral capsular thickening of the mid-third lateral capsular ligament (including the anterolateral ligament), the coronary ligament, the long head of the biceps femoris, the fabellofibular ligament, and the ITB (9). The lateral capsular thickening of the mid-third lateral capsular ligament consists of both the meniscotibial and meniscofemoral ligaments. The coronary ligament is the attachment of the posterior aspect of the lateral meniscus to the tibia. The long head of the biceps attachment is divided into a direct arm that attaches in the posterolateral aspect of the fibular head and an anterior arm that fans out superficially to the FCL. The fabellofibular ligament, a distal thickening of the short head of the biceps femoris, extends vertically from the fabella to the fibular styloid (10). The ITB is the most superficial layer of the lateral aspect of the knee and has attachments to Gerdy tubercle as well as the patella, lateral intermuscular septum, and capsule (8). All of the aforementioned structures contribute additional stability to the PLC. Importantly, the common peroneal nerve (CPN) lies posterior to the long head of the biceps femoris and crosses superficially to the lateral aspect of the fibular neck. The close proximity of the CPN to the PLC structures makes exposure and neurolysis of the nerve an essential component of the surgical approach to reconstructing the PLC.

Biomechanics

The PLC structures are the primary restraint to varus forces on the knee and posterolateral rotation of the tibia with respect to the femur. In patients with cruciate-deficient knees, the PLC structures also act as secondary stabilizers to anterior and posterior tibial translation, particularly in full extension (11–14). The primary restraint to varus stress across the knee is the FCL with the rest of the PLC structures acting as secondary stabilizers (15,16). Furthermore, the FCL and popliteus complex are primary restraints to tibial external rotation, particularly between 30 and 90 degrees of flexion with the PCL acting as a secondary restraint (17). The PLT is a minor stabilizer that plays a role in preventing internal rotation. This structure acts in conjunction with the ACL and the anterolateral ligament, which restrain internal rotation at lower and higher flexion angles, respectively (18). In addition to the PLT, the other PLC structures also function as secondary restraints to internal rotation.

DIAGNOSIS AND EVALUATION

The diagnosis and evaluation of a possible PLC injury begins with a thorough history and physical exam. A common patient-reported mechanism of injury that should increase suspicion for a PLC injury is a direct blow to the anteromedial knee, although hyperextension and noncontact varus

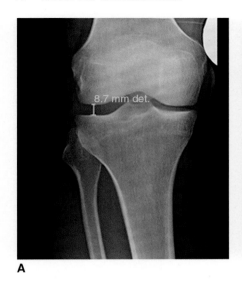 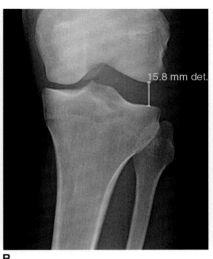 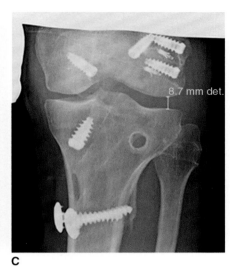

A **B** **C**

FIGURE 40-1

Varus stress radiograph of an uninjured knee **(A)** and the contralateral knee with a complete posterolateral corner injury **(B)**. Note the side-to-side difference of 7.1 mm. **C:** Varus stress radiographs at the 6-month postoperative visit following multiligament knee reconstruction including complete posterolateral corner reconstruction. The side-to-side difference between the contralateral uninjured knee has been corrected. Note that this patient also underwent anterior and posterior cruciate ligament reconstructions in addition to posterolateral corner reconstruction.

stress injuries may also lead to PLC damage (19). PLC injuries also commonly occur in the setting of cruciate ligament injury; therefore, a thorough evaluation of the PLC is mandatory when a cruciate ligament injury is detected. The patient may report symptoms such as pain, perceived side-to-side instability near extension, increased difficulty walking on uneven ground or climbing stairs, ecchymosis, and edema. Physical examination maneuvers may also be helpful in diagnosing a PLC injury. Several tests should be performed on both the injured and contralateral knee including varus stress testing, the dial test, the reverse pivot shift test, the posterolateral drawer, and external rotation recurvatum testing. CPN injuries leading to dorsal foot paresthesias and foot drop are also associated with PLC injuries and may occur in up to one third of cases (19,20), making a thorough neurologic exam mandatory in these patients.

Standard anteroposterior (AP), lateral, and flexed knee patellofemoral (sunrise) views should be obtained for all patients with knee pain or instability. Varus stress radiographs have been shown to be both reliable and reproducible in evaluating PLC injuries (21) and should also be implemented in cases in which PLC insufficiency is suspected. With the knee in 20 degrees of flexion and under an applied varus stress, a radiograph can be performed on both the injured and the contralateral knee. Measurements can then be performed on both knees and compared. Isolated FCL tears have been reported to have a side-to-side difference of 2.7 to 4.0 mm, whereas a grade III PLC injury is indicated by a difference >4.0 mm (21). Figure 40-1A–C demonstrates examples of varus stress radiographs both pre- and postoperatively in a patient with a PLC injury. In cases of suspected chronic PLC injury, a standing long-leg AP alignment radiograph will reveal the mechanical axis of the affected extremity and possible need for osteotomy to correct varus malalignment. In order to assess concomitant intra-articular or ligamentous injury and to evaluate the location of PLC injury, magnetic resonance imaging (MRI) is warranted as well.

SURGICAL TECHNIQUE

The operative extremity is exsanguinated, and a tourniquet is inflated to facilitate dissection. A lateral hockey stick incision is made extending from the distal lateral femur over the lateral femoral condyle to a point midway between Gerdy tubercle and the fibular head. Dissection is carried down sharply to the ITB (Fig. 40-2). A posteriorly based skin flap is created, and the fascia overlying the biceps femoris is identified. Next, the CPN is identified as it courses posterior and inferior to the biceps femoris tendon. Care is taken to perform a neurolysis of the CPN to the point where the

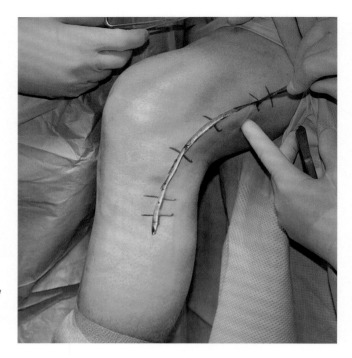

FIGURE 40-2

A hockey stick incision is made extending from the distal lateral femur over the lateral femoral condyle to a point midway between Gerdy tubercle and the fibular head. Dissection is carried down sharply to the iliotibial band.

fascia overlying the peroneus longus muscle is divided and muscle fibers of the peroneus longus are revealed (Fig. 40-3). An adequate neurolysis is a crucial component of the procedure to avoid a postoperative footdrop due to swelling around the CPN.

At this point, attention is turned to the distal aspect of the biceps femoris tendon and its attachment on the fibular head. The biceps femoris bursa is identified and split transversely in line with the femur. The FCL can be identified deep within this bursal tissue. A tag stitched is placed in the distal FCL to be used for later reference and identification of the proximal attachment of the ligament. The insertion of the FCL is then elevated sharply from the fibular head along with the direct arm of the biceps femoris tendon to reveal a "saddle" on the lateral fibular head to indicate the anatomic FCL insertion site. This point has been demonstrated to be approximately 28 mm distal to the fibular styloid and 8 mm posterior to the anterior aspect of the fibular head (8). Once this point has been appropriately identified, a guide pin is drilled through the fibular head from the FCL insertion site to a point on the posteromedial aspect of the fibular head using an aiming guide (Fig. 40-4). With the pin in place, a 7-mm cannulated reamer is used to ream a tunnel through the fibular head in line with the guide pin. Care is taken to not plunge with the guide pin or the reamer and to protect the posterior neurovascular structures with a retractor throughout this maneuver. A looped suture that will later be used to pass the graft to reconstruct the FCL is then passed through the fibular head such that the loop is facing anterolateral.

Attention is then turned to drilling the tibial tunnel. Dissection is carried anteriorly through the same skin incision by raising a full-thickness flap off the anterolateral tibia. The starting point for the

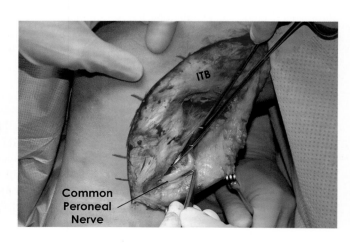

FIGURE 40-3

A common peroneal nerve neurolysis is performed distally such that the fascia overlying the peroneus longus is divided revealing the underlying muscle fibers. An adequate neurolysis is a crucial component of the procedure to avoid a postoperative footdrop due to swelling around the common peroneal nerve. ITB, iliotibial band.

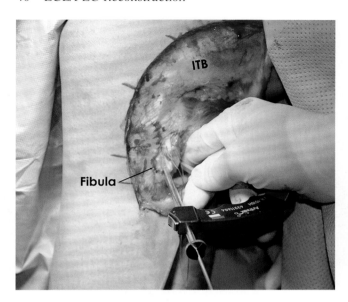

FIGURE 40-4

Once the anatomic FCL insertion site on the fibula has been appropriately identified, a guide pin is drilled through the fibular head from the FCL insertion site to a point on the posteromedial aspect of the fibular head using an aiming guide. A tag stitch is visualized in the distal aspect of the FCL that can aid in the identification of the anatomic origin and insertion of the ligament. Following pin insertion, a 7-mm cannulated reamer is used to ream a tunnel through the fibular head in line with the guide pin. ITB, iliotibial band.

tibial tunnel is then selected approximately equidistant between the tibial tubercle and Gerdy tubercle on the flat spot of the tibia in this region. Using an aiming guide, an eyelet pin is drilled posteriorly through the tibia while directed toward the musculotendinous junction of the popliteus, taking care to protect the neurovascular structures posterior to the knee (Fig. 40-5). A 9-mm reamer is then used to ream over the guide pin. Ideally, the posterior aspect of the tibial tunnel is approximately 1 cm medial and 1 cm proximal to the posteromedial exit point of the fibular tunnel. The location of the tip of the guide pin can be palpated with respect to the location of the fibular tunnel prior to reaming in order to optimize the tibial tunnel position. Once the tibial tunnel has been adequately reamed, a passing suture is placed for later graft passage such that the loop of suture is posterior.

At this point, the origin of the FCL is identified on the distal femur. Manipulating the distal aspect of the remnant FCL that was previously tagged through the biceps bursa can be helpful in identifying the trajectory of the FCL and the approximate location of the attachment of the ligament (Fig. 40-6A). An incision is then made through the ITB at this site (Fig. 40-6B). A more anterior incision through the ITB facilitates retraction of the tissue and exposure of the origin of the ligament. The FCL origin is then elevated sharply from the distal lateral femur. If the native ligament origin cannot be identified, its anatomic attachment site can be found about 1 mm proximal and 3 mm posterior to the lateral epicondyle (8). Using an aiming guide, a guide pin is then drilled through the distal femur to exit the skin on the medial side of the leg. Ideally, the guide pin will exit the medial aspect of the femur 5 cm proximal and anterior to the adductor tubercle. Care is taken to aim anteriorly and proximally

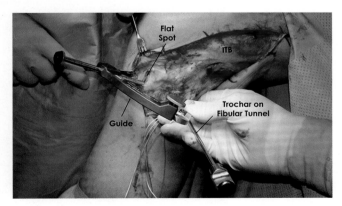

FIGURE 40-5

The tibial tunnel is created by placing an aiming guide from anterior to posterior, with the starting point for the tibial tunnel being equidistant between the tibial tubercle and Gerdy tubercle on the flat spot of the tibia in this region and aiming posterior to the musculotendinous junction of the popliteus, taking care to protect the neurovascular structures posterior to the knee. Posteriorly, the tibial tunnel should exit 1 cm proximal and 1 cm medial to the fibular tunnel. ITB, iliotibial band. (From LaPrade CM, LaPrade MD, Turnbull TL, et al. Biomechanical evaluation of the transtibial pull-out technique for posterior medial meniscal root repairs using 1 and 2 transtibial bone tunnels. *Am J Sports Med.* 2015;43(4):899–904.)

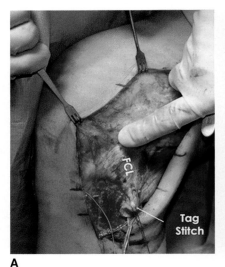
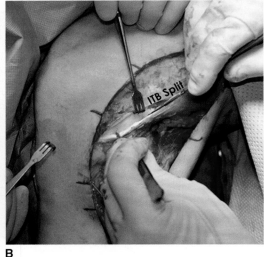

FIGURE 40-6

A: Applying tension to the tagging stitch through the FCL can help identify the course and origin of the FCL.
B: An incision is made in the ITB to identify the femoral origin of the FCL. Note the passing stitches in place through the fibular head tunnel and the tibial tunnel. FCL, fibular collateral ligament; ITB, iliotibial band.

to avoid tunnel convergence in patients who also require additional ligamentous reconstruction (22). With this pin in place, dissection is subsequently carried out approximately 18.5 mm distally to identify the origin in the PLT, which resides in the anterior fifth of the popliteus sulcus on the distal lateral femur. As the PLT insertion is intra-articular, a capsulotomy must be made to access this anatomic location. Soft tissue is elevated anteriorly to posteriorly away from the cartilage of the lateral femoral condyle until the insertion of PLT is adequately exposed (8). A second guide pin is similarly placed at this point using an aiming guide and is drilled parallel to the guide pin used to mark the site of the femoral FCL tunnel (Fig. 40-7). The anatomic locations and the distance between these two pins are subsequently confirmed. At this point, both guide pins are overreamed with a 9-mm reamer to an approximate depth of 25 mm. Finally, passing sutures are shuttled through the eyelet pins and pulled through the distal femur in order to later pass the limbs of the PLC reconstruction graft.

With all four tunnels drilled, the grafts are ready to be passed. The senior author (RFL) prefers the use of a split Achilles tendon allograft for PLC reconstruction techniques with the bone block

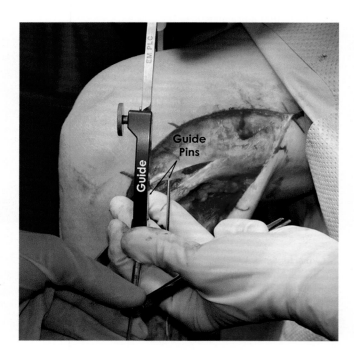

FIGURE 40-7

Using an aiming guide, a guide pin is drilled at the site of the anatomic origin of the FCL (pin alone) and the popliteus (pin with guide). A ruler is used to verify that the guide pins placed at the anatomic femoral attachments of the PLT and the FCL are 18.5 mm apart. The two pins are placed prior to reaming to ensure their parallel trajectory.

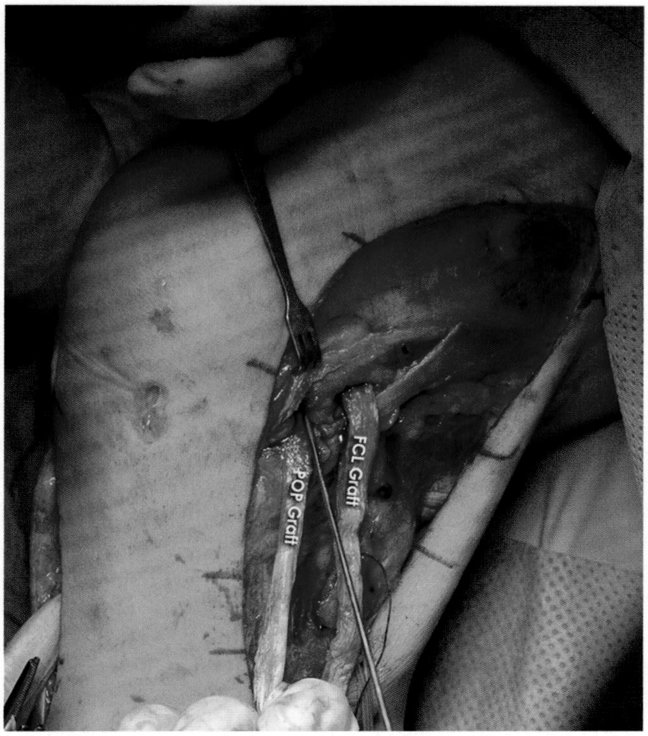

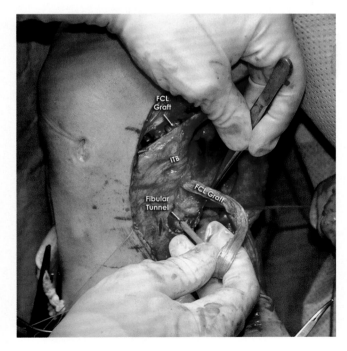

FIGURE 40-8

A 9-mm reamer is used to overream the guide pin to a depth of 25 mm at the site of the femoral attachment of the FCL. The reamer is aimed anterior and proximally to avoid tunnel convergence in the case of multiligament reconstruction. Similarly, the femoral attachment site for the PLT is reamed with a 9-mm reamer to a depth of 25 mm. The PLT and FCL grafts are fixed to the femur with cannulated titanium screws utilizing the bone blocks from the split Achilles graft in the previously drilled femoral tunnels. POP, popliteus; FCL, fibular collateral ligament.

portions of the grafts fixed into the distal femur with titanium screws and the distal soft tissue portions of the grafts fixed with bioabsorbable screws. The Achilles grafts pass from their origins in the distal femur deep to the ITB to replicate the structures of the PLC. The minimum required length of the graft is 22 cm, and the two bone blocks are fashioned to a size of 9 × 20 mm each and then passing sutures are threaded through drill holes in each bone block. The bone blocks are then fixed in the two femoral tunnels with 7- × 20-mm titanium cannulated screws (Fig. 40-8). The popliteal limb of the graft is first passed down the popliteal hiatus. The FCL graft is then passed deep to the ITB and pulled lateral to medial through the previously drilled tunnel in the fibular head (Fig. 40-9). The FCL graft is then secured in the fibular head with a 7- × 23-mm bioabsorbable

FIGURE 40-9

The FCL graft is passed through the fibular head and then fixed with a bioabsorbable screw. FCL, fibular collateral ligament; ITB, iliotibial band.

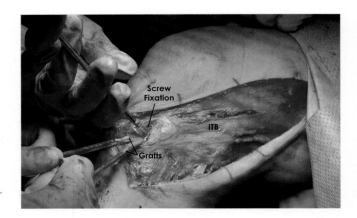

FIGURE 40-10

Ultimately, both popliteus and FCL grafts are passed posterior to anterior, and fixation is achieved by placing a biointerference screw in the tibial tunnel. ITB, iliotibial band.

screw with the knee in 20 degrees of flexion, neutral rotation, and under a gentle valgus stress in order to achieve appropriate graft tension. Finally, both remaining limbs of graft are passed posteriorly to anteriorly through the tibial tunnel, the knee is cycled through its full range of motion (ROM), and the grafts are secured with a 9- × 23-mm bioabsorbable screw with the knee in 60 degrees of flexion and neutral rotation (Fig. 40-10). If additional fixation is required, a supplemental staple can be utilized just distal to the tibial tunnel to further secure the grafts (23). At this point, the knee is examined to ensure that the prior instability has been corrected and that the knee is not overconstrained (Fig. 40-11). All wounds are then thoroughly irrigated and closed in a standard, layered fashion. Isolated FCL reconstruction can be performed in a similar manner with a semitendinosus allograft or autograft. In the case of isolated FCL reconstruction, the femoral tunnel and fibular tunnels for the FCL graft are reamed with a 6-mm reamer, and the semitendinosus graft is fixed to the femur first and then to the fibular head with the knee in 20 degrees of flexion and neutral rotation. Figures 40-12 to 40-14 demonstrate schematic illustrations of the surgical anatomy and PLC and FCL reconstructions.

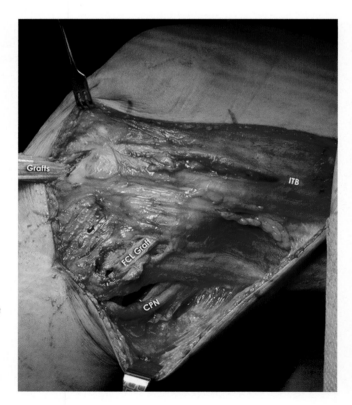

FIGURE 40-11

Posterolateral corner reconstruction with FCL fixed in the fibular tunnel and both grafts fixed on the anterolateral tibia. The common peroneal nerve that has been carefully dissected is also visualized. FCL, fibular collateral ligament; CPN, common peroneal nerve; ITB, iliotibial band.

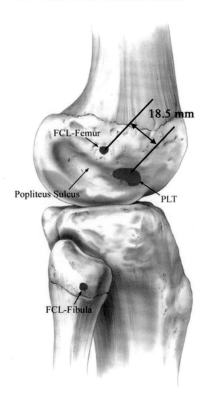

FIGURE 40-12

Illustration of a right knee showing the fibular collateral ligament (FCL) attachment sites on the femur and fibula, as well as the popliteus tendon (PLT) attachment site in the popliteus sulcus on the femur. The average distance between the femoral attachment sites is also noted. (From LaPrade RF, Ly TV, Wentorf FA, et al. The posterolateral attachments of the knee: a qualitative and quantitative morphologic analysis of the fibular collateral ligament, popliteus tendon, popliteofibular ligament, and lateral gastrocnemius tendon. *Am J Sports Med.* 2003;31(6):854–860.)

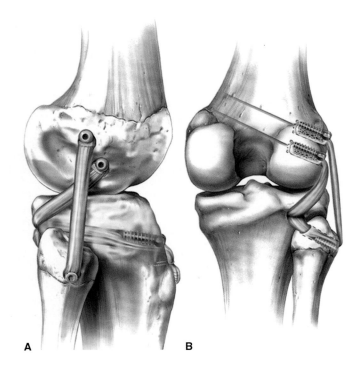

FIGURE 40-13

(A) Lateral and **(B)** posterior views of an anatomic-based posterolateral corner reconstruction utilizing two grafts to address the fibular collateral ligament, popliteus tendon, and popliteofibular ligament. (From LaPrade RF, Johansen S, Wentorf FA, et al. An analysis of an anatomical posterolateral knee reconstruction: an in vitro biomechanical study and development of a surgical technique. *Am J Sports Med.* 2004;32(6):1405–1414.)

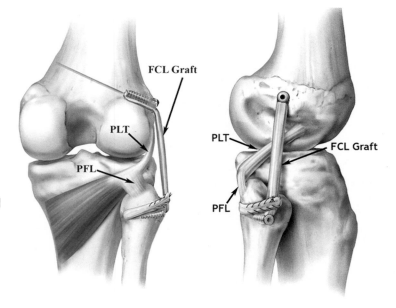

FIGURE 40-14

Posterior and lateral view of a right knee illustrating an isolated fibular collateral ligament (FCL) reconstruction procedure using a semitendinosus graft. PLT, popliteus tendon; PFL, popliteofibular ligament. (From Coobs BR, LaPrade RF, Griffith CJ, et al. Biomechanical analysis of an isolated fibular (lateral) collateral ligament reconstruction using an autogenous semitendinosus graft. *Am J Sports Med.* 2007;35(9):1521–1527.)

PEARLS AND PITFALLS (23)

Pearls and Pitfalls of Anatomic Posterolateral Corner Reconstruction

Pearls	Pitfalls
• If the common peroneal nerve (CPN) cannot be found posterior to the biceps femoris tendon, it should be dissected 2–3 cm distal to the lateral aspect of the fibular head. The CPN can usually be identified with gentle palpation.	• To avoid CPN injury, do not slide the scalpel distal to the champagne glass drop-off and always face the blade to the bone.
• When performing the neurolysis of the CPN, including the peroneus longus fascia helps prevent irritation to the nerve secondary to postoperative edema and facilitates its retraction during the procedure.	• Placing the fibular tunnel too proximal can fracture the fibular head. The pin guide should be placed slightly above the champagne glass drop-off.
• Having an assistant cut the soft tissues with a no. 15 blade while the surgeon uses a blunt clamp to dissect the CPN decreases risk of inadvertent lesion of the nerve.	• To avoid fibular head fracture in small patients, the reamer for the fibular tunnel can be downsized from 7 to 6 mm.
• After reaming the fibular tunnel, use a blunt device, such as a trocar, to pass through the tunnel and check the posteromedial exit point. The device should be left in place while drilling the tibial guide pin. The exit point on the tibia should be located 1 cm proximal and 1 cm medial to the fibular tunnel exit point.	• Drilling the tibial guide pin lateral to the flat spot increases risk of slipping the pin into the anterior compartment and also puts the proximal tibiofibular joint at risk.
• Leaving the FCL remnant in place may help preserve some proprioceptive function of the fibers.	• Splitting the ITB anterior to the FCL attachment will optimize visualization while a posterior approach will significantly decrease visualization.
• If identification of the femoral popliteal sulcus is difficult, its location can be estimated by bringing the knee to 70 degrees of flexion and making the vertical arthrotomy about 1 cm distal to the FCL attachment in a plane parallel to the fibular shaft.	• Drilling the femoral tunnels parallel to the joint can interfere with the intercondylar notch or other reconstruction tunnels. This trajectory may also place the saphenous nerve at risk. In order to avoid these issues, the guide pin should be aimed about 5 cm proximal and anterior to the adductor tubercle.
• The use of a chuck makes it easier to insert the screw guide and prevents pin bending. Additionally, if there is some difficulty inserting the screw guide pin, retracting and reinserting the bone plug along with the guide pin helps facilitate insertion of the pin.	• Because nonanatomic tunnels can compromise the reconstruction, the tunnels should only be reamed after ensuring the pins are in the proper position.
• One of the grafts can be marked with methylene blue to differentiate them from one another during surgery.	• Graft passage can be difficult if the tunnels are not completely cleared of soft tissue.
• Before fixing the distal aspect of the grafts, make sure that the popliteus is deep to the FCL in order to avoid interfering with their function.	• Proud bone plugs or interference screws can cause irritation to surrounding soft tissue and iliotibial band. Therefore, using a marking pen to demarcate the bone-tendon junction in the grafts helps ensure the bone plugs are completely within their respective tunnels.
	• Using a screw protector while placing the interference screw in the femur decreases risk of graft damage.

POSTOPERATIVE MANAGEMENT

Formal rehabilitation begins immediately following surgery with emphasis placed on tibiofemoral and patellofemoral ROM, edema, pain, and the return of quadriceps function. Patients should utilize a knee immobilizer in full extension, except during ROM exercises, and remain nonweight bearing for 6 weeks. For the first 2 weeks, passive ROM begins at 0 to 90 degrees and advances as tolerated. A goal of 90 degrees of flexion is desired by 2 weeks postoperatively. At 6 weeks, patients are encouraged to begin spinning on a stationary bike and can wean off crutches. Isolated hamstring exercises should be avoided in the first 6 weeks to avoid stretching of the grafts. Once completely off crutches and fully weight bearing, patients should begin closed chain strength exercises with a focus on initially developing muscular endurance followed by strength and power development. Running progression, along with speed and agility exercises, may be initiated once the patient has achieved adequate strength and power, which is usually approximately 6 months after surgery. Also at 6 months, varus stress radiographs should be taken to evaluate knee stability. Return to sport is possible once strength, stability, and ROM are comparable to the contralateral knee. Duration of recovery varies between patients, although typically patients can return to sport between 6 and 9 months from surgery depending on concomitant injury to the cruciates or other ligaments.

COMPLICATIONS

There are few reports of complications in the literature related to the surgical technique of PLC reconstruction in particular. The CPN is known to be a structure at risk in this anatomic location both following injury such as multiligament knee injury and knee dislocation (26,27) as well as after surgery including distal biceps femoris repair (28). Caution should be exercised to primarily identify the nerve, perform an adequate neurolysis to prevent postoperative injury from swelling, and protect the nerve throughout the duration of the procedure. In addition, care should be taken to prevent injury to the posterior neurovascular structures of the leg during drilling and reaming of the fibular head and tibia with careful use of aiming guides and retractors. Additionally, appropriate position and size of the tunnels minimizes the risk of fracture, particularly of the fibular head. A 6-mm reamer can be used instead of 7 mm to minimize the risk of iatrogenic fibular head fracture in patients with smaller fibulas.

OUTCOMES

Historically, isolated PLC injuries were often treated with primary repair and cast immobilization for 6 weeks (29,30), whereas PLC injuries with other concomitant ligament injuries were treated with immobilization alone (31). Initial reports revealed a high failure rate for primary repair (6,7) and thus began a trend toward reconstruction techniques (3,32). A recent 2-part systematic review of PLC knee injuries evaluated outcomes after both acute (33) and chronic (34) injuries. Eight studies, including 134 patients, were included in the acute injury review. Acute grade III PLC injuries that underwent repair with concomitant staged cruciate reconstruction were associated with a 38% failure rate. In contrast, similar PLC injuries treated with reconstruction techniques for both the cruciate ligaments and the PLC had a failure rate of 9%. Furthermore, the range of mean postoperative Lysholm and IKDC scores were found to be 88.7 to 90.3 (32,35–37) and 78.1 to 91.3 (3,32,38), respectively. Chronic injuries were reconstructed using a variety of techniques in all 456 patients, which demonstrated a success rate of 90%. Mean postoperative Lysholm scores ranged from 65.5 to 91.8 (32,36,39–46), while mean postoperative IKDC scores ranged from 62.6 to 86.0 (32,46–48). In addition to the varied surgical techniques of these patients, the cohort also suffered several types of combined injuries: 59% with combined PCL injury, 23% with combined ACL injury, 6% with combined ACL/PCL injury. Only 12% had isolated PLC injuries. Comparing outcomes of each surgical technique in acute and chronic injuries remains difficult due to the heterogeneity of the reported objective and subjective postoperative outcomes.

CONCLUSION

A thorough understanding of the anatomy and biomechanics of the PLC is necessary to successfully evaluate, diagnose, and treat these complex injuries. For those cases in which surgery is indicated, repair of the structures of the PLC may be an option in some settings, such as in acute (<2–3 weeks) or avulsion-type injuries; however, reconstruction is necessary in more chronic cases and for midsubstance injuries. The existing literature regarding the surgical treatment of PLC injuries has shown good results overall but is limited by the varied surgical techniques and outcome measures studied.

REFERENCES

1. Kannus P. Nonoperative treatment of grade II and III sprains of the lateral ligament compartment of the knee. *Am J Sports Med.* 1989;17(1):83–88.
2. Krukhaug Y, Molster A, Rodt A, et al. Lateral ligament injuries of the knee. *Knee Surg Sports Traumatol Arthrosc.* 1998;6(1):21–25.
3. Geeslin AG, LaPrade RF. Outcomes of treatment of acute grade-III isolated and combined posterolateral knee injuries: a prospective case series and surgical technique. *J Bone Joint Surg Am.* 2011;93(18):1672–1683.
4. Arthur A, LaPrade RF, Agel J. Proximal tibial opening wedge osteotomy as the initial treatment for chronic posterolateral corner deficiency in the varus knee: a prospective clinical study. *Am J Sports Med.* 2007;35(11):1844–1850.
5. LaPrade RF, Gilbert TJ, Bollom TS, et al. The magnetic resonance imaging appearance of individual structures of the posterolateral knee. A prospective study of normal knees and knees with surgically verified grade III injuries. *Am J Sports Med.* 2000;28(2):191–199.
6. Levy BA, Dajani KA, Morgan JA, et al. Repair versus reconstruction of the fibular collateral ligament and posterolateral corner in the multiligament-injured knee. *Am J Sports Med.* 2010;38(4):804–809.
7. Stannard JP, Brown SL, Farris RC, et al. The posterolateral corner of the knee: repair versus reconstruction. *Am J Sports Med.* 2005;33(6):881–888.
8. LaPrade RF, Ly TV, Wentorf FA, et al. The posterolateral attachments of the knee: a qualitative and quantitative morphologic analysis of the fibular collateral ligament, popliteus tendon, popliteofibular ligament, and lateral gastrocnemius tendon. *Am J Sports Med.* 2003;31(6):854–860.
9. Chahla J, Moatshe G, Dean CS, et al. Posterolateral corner of the knee: current concepts. *Arch Bone Jt Surg.* 2016;4(2):97–103.
10. Kawashima T, Takeishi H, Yoshitomi S, et al. Anatomical study of the fabella, fabellar complex and its clinical implications. *Surg Radiol Anat.* 2007;29(8):611–616.
11. Gollehon DL, Torzilli PA, Warren RF. The role of the posterolateral and cruciate ligaments in the stability of the human knee. A biomechanical study. *J Bone Joint Surg Am.* 1987;69(2):233–242.
12. Grood ES, Stowers SF, Noyes FR. Limits of movement in the human knee. Effect of sectioning the posterior cruciate ligament and posterolateral structures. *J Bone Joint Surg Am.* 1988;70(1):88–97.
13. LaPrade RF, Resig S, Wentorf F, et al. The effects of grade III posterolateral knee complex injuries on anterior cruciate ligament graft force. A biomechanical analysis. *Am J Sports Med.* 1999;27(4):469–475.
14. LaPrade RF, Tso A, Wentorf FA. Force measurements on the fibular collateral ligament, popliteofibular ligament, and popliteus tendon to applied loads. *Am J Sports Med.* 2004;32(7):1695–1701.
15. LaPrade RF. Arthroscopic evaluation of the lateral compartment of knees with grade 3 posterolateral knee complex injuries. *Am J Sports Med.* 1997;25(5):596–602.
16. LaPrade RF, Wozniczka JK, Stellmaker MP, et al. Analysis of the static function of the popliteus tendon and evaluation of an anatomic reconstruction: the "fifth ligament" of the knee. *Am J Sports Med.* 2010;38(3):543–549.
17. Ranawat A, Baker CL III, Henry S, et al. Posterolateral corner injury of the knee: evaluation and management. *J Am Acad Orthop Surg.* 2008;16(9):506–518.
18. Parsons EM, Gee AO, Spiekerman C, et al. The biomechanical function of the anterolateral ligament of the knee. *Am J Sports Med.* 2015;43(3):669–674.
19. LaPrade RF, Terry GC. Injuries to the posterolateral aspect of the knee. Association of anatomic injury patterns with clinical instability. *Am J Sports Med.* 1997;25(4):433–438.
20. Veltri DM, Deng XH, Torzilli PA, et al. The role of the cruciate and posterolateral ligaments in stability of the knee. A biomechanical study. *Am J Sports Med.* 1995;23(4):436–443.
21. LaPrade RF, Heikes C, Bakker AJ, et al. The reproducibility and repeatability of varus stress radiographs in the assessment of isolated fibular collateral ligament and grade-III posterolateral knee injuries. An in vitro biomechanical study. *J Bone Joint Surg Am.* 2008;90(10):2069–2076.
22. Moatshe G, Slette EL, Engebretsen L, et al. Intertunnel relationships in the tibia during reconstruction of multiple knee ligaments: how to avoid tunnel convergence. *Am J Sports Med.* 2016;44(11):2864–2869.
23. Serra Cruz R, Mitchell JJ, Dean CS, et al. Anatomic posterolateral corner reconstruction. *Arthrosc Tech.* 2016;5(3):e563–e572.
24. LaPrade RF, Johansen S, Wentorf FA, et al. An analysis of an anatomical posterolateral knee reconstruction: an in vitro biomechanical study and development of a surgical technique. *Am J Sports Med.* 2004;32(6):1405–1414.
25. Coobs BR, LaPrade RF, Griffith CJ, et al. Biomechanical analysis of an isolated fibular (lateral) collateral ligament reconstruction using an autogenous semitendinosus graft. *Am J Sports Med.* 2007;35(9):1521–1527.
26. Oshima T, Nakase J, Numata H, et al. Common peroneal nerve palsy with multiple-ligament knee injury and distal avulsion of the biceps femoris tendon. *Case Rep Orthop.* 2015;2015:306260.
27. Peskun CJ, Chahla J, Steinfeld ZY, et al. Risk factors for peroneal nerve injury and recovery in knee dislocation. *Clin Orthop Relat Res.* 2012;470(3):774–778.
28. Fukuda A, Nishimura A, Nakazora S, et al. Entrapment of common peroneal nerve by surgical suture following distal biceps femoris tendon repair. *Case Rep Orthop.* 2016;2016:7909805.

29. Baker CL Jr, Norwood LA, Hughston JC. Acute combined posterior cruciate and posterolateral instability of the knee. *Am J Sports Med.* 1984;12(3):204–208.

30. DeLee JC, Riley MB, Rockwood CA Jr. Acute posterolateral rotatory instability of the knee. *Am J Sports Med.* 1983;11(4):199–207.

31. Baker CL Jr, Norwood LA, Hughston JC. Acute posterolateral rotatory instability of the knee. *J Bone Joint Surg Am.* 1983;65(5):614–618.

32. Schechinger SJ, Levy BA, Dajani KA, et al. Achilles tendon allograft reconstruction of the fibular collateral ligament and posterolateral corner. *Arthroscopy.* 2009;25(3):232–242.

33. Geeslin AG, Moulton SG, LaPrade RF. A systematic review of the outcomes of posterolateral corner knee injuries, Part 1: Surgical treatment of acute injuries. *Am J Sports Med.* 2016;44(5):1336–1342.

34. Moulton SG, Geeslin AG, LaPrade RF. A systematic review of the outcomes of posterolateral corner knee injuries, Part 2: Surgical treatment of chronic injuries. *Am J Sports Med.* 2016;44(6):1616–1623.

35. Bin SI, Nam TS. Surgical outcome of 2-stage management of multiple knee ligament injuries after knee dislocation. *Arthroscopy.* 2007;23(10):1066–1072.

36. Harner CD, Waltrip RL, Bennett CH, et al. Surgical management of knee dislocations. *J Bone Joint Surg Am.* 2004;86(2):262–273.

37. Ibrahim SA, Ghafar S, Salah M, et al. Surgical management of traumatic knee dislocation with posterolateral corner injury. *Arthroscopy.* 2013;29(4):733–741.

38. Shelbourne KD, Haro MS, Gray T. Knee dislocation with lateral side injury: results of an en masse surgical repair technique of the lateral side. *Am J Sports Med.* 2007;35(7):1105–1116.

39. Fanelli GC, Edson CJ. Combined posterior cruciate ligament-posterolateral reconstructions with Achilles tendon allograft and biceps femoris tendon tenodesis: 2- to 10-year follow-up. *Arthroscopy.* 2004;20(4):339–345.

40. Fanelli GC, Fanelli DG, Edson CJ, et al. Combined anterior cruciate ligament and posterolateral reconstruction of the knee using allograft tissue in chronic knee injuries. *J Knee Surg.* 2014;27(5):353–358.

41. Kim SJ, Choi DH, Hwang BY. The influence of posterolateral rotatory instability on ACL reconstruction: comparison between isolated ACL reconstruction and ACL reconstruction combined with posterolateral corner reconstruction. *J Bone Joint Surg Am.* 2012;94(3):253–259.

42. Kim SJ, Jung M, Moon HK, et al. Anterolateral transtibial posterior cruciate ligament reconstruction combined with anatomical reconstruction of posterolateral corner insufficiency: comparison of single-bundle versus double-bundle posterior cruciate ligament reconstruction over a 2- to 6-year follow-up. *Am J Sports Med.* 2011;39(3):481–489.

43. Kim SJ, Kim SG, Lee IS, et al. Effect of physiological posterolateral rotatory laxity on early results of posterior cruciate ligament reconstruction with posterolateral corner reconstruction. *J Bone Joint Surg Am.* 2013;95(13):1222–1227.

44. Kim SJ, Kim TW, Kim SG, et al. Clinical comparisons of the anatomical reconstruction and modified biceps rerouting technique for chronic posterolateral instability combined with posterior cruciate ligament reconstruction. *J Bone Joint Surg Am.* 2011;93(9):809–818.

45. Wang CJ, Chen HS, Huang TW, et al. Outcome of surgical reconstruction for posterior cruciate and posterolateral instabilities of the knee. *Injury.* 2002;33(9):815–821.

46. Yoon KH, Lee JH, Bae DK, et al. Comparison of clinical results of anatomic posterolateral corner reconstruction for posterolateral rotatory instability of the knee with or without popliteal tendon reconstruction. *Am J Sports Med.* 2011;39(11):2421–2428.

47. LaPrade RF, Johansen S, Agel J, et al. Outcomes of an anatomic posterolateral knee reconstruction. *J Bone Joint Surg Am.* 2010;92(1):16–22.

48. Zorzi C, Alam M, Iacono V, et al. Combined PCL and PLC reconstruction in chronic posterolateral instability. *Knee Surg Sports Traumatol Arthrosc.* 2013;21(5):1036–1042.

41 Knee Dislocation

Kellie K. Middleton, Josh Chisem, and Answorth A. Allen

INTRODUCTION

Knee dislocation is an uncommon, though severe orthopaedic injury—accounting for <0.02% of all orthopaedic injuries based on prior studies (1–3). Most recently, a retrospective database review by Arom et al. found an incidence of 0.060 per 100 for closed dislocations and 0.012 per 100 for open knee dislocations from 2004 to 2009 using a national database of private insurance records (4). This is likely underestimated as authors did not account for patients who had Medicare or Medicaid or were uninsured. Furthermore, because knee dislocations can often spontaneously reduce prior to initial evaluation, the *true* incidence is unknown.

Knee dislocations are most commonly caused by high-velocity trauma or athletic injury and commonly involve injury to most of the soft tissue stabilizers of the knee resulting in multidirectional instability. Originally, an occult knee dislocation was defined as complete disruption of the femorotibial joint requiring clinical or radiographic femorotibial joint incongruity; however, multiligamentous knee injuries resulting from subluxation or unwitnessed dislocation should still be managed as a "dislocated knee" given the propensity for neurovascular compromise (5,6).

Knee dislocations often are associated with vascular and neurologic injury to the popliteal structures (7) with estimates ranging from 15% to 50% (6,8–11). As such, identification of a knee dislocation depends largely on clinical suspicion with timely diagnosis being of the utmost importance to avoid missing a potentially devastating, life-altering injury.

The number of ligaments disrupted necessary to dislocate the knee is disputed. By convention, both cruciate ligaments or central pivot and at least one collateral ligament must be torn in order for the knee to dislocate (12,13); however, some studies have shown that dislocations can still occur with one cruciate intact (14–17). In the chapter that follows, we will discuss relevant knee anatomy, the Kennedy knee dislocation classification system, clinical and radiographic workup, and management and outcomes of knee dislocations.

RELEVANT ANATOMY

A traumatic knee dislocation represents an acute insult to an inherently unstable structure (18). The knee consists of both static and dynamic soft tissue stabilizers, supported by an osseous scaffold (19). Posteromedially, the dynamic soft tissue stabilizers of the knee are the semimembranosus muscle with its anterior and direct arms inserting unto the posteromedial tibia, the medial gastrocnemius tendon inserting into the posteromedial femur, and the adductor magnus tendon that inserts into the adductor tubercle on the medial femur (20). The vastus medialis obliquus muscle offers tendinous fiber contributions to the quadriceps tendon (21).

With respect to rates of injury, studies have demonstrated that the semimembranosus tendon is partially torn in 29% to 39% of acute traumatic knee dislocations and completely torn in 0% to 6% (22) (Fig. 41-1). Partial or complete tears of the medial head of the gastrocnemius have been reported to be close to 5% (5).

The dynamic soft tissue structures of the lateral knee include the lateral gastrocnemius tendon, the popliteus tendon, and the iliotibial band (ITB). Tears of the popliteus are uncommon; however, radiologic studies have demonstrated that nearly all tears occur within the muscular belly rather than the tendon of the popliteus (23).

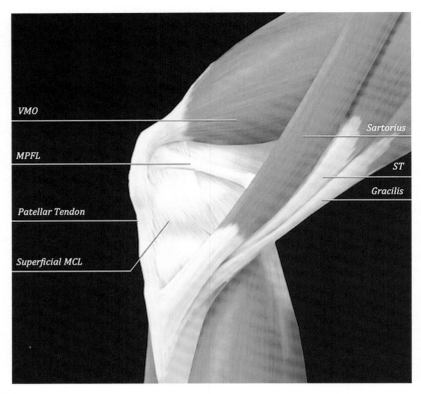

FIGURE 41-1

Medial structures of the knee. VMO, vastus medialis; MPFL, medial patella femoral ligament; MCL, medial collateral ligament; ST, semitendinosus tendon.

The static, extra-articular stabilizers of the knee are more commonly injured than the dynamic stabilizers (24). Posteromedially lies posterior oblique ligament (POL), originating on the postero-medial tibia and inserting onto the posterior femur. Slightly anterior to the POL is the superficial medial collateral ligament (MCL), which originates on the medial distal femur and has two inser-tions, one proximal and one distal (3). The proximal insertion is found on the posteromedial tibia and the distal insertion is adjacent to the pes anserine. The deep MCL originates just distally and inserts just proximally relative to the attachment sites of the superficial MCL (25). Anterior to the proximal femoral attachment of the superficial MCL lies the insertion of the medial patellofemoral ligament. Its origin is on the medial patella, and it inserts 1.9 mm anterior and 3.8 mm distal to the adductor tubercle (2,20). The lateral patellofemoral ligament is a static stabilizer, and its origin is on approximately 45% of the lateral edge of the patella. It inserts approximately 2.5 mm distal and 10.8 mm anterior to the lateral epicondyle (26,27).

The lateral collateral ligament (LCL) is important in resisting varus forces and works in con-junction with the MCL to provide stability against axial rotatory forces. Originating posterior and superior to the popliteus insertion on the lateral femoral condyle, it runs superficial to the popliteus and inserts on the fibula, anterior to the popliteofibular ligament (PFL). The LCL is included in the posterolateral corner (PLC), which works synergistically with the PCL to provide stability against external rotation and posterior translation (Fig. 41-2) (28). Other structures included in the PLC complex include the popliteus muscle and tendon, the PFL, the lateral capsule, the arcuate ligament, the ITB, and the fabellofibular ligament. The latter three structures are variably present with the fabellofibular ligament originating from the fibular head and inserting into the fabella, a sesamoid bone that is often present in the lateral gastrocnemius head (29). The PFL originates on the popliteus musculotendinous junction and inserts on the fibula head (30,31). The arcuate ligament is a ligamen-tous structure consisting of two arms. The lateral arm originates on the fibular lead and inserts into the posterolateral femur, while the medial arm inserts onto the posterior femur and blends with the fibers of the popliteal oblique ligament (32).

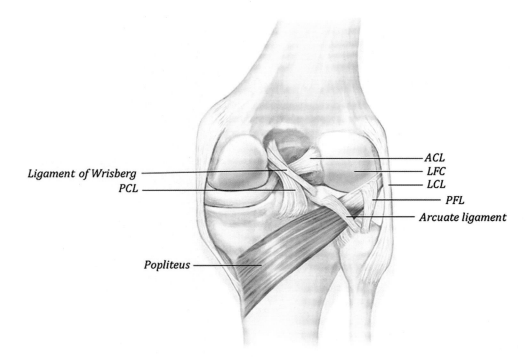

Ligament of Wrisberg
PCL

ACL
LFC
LCL
PFL
Arcuate ligament

Popliteus

FIGURE 41-2

Posterolateral structures of the knee. LCL, lateral collateral ligament; PFL, popliteofibular ligament; ACL, anterior cruciate ligament; PCL, posterior cruciate ligament; LFC, lateral femoral condyle.

The anterior cruciate ligament (ACL) and posterior cruciate ligament (PCL) are static, intra-articular stabilizers of the knee. The ACL is extrasynovial but intracapsular and provides primary restraint to anterior tibial translation and secondary restraint to varus and internal rotation stress. It is composed of two bundles (anteromedial [AM] and posterolateral [PL]), which originate on the posteromedial portion of the lateral femoral condyle and inserts on the anterior tibia between the tibial eminences (33). The PCL is also extrasynovial yet intracapsular and is composed of two bundles (anterolateral [AL] and posteromedial [PM]). It provides the primary restraint to posterior tibial translation and acts as a secondary stabilizer to valgus force and external rotation. It originates on the lateral aspect of the medial femoral condyle and inserts into the tibial sulcus posteriorly (34). The medial and lateral menisci act as secondary stabilizers. The posterior horn of the medial meniscus acts as the primary stabilizer to anterior tibial translation in an ACL-deficient knee (35). Similarly, the posterior root of the lateral meniscus contributes to dynamic rotational stability in an ACL-deficient knee. The presence of a lateral meniscal posterior root injury significantly destabilizes an ACL-deficient knee demonstrated by the pivot shift maneuver (36).

Neurovascular injuries are commonly associated with traumatic knee dislocations. The sciatic nerve has two terminal branches: the tibial nerve that courses medially superficial to popliteal vessels and the common peroneal nerve (CPN) that arises from the superolateral aspect of the popliteal fossa and courses laterally and inferiorly along the medial border of the biceps femoris (37). It then courses distally adjacent to and around the neck of the fibula prior to branching into the superficial and deep peroneal nerves. Injury to the CPN is a common sequela of traumatic knee dislocations, reportedly seen in 25% to 41% of cases (38). Popliteal artery injury is also often associated with traumatic knee dislocations as reports have estimated that arterial injury is seen in 22% to 32% of acute traumatic dislocations (18). The popliteal artery arises from the femoral artery at the level of the adductor hiatus and travels distally through the popliteal fossa (Fig. 41-3). Notably, the artery is the deepest and most anterior structure of the popliteal fossa. It contributes five genicular branches that provide blood supply to the knee. The medial genicular artery is the most commonly injured artery in traumatic knee dislocations (18).

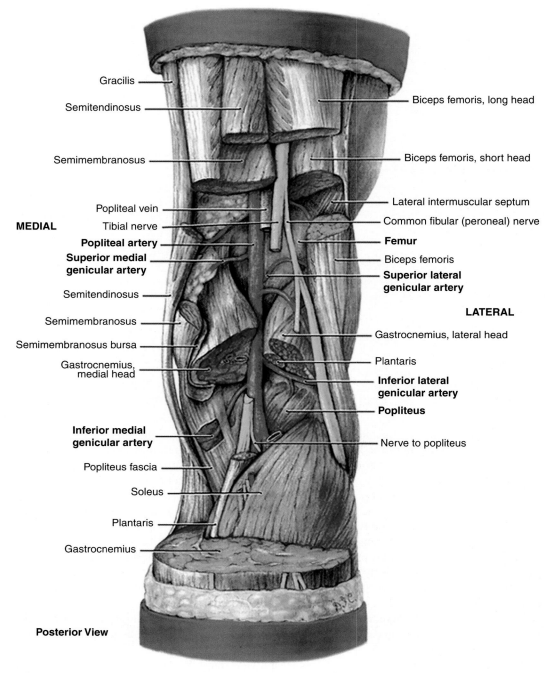

Gracilis

Semitendinosus

Semimembranosus

Popliteal vein

MEDIAL   Tibial nerve

Popliteal artery

Superior medial genicular artery

Semitendinosus

Semimembranosus

Semimembranosus bursa

Gastrocnemius, medial head

Inferior medial genicular artery

Popliteus fascia

Soleus

Plantaris

Gastrocnemius

Biceps femoris, long head

Biceps femoris, short head

Lateral intermuscular septum

Common fibular (peroneal) nerve

Femur

Biceps femoris

Superior lateral genicular artery

LATERAL

Gastrocnemius, lateral head

Plantaris

Inferior lateral genicular artery

Popliteus

Nerve to popliteus

Posterior View

FIGURE 41-3

Popliteal artery and nerve in the posterior aspect of the knee.

CLASSIFICATION

In general, knee dislocations are classified in terms of tibial displacement in relation to the femur, or the Kennedy classification system (Table 41-1) (2). In simplest terms, they are divided into five main patterns: those of the sagittal plane (anterior and posterior), the coronal plane (medial and lateral), and rotatory.

Sagittal plane dislocations typically result from an applied force in one direction. Anterior dislocations result from a hyperextension mechanism (Fig. 41-4) (2,39). Hyperextension to 30 degrees causes injury to the posterior capsule, followed by injury to PCL and the ACL. Rupture of the popliteal artery occurs after 50 degrees of hyperextension (2). Posterior dislocations result

TABLE 41-1 Schenck Classification of Knee Dislocations Based on Extent of Ligamentous Injury	
KD-I	Single cruciate + collateral injury
KD-I	Single cruciate + collateral injury
KD-II	ACL + PCL injury
KD-III M	ACL, PCL, + MCL injury
KD-III L	ACL, PCL, LCL + PLC injury
KD-IV	ACL, PCL, MCL, LCL + PLC injury
KD-V	Fracture dislocation

from a posteriorly directed force applied to the anterior tibia. This can occur while the foot is fixed on the ground during contact sports or by abrupt deceleration injuries in knee flexion when the anterior tibia abruptly strikes the dashboard during a motor vehicle collision (MVC). Posterior dislocations always disrupt the PCL, which is the primary stabilizer to posterior tibial forces. Additionally, at such high posterior loads, patellar tendon failure is also quite common followed by injury to the ACL.

Coronal plane dislocations (lateral and medial) and rotational dislocations occur far less commonly compared to sagittal plane knee dislocations (39). Such patterns are secondary to valgus and varus, respectively. Very modest coronal plane dislocations can occur following a slip off of a curb or tripping in a hole; however, more than half of reported coronal plane dislocations were caused by MVCs (40,41). Coronal plane dislocations are associated with a higher incidence of concomitant fractures and peroneal nerve injuries (41,42). Furthermore, lateral knee dislocations harbor the potential for closed irreducibility caused by interposition of the medial capsule into the knee joint. The medial femoral condyle buttonholes through the medial capsule causing a "dimple sign" of the medial soft tissue structures classically present in a patient with grossly deformed knee (Fig. 41-5).

Rotatory dislocations can be further subdivided into AM, AL, PM, and PL injuries (15,42). According to Quinlan and Sharrard, the mechanism of PL knee dislocation involves a flexed knee in a non–weight-bearing situation with a sudden applied rotatory force that abducts and internally rotates the tibia in relation to the femur (3). Similar to lateral dislocations, PL dislocations are extremely difficult—near impossible—to reduce via closed methods (3,43).

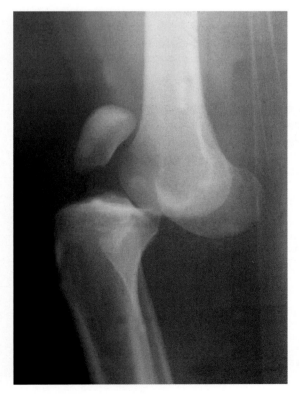

FIGURE 41-4
Anterior knee dislocation.

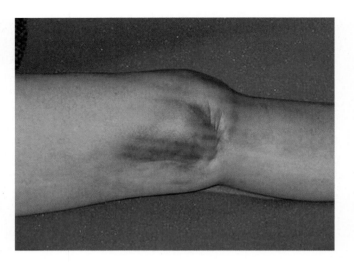

FIGURE 41-5

Dimple sign on the left knee caused by puckering of the anteromedial skin. The overlying skin is at risk of skin necrosis. (Reprinted from Harb A, Lincoln D, Michaelson J. The MR dimple sign in irreducible posterolateral knee dislocations. *Skeletal Radiol.* 2009;38(11):1111–1114. © 2009 Springer Nature, with permission.)

Knee dislocations can also be classified by high- and low-velocity categories (44). High-velocity dislocations are caused by sudden, extremely violent forces (e.g., MVC) and result in global damage to the knee, including disruption of soft tissue structures such as the joint capsule, popliteal tendon, menisci, and cartilage (44,45). Neurovascular damage can be assumed in this setting as high-velocity dislocations are more commonly associated with injury to popliteal artery and nerve and downstream branches. Low-velocity knee dislocations are commonly observed in a sports setting with almost a third of all knee dislocations being sports related, second only to MVCs (50%). According to a study evaluating the occurrence of knee dislocations in extreme sports from 2007 to 2012, the overall incidence of sports-related knee dislocations was 29.12 per 1 million person-years. The highest incidence was associated with the male sex, the age group of 10 to 19 years, and snow skiing (46).

One shortcoming to the Kennedy classification system is that often knee dislocations spontaneously reduce prior to clinical and radiographic evaluation (upward of 50% reported). Such injuries would therefore be rendered "unclassifiable" by the Kennedy system. The Schenck anatomic classification system defines knee dislocations in terms of the ligaments disrupted in the process or the Schenck anatomic classification system. This classification provides a more accurate assessment of injuries and allows for comparison of similar injures on a wide spectrum of knee dislocations (Table 41-2).

TABLE 41-2 Lateral- and Medial-Sided Classification of Knee Dislocations (Fanelli et al. (69))

Type	Clinical Manifestation	Injured Structure(s)
LATERAL-SIDED INJURIES		
A	Isolated increase in external rotation	Popliteofibular ligament (PFL) + popliteus tendon
B	Increase in external rotation + 5 mm varus laxity at 30 degrees of knee flexion	PFL, popliteus tendon + LCL
C	Increase in external rotation + 10 mm varus laxity at 30 degrees of knee flexion	PFL, popliteus tendon, LCL + tearing of lateral capsule
MEDIAL-SIDED INJURIES		
A	Isolated axial rotational laxity (anteromedial or posteromedial)	
B	Axial rotation laxity + valgus laxity at 30 degrees of flexion with a firm endpoint	
C	Gross valgus laxity with a soft endpoint	

ASSESSMENT OF KNEE DISLOCATIONS

Neurovascular Examination

Typically, the patient complains of severe pain and instability and is unable to ambulate or at minimum, continue activities. A "pop" can be heard at the time of injury—particularly during athletic injuries; however, the situation may preclude one from hearing this.

Clinical suspicion and recognition are the single most important factors of dealing with a knee dislocation. A spontaneously reduced knee dislocation can lead to underestimation of injury severity, sometimes resulting in grave consequences (e.g., missed vascular injury leading to amputation) (47). As such, vascular examination should take precedence during initial evaluation. The examination should be very thorough and involve comparison to the contralateral, uninjured limb. First and foremost, physical examination should include assessment of the dorsalis pedis and posterior tibialis artery via palpation or Doppler ultrasonography. Bilateral assessment of capillary refill, skin color, and skin temperature can also provide swift diagnostic information. Some patients may have a warm foot or palpable dorsal or pedal pulses, yet have a popliteal artery injury (8,47–49). The lack of swelling and knee effusions after dislocation can be misleading. Capsular injury and fluid extravasation may cause circulatory damage to go undetected (50). As such, ankle-brachial indexes (ABIs) can provide a more objective assessment with an ABI below 0.9 being an indication for angiography. Many experts have recommended conventional angiography and/or arteriograms for all patients presenting with knee dislocation; (51) however, others have demonstrated no gold standard and perhaps no need to do so in cases where patients have symmetrically intact distal pulses or normal ABI values (52). The debate continues regarding the optimal diagnostic method for timely detection of vascular injury; however, our institution regularly uses MR angiography to assess for vascular injury and the extent of soft tissue injury (Fig. 41-6).

Along with neurovascular examination, clinical assessment of compartments is paramount. Acute compartment syndrome is a potential complication of knee dislocation and can negatively impact functional outcomes. Regular monitoring not only of distal perfusion but of compartments should be performed for at least 72 hours following injury. The risk is so high and the complications are so significant that some surgeons advocate prophylactic fasciotomies in the setting of vascular damage.

The popliteal artery's anatomic location places it at particular risk for damage during knee dislocation. It is tethered firmly above and below the knee; hence, its susceptibility to injury. The reported frequency of vascular injury ranges from 22% to 32% (9,53) including injuries to the tunica intima, arterial occlusions, avulsion injuries, ruptures, or transections (42). The popliteal artery is injured in approximately 20% to 40% of all knee dislocations (54). Vascular impairment is most common after sagittal plane knee dislocations (54). Anterior dislocations usually result in a traction injury as the popliteal artery stretches into the intercondylar notch. In general, low-velocity injuries tend to

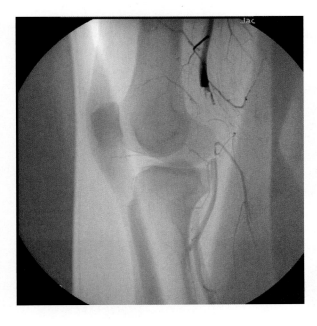

FIGURE 41-6

Arteriogram demonstrating complete disruption of the popliteal artery.

be associated with fewer vascular injuries compared to high-velocity injuries (6). Because vascular injury is potentially limb threatening, rapid recognition and resolution of any injury are critical. A delay in diagnosis increases warm ischemia time and the risk for irreversible injury.

The CPN is not tethered to the knee, though it still can be inured due to its anatomic location around the fibular neck. Peroneal nerve injury has been shown to occur in up to 35% of knee dislocations (55,56), most commonly following anterior, PL, and PM rotatory dislocations (57). The nerve is typically stretched along the posterior aspect of the lateral femoral condyle. While not as devastating an injury as the popliteal artery, a good neurologic assessment is also important. Damage to the CPN may compromise foot dorsiflexion, eversion, and gait impairment. Additionally, injury to the CPN can cause sensory changes to the anterior lateral leg and dorsum of the foot. Functional recovery after peroneal palsy after knee dislocation has a limited prognosis secondary to the energy of the insult resulting in axonotmesis over an extensive nerve segment.

Physical Examination

A thorough assessment of alignment, range of motion, extensor mechanism integrity, and grading of ligamentous injury is necessary. However, physical examination is often difficult to interpret immediately following injury—diffuse pain with and without palpation, guarding, the presence of ipsilateral fractures or polytrauma, and altered mental status make initial assessment unreliable. Additionally, the presence of minimal effusion can be misleading and may indicate a capsular injury with extravasation. Strength testing should be avoided in the acute setting; however, an orthopaedist can still evaluate the integrity of the extensor mechanism, cruciate and collateral ligaments. The extensor mechanism can be evaluated by a straight leg raise test. With a pillow placed under the knee, the Lachman test can be performed with reasonable sensitivity. Positive Lachman and pivot shift tests diagnose an ACL injury, and posterior drawer and sag tests diagnose a PCL injury. Varus and valgus stress tests performed with the leg on and hanging over the stretcher can demonstrate injury to the MCL and the LCL, respectively. The dial test can be performed at 30 degrees of flexion in most cases—90 degrees may not be possible given the instability of the knee. A positive dial test at 30 degrees of flexion raises suspicion to a PLC injury (Fig. 41-7).

Radiographic Workup

In the setting of an acute knee dislocation on the field at a sporting event—particularly with vascular compromise, an orthopaedic surgeon can reduce a dislocated knee without radiographic imaging by assessing the type of knee dislocation based on gross deformity. However, if the injury is not witnessed and the patient is transferred to a level I trauma center, an immediate radiograph should be performed to understand the type of dislocation and to assess for concomitant fractures. Prior to a formal reduction, injury films should first be obtained. Postreduction films should confirm joint congruency. If a fracture is found, computed tomography (CT) may offer additional utility. Radiographic stress testing has been described, though has mostly been abandoned given the advancement of imaging modalities. Magnetic resonance imaging (MRI) is certainly not needed in the acute setting; however, it is required for surgical planning to characterize the extent of soft tissue, ligament, and tendon injuries.

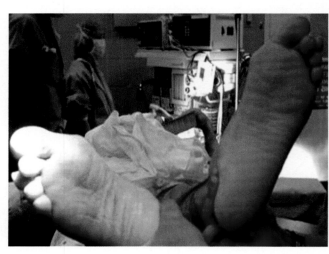

FIGURE 41-7

Positive dial test, indicator of posterolateral rotatory instability of the knee.

MANAGEMENT

Initial Management after an Acute Knee Dislocation

Patients may present immediately following a high-energy trauma or a low-energy injury during play with an acutely dislocated knee or a reduced knee with multiple ligamentous injuries. Initially, the patient should be managed with standard Advanced Trauma Life Support (ATLS) protocols to assess for concomitant trauma including head injury. A knee dislocation should be reduced as soon as possible, preferably in a controlled environment such as the emergency department with sedation. Radiographs are recommended before and after reduction.

Not all knee dislocations can be reduced by closed methods, and more injury can occur with multiple attempts. Furthermore, a dimple sign indicating a lateral or PL dislocation is a contraindication to attempted close reduction due to the high risk of skin necrosis (14). For this reason, grossly deformed limbs should be gently repositioned. Sedation can generally be provided in the emergency department and is highly recommended.

The reduction maneuver includes traction followed by gentle extension. The proximal tibia should be manipulated depending on the characteristics of the dislocation. Following reduction, limb perfusion must be confirmed. Thereafter, a detailed physical examination under anesthesia should be performed to assess for ligament integrity. If the knee is not grossly unstable and is well perfused with no neurovascular concerns, the knee can be immobilized in a long leg brace or splint (avoid a constrictive cast or brace given the risk of developing compartment syndrome). Kennedy recommended splinting with a posterior slab in 15 degrees of flexion to avoid tension of the popliteal vessels and hypervigilance with regard to repeated evaluation of skin color, capillary refill, distal pulses, temperature, and sensation (2). Compartment syndrome warrants immediate release of all four leg compartments.

In certain circumstances, immediate surgical intervention is needed in the management of acute knee dislocations. If possible, multiple issues can be addressed at the index surgery to limit the number of operations. If the knee is extremely unstable or redislocates after reduction, temporary external fixation is warranted. If the posterior capsule is compromised, posterior subluxation of the tibia ensues. Stabilizing the knee in 20 degrees of flexion during external fixation helps prevent posterior subluxation (58). External fixators can also be used if a vascular injury requires reconstruction (e.g., bypass vein grafting) and or concomitant popliteal vein repair to reduce the risk of deep venous thrombosis or pulmonary embolism. External fixators also provide structural support for soft tissue stabilization after four-compartment fasciotomy.

Open knee dislocations require emergent irrigation and debridement, soft tissue closure over drains, immobilization, and antibiotics. If associated with a fracture, antibiotics have been shown to be the most important factor preventing future infection. If possible, ligament repair can be carried out during the initial procedure. External fixation may be a helpful adjunct. In which case, care should be taken to place pins 10 cm above and below the joint line in preparation for future ligamentous reconstruction tunnels (59).

Irreducible knee dislocations require immediate surgical intervention. In many cases, soft tissue or bony incarceration is the source of irreducibility. A PL knee dislocation associated with medial femoral condyle buttonholing results in MCL invagination and a prominent "dimple sign" at the AM aspect of the knee joint, particularly when the knee is extended (the MCL gets pulled into the joint). Ligamentous repair can be performed during the index procedure particularly if irreducibility is the cause for acute surgery, as long as the knee is not grossly contaminated. Prophylactic antibiotics are recommended for all acute surgery.

Definitive Treatment of Ligamentous Injuries

Surgical and nonsurgical management both play a role in treating knee dislocations depending on the situation, patient factors, and associated injuries. Historically, knee dislocations were treated in a cast or hinged brace for several weeks to months (60). As technology and surgical procedures have evolved, the treatment paradigm has shifted in favor of surgery with the goal being to create a stable though flexible, functional knee without complications associated with prolonged immobilization and non–weight bearing.

Conservative treatment may still be pursued if the joint feels relatively stable postreduction and or depending on patient age and activity level (e.g., an older patient who is sedentary and/or nonambulatory) (14,61). Nonoperative management consists of a period of immobilization ranging from 3 to 10 weeks, with an average duration of 5.5 weeks (41,62). Immobilization >6 weeks can result in stiffness and residual functional deficits (15). As such, conservative treatment is considered unsuitable for young, active, athletic populations. Early surgical management is much more beneficial in this patient group, particularly with recent advancements in surgical techniques. Multiple studies have demonstrated a benefit to surgical management including two meta-analyses showing increased range of motion, postoperative Lysholm scores (63,64), International Knee Documentation Committee (IKDC) scores (64,65), and increased rates of return to work and return to sport (66). Ultimately, clinical judgment should be employed by all treating surgeons with regard to operative and nonoperative treatment.

Absolute indications for surgical management include irreducible dislocations, vascular injury, and open injuries with or without associated fractures. Ultimately, definitive surgical management depends on which ligaments are injured and the severity of injury to those ligaments. General recommendations are to delay surgery for 2 to 3 weeks unless there is an absolute acute surgical indication. Delaying surgery allows the soft tissues to stabilize to permit accurate intraoperative anatomic delineation and structural repair. Furthermore, delayed surgery has been shown to optimize outcomes (67,68). According to Shelbourne et al. (44), delayed surgery also reduces the risk of postoperative arthrofibrosis, which authors theorize as being associated with immediate concurrent reconstruction of the medial structures, ACL and PCL (69). Delayed surgery also has its downsides including scarring, which makes surgery, particularly PL repairs and reconstructions, increasingly difficult. For this reason, Good and Johnson suggest that repair and/or reconstruction is optimally performed between 2 and 3 weeks postdislocation (70). Some authors consider 3 weeks to be the *critical timing threshold* when capsular inflammation has resolved, thus reducing the risk of arthroscopic fluid extravasation, while no significant scar tissue has yet formed, decreasing risk to neurovascular structures including the peroneal nerve (69).

Each knee dislocation is unique to an individual, the particular mechanism, and associated neurologic, vascular, or polytrauma injuries. Nonetheless, general principles of treatment following knee dislocation have remained the same (Table 41-3). With regard to staging for surgical reconstruction, one- or two-stage procedures can be employed.

Surgical Considerations

Surgical repair and reconstruction can be achieved using a combination of arthroscopic and open techniques. Arthroscopy is a useful adjunct to assess the integrity of menisci and articular cartilage and also in preparation of the intercondylar notch for intra-articular ligament reconstructions.

TABLE 41-3 General Treatment Principles Following Knee Dislocations

1. Dislocation should always be suspected in trauma, particularly in the setting of polytrauma and when gross knee instability, swelling, and ecchymosis are present.
2. Knee reduction should be performed as soon as possible in the emergency department, preferably with sedation and prior to transfer to another hospital.
3. One should have high suspicion of vascular injury. Furthermore, all patients with a suspected knee dislocation must be closely monitored for late vascular compromise during the first week after injury.
   - Orthopaedic surgery, traumatology, and emergency department should work in close collaboration with radiology and vascular surgery.
   - The neurovascular status of the limb should be checked before and after reduction.
   - Ankle-brachial pressure index (ABI) should be obtained on all suspected knee dislocations. If normal, continued evaluation of vascular status is sufficient.
   - If vascular compromise is confirmed, vascular surgery should be consulted immediately.
4. Vascular repair should be performed as soon as possible, within 6–8 hours of injury.
5. Fasciotomies should be performed as soon as there are concerns for impending compartment syndrome or compartment syndrome.
6. Nerve exploration is generally little value, particularly in the immediate period, unless preparation has been made with a surgeon of microscopic group fascicular repair or grafting techniques.
7. If acute surgery is required, ligaments should be repaired or reconstructed during the same session unless contraindicated (e.g., contamination, compartment syndrome, threat to vascular repair).
8. Postoperatively, exercises focused on regaining motion should be initiated as soon as possible if the integrity of ligamentous procedures and vascular repair permit.

Adapted from Good L, Johnson RJ. The dislocated knee. *J Am Acad Orthop Surg.* 1995;3:284–292.

A standard AL portal is first established followed by an AM portal placed under direct visualization. In the absence of fluid extravasation, an accessory PM portal can be established just posterior to the MCL between zones A and B of the medial meniscus.

Arthroscopy can lead to extravasation of fluid into the surrounding soft tissue compartments and may cause compartment syndrome. In such circumstances, very brief arthroscopy with low-pressure flow or wrapping of the calf is preferred. The surgeon should have a low threshold for converting to an open procedure and must be prepared to do so using a long oblique anterior skin incision from proximal-lateral to distal-medial. With appropriate extension and elevation of full-thickness soft tissue flaps, this type of incision provides access to all aspects of the knee.

Generally, patients are positioned supine on a radiolucent operating table with all bony prominences well padded. A sterilely draped C-arm imaging machine run by the surgeon or an XR technologist is used to obtain fluoroscopic images throughout the case. The operating table should allow for adjustment of variable degrees of flexion at the hip and knee. For instance, the foot of the table should drop to allow for 90 degrees of knee flexion during the case. Alternatively, the senior author employs a post and distal leg positioner, which maintains the knee at 90 degrees providing access to anterior and posterior structures. Additionally, the senior author will frequently airplane the bed to better access to medial and lateral structures.

A sterile back table will allow for simultaneous graft preparation by a second assistant. Graft choices for ligament reconstructions include autografts and allografts. Excellent clinical results have been demonstrated using allografts, which have the advantage multiple graft size options with or without a bone block, no donor site morbidity, and decreased tourniquet time if no vascular procedures were performed prior (tourniquet use contraindicated after vascular repair). Furthermore, the use of allograft tissue eliminates graft site morbidity, decreases dissection time, and reduces the number and extent of incisions in an already traumatized knee (71). Cruciate reconstruction is facilitated by allograft use: bone-patellar tendon-bone (BPTB) allograft is typically recommended for ACL reconstruction. Although, Achilles tendon allograft is also an effective choice for ACL and can be used for PCL and LCL reconstructions. If allografts are unavailable in a bicruciate setting, the PCL is reconstructed using BPTB autograft and the ACL with quadrupled hamstring autograft. The senior author prefers autograft for intra-articular ligaments including contralateral BPTB for ACL reconstruction. If there is no medial-sided injury, the senior author prefers ipsilateral hamstring autograft for PCL reconstruction. In isolated injuries, studies have shown that cruciate ligament reconstructions with allografts have higher failure rates than those of autografts particularly for younger patients (72).

Techniques for Ligament Reconstruction

Certain surgical principles should be followed for a systematic approach to ligament reconstruction. One principle involves the sequence for addressing multiligamentous reconstructions (Table 41-4). Ligament wise, typically, the PCL is reconstructed first with a soft tissue graft for ease of passage, followed by the ACL, then the PLC, LCL, and MCL. However, the sequence of reconstruction is as follows: Tibial tunnels are first drilled for the PCL and the ACL. Thereafter, femoral tunnels are drilled. In the setting of a PLC or LCL injury, the femoral tunnels for the LCL are drilled next with care taken not to violate the ACL femoral tunnel using radiographic assistance, direct visualization, and tactile feedback. After the LCL graft is passed through the fibula, attention returns to the cruciates. The PCL graft is first passed given that it is the most challenging of the cruciates to reconstruct, followed by the ACL graft. After reconstruction of the cruciate ligaments and PL stability is restored, the MCL can be addressed.

Extra-articular reconstructions or repairs (e.g., extensor mechanism, ITB, and biceps tendon) can be performed after ligamentous stability is achieved. Some avulsion fractures of ligaments can also be treated with primary repair.

ACL + PCL Injuries

The details of ACL and PCL reconstruction have been well described. Arthroscopically, the femoral and tibial insertions are identified and debrided of all residual stumps and soft tissue. First, tibial tunnels are created under fluoroscopic guidance. Fluoroscopy is recommended for the tibial tunnels for safe and accurate placement of the guidewire into the posterior tibial footprint of the PCL, specifically, avoiding injury to the popliteal vessels (Fig. 41-8). The entry site for tibial PCL on the anterior cortex of the tibia is distal to the entry of the ACL tunnel. The guidewire should exit

TABLE 41-4 Surgical Principles for Multiligamentous Reconstructions

1. One suggested surgical order per Rihn et al. (71) is as follows:
   - Drill tibial tunnels for PCL, then ACL.
   - Drill femoral tunnels for ACL, then PCL.
   - Pass and fix PCL (with or without) bone block into femoral tunnel through the anterolateral portal.
   - Pass tendinous portion of PCL graft into the tibial tunnel.
   - Secure extra-articular repairs or reconstructions of the collateral ligaments.
   - Fix the PCL graft on the tibia at 90 degrees of flexion with reproduction of anteromedial step-off.
   - Fix the ACL graft on the tibial side at full extension.
2. Knee reduction should be performed as soon as possible in the emergency department, preferably with sedation and prior to transfer to another hospital.
3. One should have high suspicion of vascular injury. Furthermore, all patients with a suspected knee dislocation must be closely monitored for late vascular compromise during the first week after injury.
   - Orthopaedic surgery, traumatology, and emergency department should work in close collaboration with radiology and vascular surgery.
   - The neurovascular status of the limb should be checked before and after reduction.
   - Ankle-brachial pressure index (ABI) should be obtained on all suspected knee dislocations. If normal, continued evaluation of vascular status is sufficient.
   - If vascular compromise is confirmed, vascular surgery should be consulted immediately.
4. Vascular repair should be performed as soon as possible, within 6–8 hours of injury.
5. Fasciotomies should be performed as soon as there are concerns for impending compartment syndrome or compartment syndrome.
6. Nerve exploration is generally little value, particularly in the immediate period, unless preparation has been made
   with a surgeon of microscopic group fascicular repair or grafting techniques.
7. If acute surgery is required, ligaments should be repaired or reconstructed during the same session unless contraindicated (e.g., contamination, compartment syndrome, threat to vascular repair).
8. Postoperatively, exercises focused on regaining motion should be initiated as soon as possible if the integrity of ligamentous procedures and vascular repair permit.

8 to 10 mm distal to the level of the joint line to ensure proper tibial tunnel placement. The correct orientation of the tunnel should be parallel to the proximal tibiofibular joint, coursing just proximal to the curve of the posterior proximal tibial cortex on lateral view (Fig. 41-8). Arthroscopic placement of the PCL tibial tunnel is best accomplished using the accessory PM portal and either a 30- or 70-degree lens to visualize the posterior tibial ledge. The PCL tibial footprint can be prepared working through the AL or PM portals. The senior author prefers an all-inside PCL reconstruction technique using a Flipcutter (Arthrex, Naples, Florida, USA) reamer because of less trauma to the knee and ease of tunnel drilling.

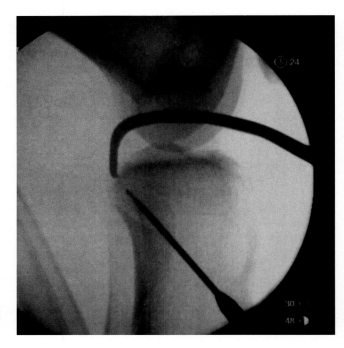

FIGURE 41-8

Fluoroscopic image of guide pin in tibial tunnel for PCL reconstruction.

After PCL femoral tunnel is established, the tibial ACL tunnel is created using an ACL drill guide set at 45 degrees. The anatomic position of the tunnel is located in line with the anterior horn of the lateral meniscus, on a virtual line splitting the distance between the medial and lateral tibial spines. Care should be taken to avoid violating ACL and PCL tunnels.

The femoral PCL insertion is anterior and proximal on the medial wall of the intercondylar notch. For single-bundle reconstructions, the goal is to reproduce the insertion of the AL bundle of the PCL. The vastus medialis is elevated from the AM femoral cortex, and the femoral drill guide is positioned in an outside-in fashion. The guidewire exits in the intercondylar notch, and an appropriately sized reamer is used over the guidewire. Alternatively, the femoral tunnel can be drilled first using an inside-out technique via a low AL portal.

Double-bundle PCL reconstructions are not typically performed after a knee dislocation. However, in isolation, double-bundle PCL reconstruction techniques have been shown to restore more normal knee kinematics compared to single-bundle techniques (73). This technique includes one tibial tunnel and two femoral tunnels to recreate both the AL and PM bundles, which are tight in flexion and extension, respectively. As mentioned above, Achilles tendon allograft can be split in its tendinous portion to create the two bundles for the femoral attachment sites.

The femoral ACL tunnel is created via the anteromedial portal (AMP). Bony landmarks such as the lateral intercondylar ridge ("resident's ridge") and the lateral bifurcate ridge help guide placement of the femoral tunnel on the lateral wall of the intercondylar notch (74–76).

Once all tunnels are drilled, the PCL graft is first passed, followed by the ACL graft. In the setting of a PLC or LCL injury, the femoral tunnel of the LCL reconstruction should be drilled prior to PCL and ACL graft passage. To pass the semitendinosus autograft for PCL reconstruction, a 22-guage wire fashioned into a loop is inserted from outside-in through the tibial tunnel. The leading edge is retrieved through the AL portal with a grasper and guided to the exit of the femoral PCL tunnel. A second grasper is passed from outside-in through the femoral PCL tunnel and into the notch, with the leading edge is brought out of the femoral tunnel. A second wire is looped through the leading edge of the first wire and brought back out of the tibial PCL tunnel. PCL draw sutures are then passed through the leading edge of the second wire and pulled up into the tibial tunnel, through the notch, and out through the femoral PCL tunnel. Next, a beath pin is used to draw the ACL graft from the AM portal into the femoral tunnel. A grasper is used in the tibial tunnel to pull the draw stitch from the femoral tunnel out through the tibial tunnel. Pulling the draw sutures will allow passage of the graft to the desired depth in the femoral tunnel.

Similar to tunnel drilling and graft passage, the PCL graft is addressed first for tensioning and final fixation. Of note, if collateral ligaments are also being reconstructed, those soft tissue grafts should first be passed and fixed prior to fixing the PCL and ACL. If a single-bundle construct is used, the PCL is tensioned at 70 degrees of knee flexion. It is vital that the knee be reduced prior to tibial fixation. The first assist can apply a manual anterior drawer to recreate the native anterior tibial step off of approximately 1 cm. Following confirmed reduction, the tibial side is fixed while applying maximal axial traction on the draw sutures. Multiple devices can be applied for additional fixation if indicated including an AO screw and washer, staple, soft tissue button, or suture anchor. Finally, the ACL graft is tensioned in full extension with maximal axial tension on the draw sutures and fixed with an interference screw. Again, secondary fixation can be employed as needed.

Lateral Structures

Next in the sequence of multiligamentous knee reconstructions is the PLC. Arthroscopy typically reveals a lateral gutter drive through sign. The open approach to PLC surgery typically involves a hockey stick–shaped incision that starts 5 cm proximal and posterior to the lateral epicondyle, ending 5 cm distal to Gerdy tubercle, just anterior to the fibular head (Fig. 41-9). Three fascial incisions are described by Terry and Laprade (Fig. 41-10) (77). The CPN must be exposed and protected from iatrogenic injury including traction (Fig. 41-11). If the CPN compromised with an intraneural hematoma, the epineurium should be opened and the hematoma evacuated.

PLC structures including the LCL, popliteus tendon, and PFL are frequently injured in knee dislocations. The proximal LCL is injured in two-thirds of knee dislocation cases and the distal LCL in one-third of the cases. The popliteus tendon similarly is disrupted at its proximal insertion in two-thirds of the cases and at the musculotendinous junction in one-third of the cases. The PFL is almost always injured and can be repaired primarily in cases of bony avulsion and when there is an adequate ligamentous remnant.

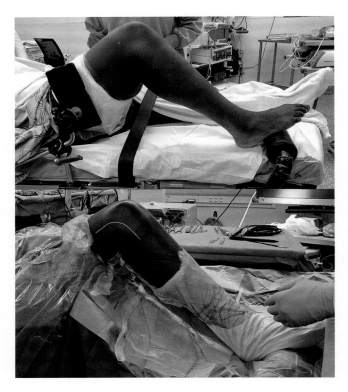

FIGURE 41-9

Lateral hockey-shaped incision
for approach to the posterolateral knee.

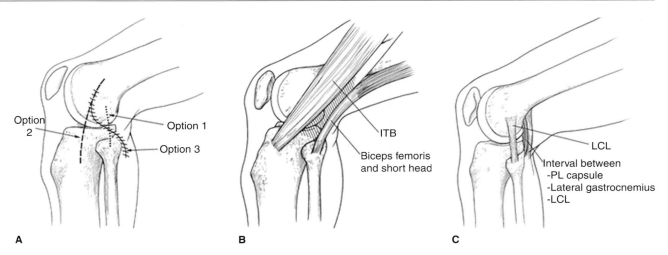

A   **B**   **C**

FIGURE 41-10

Posterolateral approach to the knee. **A:** Multiple options for lateral incisions including (*1*) a 3-cm vertical incision made at the joint
line, just posterior to the lateral collateral ligament (LCL). (*2*) A gently curved lateral incision centered over the lateral joint line and
extended distally to expose the fibular head. (*3*) An S-shaped incision can be curved to the posterior aspect of the fibular head for
more posterior access. **B:** Open the interval between the short head of the biceps femoris and the iliotibial band (ITB). **C:** Retracting
the biceps femoris protects the underlying peroneal nerve and exposes the interval between the posterolateral capsule, LCL, biceps
tendon, and lateral gastrocnemius head. (Reprinted from Medvecky MJ, Noyes FR. Surgical approaches to the posteromedial and
posterolateral aspects of the knee. *J Am Acad Orthop Surg.* 2005;13(2):121–128, with permission.)

The popliteus tendon is addressed prior to LCL reconstruction. In some cases, its integrity is
maintained and adequate for repair; that is reattachment to its femoral insertion or advancement if
the tendon is intact yet attenuated. In cases of complex tears located at the musculotendinous junction with concomitant injury to the PFL, the popliteus tendon can be tenodesed to the PLC of the
tibia or posterior fibular head at the insertion of the PFL. The popliteus insertion on the fibular head
is situated on the posteriorly sloped surface of the head, 8 to 10 mm posterior and 3 to 5 mm medial to the insertions of the LCL and biceps tendons. The reconstruction is carried out by detaching

FIGURE 41-11

Intraoperative photo of a lateral collateral ligament reconstruction with a white Penrose drain around the common peroneal nerve. Note the two limbs of the semitendinosus allograft used for the LCL reconstruction.

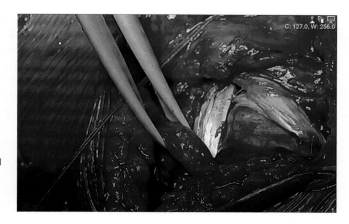

the popliteus tendon from its muscular junction, controlling it with a no. 2 Ethibond (Ethicon Inc., Somerville, New Jersey), and attaching it through a K-wire tunnel over a suture button on the fibula, tensioned in 70 degrees of knee flexion while the lateral tibia is drawn anteriorly to its neutral position. If the popliteus tendon quality is compromised, it can be augmented with a thin strip of ITB left attached to Gerdy tubercle and routed along the popliteus tendon through drill holes in the proximal tibia from anterior to posterior.

Hamstring autograft or allograft can be used for combined fibula-based reconstructions (Larson technique) of the popliteus and PFL. First, the fibula tunnel is created at the insertion of the PFL with the use of a retractor posteriorly to protect the CPN. The fibula tunnel is then reamed over a 6- to 7-mm guidewire from anterior to posterior. The femoral insertion of the popliteus tendon can be found approximately 18 mm anterior and inferior from the LCL femoral insertion. The femoral tunnel is then reamed over a guidewire to a depth of 25 mm. The graft is passed through the fibula. Both limbs of the graft are truncated ensuring no more than 25 mm of graft length in the tunnel and are then passed into the femoral tunnel by pulling on the draw sutures medially. The graft is fixed with an interference screw at 30 degrees of knee flexion with manually applied internal rotation and valgus.

After fixing the popliteus and PFL, the LCL can be addressed either by primary repair, partial reconstruction using biceps tendon or semitendinosus allograft (senior authors preference), or through a combined fibula-based PCL reconstruction (Fig. 41-11). Care must be taken to avoid tunnel convergence, especially on the lateral side. Primary repair is an option in the setting of an LCL femoral avulsion if performed within 21 days following injury. LCL can be reattached through a shallow bone tunnel at the insertion site on the lateral epicondyle and secured with a suture button on the medial femoral condyle. A guidewire is placed 25 mm proximal to the joint line on the lateral femoral condyle. With the knee at 30 degrees of flexion, ligament excursion is assessed and the guidewire is adjusted to the point of lowest ligament excursion. Next, a 5- to 10-mm shallow bone tunnel is drilled, followed by a 6-mm reamer at the predetermined site. A beath pin is driven through the tunnel across the femur exiting medially through the medial femoral condyle. Draw sutures placed on the free end of the ligament are passed, and the LCL is drawn into the bone tunnel and secured medially over a suture button.

If direct LCL repair is not possible, LCL reconstruction can be carried out with the use of the biceps femoris tendon as a graft or a soft tissue allograft, which is the senior author's preference to avoid trauma to the biceps tendon. If the biceps tendon is used, a 20 × 80-mm strip is elevated from underlying muscle with a no. 15 blade, leaving the attachment on the fibular head intact. The biceps tendon strip is then tubularized by rolling one longitudinal half to the midline and rolling the other half around it, secured with simple stitches passing through the tendon. A screw and washer construct can be used to fix the tendon strip at the LCL femoral insertion, thus restoring the PLC of the knee.

Medial Structures

In cases of combined cruciate and medial knee structure reconstructions, the cruciates should be reconstructed first to restore the functional central pivot. The central pivot is necessary to accurately determine the isometry of planned reconstructions. In rare situations of an MCL avulsion from its tibial insertion, it can be primarily reattached—after debridement of the distal insertion—with a screw and washer construct, staple, or suture anchors. Most MCL injuries (80% of cases) occur at the femoral insertion (78). Primary repair is frequently complicated by poor tissue integrity of the proximal stump. Nonetheless, primary repair can be carried out if the posterior portion of the MCL, POL, and the PM capsule are of decent quality. The posterior capsuloligamentous tissues are advanced anteriorly and reefed with the MCL stump secured to the femoral insertion with suture anchors.

Knee dislocations usually result in complete severance of the MCL and POL with irreparable injury to the posterior capsule. In this case, reconstruction with hamstring or Achilles tendon allograft is necessary. The semitendinosus tendon can be used to augment the reconstruction as described by Bosworth: the semitendinosus tendon remains attached to the pes anserinus on the tibia and is dissected free proximally (79). The isometry point is determined by placing a guidewire in the medial femoral epicondyle and assessing excursion of the semitendinosus tendon over the guidewire. At the point of minimal excursion, the tendon is advanced to the predetermined MCL center of rotation on the femur. The MCL is then fixed with a screw and washer at 30 degrees of knee flexion and a manually applied varus stress. MCL remnants on the tibia are secured to the semitendinosus tendon.

Because the MCL has two separate tibial insertions, anatomic double-bundle MCL reconstruction is another method of fixation and is actually preferred over nonanatomic semitendinosus tenodesis to more closely reproduce the biomechanics of the native MCL. A semitendinosus autograft or allograft is fixed with a staple or interference screw on the femur and two separate interference screws on the tibia. The graft is tensioned at 30 degrees of knee flexion with maximal axial traction on the draw sutures. Manual internal rotation and varus forces are applied during fixation. If present, the remnant of the native MCL is reefed over the graft, thus restoring the PM corner of the knee.

POSTOPERATIVE MANAGEMENT AND REHABILITATION

Immediate postoperative management occurs in an inpatient setting for regular neurovascular checks and evaluation of pain management. Additionally, wounds and soft tissue evaluation are a priority and can easily be followed as an inpatient. Some advocate prophylactic release of the anterior and lateral compartments of the leg to decrease the risk of compartment syndrome following multiligamentous reconstructions, particularly PLC surgery. Whether or not fasciotomies are performed, surgical dressings should be loosely applied to negate neurovascular compromise. The knee is then placed in a hinged knee brace locked in full extension. Patients can typically be observed for the first 24 to 48 hours following surgery for neurovascular and compartment checks, hematoma formation, incision drainage, and for intravenous antibiotics and cold therapy.

In general, bracing and early motion are the hallmarks of postoperative knee rehabilitation. Obviously, patients with multiligamentous reconstructions should be rehabbed slower than those with isolated reconstructions with progression determined on an individual basis based on the ligaments reconstructed. For instance, after LCL reconstruction, the knee should be splinted in 30 degrees of flexion. Patients are typically non–weight bearing for 2 weeks and gradually progressed. Deep venous thrombosis prophylaxis is also provided for a minimum of 4 weeks, which the patient is non–weight bearing. Some form of chemoprophylaxis with or without mechanical measures should be utilized.

No studies to date have clarified how aggressive rehabilitation should be, in part because of the variation of reconstructions following a knee dislocation. The most well-known common complication following surgical treatment of knee dislocations is loss of motion. There is a high risk of arthrofibrosis in knee dislocation patients. If possible, early continuous passive motion can be initiated from 0 to 30 degrees until a 0- to 70-degree arc of motion is comfortably maintained. If 90 degrees of flexion is not established by 8 to 10 weeks postoperatively, manipulation should be carried out under anesthesia. An example of a postoperative rehabilitation protocol is found in Table 41-5.

Though stiffness is a major concern following ligamentous reconstruction of a knee dislocation, the alternative being some degree of instability is not well tolerated by patients resulting in both functional disability and pain.

CLINICAL OUTCOMES

Knee dislocations cause severe soft tissue injuries that can preclude return of normal knee function. Clinical outcome is generally better following lower-energy mechanisms such as sports injuries (80). Patients who are treated acutely (between 2 and 3 weeks) achieve superior clinical outcomes compared to those patients treated chronically (67,81). Activities of daily living can be more predictably achieved than high-demand sporting activities or heavy manual labor (81).

TABLE 41-5 Rehabilitation Protocol Example

Week 1–3	Non–weight bearing on surgical extremity
	Brace locked in extension
	Ambulation with crutches
	No physical therapy (PT)
Week 4–6	Progression to partial weight bearing
	Brace locked in extension
Week 7–12	Gradually discard crutches
	Unlock brace from 0 to 30 degrees, gradually increasing arc of motion
	Supervised gait training
	More aggressive ROM therapy with PT
	Begin closed-kinetic chain exercises: leg press, half squats, stair exercises
	Avoid open-kinetic chain active isolated quadriceps and hamstring exercises
	Stationary bicycle exercises permitted
Week 13–16	Full range of motion should be established
	Closed-kinetic chain exercises continued
	Elliptical trainer exercises started
Week 17–24	Increase resistance, proprioceptive, and agility training
	Return to full activity NOT recommended before 36–48 weeks (9–12 months)

CONCLUSION

The management of knee dislocations requires a team approach including but not limited to orthopaedic surgery traumatology and sports medicine, general surgery trauma, vascular surgery, interventional and musculoskeletal radiologist, and physical therapist and rehabilitation specialists. A systematic management strategy consisting of emergent safe reduction, stabilization of the joint, and neurovascular assessment is of the utmost importance, followed by thorough physical examination, radiographic imaging, and examination under anesthesia. With regard to surgery, a carefully calculated preoperative plan for surgical reconstruction versus repair is critical for optimal clinical outcome.

REFERENCES

1. Hoover N. Injuries of the popliteal artery associated with dislocation of the knee. *Surg Clin North Am.* 1961;41:1099–1112.
2. Kennedy JC. Complete dislocations of the knee joint. *J Bone Joint Surg Am.* 1963;45:889–904.
3. Quinlan AG, Sharrard WJW. Posterolateral dislocation of the knee with capsular interposition. *J Bone Joint Surg Br.* 1958;40:660–663.
4. Aron GA, Yeranosian MG, Petrigliano FA, et al. The changing demographics of knee dislocation: a retrospective database review. *Clin Orthop Relat Res.* 2014;472:2609–2614.
5. Frykberg ER. Popliteal vascular injuries. *Surg Clin North Am.* 2002;82(1):67–89.
6. Shelbourne KD, Klootwyk TE. Low-velocity knee dislocation with sports injuries. Treatment principles. *Clin Sports Med.* 2000;19(3):443–456.
7. Henrichs A. A review of knee dislocations. *J Athl Train.* 2004;39:365–369.
8. Green NE, Allen BL. Vascular injuries associated with dislocation of the knee. *J Bone Joint Surg Am.* 1977;59:236–239.
9. Wascher DC, Dvirnak PC, DeCoster TA. Knee dislocation: initial assessment and implications for treatment. *J Orthop Trauma.* 1997;11:525–529.
10. Stannard JP, Sheils TM, Lopez-Ben RR, et al. Vascular injuries in knee dislocations: the role of physical examination in determining the need for arteriography. *J Bone Joint Surg Am.* 2001;86-A(5):910–915.
11. Wascher DC. High-velocity knee dislocation with vascular injury. Treatment principles. *Clin Sports Med.* 2000;19(3):457–477.
12. Meyers MH, Harvey JP Jr. Traumatic dislocation of the knee joint: a study of eighteen cases. *J Bone Joint Surg Am.* 1971;53:16–29.
13. Hill JA, Rana NA. Complications of posterolateral dislocation of the knee: case report and literature view. *Clin Orthop.* 1981;154:212–215.
14. Holmes CA, Bach BR Jr. Knee dislocations: immediate and definitive care. *Phys Sportsmed.* 1995;23(11):69–83.
15. Cole BJ, Harner CD. The multiple ligament injured knee. *Clin Sports Med.* 1999;18:241–262.
16. Reckling FW, Peltier LF. Acute knee dislocations and their complications. *J Trauma.* 1969;9:181–191.
17. Cooper DE, Speer KP, Wickiewicz TL, et al. Complete knee dislocation without posterior cruciate ligament disruption: a report of four cases and review of the literature. *Clin Orthop.* 1992;284:228–233.
18. Zlotnicki JP, Naendrup JH, Ferrer GA, et al. Basic biomechanic principles of knee instability. *Curr Rev Musculoskelet Med.* 2016;9(2):114–122.
19. Higuchi H, Terauchi M, Kimura M, et al. The relation between static and dynamic knee stability after ACL reconstruction. *Acta Orthop Belg.* 2003;69(3):257–266.
20. LaPrade RF, Engebretsen AH, Ly TV, et al. The anatomy of the medial part of the knee. *J Bone Joint Surg Am.* 2007;89(9):2000–2010.

21. Lefebvre R, Leroux A, Poumarat G, et al. Vastus medialis: anatomical and functional considerations and implications based upon human and cadaveric studies. *J Manipulative Physiol Ther.* 2006;29(2):139–144.

22. Werner BC, Hadeed MM, Gwathmey FW, et al. Medial injury in knee dislocations: what are the common injury patterns and surgical outcomes? *Clin Orthop Relat Res.* 2014;472(9):2658–2666. doi:10.1007/s11999-014-3483-3.

23. Jadhav SP, More SR, Riascos RF, et al. Comprehensive review of the anatomy, function, and imaging of the popliteus and associated pathologic conditions. *Radiographics.* 2014;34(2):496–513. doi:10.1148/rg.342125082.

24. Schenck RC, Richter DL, Wascher DC. Knee dislocations: lessons learned from 20-year follow-up. *Orthop J Sports Med.* 2014;2(5):2325967114534387.

25. Chen L, Kim PD, Ahmad CS, et al. Medial collateral ligament injuries of the knee: current treatment concepts. *Curr Rev Musculoskelet Med.* 2008;1(2):108–113. doi:10.1007/s12178-007-9016-x.

26. Kozanek M, Fu EC, Van de Velde SK, et al. Posterolateral structures of the knee in posterior cruciate ligament deficiency. *Am J Sports Med.* 2008;37(3):534–541.

27. Shah KN, DeFroda SF, Ware JK, et al. Lateral patellofemoral ligament: an anatomic study. *Orthop J Sports Med.* 2017;5(12):1–6.

28. LaPrade RF, Bollom TS, Wentorf FA, et al. Mechanical properties of the posterolateral structures of the knee. *Am J Sports Med.* 2005;33(9):1386–1391.

29. Dalip D, Iwanaga J, Oskouian RJ, et al. A comprehensive review of the fabella bone. *Cureus.* 2018;10(6):e2736. doi:10.7759/cureus.2736.

30. Sudasna S, Harnsiriwattanagit K. The ligamentous structures of the posterolateral aspect of the knee. *Bull Hosp Jt Dis Orthop Inst.* 1990 Spring;50(1):35–40.

31. Wadia FD, et al. An anatomic study of the popliteofibular ligament. *Int Orthop.* 2003;27(3):172–174.

32. Thaunat M, Pioger C, Chatellard R, et al. The arcuate ligament revisited: role of the posterolateral structures in providing static stability in the knee joint. *Knee Surg Sports Traumatol Arthrosc.* 2014;22(9):2121–2127. doi:10.1007/s00167-013-2643-4.

33. Dargel J, Gotter M, Mader K, et al. Biomechanics of the anterior cruciate ligament and implications for surgical reconstruction. *Strategies Trauma Limb Reconstr.* 2007;2(1):1–12.

34. Amis AA, Gupte CM, Bull AM, et al. Anatomy of the posterior cruciate ligament and the meniscofemoral ligaments. *Knee Surg Sports Traumatol Arthrosc.* 2006;14(3):257–263.

35. Makris EA, Hadidi P, Athanasiou KA. The knee meniscus: structure-function, pathophysiology, current repair techniques, and prospects for regeneration. *Biomaterials.* 2011;32(30):7411–7431.

36. Hoshino Y, Miyaji N, Nishida K, et al. The concomitant lateral meniscus injury increased the pivot shift in the anterior cruciate ligament-injured knee. *Knee Surg Sports Traumatol Arthrosc.* 2019;27(2):646–651.

37. Garg K. Chapter 6: Popliteal fossa. In: *BD Chaurasia's Human Anatomy (Regional and Applied Dissection and Clinical) Volume 2—Lower Limb, Abdomen, and Pelvis.* 5th Ed. India: CBS Publishers and Distributors Pvt Ltd; 2010:87,88. ISBN 978-81-239-1864-8.

38. Medina O, Arom GA, Yeranosian MG, et al. Vascular and nerve injury after knee dislocation: a systematic review. *Clin Orthop Relat Res.* 2014;472(9):2621–2629.

39. Gustilo RB, Cabatan DM. Traumatic dislocation of the knee. In: Gustilo RB, Kyle R, Templeman D, eds. *Fractures and Dislocations.* St. Louis, MO: 1993:885–895.

40. Roman PD, Hopso CN, Zenni EJ Jr. Traumatic dislocation of the knee: a report of 30 cases and literature review. *Orthop Rev.* 1987;16:917–924.

41. Taylor AR, Arden GP, Rainey HA. Traumatic dislocation of the knee: a report of forty-three cases with special reference to conservative treatment. *J Bone Joint Surg Br.* 1972;54:96–102.

42. Brautigan B, Johnson DL. The epidemiology of knee dislocations. *Clin Sports Med.* 2000;19(3):387–397.

43. Pardiwala DN, Rao NN, Anand K, et al. Knee dislocations in sports injuries. *Indian J Orthop.* 2017;51(5):552–562.

44. Shelbourne KD, Porter DA, Clingman JA, et al. Low-velocity knee dislocation. *Orthop Rev.* 1991;20:995–1004.

45. Montgomery JB. Dislocation of the knee. *Orthop Clin North Am.* 1987;18:149–156.

46. Sabesan V, Lombardo JD, Sharma V, et al. Hip and knee dislocations in extreme sports: a six year national epidemiologic study. *J Exerc Sports Orthop.* 2015;2:1–4.

47. Swenson TM. Physical diagnosis of the multiple-ligament-injured knee. *Clin Sports Med.* 2000;19:415–423.

48. McCuthan JD, Gillham NR. Injury to the popliteal artery associated with dislocation of the knee: palpable distal pulses do not negate the requirement for arteriography. *Injury.* 1989;20:307–310.

49. McCoy GF, Hannon DG, Barr RJ, et al. Vascular injury associated with low-velocity dislocation of the knee. *J Bone Joint Surg Br.* 1987;69:285–287.

50. Hegyes MS, Richardson MW, Miller MD. Knee dislocation: complications of nonoperative and operative management. *Clin Sports Med.* 2000;9:519–543.

51. Mills WJ, Barei DP, McNair P. The value of the ankle-brachial index for diagnosing arterial injury after knee dislocation: a prospective study. *J Trauma.* 2004;56:1261–1265.

52. Hollis JD, Daley BJ. 10-year review of knee dislocations: is arteriography always necessary? *J Trauma.* 2005;59(3):672–675.

53. Green NE, Allen BL. Vascular injuries associated with dislocation of the knee. *J Bone Joint Surg Am.* 1997;59:236–239.

54. Kaufman SL, Martin LG. Arterial injuries associated with complete dislocation of the knee. *Radiology.* 1992;184:153–155.

55. Hegyes MS, Richardson MW, Miller MD. Knee dislocation. Complications of nonoperative and operative management. *Clin Sports Med.* 2000;19(3):519–543.

56. Niall DM, Nutton RW, Keating JF. Palsy of the common peroneal nerve after traumatic dislocation of the knee. *J Bone Joint Surg Br.* 2005;87:664–667.

57. Bratt HD, Newman AP. Complete dislocation of the knee without disruption of both cruciate ligaments. *J Trauma.* 1993;34(3):383–389.

58. Seroyer ST, Musahl V, Harner CD. Management of acute knee dislocation: the Pittsburgh experience. *Injury.* 2008;39:710–718.

59. Howells NR, Brunton LR, Robinson J, et al. Acute knee dislocation: an evidence based approach to the management of the multiligament injured knee. *Injury.* 2011;42:1198–1204.

60. Meyers MH, Moore TM, Harvey JP Jr. Traumatic dislocations of the knee joint. *J Bone Joint Surg Am.* 1975;57:430–433.

61. Windsor RE. Dislocation. In: Insall JN, ed. *Surgery of the Knee.* 2nd Ed. New York: Churchill Livingstone; 1993:555–560.

62. Frassica FJ, Sim FH, Staeheli JW, et al. Dislocation of the knee. *Clin Orthop.* 1991;263:200–205.

63. Richter M, Bosch U, Wippermann B, et al. Comparison of surgical repair or reconstruction of the cruciate ligaments versus nonsurgical treatment in patients with traumatic knee dislocations. *Am J Sports Med*. 2002;30(5):718–727.

64. Dedmond BT, Almekinders LC. Operative versus nonoperative treatment of knee dislocations: a meta-analysis. *Am J Knee Surg*. 2001;14(1):33–38.

65. Levy BA, Dajani KA, Whelan DB, et al. Decision making in the multiligament-injured knee: an evidence-based systematic review. *Arthroscopy*. 2009;25(4):430–438.

66. Peskun CJ, Whelan DB. Outcomes of operative and nonoperative treatment of multiligament knee injuries: an evidence-based review. *Sports Med Arthrosc Rev*. 2011;19(2):167–173.

67. Liow RY, McNicholas MJ, Keating JF, et al. Ligament repair and reconstruction in traumatic dislocation of the knee. *J Bone Joint Surg Br*. 2003;85(6):845–851.

68. Fanelli GC, Edson CJ. Arthroscopically assisted combined anterior and posterior cruciate ligament reconstruction in the multiple ligament injured knee: 2- to 10-year follow-up. *Arthroscopy*. 2002;18(7):703–714.

69. Fanelli GC. Multiple ligament-injured (dislocated) knee. *Sports Med Arthrosc Rev*. 2011;19(2):81.

70. Good L, Johnson RJ. The dislocated knee. *J Am Acad Orthop Surg*. 1995;3:284–292.

71. Rihn JA, Cha PS, Groff YJ, et al. The acutely dislocated knee: evaluation and management. *J Am Acad Orthop Surg*. 2004;12:334–346.

72. Van Eck CF, Schkrohowsky JG, Ramirez C, et al. Failure rate and predictors of failure after anatomic ACL reconstruct with allograft (SS-61). *Arthroscopy*. 2011;27(5):e62–e63.

73. Harner CD, Janaushek MA, Kanamori A, et al. Biomechanical analysis of a double-bundle posterior cruciate ligament reconstruction. *Am J Sports Med*. 2000;28(2):144–151.

74. Ferretti M, Ekdahl M, Shen W, et al. Osseous landmarks of the femoral attachment of the anterior cruciate ligament: an anatomic study. *Arthroscopy*. 2007;23:1218–1225.

75. Iwahashi T, Shino K, Nakata K, et al. Direct anterior cruciate ligament insertion to the femur assessed by histology and 3-dimensional volume-rendered computed tomography. *Arthroscopy*. 2010;26(9 Suppl):S13–S20.

76. Shino K, Suzuki T, Iwahashi T, et al. The residents ridge as an arthroscopic landmark for anatomic femoral tunnel drilling in ACL reconstruction. *Knee Surg Sports Traumatol Arthrosc*. 2010;18:1164–1168.

77. Terry GC, LaPrade RF. The posterolateral aspect of the knee. Anatomy and surgical approach. *Am J Sports Med*. 1996;24(6):732–739.

78. Potter HG, Weinstein M, Allen AA, et al. Magnetic resonance imaging of the multiple-ligament injured knee. *J Orthop Trauma*. 2002;16(5):330–339.

79. Bosworth DM. Transplantation of the semitendinosus for repair of laceration of medial collateral ligament of the knee. *J Bone Joint Surg Am*. 1952;34-A(1):196–202.

80. Richter M, Lobenhoffer P, Tscherne H. Knee dislocation. Long-term results after operative treatment. *Chirurg*. 1999;70(11):1294–1301.

81. Harner CD, Waltrip RL, Bennett CH, et al. Surgical management of knee dislocations. *J Bone Joint Surg Am*. 2004;86-A(2):262–273.

42 Cartilage: Débridement and Microfracture

Spencer M. Stein, Alexander M. Satin, Daniel Grande, and Nicholas A. Sgaglione

INTRODUCTION

Achieving a predictable and durable repair after an articular cartilage injury has remained a clinical challenge. Advancements in arthroscopy and magnetic resonance imaging (MRI) have led to an increase in the acute recognition of articular cartilage injuries. Several investigators have reported on the incidence of such lesions. Curl et al. retrospectively reviewed 31,516 knee arthroscopies and reported lesions in 63% of patients (1). Similarly, Aroen et al. published a survey of 993 consecutive knee arthroscopies, which revealed articular cartilage pathology in 66%, with a localized full-thickness lesion in 11% (2). Hjelle et al. reported chondral or osteochondral lesions in 61% of 1,000 knee arthroscopies, 5% of which were full thickness (3).

Articular cartilage defects can result in pain, swelling, clicking, instability, and ultimately, progression to a more diffuse, degenerative process (4). The response of articular cartilage to injury, and thus healing, depends upon the type, location, and mechanism of the injury as well as numerous clinical patient factors. Due to the avascular nature of cartilage, superficial injuries fail to stimulate a predictable healing response (4). However, full-thickness injuries that penetrate subchondral bone may have more direct vascular access and, consequently, have a greater capacity for healing. The repair tissue, in general, has the structure, histology, and biomechanical properties of a fibrocartilaginous mosaic with potential variable islands of hyaline-like cartilage. Despite the altered biomechanics and potentially inferior long-term durability, some clinical studies have reported symptomatic and functional improvement in subsets of patients (4–7).

Current surgical options broadly include palliative, reparative, replacement, and regenerative approaches. Palliative techniques include arthroscopic debridement and lavage using mechanical shavers or radiofrequency devices. Reparative options include arthroscopic marrow stimulation and microfracture techniques. These techniques necessitate the deliberate penetration of subchondral bone at the base of the lesion in order to elicit bleeding and subsequent bone marrow-mediated repair. Replacement methodologies include osteochondral autograft transplantation (OAT) or osteochondral allograft transplantation (OCA). Regenerative techniques include cell-based therapies, such as autologous chondrocyte implantation (ACI), and next-generation approaches, such as three-dimensional ACI scaffold augmentation—The tissue repair response after marrow stimulation has been shown to be composed of primarily type I collagen with poorer proteoglycan and type II collagen content than found in normal hyaline cartilage (5,8–10). In addition, some authors have questioned the utility of the traditional microfracture techniques in light of the reported potential complications and/or adverse events as well as short-term benefits (11–13). More recently, interest in next-generation "augmented" marrow stimulation techniques has increased to address these limitations. These newer methodologies are based upon efforts to stabilize the mesenchymal clot produced by marrow stimulation and to improve mesenchymal stem cell (MSC) differentiation into more hyaline-like repair tissue. Of note, augmented microfracture techniques are usually carried out using a single-stage, minimally invasive approach performed in a similar manner to traditional microfracture.

This chapter will focus on the surgical techniques and outcomes of two primary treatment methods, debridement and marrow stimulation, and will provide an evidence-based review of the latest developments of augmented marrow stimulation techniques.

PREOPERATIVE PLANNING

A comprehensive history should be taken with any patient presenting with a possible articular cartilage injury and clinically correlative symptoms. Treatment indications optimally include those patients with defined symptoms and whose potential confounding pathology can be precisely characterized. Historically, clinical results for both debridement and microfracture vary depending on the type of chondral injury (degenerative vs. acute), as well as the age, body mass index (BMI), surgical history, and activity level and functional goals of the patient. Thus, the timing, symptoms, mechanism of injury, occupation, and activity level of the patient should be ascertained. In an effort to distinguish traumatic or focal lesions from degenerative lesions associated with osteoarthritis (OA), the type, timing, and location of symptoms as they relate to the injury must be defined, with distinction between focal mechanical symptoms from those that are more diffuse and longstanding. Traumatic chondral and osteochondral lesions commonly present acutely with a hemarthrosis, pain, and often, mechanical symptoms suggestive of a loose body, while a subset of patients will describe a more chronic indolent scenario. A complete exam should follow, specific for the affected joint, and assessed relative to the unaffected limb. General appearance and focal tenderness to palpation should be noted, as well as an evaluation of generalized ligamentous laxity. Range of motion should be measured in addition to the presence of joint crepitus. Furthermore, the mechanical and anatomical axis of the lower extremity as well as gait analysis should be assessed and measured.

Plain radiography should always be obtained including weight-bearing radiographs of the affected limb as well as a standing hip to ankle radiographs for determination of the lower extremity mechanical axis. Additional views, such as a patellar skyline, notch or tunnel views, and 45-degree flexion weight-bearing posteroanterior views, are essential. MRI offers the ability to evaluate for coexistent meniscal or ligamentous injuries, and modern advancements in articular cartilage-specific MRI techniques, such as modified fast spin-echo sequence, can increase the detection of cartilage lesion size and depth. Additionally, the use of three-dimensional pulse sequences and the addition of isotropic voxels allow for a more precise measurement of lesion size, cartilage volume, and for postoperative tissue fill analysis (14).

Traditional grading systems for articular cartilage lesions are commonly based upon the arthroscopic assessment of the lesion. The most commonly used classification systems are the Outerbridge (15), Modified Outerbridge, and International Cartilage Repair Society (ICRS) (16) grading systems (Table 42-1).

In those patients who remain symptomatic after a trial of nonoperative treatment, surgical intervention may be considered. The criteria used to indicate a patient for any osteochondral resurfacing procedure is multifactorial. The age and preinjury activity level of the patient must be considered, and patient expectations and goals should be addressed and discussed. Patients should be counseled as to the potential benefit and risks of the proposed procedure. It is important to explain that while surgical interventions are often successful in providing pain relief and resumption of activities, the ability to consistently reproduce the pre-injury articular surface at long-term follow-up remains elusive.

TABLE 42-1 Modified Outerbridge Classification Versus ICRS[a] Classification System

	Modified Outerbridge (15)	ICRS[a] (16)
Grade 0	Normal	Normal
Grade I	Softening and swelling	Nearly Normal: Soft indentation and/or superficial fissures and cracks
Grade II	Partial-thickness defect: Fissuring within softened areas	Abnormal: Lesion extending to <50% of cartilage depth
Grade III	Full-thickness defect: Breakdown of the surface: Fibrillation	Severely Abnormal: Lesion extending to A. >50% of cartilage depth B. Calcified layer C. To subchondral bone D. Includes blisters
Grade IV	Complete loss of cartilage Erosive changes and exposure of subchondral bone	Severely Abnormal: Lesion extending through subchondral bone

[a]International Cartilage Repair Society.

DEBRIDEMENT

Indications/Contraindications

Arthroscopic debridement has gained popularity as a technically simple and efficient method to treat articular cartilage lesions and arthritic knees. Using high-speed arthroscopic rotary shavers, handheld basket punches, arthroscopic curettes, and radiofrequency (RF) ablative devices, the procedure consists primarily of the removal of incongruent, unstable delaminated cartilaginous flaps; the shaving of fibrillated tissue; the removal of all loose bodies; and the resection of any unstable meniscal tears. RF devices utilize modulated thermal energy on cartilage injury to produce a uniform biological scar. While RF instruments have been shown to effectively remove injured cartilage, the utilization of RF techniques has declined in recent years due to concerns regarding unpredictable adverse effects on adjacent native tissue. Interestingly, a recent systematic review noted that despite concerns regarding subchondral bone necrosis, low complication rates are reported in the literature. However, the authors concluded that the heterogeneity of RF devices reported and the lack of evidence on the long-term effects make the use of RF chondroplasty a controversial topic among orthopedic surgeons (17,18).

In 2008, the American Academy of Orthopaedic Surgery (AAOS) published clinical practice guidelines (CPGs) for the treatment of symptomatic knee OA. The second edition was published in 2013, with more stringent inclusion criteria regarding evidence; systematic reviews were removed because of significant variability, additional potential for bias, and variable clinical applicability. The AAOS guidelines recommend against performing an arthroscopic debridement and lavage, for patients with a primary diagnosis of OA (19). However, these recommendations do not apply to patients with a primary diagnosis of loose body, meniscal tear, or other mechanical symptoms (20).

Arthroscopic debridement is a clinically useful and practical first-line treatment for focal, unstable osteochondral lesions, with minimal morbidity and few complications. The clinical benefits of arthroscopic chondroplasty for professional athletes and the general population have been reported. Furthermore, arthroscopic chondroplasty may be a more effective option than marrow stimulation for high-level athletes with articular cartilage lesions who are focused on expeditious return to activities. Scillia et al. retrospectively reviewed NFL players who underwent arthroscopic chondroplasty to determine rate of return to play and factors influencing successful return. The authors found that a majority of players (67%) were able to return to regular season play and that players who underwent concomitant microfracture were 4.4 times less likely to return to the NFL. Furthermore, there was no difference regarding age at surgery, lesion location, lesion size, lesion grade, and position (21). These results highlight the need for careful evaluation of each patient's functional goals when deciding upon treatment choices.

Focal osteochondritis dissecans (OCD) lesions treated solely with excision demonstrate radiographic progression of degenerative joint disease on long-term follow-up (22,23). Furthermore, Shelbourne et al. found inferior results for patients undergoing anterior cruciate ligament (ACL) reconstruction with articular cartilage defects of average size 1.7 cm^2 after an average of 8.7-year follow-up as compared with patients without cartilage defects. The clinical outcome scores were similar and likely not clinically significant (i.e., IKDC 95.2 vs. 94 for medial compartment defects) (24). Therefore, some OCD or posttraumatic lesions may benefit from a more conservative approach, although adjuvant debridement or lavage in association may have a role in lesions with unstable tissue.

In summary, the indications for the procedure include those symptomatic patients with well-aligned knees presenting with unstable focal articular cartilage lesions (<2 cm^2) and lesions with associated flaps or loose bodies, including those associated with OCD or fractures. Contraindications include end-stage diffusely arthritic knees, BMI > 25 to 30, underlying ligamentous instability, rheumatologic and systemic disorders, sepsis, and joint malalignment. The role of debridement in patients with mild to moderate knee OA remains controversial.

Surgical Technique and Pearls and Pitfalls

Debridement and Lavage

Standard anterolateral and anteromedial portals are used and a diagnostic arthroscopy is performed. All loose bodies, which typically settle in the medial and lateral gutters or the suprapatellar pouch, should be identified and removed using an arthroscopic grasper. Cartilage fibrillations and

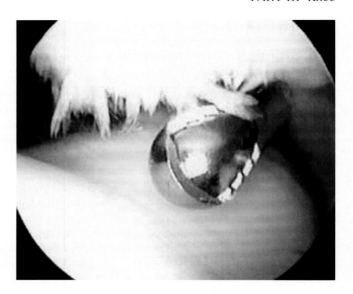

FIGURE 42-1

Shaver debridement of fibrillated cartilage, with the blade directed just off of the surface. Suction should be used to bring the fibrillations to the shaver.

delaminating flaps should be debrided to eliminate any mechanical symptoms or pain as well as to reduce propagation of the defect. Shavers, ring curettes, or electrocautery can be used to trim loose cartilage with care taken not to damage adjacent healthy tissue or to expose underlying bone (Fig. 42-1). Sharp curettes, either domed or ringed, can be effective to remove larger flaps.

Postoperative Care and Rehabilitation

Modified weight bearing to comfort with immediate range of motion is encouraged. Inflammation reduction measures and the use of cryotherapy are advised throughout the rehabilitation process. The patient is instructed to perform a low-impact exercise regimen consisting of quadriceps setting, straight leg raising, active-assisted range of motion exercises, and cycling. The goal of rehabilitation is to achieve balanced muscle strength, flexibility, and full range of motion.

Results

Arthroscopic joint debridement for arthritis without specific mechanical symptoms remains a controversial topic. Moseley et al. performed a level I randomized controlled trial of 180 patients with OA who failed medical management, comparing arthroscopic debridement, lavage alone, and placebo "sham" surgery. The results were similar in all three groups, with no surgical benefit proven (25). A level I randomized control study by Kirkley et al. of 188 patients treated with either arthroscopic debridement and lavage or physical therapy and medical management demonstrated no significant improvement in the surgical group (26).

Several other investigators have reported that arthroscopic treatment of cartilage lesions can provide symptomatic relief in certain patients. Steadman et al. retrospectively reviewed 61 patients (69 knees) with moderate to severe knee OA treated with an arthroscopic treatment regimen focused on increasing joint volume. The majority of patients (87%) in their study had a satisfactory result, and the authors concluded that their arthroscopic treatment regimen and rehabilitation protocol can improve function and activity levels in patients with moderate to severe OA (27). In 2013, Spahn et al. published a meta-analysis that reviewed 30 published reports of arthroscopic debridement. The authors found good to excellent outcomes in 66% of patients at middle term (3–5 year) follow-up (28). They also reported on a delay in the progression to arthroplasty for about 4 years after arthroscopic debridement. High-grade lesions with more advanced OA were noted to have worse outcomes after debridement. Other factors that were identified as risk factors for poor outcomes included smoking, obesity, limb malalignment, retropatellar crepitus, tibial osteophytes, calcifications and prior meniscectomy (28).

Bert and Maschka compared debridement and lavage to abrasion arthroplasty and showed little clinical difference between the two procedures (29). In 2013, Gudas et al. randomized 102 patients undergoing ACL with articular cartilage damage in the medial femoral condyle to receive a concomitant OAT procedure, microfracture, or debridement. They found patients who underwent OAT had significantly improved outcome scores compared to the microfracture and debridement groups.

Of note, the authors found compelling evidence that here was no significant difference between the microfracture and debridement at 3-year follow-up (30).

Arthroscopic debridement remains a popular first-line treatment method for focal osteochondral injuries. In appropriately indicated patients, it remains a relevant, simple, first-line treatment of articular cartilage defects. Debridement as a treatment for knee OA without mechanical symptoms continues to remain a controversial topic due to conflicting results and a lack of high-level, long-term evidence. The most recent AAOS CPGs do not support arthroscopic debridement and lavage for patients with a primary diagnosis of OA (19).

MARROW STIMULATION

Introduction

The concept behind marrow stimulation techniques was introduced in 1959 when Pridie noted that a fibrocartilage tissue repair response developed in lesions where subchondral bone was eburnated following drilling (31). In 1986, Johnson introduced arthroscopic abrasion arthroplasty of chondral defects with the use of a high-speed burr to superficially abrade subchondral bone and create a bleeding surface. Initial clinical improvement was reported in 77% of patients and, at a 2-year follow-up, widened joint space on AP x-rays was noted in nearly 50% (32). However, Johnson many years later acknowledged that the fibrocartilage infill lacks the biomechanical properties of articular cartilage and may require biological augmentation to enhance the tissue repair response (33). More recently, Sansone et al. presented their long-term (mean follow-up 20 years) results of abrasion arthroplasty for full-thickness cartilage lesions of the medial femoral condyle. The authors found a 71.4% survivorship (no reoperation) with the best results in younger patients (<50 years) with smaller lesions (<4 cm^2) (34).

In the 1980s, Steadman coined the term "microfracture" and later popularized the procedure when he described the surgical technique and favorable results in a series of patients in 1997 (35). The technique employs the controlled and systematic use of arthroscopic awls rather than high-speed drills or burrs, thus negating the concern for thermal necrosis. Microfracture also offered superior control and improved arthroscopic access to the articular surfaces of the knee. The careful debridement of chondral lesions to a stable peripheral rim prior to creating the perforations ("microfractures") allowed for the adherence of a "superclot," composed of marrow stromal progenitor cells, which ultimately filled the defect (35,36). However, the tissue infill produced after marrow stimulation has been shown to be composed of primarily type I collagen (fibrocartilage) with poorer proteoglycan and type II collagen content than found in normal cartilage (5,8–10,37). In recent years, some authors have advocated for the abandonment of microfracture given the potential complications (subchondral cysts, subchondral bone hypertrophy, etc.) and shorter-term outcomes in more active patients (11–13). Interest in next-generation "augmented" marrow stimulation techniques has increased to address the limitations of traditional microfracture. These newer techniques are designed to stabilize the mesenchymal clot produced by marrow stimulation and to potentially improve MSC differentiation into more hyaline-like articular cartilage.

Augmented microfracture marrow stimulation techniques to improve upon the success of the traditional microfracture procedure have been recently introduced and are being studied to assess efficacy. These augmentation strategies are purported to produce a more predictable quality repair tissue. Numerous strategies and techniques have been reported on and include use of scaffold enhancement, hyaluronic acid (HA) viscosupplementation, morphogenic growth factors, and cytokine modulation techniques (38–43).

Indications/Contraindications

The published results of marrow stimulation procedures have provided more precise guidelines regarding clinical indications. In their initial series of 1,200 patients treated with microfracture, Steadman et al. noted worse results in patients presenting with chronic lesions and advanced age and in those who failed to use a continuous passive motion machine (CPM) postoperatively (35). In a later 11-year follow-up of patients treated with microfracture, age <35 years was a predictor of better clinical outcome. More optimal results were reported, although not statistically significant, with lesions smaller than 400 mm^2 compared with larger lesions (44). Mithoefer et al. found, in a study of high-impact pivoting athletes treated with microfracture, that a significantly higher rate of return to high-impact sports (64%) was noted in those patients with lesions <200 mm^2 as compared to those

TABLE 42-2 Indications/Contraindications for the Microfracture Procedure	
Microfracture	
Optimal Indications	**Contraindications**
Full-thickness cartilage defects	BMI >30
Small, contained defect (<200 mm²)	Age >55
Posttrauma	Inability to comply with postoperative rehab
Young, active patient (<35 y)	Ligamentous instability
<1 year from time of injury	Malaligned knee
Femoral condyle lesions	Coagulopathy
	Advanced degenerative changes
	Underlying avascular necrosis
	Collagen vascular disease
	Sepsis

with larger lesions (22%). An increased time interval from injury was also found to be a negative prognostic factor, with return to sport increasing from 44% to 67% if microfracture was performed within 1 year of injury (45). Less optimal results have been associated with obese patients, as shown in a prospective cohort study by Mithoefer et al., where lower clinical scores and lesion fill grades were reported in patients with a BMI >30 (46). Furthermore, it appears that lesions of the femoral condyles were associated with better clinical and defect-filing results, as measured by MRI, when compared to patellofemoral lesions (47).

Enhanced marrow stimulation techniques have similar indications and contraindications as first-generation marrow stimulation methods. Contraindications include bipolar cartilage lesions, inflammatory arthritis, diffuse degenerative OA, ligamentous laxity, and uncorrected mechanical malalignment. In addition, patients who are unable to comply with postoperative rehabilitation and weight-bearing restrictions should not undergo advanced marrow stimulation techniques.

In summary, microfracture is indicated in younger patients with posttraumatic, full-thickness, symptomatic, articular cartilage lesions and, in some cases, mildly degenerative knees with focal, full-thickness cartilage lesions (36) (Table 42-2).

Surgical Technique and Pearls and Pitfalls

The surgical approach begins with preoperative counseling to assess patient expectations and to prepare patients for postoperative protocols and a potentially more extensive and extended recovery compared to arthroscopic debridement. The patient should be educated as to the potential need and importance of modified weight bearing and the need to strictly adhere to physical therapy protocols. Once the lesion is identified, the periphery of loose, unstable cartilage is debrided back to a stable, perpendicular edge of viable cartilage using either an arthroscopic shaver or, preferably, a sharp domed or ringed curette (Fig. 42-2). This technique allows for the marrow clot to maximally adhere to the defect base and mature into reparative fibrous tissue.

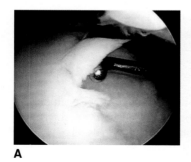 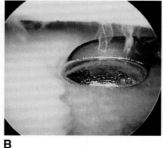 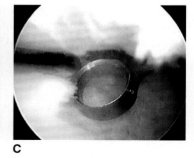

A   **B**   **C**

FIGURE 42-2

Microfracture lesion preparation. **A:** Unstable, nonviable cartilage should be debrided back to a stable, vertical rim to which the marrow clot can adhere. **B:** Use of a curette for debridement. **C:** Use of a loop curette for debridement.

Once the lesion perimeter is defined, the existing calcified cartilage layer is removed using a curette (Fig. 42-3). This has been shown to improve the adhesion of the superclot and subsequent bonding of the repair tissue to the defect site (5,48). However, excessive removal of the calcified cartilage can lead to overpenetration of the subchondral bone. This can lead to subsequent boney overgrowth, which can result in thin, biomechanically inferior repair tissue (46). The microfracture perforations should be made perpendicular to the surface of the lesion, avoiding skiving. The proprietary awls are typically available in 30, 45, and 90 degrees and allow perpendicular placement to most areas of the knee joint, with the 90-degree awl generally reserved for patellar lesions (Fig. 42-4). The microfracture holes are made initially along the perimeter of the lesion to address peripheral integration of the repair tissue with the native hyaline cartilage. The perforations are made sequentially from the periphery to the center of the lesion. The holes are made as close together as possible without creating or propagating a fracture of the subchondral bone bridge with subsequent confluence of holes (which should be at least 3–4 mm apart) (Fig. 42-5A and B). Some microfracture awls have laser-lined depth markers on the tip, though appropriate depth can be assured by turning off the irrigation fluid (and letting down the tourniquet if used) and observing fat droplets and blood extruding from the microfracture holes (Fig. 42-5C). Adequate preparation of the lesion perimeter and shoulders results in a stable bleeding bed to which the marrow clot can adhere to (Fig. 42-6).

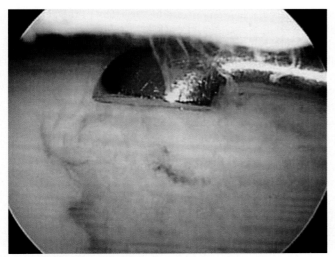

FIGURE 42-3
Curettage of calcified cartilage layer.

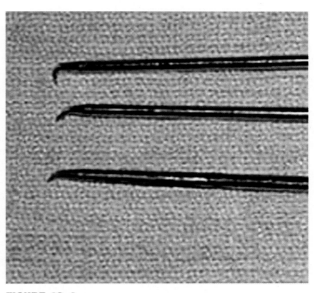

FIGURE 42-4
Microfracture awls.

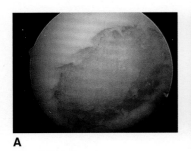 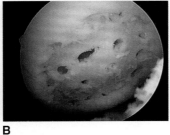 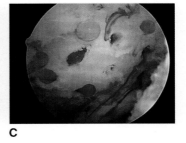

A **B** **C**

FIGURE 42-5

Microfracture sequence. **A:** Postdebridement of calcified cartilage layer. **B:** The microfracture should proceed in a periphery to central direction. **C:** Marrow elements including fat droplets and blood extruding from the microfracture holes assuring adequate penetration depth.

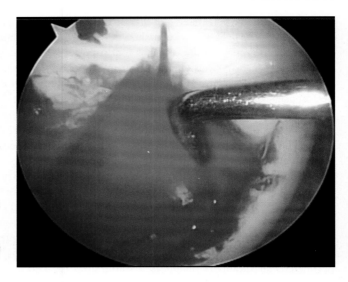

FIGURE 42-6

Adherent superclot to a stable rim of viable cartilage.

While the most common methods of performing microfracture use awls, other devices have been described. These methods have been investigated to address shortcomings of traditional microfracture, including boney hypertrophy, the production of fibrocartilaginous tissue, and the deterioration of clinical results at long-term follow-up. Research is ongoing regarding the effect of the geometry of the microfracture device. Conical tips, as seen on Kirschner wires (K-wires), may produce undesirable subchondral bone impaction while polyhedral tips, typical of traditional awls, may precipitate extensive fractures of subchondral bone (49,50). Chen et al. hypothesized that drilling would remove bone debris while proceeding less trauma to subchondral bone. They compared marrow stimulation using a 0.9-mm drill with cooled irrigation and traditional awl technique in rabbits (51). Microdrilling produced less bone debris, compaction, and osteocyte necrosis adjacent to the defect channel with no evidence of thermal necrosis after microdrilling.

Over variations of the microfracture technique have been proposed to reduce trauma to subchondral bone. Mechanical power awls (PowerPick, Arthrex, FL) with a cannulated guide may achieve adequate penetration into subchondral bone with reduced damage to subchondral bone architecture (52). K-wire drilling (Fig. 42-7) and 1-mm nitinol wire drilling (Nanofracture Arthrosurface, MA) have also been described as less traumatic, technically simple techniques with uniform defect penetration (49,53). Ultimately, multiple techniques are available to facilitate the ease of marrow stimulation, each with its proposed benefits and limitations.

However, the ideal clinical technique that offers uniform subchondral bone penetration with minimal trauma to adjacent tissue remains to be determined.

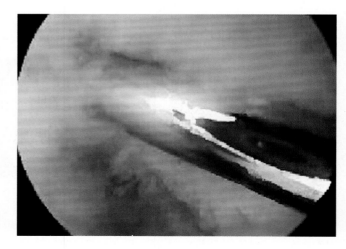

FIGURE 42-7

K-wire drilling for a chondral defect with bone marrow visible after drilling.

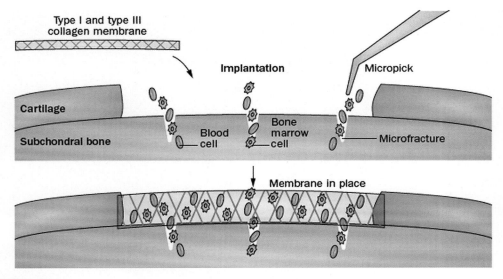

FIGURE 42-8

A collagen membrane is used in conjunction with microfracture to allow blood and bone marrow cells to migrate into the scaffold. (Reprinted from Smith BD, Grande DA. The current state of scaffolds for musculoskeletal regenerative applications. *Nat Rev Rheumatol.* 2015;11(4):213–222. Copyright © 2015 Springer Nature, with permission from Nature.)

Several adjuvant technique methodologies have been introduced in an effort to develop a matrix biomaterial that can provide the appropriate biologic, structural, and architectural cues to facilitate cell attachment, proliferation, and chondrogenic differentiation (54). (Fig. 42-8) Ideally, a scaffold can initially provide a volume stable load-bearing mechanical support and then gradually be replaced by regenerative tissue, as it matures and takes on a higher proportion of load sharing (38,41). Unlike two-stage cartilage restoration procedures, augmented microfracture techniques are performed using a single-stage technique that is similar to traditional microfracture. Before completing augmentation of the microfracture site, the operative leg should be lifted such that the defect is in a horizontal position. When mini-open techniques are utilized, the arthroscopy fluid should be drained following microfracture and prior to augmentation (scaffold, membrane, etc.). Finally, techniques that utilize autologous blood products (platelet-rich plasma, partially autologous fibrin glue, etc.) require coordination with the anesthesia team.

Collagen Scaffold/Membrane Augmentation

Autologous matrix-induced chondrogenesis (AMIC) with Chondro-Gide (Geistlich, Switzerland) is a technique used in Europe that combines microfracture with a type I/III porcine collagen membrane. Originally described by Benthien et al., AMIC is a one-step microfracture augmentation technique performed through a mini-open arthrotomy (55,56). The matrix covers the mesenchymal clot and allows MSCs to differentiate to chondrocytes. An aluminum template is used to size the defect and prepare the membrane. Benthien et al. recommend slightly undersizing the membrane to avoid dislocation after movement. Incorrect membrane sizing can result in overstuffing the defect and subsequent dissociation of the product. The collagen membrane is fixed with fibrin glue. Although allogenic fibrin glue products are commercially available, partially autologus fibrin glue can be generated by centrifuging the patient's blood and mixing the resulting thrombin with allogenic fibrinogen. Alternatively, sutures can be used to fix the membrane but can cause cartilage damage (47,48,57). Dhollander et al. described a modification of this technique named "AMIC Plus," which uses AMIC combined with a platelet-rich plasma (PRP) gel inserted deep to the collagen membrane (58) (Fig. 42-9).

CartiFill (atelocollagen; Sewon Cellontech Co Ltd, Korea) was developed to increase matrix stability following marrow stimulation and maintain progenitor cells at the cartilage defect site. Atelocollagen is a purified porcine-derived type I collagen matrix that is slightly modified (removal of telopeptides) to eliminate the risk of rejection. The collagen matrix provides a three-dimensional structure for chondrogenic differentiation and mechanical support. Following marrow

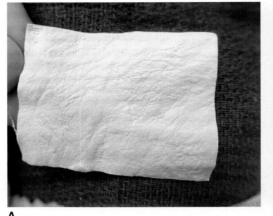

A

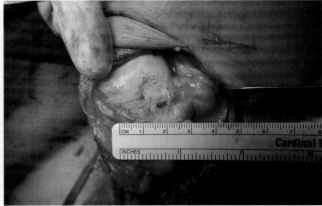

B

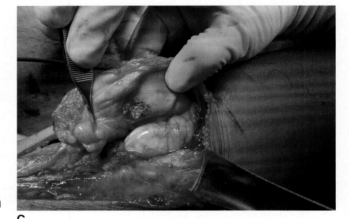

C

FIGURE 42-9

The AMIC technique with Chondro-Gide (Geistlich, Switzerland) uses a type I/III collagen bilayer membrane **(A)**. The defect can be seen in **(B)**. The scaffold can be fixed with suture or fibrin glue though a mini-open arthrotomy **(C)**.

stimulation, CartiFill is prepared using two 1-mL syringes and a Y-shaped mixing catheter connected to a 20-gauge needle. One syringe is filled with 1 mL of fibrinogen and the other is filled with 0.9 mL of CartiFill and 50 IU of thrombin. Under arthroscopic vision from the anterolateral portal, the gel is slowly applied into the defect using an extended anteromedial portal. One to two minutes after an initial layer is generated, an additional gel layer is added to fully seal the defect. The atelocollagen hardens in 5 minutes and then matrix stability can be checked by flexion and extension maneuvers (59).

Chitosan-Based Scaffold Augmentation

BST-CarGel (Smith and Nephew, London, UK), a chitosan-glycerol phosphate scaffold, was developed to stabilize the microfracture clot. Chitosan, a glucosamine polysaccharide found in the exoskeleton of crustaceans, is an ideal scaffold due to its adhesive properties and availability (60). The cytocompatible liquid solution reinforces the implanted superclot, without impairing normal coagulation, by impeding its retraction, and thus maintaining critical blood factors at the marrow penetration sites (61,62). The matrix is manually prepared with autologous whole blood (at least 5 mL are needed). As such, a surgical assistant prepares the BST-CarGel/blood mixture while the defect is microfractured. This technique is performed arthroscopically or through a mini-open approach and depends on surgeon preference, defect location, and defect size.

A sterile vented dispensing pin is inserted into the prepackaged BST-CarGel mixing vial. A nonsterile assistant then attaches the syringe with the peripheral blood to the pin and injects 4.5 mL of blood. The mixing vial is then shaken vigorously. A new, sterile vented dispensing pin is then inserted into the vial, and 2 mL of the BST-CarGel/blood mixture is withdrawn. The 2 mL mixture is injected into the lesion bed in a drop-wise manner over each microfracture hole, and then over the entire lesion, without overfilling. Careful drying of the defect with suction or a gauze swab is critical to the adhesion of BST-CarGel. A stable clot is formed after a 15-minute period in which the leg is held still (57,63,64) (Fig. 42-10).

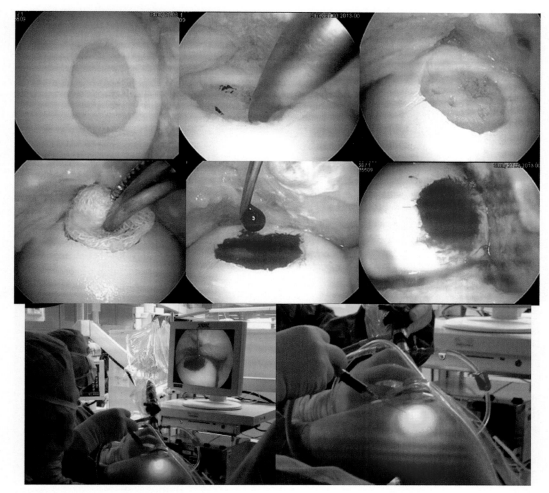

FIGURE 42-10

BST-CarGel (Smith and Nephew, London, UK) is a chitosan-based scaffold that is combined with 5 mL of whole blood. After standard microfracture, 2 mL of the mixture is injected into the lesion after microfracture is performed. (Reprinted with permission from Prof. Matthias Steinwachs, SportClinic Zurich, Switzerland.)

Polymer-Based Scaffold Augmentation

Chondrotissue (BioTissue AG, Switzerland) is a cell-free polyglycolic acid (PGA) scaffold with freeze-dried HA. The technique has been described as a microfracture augmentation technique performed using a miniarthrotomy. The polymer is immersed in 3 milliliter (mL) of autologous serum for 10 minutes and then secured over the defect using transosseous bioresorbable pins after standard debridement, and microfracture is performed (65–67). Siclari et al. have described a successful chondroinductive augmentation to this technique using 5 to 10 minutes of autologous PRP immersion prior to implantation (68) (Fig. 42-11).

Hydrogel-Based Scaffold Augmentation

Polyethylene glycol (PEG) diacrylate bound to fibrinogen (GelrinC, Regentis Biomaterials, Israel) is a photopolymerizable hydrogel that is also under investigation as a microfracture augmentation technique. It can be injected as a gel into a microfractured defect and polymerized in situ during a 90-second period using a prepackaged ultraviolet (UV) light apparatus. Following exposure to UV light, the hydrogel becomes a semisolid material that integrates with the surrounding tissue. This technique allows for congruent resurfacing of the defect. In the 6 to 12 months following implantation, the hydrogel degrades synchronously with the development of hyaline-like cartilage tissue (57,69–71) (Fig. 42-12).

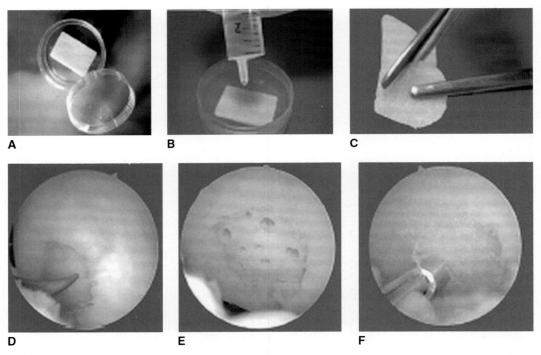

FIGURE 42-11

Chondrotissue (BioTissue AG, Switzerland), a cell-free polyglycolic acid (PGA) scaffold with freeze-dried hyaluronic acid **(A)**, **(B)** reconstituted with autologous blood serum, **(C)** cut to fit the **(D)** defect, and **(F)** implanted with pin fixation after **(E)** microfracture preparation of the cartilage defect. (Reprinted with permission from BioTissue AG, Switzerland.)

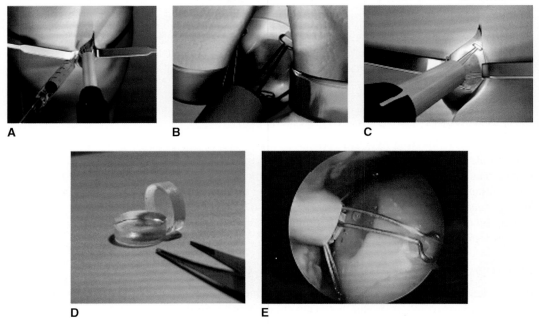

FIGURE 42-12

GelrinC (Regentis Biomaterials, Israel) is a PEG diacrylate fibrinogen scaffold. As shown in the renderings **(A-C)**, it is injected as a gel with the use of a chondroitin sulfate adhesive. It is polymerized in situ using UV light. **(D)** shows GelrinC in solidified and **(E)** shows in vivo curing of the hydrogel during arthroscopy. (Reprinted from Regentis Biomaterials Ltd., with permission.)

In order to stabilize the viscous PEG hydrogel material, the use of a chondroitin sulfate adhesive applied to the chondral defect after marrow stimulation but before application of the scaffold has been developed (Chondux, Biomet, Warsaw, IN) (72,73). The chondroitin sulfate primer simultaneously bonds tissue amines and the PEG hydrogel prior to in situ polymerization and curing.

Micronized Allograft/PRP Scaffold Augmentation

BioCartilage (Arthrex, Naples, Florida) is micronized allograft cartilage that is hydrated with PRP and placed over a microfractured cartilage defect. The allogenic cartilage extracellular matrix contains proteoglycans and type II collagen. The cartilage is dehydrated and micronized prior to packaging and has a 5-year shelf life. The surgeon's preferred PRP system should be available in the operating room at the time of surgery. Prepackaged micronized allograft (1 mL) is combined with 1 mL of PRP into a syringe to create a homogenous solution. Care should be taken to not overhydrate (use >1 mL PRP) the mixture. A Tuohy needle is inserted into the joint following microfracture of the cartilage defect. Suction is applied to the needle to keep the defect bed as dry as possible. The syringe containing the PRP-micronized allograft mixture is then attached and the product is injected into the microfractured defect. Fibrin glue is placed over the mixture and allowed to dry for 10 minutes. The knee is ranged to evaluate implant stability (52,57,74).

Porated Osteochondral Allograft Augmentation

A cryopreserved osteochondral allograft (Cartiform, Arthrex, Naples, FL) has been developed with the goal of providing 3D architecture, viable cells, and growth factors for marrow stimulation augmentation (75,76). The graft maintains all layers of hyaline cartilage, has viable chondrocytes, and eludes chondrogenic growth factors in culture. Additionally, the osteochondral allograft is porated to allow for cellular infiltration as well as improve the cryopreservation and flexibility of the graft. During the single-stage procedure, it is contoured to the shape of the defect and fixed with fibrin glue or sutures after microfracture is performed. It is important to note that fibrin glue should only be used on the periphery of the lesion, as the docking site should be should be unobstructed to allow MSC infiltration of the graft. This graft has the advantage of being cryopreserved with a shelf life of 2 years when stored between $-75°C$ and $-85°C$.

Biologic Augmentation

In addition to scaffold augmentation, the use of biologic augmentation is also under investigation. In rabbit models, growth factors have been used to guide MSCs towards a chondrogenic cell lineage. Improved quality of microfractured defects has been described with bone morphogenetic protein (BMP)-2, BMP-4, osteogenic protein (OP)-1 with thrombospondin-1, insulin-like growth factor (IGF)-1 and IL-1ra (77–84). Chemotactic agents such as stromal derived factor-1 (SDF-1) and transforming growth factor β-3 (TGFβ-3) have been used to preferentially hone MSCs to the defect site (85,86). Hyaluronic acid may be utilized both as a postprocedure injection treatment modality and as an adjuvant augmentation treatment during the microfracture procedure (87–90).

Bone marrow aspirate concentrate (BMAC), a concentrated source of MSCs and growth factors, has emerged as a means to enhance cartilage regeneration following marrow stimulation (91,92). Gigante et al. described augmented microfracture and bone marrow concentrate (CMBMC), a novel arthroscopic technique that combines microfracture, BMAC, and a protective scaffold for the treatment of focal cartilage lesions. BMAC is obtained from iliac crest and prepared according to manufacturer's protocol. Using a long needle, a 10:1 mixture of 1 to 2 mL of fibrin glue (off-the-shelf) and BMAC is placed in the microfractured defect. The previously measured and prepared collagen membrane (MeRG collagen membrane, Bioteck, Vicenza, Italy) is inserted through the medial portal with a grasper and fitted into place with a probe. Next, 2 to 3 mL of the fibrin glue-BMC mixture is deposited on the membrane left to solidify for 2 to 3 minutes. Extraneous mixture is removed and membrane stability is checked through repeated extension and flexion. Enea et al. expanded on the original CMBMC technique by replacing the collagen membrane with a resorbable polyglycolic acid/hyaluronan (PGA-HA) matrix (Chondrotissue, BioTissue AG, Zurich, Switzerland). In this technique, termed PGA-HA-CMBMC, the PGA-HA matrix is soaked in BMAC until implantation (93).

Kim et al. described autologous bone marrow mesenchymal cell-induced chondrogenesis (MCIC), a technique that augments microfracture with BMAC, HA, and fibrin glue. Saline is drained from the joint following arthroscopy and microfracture, and carbon dioxide (CO_2) is introduced into the joint at 20 mm Hg through the superolateral portal. Two 1-mL syringes are connected to a Y-shaped common mixing catheter. One syringe contains 0.8 mL of fibrinogen (off-the-shelf) and 0.2 mL of HA. The second syringe contains 0.8 mL of BMAC, prepared according to manufacturer protocol, and 0.2 mL of thrombin (off-the-shelf). The microfractured lesion is dried and a 20-gauge needle spinal needle is inserted into the joint through an appropriate portal. Under arthroscopic guidance, the BMAC, HA, and fibrin-gel mixture is gently applied via the double syringe and uniformly over the lesion. The tamponade effect of the CO_2 coupled with the adhesiveness of the gel, allows the graft to securely adhere to the lesion, even against gravity. If necessary, a second layer can be added. The graft hardens after 5 minutes and the knee is moved through several range of motion cycles to anatomically sculpt the graft and test its stability (94).

Broyles et al. describe a long-term protocol for microfracture augmentation using BMAC, PRP, and HA to treat full-thickness chondral damage. BMAC and PRP are prepared according to manufacturer protocol. Care is taken to coordinate positioning and preparation of the autologous samples with the anesthesia team. The outlined protocols typically yield 3 to 5 mL of BMAC and 7 mL of PRP. The autologous solutions are combined with 25 mg of HA. Following microfracture, all saline is removed from the joint. Next, an 18-gauge spinal needle is inserted percutaneously into the primary chondral lesion. The 20-mL syringe containing the BMAC, PRP, and HA is attached to the spinal needle, and the mixture is then injected into the knee. Their protocol consists of 11 additional outpatient BMAC/PRP/HA injections (12 total) over the next 12 months. If an effusion is present, it is aspirated prior to repeat injection. The outpatient protocol begins at 1 week postoperatively and consists of weekly injections for 5 weeks. At 4 months and at 1 year postoperatively, three more weekly injections are performed (95).

Postoperative Care and Rehabilitation

The initial goals of physical therapy emphasize maximal protection of the treated lesion site. Standard postoperative marrow stimulation protocols are employed after augmentation techniques as well. For tibiofemoral defects, initial weight bearing is toe-touch (<5 lbs) with the use of crutches for 4 to 6 weeks. Patients with patellofemoral defects can weight bear as tolerated in extension with limitations while the knee is in flexion commonly implemented by weight bearing in a hinged brace orthosis locked at 15 to 20 degrees of flexion. Gentle passive range of motion exercises is encouraged immediately following surgery to reduce pain and edema. Despite mixed results regarding its use, CPM is typically initiated immediately following surgery, with initial settings of 0 to 90 degrees and progression as tolerated for 6 to 8 weeks (96,97). Some surgeons prefer delaying the initiation of CPM for 2 to 5 days postoperatively in order to stabilize clot formation. Those patients for whom CPM machines are not available are instructed to perform 500 knee flexion bends, three times daily, to maintain range of motion. Bilateral leg presses and one-third squats are used, with range of motion and weight gradually increased. Stationary biking with variable resistance, treadmills, and elliptical trainers are all used to achieve early progressive strengthening and range of motion gains (98). The patient is also encouraged to perform active-assisted range of motion exercises several times daily. Achieving full passive extension is an important early goal. Active-assisted range of motion exercises is progressed as tolerated with an emphasis on closed-chain exercises.

Knee range of motion in a hinged brace is progressed over a period of 6 to 8 weeks. In cases in which condylar lesions are treated, crutches are weaned and a return to full weight bearing is begun at 6 weeks. Patients are then advised to begin progressive return to normal activities of daily living. Sport-specific protocols and agility drills focusing on acceleration, deceleration, and cutting maneuvers are slowly added at around 4 to 6 months. While low-impact activities such as golfing, walking, and bicycling are recommended at this point, return to high-impact activities are typically delayed until 6 to 9 months postsurgery (99). Patellofemoral microfracture patients differ in that initial weight bearing is 50%, progression to weight bearing as tolerated is at week 2, and a brace is employed to initially permit only 0 to 20 degrees of motion to avoid flexion overload, thus preventing shearing at the microfracture site.

Results

Clinical outcomes of patients with full-thickness chondral lesions treated with microfracture have yielded good to excellent results in 60% to 80% of patients (35,44,46). A pooled meta-analysis by Negrin et al. demonstrated that a mean improvement in 22 Knee Injury and Osteoarthritis Outcome

Score (KOOS) points after microfracture correlates to a clinically significant improvement at middle term follow-up (100). In a systematic review of 15 level I and II studies, Goyal et al. reported significant improvement from baseline with better outcomes in smaller lesions (<4 cm²) at 5-year follow-up. However, after 5 years, failure rates were reported at 23% and were up to 38% at 10-year follow-up (101). A systematic review by Mithoefer et al. reported on longer-term results following microfracture. All 28 studies included in their review showed symptomatic improvement in the first 24 months following microfracture. However, several studies revealed a functional deterioration of patients (47% to 80% of patients) between 18 and 36 months postmicrofracture. The authors concluded that the observed decline in functional status is inherent to the shortcomings of microfracture and is associated with incomplete defect filling, poor integration with normal hyaline cartilage, and inferior wear characteristic of fibrocartilage (102–104).

Clinical outcomes in high-level athletes undergoing marrow stimulation have been reported. Steadman et al. in 2003 reported that 76% of professional football players returned to competition (105). Gobbi et al. recently reported on competitive athletes with an average age of 31 years and similarly found 78% of patients experienced improvement in symptoms at 2 years. However, at 5-year and final (average 15 years) follow-up, there was a significant deterioration in clinical outcome scores (106,107). Mithoefer et al. published a prospective evaluation of microfracture in athletes who participate in high-impact pivoting sports. Forty-four percent of the athletes were able to return to regular participation in high-impact pivoting sports, 71% of which were at a competitive level. Only 57% of returning athletes achieved their preoperative level of play (45). These results indicate that microfracture surgery performed in high-intensity athletes may be less predictable and durable than for those low-demand patients.

Recently, there has been an increase in the number of studies comparing microfracture to other cartilage biorestoration techniques. Gudas et al. reported on a prospective randomized study of 60 young athletes (mean age of 24.3 years) receiving either osteochondral autologous transplantation (OAT) or microfracture. At 10-year follow-up, both groups had significant improvement of ICRS clinical score from baseline. However, patients who underwent OAT procedures had significantly better clinical scores and higher rate of return to preinjury sport activities. There was a significant decrease in ICRS scores in both groups during the 3- to 10-year follow-up period (108). Ulstein et al. also compared microfracture to OATs in a 10-year follow-up study and reported no significant difference between clinical outcomes, muscle strength, and radiographic advancement in OA (109).

In a level II prospective cohort study, Gobbi et al. compared the medium-term (5 years) clinical outcomes of cartilage repair using a one-stage technique of a HA-based scaffold with activated BMAC to microfracture. While both groups demonstrated significant clinical improvement at 2 years postoperatively, the microfracture group exhibited a significant decline in objective and subjective clinical outcome measures by 5 years. Patients in the HA-BMAC group did not experience a similar decline in outcome scores. The authors concluded that HA-BMAC provides better clinical outcomes with more durable cartilage repair compared with microfracture. Of note, patient treatment was determined by insurance coverage and not randomization. The patients in the HA-BMAC group were significantly older than those in the microfracture group (110).

In a level I prospective randomized controlled series, Knutsen et al. compared microfracture and ACI in 80 patients. At 2-year follow-up, the microfracture group had significantly better clinical improvement than the ACI group. However, at 5- and 15-year follow-up, there was no significant difference between microfracture and ACI with regard to clinical outcome and rates of failure (6,7,111). Comparisons between second-generation ACI with scaffold augmentation have shown improved outcomes as compared to microfracture (112–115). However, these reports are limited to 2- to 5-year follow-up. Microfracture has also been compared to characterized chondrocyte implantation (CCI), which utilizes cell marker-specific selected autologous chondrocytes for ACI. On second-look biopsies, the CCI group demonstrated improved histologic outcomes, but in a 5-year follow-up study there was no significant clinical benefit from CCI as compared to microfracture (116,117) (Table 42-3).

Scaffold Augmentation

Gille et al. used AMIC with Chondro-Gide, a collagen I/III scaffold, to treat 32 grade IV chondral lesions in 27 patients with an average age of 39 years (16–50 years) (118). The average defect size was 4.2 cm (1.3–8.8 cm) and the average follow-up was 37 months (24–62 months). They reported significant improvement in clinical outcomes scores at 1 year with continued improvement at up to 2-year follow-up. On MRI follow-up, 10 of 15 patients had >50% of their defect filled. A more recent analysis of the AMIC registry demonstrated significant improvement in clinical scores at 1 and 2 years (42).

TABLE 42-3 Microfracture Versus Other Chondral Resurfacing Procedures

Microfracture Comparison	Study Design	Follow up	Author	Comments
vs. ACI	Level I Prospective Randomized 80 pts	2 y	Knutsen (2004)	Microfracture significantly better clinical improvement (SF-36 Physical Component) Histologically no significant difference No correlation between histological and clinical results Younger, more active patients with better clinical results
	Level I Prospective Randomized 80 pts	5 y	Knutsen (2007)	No difference in radiographic or clinical results 23% failure rate in each group Improved histology associated with reduced risk of failure
	Level I Prospective Randomized 80 pts	15 y	Knutsen (2016)	Significant improvement from baseline clinical scores in both groups Failure rate 42% in ACI, 32.5% in MFx groups ($p = 0.356$) No significant difference in clinical score or failure rate between groups
vs. Second-generation ACI (Hyalograft C)	Level II Prospective Cohort Study 80 pts	5 y	Kon (2009)	Second-generation ACI with better clinical results (IKDC) Second-generation ACI with more prolonged resumption of sports
vs. Second-generation ACI (MACI)	Level I Prospective Randomized 60 pts	2 y	Basad (2010)	Larger defects (4–10 cm²) Improvement in both groups form baseline at 2 y Second-generation ACI with better clinical scores over time than microfracture using Lysholm, Tegner, ICRS scores
	Level I Prospective Randomized 137 pts	2 y	Saris (2014)	Mean defect size 4.8 cm² MACI with significantly better clinical results (KOOS) No significant difference in histology or MRI assessment
vs. Second-generation ACI (NeoCart)	Level I Prospective Randomized 30 pts	2 y	Crawford (2012)	FDA phase II trial NeoCart and MFx significant clinical improvement from baseline NeoCart significant more improvement in clinical scores vs. MFx
vs. OAT	Level I Prospective Randomized 25 pts	9.8 y	Ulstein (2014)	No significant difference between groups (Lysholm, KOOS) No significant difference in muscle strength between groups No significant difference in radiographic advancement of osteoarthritis
	Level I Prospective Randomized 60 pts	10 y	Gudas (2012)	OAT with significantly better ICRS score OAT with significantly higher return to preinjury sports activities However, significant decrease in sports activities in both groups from 3 to 10 y Nonsignificant decrease in ICRS scores in both groups from 3 to 10 y Both groups with significant ICRS improvement from baseline OAT with better defect filling and integration on MRI evaluation
vs. CCI	Level I Prospective Randomized 112 pts	5 y	Vanlauwe (2011)	No significant difference in clinical benefit (KOOS) CCI better clinical outcome in patients with <3 y of symptoms

ACI, Autologous Chondrocyte Implantation; CCI, Characterized Chondrocyte Implantation; MACI, Matrix-induced autologous chondrocyte implantation; OAT, Osteochondral autograft transplantation; KOOS, Knee Injury and Osteoarthritis Outcome Score; IKDC, International Knee Documentation Committee—objective score; HSS, Hospital for Special Surgery Knee Score; ICRS, International Cartilage Repair Society Score; Short Form-36.

Kim et al. completed a randomized clinical trial to compare microfracture augmented with collagen gel augmentation (CartiFill) to microfracture alone in patients undergoing high tibial osteotomy (HTO). The authors analyzed 40 patients <65 years of age with isolated medial compartment OA. Second-look arthroscopy with biopsy of repair tissue was performed at 1 year postoperatively in conjunction with HTO plate removal. The authors found the quality of cartilage repair (mean ICRS II score) after microfracture with collagen augmentation to be significantly ($p = 0.002$) superior to that after microfracture alone. In addition, imaging outcomes based on the magnetic resonance observation of cartilage repair tissue (MOCART) score were significantly ($p = 0.001$) superior in the group treated with collagen augmentation. However, clinical results at 1 year did not reflect the difference in tissue repair quality (59).

Erggelet et al. evaluated microfracture augmentation using a cell-free, polymer-based freeze-dried scaffold composed of poly-glycolic acid (PGA) and hyaluronan in a sheep articular defect model (66). Histologic analysis performed 6 months postoperatively demonstrated that the scaffold-augmented repair tissue had greater and more evenly distributed type II collagen and proteoglycan content and more normal appearing chondrocytes than the microfracture-alone group. A pilot clinical series of five patients with 24-month follow-up demonstrated improved clinical scores and stable cartilage appearance on MRI evaluation (65).

Using an ovine model, Hoemann et al. examined the effect of a chitosan-glycerol phosphate blood scaffold on the repair tissue after microfracture (61). One hour postprocedure, clots in the augmented group showed increased adhesion to the walls of the defect compared with controls (microfracture alone). Analysis of repair tissue performed 6 months postoperatively showed that use of the scaffold resulted in higher type II collagen and glycosaminoglycan content, more complete defect filling, and a higher percentage of hyaline repair than controls.

In 2007, Buschmann et al. published preliminary clinical results from 33 patients treated with in situ augmentation of the microfracture clot with chitosan-glycerol phosphate (BST-CarGel, Biosyntec Inc., Laval, Quebec, Canada) (119). This study demonstrated the safety of the technique as well as improved tissue repair quality compared with controls. Tissue biopsies from the knees of 22 patients from the chitosan-treated group compared to microfracture alone showed better cell morphology, cell viability, superficial zone morphology, repair tissue thickness, surface architecture, and collagen structure, resulting in significantly better overall ICRS II scores (64.5 vs. 36.9; $p = 0.045$). Macroscopic grading of the cartilage repair was also significantly improved ($p = 0.016$).

In an international, multicenter randomized control trial, Stanish et al. reported on 80 patients with grade III and IV focal femoral condyle lesions who were randomized to BST-CarGel versus microfracture. They showed that augmented lesions had significantly more repair tissue filling based on MRI than microfracture lesions alone at 1-year follow-up. However, there were no significant differences between the groups regarding clinical outcome scales. Regardless, the authors suggest the improved defect filling is critical, as prior studies have demonstrated the importance of defect filling at longer follow-up (64). The results of this study were used as the basis for marketing approval for the product in Canada and Europe. The authors, under an extension protocol, followed patients for long-term follow-up for 5 years posttreatment. At 5 years, blinded MRI analysis showed that patients treated with BST-CarGel had significantly increased lesion filling and repair tissue that more closely resembled native cartilage compared with microfracture alone. Both groups experienced statistically significant clinical improvement (WOMAC subscale) above baseline, but there was no significant difference between groups. The authors concluded that BST-CarGel treatment resulted in significantly superior repair tissue quantity and quality over microfracture at 5 years posttreatment. However, there was no significant clinical (WOMAC) difference between the groups (120).

Frappier et al. performed an economic evaluation of BST-CarGel and microfracture alone to assess the economic value of the augmented technique. Using a decision tree model, the authors showed that BST-CarGel yields a positive return on investment at year 4. The cost savings were the greatest in patients with larger lesions. In this model, the cost savings resulted from a reduced risk of undesirable clinical events (121).

Wang et al. developed a novel microfracture augmentation method that combines chondroitin sulfate with a hydrogel scaffold (73). Chondroitin sulfate enhances peripheral adhesion while the injectable, biodegradable hydrogel scaffold enhances microfracture repair. The hydrogel is photopolymerized for rapid stabilization (ChonDux, Biomet Inc., Warsaw, IN). A preliminary report suggests that this technique can produce >75% defect fill in 90% of patients based on MRI (122).

A biodegradable scaffold to augment microfracture is created by crosslinking PEG polymer hydrogel with <1% fibrinogen chains (GelrinC, Regentis Biomaterials Ltd., Or Akiva, Israel). This matrix can also be modified as a delivery vehicle for inductive growth factors. Preclinical animal studies of this scaffold demonstrated increased hyaline differentiation of the resulting cartilage repair tissue (69,70).

Zantop and Petersen described two clinical cases where microfracture was successfully augmented by the arthroscopic implantation of a three-dimensional matrix coupled with a cell-free chondroinductive cover (Chondrotissue, BioTissue AG, Zurich, Switzerland) composed of a resorbable polymer felt and sodium hyaluronan. Following surgical microfracture, the matrix was soaked in autologous serum for 10 minutes, fashioned to the size and shape of the defect, and inserted into the knee through a cannula. Fixation of the implant was achieved using two 1.5-mm bioabsorbable polylactic acid (PLA) pins. At 1 year postoperatively, both patients were symptom-free, and follow-up MRI demonstrated excellent defect fill with repair tissue (123).

Using an animal model, Geraghty et al. showed that porated osteochondral allograft (Cartiform, Arthrex, Naples, FL) augmentation improves the histologic appearance of cartilage repair as compared to marrow stimulation alone at 3 months (76). The defect edges were completely integrated with the graft by 12 months and showed better organization and lesion filling than defects treated with marrow stimulation alone. In a published case report, a 5 × 10 mm trochlear defect was treated with marrow stimulation augmented with porated osteochondral allograft (75). The authors report good clinical outcome with no pain by 5 months and return to sports by 9 months. At 9 months, second-look arthroscopy demonstrated good lesion filling and incorporation, and on MRI imaging, the lesion was isointense with the surrounding articular cartilage. Histologic analysis of the biopsy taken 9 months postoperatively demonstrated 85% articular cartilage with a high composition of type II collagen and a limited amount of type I collagen. Further investigations will be required to confirm these promising preliminary results.

Scaffold and Chondrocyte Augmentation

Dorotka et al. studied the augmentation of microfracture with an implanted matrix (Geistlich Biomaterials, Wolhusen, Switzerland) composed of types I, II, and III collagen seeded with cultured autologous chondrocytes (124). Their in vitro analysis showed that viable, active chondrocytes were present within the matrix up to 3 weeks following seeding. The authors also investigated the cell-seeded matrix in a sheep articular defect model (125). At 4 months postoperatively, the specimens that received the seeded matrix following microfracture generated repair tissue with the greatest defect fill and largest quantity of hyaline-like tissue. At 12 months, the authors noted that the specimens augmented with the cell-seeded matrix had greater defect fill and better integration with the adjacent cartilage compared to what was seen at 4 months. However, at 12 months, the amount of hyaline tissue present had decreased, and specimens displayed histological evidence of deterioration.

Bone Marrow Aspirate Concentrate Augmentation

Using an equine model, Fortier et al. compared microfracture augmented with BMAC to microfracture alone. At 8 months, the lesions treated with BMAC and microfracture demonstrated a significant improvement in repair tissue compared with microfracture alone. MRI data indicated that BMAC increased the fill of defects and improved integration of repair tissue into surrounding normal cartilage. There was greater type II collagen content and improved orientation of the collagen as well as significantly more glycosaminoglycan in the BMAC-treated defects (91).

Kim et al. retrospectively compared patient satisfaction and cost in patients undergoing total knee arthroplasty (TKA) to MCIC. All patients were over 50 years of age and showed grade IV chondral lesions. However, patients in the TKA group were older and predominately female. Nevertheless, their analysis showed equivalent satisfaction and a lower monetary cost in the MCIC group (94).

Broyles et al. evaluated 18 patients who underwent microdrilling of full-thickness chondral lesions followed by 12 injections of BMAC, PRP, and HA. At 24 months postoperatively, there was a significant improvement ($p < 0.0001$) in International Knee Documentation Committee (IKDC) and Knee Society (KS) scores. Furthermore, there was a 0.7 ± 0.3 mm overall increase in joint space at 24 months. The authors concluded that microdrilling of chondral defects augmented with a long-term BMAC/PRP/HA aspiration-injection protocol may be a viable treatment for chondral disease with good early clinical and radiological results (126).

Enea et al. retrospectively assessed nine patients who underwent PGA-HA-CMBMC for focal lesions of the condylar articular cartilage. Five of these patients elected to undergo second look arthroscopy. All but one patient in their series showed improvement at latest follow-up (average 22 ± 2 months). Macroscopic assessment at 12 months revealed that one repair appeared normal, three appeared almost normal, and one appeared abnormal. MRI at 8 to 12 months showed complete defect filling. The authors concluded that PGA-HA-CMBMC is safe, improves knee function, and has the potential to regenerate hyaline-like cartilage (93).

Hyaluronic Acid Augmentation

HA is a high molecular weight glycosaminoglycan component of joint synovial fluid that is produced endogenously by hyaluronan synthase. It plays a key role in the structure and organization of the articular extracellular matrix (127). Interest in HA augmentation of microfracture stems from in vitro and animal studies suggests that HA viscosupplementation promotes chondrocyte differentiation and proliferation while increasing cartilage proteoglycan content (128–130). The authors believe that HA augmentation following cartilage repair creates an environment favorable for cartilage regeneration (89,131). HA provides a framework for mesenchymal cells introduced by microfracture and potentially promotes chondrocyte differentiation and proliferation (39).

Using a rabbit chondral defect model, Strauss et al. evaluated the efficacy of HA augmentation following surgical microfracture (87). In their model, HA augmentation resulted in improved repair tissue compared to controls. After 3 months, the specimens treated with microfracture followed by HA injections demonstrated significantly better defect fill with more hyaline-like tissue with higher mean ICRS scores than control specimens (microfracture alone). In this study, postoperative HA viscosupplementation also provided an anti-inflammatory effect, limiting the development of degenerative changes within the knee at the 6-month evaluation.

Using a similar rabbit model, Legovic et al. evaluated the effect of weekly HA supplementation following microfracture (88). At 6 weeks posttreatment, they found the repair tissue in specimens treated with HA to have a smoother surface and more organized histological appearance. At 10 weeks postmicrofracture, HA supplementation had a more significant effect. HA supplementation resulted in repair tissue with significantly higher ICRS scores than controls, with more complete defect fill and better integration with the surrounding articular cartilage.

Kang et al. also demonstrated a positive effect of exogenous HA following microfracture in their rabbit model (89). In their study, HA gel with or without the addition of transforming growth factor (TGF)–β3 was applied to microfractured chondral defects. No effect of TGF-β3 was noted. However, repair tissue in the specimens receiving HA supplementation showed greater defect fill, with a more hyaline-like tissue than that seen in the control specimens. Additionally, histological evaluation demonstrated that repair tissue from defects treated with the HA gel had a greater glycosaminoglycan content than those treated with microfracture alone.

In a level II prospective cohort study, Gobbi et al. compared the medium-term (5 year) clinical outcomes of cartilage repair using a one-stage technique of a HA-based scaffold with activated BMAC to microfracture. While both groups demonstrated significant clinical improvement at 2 years postoperatively, the microfracture group exhibited a significant decline in objective and subjective clinical outcome measures by 5 years. Patients in the HA-BMAC group did not experience a similar decline in outcome scores. The authors concluded that HA-BMAC provides better clinical outcomes with more durable cartilage repair compared with microfracture. The patients in the HA-BMAC group were significantly older than those in the microfracture group (110). See table 42-4 for a summary of microfracture augmentation scaffolds.

Growth Factor Augmentation

The addition of growth factors is another potential method of augmenting cartilage repair following microfracture. Growth factors can stimulate MSCs within the fibrin clot to create repair tissue that is closer in appearance and biomechanical properties to normal articular cartilage (39).

Bone morphogenetic protein 7 (BMP-7), also known as osteogenic protein-1, is a growth factor found in normal articular cartilage that has been shown to induce chondrocyte proliferation, differentiation, and stimulate metabolism (132–135). These effects make BMP-7 an attractive target for microfracture augmentation. Jelic et al. showed that BMP-7 delivery via a mini-osmotic pump improved articular cartilage repair in a sheep model (136).

Kuo et al. investigated the use of BMP-7 in a rabbit model consisting of full-thickness defects in the articular cartilage of the patellar groove (82). BMP-7 alone increased the amount of repair tissue without compromising the quality of repair tissue. When BMP-7 was combined with microfracture, both the quality and quantity of repair tissue increased. The observed synergistic reaction between BMP-7 and microfracture is likely related to BMP-7's ability to act directly on the pluripotent MSCs introduced into the defect (39).

Bone morphogenetic protein 4 (BMP-4), another member of the BMP superfamily, has also been studied as an adjuvant morphogen to microfracture and cartilage repair. Kuroda et al. examined the effect of BMP-4 on full-thickness articular cartilage defects in a rat model. They found that local delivery of BMP-4 enhanced muscle-derived stem cell chondrogenesis and improved articular cartilage repair (79). The augmentation of microfracture with BMP-4 has also been reviewed in a rabbit model. Following the creation of a full-thickness cartilage defect in trochlear groove, an adenovirus-BMP-4 was placed in a biomaterial scaffold of perforated decalcified cortical bone matrix (DCBM) and delivered to the microfracture site. When compared with controls, the addition of adenovirus-BMP-4 led to a more vigorous and rapid repair, with regeneration of hyaline articular cartilage at 6 weeks and complete repair of articular cartilage and subchondral bone by 12 weeks (80).

Cytokine Modulation

Inflammatory cytokines such as interleukin-1 (IL-1) can lead to matrix degradation and loss of articular cartilage (83). Inhibition of IL-1 by interleukin 1 receptor antagonist (IL-1ra) has been shown to reduce proteoglycan breakdown in animal models (137). Given these results, inhibition of inflammatory cytokines has emerged as a potential target for improved cartilage repair. Morisset et al. combined IL-1ra and IGF-1 with microfracture in an equine chondral defect model (83). The authors sought to combine mesenchymal cell proliferation (microfracture) with a potent growth factor (IGF-1) and an inflammatory inhibitor (IL-1ra). This treatment was injected as an IL-1ra/IGF-1 adenoviral preparation and resulted in increased proteoglycan content and augmented type II collagen when compared with controls. A combination of growth factors and inflammatory inhibitors may result in improved cartilage repair. The inhibition of matrix metalloproteinases (MMPs), which normally play a role in the degradation of articular cartilage extracellular matrix, has been proposed as a method to improve marrow stimulation techniques. Oral administration of doxycycline, a potent MMP inhibitor, has been shown to improve the thickness and quality of repair tissue in a microfracture model in rats (138).

COMPLICATIONS

Surgical complications from microfracture may be categorized into preoperative, intraoperative or procedure-specific, and postoperative. Preoperative complications include poor patient selection, imprecise surgical indications, and incomplete preoperative counseling. Intraoperative complications include broken microfracture awls and fracturing of the subchondral bridge. Osseous overgrowth has been described by Mithoefer et al. in 6 of 24 patients at an average of 12 months postsurgery. Others have reported complications after microfracture including subchondral cysts, sclerosis, and intralesional osteophytes (44,47,139). Osteophytes also regrow in 40% of patients undergoing ACI, however that number is significantly reduced when a membrane is used (139). Reported in 30% to 60% of microfracture patients, this is thought result from metaplasia of the deep layer of repair cartilage, possibly due to excessive removal of the subchondral bone plate during debridement of the calcified cartilage layer. Damage to the subchondral bone and subsequent adverse events can result in a relative thinning of the repair tissue with potential implications on long-term repair durability and possible revision with ACI (46). Minas et al. noted that previous marrow stimulation surgery negatively affected subsequent cartilage repair with ACI, producing a failure rate three times that of untreated knees (140).

CONCLUSION

In summary, both articular debridement and marrow stimulation, using marrow stimulation and microfracture techniques, offer the surgeon a cost-effective, practical, arthroscopic primary treatment for symptomatic osteochondral defects. These techniques are technically simple and are associated with few complications and minimal morbidity. Current literature demonstrates that debridement and marrow stimulation can produce satisfactory subjective and functional outcomes in most patients. However, clinical results appear to deteriorate at long-term follow-up, which is likely due to the inability of marrow stimulation techniques to reproduce the biomechanical characteristics of the articular cartilage preinjury joint surface. In order to address the shortcomings of microfracture, augmentation methods are under investigation, but the literature is still limited in terms of valid long-term outcome data to provide conclusions regarding efficacy. Multiple scaffold augmentation techniques have been studied and have shown good short-term outcomes. The ability for marrow stimulation augmentation techniques to alter the natural course of articular cartilage disease will likely depend on the quality and integration of the resultant repair tissue. The ultimate goal in the quest for cartilage repair is to develop a simple technique that can produce well-integrated hyaline cartilage and can delay the progression of degenerative joint disease.

TABLE 42-4 Microfracture Augmentation Scaffolds: Composition and Summary of Results

Augment	Composition	Results
Autologous matrix-induced chondrogenesis (AMIC) with Chondro-Gide	Collagen I/III bilayer	Significant improvement in Lysholm scores at 1- and 2-year follow-up with average defect size 3.4 cm^2 (42) MRI with moderate to complete defect fill (118) Clinical trial with 80 patients enrolled, estimated completion 2024 (141)
BST-CarGel	Chitosan-glycerol	Significantly more repair tissue and better quality repair tissue than microfracture-treated lesions on MRI No difference in WOMAC scores at 12 mo (64)
CartiFill	Atelocollagen (purified porcine-derived collagen I)	Significantly higher histologic and MRI outcome as compared to microfracture alone. Clinical outcome scores improved significant among both groups without significant difference between groups at 1-year follow-up (59).
Chondrotissue	Cell-free, freeze-dried polyglycolic acid (PGA) with hyaluron	Improved clinical scores at 24 mo (65) Improved KOOS scores at 3–12 mo, good repair integration with hyaline cartilage morphology on biopsy (with PRP) (68) MRI follow-up at 6–9 mo significantly improved compared to controls. 86% of defect filled with no osseous overgrowth (72).
ChonDux	Chondroitin sulfate adhesive with photopolymerizable hydrogel scaffold	Pilot study shows improved IKDC scores, with 75% defect filling on MRI (13 patients) (122)
GelrinC	Polyethylene glycol (PEG)-fibrinogen hydrogel	Ovine models demonstrate collagen II and proteoglycans in defects (69) Significant improvement in KOOS, IKDC, SF-36 scores in pilot study (142)
Osteochondral Allograft	Osteochondral allograft modified with poration and cryopreserved	Goat model with improved histologic appearance compared to marrow stimulation alone (76). Case report with good clinical outcome, good integration, MRI isointense with articular cartilage, and 85% articular cartilage on biopsy (75).
Hyalofast with BMAC	Hyaluronic acid-based scaffold with activated BMAC	HA-BMAC group and microfracture both significantly improved from baseline at 2-year follow-up. At 5-year follow-up, the HA-BMAC group had significantly better clinical outcome scores than the microfracture-alone group (110).

REFERENCES

1. Curl WW, Krome J, Gordon ES, et al. Cartilage injuries: a review of 31,516 knee arthroscopies. *Arthroscopy*. 1997;13(4):456–460.
2. Aroen A, Loken S, Heir S, et al. Articular cartilage lesions in 993 consecutive knee arthroscopies. *Am J Sports Med*. 2004;32(1):211–215.
3. Hjelle K, Solheim E, Strand T, et al. Articular cartilage defects in 1,000 knee arthroscopies. *Arthroscopy*. 2002;18(7):730–734.
4. Mankin HJ. The response of articular cartilage to mechanical injury. *J Bone Joint Surg Am*. 1982;64(3):460–466.
5. Frisbie DD, Oxford JT, Southwood L, et al. Early events in cartilage repair after subchondral bone microfracture. *Clin Orthop Relat Res*. 2003;(407):215–227.
6. Knutsen G, Engebretsen L, Ludvigsen TC, et al. Autologous chondrocyte implantation compared with microfracture in the knee. A randomized trial. *J Bone Joint Surg Am*. 2004;86-A(3):455–464.
7. Knutsen G, Drogset JO, Engebretsen L, et al. A randomized multicenter trial comparing autologous chondrocyte implantation with microfracture: long-term follow-up at 14 to 15 years. *J Bone Joint Surg Am*. 2016;98(16):1332–1339.
8. Furukawa T, Eyre DR, Koide S, et al. Biochemical studies on repair cartilage resurfacing experimental defects in the rabbit knee. *J Bone Joint Surg Am*. 1980;62(1):79–89.
9. Hjertquist SO, Lemperg R. Histological, autoradiographic and microchemical studies of spontaneously healing osteochondral articular defects in adult rabbits. *Calcifi Tissue Res*. 1971;8(1):54–72.
10. Mitchell N, Shepard N. The resurfacing of adult rabbit articular cartilage by multiple perforations through the subchondral bone. *J Bone Joint Surg Am*. 1976;58(2):230–233.
11. Bert JM. Abandoning microfracture of the knee: has the time come? *Arthroscopy*. 2015;31(3):501–505.
12. Lubowitz JH. Arthroscopic microfracture may not be superior to arthroscopic debridement, but abrasion arthroplasty results are good, although not great. *Arthroscopy*. 2015;31(3):506.
13. Johnson LL, Spector M. The new microfracture: all things considered. *Arthroscopy*. 2015;31(6):1028–1031.

14. Potter HG, Black BR. New techniques in articular cartilage imaging. *Clin Sports Med.* 2009;28(1):77–94.
15. Outerbridge R. The etiology of chondromalacea patellae. *J Bone Joint Surg* 1961;43B:752–757.
16. Brittberg M. ICRS Clinical Cartilage Injury Evaluation System. *Third International Cartilage Repair Society Meeting*; April 28, 2000.
17. Horton D, Anderson S, Hope NG. A review of current concepts in radiofrequency chondroplasty. *ANZ J Surg.* 2014;84(6):412–416.
18. Rocco P, Lorenzo DB, Guglielmo T, et al. Radiofrequency energy in the arthroscopic treatment of knee chondral lesions: a systematic review. *Br Med Bull.* 2016;117(1):149–156.
19. American Academy of Orthopaedic Surgeons. *Treatment of Osteoarthritis of the Knee: Evidence-Based Guideline.* 2nd Ed. Available at: http://www.aaos.org/research/guidelines/TreatmentofOsteoarthritisoftheKneeGuideline.pdf. Accessed December 21, 2016.
20. Lee GW, Son JH, Kim JD, et al. Is platelet-rich plasma able to enhance the results of arthroscopic microfracture in early osteoarthritis and cartilage lesion over 40 years of age? *Eur J Orthop Surg Traumatol.* 2013;23(5):581–587.
21. Scillia AJ, Aune KT, Andrachuk JS, et al. Return to play after chondroplasty of the knee in National Football League Athletes. *Am J Sports Med.* 2015;43(3):663–668.
22. Anderson AF, Pagnani MJ. Osteochondritis dissecans of the femoral condyles. Long-term results of excision of the fragment. *Am J Sports Med.* 1997;25(6):830–834.
23. Lim HC, Bae JH, Park YE, et al. Long-term results of arthroscopic excision of unstable osteochondral lesions of the lateral femoral condyle. *J Bone Joint Surg Br.* 2012;94(2):185–189.
24. Shelbourne KD, Jari S, Gray T. Outcome of untreated traumatic articular cartilage defects of the knee: a natural history study. *J Bone Joint Surg Am.* 2003;85-A(suppl 2):8–16.
25. Moseley JB, O'Malley K, Petersen NJ, et al. A controlled trial of arthroscopic surgery for osteoarthritis of the knee. *N Engl J Med.* 2002;347(2):81–88.
26. Kirkley A, Birmingham TB, Litchfield RB, et al. A randomized trial of arthroscopic surgery for osteoarthritis of the knee. *N Engl J Med.* 2008;359(11):1097–1107.
27. Steadman JR, Ramappa AJ, Maxwell RB, et al. An arthroscopic treatment regimen for osteoarthritis of the knee. *Arthroscopy.* 2007;23(9):948–955.
28. Spahn G, Hofmann GO, Klinger HM. The effects of arthroscopic joint debridement in the knee osteoarthritis: results of a meta-analysis. *Knee Surg Sports Traumatol Arthrosc.* 2013;21(7):1553–1561.
29. Bert JM, Maschka K. The arthroscopic treatment of unicompartmental gonarthrosis: a 5-year follow-up study of abrasion arthroplasty plus arthroscopic debridement and arthroscopic debridement alone. *Arthroscopy.* 1989;5(1):25–32.
30. Gudas R, Gudaite A, Mickevicius T, et al. Comparison of osteochondral autologous transplantation, microfracture, or debridement techniques in articular cartilage lesions associated with anterior cruciate ligament injury: a prospective study with a 3-year follow-up. *Arthroscopy.* 2013;29(1):89–97.
31. Pridie A. The method of resurfacing osteoarthritic joints. *J Bone Joint Surg.* 1959;41B:618–623.
32. Johnson LL. Arthroscopic abrasion arthroplasty historical and pathologic perspective: present status. *Arthroscopy.* 1986;2(1):54–69.
33. Johnson LL. Arthroscopic abrasion arthroplasty: a review. *Clin Orthop Relat Res.* 2001;(391 suppl):S306–S317.
34. Sansone V, de Girolamo L, Pascale W, et al. Long-term results of abrasion arthroplasty for full-thickness cartilage lesions of the medial femoral condyle. *Arthroscopy.* 2015;31(3):396–403.
35. Steadman JR, Rodkey WG, Singleton SB, et al. Microfracture technique for full-thickness chondral defects: technique and clinical results. *Oper Tech Orthop.* 1997;7:300–304.
36. Steadman JR, Rodkey WG, Rodrigo JJ. Microfracture: surgical technique and rehabilitation to treat chondral defects. *Clin Orthop Relat Res.* 2001;(391 Suppl):S362–S369.
37. Shapiro F, Koide S, Glimcher MJ. Cell origin and differentiation in the repair of full-thickness defects of articular cartilage. *J Bone Joint Surg Am.* 1993;75(4):532–553.
38. Gomoll AH. Microfracture and augments. *J Knee Surg.* 2012;25(1):9–15.
39. Strauss EJ, Barker JU, Kercher JS, et al. Augmentation strategies following the microfracture technique for repair of focal chondral defects. *Cartilage.* 2010;1(2):145–152.
40. Lee HH, O'Malley MJ, Friel NA, et al. Effects of doxycycline on mesenchymal stem cell chondrogenesis and cartilage repair. *Osteoarthritis Cartilage.* 2013;21(2):385–393.
41. Lee YH, Suzer F, Thermann H. Autologous matrix-induced chondrogenesis in the knee: a review. *Cartilage.* 2014;5(3):145–153.
42. Gille J, Behrens P, Volpi P, et al. Outcome of Autologous Matrix Induced Chondrogenesis (AMIC) in cartilage knee surgery: data of the AMIC Registry. *Arch Orthop Trauma Surg.* 2013;133(1):87–93.
43. Goldstein T, Schwartz J, Mullen J, et al. Differential Chondrogenesis and Chondrocyte Expression in Collagen Gels & Scaffolds. Abstract Presented at 2014 Annual Meeting of the Orthopaedic Research Society, New Orleans, LA, March 2014.
44. Steadman JR, Briggs KK, Rodrigo JJ, et al. Outcomes of microfracture for traumatic chondral defects of the knee: average 11-year follow-up. *Arthroscopy.* 2003;19(5):477–484.
45. Mithoefer K, Williams RJ III, Warren RF, et al. High-impact athletics after knee articular cartilage repair: a prospective evaluation of the microfracture technique. *Am J Sports Med.* 2006;34(9):1413–1418.
46. Mithoefer K, Williams RJ III, Warren RF, et al. The microfracture technique for the treatment of articular cartilage lesions in the knee. A prospective cohort study. *J Bone Joint Surg Am.* 2005;87(9):1911–1920.
47. Kreuz PC, Steinwachs MR, Erggelet C, et al. Results after microfracture of full-thickness chondral defects in different compartments in the knee. *Osteoarthritis Cartilage.* 2006;14(11):1119–1125.
48. Frisbie DD, Morisset S, Ho CP, et al. Effects of calcified cartilage on healing of chondral defects treated with microfracture in horses. *Am J Sports Med.* 2006;34(11):1824–1831.
49. Benthien JP, Behrens P. Reviewing subchondral cartilage surgery: considerations for standardised and outcome predictable cartilage remodelling: a technical note. *Int Orthop.* 2013;37(11):2139–2145.
50. Orth P, Duffner J, Zurakowski D, et al. Small-diameter awls improve articular cartilage repair after microfracture treatment in a translational animal model. *Am J Sports Med.* 2016;44(1):209–219.
51. Chen H, Sun J, Hoemann CD, et al. Drilling and microfracture lead to different bone structure and necrosis during bone-marrow stimulation for cartilage repair. *J Orthop Res.* 2009;27(11):1432–1438.
52. Abrams GD, Mall NA, Fortier LA, et al. BioCartilage: background and operative technique. *Oper Tech Sports Med.* 2013;21(2):116–124.

53. Gianakos AL, Yasui Y, Fraser EJ, et al. The effect of different bone marrow stimulation techniques on human talar subchondral bone: a micro-computed tomography evaluation. *Arthroscopy.* 2016;32(10):2110–2117.

54. Smith BD, Grande DA. The current state of scaffolds for musculoskeletal regenerative applications. *Nat Rev Rheumatol.* 2015;11(4):213–222.

55. Benthien J, Behrens P. Autologous matrix-induced chondrogenesis (AMIC) combining microfracturing and a collagen I/III matrix for articular cartilage resurfacing. *Cartilage.* 2010;1(1):65–68.

56. Benthien JP, Behrens P. The treatment of chondral and osteochondral defects of the knee with autologous matrix-induced chondrogenesis (AMIC): method description and recent developments. *Knee Surg Sports Traumatol Arthrosc.* 2011;19(8):1316–1319.

57. Frank RM MK, Bhatia S, Cole BJ. Enhanced marrow-stimulation techniques. In: Cole BJ HJ, ed. *Biologic Knee Reconstruction: A Surgeon's Guide.* Thorofare, NJ: SLACK Inc.; 2015.

58. Dhollander A, De Neve F, Almqvist K, et al. Autologous matrix-induced chondrogenesis combined with platelet-rich plasma gel: technical description and a five pilot patients report. *Knee Surg Sports Traumatol Arthrosc.* 2011;19(4):536–542.

59. Kim MS, Koh IJ, Choi YJ, et al. Collagen augmentation improves the quality of cartilage repair after microfracture in patients undergoing high tibial osteotomy. *Am J Sports Med* 2017;45:1845–1855.

60. Kumar MN, Muzzarelli RA, Muzzarelli C, et al. Chitosan chemistry and pharmaceutical perspectives. *Chem Rev.* 2004;104(12):6017–6084.

61. Hoemann CD, Hurtig M, Rossomacha E, et al. Chitosan-glycerol phosphate/blood implants improve hyaline cartilage repair in ovine microfracture defects. *J Bone Joint Surg Am.* 2005;87(12):2671–2686.

62. Hoemann CD, Sun J, McKee MD, et al. Chitosan-glycerol phosphate/blood implants elicit hyaline cartilage repair integrated with porous subchondral bone in microdrilled rabbit defects. *Osteoarthritis Cartilage.* 2007;15(1):78–89.

63. Shive MS, Hoemann CD, Restrepo A, et al. BST-CarGel: in situ chondroinduction for cartilage repair. *Oper Tech Orthop.* 2006;16(4):271–278.

64. Stanish WD, McCormack R, Forriol F, et al. Novel scaffold-based BST-CarGel treatment results in superior cartilage repair compared with microfracture in a randomized controlled trial. *J Bone Joint Surg Am.* 2013;95(18):1640–1650.

65. Dhollander A, Verdonk P, Lambrecht S, et al. The combination of microfracture and a cell-free polymer-based implant immersed with autologous serum for cartilage defect coverage. *Knee Surg Sports Traumatol Arthrosc.* 2012;20(9):1773–1780.

66. Erggelet C, Endres M, Neumann K, et al. Formation of cartilage repair tissue in articular cartilage defects pretreated with microfracture and covered with cell-free polymer-based implants. *J Orthop Res.* 2009;27(10):1353–1360.

67. Patrascu J, Freymann U, Kaps C, et al. Repair of a post-traumatic cartilage defect with a cell-free polymer-based cartilage implant. *J Bone Joint Surg Br.* 2010;92(8):1160–1163.

68. Siclari A, Mascaro G, Gentili C, et al. A cell-free scaffold-based cartilage repair provides improved function hyaline-like repair at 1 year. *Clin Orthop Relat Res.* 2012;470(3):910–919.

69. McNickle AG, Provencher MT, Cole BJ. Overview of existing cartilage repair technology. *Sports Med Arthrosc Rev.* 2008;16(4):196–201.

70. Ahmed TA, Hincke MT. Strategies for articular cartilage lesion repair and functional restoration. *Tissue Eng Part B Rev.* 2010;16(3):305–329.

71. Seliktar D, Peled E, Livnat M. Articular Cartilage repair using in situ polymerizable hydrogel implant in osteochondral defects. *International Cartilage Repair Society*; 2007; Warsaw, Poland.

72. Sharma B, Fermanian S, Gibson M, et al. Human cartilage repair with a photoreactive adhesive-hydrogel composite. *Sci Transl Med.* 2013;5(167):167ra166–167ra166.

73. Wang DA, Varghese S, Sharma B, et al. Multifunctional chondroitin sulphate for cartilage tissue-biomaterial integration. *Nat Mater.* 2007;6(5):385–392.

74. Fortier LA, Chapman HS, Pownder SL, et al. BioCartilage improves cartilage repair compared with microfracture alone in an equine model of full-thickness cartilage loss. *Am J Sports Med.* 2016;44(9):2366–2374.

75. Hoffman JK, Geraghty S, Protzman NM. Articular cartilage repair using marrow stimulation augmented with a viable chondral allograft: 9-month postoperative histological evaluation. *Case Rep Orthop.* 2015;2015:617365.

76. Geraghty S, Kuang JQ, Yoo D, et al. A novel, cryopreserved, viable osteochondral allograft designed to augment marrow stimulation for articular cartilage repair. *J Orthop Surg Res.* 2015;10:66.

77. Sellers RS, Zhang R, Glasson SS, et al. Repair of articular cartilage defects one year after treatment with recombinant human bone morphogenetic protein-2 (rhBMP-2). *J Bone Joint Surg Am.* 2000;82(2):151–160.

78. Steinert A, Weber M, Dimmler A, et al. Chondrogenic differentiation of mesenchymal progenitor cells encapsulated in ultrahigh-viscosity alginate. *J Orthop Res.* 2003;21(6):1090–1097.

79. Kuroda R, Usas A, Kubo S, et al. Cartilage repair using bone morphogenetic protein 4 and muscle-derived stem cells. *Arthritis Rheum.* 2006;54(2):433–442.

80. Zhang X, Zheng Z, Liu P, et al. The synergistic effects of microfracture, perforated decalcified cortical bone matrix and adenovirus-bone morphogenetic protein-4 in cartilage defect repair. *Biomaterials.* 2008;29(35):4616–4629.

81. Gelse K, Klinger P, Koch M, et al. Thrombospondin-1 prevents excessive ossification in cartilage repair tissue induced by osteogenic protein-1. *Tissue Eng Part A.* 2011;17(15-16):2101–2112.

82. Kuo AC, Rodrigo JJ, Reddi AH, et al. Microfracture and bone morphogenetic protein 7 (BMP-7) synergistically stimulate articular cartilage repair. *Osteoarthritis Cartilage.* 2006;14(11):1126–1135.

83. Morisset S, Frisbie DD, Robbins PD, et al. IL-1ra/IGF-1 gene therapy modulates repair of microfractured chondral defects. *Clin Orthop Relat Res.* 2007;462:221–228.

84. Fortier LA, Mohammed HO, Lust G, et al. Insulin-like growth factor-I enhances cell-based repair of articular cartilage. *J Bone Joint Surg Br.* 2002;84(2):276–288.

85. Chinitz N, Catanzano A, Razzano P, et al. *Novel Strategies to Enhance the Quality of Microfracture Surgery: Use of SDF-1 and Sphingosine in Isolated Cartilaginous Defects AAOS*; 2013.

86. Mendelson A, Frank E, Allred C, et al. Chondrogenesis by chemotactic homing of synovium, bone marrow, and adipose stem cells in vitro. *FASEB J.* 2011;25(10):3496–3504.

87. Strauss E, Schachter A, Frenkel S, et al. The efficacy of intra-articular hyaluronan injection after the microfracture technique for the treatment of articular cartilage lesions. *Am J Sports Med.* 2009;37(4):720–726.

88. Legovic D, Zorihic S, Gulan G, et al. Microfracture technique in combination with intraarticular hyaluronic acid injection in articular cartilage defect regeneration in rabbit model. *Coll Antropol.* 2009;33(2):619–623.

89. Kang SW, Bada LP, Kang CS, et al. Articular cartilage regeneration with microfracture and hyaluronic acid. *Biotechnol Lett.* 2008;30(3):435–439.

90. Tuncay I, Erkocak OF, Acar MA, et al. The effect of hyaluronan combined with microfracture on the treatment of chondral defects: an experimental study in a rabbit model. *Eur J Orthop Surg Traumatol.* 2013;23(7):753–758.

91. Fortier LA, Potter HG, Rickey EJ, et al. Concentrated bone marrow aspirate improves full-thickness cartilage repair compared with microfracture in the equine model. *J Bone Joint Surg Am.* 2010;92(10):1927–1937.

92. Gigante A, Cecconi S, Calcagno S, et al. Arthroscopic knee cartilage repair with covered microfracture and bone marrow concentrate. *Arthrosc Tech.* 2012;1(2):e175–e180.

93. Enea D, Cecconi S, Calcagno S, et al. Single-stage cartilage repair in the knee with microfracture covered with a resorbable polymer-based matrix and autologous bone marrow concentrate. *Knee.* 2013;20(6):562–569.

94. Kim JM, Han JR, Shetty AA, et al. Comparison between total knee arthroplasty and MCIC (autologous bone marrow mesenchymal-cell-induced-chondrogenesis) for the treatment of osteoarthritis of the knee. *Tissue Eng Regen Med.* 2014;11(5):405–413.

95. Broyles JE, O'Brien MA, Stagg MP. Microdrilling surgery augmented with intra-articular bone marrow aspirate concentrate, platelet-rich plasma, and hyaluronic acid: a technique for cartilage repair in the knee. *Arthrosc Tech.* 2017;6(1):e201–e206.

96. Rodrigo J, Steadman J, Silliman J, et al. Improvement of full-thickness chondral defect healing in the human knee after debridement and microfracture using continuous passive motion. *Am J Knee Surg.* 1994;7(3):109–116.

97. Marder RA, Hopkins G Jr, Timmerman LA. Arthroscopic microfracture of chondral defects of the knee: a comparison of two postoperative treatments. *Arthroscopy.* 2005;21(2):152–158.

98. Cavanaugh JSN. Cartilage repair: chondroplasty, abrasion arthroplasty and microfracture. In: Manske RC, ed. *Postsurgical Orthopedic Sports Rehabilitation: Knee & Shoulder.* St. Louis, MO: Mosby; 2006:365–382.

99. Wilk KE, Macrina LC, Reinold MM. Rehabilitation following Microfracture of the Knee. *Cartilage.* 2010;1(2):96–107.

100. Negrin L, Kutscha-Lissberg F, Gartlehner G, et al. Clinical outcome after microfracture of the knee: a meta-analysis of before/after-data of controlled studies. *Int Orthop.* 2012;36(1):43–50.

101. Goyal D, Keyhani S, Lee EH, et al. Evidence-based status of microfracture technique: a systematic review of level I and II studies. *Arthroscopy.* 2013;29(9):1579–1588.

102. Mithoefer K, McAdams T, Williams RJ, et al. Clinical efficacy of the microfracture technique for articular cartilage repair in the knee: an evidence-based systematic analysis. *Am J Sports Med.* 2009;37(10):2053–2063.

103. Gudas R, Kalesinskas RJ, Kimtys V, et al. A prospective randomized clinical study of mosaic osteochondral autologous transplantation versus microfracture for the treatment of osteochondral defects in the knee joint in young athletes. *Arthroscopy.* 2005;21(9):1066–1075.

104. Kreuz PC, Erggelet C, Steinwachs MR, et al. Is microfracture of chondral defects in the knee associated with different results in patients aged 40 years or younger? *Arthroscopy.* 2006;22(11):1180–1186.

105. Steadman JR, Miller BS, Karas SG, et al. The microfracture technique in the treatment of full-thickness chondral lesions of the knee in National Football League players. *J Knee Surg.* 2003;16(2):83–86.

106. Gobbi A, Nunag P, Malinowski K. Treatment of full thickness chondral lesions of the knee with microfracture in a group of athletes. *Knee Surg Sports Traumatol Arthrosc.* 2005;13(3):213–221.

107. Gobbi A, Karnatzikos G, Kumar A. Long-term results after microfracture treatment for full-thickness knee chondral lesions in athletes. *Knee Surg Sports Traumatol Arthrosc.* 2014;22(9):1986–1996.

108. Gudas R, Gudaite A, Pocius A, et al. Ten-year follow-up of a prospective, randomized clinical study of mosaic osteochondral autologous transplantation versus microfracture for the treatment of osteochondral defects in the knee joint of athletes. *Am J Sports Med.* 2012;40(11):2499–2508.

109. Ulstein S, Aroen A, Rotterud JH, et al. Microfracture technique versus osteochondral autologous transplantation mosaicplasty in patients with articular chondral lesions of the knee: a prospective randomized trial with long-term follow-up. *Knee Surg Sports Traumatol Arthrosc.* 2014;22(6):1207–1215.

110. Gobbi A, Whyte GP. One-stage cartilage repair using a hyaluronic acid-based scaffold with activated bone marrow-derived mesenchymal stem cells compared with microfracture: five-year follow-up. *Am J Sports Med.* 2016;44(11):2846–2854.

111. Knutsen G, Drogset JO, Engebretsen L, et al. A randomized trial comparing autologous chondrocyte implantation with microfracture. Findings at five years. *J Bone Joint Surg Am.* 2007;89(10):2105–2112.

112. Kon E, Gobbi A, Filardo G, et al. Arthroscopic second-generation autologous chondrocyte implantation compared with microfracture for chondral lesions of the knee: prospective nonrandomized study at 5 years. *Am J Sports Med.* 2009;37(1):33–41.

113. Saris D, Price A, Widuchowski W, et al. Matrix-applied characterized autologous cultured chondrocytes versus microfracture: two-year follow-up of a prospective randomized trial. *Am J Sports Med.* 2014;42(6):1384–1394.

114. Basad E, Ishaque B, Bachmann G, et al. Matrix-induced autologous chondrocyte implantation versus microfracture in the treatment of cartilage defects of the knee: a 2-year randomised study. *Knee Surg Sports Traumatol Arthrosc.* 2010;18(4):519–527.

115. Crawford DC, DeBerardino TM, Williams RJ III. NeoCart, an autologous cartilage tissue implant, compared with microfracture for treatment of distal femoral cartilage lesions: an FDA phase-II prospective, randomized clinical trial after two years. *J Bone Joint Surg Am.* 2012;94(11):979–989.

116. Saris DB, Vanlauwe J, Victor J, et al. Characterized chondrocyte implantation results in better structural repair when treating symptomatic cartilage defects of the knee in a randomized controlled trial versus microfracture. *Am J Sports Med.* 2008;36(2):235–246.

117. Vanlauwe J, Saris DB, Victor J, et al. Five-year outcome of characterized chondrocyte implantation versus microfracture for symptomatic cartilage defects of the knee: early treatment matters. *Am J Sports Med.* 2011;39(12):2566–2574.

118. Gille J, Schuseil E, Wimmer J, et al. Mid-term results of autologous matrix-induced chondrogenesis for treatment of focal cartilage defects in the knee. *Knee Surg Sports Traumatol Arthrosc.* 2010;18(11):1456–1464.

119. Buschmann MD, Hoemann CD, Hurtig MB, et al. Cartilage repair with chitosan-glycerol phosphate-stabilized blood clots. *Cartilage Repair Strategies.* Totowa, NJ: Humana Press; 2007:85–104.

120. Shive MS, Stanish WD, McCormack R, et al. BST-CarGel(R) treatment maintains cartilage repair superiority over microfracture at 5 years in a multicenter randomized controlled trial. *Cartilage.* 2015;6(2):62–72.

121. Frappier J, Stanish W, Brittberg M, et al. Economic evaluation of BST-CarGel as an adjunct to microfracture vs microfracture alone in knee cartilage surgery. *J Med Econ.* 2014;17(4):266–278.

122. Sharma B, Taminiau L, Stibbe A, et al. A clinical feasibility study evaluating biomaterial guided cartilage repair in the knee. *Orthopaedic Research Society Annual Meeting February 23, 2009, 2009;* Las Vegas, NV.

123. Zantop T, Petersen W. Arthroscopic implantation of a matrix to cover large chondral defect during microfracture. *Arthroscopy.* 2009;25(11):1354–1360.

124. Dorotka R, Windberger U, Macfelda K, et al. Repair of articular cartilage defects treated by microfracture and a three-dimensional collagen matrix. *Biomaterials.* 2005;26(17):3617–3629.

125. Dorotka R, Bindreiter U, Macfelda K, et al. Marrow stimulation and chondrocyte transplantation using a collagen matrix for cartilage repair. *Osteoarthritis Cartilage.* 2005;13(8):655–664.

126. Broyles JE, O'Brien MA, Broyles ST, et al. Biologic augmented micro-drilling surgery for multiple and large full-thickness cartilage lesions in the knee: early clinical and radiological results. *Surg Sci* 2017;8:102–117.

127. Laurent TC, Laurent UB, Fraser JR. The structure and function of hyaluronan: an overview. *Immunol Cell Biol.* 1996;74(2):A1–A7.

128. Kujawa MJ, Caplan AI. Hyaluronic acid bonded to cell-culture surfaces stimulates chondrogenesis in stage 24 limb mesenchyme cell cultures. *Dev Biol.* 1986;114(2):504–518.

129. Miyakoshi N, Kobayashi M, Nozaka K, et al. Effects of intraarticular administration of basic fibroblast growth factor with hyaluronic acid on osteochondral defects of the knee in rabbits. *Arch Orthop Trauma Surg.* 2005;125(10):683–692.

130. Kawasaki K, Ochi M, Uchio Y, et al. Hyaluronic acid enhances proliferation and chondroitin sulfate synthesis in cultured chondrocytes embedded in collagen gels. *J Cell Physiol.* 1999;179(2):142–148.

131. Solchaga LA, Yoo JU, Lundberg M, et al. Hyaluronan-based polymers in the treatment of osteochondral defects. *J Orthop Res.* 2000;18(5):773–780.

132. Chubinskaya S, Merrihew C, Cs-Szabo G, et al. Human articular chondrocytes express osteogenic protein-1. *J Histochem Cytochem.* 2000;48(2):239–250.

133. Klein-Nulend J, Louwerse RT, Heyligers IC, et al. Osteogenic protein (OP-1, BMP-7) stimulates cartilage differentiation of human and goat perichondrium tissue in vitro. *J Biomed Mater Res.* 1998;40(4):614–620.

134. Klein-Nulend J, Semeins CM, Mulder JW, et al. Stimulation of cartilage differentiation by osteogenic protein-1 in cultures of human perichondrium. *Tissue Eng.* 1998;4(3):305–313.

135. Nishida Y, Knudson CB, Kuettner KE, et al. Osteogenic protein-1 promotes the synthesis and retention of extracellular matrix within bovine articular cartilage and chondrocyte cultures. *Osteoarthritis Cartilage.* 2000;8(2):127–136.

136. Jelic M, Pecina M, Haspl M, et al. Regeneration of articular cartilage chondral defects by osteogenic protein-1 (bone morphogenetic protein-7) in sheep. *Growth Factors.* 2001;19(2):101–113.

137. Hung GL, Galea-Lauri J, Mueller GM, et al. Suppression of intra-articular responses to interleukin-1 by transfer of the interleukin-1 receptor antagonist gene to synovium. *Gene Ther.* 1994;1(1):64–69.

138. Stein S, Liang H, Grande D. MMP Inhibition and its Effects on Cartilage Repair. *Paper presented at: Orthopaedic Research Society* 2017; San Diego, CA.

139. Demange MK, Minas T, von Keudell A, et al. Intralesional osteophyte regrowth following autologous chondrocyte implantation after previous treatment with marrow stimulation technique. *Cartilage.* 2017;8(2):131–138.

140. Minas T, Gomoll AH, Rosenberger R, et al. Increased failure rate of autologous chondrocyte implantation after previous treatment with marrow stimulation techniques. *Am J Sports Med.* 2009;37(5):902–908.

141. Clinicaltrials.gov. *ACI-C Versus AMIC. A Randomized Trial Comparing Two Methods for Repair of Cartilage Defects in the Knee.* 2016. Available at: https://clinicaltrials.gov/ct2/show/NCT01458782?term=amic&rank=1. Accessed April 15, 2017.

142. Almqvist K, Cole B, Bellemans R. The treatment of cartilage defects of the knee with microfracture augmented with a biodegradable scaffold: outcomes at 12 months. *11th World Congress of the International Cartilage Repair Society September 15-18, 2013;* Izmir, Turkey.

43 Osteochondral Autograft and Allograft Transplantation for Knee Cartilage Defects

Humza S. Shaikh, Kellie K. Middleton, and Bryson P. Lesniak

INTRODUCTION

Large case studies have found a high prevalence of complex knee cartilage pathologies including large chondral or osteochondral lesions, focal osteonecrosis, traumatic arthritis, and degenerative changes, with reported incidences >65% for osteochondral lesions found during arthroscopy for various procedures (1–4). Though these lesions are most prevalent in younger, active patients (age 20–40 years), they can impede return to sports and significantly interfere with activities of daily living across all demographics. As such, knee chondral lesions pose a major challenge to the orthopaedic community.

Treatment for these pathologies is of particular interest because of the inability of cartilage to heal without intervention. Cartilage has a low potential for regeneration, and injuries that disrupt the joint surface invariably alter biomechanics, leading to accelerated joint degeneration and associated injuries. Partial-thickness chondral tears tend not to heal, while full-thickness osteochondral defects fill with biomechanically inferior fibrocartilage (primarily type I collagen), in contrast to the native type II hyaline cartilage.

Treatments of articular lesions range from conservative measures like weight loss, activity modification, physical therapy with muscle strengthening, unloader bracing, systemic medications including nonsteroidal anti-inflammatory drugs (NSAIDs), and intra-articular corticosteroid and viscosupplementation injections (5). Unfortunately, nonoperative treatment results are less than favorable. Surgical modalities range from palliative procedures with short-term relief of pain and mechanical symptoms to more advanced restorative techniques. Palliative procedures, which have little influence on the potential progression to degenerative joint disease, include arthroscopic lavage, debridement, and chondroplasty. Additional surgical options include marrow stimulating techniques such as microfracture and osteochondral drilling (6,7). More definitive, restorative techniques include osteochondral autograft transplantation (OAT), autologous chondrocyte implantation (ACI), and osteochondral allograft (OCA) transplantation. Currently, there is no agreed-upon gold standard technique in the armamentarium of the arthroscopist to treat osteochondral defects.

This chapter focuses on OAT and OCA procedures that aim to treat the loss of articular cartilage with biomechanically identical hyaline cartilage.

INDICATIONS

Ideal candidates for osteochondral transplantation are young (between 20 and 30 years), thin (BMI < 25), athletic patients who suffer symptomatic, focal, type IV Outerbridge chondral defects with exposed subchondral bone (Fig. 43-1). Pathogenesis of these injuries can be either traumatic or

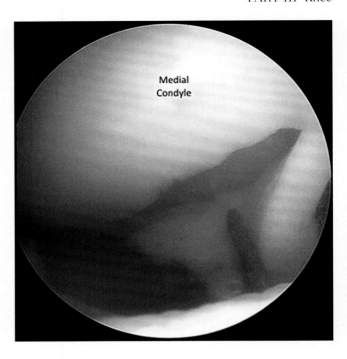

FIGURE 43-1

Posteromedial femoral condyle viewed through the medial portal shows 12 × 5 mm full thickness chondral defect.

degenerative, from osteochondritis dissecans, or secondary to avascular necrosis. Instability due to meniscal or ligamentous insufficiency, or mechanical malalignment also predisposes patients to osteochondral injury.

Indications for osteochondral transplantation are limited predominately by donor-site availability and recipient healing response. Thus, most treatment algorithms differentiate between auto and allograft based on defect size. Smaller defects (<2–4 cm^2) are amenable to single plug or multiple plug (mosaicplasty) autograft transplantation. Large defects (>2–4 cm^2) tend to require allograft transplants given higher risk of donor site morbidity with large autografts, although Mega-OATs procedures have been described for 6 to 9 cm^2 lesions in young adults who can avoid knee hyperflexion and are not indicated for total knee arthroplasty (8). OCAs are also useful as salvage following failed microfracture, ACI, or OATs, as well as for salvage reconstructions following intra-articular fractures with extensive osteochondral damage.

CONTRAINDICATIONS

Contraindications for both OATs and OCA procedures include

- Uncorrected joint instability/malalignment
- Infections or tumor defects
- Nonfocal uni-/multicompartment osteochondral lesions
- Generalized rheumatoid and/or degenerative arthritis (acute or chronic)
- Chondrocalcinosis
- Age and activity level suitable for arthroplasty

    Relative contraindications include

- Age 40 to 55 years
- BMI > 40 kg/m^2
- Grade III–IV osteoarthritis
- Altered bone metabolism (e.g., smokers, chronic steroid use)
- Ipsilateral compartment meniscal deficiency (unless performing concomitant meniscal transplant)

Patients older than 50 years generally begin to exhibit diminished biologic healing and tend to be poor candidates, although one study by Baltzer et al. found improved pain and quality of life measures at 26-month follow-up in a study of 112 patients who underwent OATs for focal nontraumatic lesions with a mean age 48 years (9). This suggests that patients approaching 50 years of age may still benefit from OATs procedure.

Finally, certain patients may be poor candidates for OATs; however, they may be well served with OCA procedures. Such patients include those with the following characteristics:

- Thin donor site cartilage
- Large, deep (>8 mm) defects make it difficult to reconstruct subchondral bone while maintaining cartilage surface congruency and achieving complete coverage

CASE EXAMPLE OF OSTEOCHONDRAL AUTOGRAFT TRANSPLANTATION

A 37-year-old male recreational athlete with no significant past medical or surgical history presents with 3 months of worsening right knee pain. He notes no specific injury but reports that the pain worsens after softball, racquetball, and climbing stairs. The pain is described as being in the front and medial aspect of the knee. He also reports episodes of instability ("giving out") and subjective weakness. Most recently, he experienced an instability episode after physical activity with substantial knee pain and swelling. Otherwise, he denies catching and locking. He has tried topical analgesics and neoprene sleeves in the past without relief.

Examination was unremarkable except for mild tenderness to palpation over the anteromedial joint line and medial patellar facet, 2+ patellar crepitation, and negative flexion McMurray's. The patient was initially diagnosed with patellofemoral syndrome and prescribed physical therapy, with acute worsening of symptoms during his first PT session. On repeat clinic visit, MRI obtained to work up his recurrent knee effusions demonstrated bone edema in the medial femoral condyle and an underlying 12 mm (AP) by 5 mm (ML) osteochondral lesion in the posteromedial femoral condyle. No loose bodies or other pathology to the menisci, collateral, or cruciate ligaments was identified.

The patient was diagnosed with an osteochondral lesion of the medial femoral condyle. Given recurrent symptoms and size of osteochondral lesion, patient and surgeon chose to proceed with OAT.

PREOPERATIVE PREPARATION

Following patient selection, preoperative planning includes radiographs and magnetic resonance imaging (MRI) of the knee. Flexion, weight-bearing posteroanterior, anteroposterior, lateral, and sunrise views are necessary to assess extent of degenerative disease if present. Standing, full-length, mechanical axis films are useful to assess malalignment, though there are no specific cutoff parameters. MRI is ultimately the best preoperative modality to determine the size and location of chondral lesions and to rule out concomitant meniscal and ligamentous injury (Fig. 43-2A–C).

SURGICAL TECHNIQUE

Osteochondral transplant can be performed either arthroscopically or open, including mini-open techniques, depending on the size of the defect and surgeon preference. Studies comparing quality of the grafts following arthroscopic versus mini-open harvest found no difference with regard to usability (graft cartilage quality, axis angle, or articular congruency), except for grafts harvested from the medial supracondylar ridge, for whom mini-open allowed for more perpendicular graft harvest (10,11). A tourniquet should be placed around the thigh. The patient should be positioned to the surgeon's preference. Our preference is to drape the operative leg out free on the bed with a side post laterally and a bump on the table to allow flexion of 90 degrees (Fig. 43-3).

Early steps are identical for both autologous and allograft osteochondral transplants. To ensure proper harvest and insertion of the grafts, perpendicular access to the articular cartilage/lesion is crucial. When performing the procedure arthroscopically, a spinal needle can be used to visualize orientation of the tube harvester. The anterolateral (AL) portal is commonly used for assessment of cartilage lesions, while a working, medial portal (MP) is often used to perform cartilage repair. If concomitant pathology needs to be addressed, the OATs procedure is performed last to avoid iatrogenic damage to the graft.

When the arthroscopic approach is not feasible due to defect location or size, medial and lateral parapatellar arthrotomies can be used to improve defect exposure, preparation, graft harvest (if autograft), and graft insertion.

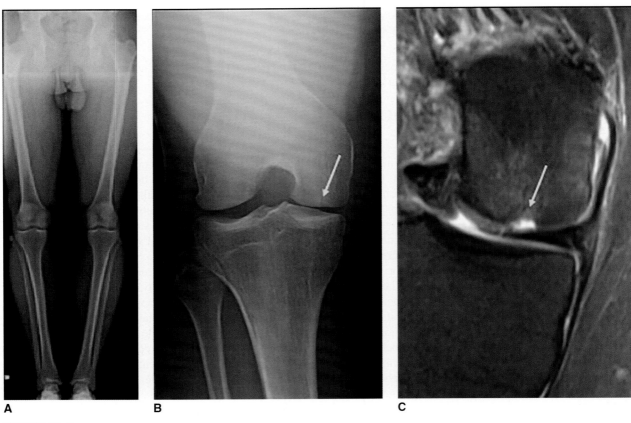

FIGURE 43-2

A: Standing, full-length, mechanical axis radiographs reveal 4 degrees varus alignment of right lower extremity. **B:** Flexion, weight-bearing AP radiographs reveal focal medial femoral condyle defect without additional degenerative changes. **C:** Magnetic resonance imaging of the right knee reveals focal, 12 × 5 mm, full thickness chondral defect along the posteromedial femoral condyle.

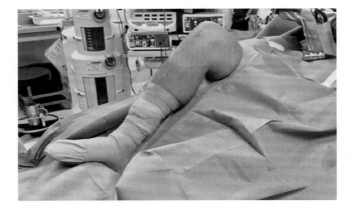

FIGURE 43-3

Patient positioning with operative knee stabilized using a post. Contralateral leg is laid flat and draped out.

Open Exposure

A longitudinal incision is made along the medial aspect of the patellar tendon from the inferior pole of the patella to the medial attachment of the patellar tendon on the tibia tubercle (Fig. 43-4). This can be extended either proximally or distally as required to expose the femoral condyle. The arthrotomy is made medial to the patellar tendon, parallel to the skin incision. Appropriate subcutaneous flaps are made to identify the patellar tendon edge medially so as not to violate it. Care should be taken to avoid damaging the anterior horn of the medial meniscus as the arthrotomy is carried distally. Once the arthrotomy is made, excision of the fat pad is performed sharply to improve

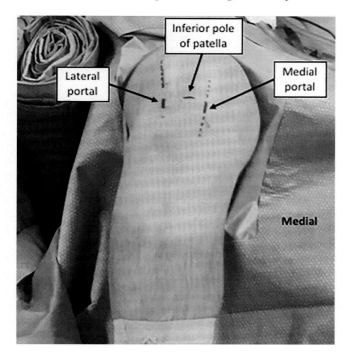

FIGURE 43-4

Using the inferior pole of the patella as our landmark, we mark the medial and lateral portals on their respective sides of the patellar tendon. These portals can be elongated for open approaches requiring medial or lateral parapatellar arthrotomies.

visualization of the femoral articular cartilage. For lateral condyle lesions, the same principles are applied to a lateral arthrotomy. Exposure to the articular defect is maximized with the use of Z retractors or Homan retractors once the ideal degree of knee flexion or extension is achieved.

Defect Preparation

The edges of the lesion must be debrided removing all unstable cartilaginous flaps. This can be performed during arthroscopy or after an arthrotomy is made. The use of curettes is useful in obtaining clean edges, and the shaver or a curette is used to debride the base of the lesion. The defect should be left surrounded by well-defined walls of stable, normal hyaline cartilage to receive the plugs and stop progression of the lesion (Fig. 43-5).

The size of the lesion determines the number of plugs required to fill the defect. Defects should receive >70% coverage to achieve optimal outcomes as unfilled defect will heal with biomechanically inferior fibrocartilage (12).

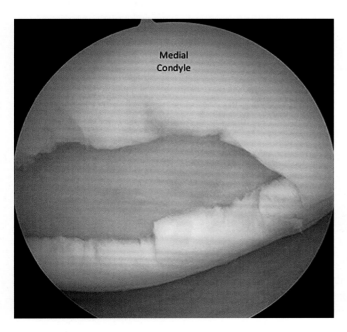

FIGURE 43-5

Viewed through the medial portal: the full-thickness chondral defect should be left surrounded by well-defined walls of stable, normal hyaline cartilage to receive the plugs and stop progression of the lesion.

Depending on whether the procedure is done open or arthroscopically, the size of the defect can be measured using a ruler or drill guide/sizer. Commercially available systems include variable diameter harvesters, ranging from 2.7 to 14 mm. The goal is to maximize congruency between graft and the healthy cartilage border, limiting the amount of fibrocartilage while recreating a flush, congruent articular surface.

AUTOGRAFT

Donor Site Selection and Harvesting

There are several cartilage donor regions that can be selected depending on shape, size, and congruency required to fill the defect. The shape of the donor site must also be taken into account to match the recipient site curvature. Normally, the periphery of the femur provides grafts with a convex articular surface, while the notch area provides concave surfaces. To aid in the harvest, the knee can be extended and flexed to access the more superior and inferior donor sites. The sulcus terminalis of the femur is typically considered the inferior limit for graft harvest on both femoral condyles. The originators of the technique, Hangody et al., suggested that donor sites be at the periphery of the articular surface of the femur above the sulcus terminalis, including the medial, lateral, and superior edges (13). They studied 10 different harvest sites and found that the superolateral aspect of the lateral femoral condyle and the superomedial aspect of the intercondylar notch experienced the least contact pressures.

Once the desired graft harvest site is selected, the tubular graft harvester is placed perpendicular to the donor cartilage. Once positioned, the harvester is malleted to a depth of 15 mm for chondral defects and up to 25 mm for osteochondral defects. This 10-mm difference provides additional cancellous bone for deep defects. Since depth is important, markings must be clear to ensure accurately sized grafts. In general, grafts should ideally be twice as deep as their diameter.

Graft spacing is also important to avoid communication of harvest sites at depth. The donor sites will eventually fill with cancellous bone and fibrocartilage, but care should be taken when harvesting grafts to avoid patellar maltracking or iatrogenic injury to the donor condyle.

Receiver Socket Preparation and Graft Insertion

As osteochondral autografts use press-fit fixation, preparation of the bed is critical.

Several commercially available devices and accompanying techniques are commonly used to prepare the recipient site. A drill, dilator, and specific delivery technique is utilized by *Mosaicplasty*, the Smith & Nephew Autogenous Osteochondral Graft System (Smith & Nephew, Memphis, TN). This system facilitates lesion coverage using a combination of 2.7, 3.5, 4.5, 6.5, and 8.5 mm grafts. First, a universal drill guide is tapped into the subchondral bone, perpendicular to the prepared defect (Fig. 43-6A). The appropriately sized drill bit is then inserted and drilled to the desired depth.

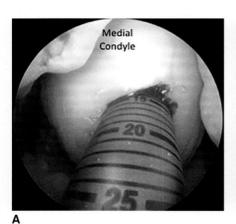
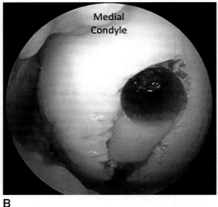
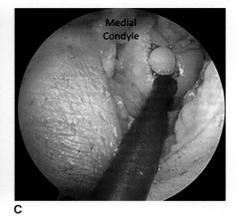

A   B   C

FIGURE 43-6

Viewed through the medial portal. **A:** A universal drill guide is tapped into the subchondral bone, perpendicular to the prepared defect, to a depth of 15 mm. **B:** The length of the recipient hole should be a few millimeters deeper than the length of the graft, with a stable chondral border. **C:** The grafts are delivered under direct visualization, using a tamp until flush with the native articular surface.

The length of the recipient hole should be a few millimeters deeper than the length of the graft (Fig. 43-6B). This minimizes high intraosseous pressure that can be damaging to cartilage. At this point, inflow should be reduced in order to minimize leakage. Once the drill is removed, a dilator is advanced through the drill guide to the desired depth. Using a delivery tamp, the graft is then seated left slightly higher than the depth of the defect to prevent overpenetration. At this point, inflow is stopped to prevent graft extrusion. The graft is then delivered under direct visualization using the tamp until it is flush with the native articular surface (Fig. 43-6C). Additional grafts are inserted adjacently and in identical fashion until the defect is maximally filled (Fig. 43-7A).

The Arthrex OATs system utilizes the manual punch technique and facilitates lesion coverage with 6, 8, and 10 mm grafts. The recipient harvester tube is 1 mm shorter in diameter than the donor tube to allow for press-fit fixation. With the donor harvester placed perpendicular to the articular cartilage, it is malleted into a depth of 15 mm. Once proper depth is obtained, an abrupt twisting of the device handle in 180 degrees in a clockwise and then counterclockwise direction is performed to separate the plug from the surround subchondral bone. The edges of the donor harvester are designed to separate the graft from subchondral bone while the core depth is measured through windows in the device. The recipient harvester is then malleted to a depth of 13 mm, or 2 mm shorter than graft, to ensure transplanted grafts are flushed with the articular cartilage. The harvester is then abruptly rotated to separate the plug from the surround condyle and then pulled out, rather than levered out, to remove the cancellous bone. Alignment rods are used to measure the depth of the socket and to confirm alignment for graft insertion. The donor harvester with the core graft is reinserted into the driver assembly. The impaction cap is unscrewed and a collared pin exposed, advancing the graft into the socket. The harvester has a beveled edge that allows easy insertion in the socket. This seats the harvester and stabilizes final graft position. A mallet is used to gently tap the pin for seating of the graft. Ideally, the graft should be left approximately 1 mm proud, and final seating should be performed with an oversized tamp. Once donor graft seating is complete, donor sites can be filled with unusable subchondral bone excised from the recipient sites (Fig. 43-7B).

The stability of OATs procedures has been evaluated in the porcine model (14). Findings suggest that 15 and 20 mm grafts were significantly more stable than 10-mm–deep grafts. When diameter is taken into account, larger diameter grafts are more stable, and reinsertion after pullout significantly reduces primary fixation strength. Interestingly, stability is compromised when the harvest is performed, and levering is used compared to the rotation system (14). Additionally, drilling can lead to thermal damage to surrounding cartilage. Manual punch techniques for graft harvest and socket creation have shown to improve chondrocyte survival over power techniques (15).

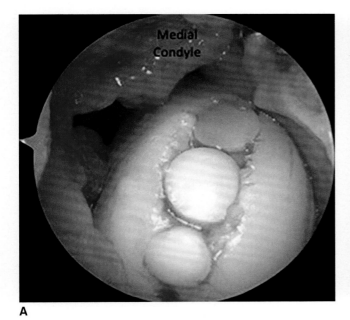
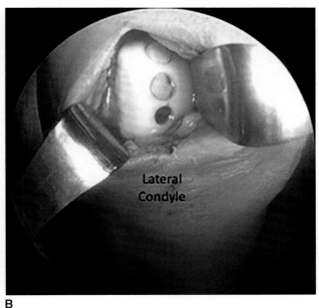

A   **B**

FIGURE 43-7

A: Recipient site after grafts has been inserted adjacently and in identical fashion until the defect is maximally filled. **B:** Once donor graft seating is complete, donor sites can be filled with unusable subchondral bone excised from the recipient sites.

OSTEOCHONDRAL ALLOGRAFT

Defect Exposure and Sizing

The defect is exposed using the aforementioned open or arthroscopic methods. The chondral or osteochondral defect is then measured at its widest points to determine appropriate donor diameter. Based on the defect size, a guide pin is placed through the appropriate sizing guide. The guide is then placed perpendicularly against the defect, the guide pin is advanced 3 cm into the condyle, and the sizing block is removed.

The appropriately sized reamer is then advanced over the guide pin (Fig. 43-8A). Though the recommended depth varies, we recommend drilling the recipient subchondral bone to a depth of 7 to 10 mm (Fig. 43-8B). This allows for easy plug insertion and provides a big enough graft for a press fit. Care should be taken to maximize exposure of the condyle to allow safe reaming without iatrogenic injury to the anterior horn of the meniscus or the patellar tendon.

Using a depth gauge, we measure depth at the 12, 3, 6, and 9 o'clock positions. The 12 o'clock position on the defect is noted with an indelible marker as a reference point. Using the same guide pin, a dilator is malleted into the recipient site, flush to the bottom of the socket as determined by the depth gauge.

The donor plug is preoperatively matched for condyle size and radius of curvature based on the patient's MRI. The expected donor condyle is thawed and washed with sterile saline. The allograft is then placed in the commercially available jig that secures the allograft in place to allow for accurate harvesting (Fig. 43-9). A sizing guide is placed perpendicular against the planned donor site as determined by the radius of curvature and contour of the condyle. We prefer to always use a medial hemicondyle for a medial recipient condyle and a lateral hemicondyle for a lateral recipient condyle, although it has been described to do otherwise. Once the location of the donor is confirmed, the jig is adjusted and secured appropriately.

A reamer of appropriate size is then introduced, and the plug is reamed. For the authors' preferred system, the donor plug is created 1 mm larger than the recipient socket to allow for an optimal press fit. We create a plug deeper than necessary for the recipient socket and then transect the plug with an orthogonal cut with a sagittal saw. Once the two cuts are completed, the plug can be withdrawn from the donor hemicondyle and gently extruded from the reamer. Of note, care is taken not to destroy the hemicondyle when extracting the donor plug. This ensures that adequate articular surface is available in the event that a second plug is needed (i.e., if the first plug becomes damaged or contaminated or rendered unusable in any way).

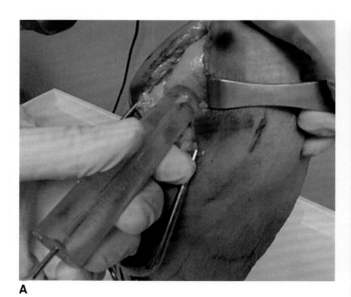
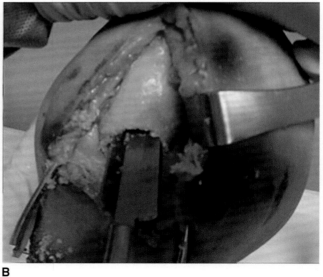

A   **B**

FIGURE 43-8

Lateral condyle. **A:** Based on defect size, a guide pin is placed through the appropriate sizing guide perpendicularly against the defect, and advanced 3 cm into the condyle. **B:** The appropriately sized reamer is then advanced over the guide pin and drilled to a depth of 7 to 10 mm.

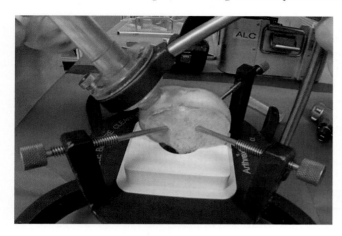

FIGURE 43-9

Lateral condyle, once marked according to the measurements taken from the recipient socket, the allograft is placed in a commercially available jig that secures the allograft in place to allow for accurate harvesting.

The donor plug depth is then marked at the 12, 3, 6, and 9 o'clock positions as determined by the recipient socket (Fig. 43-10A). A matching mark at the 12 o'clock position is made on the articular cartilage of the plug to maintain graft orientation when preparing the donor. The plug is then prepared with a sagittal saw based on the depth markings. Once cut to the appropriate dimensions, the edges of the plug are then gently beveled to facilitate graft placement. Next, the deep surface of the plug is gently scored with a sagittal saw to create a waffle or "tic-tac-toe" type of pattern. This allows the graft to be more gently pressed into place if the plug is slightly proud. To insert the plug into the recipient site, the two 12 o'clock articular cartilage marks should be aligned as closely as possible to ensure the most symmetric contour (Fig. 43-10B). On some plugs, these lines are slightly offset to maximize contour symmetry. If needed, the plug can be gently malleted into place using an oversized tamp to minimize contact pressure on the cartilage. Again, if slightly proud, malleting the plug into position is more easily achieved after creating the waffle pattern on the plug. If the plug is recessed and not flush with the condyle, the plug can be gently removed and some cancellous bone from the initial socket reaming can be obtained and packed deep into the socket to allow for a flush plug on the recipient condyle. Cancellous bone from the donor hemicondyle can also be used for this purpose, but we prefer to use autograft when it is available.

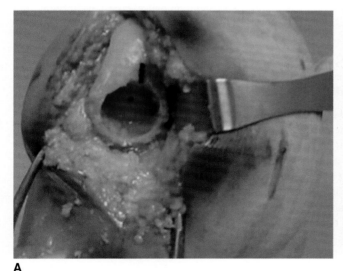

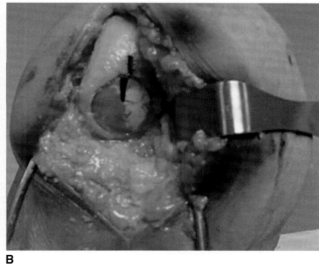

A   **B**

FIGURE 43-10

Lateral condyle. **(A)** The recipient site is marked at 12 o'clock position and **(B)** the matching donor plug is delivered, ensuring the two marks align as closely as possible to ensure the most symmetric contour.

PEARLS AND PITFALLS

- Guide pin insertion and harvesters must be perpendicular and central at both the donor and recipient sites. Nonperpendicular sockets or plugs can lead to poor contour of the plugs with final insertion, which has been shown to have inferior results.
- Care must be taken when harvesting autograft from the donor site, whether using the "pry-off" or "twist-off" technique.
- Appropriate dimension and orientation of harvested autograft/allograft is ensured with preoperative (on MRI) and intraoperative measurements (arthroscopically or using an open technique) as well as appropriate marking of the donor graft with respect to the recipient site.

CLOSURE AND POSTOPERATIVE MANAGEMENT

Once the osteochondral defect is filled and the grafts are in place, the knee should be ranged through its full arc of motion and varus/valgus stress should be applied. This confirms the stability of the plug or plugs and helps the osteochondral graft sit properly. After irrigating and draining the knee, a standard closure should be performed and dressing applied including a soft compressive ace bandage wrap. Patients are placed in a hinged knee brace with non–weight-bearing restrictions.

Postoperatively, the patient follows a non–weight-bearing protocol for 2 weeks, progressing to partial weight bearing for an additional 4 weeks. Range of motion and isometric quadriceps exercises and swimming are encouraged during this period. Barring complications, return to activities can take place at approximately 3 to 4 months.

COMPLICATIONS

No orthopaedic procedure is without complication. In the largest series published of 1,097 mosaic-plasties, Hangody et al. reported four deep infections and four deep vein thromboses (16). They also reported 56 painful hemarthroses (8%) following the chondral procedure. All deep infections and 12 hemarthroses (1.7%) were treated by means of arthroscopic or open debridement. The remaining articular hemorrhages were only treated by aspiration and cryotherapy.

Technical complications can arise during surgery and be a major source of postoperative problems. At the donor site, mobilization of the graft and loosening can occur as early as 4 months postoperatively (17). At the recipient side, breakage of the autograft and the creation of a loose body can occur. Malposition of the plug, both too deep and too proud, can cause excess wear, pain, and impair healing.

SURGICAL OUTCOMES

Autologous Transplantation

References to the results of autologous osteochondral transplantation can be found as early as 1952 when Wilson and Jacobs published their results for depressed lateral tibial plateau fractures treated with patellar autograft, with successful outcomes from 6 months to over 10 years (18). They demonstrated that hyaline cartilage survives after transplantation over this time period.

Short-term results on osteochondral transplantation have been promising. Bobic found good clinical results in 10 of 12 patients undergoing simultaneous first-generation OATs and ACL reconstruction. Their histologic studies also demonstrated no histologic degeneration of the articular cartilage (19). A fibrocartilage border spanned the recipient and donor cartilage, with hypercellularity of the transplanted hyaline cartilage.

In a retrospective study involving 16 knees, Wang et al. found "good" and "excellent" results (80%) at 2- and 4-year follow-up after OCA (20). No progression of the lesion was noted radiographically after treatment at both 2- and 4-year follow-up visits. These findings support the results of other short-term studies (21,22).

With longer follow-up, positive outcomes following chondral procedures persisted. In a consecutive series of 52 patients treated with osteochondral autografts of the knee, the level of knee function improved from 86% at 2 years to 92% at 5 years (23). At 40 months, Lahav et al. demonstrated that 15 patients were able to return to their preinjury levels of IKDC score. Additionally, patient quality of life as measured by the Knee Injury and Osteoarthritis Outcome Score (KOOS) was 93.4 for activities of daily living, with reported knee function improving in 86% of patients (24).

A large, prospective, multicenter study was conducted to further elucidate long-term clinical outcomes following a chondral procedure. Hangody et al. evaluated 831 patients who underwent either a knee or talar mosaicplasty procedure at 10-year follow-up. Authors found good to excellent results in 92% of patients treated with femoral condylar implantations, 87% of those treated with tibial resurfacing, and 79% of those treated with patellar and/or trochlear mosaicplasty with regard to the knee (12,25). Results from another long-term systematic review indicated that 72% of OATs cases had a successful outcome. With a total sample size of 610 patients at a mean of 10.2 years, Pareek et al. also found increased age at surgery, prior surgeries, and defect size all positively correlated with the failure rate, while concomitant procedures improved outcomes (26).

Microfracture has been considered the gold standard in the treatment of chondral defects due to its good results and uncomplicated technique (27). However, when compared to osteochondral autografts in young competitive players in a randomized clinical trial at 3 years, OATs was found to have better clinical results at 12, 24, and 36 months (7). Patients in the OATs group had 96% of good and excellent results versus 52% in the microfracture group, using the Hospital for Special Surgery (HSS) and International Cartilage Repair Society (ICRS) outcome scores. The number of patients able to return to their preinjury level of sports activity at 6.5 months was higher in the OATs group (93% vs. 52%). When taking into account the level of integration shown in MRI studies, the OATs group had excellent or good repairs in 94% of the patients compared to 49% in the microfracture group. OATs also did better in the histologic analysis. A meta-analysis of prospective studies comparing OATs and microfracture by Pareek et al. included 249 patients, reported similar results, noting that the difference in outcomes disappeared for lesions <3 cm^2 (28).

The other option that surgeons have when treating osteochondral defects is the ACI. There are three studies comparing the results of OATs and ACI in a prospective randomized manner, with discrepant conclusions. Bentley et al. found, at 1-year follow-up, ACI had better clinical and arthroscopic results using the Cincinnati and Stanmore scoring system (88% vs. 69%) and the ICRS score (82% vs. 35%). These results should be viewed with caution due to the different rehabilitation protocols used and also due to the fact that the mean size of the defects treated were greater than the ideal indication (29). In contrast, Horas et al. reported their results at 2 years in 40 patients with lesions in the femoral condyle (30). They used the Lysholm and Tegner scores finding no clinical differences between the techniques, although the ACI group showed a slower recovery. Histologically, there was more viable hyaline cartilage in the OATs group, although there was lack of complete integration of the core grafts and that surrounding the articular surface.

Allograft Transplantation

The overall success rates for fresh frozen allografts in the literature range from 10% to 95%, varying based on pathologies and indications (31–37). The least favorable results have been found when performing bipolar reconstruction of the femur and tibia, as well as the patellofemoral joint (32,38,39).

Chondrocyte stability following an allograft procedure has been found as late as 25 and 29 years. Case reports of two patients undergoing total knee arthroplasty performed histologic analysis and in situ hybridization on transplanted chondrocytes demonstrating continued survival of transplanted cells at those timepoints (40,41). Another study by Gross et al. found that long-term allograft survival depends on the stability of host-graft bone interface, with a stable interface supporting graft survival at 25 years (33).

Unfortunately, there are no studies comparing fresh osteochondral autografts with allografts in humans. However, in a canine model comparing outcomes of fresh autograft versus allograft transplantation in dogs, both showed "excellent" bony incorporation with no significant biomechanical differences detected at 3 or 6 months post procedure (42). Furthermore, authors demonstrated no difference in articular cartilage composition after 6 months of implantation.

CONCLUSION

OAT and OCA procedures are useful tools for the sports arthroscopist for the treatment of articular cartilage loss, replacing it with biomechanically identical hyaline cartilage. These strategies can restore function in patients with focal lesions who are not yet suited for knee arthroplasty. When used in appropriately selected patients, osteochondral transplants have proven viability and good outcomes at long-term follow-up.

REFERENCES

1. Curl WW, Krome J, Gordon ES, et al. Cartilage injuries: a review of 31,516 knee arthroscopies. *Arthroscopy.* 1997;13(4):456–460.
2. Aroen A, Loken S, Heir S, et al. Articular cartilage lesions in 993 consecutive knee arthroscopies. *Am J Sports Med.* 2004;32(1):211–215.
3. Flanigan DC, Harris JD, Trinh TQ, et al. Prevalence of chondral defects in athletes' knees: a systematic review. *Med Sci Sports Exerc.* 2010;42(10):1795–1801.
4. Hjelle K, Solheim E, Strand T, et al. Articular cartilage defects in 1,000 knee arthroscopies. *Arthroscopy.* 2002;18(7):730–734.
5. Detterline AJ, Goldberg S, Bach BR Jr., et al. Treatment options for articular cartilage defects of the knee. *Orthop Nurs.* 2005;24(5):361–366; quiz 7–8.
6. Gudas R, Gudaite A, Mickevicius T, et al. Comparison of osteochondral autologous transplantation, microfracture, or debridement techniques in articular cartilage lesions associated with anterior cruciate ligament injury: a prospective study with a 3-year follow-up. *Arthroscopy.* 2013;29(1):89–97.
7. Gudas R, Kalesinskas RJ, Kimtys V, et al. A prospective randomized clinical study of mosaic osteochondral autologous transplantation versus microfracture for the treatment of osteochondral defects in the knee joint in young athletes. *Arthroscopy.* 2005;21(9):1066–1075.
8. Brucker PU, Braun S, Imhoff AB. [Mega-OATS technique—autologous osteochondral transplantation as a salvage procedure for large osteochondral defects of the femoral condyle]. *Oper Orthop Traumatol.* 2008;20(3):188–198.
9. Baltzer AW, Ostapczuk MS, Terheiden HP, et al. Good short- to medium-term results after osteochondral autograft transplantation (OAT) in middle-aged patients with focal, non-traumatic osteochondral lesions of the knee. *Orthop Traumatol Surg Res.* 2016;102(7):879–884.
10. Keeling JJ, Gwinn DE, McGuigan FX. A comparison of open versus arthroscopic harvesting of osteochondral autografts. *Knee.* 2009;16(6):458–462.
11. Epstein DM, Choung E, Ashraf I, et al. Comparison of mini-open versus arthroscopic harvesting of osteochondral autografts in the knee: a cadaveric study. *Arthroscopy.* 2012;28(12):1867–1872.
12. Hangody L, Fules P. Autologous osteochondral mosaicplasty for the treatment of full-thickness defects of weight-bearing joints: ten years of experimental and clinical experience. *J Bone Joint Surg Am.* 2003;85-A(suppl 2):25–32.
13. Hangody L, Kish G, Karpati Z, et al. Arthroscopic autogenous osteochondral mosaicplasty for the treatment of femoral condylar articular defects. A preliminary report. *Knee Surg Sports Traumatol Arthrosc.* 1997;5(4):262–267.
14. Duchow J, Hess T, Kohn D. Primary stability of press-fit-implanted osteochondral grafts. Influence of graft size, repeated insertion, and harvesting technique. *Am J Sports Med.* 2000;28(1):24–27.
15. Evans PJ, Miniaci A, Hurtig MB. Manual punch versus power harvesting of osteochondral grafts. *Arthroscopy.* 2004;20(3):306–310.
16. Hangody L, Vasarhelyi G, Hangody LR, et al. Autologous osteochondral grafting—technique and long-term results. *Injury.* 2008;39(suppl 1):S32–S39.
17. Kim SJ, Shin SJ. Loose bodies after arthroscopic osteochondral autograft in osteochondritis dissecans of the knee. *Arthroscopy.* 2000;16(7):E16.
18. Wilson WJ, Jacobs JE. Patellar graft for severely depressed comminuted fractures of the lateral tibial condyle. *J Bone Joint Surg Am.* 1952;34-a(2):436–442.
19. Bobic V. Arthroscopic osteochondral autograft transplantation in anterior cruciate ligament reconstruction: a preliminary clinical study. *Knee Surg Sports Traumatol Arthrosc.* 1996;3(4):262–264.
20. Wang CJ. Treatment of focal articular cartilage lesions of the knee with autogenous osteochondral grafts. A 2- to 4-year follow-up study. *Arch Orthop Trauma Surg.* 2002;122(3):169–172.
21. Koulalis D, Schultz W, Heyden M, et al. Autologous osteochondral grafts in the treatment of cartilage defects of the knee joint. *Knee Surg Sports Traumatol Arthrosc.* 2004;12(4):329–334.
22. Delcogliano A, Caporaso A, Menghi A, et al. Results of autologous osteochondral grafts in chondral lesions of the knee. *Minerva Chir.* 2002;57(3):273–281.
23. Jakob RP, Franz T, Gautier E, et al. Autologous osteochondral grafting in the knee: indication, results, and reflections. *Clin Orthop Relat Res.* 2002;(401):170–184.
24. Lahav A, Burks RT, Greis PE, et al. Clinical outcomes following osteochondral autologous transplantation (OATS). *J Knee Surg.* 2006;19(3):169–173.
25. Hangody L, Rathonyi GK, Duska Z, et al. Autologous osteochondral mosaicplasty. Surgical technique. *J Bone Joint Surg Am.* 2004;86(suppl 1):65–72.
26. Pareek A, Reardon PJ, Maak TG, et al. Long-term outcomes after osteochondral autograft transfer: a systematic review at mean follow-up of 10.2 years. *Arthroscopy.* 2016;32(6):1174–1184.
27. Steadman JR, Rodkey WG, Briggs KK. Microfracture: its history and experience of the developing surgeon. *Cartilage.* 2010;1(2):78–86.
28. Pareek A, Reardon PJ, Macalena JA, et al. Osteochondral autograft transfer versus microfracture in the knee: a meta-analysis of prospective comparative studies at midterm. *Arthroscopy.* 2016;32(10):2118–2130.
29. Kish G, Hangody L. A prospective, randomised comparison of autologous chondrocyte implantation versus mosaicplasty for osteochondral defects in the knee. *J Bone Joint Surg Br.* 2004;86(4):619; author reply 620.
30. Horas U, Pelinkovic D, Herr G, et al. Autologous chondrocyte implantation and osteochondral cylinder transplantation in cartilage repair of the knee joint. A prospective, comparative trial. *J Bone Joint Surg Am.* 2003;85-a(2):185–192.

31. Lattermann C, Romine SE. Osteochondral allografts: state of the art. *Clin Sports Med.* 2009;28(2):285–301, ix.
32. Bugbee WD, Convery FR. Osteochondral allograft transplantation. *Clin Sports Med.* 1999;18(1):67–75.
33. Gross AE, Kim W, Las Heras F, et al. Fresh osteochondral allografts for posttraumatic knee defects: long-term followup. *Clin Orthop Relat Res.* 2008;466(8):1863–1870.
34. Gross AE, Shasha N, Aubin P. Long-term followup of the use of fresh osteochondral allografts for posttraumatic knee defects. *Clin Orthop Relat Res.* 2005;(435):79–87.
35. Emmerson BC, Gortz S, Jamali AA, et al. Fresh osteochondral allografting in the treatment of osteochondritis dissecans of the femoral condyle. *Am J Sports Med.* 2007;35(6):907–914.
36. Garrett JC. Fresh osteochondral allografts for treatment of articular defects in osteochondritis dissecans of the lateral femoral condyle in adults. *Clin Orthop Relat Res.* 1994;(303):33–37.
37. Garrett JC. Osteochondral allografts for reconstruction of articular defects of the knee. *Instr Course Lect.* 1998;47:517–522.
38. Chu CR, Convery FR, Akeson WH, et al. Articular cartilage transplantation. Clinical results in the knee. *Clin Orthop Relat Res.* 1999;360:159–168.
39. Jamali AA, Emmerson BC, Chung C, et al. Fresh osteochondral allografts: results in the patellofemoral joint. *Clin Orthop Relat Res.* 2005;437:176–185.
40. Jamali AA, Hatcher SL, You Z. Donor cell survival in a fresh osteochondral allograft at twenty-nine years. A case report. *J Bone Joint Surg Am.* 2007;89(1):166–169.
41. Maury AC, Safir O, Heras FL, et al. Twenty-five-year chondrocyte viability in fresh osteochondral allograft. A case report. *J Bone Joint Surg Am.* 2007;89(1):159–165.
42. Glenn RE Jr., McCarty EC, Potter HG, et al. Comparison of fresh osteochondral autografts and allografts: a canine model. *Am J Sports Med.* 2006;34(7):1084–1093.

44 Autologous Chondrocyte Implantation

Brian T. Feeley, Christina Allen, Hubert Kim, and Thierry Pauyo

INTRODUCTION

Autologous chondrocyte implantation (ACI) was first described in the *New England Journal of Medicine* in 1994 (1). At that time, ACI was a truly pioneering application of tissue engineering to treat full-thickness cartilage defects. In this two-stage technique, chondrocytes are first isolated from the patients' own articular cartilage and expanded ex vivo. During the second stage, the chondrocytes are implanted into the defect under a periosteal patch. Recently, third-generation ACI called matrix-induced autologous chondrocyte implantation (MACI) has been developed. During MACI, chondrocytes are harvested in the first stage of the procedure and are then cultured and embedded in a matrix or scaffold and finally directly implanted in the second stage of the procedure (2). The primary advantages of ACI and MACI are the ability to address relatively large defects and the development of mature, organized hyaline or hyaline-like cartilage within the repair site (3). Theoretically, the presence of mature, organized hyaline or more hyaline-like cartilage will enhance the long-term durability and performance of the repair tissue.

Indications

The indications for ACI are similar to those of other cartilage procedures. The appropriate patient has a symptomatic grade III to IV lesions on the weight-bearing portion of the femoral condyle(s) or trochlea, between the ages of 15 and 55 years (Fig. 44-1). The typical size of the lesion is between 2 and 12 cm². Larger lesions and/or multiple lesions are also amenable to ACI treatment. Many

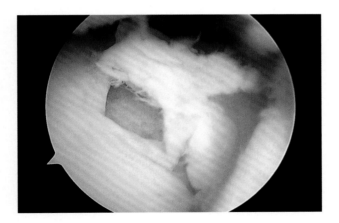

FIGURE 44-1

The patient is an active 37-year-old man with a 1-year history of activity-related knee pain and swelling after a direct blow to his knee. He has been unable to return to his usual sports activities in spite of standard conservative management. This intraoperative photograph taken at the time of the index procedure shows a large cartilage lesion involving the anterior aspect of the lateral femoral condyle. The articular cartilage had delaminated from the underlying bone, and the area of involvement was estimated to be at least 5 cm². The loose cartilage flaps were debrided. A cartilage biopsy specimen was performed in preparation for possible ACI. To be safe, sufficient cartilage (four Tic Tac size pieces) was harvested for the preparation of two vials of expanded chondrocytes. No microfracture was performed.

patients would have had one or more prior cartilage procedure (i.e., debridement or microfracture). It is generally our preference to avoid performing microfracture in patients who are likely to undergo ACI. The outcomes of ACI as a revision surgery are not as good as for ACI as an initial procedure (4).

The usual ACI and MACI procedures involved the restoration of cartilaginous lesion without subchondral bone involvement (5). Although bony involvement is not a strict contraindication, bone loss of more than 6 mm in-depth generally precludes the use of traditional ACI and MACI. However, significant bone involvement can be addressed by combining ACI with staged or concurrent bone grafting. Patients with grade III or grade IV reciprocal "kissing" lesions on the femur or tibia are not good candidates for ACI and MACI nor are patients with degenerative disease with more than 50% joint space narrowing. Relative contraindications include inflammatory arthritis, body mass index (BMI) of >35, and tobacco use (6–8). Patients who are unable to be compliant with the postoperative restrictions and rehabilitation program should not undergo this procedure. Malalignment or instability of the affected limb that would overload the repair tissue should be corrected either before or at the time of ACI and MACI. It is our usual practice to perform any necessary corrective surgeries first and allow for recovery prior to any ACI and MACI procedures; however, other surgeons regularly perform ACI and MACI in conjunction with concurrent osteotomy and/or ligament reconstruction with good results.

Surgical Technique

The technique for standard ACI has remained essentially unchanged since its original description (Figs. 44-2–44-5). The initial phase is identical for ACI and MACI, and it consists of arthroscopically harvesting of the patient's articular cartilage. During the arthroscopy, areas of grade III to IV cartilage change are identified, and the size of the lesion is determined. Care is taken to identify any reciprocal grade III or IV "kissing" lesions, as this would be a contraindication to proceeding with ACI. Cartilage biopsies are usually obtained from the superomedial or superolateral aspect of the femoral condyles along the peripheral margin of articular cartilage. Alternatively, cartilage biopsies can be taken from the intercondylar notch. There are no data to suggest that any of these sites is clearly superior to the others. The cartilage biopsy is obtained using a gouge or ringed curette to remove approximately 200 to 300 mg (two "Tic Tacs") of tissue. A sharp gouge is frequently easier and more efficient to use than a curette. Inclusion of a small amount of bone with the cartilage specimen is common and not a problem, as subsequent processing prior to in vitro expansion will remove the contaminating bone component. While it may be tempting in some cases to harvest

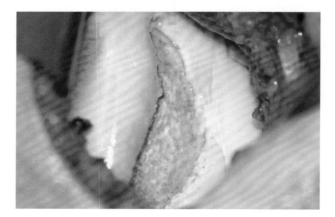

FIGURE 44-2

Eight weeks after the index procedure, the patient underwent the second stage of ACI. Based upon the location of the lesion, a limited lateral parapatellar arthrotomy was made. For the most part, there was a clear demarcation between the damaged area and surrounding normal cartilage. The margins of the lesion were cleanly outlined with a scalpel. Attention to tactile feedback is important during this step as the cut cartilage should feel relatively firm; otherwise, it is unlikely to hold a suture, and the margin should be extended in that area. The damaged cartilage was removed with a ringed curette down to subchondral bone. Punctate bone bleeding was controlled using small thrombin soaked sponges.

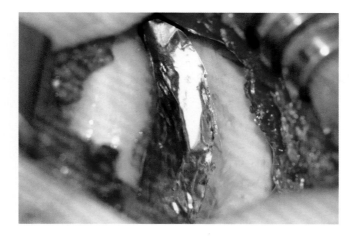

FIGURE 44-3

Sterile foil from a scalpel blade wrapper was cut to match the size and shape of the defect. This step requires some trial and error but must be performed precisely as a poorly sized or shaped template will make the rest of the procedure much more difficult.

mildly degenerative cartilage, we believe this should be avoided. The harvested tissue is placed into a sterile transport container that is shipped to the cell processing facility. In the United States, almost all cartilage tissue processing for ACI is performed by Genzyme Corporation (Cambridge, MA). Chondrocytes are released from the cartilage matrix by enzymatic digestion and are then expanded under standard tissue culture conditions. The details of this process are considered proprietary and may vary slightly from one facility to another. The end product is a cell suspension of partially dedifferentiated chondrocytes. Typically, one vial of cells containing approximately 12 million cells is sufficient to treat a defect up to 7 cm^2 in size. Larger lesions may require more than one vial of cells, and this must be taken into account when sizing the defect(s), harvesting cartilage, and ordering cells for implantation.

The second procedure for implantation of the expanded chondrocyte cells is performed in a minimum of 4 weeks following the index procedure to allow for in vitro expansion of the harvested chondrocytes. The procedure can be performed under either general or regional anesthesia. The patient is positioned supine on a standard operating table. It is helpful to tape a sand bag or 3-L saline bag

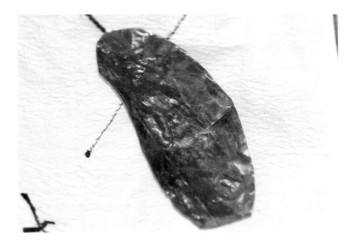

FIGURE 44-4

For this case, a synthetic collagen I/III collagen membrane (Bio-Gide) was used in lieu of an autologous periosteal patch. Prior to surgery, this modification to the standard ACI procedure was discussed with the patient in depth as this treatment is "off-label." This membrane has smooth and rough sides. The rough side is treated like the cambium side of a periosteal patch. A standard skin marking pen is used to mark the smooth side to maintain orientation. The collagen membrane is easier to manipulate and cut to shape when dry. Suture passes through this material more smoothly than through periosteum, so the use mineral oil is not necessary.

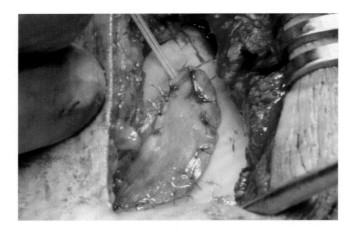

FIGURE 44-5

The membrane is secured to the margins of the cartilage defect using 6-0 Vicryl sutures spaced approximately 4 mm apart. Saline is injected under to patch to check for watertightness, and additional sutures as placed as necessary. We strive for watertightness with sutures alone, but a small amount of leakage can be managed with fibrin glue. The cultured chondrocytes are gently resuspended in the transport vial and then injected under the patch. The opening is closed with an additional suture and sealed with fibrin glue.

to the table at the midcalf level so that the knee can be held flexed to approximately 90 degrees. An Alvarado positioner can be used instead, and it has the added benefit of being able to fine-tune the knee position for optimal exposure. A lateral post is also useful to keep the leg vertically positioned. The leg is prepped distal to a nonsterile tourniquet, which is not typically inflated. For most cases, we prefer a midline skin incision, which can most easily be incorporated into any future surgical procedures on the knee. Alternatively, a parapatellar skin incision can be used and is equally effective. The arthrotomy is performed based on the location of the lesion. For trochlear lesions, we favor a medial parapatellar arthrotomy with a "midvastus" extension as necessary. Any dissection distally along the tibial plateau should be performed carefully in order not to damage the anterior horn of the medial or lateral meniscus.

For defects involving the medial or lateral femoral condyles, bent Homan retractors are placed on either side of the affected condyle. Knee flexion is adjusted to an appropriate angle to best expose the lesion in the operative field. For trochlear lesions, typically less flexion or even full extension provides optimal exposure. Once the defect is well visualized, the perimeter of the lesion is demarcated with a fresh no. 15 blade cutting perpendicular to the articular surface down to the subchondral bone. Although some surgeons use a sharp curette for this step, we believe a scalpel minimizes iatrogenic damage and cell death in the surrounding cartilage that may affect repair tissue integration. Straight, angled, and ring curettes are used to remove all remaining cartilage within the outlined lesion. The goal is to create a sharp line of demarcation with vertical walls of surrounding articular cartilage. Care should be taken to avoid penetration of the subchondral bone so as to prevent bleeding that may have an adverse effect on the implanted cells. If some bleeding in the prepared bed is identified, hemostasis can usually be obtained by placing a thrombin-soaked sponge in the defect during the harvesting of the periosteal graft and/or with the use of fibrin glue. Ideally, the repair site is prepared such that the entire perimeter of surrounding cartilage is completely normal. However, "real-world" lesions frequently are bordered by some areas of slightly softened articular cartilage. Our experience is that ACI can be performed successfully in these situations as long as the cartilage is firmly fixed to the underlying bone and that sutures can be placed securely into the surrounding cartilage. If not, the area to be repaired must be enlarged.

The defect is then measured to determine the proper size of the periosteal patch. Either sterile paper or a small piece of aluminum is placed over the lesion site and marked with a surgical marker as a template for periosteal graft harvest. We typically use the aluminum foil from the sterile scalpel blades as this is easy to manipulate as a template for the graft. The template should be sized 1 to 2 mm larger than the defect around the entire circumference.

The periosteal graft can be obtained from multiple sites. The most common location is the proximal medial tibia, just distal to the pes insertion. The periosteum at this site is particularly well suited for implantation. The incision can be extended, or a separate incision can be made. The dissection is carried down to the periosteum sharply, and all fat and subcutaneous tissue is removed from the harvest site. The periosteum to be harvested is marked from the template, and a fresh no. 15 blade or sharp and thin periosteal elevator is used to elevate the periosteum from the underlying bone. Prior to harvesting, it is useful to mark the exposed surface of the graft with a standard marking pen so that there will be no confusion as to which side is the cambium surface. Electrocautery should not be used to harvest the periosteal graft as this will kill cells that potentially contribute to the repair. It is important to handle the periosteal graft gently and not allow it to dry out. Although every attempt should be made to harvest the periosteum as an intact sheet, perforations do occur and can be repaired using interrupted or running 6-0 Vicryl suture.

The graft is fixed over the lesion to the surrounding cartilage using a 6-0 Vicryl suture with a cutting needle, cambium layer down. Sutures are placed at 3- to 4-mm intervals around periphery of the lesion. Using a dyed suture, though not necessary, makes visualization of the suture material considerably easier during graft fixation. The use of magnifying loupes during this portion of the procedure may also be helpful. Sterile mineral oil can be used to coat the suture prior to passage through the periosteum in order to prevent binding of the suture to the periosteum. The needle is first passed through the periosteum, 2 mm from the edge, and then into the cartilage edge, exiting approximately 4 mm from the edge. It is sometimes helpful to decrease the needle's radius of curvature by carefully bending it with needle drivers, maintaining a smooth curve. Simple instrument tying techniques are used to secure the sutures. The knot should be placed over the periosteum, not the adjacent native cartilage. It is often easiest to place the first four sutures at the 12, 6, 3, and 9 o'clock positions, respectively, for round or oval defects. For more rectangular-shaped defects, the first four sutures are best placed in the "corners." It is also possible to address lesions that are not completely bordered by articular cartilage by securing the periosteal patch using small suture anchors. In these cases, anchors should be placed not more than 5 mm apart. Alternatively, sutures can be placed through transosseous tunnels made with a small K-wire. A potential downside to the use of either anchors or transosseous tunnels is the risk of increased bleeding at the repair site. However, bleeding from the bone holes usually can be controlled using fibrin glue. Regardless of fixation method, secure graft fixation is paramount.

A small area at the most superior aspect of the repair site is left open to accommodate an 18-gauge angiocatheter through which the cells will be injected. Otherwise, the repair must be essentially watertight prior to cell implantation, which should be verified by injecting saline under the patch. Additional sutures are placed as necessary. Any fluid beneath the patch is aspirated. The chondrocyte cell suspension is then drawn into a syringe and injected under the periosteal patch. The angiocatheter is removed, and additional sutures are placed to complete the watertight seal. We routinely seal the edges of the repair site with fibrin glue, which may decrease the chances of subsequent leakage. The use of fibrin glue may be especially prudent if the quality of the surrounding cartilage is less than ideal or if suture anchors were used to secure part of the patch. If the tourniquet was inflated, it should be released and meticulous hemostasis obtained prior to wound closure. We prefer not to use intra-articular anesthetics based on reports of toxicity to chondrocytes, particularly when they lack the protective barrier of their native extracellular matrix.

Recent modifications to the original ACI procedure have made the procedure substantially simpler. Third-generation ACI or MACI has newly been cleared by the U.S. Food and Drug Administration (FDA) for use in the general population. The primary benefits of MACI include decreased morbidity and complications associated with the suturing a cover over the repair (9). The surgical technique allows for the second stage to be minimally invasively, through arthroscopy where the chondrocyte-seeded biocompatible scaffold is inserted in the articular defect and fixed in place with fibrin glue and no sutures or membrane cover are necessary (10). This fixation technique allows for a simplified surgical technique, decreased operative time, and accelerated rehabilitation of the patients.

POSTOPERATIVE CARE

Postoperative rehabilitation following ACI is felt to be critical to achieving optimal results. Immediately after surgery, patients are immobilized for 6 to 12 hours to allow the cells to adhere to the subchondral bone. The first phase of the rehabilitation process, lasting approximately 6 weeks, focuses on protection of the repair site to allow for initial filling of the defect with repair tissue.

Typically, patients are instructed to remain non–weight bearing during this phase, particularly for lesions involving the central weight-bearing areas of the femoral condyles. Patients with trochlear lesions or femoral lesions outside of the central weight-bearing areas may be advanced more rapidly, with range of motion limits set to prevent engaging the defect during weight bearing. A CPM is initiated from postoperative day 1 and used 6 to 12 hours per day for 4 to 6 weeks if possible. The second phase, lasting through week 12, focuses on a gradual increase in functional activities while protecting the repair tissue, which remains soft and highly susceptible to damage. Low-impact exercises such as stationary bicycling and treadmill walking are initiated, and transition to full weight bearing is allowed as tolerated. The third phase, lasting through the 6th postoperative month, focuses on achieving full functional capacity other than sports. The goal should be normal knee motion, leg strength, balance, and stability. By this point, the repair tissue is more durable and tolerant to impact activities. Full activities, particularly high-impact sports, are limited for the first 12 to 18 months postoperatively to allow for further repair tissue maturation.

RESULTS

The initial outcomes of ACI were reported in 1994 by Brittberg et al. (1). The 23 patients ranged from 14 to 48 years of age, and the lesions ranged from 1.6 to 6.5 cm^2. The average follow-up was 39 months. A majority of the patients underwent multiple "second-look" arthroscopies. At 3 months, the grafts were leveled with the surrounding tissue and spongy when probed. At the second arthroscopy, the grafts looked similar but had significantly more firmness. Biopsies showed that 11 of the 15 femoral transplants and 1 of the 7 patellar transplants had the appearance of hyaline cartilage. Fourteen of the sixteen patients with femoral condylar lesions had good or excellent results. The other two patients required a second operation due to severe central wear and persistent locking and pain. Recently, these authors reported long-term 10- to 20-year results demonstrating maintained clinical and functional benefits based on patient-completed questionnaires (11). There have been very few well-controlled studies that have evaluated the outcomes of ACI. Zaslav et al. (12) recently performed a prospective clinical study to determine the effectiveness of ACI in patients who failed prior treatments for articular cartilage defects in the knee. There were 154 patients with a mean follow-up of 4 years in this multicenter trial. At the time of follow-up, 76% of the patients were deemed a clinical success based on knee pain, quality of life, and overall health. The results did not differ if the patients had a marrow stimulation procedure prior or a debridement alone. Seventy-six (49%) of the patients had a subsequent surgical procedure. The authors concluded that ACI was effective in providing pain relief as well as improved quality of life in patients who had undergone a previous knee cartilage procedure.

However, in a recent study, Minas et al. (4) evaluated the effectiveness of ACI as an initial procedure compared to ACI as a revision procedure in a cohort study. They followed 321 patients prospectively over 2 years. They found that the failure rate was three times higher following ACI performed after a failed microfracture (26%) than it was following ACI performed as a primary procedure (8%). This failure rate of ACI as a revision surgery (26%) is similar to the failure rate of Zaslav et al. (12) (24%) mentioned above (5).

Several studies have compared ACI to other cartilage restoration techniques. Anderson et al. (13) compared ACI to microfracture in a prospective study. There were 23 patients in each group, and all lesions were >2 cm^2. There were mean improvements in overall condition scores in both groups (microfracture: 1.3; ACI 3.1, $p < 0.05$). Two patients in the ACI group and six in the microfracture group were categorized as treatment failures. Brittberg et al. (14) evaluated the effectiveness of MACI compared to microfracture in a randomized controlled trial evaluating 128 patients with 5 years of follow-up. The MACI group comprised of 65 patients, and the microfracture group had 63 patients. At the 5-year follow-up, the improvement in the Knee Injury and Osteoarthritis Outcome Score was statistically higher for MACI over microfracture in the co-primary end point of pain and function. Both techniques demonstrated similar results with magnetic resonance imaging evaluation in cartilage defect filling.

Bentley et al. (15) performed a prospective, randomized study comparing ACI to mosaicplasty, with 50 patients in each treatment group. The patients were young (average age: 31 years), and the lesions were an average of 4.7 cm^2. The patients typically had a long duration of symptoms (mean: 7.2 years), and many had a previous surgery. At 19-month average follow-up, 88% of the ACI patients and 69% of the mosaicplasty patients had a good to excellent result with clinical outcome scores. Arthroscopy at 1 year demonstrated excellent or good repairs in 82% after ACI and in 34% after mosaicplasty. The authors concluded that there was a significant advantage of using ACI compared to mosaicplasty, as it appeared to offer better clinical outcomes with better repairs as visualized by arthroscopy.

There are several limitations to ACI. Many patients are unwilling to undergo two procedures and the long recovery time necessary in order to allow the cartilage to mature. The additional cost of a second surgery, along with the cost of ex vivo chondrocyte expansion, is substantial and may negate any clinical benefit from a cost-utility standpoint. In the United States, insurance authorization can be problematic, but is greatly facilitated with good clinical documentation. Wood et al. (16) reviewed the adverse outcomes of ACI reported to the FDA from 1996 to 2003. During this time, there were 7,500 lots of Carticel (Genzyme Tissue Repair, Cambridge, MA) distributed to physicians and 294 adverse event reports. More than one adverse event were reported for 135 of the 294 (46%) patients. The median interval from implantation to the diagnosis of an adverse event was 240 days (range: 1–2, 105). The most common adverse event was graft failure, accounting for 24.8% of all adverse events. Delamination represented 22.1% of adverse events, and tissue hypertrophy accounted for 17.7% of adverse events. Of the 294 patients who had an adverse event, 273 (93%) had 389 surgical revisions subsequent to implantation. Most of the revisions (48%) involved subsequent cartilage procedures and included debridement, chondroplasty, and microfracture. Almost 25% of the reoperations were periarticular procedures such as a lysis of adhesions, lateral release, or synovectomy. Eight patients required a total knee replacement. The data from this study reflect the outcomes of previous studies examining the outcomes of ACI.

Peterson et al. reported 52 adverse events in 101 patients, including 26 instances of periosteal hypertrophy and seven graft failures. Similarly, Minas describes 5 of 70 patients requiring additional surgical intervention following ACI (17). While the overall complication rate and need for reoperation for ACI have been relatively high, addressing these problems typically involves simple debridement and yields excellent results. Furthermore, procedure modifications including the substitution of a collagen matrix patch for the traditional periosteal patch markedly decreased the need for reoperation. Nevertheless, it is prudent to specifically discuss with each patient the possible need for an additional, but straightforward, arthroscopic surgery after ACI.

REFERENCES

1. Brittberg M, Lindahl A, Nillson A, et al. Treatment of deep cartilage defects in the knee with autologous chondrocyte transplantation. *N Engl J Med.* 1994;331(14):889–895.
2. Sacolick DA, Kirven JC, Abouljoud MM, et al. The treatment of adult osteochondritis dissecans with autologous cartilage implantation: a systematic review. *J Knee Surg.* 2018.
3. Knutsen G, Drogset JO, Engebretsen L, et al. A randomized trial comparing autologous chondrocyte implantation with microfracture. Findings at five years. *J Bone Joint Surg Am.* 2007;89(10):2105–2112.
4. Minas T, Gomoll AH, Rosenberger R, et al. Increased failure rate of autologous chondrocyte implantation after previous treatment with marrow stimulation techniques. *Am J Sports Med.* 2009;37(5):902–908.
5. Krill M, Early N, Everhart JS, et al. Autologous Chondrocyte Implantation (ACI) for knee cartilage defects: a review of indications, technique, and outcomes. *JBJS Rev.* 2018;6(2):e5.
6. Alford JW, Cole BJ. Cartilage restoration, part 2: techniques, outcomes, and future directions. *Am J Sports Med.* 2005;33(3):443–460.
7. Mithoefer K, Williams RJ III, Warren RF, et al. The microfracture technique for the treatment of articular cartilage lesions in the knee. A prospective cohort study. *J Bone Joint Surg Am.* 2005;87(9):1911–1920.
8. Jaiswal PK, Macmull S, Bentley G, et al. Does smoking influence outcome after autologous chondrocyte implantation? A case-controlled study. *J Bone Joint Surg.* 2009;91(12):1575–1578.
9. Niethammer TR, Holzgruber M, Gulecyuz MF, et al. Matrix based autologous chondrocyte implantation in children and adolescents: a match paired analysis in a follow-up over three years post-operation. *Int Orthop.* 2017;41(2):343–350.
10. Ruta DJ, Villarreal AD, Richardson DR. Orthopedic surgical options for joint cartilage repair and restoration. *Phys Med Rehabil Clin N Am.* 2016;27(4):1019–1042.
11. Peterson L, Vasiliadis HS, Brittberg M, et al. Autologous chondrocyte implantation: a long-term follow-up. *Am J Sports Med.* 2010;38(6):1117–1124.
12. Zaslav K, Cole B, Brewster R, et al. A prospective study of autologous chondrocyte implantation in patients with failed prior treatment for articular cartilage defect of the knee: results of the Study of the Treatment of Articular Repair (STAR) clinical trial. *Am J Sports Med.* 2009;37(1):42–55.
13. Anderson AF, Fu F, Mandelbaum B. A controlled study of autologous chondrocyte implantation vs microfracture for articular cartilage lesions of the femur. Paper presented at Annual Meeting of the American Academy of Orthopaedic Surgeons, Dallas, TX, 2002.
14. Brittberg M, Recker D, Ilgenfritz J, et al. Matrix-applied characterized autologous cultured chondrocytes versus microfracture: five-year follow-up of a prospective randomized trial. *Am J Sports Med.* 2018;46(6):1343–1351.
15. Bentley G, Biant LC, Carrington RW, et al. A prospective, randomised comparison of autologous chondrocyte implantation versus mosaicplasty for osteochondral defects in the knee. *J Bone Joint Surg Br.* 2003;85(2):223–230.
16. Wood JJ, Malek MA, Frassica FJ, et al. Autologous cultured chondrocytes: adverse events reported to the United States Food and Drug Administration. *J Bone Joint Surg Am.* 2006;88(3):503–507.
17. Minas T. Autologous chondrocyte implantation for focal chondral defects of the knee. *Clin Orthop Relat Res.* 2001;391:S349–S361.

45 Osteochondritis Dissecans

Taylor M. Southworth, Mark Slabaugh, Tracy M. Tauro, Neal B. Naveen, Nicole A. Friel, Benedict U. Nwachukwu, and Brian J. Cole

INTRODUCTION

Osteochondritis dissecans (OCD) results in the destruction of subchondral bone with secondary damage to overlying articular cartilage (1,2). The prevalence of this condition is estimated to be between 11.5 and 21 per 100,000 (3,4). OCD is classically divided into juvenile and adult forms based on the patient's skeletal maturity (1). Juvenile OCD (JOCD) lesions occur in children and young adolescents with open growth plates. Although adult OCD lesions may arise de novo, they more commonly result from an incompletely healed and previously asymptomatic JOCD lesion (5). JOCD lesions have a better prognosis and higher rates of spontaneous healing with conservative treatment than do adult OCD lesions (6). Adult OCD lesions have a greater propensity for instability and, once symptomatic, typically follow a clinical course that is progressive and unremitting (7). While lesions most frequently occur on the femoral condyles, they are also found in the elbow, wrist, ankle, and femoral head (8–12). The highest incidence rates in JOCD are among patients ages 10 and 15 years old, ranking among the most common causes of knee pain and dysfunction in young adults (6,7,13) (Fig. 45-1).

The typical presentation of OCD in the knee includes pain and swelling related to activity. Instability is not usually reported, though mechanical symptoms, such as catching and locking, usually occur in the presence of a loose body and are frequently the initial presenting symptoms. The patient may walk with an antalgic gait or with the leg externally rotated to decrease pressure over the lesion, known as Wilson sign (14). Effusion, decreased range of motion, and quadriceps atrophy are variably present depending upon the severity and duration of the lesion (15). Patients typically have tenderness localized over the lesion. More than 70% of OCD lesions are found in the lateral aspect of the medial femoral condyle (MFC), intersecting the intercondylar notch near the posterior cruciate ligament (PCL). Central lateral condylar lesions account for 15% to 20% and femoral trochlear lesions for <1%. Patellar involvement is uncommon (5%–10%) and, if present, is typically located in the inferior medial area (7).

INDICATIONS

Operative treatment for OCD lesions is focused on improving the blood supply to the lesion, restoring the joint surface, and providing rigid fixation (16). Surgery is indicated both for young patients with detached or unstable lesions as well as for those approaching physeal closure whose lesions have been unresponsive to nonoperative management (1,17). Operative treatment may also be considered in patients who are unable to participate in a prolonged nonoperative course.

Specifically, interventions such as drilling or internal fixation are indicated for the symptomatic juvenile patient who has failed a course of 3 to 6 months of nonoperative treatment. However, when the presence of significant mechanical symptoms dominates the clinical presentation, the decision to operate might occur earlier. Drilling is generally limited to young patients with open physes and low-grade lesions, Guhl grades I and II, that are not grossly unstable with palpation.

Higher grade OCD lesions with articular cartilage flaps or loose bodies, Guhl grades III and IV respectively, are generally not amenable to conservative treatment. Ananthaharan and Randsborg

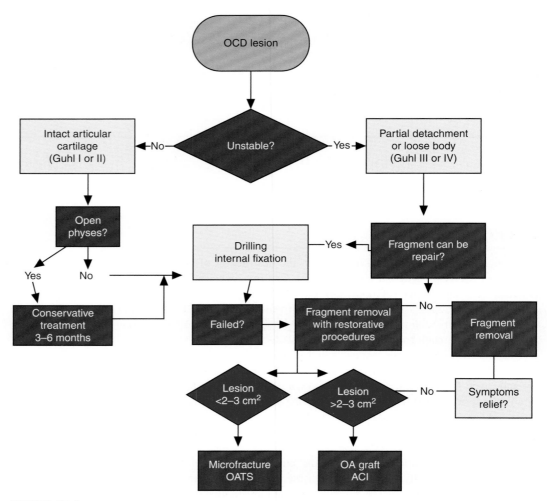

FIGURE 45-1

Algorithm for surgical treatment of JOCD/OCD. Surgical goals should always try to reestablish the joint surface and conserve the osteochondral fragment. If not, restorative treatment should be implemented.

found that patients with grade III and IV lesions were five times more likely to fail conservative treatment when compared to those with grades I and II lesions (3). Thus, fixation of partially detached lesions or loose bodies is appropriate for large fragments containing sufficient subchondral bone to provide union and support of the fixation system. Lower grade lesions, Guhl grades I or II, may also be fixed if conservative treatment has failed or there is clinical suspicion of instability. Additionally, unstable "trap door" lesions that are partially elevated from the subchondral bed require fixation (18,19).

Many patients function well despite having OCD lesions and only become symptomatic when the OCD fragment becomes unstable. In these cases, fragment removal is indicated and can lead to symptomatic relief. For example, if the defect is relatively small, from an area with less contact pressure (20), such as the "classic" OCD lesion located near the PCL origin on the "upslope" of the MFC, and is associated with the acute onset of mechanical symptoms in a skeletally mature adult, fragment removal and observation are indicated. In contrast, complaints of "achy discomfort," effusions unrelated to mechanical symptoms, and weight-bearing pain over the lesion may be indicative of symptoms that are due to the defect itself rather than the unstable or displaced fragment. These lesions are an indication for a cartilage restoration procedure, such as a marrow stimulation technique, osteochondral autograft, osteochondral allograft (OCA), or autologous chondrocyte implantation (ACI). Specifically, microfracture is indicated in patients with a localized cartilage defect (<2–4 cm²). Patients with low demand

and bigger lesions can also improve with this technique. The indications and optimal patient population for osteochondral autograft remain narrow. A single plug autograft is preferred for defects smaller than 1 cm^2. However, some authors perform mosaicplasty with multiple smaller plugs on defects as large as 4 cm^2 with encouraging results (21). Larger OCD lesions (>2 cm^2) may be treated with OCA transplantation (22). OCA transplantation provides the ability to resurface larger and deeper defects with mature hyaline cartilage, while addressing the underlying bone deficiency. ACI is ideal for symptomatic, unipolar, well-contained chondral and osteochondral defects measuring between 2 and 10 cm^2 with bone loss <6 to 8 mm (Fig. 45-1).

In contrast to JOCD where nonoperative treatment is usually first line, adult OCD typically requires early surgical intervention (5). Additionally, in cases of chondral separation, surgical results are better than those with nonsurgical treatments (23,24).

CONTRAINDICATIONS

Surgical decision-making is based on patient age, skeletal maturity, lesion appearance, and clinical symptoms. The ideal goal of conservative treatment is to obtain lesion healing before physeal closure. Stable OCD lesions in young patients have a favorable prognosis when treated initially with nonoperative treatment. A large multicenter review of the European Pediatric Orthopedic Society study (509 knees, 318 juvenile, and 191 adult in 452 patients) suggests an improved prognosis with conservative treatment in young patients with a small lesion (<2 cm^2) in the classic location with no signs of dissection or effusion (23). Ananthaharan and Randsborg noted that 78% of grade I and II lesions were successfully treated with conservative management (3). Moreover, spontaneous healing of JOCD lesions has been reported when the lesion is not in the classical location of the lateral aspect of the MFC (25).

Traditional nonoperative treatment for JOCD consists of an initial phase of knee immobilization with partial weight bearing (4–6 weeks) in those patients in whom no detachment is noted on MRI. Once the patient is pain free, weight bearing as tolerated is permitted and a rehabilitation program emphasizing knee range of motion and low-impact strengthening exercises ensues. If there are radiographic and clinical signs of healing at 3 or 4 months after the initial diagnosis, patients may participate in a gradual return to sports with increasing intensity allowed in the absence of knee symptoms. The likelihood that the lesion will heal with this management is approximately 50% at 10 to 18 months (9).

Neither the literature nor our experience allows us to definitively determine whether an untreated OCD lesion with the fragment in situ or treatment via fragment excision has a more significant likelihood of developing into symptomatic degenerative joint disease in the future when compared to cartilage restoration procedures. Linden performed a long-term retrospective study of patients with OCD of the femoral condyles with an average follow-up of 33 years after initial diagnosis (13). It was concluded that while individuals who are older when the OCD manifests, such as those with adult OCD, have an increasing incidence of knee osteoarthritis (OA), JOCD is not associated with an increased risk of OA compared to the normal population. In contrast, Twyman et al. prospectively followed 22 knees with JOCD into middle age and found that 50% had some radiographic signs of OA (26). The likelihood of OA development was found to be proportional to the size of the area involved.

PREOPERATIVE PREPARATION

Standard anteroposterior and lateral radiographs of the knee permit localization of the lesion and assessment of the physeal status of the patient. Additional images such as tunnel or sunrise views are useful for suspected distal MFC or patellar lesions, respectively. By convention, lesions may be anatomically localized using the Cahill classification (1) (Fig. 45-2). Magnetic resonance imaging (MRI) is the mainstay in diagnosis of OCD lesions. Lesion qualities including bone edema, subchondral separation, and cartilage condition may be evaluated prior to determining treatment course (Fig. 45-3). Intraoperatively, OCD lesions may be classified using the criteria suggested by Guhl (27) (Table 45-1).

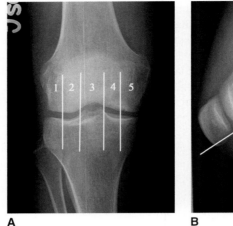
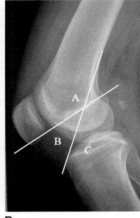

A   **B**

FIGURE 45-2

A: Anteroposterior radiograph of a 35-year-old male with an OCD lesion occupying the weight-bearing area of the femoral condyle. As per Cahill's classification for medio-lateral localization of the lesion, numbering of the five anatomic areas is as follows: the condyles are bisected, and area 3 is bounded by the walls of the intercondylar notch. **B:** Lateral radiograph of the same OCD lesion. The line separating *A* and *B* represents the roof of the intercondylar notch. The line separating *B* and *C* is a continuation of the posterior femoral cortex.

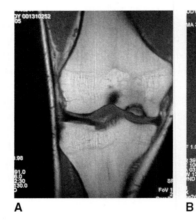
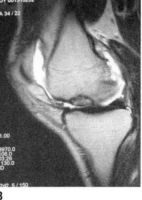

A   **B**

FIGURE 45-3

A: Coronal MRI of the knee of an OCD lesion of the MFC of the left knee. Note the low-intensity signal between the osteochondral fragment and the subchondral bone, suggesting an unstable fragment. **B:** Sagittal MRI through the MFC.

TABLE 45-1 Description of the Guhl Classification	
Grade	**Intraoperative Finding**
I	Normal articular cartilage
II	Fragmentation in situ
III	Partial detachment
IV	Complete detachment, loose body present

Source: Reprinted from Guhl JF. Arthroscopic treatment of osteochondritis dissecans. *Clin Orthop Relat Res.* 1982;167:65–74, with permission.

OCD LESION TREATMENT TECHNIQUES

Reparative Treatments

The goal of reparative procedures is to restore the integrity of the native subchondral interface and preserve the overlying articular cartilage (28).

Drilling

The disruption of subchondral blood supply is thought to be an important factor in the development of OCD (29). Drilling involves the creation of vascular channels to the devitalized region in order to restore blood flow and enhance healing.

Antegrade drilling involves drilling through the articular surface and into the femoral epiphysis. It is done arthroscopically under direct visualization (30–32). If the lesion is not accessible via standard portals, accessory portals are created to obtain an orthogonal drilling angle. A K-wire 2 cm longer than a small cannula facilitates the direction and depth of the channels (29). Return of blood and fat droplets through the articular surface confirms penetration of cancellous bone.

More commonly, drilling is performed by entering at a nonarticular location. For example, the classic OCD lesion is located along the lateral aspect of the MFC and can be accessed at the anterior aspect of the PCL origin along the inner margin of the MFC with a K-wire introduced percutaneously or through the inferolateral portal.

Retrograde drilling is inherently more difficult when targeting the lesion base. C-arm visualization is needed to help avoid joint penetration or dislodgement of the OCD fragment. Alternative methods, including sonography (33) and the use of an ACL guide (34), have been proposed. Large-diameter drilling with iliac crest bone graft supplementation has also been described (35).

Internal Fixation

Fixation can be accomplished with bone pegs, osteochondral grafts, or metal or bioabsorbable devices (29,36,37). As mentioned previously, unstable "trap door" lesions that are partially elevated from the subchondral bed require fixation (11,19). If accessible, the base of the lesion and bony surface of the flap are debrided. Microfracture awls can be used to penetrate the base and allow improved access to the subchondral blood supply. The fragment is reduced and temporarily fixed with K-wires to facilitate the final placement of the fixation device. In most cases, fixation is accomplished at two or more locations to impart compression and rotational stability to the fragment. This is important as in vitro studies suggest that compression results in friction between the fragment and the base, thus improving stability and resistance to shear loading. All devices should be recessed beneath the cartilage surface with metal screws removed postoperatively when evidence of union is seen (Fig. 45-4), typically 6 to 8 weeks later. Hardware removal allows for second-look arthroscopy, which provides the benefit of verifying defect healing. Additionally, hardware removal is an added plus as the screws may become prominent and bothersome should the fragment settle around the fixation device. Bioabsorbable fixation is also an option, especially when patients desire

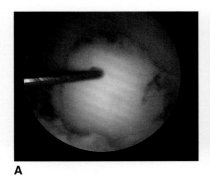   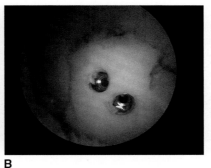

A   B

FIGURE 45-4

A: Intraoperative, arthroscopic view of OCD lesion of the MFC in a 20-year-old male. **B:** Anatomic reduction and fixation of the osteochondral fragment was performed with compression screw fixation.

to avoid a second surgery. Bioabsorbable screws are often made from biphasic calcium phosphate and poly-L,D-lactic acid or amorphous poly-L-lactic acid, which allows for controlled degradation over time.

Restorative Treatments

Restorative procedures attempt to replace damaged cartilage with hyaline or hyaline-like tissue (30,38,39). In the event either that the OCD fragment cannot be initially stabilized and requires excision or that the fragment fails to heal after initial fixation, it is important to determine the clinical relevance of the remaining defect to decide if a cartilage restoration procedure is the best next step. Most importantly, identifying and treating each patient with relevant comorbidities such as malalignment and meniscal and ligament deficiency is imperative to render successful treatment.

Marrow Stimulation Techniques

Abrasion chondroplasty, subchondral drilling, and microfracture involve breaching the subchondral bone to allow the influx of pluripotent stem cells from the marrow into the osteochondral defect resulting in fibrocartilage formation (40). The calcified cartilage layer is carefully debrided, and surgical awls are used to penetrate the subchondral bone to enhance defect fill (41) (Fig. 45-5).

Osteochondral Autograft Transplantation

Osteochondral autograft transplantation involves transplanting osteochondral tissue from a non–weight-bearing region of the patient's own knee to restore the articular surface. The technique has been well described (27) and includes the careful consideration of minimizing donor-site morbidity during graft harvest. When treating the defect with an osteochondral autograft, specific attention should be paid to recreating the natural contour of the condyle with accurate depth and plug placement to avoid graft instability due to relative noncontainment. These steps are critical to avoid early failure.

Osteochondral Allograft Transplantation

Osteochondral allograft transplantation, in contrast to autograft, involves transplanting osteochondral tissue from a donor cadaver. From the donor, an osteochondral plug is able to be harvested. Commercially available instrumentation systems permit accurate sizing and matching of a cylindrical allograft plug to the defect. To do this, a 2.4-mm guide pin is driven through the cannulated sizing guide into the base of the defect. The guide is then removed and used to size the allograft at the appropriate topographic location on the donor. A cannulated cutting reamer of the same size is used to ream to a depth of approximately 6 to 8 mm. Usually, it is possible to press fit the graft with the use of an oversized tamp to secure it. However, if necessary, fixation of the allograft with bioabsorbable compression screws or headless differentially pitched titanium screws is performed.

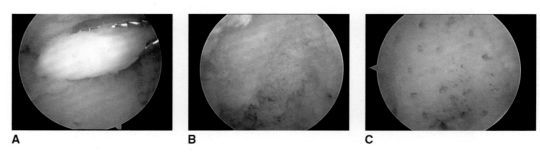

A   **B**   **C**

FIGURE 45-5

A: Intraoperative, arthroscopic view of an unstable osteochondral fragment. **B:** Removal of the unstable lesion, revealing the underlying subchondral bone. **C:** Microfracture holes throughout the entire area of the OCD lesion.

Autologous Chondrocyte Implantation

In ACI, healthy chondrocytes are biopsied from a non–weight-bearing region and expanded in vitro over 4 to 6 weeks. Alternatively, the cells may be cryopreserved for up to 5 years and utilized when necessary. At implantation, defect preparation involves debriding to the calcified cartilage base and creating vertical walls of healthy cartilage to shoulder the lesion. A periosteal patch from the proximal tibia or a synthetic collagen membrane is attached to the perimeter using interrupted 5-0 or 6-0 Vicryl sutures. The edges of the patch are sealed with fibrin glue and the cells injected beneath the patch into the virtual chamber. In third-generation ACI, or matrix-induced ACI (MACI), the chondrocytes are added to a collagen membrane prior to implantation, thus removing the need for a periosteal patch or injection of cells.

Defects deeper than 8 to 10 mm can be approached by concomitant or staged bone grafting. Bone grafting should be performed up to the level of the subchondral bone (42). Prior to bone grafting, drilling through the bed following debridement allows appropriate blood flow into the defect, ensuring subsequent bone graft incorporation. When bone grafting is performed as a primary procedure in an effort to stage for definitive treatment with ACI, most surgeons will wait for a minimum of 6 months to allow for bone graft incorporation. Limited experience exists with anecdotal results of a "sandwich" technique where bone grafting is performed in combination with ACI using a "periosteal sandwich" with both cambium layers facing one another and the cells injected in between.

PEARLS AND PITFALLS

Important pearls and pitfalls involve the clinical decision of the appropriate disease management.

- If a too advanced procedure is performed too early, it limits the options for future procedures.
- Nonoperative course should be first-line treatment in the majority of cases.
- Detached or unstable lesions require surgical intervention.
- Adult OCD lesions often require early surgical intervention.
- Guhl grades III and IV do not respond well to conservative management.
- Be careful to differentiate between symptoms caused by the fragment versus symptoms caused by the defect to determine if a cartilage restoration procedure is needed.

POSTOPERATIVE MANAGEMENT

Authors who focus on the biology of the fragment–subchondral bone interface argue that the knee should be protected in a knee immobilizer and treated similarly to an intra-articular fracture (1). Alternatively, some authors place a premium on the health of the articular cartilage and note the value of continuous motion (1). Hughston et al. demonstrated the detrimental effects of prolonged immobilization, including stiffness, atrophy, osteopenia, and, potentially, chondropenia (4).

In the senior author's practice, after internal fixation, patients may heel-touch weight bear and utilize continuous passive motion (CPM) machines for 4 to 6 hours per day. For postoperative management after a marrow stimulation procedure, instructions depend on the location of the lesion. For microfracture of the femoral condyle, no brace is usually required, but a CPM machine is recommended for 6 to 8 hours per day. Patients begin initially on crutches with 20% to 30% weight bearing. For microfracture of the patella or trochlea, patients are instructed to wear a brace locked to achieve up to 40 degrees of flexion until the first postoperative visit. These patients also are able to weight bear as tolerated and are recommended to use CPM machines for 6 hours per day. After osteochondral autograft transplantation, protected weight bearing is encouraged for up to 6 weeks postoperatively. For OCAs, restricted weight bearing is recommended for at least 8 weeks. The senior author's preferred postoperative management program for OCA has been previously described (43). Patients use a hinged-brace locked in extension for 2 weeks followed by an additional use of 2 to 4 weeks. During this time, the patient is restricted to touch-down weight-bearing protocol. The brace is discontinued after the patient is able to demonstrate a straight leg raise without extension lag. Partial weight bearing begins at 6 weeks post-operatively and is gradually progressed to full weight bearing. Patients are able to begin higher impact activities beginning at 6 to 8 months. For ACI postoperative management, similar to many other procedures, non–weight bearing status and CPM are indicated.

Complications

Complications, like indications, are both general and specific to each surgical technique. General complications include technique failure or failure to relieve patients' symptoms requiring an additional reoperation. Interestingly, Kramer et al. found that female sex, prolonged duration of symptoms, and internal fixation may be associated with worse outcomes in terms of residual pain, rates of reoperation, and return to sport. Kramer et al. also found that of 26 patients who underwent transarticular drilling, drilling with fixation, or a marrow stimulation procedure with excision, 14% required unplanned reoperation (44). Complications associated with OCD fixation include damage to opposing cartilage surfaces from proud hardware, broken hardware, loose bodies, and synovitis (24,45,46). Osteochondral autograft transplantation complications include donor site morbidity, which is why lesion size is one of the limiting factors in using this technique. Potential complications of OCAs include poor graft contour matching, immunogenicity, and possible disease transmission, the risk for the latter two being exceedingly uncommon.

Results

Early studies evaluating the results of treatment of these lesions focused on fragment excision. Denoncourt et al. treated 37 patients with arthroscopic removal of the fragment and curettage of the lesion (47). They reported complete "healing" in 10 cases by second-look arthroscopy. They recommended this treatment in adults and children who have failed initial attempts at nonoperative treatment. Similarly, Ewing and Voto excised the fragments and drilled the defect in 29 patients (17). They reported a satisfactory result in 72% of their patients with short-term (<1 year) follow-up. Recent reports suggest that fragment excision may provide short-term pain relief but not provide long-term success with further follow-up. Anderson et al. evaluated 19 patients with 20 OCD lesions who were treated with fragment excision (29). Follow-up between 2 and 20 years showed that only five patients could participate in strenuous activity without significant symptoms. Eleven patients had pain with activities of daily living, and the remaining three patients had pain with light activities. It was concluded that fragment excision may show improvement of the symptoms in the short term, but the remaining defect and involved compartment may worsen with time.

Outcomes of OCD drilling are generally favorable, with patient age being the best prognostic factor. Individuals with OCD diagnosed and treated with drilling as an adult have decreased radiographic healing and less favorable symptom outcomes (48). Louisia et al. noted 71% (12/17) radiographic healing and two poor results in JOCD compared with 25% (2/8) healing and four poor results in adult OCD patients (32). Overall, good to excellent results are observed in >80% of adolescent patients, with 70% or more being able to return to sports (7,8,32,34). It is our opinion that the ideal patient with symptomatic OCD to treat with drilling is when the defect is grossly stable to palpation despite some MRI evidence of fluid behind the fragment indicating biologic instability. Occasionally, we will augment the treatment of these lesions with the placement of a bioabsorbable differentially pitched threaded compression screw (Arthrex, Inc., Naples, FL).

Favorable outcomes after internal fixation of OCD fragments have been reported for both metallic and bioabsorbable devices. Kivistö et al. noted good to excellent results in 86% of young patients treated with staple fixation (53% radiographic healing) (46). A study of Herbert compression screw fixation yielded 13/15 (87%) normal knees by IKDC grading and radiographic healing in 93% (49). Gomoll et al. evaluated 12 adolescent patients with unstable Cahill Type 2C lesions treated with compression screw fixation with average 6-year follow-up (36). All lesions healed without clinical or radiographic evidence of degenerative disease. Fixation with self-reinforced poly-L-lactic acid nails and pins permits radiographic healing in 60% to 100% of cases (50,51). A cohort study by Weckström et al. suggests that implant geometry (i.e., presence of barbs or a flared head) is a factor in successful outcomes (52).

Ishikawa et al. studied 13 knees in 13 patients with open physes who were treated with internal fixation with an average follow-up of 22.92 +/- 10.95 months. The study found that 76.9% patients significantly improved in Lysholm score postoperatively. Twenty-three percent of these patients required revision surgery, all of which were considered Guhl grade II arthroscopically but grade III on MRI on the grading system described by Dipaola (53). Kubota et al. evaluated

22 patients who underwent internal fixation for OCD fragments, 14 of which were skeletally mature, and found Lysholm score was significantly improved from baseline at both short-term (35.4 months) and mid–long-term (142.5 months) follow-up. It should be noted that outcomes were significantly better at short-term follow-up when compared to mid–long-term follow-up. In contrast to Lysholm scores, Tegner activity scale was deteriorated at mid–long-term follow-up compared to preoperative scores and short-term scores. The authors noted this was likely due to patients discontinuing sports due to age rather than knee symptoms (54). In a retrospective cohort study, Wu et al. studied 87 patients with unstable lesions who underwent internal fixation for a mean follow-up of 60 months and found that 76% of the lesions showed healing beyond 2 years postoperatively. The study noted 24% of these fixations were considered failures based on the need for further surgical management but found no difference in failure rates between patients with open versus closed physes (55).

Chadli et al. evaluated nine patients with either ICRS grade II or III lesions who were treated with hybrid fixation, which involves the addition of a biologic fixation to the mechanical fixation, such as an osteochondral graft, with a median follow-up of 10.1 years (7–14 years). While this study did not compare preoperative and postoperative outcomes, it did evaluate the incorporation of the graft during hardware removal and noted the plugs were integrated but with a superficial peripheral chondral gap (56).

Gudas et al. suggested that OCD lesions treated with microfracture have a significantly worse clinical outcome than do traumatic cartilage lesions (57). Normally, large lesions (more than 2 cm^2) treated with microfracture demonstrate deterioration with time due to decreased fibrocartilage resilience and stiffness (58). Knutsen et al. compared results at 2- and 5-year follow-up in 80 patients who had a single chronic symptomatic cartilage defect on the femoral condyle of the knee, treated randomly with microfracture or ACI (59). Twenty-eight percent of these lesions were due to OCD. Both treated groups showed satisfactory results in 77% of the patients at 5 years. No significant difference between the two treatments groups was evident. They proposed that microfracture should be preferred as first-line treatment option for defects located on the medial or lateral femoral condyle of the knee. Microfracture should therefore be considered as the first-line treatment in lesions <2 cm^2 with subchondral bone integrity and in patients with lower physical demand levels and slightly larger lesions (2–4 cm^2).

The advantages of the osteochondral autograft transplantation technique include absence of disease transmission risk and the lower cost of a single-stage procedure. Disadvantages include donor site morbidity and limited available graft volume. In addition, it is technically difficult to position the plugs to recreate the exact contour of the condylar surfaces. Despite these limitations, results from isolated small to medium-sized lesions of the femoral condyle have been good: 91% good to excellent results at >3 years (21). Interestingly, Miniaci et al. have suggested using the OATS technique for the fixation of unstable OCD lesions of the knee. Twenty patients with OCD lesions were fixed in situ by using multiple 4.5-mm osteochondral dowel grafts harvested from the edges of the trochlea. At 18 months postoperatively, all knees were scored as normal and radiographically healed at 6 months postoperatively (37). Advantages of this technique include the fact that a considerable volume of the original lesion is replaced by autologous bone graft. This technique was used to provide stable biologic fixation using autogenous bone graft. Outerbridge et al. reported favorable short-term results using autografts harvested from the lateral facet of the patella in 10 patients with large femoral OCD lesions (60).

In a cohort of 64 patients treated with fresh OATS, 72% had good to excellent clinical outcomes at 7.7 years after surgery (61). Garret et al. reported on a series of 17 patients treated with a OAs with 94% clinical success at a mean follow-up of 3 years (5). McCulloch et al. studied the clinical outcomes on 25 patients who underwent prolonged fresh OA (these grafts are harvested and are typically maintained refrigerated at 4°C for up to 28 days). Six of these patients were diagnosed with OCD. They reported 84% patient satisfaction and 88% radiographic incorporation of prolonged fresh allografts to the femoral condyle (58). Convery et al. reviewed retrospectively 12 patients treated with OA grafts with a mean follow-up of 5 years. Four of these patients had OCD. Overall, outcomes were rated as excellent in all but one patient, who had a gross technical deficiency. The need for technical proficiency in performing fresh osteochondral allografting was assessed (62). In summary, treatment of OCD with osteochondral allografting provides subjective improvement in 75% to 85% of patients and has the longest-term follow-up in the literature (36) (Fig. 45-6).

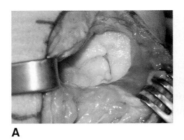 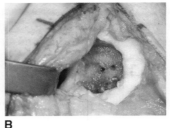 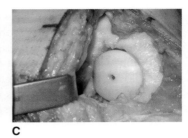

A   B   C

FIGURE 45-6

A: Intraoperative photo demonstrating a large OCD lesion located on the MFC. **B:** The OCD fragment was removed, and the recipient site was cored. **C:** The lesion was treated with a fresh OA.

In a case series, Cotter et al. studied 37 skeletally mature patients (39 knees) who underwent OCA after failure of initial OCD treatment with an average follow-up of 7.29 +/− 3.30 years. The study found significant improvement in all patient-reported outcome scores, except the Short Form 12 mental subscale. Of note, 81.8% of these patients returned to sport at an average of 14.0 +/− 8.7 months; 35.9% of patients underwent subsequent surgery, and 5% reported OCA failure (43).

In another case series, Sadr et al. followed 135 patients, 149 knees, with OCD treated with OCA with a median follow-up of 6.3 years (1.9–16.8 years). These patients displayed significant improvement in pain and function scores, and 95% stated they were satisfied with the procedure. Of the 149 OCAs performed, 23% underwent reoperation and 8% were classified as failures. Graft survivorship was noted to be 93% at 10-year follow-up (63). Along with Cotter et al., these studies show that although there is a relatively high reoperation rate, failure rates are low when OCA is used as treatment for OCD.

Peterson et al. evaluated 58 patients (mean age: 26.4) with OCD who underwent ACI after a mean follow-up of 2 to 10 years. Thirty-five patients had JOCD and 23 adult OCD. Integrated nonarticular cartilage repair tissue had formed (46), and successful clinical results were noted in more than 90% of patients. Only 30% of the 27 patients with preoperative and postoperative radiographs showed joint space narrowing. ACI appears to be a reasonable alternative in OCD lesions (64). Results evaluated at a minimum 2-year follow-up essentially mirror that reported in the literature: 76% successful outcomes at 4-year follow-up (65) (Fig. 45-7).

SUMMARY

OCD of the knee requires a timely diagnosis in order to prevent compromise to the articular cartilage and maximize opportunity to perform a restorative procedure. Indications for surgical treatment are based on lesion stability, skeletal maturity, and clinical symptoms. Reestablishing the joint surface, improving the blood supply of the fragment, rigid fixation, and early motion are primary goals for osteochondral fragment preservation. When the fragment is not suitable for preservation, careful consideration of defect location and the patient's clinical presentation will determine when cartilage restoration procedures should be utilized. Successful restorative options should relieve pain, restore function, and prevent the development of secondary OA.

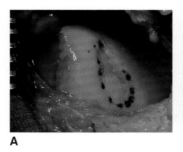 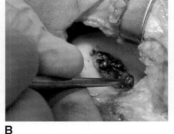 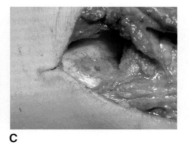

A   B   C

FIGURE 45-7

A: Lesion of the lateral femoral condyle, circled to define the borders for ACI. **B:** Preparation of the defect.
C: Lesion following injection of cultured chondrocytes and suturing of periosteal graft in place.

REFERENCES

1. Cahill B. Osteochondritis dissecans of the knee: treatment of juvenile and adult forms. *J Am Acad Orthop Surg.* 1995;3(4):237–247. Available at: http://www.ncbi.nlm.nih.gov/pubmed/10795030
2. Detterline A, Goldstein J, Rue J, et al. Evaluation and treatment of osteochondritis dissecans lesions of the knee. *J Knee Surg.* 2008;21(2):106–115.
3. Ananthaharan A, Randsborg PH. Epidemiology and patient-reported outcome after juvenile osteochondritis dissecans in the knee. *Knee.* 2018;25(4):595–601. doi:10.1016/j.knee.2018.02.005.
4. Hughston J, Hergenroeder P, Courtenay B. Osteochondritis dissecans of the femoral condyles. *J Bone Joint Surg Am.* 1984;66(9):1340–1348.
5. Garrett J. Fresh osteochondral allografts for treatment of articular defects in osteochondritis dissecans of the lateral femoral condyle in adults. *Clin Orthop Relat Res.* 1994;303:33–37.
6. Bradley J, Dandy D. Osteochondritis dissecans and other lesions of the femoral condyles. *J Bone Joint Surg Br.* 1989;71(3):518–522.
7. Kocher M, Micheli L, Yaniv M, et al. Functional and radiographic outcome of juvenile osteochondritis dissecans of the knee treated with transarticular arthroscopic drilling. *Am J Sports Med.* 2001;29(5):562–566.
8. Bauer M, Jonsson K, Lindén B. Osteochondritis dissecans of the ankle. A 20-year follow-up study. *J Bone Joint Surg Br.* 1987;69(1):93–96.
9. Cahill B. Editorial commentary: current concepts review. Osteochondritis dissecans. *J Bone Joint Surg Am.* 1997;79(3):471–472.
10. Fowler J, Wicks M. Osteochondritis dissecans of the lunate. *J Hand Surg [Am].* 1990;15(4):571–572.
11. Mitsunaga M, Adishian D, Bianco A Jr. Osteochondritis dissecans of the capitellum. *J Trauma.* 1982;22(1):53–55.
12. Pappas A. Osteochondrosis dissecans. *Clin Orthop Relat Res.* 1981;158:59–69.
13. Linden B. Osteochondritis dissecans of the femoral condyles: a long-term follow-up study. *J Bone Joint Surg Am.* 1977;59(6):769–776.
14. Mandelbaum B, Browne J, Fu F, et al. Articular cartilage lesions of the knee. *Am J Sports Med.* 1998;26(6):853–861.
15. Flynn J, Kocher M, Ganley T. Osteochondritis dissecans of the knee. *J Pediatr Orthop.* 2004;24(4):434–443.
16. Pascual-Garrido C, Moran CJ, Green DW, et al. Osteochondritis dissecans of the knee in children and adolescents. *Curr Opin Pediatr.* 2013;25(1):46–51. doi:10.1097/MOP.0b013e32835adbf5.
17. Ewing J, Voto S. Arthroscopic surgical management of osteochondritis dissecans of the knee. *Arthroscopy.* 1988;4(1):37–40.
18. Morelli M, Poitras P, Grimes V, et al. Comparison of the stability of various internal fixators used in the treatment of osteochondritis dissecans—a mechanical model. *J Orthop Res.* 2007;25(4):495–500.
19. Wouters D, Bos R, Mouton L, et al. The meniscus Arrow or metal screw for treatment of osteochondritis dissecans? In vitro comparison of their effectiveness. *Knee Surg Sports Traumatol Arthrosc.* 2004;12(1):52–57.
20. Simonian P, Sussmann P, Wickiewicz T, et al. Contact pressures at osteochondral donor sites in the knee. *Am J Sports Med.* 1998;26(4):491–494.
21. Hangody L, Fules P. Autologous osteochondral mosaicplasty for the treatment of full-thickness defects of weight-bearing joints: ten years of experimental and clinical experience. *J Bone Joint Surg Am.* 2003;85-A(suppl 2):25–32.
22. Gross A. Repair of cartilage defects in the knee. *J Knee Surg.* 2002;15(3):167–169.
23. Hefti F, Beguiristain J, Krauspe R, et al. Osteochondritis dissecans: a multicenter study of the European Pediatric Orthopedic Society. *J Pediatr Orthop B.* 1999;8(4):231–245.
24. Scioscia T, Giffin J, Allen C, et al. Potential complication of bioabsorbable screw fixation for osteochondritis dissecans of the knee. *Arthroscopy.* 2001;17(2):E7.
25. Crawfurd E, Emergy R, Aichroth P. Stable osteochondritis dissecans—does the lesion unite? *J Bone Joint Surg Br.* 1990;72(2):320.
26. Twyman R, Desai K, Aichroth P. Osteochondritis dissecans of the knee. A long-term study. *J Bone Joint Surg Br.* 1991;73(3):461–464.
27. Guhl J. Arthroscopic treatment of osteochondritis dissecans. *Clin Orthop Relat Res.* 1982;167:65–74.
28. Mandelbaum BR. Editorial commentary: focal cartilage defects in young patients indicate autologous chondrocyte implantation sooner rather than later. *Arthroscopy.* 2016;32(9):1917–1918. doi:10.1016/j.arthro.2016.07.011.
29. Anderson A, Pagnani M. Osteochondritis Dissecans of the femoral condyles: long-term results of excision of the fragment. *Am J Sports Med.* 1997;25(6):830–834.
30. Cain E, Clancy W. Treatment algorithm for osteochondral injuries of the knee. *Clin Sports Med.* 2001;20(2):321–342. doi:10.1016/S0278-5919(05)70309-4.
31. Kocher M, Tucker R, Ganley T, et al. Management of osteochondritis dissecans of the knee: current concepts review. *Am J Sports Med.* 2006;34(7):1181–1191.
32. Louisia S, Beaufils P, Katabi M, et al. Transchondral drilling for osteochondritis dissecans of the medial condyle of the knee. *Knee Surg Sports Traumatol Arthrosc.* 2003;11(1):33–39.
33. Berna-Serna J, Martinez F, Reus M, et al. Osteochondritis dissecans of the knee: sonographically guided percutaneous drilling. *J Ultrasound Med.* 2008;27(2):255–259.
34. Kouzelis A, Plessas S, Papadopoulos A, et al. Herbert screw fixation and reverse guided drillings, for treatment of types III and IV osteochondritis dissecans. *Knee Surg Sports Traumatol Arthrosc.* 2006;14(1):70–75.
35. Lebolt J, Wall E. Retroarticular drilling and bone grafting of juvenile osteochondritis dissecans of the knee. *Arthroscopy.* 2007;23(7):791–794.
36. Gomoll A, Flik K, Hayden J, et al. Internal fixation of unstable Cahill type-2C osteochondritis dissecans lesions of the knee in adolescent patients. *Orthopedics.* 2007;30(6):487–490.
37. Miniaci A, Tytherleigh-Strong G. Fixation of unstable osteochondritis dissecans lesions of the knee using arthroscopic autogenous osteochondral grafting (mosaicplasty). *Arthroscopy.* 2007;23(8):845–851.
38. Lewis P, McCarty LI, Kang R, et al. Basic science and treatment options for articular cartilage injuries. *J Orthop Sports Phys Ther.* 2006;36(10):717–727.
39. McCarty L. Primary repair of osteochondritis dissecans in the knee. In: Cole B, Sekiya J, eds. *Surgical Techniques of the Shoulder, Elbow and Knee in Sports Medicine.* Philadelphia, PA: Elsevier; 2008.
40. Steadman JR, Briggs KK, Rodrigo JJ, et al. Outcomes of microfracture for traumatic chondral defects of the knee: average 11-year follow-up. *Arthroscopy.* 2003;19(5):477–484. doi:10.1053/jars.2003.50112.

41. Frisbie DD, Lu Y, Kawcak CE, et al. In vivo evaluation of autologous cartilage fragment-loaded scaffolds implanted into equine articular defects and compared with autologous chondrocyte implantation. *Am J Sports Med.* 2009; 37(1_suppl):71S–80S. doi:10.1177/0363546509348478.

42. Minas T, Peterson L. Advanced techniques in autologous chondrocyte transplantation. *Clin Sports Med.* 1999;18(1):13–44.

43. Cotter EJ, Frank RM, Wang KC, et al. Clinical outcomes of osteochondral allograft transplantation for secondary treatment of osteochondritis dissecans of the knee in skeletally mature patients. *Arthroscopy.* 2018;34(4):1105–1112. doi:10.1016/j.arthro.2017.10.043.

44. Kramer DE, Yen YM, Simoni MK, et al. Surgical management of osteochondritis dissecans lesions of the patella and trochlea in the pediatric and adolescent population. *Am J Sports Med.* 2015;43(3):654–662. doi:10.1177/0363546514562174.

45. Friederichs M, Greis P, Burks R. Pitfalls associated with fixation of osteochondritis dissecans fragments using bioabsorbable screws. *Arthroscopy.* 2001;17(5):542–545.

46. Kivistö R, Pasanen L, Leppilahti J, et al. Arthroscopic repair of osteochondritis dissecans of the femoral condyles with metal staple fixation: a report of 28 cases. *Knee Surg Sports Traumatol Arthrosc.* 2002;10(5):305–309.

47. Denoncourt P, Patel D, Dimakopoulos P. Arthroscopy update #1. Treatment of osteochondrosis dissecans of the knee by arthroscopic curettage, follow-up study. *Orthop Rev.* 1986;15(10):652–657.

48. Anderson A, Richards D, Pagnani M, et al. Antegrade drilling for osteochondritis dissecans of the knee. *Arthroscopy.* 1997;13(3):319–324.

49. Makino A, Muscolo D, Puigdevall M, et al. Arthroscopic fixation of osteochondritis dissecans of the knee: clinical, magnetic resonance imaging, and arthroscopic follow-up. *Am J Sports Med.* 2005;33(10):1499–1504.

50. Dines JS, Fealy S, Potter HG, et al. Outcomes of osteochondral lesions of the knee repaired with a bioabsorbable device. *Arthroscopy.* 2008;24(1):62–68. doi:10.1016/j.arthro.2007.07.025.

51. Nakagawa T, Kurosawa H, Ikeda H, et al. Internal fixation for osteochondritis dissecans of the knee. *Knee Surg Sports Traumatol Arthrosc.* 2005;13(4):317–322.

52. Weckström M, Parviainen M, Kiuru M, et al. Comparison of bioabsorbable pins and nails in the fixation of adult osteochondritis dissecans fragments of the knee: an outcome of 30 knees. *Am J Sports Med.* 2007;35(9):1467–1476.

53. Ishikawa M, Nakamae A, Nakasa T, et al. Limitation of in-situ arthroscopic fixation for stable juvenile osteochondritis dissecans in the knee. *J Pediatr Orthop B* 2018;27(6):516–521. doi:10.1097/BPB.0000000000000531.

54. Kubota M, Ishijima M, Ikeda H, et al. Mid and long term outcomes after fixation of osteochondritis dissecans. *J Orthop.* 2018;15(2):536–539. doi:10.1016/j.jor.2018.01.002.

55. Wu IT, Custers RJH, Desai VS, et al. Internal fixation of unstable osteochondritis dissecans: do open growth plates improve healing rate? *Am J Sports Med.* 2018;46(10):2394–2401. doi:10.1177/0363546518783737.

56. Chadli L, Steltzlen C, Beaufils P, et al. Neither significant osteoarthritic changes nor deteriorating subjective outcomes occur after hybrid fixation of osteochondritis dissecans in the young adult. *Knee Surg Sports Traumatol Arthrosc.* 2018:1–5. doi:10.1007/s00167-018-5025-0.

57. Gudas R, Stankevicius E, Monastyreckiene E, et al. Osteochondral autologous transplantation versus microfracture for the treatment of articular cartilage defects in the knee joint in athletes. *Knee Surg Sports Traumatol Arthrosc.* 2006;14(9):834–842.

58. McCulloch P, Kang R, Sobhy M, et al. Prospective evaluation of prolonged fresh osteochondral allograft transplantation of the femoral condyle: minimum 2-year follow-up. *Am J Sports Med.* 2007;35(3):411–420.

59. Knutsen G, Drogset J, Engebretsen L, et al. A randomized trial comparing autologous chondrocyte implantation with microfracture. *J Bone Joint Surg Am.* 2007;89(10):2105–2112.

60. Outerbridge H, Outerbridge A, Outerbridge R. The use of a lateral patellar autologous graft for the repair of a large osteochondral defect in the knee. *J Bone Joint Surg Am.* 1995;77(1):65–72.

61. Emmerson BC, Görtz S, Jamali AA, et al. Fresh osteochondral allografting in the treatment of osteochondritis dissecans of the femoral condyle. *Am J Sports Med.* 2007;35(6):907–914. doi:10.1177/0363546507299932.

62. Convery F, Meyers M, Akeson W. Fresh osteochondral allografting of the femoral condyle. *Clin Orthop Relat Res.* 1991;273:139–145.

63. Sadr KN, Pulido PA, McCauley JC, et al. Osteochondral allograft transplantation in patients with osteochondritis dissecans of the knee. *Am J Sports Med.* 2016;44(11):2870–2875. doi:10.1177/0363546516657526.

64. Peterson L, Minas T, Brittberg M, et al. Treatment of osteochondritis dissecans of the knee with autologous chondrocyte transplantation: results at two to ten years. *J Bone Joint Surg Am.* 2003;85(suppl 2):17–24.

65. Cole BJ, Lee SJ. Complex knee reconstruction: articular cartilage treatment options. *Arthroscopy.* 2003;19(10 suppl 1): 1–10. doi:10.1016/j.arthro.2003.09.025.

46 Osteotomies about the Knee

Jeremy M. Burnham, Jonathan D. Hughes, Jason P. Zlotnicki, and Volker Musahl

INTRODUCTION

Before total knee arthroplasty (TKA) became a successful technique in the 1970s, osteotomies were the main treatment option for unicompartmental arthritis, especially in the older population (1). As techniques improved, TKA became the definitive surgical option for an aging patient with symptomatic osteoarthritis (OA), while osteotomies were performed less frequently due to unpredictable outcomes and the demanding nature of the procedure. However, osteotomies reemerged in the early 1990s as a treatment option for young patients with unicompartmental arthritis after various studies showed good results from high tibial osteotomy (HTO) (2,3).

The knee joint experiences two to four times body weight when ambulating. Approximately 75% of this load is on the medial compartment in the single leg stance phase of gait, and this is exacerbated with varus deformity. On the other hand, with 6 degrees of mechanical valgus, only 40% of this load is transmitted through the medial compartment. Thus, the goal of the osteotomy is to correct the angular deformity of the knee (whether valgus or varus deformity) and decrease the abnormal load on the affected tibiofemoral compartment, thereby allowing the young patient to return to activities, while hopefully avoiding or at least delaying TKA. Even minimal angular deformities in the coronal and sagittal planes can cause a significant increase in forces to the tibiofemoral compartments (4,5). It has been shown that offloading the affected compartment leads to articular cartilage recovery and a decrease in symptoms (6). In this chapter, HTO and distal femur osteotomy (DFO) for treatment of varus and valgus knee conditions, respectively, are discussed.

HIGH TIBIAL OSTEOTOMY

Indications

The primary indication for HTO is symptomatic isolated medial compartment OA in a young, physically active patient with varus knee malalignment (7–9), and a successful outcome depends on proper patient selection. Important factors to consider when considering HTO are age, smoking status, knee range of motion, degree of deformity, body mass index (BMI), and quality of the menisci and cartilage. Classic indications for HTO include patients aged 40 to 60 years, at least 10 degrees of proximal tibial varus, good knee range of motion with <10 degrees flexion contracture, BMI of <30, nonsmokers, and relatively well-preserved lateral compartment cartilage and menisci. In 2005, the International Society of Arthroscopy, Knee Surgery, and Orthopaedic Sports Medicine (ISAKOS) created guidelines for patient selection when considering an HTO (Table 46-1) (10). Since that time, guidelines have evolved and expanded to include patients <40 years of age or >60 years of age, patients with flexion contractures up to 25 degrees, and overweight patients (13,14). Additionally, studies have demonstrated that a tibial bone varus angle (TBVA) > 5 degrees is a good prognostic factor for success (15). HTO can be performed concomitantly with ligamentous reconstruction, cartilage restoration, and meniscal transplant (16–19).

Contraindications

There are strict criteria when selecting the ideal patient for an HTO. The contraindications are listed in Table 46-1. Although indications continue to expand, age >65 to 70 years is a relative

TABLE 46-1 Patient Selection Criteria for High Tibial Osteotomy (HTO)

Indications (10)	Relative Indications (11)	Contraindications (10–12)
Young age (40–60 y)	ACL, PCL, or PLC insufficiency	Obesity (BMI > 30)[a]
Isolated medial joint line pain	Age (60–70 y or <40 y)	Bi- or tricompartmental osteoarthritis
Body mass index (BMI) < 30	Moderate patellofemoral arthritis	Flexion contracture >25 degrees
High activity level	Flexion contracture of 15–25 degrees	Prior lateral meniscectomy
Tibial mechanical axis deformity >5 degrees		Knee arc of motion <120 degrees
Nonsmoker		Inflammatory osteoarthritis
No lateral or patellofemoral pain		
Flexion contracture <15 degrees		

A chart demonstrating the indications, relative indications, and contradictions for osteotomy set forth by the International Society of Arthroscopy, Knee Surgery, and Orthopaedic Sports Medicine (ISAKOS), as well as various recent studies (10–12).
[a]Relative contraindication.

contraindication. Smoking cessation should be encouraged before surgery due to risk of nonunion and wound breakdown (20). An arc of motion <120 degrees is a risk factor for early failure, especially flexion contractures >10 degrees (21), as well as inflammatory arthritis. BMI remains a controversial contraindication, as some studies have indicated greater failure rates in heavier patients, while others have reported higher failure rates in lean patients (1,21–23). However, since obesity has a negative effect on orthopedic surgery in general, a BMI > 30 is considered a relative contraindication, and other aspects of the patient's health should be taken into consideration. Lastly, arthritis or prior total meniscectomy in the lateral compartment is a contraindication, since the procedure will offload the medial compartment and place more stress on the lateral compartment (21).

Preoperative Planning

Precise preoperative planning is crucial to obtain satisfactory outcomes and avoid undercorrection or overcorrection. The degree of correction will rely on the amount of mechanical axis deviation in the lower extremity, as determined preoperatively via full-length standing radiographs. This includes selecting a specific wedge angle to match the angular deformity and adding this specific angle to the desired overcorrection or undercorrection (24). Additionally, the condition of the three compartments, as well as the bony morphology of the patient, will help determine whether an opening-wedge or closing-wedge osteotomy is performed. Magnetic resonance imaging can be very helpful to determine the extent of cartilage damage, as well as concomitant ligamentous injuries.

A complete radiographic evaluation should be obtained, including weight-bearing anteroposterior or posteroanterior views, sunrise view, lateral radiograph of the involved knee, intercondylar notch view, and full-length hip-to-ankle standing views of both lower extremities. All three compartments must be checked for signs of OA. The patella height needs to be assessed preoperatively on the lateral view, as patella baja can occur after both medial opening-wedge and lateral closing-wedge HTO (25). Additionally, tibial slope must be measured on this view to ensure that a biplanar osteotomy does not need to be performed, especially in combination with anterior cruciate ligament (ACL) or posterior cruciate ligament (PCL) injuries. Lateral tibial plateau slope has been found to average between 5 and 7 degrees (26), and a recent study demonstrated that increasing the tibial slope causes an anterior shift in the tibial resting position under axial loads (27,28). Thus, an ACL-deficient knee would benefit from a decreased tibial slope, while increasing tibial slope would help protect a PCL-deficient knee.

The full-length standing radiographs will assist with calculating the mechanical axis (24). Many methods have been described, but most aim to correct the mechanical femorotibial axis to 3 to 6 degrees of valgus, or the anatomic femorotibial axis to 6 to 15 degrees of valgus. The authors' preferred technique is to use the weight-bearing line (WBL) method to correct the angular deformity, as described by Noyes et al. and Miniaci et al. This technique appropriately accounts for the tibial and femoral length using full-length weight-bearing films (29). To use this method, the mechanical axis WBL is first drawn, which goes from the center of the femoral head to the center of the talus. In a normally aligned knee, this line passes through the medial aspect of the lateral tibial spine, although in patients with varus deformity, the WBL will pass through or medial to the medial compartment. Next, the WBL is adjusted such that it passes through the tibial plateau at approximately 62% to 66% of the medial to lateral width of the plateau. This usually corresponds with the lateral aspect of the lateral tibial spine (29), which approximates a desired 3 to 5 degrees valgus mechanical axis. A line is then drawn from the distal point of that line, at the level of the tibiotalar joint, up to the proximal tibial hinge point of the planned osteotomy, and back down to the center of the talus. The angle subtended by these lines represents the degree of correction needed to correct the angular deformity (Fig. 46-1). This degree of correction is then templated on the proximal tibia, and the distance of wedge opening (or closing) is measured. Several authors have suggested slight overcorrection into valgus due to reports of loss of reduction into varus with undercorrection (1,24,30). However, it is important to consider the anatomic alignment of the contralateral limb. Overcorrection without addressing the contralateral knee could result in a windswept deformity, which is poorly tolerated by patients. If biplanar correction is warranted, the sagittal plane correction should be taken into consideration with the final wedge angle to address both deformities with one corrective surgery.

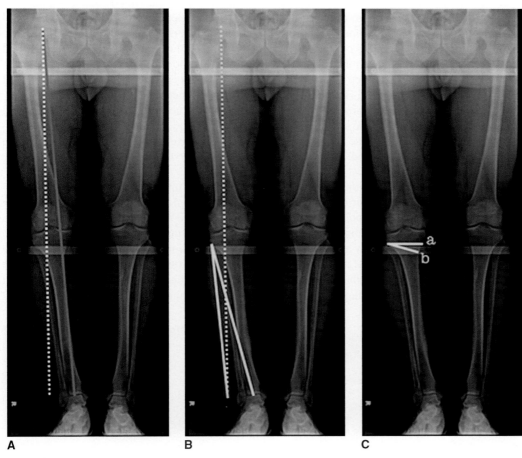

A   B   C

FIGURE 46-1

Preoperative planning for opening-wedge high tibial osteotomy. Full-length, weight-bearing alignment films show varus malalignment of the right knee. **A:** The weight-bearing line is shown in *blue* and passes through the medial compartment, consistent with this patient's varus deformity. The *dashed line* shows the preferred weight-bearing line passing through the lateral aspect of the lateral tibial spine, or about 62% to 66% of the medial to lateral distance of the proximal tibia. **B:** Lines are drawn from the modified weight-bearing line at the level of the tibiotalar joint, to the planned hinge point at the lateral proximal tibia, and back down to the center of the tibiotalar joint. The angle formed by these lines (shown in *yellow*) is the correction angle needed to restore ideal knee alignment. **C:** The correction angle is superimposed over the osteotomy site, and the needed distraction distance of the medial tibia can be calculated as the distance from point "*a*" to point "*b*."

Surgical Technique

The medial opening-wedge and lateral closing-wedge HTO are ideal for valgization of proximal tibia varus. Diagnostic arthroscopy can be utilized to verify meniscal, chondral, and ligamentous structures prior to initiating the osteotomy.

Osteotomy-specific instruments needed:

- Oscillating saw with wide saw blade and a blade length of approximately 9 cm
- Several flat osteotomes from 10 to 20 mm in width
- 2.3-mm guidewires
- Caliper
- Lamina spreader
- Osteotomy spreader (optional)
- Allograft bone wedges (optional)

Medial Opening-Wedge High Tibial Osteotomy

The patient is positioned supine with a tourniquet, and a lateral leg holder and footrest. The authors prefer performing the procedure without tourniquet inflated. The knee is positioned at 70 to 90 degrees of flexion during portions of the case. After optional diagnostic arthroscopy, anatomic landmarks are drawn: medial joint line, pes anserinus, and tibial tuberosity. The incision is made longitudinally approximately 6 to 8 cm in length between the medial edge of the tibial tuberosity and posteromedial edge of the tibia, inferior to the joint surface (Fig. 46-2A). The superior border of the pes anserinus is dissected and retracted distally to expose the superficial fibers of the MCL. Blunt dissection allows placement of a Hohmann retractor under the superficial MCL and behind the posterior tibial ridge, safely retracting the MCL and protecting the neurovascular structures. Limited release of the distal portion of the superficial MCL helps to relieve joint tension and improve medial compartment unloading (29). The superior edge of the patellar insertion at the tubercle should also be identified and bluntly exposed. This can be marked with a curved hemostat placed between the tibia and tendon at the insertion.

With the knee in full extension, two 2.3-mm guidewires are inserted into the medial tibia 3.5 to 4.0 cm below the medial joint line and aimed obliquely toward the most superior aspect of the fibular head (the planned hinge point). The posterior wire is placed first, and a second wire is placed parallel in the coronal plane, with a 2- to 3-cm anteroposterior distance between them (Fig. 46-2B). The starting points and trajectory are checked on intraoperative fluoroscopy. It is paramount that the fluoroscopy image is a true AP of the knee, with the knee in full extension, and overlap of the tib-fib joint such that one third of the fibular head is overlapped by the tibia. Each wire should be docked in the far cortex but not protruding through it. The wires and planned saw cut should be positioned

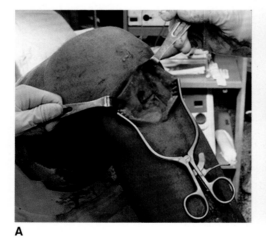
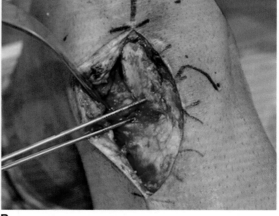

A   **B**

FIGURE 46-2

Opening-wedge high tibial osteotomy. Intraoperative picture of a right knee during high tibial osteotomy. **A:** The exposure has provided adequate access to the tibia, and the planned bone cuts of a biplanar osteotomy are sketched with a surgical marker. **B:** Two parallel pins provide a cutting template for the saw blade. The pins are placed parallel and 2 to 3 cm apart.

such that there is adequate room proximally for the proximal row of locking screws and the most proximal shaft screw of the plate. The approximate distance of the osteotomy cut can be measured using a third guide pin, which is placed adjacent to one or both of the existing guide pins, just touching the near cortex. The distance between the exposed ends, <1 cm, is marked on the saw blade.

The knee should now be placed in 90 degrees of flexion, and the planned cut line should be marked out with a Bovie or surgical marker on the medial tibia prior to initiating the cut. The anterior ascending osteotomy should be marked at an angle of approximately 110 degrees and should exit the anterior tibia just proximal to the patellar insertion. This anterior ascending cut should intersect the main cut line 1.5 to 2 cm posterior to the anterior border.

The osteotomy is started with an oscillating saw directly below the guidewires, using the wires as a saw guide to direct the blade. It is important to stop the cut 1 cm medial to the lateral cortex, as breach of this cortex leads to instability and higher nonunion rates. Judicious use of irrigation with sterile saline can prevent heat osteonecrosis from the saw. The posterior two thirds of the tibia is cut first, with Hohmann retractors protecting the posterior neurovascular structures. When the posterior cortical cut is complete, there will be noticeable loss of resistance to the saw blade. The anterior ascending cut is then completed. To avoid excessive opening or fracture of the lateral cortex, osteotomes should be added in a stepwise fashion to distract and open the osteotomy. Most osteotomy systems provide instrumentation that allows for precise opening of the osteotomy to correspond with the preoperative templating. If the tibial slope is to remain unchanged, it is important to distract the osteotomy equally in the anterior and posterior sections of the cut. In cases of biplanar correction, the degree of distraction can be varied to achieve the desired level of tibial slope adjustment. For instance, in the ACL-injured knees with increased tibial slope, the osteotomy can be distracted more posteriorly than anteriorly, effectively decreasing the tibial slope. Bone graft can be contoured accordingly or placed only in the posterior portion of the osteotomy. The opposite approach can be used in patients with PCL deficiency and decreased tibial slope. The knee is once again placed into full extension, and intraoperative fluoroscopy or radiographs are used to evaluate the alignment. Fine adjustments are made as needed.

Once correction is achieved, internal plate fixation is performed. A pin is placed through the middle proximal hole, and position of the plate is confirmed under C-arm. A bicortical screw is placed through the first hole distal to the osteotomy to reduce the plate to the bone. The proximal screws are placed under fluoroscopy to avoid violation of the plateau. Often, plates will include a spacer component that provides rigid distraction at the cortical region of the osteotomy, though selection of hardware is based on surgeon preference. Bone grafting is then performed in cases of large defects (>8–10 mm). The authors' preferred method of fixation is a large fragment proximal tibial plate with a row of locking screws proximally and locking and cortical screw options in the shaft portion of the plate (Fig. 46-3). These larger plates have shown improved performance in biomechanical testing than the shorter "spacer" plates, as they provide a long, rigid lever arm with angle-stable locking screws (29). The locking screws should not protrude past the lateral cortex to prevent hardware irritation (Fig. 46-4).

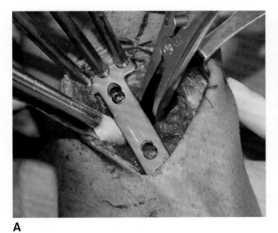
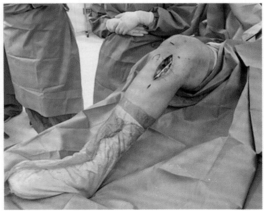

A   B

FIGURE 46-3

Opening-wedge high tibial osteotomy. **A:** Insertion of bone graft into posterior aspect of the left knee high tibial osteotomy. An osteotomy spreader is located anterior to the plate and maintaining adequate distraction for graft placement. **B:** Final result after graft placement and hardware fixation of right knee high tibial osteotomy.

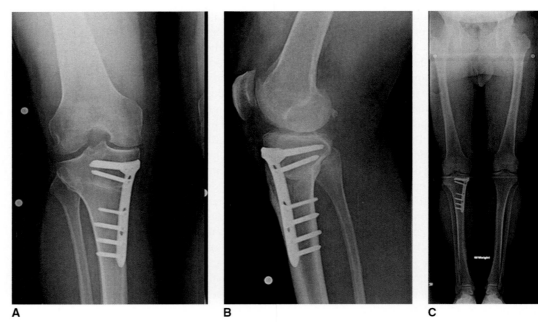

A   **B**   **C**

FIGURE 46-4

Postoperative images from opening-wedge high tibial osteotomy. Anteroposterior **(A)** and lateral **(B)** radiographs 9 months after high tibial osteotomy demonstrating complete healing of the osteotomy and incorporation of bone graft. **C:** Full-length alignment films demonstrate correction of preoperative varus and symmetry with the contralateral knee.

Lateral Closing-Wedge High Tibial Osteotomy

An anterolateral L-shaped incision is made centered over Gerdy tubercle; the vertical aspect runs distally along the tibia, and the horizontal aspect runs parallel to, and approximately 1 cm distal to, the joint line toward the fibular head. Exposure of the lateral edge of the tibia is performed with subperiosteal elevation of the proximal anterior leg musculature, ensuring adequate hemostasis throughout the dissection. The peroneal nerve is identified and protected throughout the duration of the case. To further expose the osteotomy site, the proximal tibiofibular joint must be addressed. Various options exist, including producing an oblique osteotomy of the fibular head with a curved osteotome, fibular shaft osteotomy (~10 cm distal to the fibular head), excising the tibiofibular joint, or fibular head excision. Under fluoroscopic guidance, a guidewire is placed transversely from lateral to medial, 2 cm distal to the joint line, until the medial cortex is reached. A second guidewire is then placed at a predetermined distance distal to the first guidewire on the lateral cortex (this distance will correlate with the overall correction required). It is driven medially in an oblique direction and connected with the prior guidewire approximately 1 cm lateral to the medial cortex. This will allow a wedge of bone to be removed while leaving the medial cortex intact during cutting. Cuts are then made with an oscillating saw and osteotomes along these guidewires, while protecting the soft tissues anteriorly and posteriorly. Once the bone wedge is removed, mild valgus stress should be applied to the site resulting in deformation of the medial cortex and closing of the osteotomy site. If resistance is met, a 2.0 drill can be used to perforate and increase the plasticity of the medial cortex without causing overt fracture. The plate is then applied in submuscular fashion and secured into place.

DISTAL FEMUR OSTEOTOMY

Indications

The primary indication for opening- or closing-wedge DFO is a patient with considerable valgus and isolated lateral compartment arthritis (12). The goals of this varus-producing procedure are to correct the knee to within 0 to 2 degrees difference between the mechanical and anatomic alignment without overcorrecting into varus, minimizing pain and restoring function (12,31). Similar to HTO,

TABLE 46-2 Patient Selection Criteria for Distal Femur Osteotomy (DFO)

Indications (10,12,32)	Relative Indications	Contraindications (10,12,32)
Young age (40–60 y) Isolated lateral joint line pain	Moderate patellofemoral arthritis Age (60–70 y or <40 y)	Extension deficit >10 degrees Loss of significant portion of medial meniscus
Body mass index (BMI) < 30	ACL, PCL, or PLC insufficiency	Medial compartment degenerative joint disease
High activity level Valgus deformity >10 degrees Unicompartmental gonarthrosis		Bi- or tricompartmental osteoarthritis Inflammatory osteoarthritis Valgus deformity >20 degrees with subluxation of the tibia
Reconstructive cartilage procedure in lateral compartment Nonsmoker		Osteonecrosis of lateral femoral condyle Obesity (BMI > 30)[a]

A chart demonstrating the indications, relative indications, and contradictions for osteotomy set forth by the International Society of Arthroscopy, Knee Surgery, and Orthopaedic Sports Medicine (ISAKOS), as well as various recent studies (10,12,32).
[a]Relative contraindication.

proper patient selection is crucial for optimal success (Table 46-2). Although older age is often cited as a contraindication, the patient's lifestyle, overall health, and goals must be taken into consideration. Overall, most studies suggest that a DFO should be utilized to treat lateral unicompartmental OA in relatively young patients with well-maintained range of motion and early stages of OA with a valgus knee deformity (33). Similar to an HTO, ligamentous reconstruction and DFO can be performed concomitantly.

Contraindications

As with an HTO, the strict criteria for a DFO allow for improved long-term outcomes and implant survival. Contraindications are listed in Table 46-2. When planning this procedure, the most crucial factors to consider are age, smoking status, degree of deformity, and condition of cartilage and meniscus in the medial compartment. There is no definite age at which an osteotomy cannot be performed; however, numerous studies have demonstrated that age >70 years is associated with early failure after osteotomy (12,21,31–33). Severe valgus deformity >20 degrees can be associated with subluxation of the tibia and, when present, is an absolute contraindication to DFO (12,31,33). Lateral femoral condyle osteonecrosis will continue to cause the patient pain after a DFO, even with the resultant balanced load distribution, and hence is an absolute contraindication (12,31). Since the goal of a DFO is to offload the lateral compartment and improve pain, the meniscus and cartilage in the medial compartment must be relatively preserved in order to bear a greater load.

Preoperative Planning

Careful and meticulous preoperative planning are paramount for successful outcomes after DFO. The valgus extremity should not be overcorrected into varus, with a goal of 0 to 2 degrees difference between the mechanical and anatomic axes (31). A full radiographic evaluation, as described in the section above, should be performed. Full-length standing radiographs are needed to fully assess the deformity. The mechanical axis line, or WBL, is first drawn, which indicates where the majority of the load is concentrated in the knee. Then, as described previously, a reference point is chosen on the tibial plateau that approximates neutral alignment (24). This reference point is 48% to 50% the width of the tibial plateau as measured from the medial aspect. Two lines are drawn, one from the center of the femoral head to the reference point and the second one from the reference point to the center of the talus. The angle at which these two lines intersect represents the degree of fixation needed without overcorrecting into varus (Fig. 46-5). The size of the wedge can then be determined by measuring the width of the femur at the site of the proposed osteotomy. Both a lateral opening-wedge and medial closing-wedge osteotomy can be performed, although the lateral opening-wedge is more common. However, one study demonstrated that a medial closing-wedge osteotomy decreases the risk of nonunion in smokers and obese patients (34). Fixation of femoral deformities in the sagittal plane have yet to be described.

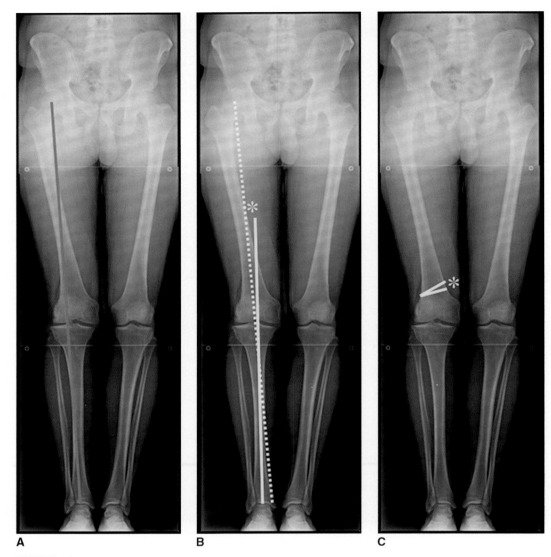

FIGURE 46-5

Preoperative planning for closing-wedge distal femoral osteotomy. **A:** The weight-bearing line (*blue line*) passes through the lateral compartment in this patient with valgus malalignment and symptomatic isolated lateral compartment arthritis. **B:** The correction angle is calculated by drawing a line (*dotted line*) from the center of the femoral head that passes through a point located at 50% of the medial to lateral width of the tibial articular surface. A separate line (*yellow line*) is drawn from the center of the tibial talar joint and passing through 50% of the tibial articular surface width at the knee. The angle (*) subtended by these lines can then be measured out on the planned osteotomy site **(C)** to identify the planned bone cuts.

Surgical Technique

Optimal surgical technique starts with thorough preoperative planning, including review of full-length weight-bearing films and plan for amount of surgical correction, as well as reversal of any patient-modifiable risk factors. A preoperative decision should also be made regarding the intended fixation strategy; whether a T-shaped tooth plate, a more robust locking plate, or a fixed angle blade plate is used will depend upon surgeon preference, whether the patient has sufficient soft tissue coverage such that a higher profile plate will not be symptomatic, and/or whether earlier weight bearing will be allowed.

Medial Closing-Wedge Distal Femur Osteotomy

The patient is placed in the supine position. A longitudinal incision of approximately 10 cm is made just medial to the anterior midline of the knee. A large medial flap of skin and soft tissue superficial to the fascia is created with blunt dissection and electrocautery, isolating the vastus medialis muscle. Once isolated, the fascia is opened in longitudinal fashion. Utilizing this approach, the medial patellofemoral ligament must be split and subsequently repaired at the conclusion of the case, prior to layered closure. The vastus medialis is elevated, and a Hohmann retractor is placed across the anterior aspect of the femur. A key to this procedure is to dissect in a precise, layered fashion as the muscles are elevated to avoid aberrant bleeding from deep perforating arteries of the muscle. Once the distal femur is exposed, a guide pin is inserted under fluoroscopic guidance. The pin should be aiming at the metaphyseal corner of the lateral condyle and reach, but not perforate, the far cortex. A second pin is inserted parallel and just posterior to the first pin. These pins provide the plane for the oscillating saw to create the osteotomy. Before making the osteotomy cut, rotation needs to be established and marked on the bone to avoid malrotation. This can be done by using the Bovie and making a vertical line along the bone, crossing the osteotomy site, allowing the lines to be realigned after the cut. The cut should stop 1 cm short of the far cortex. The second cut is made at a predetermined distance proximal to the original cut (this distance will correlate with the overall correction required). The saw should connect with the original osteotomy cut, so that a wedge of bone can be removed while leaving the lateral cortex intact. This conversion point should be approximately 1 cm medial to the lateral cortex. Once the bone wedge is removed, mild varus stress should be applied to the site resulting in deformation of the lateral cortex and closing of the osteotomy site. If resistance is met, a 2.0 drill can be used to perforate and increase the plasticity of the lateral cortex without causing overt fracture. The plate is then applied in submuscular fashion, and a smooth k-wire used to hold the plate in place. Typically, a cortical screw is applied to a proximal hole in the plate permitting for the plate to sit flush along the femoral shaft. Then, locking screws are inserted in the distal segment, securing the plate. Remaining holes are filled with locking or cortical screws as indicated (Figs. 46-6 and 46-7). Final screw length and location is confirmed on fluoroscopy at the conclusion of the case.

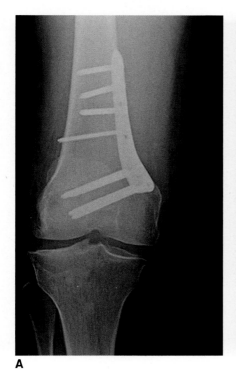
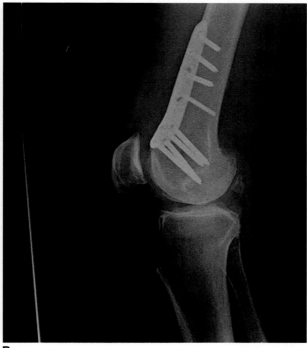

A   **B**

FIGURE 46-6

Postoperative radiographs after closing-wedge distal femoral osteotomy. **(A)** Anteroposterior and **(B)** lateral radiographs after a medial closing-wedge distal femoral osteotomy, demonstrating correction of the valgus malalignment. The distal screws are locking screws to increase pullout strength in soft metaphyseal bone. The most distal shaft screw is a cortical screw used to reduce the plate to the bone. The proximal shaft screws can be locking or nonlocking screws.

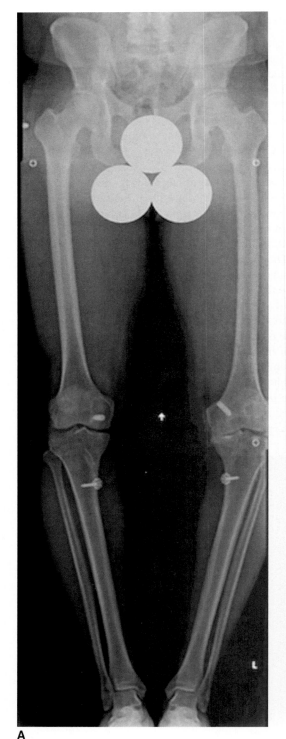
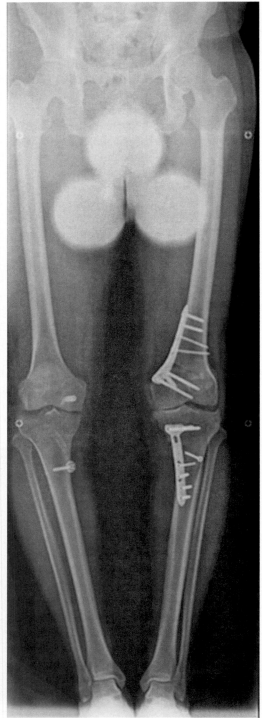

A   B

FIGURE 46-7

Pre- and postoperative radiographs after combined femoral and tibial osteotomy. **A:** Preoperative radiographs demonstrate a severe varus deformity that includes the distal femur and the proximal tibia. In these cases of severe deformity, addressing either the femur or tibia in isolation will not adequately correct the alignment. **B:** Postoperative radiographs demonstrating the medial opening-wedge distal femoral osteotomy and the medial opening-wedge high tibial osteotomy. Addressing both the tibial and femoral deformities resulted in correction of the patient's significant varus.

Lateral Opening-Wedge Distal Femur Osteotomy

Surgery is initiated with an approximately 12-cm incision starting from the lateral femoral epicondyle. Once the lateral femoral cortex is located, leaving the joint capsule intact, a freehand guidewire is drilled in a proximal to distal trajectory with the acuity of the angle based on the amount of correction required. Under fluoroscopic guidance, an oscillating saw should be used to start the osteotomy while wedge osteotomes are used in progressive fashion to "open" the osteotomy site. Depending on host factors, approximately 1 cm of medial hinge should be left intact to preserve stability at the osteotomy site and decrease rate of nonunion with a lateral-based plate for final fixation. Postoperative protocols are variable depending upon host factors and surgeon preference, but should generally consist of venous thromboembolism (VTE) prophylaxis, early range of motion and/or continuous passive motion (CPM) device, and non–weight bearing for approximately 6 to 8 weeks with resolution of full weight bearing at 8 to 10 weeks.

POSTOPERATIVE COURSE

Patients are made limited weight bearing for 6 weeks after surgery. Recent studies have suggested improved outcomes with early weight bearing (35), although this should be avoided in cases where the far cortex (hinge point) is breached. Mobilization and range of motion exercises are initiated on postoperative day 1, and sutures are removed after 7 to 10 days. Chemical thromboembolism prophylaxis is prescribed for 3 to 6 weeks. Bone healing can be assessed radiographically, and usually occurs from the bony hinge outward in opening-wedge osteotomies. Some bone resorption may be present around weeks 3 to 4, but approximately 33% of the osteotomy surface area should be healed at 6 weeks, and over 50% at 3 months. Hardware removal is safe after 90% healing, and not prior to 6 months. Nicotine use will significantly prolong these milestones (29).

PEARLS AND PITFALLS

"Pearls" for success with corrective osteotomies center upon use of a repeatable and consistent pre-, intra- and postoperative plan. Firstly, thorough examination and patient selection must be performed prior to surgery. Strict indications (see above) must be adhered to for the optimization of pain relief and functional outcome, and the overall success of the procedure. Once the patient has been carefully selected, all modifiable risk factors (smoking, blood glucose, weight loss, etc.) should be addressed and the patient should be optimized for surgery. Careful preoperative planning should take into account the overall magnitude of deformity, the desired correction, and the location of osteotomy to reduce intraoperative adjustments and operative time. Once this plan has been carefully established, there should be no deviation during the surgery. This may lead to an increased rate of under- or overcorrection, and/or increase the risk of medial cortex disruption. Finally, adherence to the Arbeitsgemeinschaft für Osteosynthesefragen (AO) principles for fracture fixation, including restoration of anatomy, stable fracture fixation, preservation of blood supply, and early mobilization of the limb and patient will improve the repeatability and overall success of this procedure while reducing complication rates.

COMPLICATIONS

With completion of closing- and opening-wedge osteotomies, close attention must be paid to the avoidance and/or correction of any intra- or postoperative complications. As noted in the technique section, it is desirable for the surgeon to maintain a medial/lateral bone bridge or intact cortex to "hinge" the osteotomy—this provides for enhanced rigidity and decreased rates of nonunion. However, fracture of the cortex may occur during the operative cuts or during the opening/closing of the osteotomy site. Addressing this fracture requires close attention to cortical reads on intra-op fluoroscopy, avoiding malreduction and/or rotation by visualizing the osteotomy site and checking the reduction at multiple intervals during plate and screw application. Weight-bearing protocols may vary on a surgeon-to-surgeon basis after disruption of the far cortex. In some cases, a separate incision and fixation of the cortical breach is needed. Under- or overcorrection at the osteotomy site may occur. Close attention must be paid to preoperative planning principles, as well as during intraoperative pin and guidewire placement prior to making final cut and applying lateral-based plates. Iatrogenic injury to the articular surface or lateral-based ligaments is rare but must be addressed intraoperatively and repaired as appropriate. Deep vein thrombosis (DVT) is a significant compli-cation that must be treated in the event of postoperative occurrence. Appropriate mechanical and chemical prophylaxis must be used in the immediate postoperative period, and early mobilization protocols may also reduce the overall risk. Low molecular weight heparin (Lovenox) may be used for 30 days post-op as indicated in patients with increased risk of DVT.

OUTCOMES

Long-term follow-up studies have shown that HTO results in good outcomes and overall survival of >50% at 18 years (9). Furthermore, over 85% of patients return to work and/or sports, and most return to the same or greater level of activity. Of those returning to sports, 78.6% returned at an equal or greater level. Among competitive athletes, 54% returned to competition (36), 90% of patients returning to work or sport did so by 1 year, and 65.5% returned at an equal or greater level (36). However, other studies have suggested excellent early results that deteriorate a 10-year time period, especially when performed with concomitant cartilage procedures (37). A comparison of patients with TKA performed after a previous HTO reported similar results to patients with primary TKA and no history of HTO (38). In young patients with varus deformity and medial compartment arthri-tis, HTO has been shown to be cost-effective compared to TKA. Similarly, studies have shown good functional outcomes and improvements in patient-reported outcomes at 10 years, with an approxi-mately 25% conversion to TKA at a mean of 6 years (39). A systematic review of both closing- and opening-wedge DFO reported 80% survivorship at 10 years with a low complication rate (40). A systematic review comparing standard HTO to HTO with computer navigation found that navi-gated HTO resulted in improved mechanical axis correction, although there were no significant differences in clinical outcomes (41).

SUMMARY

Distal femoral or proximal tibial osteotomy is a good option for knee preservation in patients with unicompartmental gonarthritis with associated tibiofemoral malalignment. While patient selection and technical precision is key, osteotomy of the knee can improve patient function, decrease pain symptoms, facilitate return to work or sport, and provide a meaningful delay (or complete avoid-ance) of a more complex arthroplasty procedure. Knee osteotomy procedures should be strongly considered in young, active patients with knee arthritis isolated to a single compartment and an accompanying varus or valgus deformity.

REFERENCES

1. Coventry MB. Osteotomy of the upper portion of the tibia for degenerative arthritis of the knee. A preliminary report. *J Bone Joint Surg Am.* 1965;47(5):984–990.
2. Holden DL, James SL, Larson RL, et al. Proximal tibial osteotomy in patients who are fifty years old or less. A long-term follow-up study. *J Bone Joint Surg Am.* 1988;70(7):977–982.
3. Morrey BF. Upper tibial osteotomy for secondary osteoarthritis of the knee. *J Bone Joint Surg Br.* 1989;71(4):554–559.
4. Levine HB, Bosco JA III. Sagittal and coronal biomechanics of the knee: a rationale for corrective measures. *Bull NYU Hosp Jt Dis.* 2007;65(1):87–95.
5. Wu DD, Burr DB, Boyd RD, et al. Bone and cartilage changes following experimental varus or valgus tibial angulation. *J Orthop Res.* 1990;8(4):572–585.
6. Parker DA, Beatty KT, Giuffre B, et al. Articular cartilage changes in patients with osteoarthritis after osteotomy. *Am J Sports Med.* 2011;39(5):1039–1045.
7. Shaw JA, Moulton MJ. High tibial osteotomy: an operation based on a spurious mechanical concept. A theoretic treatise. *Am J Orthop (Belle Mead NJ).* 1996;25(6):429–436.
8. Jackson JP, Waugh W, Green JP. High tibial osteotomy for osteoarthritis of the knee. *J Bone Joint Surg Br.* 1969;51(1):88–94.
9. Michaela G, Florian P, Michael L, et al. Long-term outcome after high tibial osteotomy. *Arch Orthop Trauma Surg.* 2008;128(1):111–115.
10. Rand J, Neyret P, eds. ISAKOS meeting on the management of osteoarthritis of the knee prior to total knee arthroplasty. ISAKOS Congress; 2005.
11. Lobenhoffer P, Agneskirchner JD. Improvements in surgical technique of valgus high tibial osteotomy. *Knee Surg Sports Traumatol Arthrosc.* 2003;11(3):132–138.
12. Uquillas C, Rossy W, Nathasingh CK, et al. Osteotomies about the knee. *J Bone Joint Surg Am.* 2014;96(24):e199.
13. Seil R, van Heerwaarden R, Lobenhoffer P, et al. The rapid evolution of knee osteotomies. *Knee Surg Sports Traumatol Arthrosc.* 2013;21(1):1–2.
14. Brinkman JM, Lobenhoffer P, Agneskirchner JD, et al. Osteotomies around the knee: patient selection, stability of fixa-tion and bone healing in high tibial osteotomies. *J Bone Joint Surg Br.* 2008;90(12):1548–1557.

15. Bonnin M, Chambat P. Current status of valgus angle, tibial head closing wedge osteotomy in media gonarthrosis. *Orthopade*. 2004;33(2):135–142.
16. Imhoff AB, Linke RD, Agneskirchner J. Corrective osteotomy in primary varus, double varus and triple varus knee instability with cruciate ligament replacement. *Orthopade*. 2004;33(2):201–207.
17. Noyes FR, Barber SD, Simon R. High tibial osteotomy and ligament reconstruction in varus angulated, anterior cruciate ligament-deficient knees. A two- to seven-year follow-up study. *Am J Sports Med*. 1993;21(1):2–12.
18. Dejour D, Khun A, Dejour H. Osteotomie tibiale de déflexion et laxité chronique antérieure à propos de 22 cas. *Rev Chir Orthop Reparatrice Appar Mot*. 1998;84:28.
19. Sonnery-Cottet B, Mogos S, Thaunat M, et al. Proximal tibial anterior closing wedge osteotomy in repeat revision of anterior cruciate ligament reconstruction. *Am J Sports Med*. 2014;42(8):1873–1880.
20. van Houten AH, Heesterbeek PJ, van Heerwaarden RJ, et al. Medial open wedge high tibial osteotomy: can delayed or nonunion be predicted? *Clin Orthop Relat Res*. 2014;472(4):1217–1223.
21. Naudie D, Bourne RB, Rorabeck CH, et al. The Install Award. Survivorship of the high tibial valgus osteotomy. A 10- to 22-year followup study. *Clin Orthop Relat Res*. 1999;367(367):18–27.
22. Akizuki S, Shibakawa A, Takizawa T, et al. The long-term outcome of high tibial osteotomy: a ten- to 20-year follow-up. *J Bone Joint Surg Br*. 2008;90(5):592–596.
23. Matthews LS, Goldstein SA, Malvitz TA, et al. Proximal tibial osteotomy: factors that influence the duration of satisfactory function. *Clin Orthop Relat Res*. 1988;229:193–200.
24. Dugdale TW, Noyes FR, Styer D. Preoperative planning for high tibial osteotomy. The effect of lateral tibiofemoral separation and tibiofemoral length. *Clin Orthop Relat Res*. 1992;274(274):248–264.
25. El-Azab H, Glabgly P, Paul J, et al. Patellar height and posterior tibial slope after open- and closed-wedge high tibial osteotomy: a radiological study on 100 patients. *Am J Sports Med*. 2010;38(2):323–329.
26. Hashemi J, Chandrashekar N, Gill B, et al. The geometry of the tibial plateau and its influence on the biomechanics of the tibiofemoral joint. *J Bone Joint Surg Am*. 2008;90(12):2724–2734.
27. Giffin JR, Vogrin TM, Zantop T, et al. Effects of increasing tibial slope on the biomechanics of the knee. *Am J Sports Med*. 2004;32(2):376–382.
28. Neyret P, Zuppi G, Selmi TAS. Tibial deflexion osteotomy. *Oper Tech Sports Med*. 2000;8(1):61–66.
29. Lobenhoffer P, Van Heerwaarden R, Staubi A, et al. *Osteotomies around the Knee*. Switzerland: AO Publishing; 2008.
30. Tjornstrand B, Egund N, Hagstedt B, et al. Tibial osteotomy in medial gonarthrosis. The importance of over-correction of varus deformity. *Arch Orthop Trauma Surg*. 1981;99(2):83–89.
31. Puddu G, Cipolla M, Cerullo G, et al. Osteotomies: the surgical treatment of the valgus knee. *Sports Med Arthrosc*. 2007;15(1):15–22.
32. Van Heerwaarden RJ, Wymenga AB, Freiling D, et al. Supracondylar varization osteotomy of the femur with plate fixation. In: Lobenhoffer P, van Heerwaarden RJ, Staubli AE, Jakob RP, eds. *Osteotomies around the Knee*. Stuttgart, Germany: Thieme. AO Foundation Publishing; 2008:147–166.
33. Puddu G, Cipolla M, Cerullo G, et al. Which osteotomy for a valgus knee? *Int Orthop*. 2010;34(2):239–247.
34. Healy WL, Anglen JO, Wasilewski SA, et al. Distal femoral varus osteotomy. *J Bone Joint Surg Am*. 1988;70(1):102–109.
35. Lee OS, Ahn S, Lee YS. Effect and safety of early weight-bearing on the outcome after open-wedge high tibial osteotomy: a systematic review and meta-analysis. *Arch Orthop Trauma Surg*. 2017;137(7):903–911.
36. Ekhtiari S, Haldane CE, de Sa D, et al. Return to work and sport following high tibial osteotomy: a systematic review. *J Bone Joint Surg Am*. 2016;98(18):1568–1577.
37. Harris JD, McNeilan R, Siston RA, et al. Survival and clinical outcome of isolated high tibial osteotomy and combined biological knee reconstruction. *Knee*. 2013;20(3):154–161.
38. W-Dahl A, Robertsson O. Similar outcome for total knee arthroplasty after previous high tibial osteotomy and for total knee arthroplasty as the first measure. *Acta Orthop*. 2016;87(4):395–400.
39. Ekeland A, Nerhus TK, Dimmen S, et al. Good functional results of distal femoral opening-wedge osteotomy of knees with lateral osteoarthritis. *Knee Surg Sports Traumatol Arthrosc*. 2016;24(5):1702–1709.
40. Chahla J, Mitchell JJ, Liechti DJ, et al. Opening- and closing-wedge distal femoral osteotomy: a systematic review of outcomes for isolated lateral compartment osteoarthritis. *Orthop J Sports Med*. 2016;4(6):2325967116649901.
41. Yan J, Musahl V, Kay J, et al. Outcome reporting following navigated high tibial osteotomy of the knee: a systematic review. *Knee Surg Sports Traumatol Arthrosc*. 2016;24(11):3529–3555.

47 Hip Arthroscopy

Christopher Potts and Vonda Joy Wright

The arthroscopic approach to hip pathology has rapidly expanded in scope and practice in the last decade to become an accepted and common tool in the orthopedic surgeons' armamentarium. Improvements in instrumentation, technique, and surgeons' experience have made the minimally invasive treatment of multiple hip derangements possible. This chapter provides the novice hip arthroscopist with a detailed description of the indications, operative setup, and technique for performing hip arthroscopy.

BACKGROUND, PRESENTATION, AND INDICATIONS FOR HIP ARTHROSCOPY

Hip arthroscopy is not a new procedure. For decades, however, few surgeons approached the hip arthroscopically as the procedure itself requires significant technical acumen, and definitive diagnosis of hip pathology is sometimes difficult. The clinical symptoms and physical finding associated with hip pain may be varied and subtle. These historical barriers to access to definitive hip care have diminished as the availability of formal training via fellowships and society educational offerings have expanded, and more surgeons have acquired these skills. This being said, knowledge of the arthroscopic approach to the hip is still not ubiquitous, and diagnosis is often delayed by an average of 21 months as patients are referred to an average of 3.3 health care providers before reaching a hip arthroscopist. During that period, they have often undergone a variety of treatments including physical therapy, nonsteroidal anti-inflammatory or narcotic medications, or other surgery including spine, ovary, or hernia exploration.

Not all pain believed to be emanating from the hip is actually intra-articular hip pain. The numerous anatomic structures in the vicinity of the hip joint may confuse the clinical presentation. Presentation of intra-articular hip pain is most commonly groin pain with or without radiation to the knee, pain localized by the patient with his or her hand encircling the lateral hip above the greater trochanter with the thumb posterior and fingers in a C-shape (C-sign), mechanical clicking or pinching in the groin, or pain with sitting and getting in and out of a car. The presence of mechanical symptoms in addition to groin pain is a favorable prognostic factor with more than 85% improvement postoperatively (1). Typically, intra-articular hip pain is not lateral pain over the greater trochanter, buttock/posterior leg pain, or palpable hip girdle tenderness (Table 47-1).

Proper patient selection is paramount in achieving a successful outcome from arthroscopic hip surgery. In addition to the history and physical examination, a focused examination, as summarized in Table 47-2, provides valuable clues for localizing pathology.

Perhaps, the most important imaging tools in evaluating the hip are plain radiographs. Table 47-3 summarizes important radiographs and the measurements they provide.

TABLE 47-1 Summary of Hip Symptoms Associated with Labral Tears

Onset of symptoms	Insidious	61%
	Acute	30%
	Trauma	9%
Intensity	Moderate/severe	86%
Location	Groin	92%
	Anterior thigh/lateral hip/buttock	
Quality of pain	Sharp	86%
	Dull	80%
	Combination sharp/dull	70%
	Activity related	91%
	Night pain	71%
	Mechanical symptoms	53%–77%
	Pain during walking	70%
	Pain during pivot	70%

Adapted from *J Bone Joint Surg.* 2005;88-A:1450.

TABLE 47-2 Focused Physical Examination of the Hip

Examination Name	Examination Indication
Gait	Antalgic—pain/Trendelenburg—gluteal weakness
Trendelenburg sign	Gluteal weakness
Palpation (groin, lateral hip, buttocks)	Intra-articular pathology generally not palpable
Strength (hip flexors/abd/add)	
Thomas sign	Tight hip flexors
Range of motion	Flex—FAI, ER—tight hip capsule, IR—OA
Log roll/heel strike	Intra-articular pathology/fracture
Scour test	Labral tear
FADIR	Impingement ± popping/clicking
FABER (location important)	SI joint/iliopsoas/FAI

TABLE 47-3 Radiographic Evaluation of the Hip

Radiograph	Measurement
AP WB pelvis	CEA—dysplasia
	<20 under coverage
	20–40 normal
	>40 pincer lesion
AP hip	Tonnis angle
	<10 degrees normal
	>10 degrees increased lateral contact pressures
	Crossover sign—anterior rim crosses in front of posterior rim indicating retroversion of the acetabulum
Cross table lateral	cam—decreased femoral neck offset

In addition, the Dunn or elongated-neck lateral (performed with the hip in 90 degrees of flexion and 20 degrees of abduction) may be used to further identify femoral neck offset. The false profile radiograph, with the patient rotated 65 degrees and the beam perpendicular to the hip, demonstrates anterior osseous coverage of the hip.

When history, physical examination, and plain radiographs indicate intra-articular pathology, the final two steps in preoperative diagnosis are magnetic resonance arthrogram (MRA) and possible diagnostic injection with analgesics (Figs. 47-1–47-3). Soft tissues of the hip should be visualized using MRA in most clinical settings. Figures 47-4 to 47-6 demonstrate common

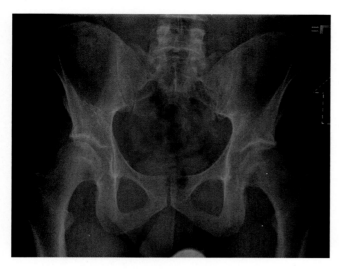

FIGURE 47-1
AP pelvis without crossover sign.

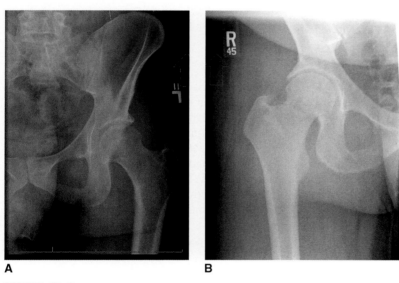

A   **B**

FIGURE 47-2
A: AP hip with normal CEA. **B:** AP hip with Pincer lesion.

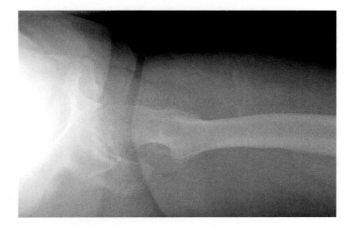

FIGURE 47-3
Cross table lateral with cam lesion.

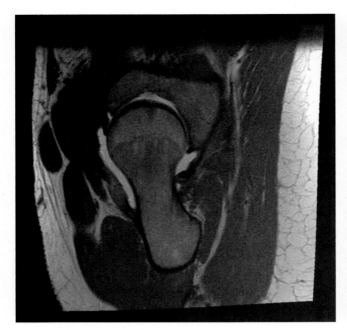

FIGURE 47-4

MRA axial oblique with labral tear.

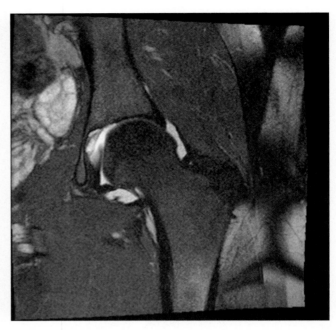

FIGURE 47-5

MRA coronal.

MRA views. While some institutions report the ability to visualize these structures adequately without the addition of contrast, in most settings, the addition of contrast is vital. MRA has 90% sensitivity and 91% accuracy for detecting hip pathology, while plain MRI has only 30% and 36%, respectively (2). Finally, confirmation of intra-articular pathology as the source for hip pain can be obtained via intra-articular injection. At the time of MRA, a mixture of lidocaine (6 mL 1%), Marcaine (6 mL 0.25%), and Kenalog (80 mg) is injected into the joint. The patient is then asked to perform the activities that normally cause pain to the hip and report the degree of relief from these symptoms within the first 3 hours following injection. The amount of relief from this diagnostic injection within the first 3 hours following injection is 90% predictive of the relief the patient can expect postoperatively.

Hip arthroscopy is indicated when patients present with persistent pain that is unrelieved by thorough physical therapy, reproducible by physical examination, and unresponsive to other

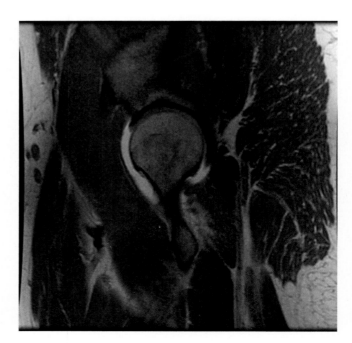

FIGURE 47-6

MRA sagittal.

conservative measures. Another useful diagnostic tool used by some is an intra-articular injection with pain relief within the first 3 hours after injection.

In recent years, much focus has illuminated the pathology behind labral tears. Though the pain associated with a torn labrum is often the inciting reason patients seek medical care, labral pathology itself is typically the consequence of the primary underlying hip derangement. These pathologies include femoral acetabular impingement (FAI), major or athletic hip trauma, capsular laxity/hip hyper mobility, hip dysplasia and subsequent hypertrophic labrum, iliopsoas impingement, and degenerative joint disease (DJD) with degeneration of the labrum as well as the articular cartilage. Detailed coverage of several of these topics appears in subsequent chapters and will be described in brief here.

Femoral Acetabular Impingement

First described in 1965 (3), FAI describes the repetitive abutment and subsequent microtrauma between the femoral neck and acetabular rim (Table 47-4). The impingement occurs as the femoral neck cam lesion flexes against a normal or overhanging acetabulum and pushes the labrum up and away from the acetabular edge. This leads to labral tearing or fraying and to peel back the acetabular cartilage at the area of impact. This repetitive impact of the cartilage then leads to early hip arthritis. The concept of optimal femoral neck offset is well known from the arthroplasty literature with too little offset leading to hip instability where the femoral head levers out of the cup, which causes impingement and wear. Historically, surgical management of FAI included periacetabular osteotomy (4) and surgical dislocation (5). Now FAI, including osteoplasty of the acetabular rim and femoral cam lesion, is performed arthroscopically as described in the following chapters.

Acetabular Dysplasia

Acetabular dysplasia is a part of a continuum of developmental disorders that includes FAI. While severe dysplasia cannot be treated by arthroscopy alone and requires open osteotomy, mild and moderate dysplasia may be amenable to an arthroscopic approach. Acetabulum with center edge angle (CEA) of 16 to 28 degrees is amenable to arthroscopic labral surgery (6). With dysplasia, the labrum becomes hypertrophic in the anterior and superior regions and is more susceptible to tearing (7). In these cases, the labrum is repaired back down to acetabular rim. Developmental dysplasia is also associated with hypertrophy of the ligamentum teres and increased wear with time causing impingement and pain. Débridement of the ligamentum and repair of the labrum in dysplasia have demonstrated improved clinical outcomes (8,9).

Avascular Necrosis of Femoral Head

Osteonecrosis of the femoral head can present in the pediatric and adult populations. In children, avascular necrosis (AVN) may present as Perthes disease or as a sequela of slipped capital femoral epiphysis disorder. Treatment of these conditions by routine arthroscopic procedures for débridement of loose bodies and chondroplasty demonstrated positive outcomes in children and adolescents (10). For adults, hip arthroscopy can be used for treatment of AVN in its early stages. Patients who fail conservative therapy and have chondral flaps, loose bodies and/or labral tears may benefit from arthroscopic débridement and repair (11). Additionally, hip arthroscopy can be performed simultaneously with other surgical treatments of AVN, such as core decompression, to evaluate the joint surface and accurately stage the severity of AVN.

TABLE 47-4 Functional of the Acetabular Labrum
The labrum runs circumferentially around the acetabular perimeter to the base of the fovea and then attaches anterior and posterior to the transverse acetabular ligament. Blood supply is provided peripherally
Decreased cartilage surface pressure
Participates in load bearing in flexion
Stability in capsular laxity and dysplasia
Performs a sealing function
Structural resistance to altered motion of the femoral head
Provides proprioception
Adapted from Kelly BT, Shapiro GS, Digiovanni CW, et al. Vascularity of the hip labrum: a cadaveric investigation. *Arthroscopy.* 2005;21(1):3–11.

Septic Hip

The standard treatment for septic arthritis of the hip is a formal arthrotomy with irrigation. However, open arthrotomies that may require dislocation of the femoral head can result in higher morbidity, with an increased risk for AVN or pain and a longer hospital stay. An alternative to an arthrotomy is to perform hip arthroscopy with ample irrigation and débridement of infected tissue. A study by Nusem demonstrated that the three-portal technique with the patient in the supine position (12) can adequately treat infections and provides rapid postoperative recovery with minimal complications (13).

Degenerative Disease

Osteoarthritis (OA) in the hip often occurs in association with labral tears as anterior tears are associated with cartilaginous lesions in the femoral head or acetabulum (14). With time and wear, these cartilage lesions erode and result in OA. In general, it is not recommended to perform hip arthroscopies in patients with severe degenerative disease, where the articular cartilage is fully denuded and is unable to be restored. However, in cases of early and mild OA, studies have shown that arthroscopic intervention may decrease pain after performing capsular release, débridement, synovectomy, and/or microfracture (15). In patients who have anatomic deformities that lead to OA, such as FAI and pistol grip deformities of the femoral neck, treatments by osteoplasty and chondroplasty through arthroscopy can also be beneficial (16–18).

Trauma

Using hip arthroscopy to remove loose bodies is a well-established indication. This has traditionally been employed in removing chondral fragments (19). Two additional uses of hip arthroscopy in the setting of trauma include removal of entrapped bony fragments after traumatic hip dislocations and acetabular wall fractures as well as the removal of foreign bodies as a result of trauma. Bullet fragments within the hip joint may be removed arthroscopically (15). For traumatic hip dislocations, the femoral head impinges against the acetabular lip, and the trauma may result in bony and cartilaginous fracture fragments. In a study by Mullis and Dahners, 36 patients underwent hip arthroscopy after hip dislocation, and 92% of patients were found to have loose bodies. Of note, these fragments were not all seen on radiographs or computed tomography scans (20). This finding highlights the importance of direct visualization of fracture fragments with hip arthroscopy.

Adhesive Capsulitis

Adhesive capsulitis is a condition defined by capsular fibrosis that is diagnosed on physical examination under anesthesia by decreased range of internal and external rotation with the hip in 90 degrees of flexion. To release the adhesions, the affected hip is placed in the figure-of-four position, and a downward force is placed on the medial aspect of the knee. Arthroscopic débridement is performed to remove debris within the joint. Surgical intervention is indicated for patients who have unremitting hip pain and patients who do not have severe degenerative changes (20).

Peritrochanteric Disorders

Peritrochanteric disorders encompass a variety of conditions that are associated with greater trochanteric pain, which is often found in young athletic female patients. Historically, surgical interventions were performed through open incisions, but with arthroscopy, these procedures may be performed with decreased morbidity. These conditions include trochanteric bursitis, external snapping of the iliotibial band, and gluteus medius and minimus tears. Trochanteric bursas may be debrided arthroscopically, and recalcitrant trochanteric bursitis may require a concomitant release of the iliotibial band (21). Snapping of the posterior one third of the iliotibial band, or coxa saltans externus, may also be relieved by release of the iliotibial band (22). Additionally, gluteus medius and minimus tears may either be repaired or debrided arthroscopically.

Synovial Abnormalities

The synovial lining of the hip degenerates over time as a result of inflammatory arthropathies, trauma, and/or repetitive stresses to the joint. Early treatment of conditions by arthroscopic débridement may slow the deterioration of articular cartilage. Primary synovial chondromatosis is a benign condition of cartilaginous metaplasia that produces intracapsular and extracapsular loose bodies. Studies have shown that treating primary synovial chondromatosis arthroscopically produces good to excellent results, as measured by patient satisfaction questionnaires, visual analogue scale for pain, and mobility scales (23). Arthroscopy can also be used to treat pigmented villonodular synovitis as a diagnostic tool to obtain tissue for pathology analysis, a prognostic tool to assess the cartilage and a therapeutic tool to perform partial synovectomies. Similarly, arthroscopy can have a role in treating the early stages of rheumatoid arthritis by debulking inflamed synovium to provide pain relief and improve mobility (24).

Total Hip Arthroplasty

Hip arthroscopy also plays a role in total hip arthroplasty (THA) revisions, as well as complications from THAs. Infected THAs can be irrigated and debrided arthroscopically, especially in patients who are unable to tolerate an arthrotomy. Debris from polyethylene wear and pelvic osteolysis can be debrided arthroscopically with less morbidity than open procedures (25). Arthroscopy can also be used for diagnostic purposes when assessing the need for revision surgery. Acetabular cup loosening can be evaluated arthroscopically before proceeding to a revision THA. In cemented THAs, the femoral cement mantle can be assessed, removal of the distal cement centralizer can be examined, and preparation of the cement mantle for recementing can be performed (1). Also useful could be an endoscopic iliopsoas lengthening secondary to iliopsoas impingement due to an anteverted or oversized acetabular prosthesis. A diagnostic anesthetic injection into the iliopsoas sheath is a useful tool in evaluating this issue.

PROCEDURE

The importance of setup is to facilitate the procedure being performed in order to correct the diagnosed pathology. Careful consideration must be used when positioning patients and placing portals. Erroneous portal placement may cause chondral scuffing or may not allow adequate access to certain compartments of the hip. Incorrect patient positioning may require prolonged distraction time and may result in pudendal or peroneal nerve injury. The following sections describe various patient positioning and portal placement in depth.

Setup

The patient is identified and the operative site verified by the surgeon, patient, and operating room staff. The patient is then brought back to the operating room and carefully placed on the operating room table. Anesthesia is induced at this time with general anesthesia most commonly employed; an laryngeal mask airway (LMA) is typically sufficient, but an endotracheal tube may be required in situations where paralysis is necessary. If a sufficient motor block is established, a spinal anesthesia may be used. In addition, a quadratus lumborum block may be administered at this time by the anesthesia team to aid in postoperative pain management. Preoperative antibiotics are administered.

Supine

Supine positioning is the most common approach to the hip joint for arthroscopy. Specially designed beds such as traction tables, Hanna tables, and more recently postless traction tables, are utilized to aid in hip distraction during the procedure. The patient is positioned with his or her perineum against a well-padded perineal post, and the feet are placed in well-padded boots or padded with Webril prior to being secured to the traction table. Initially, the traction cranks are fully unloaded. Many traction tables allow lateralization of the bed toward the operative leg. The patient's arms are draped out of the field. The author's preference is to place the arm on the operative side over the chest, resting in foam padding and secured with a strap and/or tape. This ensures that the arm will not hinder the surgeon's maneuverability or positioning of intraoperative fluoroscopy (Fig. 47-7).

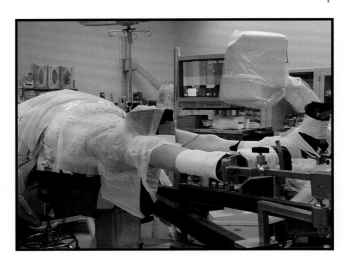

FIGURE 47-7

Patient positioning for supine hip arthroscopy.

Both legs are extended straight in the fracture boots without engaging the traction mechanism. A C-arm fluoroscan is placed across the table, opposite to the operative leg, and traction is pulled through the pelvis under direct fluoroscopic guidance. Patient positioning is key as the ability to adduct the hip around the peroneal post is as important as in-line traction for hip distraction. The patient's pelvis is positioned abutting the peroneal post and as far toward the nonoperative side as possible. Next, traction is gently pulled manually through the nonoperative leg first to both stabilize and level the pelvis and then attention can be turned to the operative leg. On the operative side, the hip is flexed 10 degrees to relax the iliofemoral ligament; the leg is abducted approximately 30 degrees and placed in 30 degrees of internal rotation. Next, gross traction is applied to the leg until it is tight, and the leg is then adducted around the post to a position of 5 degrees of abduction. Often, this alone will allow for adequate distraction of the hip, but if further distraction is required, fine traction can be applied to the desired level. Additionally, the foot may be internally rotated to eliminate the effect of femoral anteversion during the approach (26). When the surgeon is satisfied that the hip can be adequately distracted to perform arthroscopy, the traction is released and the operative leg prepped and draped. The goal is to minimize traction pressure against the perineum and thereby minimize pudendal nerve neuropraxia. This author prefers to drape out the operative field with four 1,000 drapes placed proximal to the umbilicus, as midline as possible, just proximal to the knee and one posterior. This area is then cleansed and draped with a shower curtain–type drape. The C-arm is draped sterilely and brought in over the field. Traction is then reestablished.

Anatomic landmarks are made marked at this time and include the anterior superior iliac spine (ASIS) with a line drawn sagittally from this point to distal in the field and the superior and anterior edges of the greater trochanter. The vertical ASIS line is a visual reminder of the most medial extent of the safe field as the femoral neurovascular structure lies within 3 to 4 cm of this line (27) (Fig. 47-8).

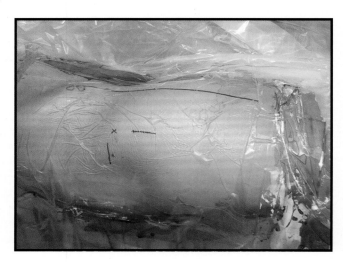

FIGURE 47-8

Hip arthroscopy anatomic landmarks.

The supine approach is more difficult with obese patients with a large pannus and in patients with large anterolateral osteophytes. For these patients, the lateral approach allows gravity to pull the pannus and buttocks away from the field. The lateral position is also thought to allow more easy access to the posterior portion of the hip. The lateral approach, however, may be more time consuming to set up as it requires multiple adjustments to the perineal traction posts. A perineal post is placed against the medial thigh of the surgical leg, and the hip is slightly flexed and abducted to relax the hip capsule. Special traction devices may be used to distract the leg and allow visualization of the hip joint. However, if traction devices are not available, a traction post may also be used. The contralateral leg is padded and may be secured to the table (28).

Portals

Correct portal placement is crucial to adequate visualization of the hip. Three main portals typically utilized are the anterolateral portal (ALP), modified mid-anterior portal (MMAP), and the distal anterolateral accessory (DALA) portal. These three portals allow for adequate mobility around the joint, which helps facilitate many necessary steps including a thorough evaluation of the central compartment, carrying out any bone or cartilage work, and affording a safe trajectory to the acetabular rim for anchor placement. The ALP is often created first and is placed approximately 2 cm anterior and 2 cm distal from the tip of the greater trochanter. The ALP enters the lateral capsule at the anterior margin through the gluteus medius muscle (29). Less commonly, the posterolateral portal is established 2 cm posterior to the tip of the greater trochanter if access to the posterior joint is necessary to remove a loose body or aid in synovial excision.

Next, the modified mid-anterior portal is then placed under direct visualization once the ALP is established. The MMAP is typically placed 3 cm anterior and 4 to 5 cm distal to the ALP with necessary adjustments made based on the size of the patient. Advantages of this portal include a more favorable angle of approach to the central compartment for bone work, access to the acetabular rim, and facilitation of transcapsular iliopsoas release. Caution must be taken when placing this portal, as the lateral femoral cutaneous nerve and a terminal branch of the lateral circumflex femoral artery may be at risk of injury. However, the more lateral location of this portal compared to the traditional direct anterior portal helps minimize this risk (30).

The DALA portal is typically the third portal established at a location about 6 cm distal to the ALP under direct visualization. This portal is beneficial as it allows access to a significant portion of the acetabular rim and provides safe access for anchor placement as it can decrease the risk of articular cartilage perforation. Literature has shown cartilage perforation occurs at a rate of about 5% when this portal is used for labral anchor drilling and placement. It is the author's preference to place most of the labral anchors through this portal with the use of a curved drill guide while utilizing this portal as well as the MMAP for suture passage.

The posterolateral portal is placed posterior and superior to the greater trochanter. It is approximately 4 cm from the gluteal nerve and 2.9 cm from the lateral edge of the sciatic nerve (27). This portal enters the posterior margin of the lateral capsule by going anterior and superior to the piriformis tendon and piercing through the gluteus medius and minimus.

After the patient is prepped and draped, traction is reestablished, to distract the joint approximately 1 cm, and the ALP is established first under direct fluoroscopic visualization using a spinal needle. The needle is directed slightly posterior and cephalad into the joint with the goal of establishing a portal that does not violate the femoral head cartilage or the labrum. Also of note is to angle the bevel of the spinal needle up in an attempt to decrease labral penetration. Once the needle has entered the joint, this can be confirmed on fluoroscopy with the presence of an air arthrogram. The need for fluoroscopic visualization of this entry is minimized by experience. Recent studies have highlighted the usefulness of ultrasound for guiding the placement of portals in real time, without the need for radiation from fluoroscopy (31). At this point, some surgeons opt to distend the joint with 30 to 60 mL of saline although this is not mandatory (Fig. 47-9).

Once in the joint, the needle is exchanged for a nitinol wire, a small vertical skin incision is made with a no. 11 blade, and a 4.5 cannula/obturator is slowly advanced along the wire, through the thick capsule and into the joint. Gently pronating and supinating the wrist increases ease of passage through the soft tissue. The obturator and the wire are removed together to prevent breakage

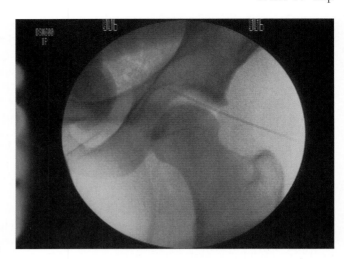

FIGURE 47-9

Anterolateral portal placement.

of the wire. Many surgeons place a 5-mm cannula directly over the wire into the joint instead of the 4.5 and scope using this portal. This author prefers to use a blunt, plastic cannula to minimize any potential cartilage injury to the femoral head, with both an inflow port and an outflow port (as in shoulder arthroscopy). Next, a 70-degree scope is inserted into the joint which is then irrigated as needed (Fig. 47-10).

With the 70-degree scope in place, it is possible to visualize the anterior triangle made by the femoral head distally, the labrum and acetabulum superiorly, and the hip capsule superiorly. If visualization of this triangle is difficult it is likely that the cannula has either been inserted through the labrum (which will restrict mobility) or the patient has an overlying hypertrophic labrum. The medial wall of this triangle is the anterior capsule that overlays the iliopsoas tendon (Fig. 47-11). This capsule is often red and inflamed when the iliopsoas tendon is tight or popping over the anterior acetabulum yielding a positive "iliopsoas sign."

With the anterior triangle in view, the modified mid-anterior portals established under direct visualization with needle localization 3 cm anterior and 4 to 5 cm distal to the ALP. The spinal needle is directed approximately 45 degrees cephalad and 45 degrees medial. The needle should be visualized entering the joint adjacent to but not through the anterior superior labrum. The hip joint is sometimes filled with serosanguinous joint fluid necessitating that this portal may need to be established without visualization. In this instance, fluoroscopy can be of assistance and when the needle is in the joint, there will be outflow once the stylus is removed allowing for clearing of the visual field. After the anterior portal is established, a blunt, plastic cannula is placed into the joint as previously described. The MMAP then becomes the working portal, and a probe is placed intra-articularly. Once these first two portals are established, an interportal capsulotomy is created with arthroscopic knife or cautery wand to allow for adequate mobilization around the joint. It is the preference of the author to do an interportal capsulotomy as opposed to a T-capsulotomy unless specific pathology

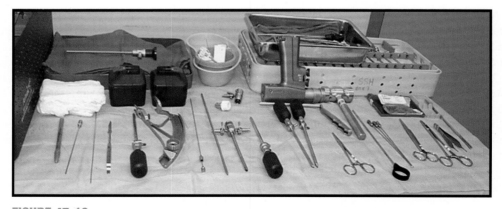

FIGURE 47-10

Standard hip arthroscopy equipment.

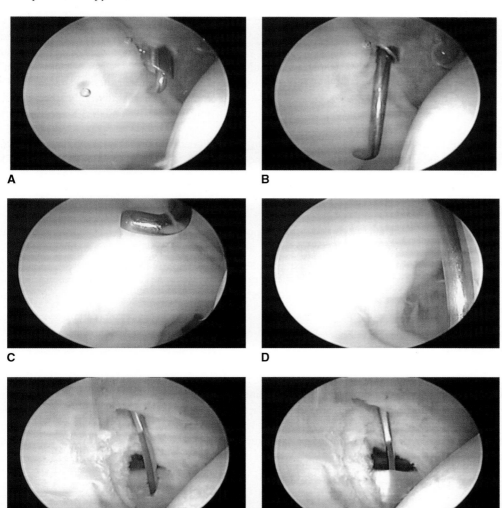

FIGURE 47-11

Intra-articular hip anatomy. Anterior labrum **(A)**; acetabulum **(B)**; labrum **(C)**; acetabular cartilage **(D)**; anterior capsulotomy **(E)**; iliopsoas tendon **(F)**.

necessitates the use of the latter. Also, with an interportal capsulotomy, capsular traction stitches can be placed both medially and laterally during bony work to facilitate visualization of the acetabulum and femoral head, respectively.

Once the portals are established, either the 30- or 70-degree scope may be used. Literature supports the use of the 70-degree scope in all portals and the 30-degree scope in posterolateral and superior trochanteric portals where wider visualization may be obtained (32).

Diagnostic Scope

Evaluation of the hip begins with placement of the 70-degree camera through the ALP. This allows the greatest visualization of the more peripheral portions of the joint and the best view of the anterior/superior hip. The 70-degree camera also allows for direct visualization of the anterior and posterior joint for accessory portal placement. The modified mid-anterior portals are placed under direct visualization, and a probe is introduced. The intra-articular structures including the anterior and superior labrum, acetabular cartilage, femoral head cartilage, anterior capsule overlying the iliopsoas tendon, transverse acetabular ligament, and the fovea and its contents are easily evaluated. Introduction of the 30-degree scope through the ALP allows a more direct view of the fovea and its contents (Fig. 47-11).

The camera can then be placed in the modified mid-anterior portal to evaluate the position of the ALP and the most inferior margin of the anterior labrum (33). Finally, if a posterior lateral portal was established, the camera is placed there for viewing the posterior labrum. For extra-articular pathology that is still intracapsular, patients should be placed in 30 to 45 degrees of hip flexion to relax the anterior capsule. This allows for access to the peripheral compartment of the hip and allows treatment of synovial disease, loose bodies in the peripheral recess, and adhesive capsulitis (24). Problems with excessive flexion include potential sciatic nerve palsy and may obstruct anterior portal entry.

Following thorough evaluation of the hip joint, the intended surgery is initiated. The following chapters will address the arthroscopic management of labral tears of the hip and osteoplasty for femoral-acetabular impingement.

Complications

Complication rates associated with hip arthroscopy are low and range between 0.5% and 6.4% in the literature (28). The most common complications are neuropraxias of the pudendal nerve secondary to traction and lateral femoral cutaneous nerve secondary to anterior portal placement. Other complications include infection, damage to the femoral neurovascular structures, deep vein thrombosis (DVT), fluid extravasations, iatrogenic chondral or labral damage, postoperative hip dislocation, and intra-articular instrument breakage.

CONCLUSION

Hip arthroscopy has expanded as a field over the last 20 years. The indications for performing hip arthroscopy have grown, as have the surgical techniques to treat these conditions. Newer indications are being developed in other areas of orthopedics, such as arthroplasty and trauma. Further studies will need to be conducted to evaluate the long-term effectiveness and sequelae of these newer procedures. Overall, the field of hip arthroscopy continues to grow and will continue to provide promising treatments to disease processes.

REFERENCES

1. Voos JE, Rudzki JR, Shindle MK, et al. Arthroscopic anatomy and surgical techniques for peritrochanteric space disorders in the hip. *Arthroscopy*. 2007;23(11):1246.e1–1246.e5.
2. Armfield DR, Towers JD, Robertson DD. Radiographic and MR imaging of the athletic hip. Clin Sports Med. 2006;25(2):211–239.
3. Murray. *Br J Radiol*. 1965.
4. Siebenrock KA, Schoeniger R, Ganz R. Anterior femoro-acetabular impingement due to acetabular retroversion. Treatment with periacetabular osteotomy. *J Bone Joint Surg Am*. 2003;85:278–286.
5. Peters CL, Erickson JA. Treatment of femoro-acetabular impingement with surgical dislocation and debridement in young adults. *J Bone Joint Surg Am*. 2006;88:1735–1741.
6. Massie WK, Howorth MB. Congenital dislocation of the hip: Part I. Method of grading results. *J Bone Joint Surg Am*. 1950;32A:519–531.
7. Fujii M, Nakashima Y, Jingushi S, et al. Intraarticular findings in symptomatic developmental dysplasia of the hip. *J Pediatr Orthop*. 2009;29(1):9–13.
8. Byrd JW, Jones KS. Hip arthroscopy in the presence of dysplasia. *Arthroscopy*. 2003;19(10):1055–1060.
9. Byrd JW. Hip arthroscopy: surgical indications. *Arthroscopy*. 2006;22(12):1260–1262.
10. Kocher MS, Kim YJ, Millis MB, et al. Hip arthroscopy in children and adolescents. *J Pediatr Orthop*. 2005;25(5): 680–686.
11. McCarthy J, Puri L, Barsoum W, et al. Articular cartilage changes in avascular necrosis: an arthroscopic evaluation. *Clin Orthop Relat Res*. 2003;406:64–70.
12. Byrd JW. Hip arthroscopy. The supine position. *Clin Sports Med*. 2001;20(4):703–731.
13. Nusem I, Jabur MKA, Playford EG. Arthroscopic treatment of septic arthritis of the hip. *Arthroscopy*. 2006;22(8): 902.e1–902.e3.
14. McCarthy JC, Lee JA. Arthroscopic intervention in early hip disease. *Clin Orthop Relat Res*. 2004;429:157–162.
15. Jerosch J, Schunck J, Khoja A. Arthroscopic treatment of the hip in early and midstage degenerative joint disease. *Knee Surg Sports Traumatol Arthrosc*. 2006;14(7):641–645.
16. Campbell DG, Rietveld JA. Technique for arthroscopic assisted revision hip arthroplasty. *Int Orthop*. 2001;25(4): 236–238.
17. Diulus CA, Krebs VE, Hanna G, et al. Hip arthroscopy technique and indications. *J Arthroplasty*. 2006;21(4 suppl 1): 68–73.
18. Kim KC, Hwang DS, Lee CH et al. Influence of femoroacetabular impingement on results of hip arthroscopy in patients with early osteoarthritis. *Clin Orthop Relat Res*. 2007;456:128–132.
19. Byrd JW, Jones KS. Hip arthroscopy in athletes: 10-year follow-up. *Am J Sports Med*. 2009;37(11):2140–2143.

20. Kim YJ. Nonarthroplasty hip surgery for early osteoarthritis. *Rheum Dis Clin North Am.* 2008;34(3):803–814.
21. Tanzer M, Noiseux N. Osseous abnormalities and early osteoarthritis: the role of hip impingement. *Clin Orthop Relat Res.* 2004;429:170–177.
22. Meyer NJ, Thiel B, Ninomiya JT. Retrieval of an intact, intraarticular bullet by hip arthroscopy using the lateral approach. *J Orthop Trauma.* 2002;16:51–53.
23. Mullis BH, Dahners LE. Hip arthroscopy to remove loose bodies after traumatic dislocation. *J Orthop Trauma.* 2006;20(1):22–26.
24. Byrd JW, Jones KS. Adhesive capsulitis of the hip. *Arthroscopy.* 2006;22(1):89–94.
25. Farr D, Selesnick H, Janecki C. Arthroscopic bursectomy with concomitant iliotibial band release for the treatment of recalcitrant trochanteric bursitis. *Arthroscopy.* 2007;23(8):905.e1–905.e5.
26. Byrd JW. Hip arthroscopy utilizing the supine position. *Arthroscopy.* 1994;10:275–280.
27. Byrd JW, Pappas JN, Pedley MJ. Hip arthroscopy: an anatomic study of portal placement and relationship to the extra-articular structures. *Arthroscopy.* 1995;11(4):418–423.
28. Smart LR, Oetgen M, Noonan B, et al. Beginning hip arthroscopy: indications, positioning, portals, basic techniques, and complications. *Arthroscopy.* 2007;23(12):1348–1353.
29. Byrd JW. Hip arthroscopy. *J Am Acad Orthop Surg.* 2006;14:433–444.
30. Robertson WJ, Kelly BT. The safe zone for hip arthroscopy: a cadaveric assessment of central, peripheral, and lateral compartment portal placement. *Arthroscopy.* 2008;24(9):1019–1026.
31. Hua Y, Yang Y, Chen S. Ultrasound-guided establishment of hip arthroscopy portals. *Arthroscopy.* 2009;25(12):1491–1495.
32. McCarthy JC, Lee J. Hip arthroscopy: indications and technical pearls. *Clin Orthop Relat Res.* 2005;441:180–187.
33. Bond JL, Knutson ZA, Ebert A, et al. The 23-point arthroscopic examination of the hip: basic setup, portal placement, and surgical technique. *Arthroscopy.* 2009;25(4):416–429.

48 Acetabular Labrum: Debridement and Repair

Simon Lee, Neil Bakshi, Jacob M. Kirsch,
Jon K. Sekiya, and Asheesh Bedi

INTRODUCTION

The acetabular labrum has been widely recognized as a source of hip pain, particularly in young and active populations (1–4). Labral injury has increasingly been identified as a source of hip pain and mechanical symptoms and has been implicated in the accelerated development of degenerative osteoarthritis (5). Labral injury can result from a variety of traumatic or atraumatic mechanisms including femoroacetabular impingement (FAI), hip dysplasia, hip dislocation, or athletic injuries (1–4). As more has been learned about hip labral pathology, significant advances have been made in the surgical treatment of labral tears. Early techniques of addressing labral pathology included surgical hip dislocation with labral debridement and management of associated pathology. However, this open approach requires a larger incision, increased soft tissue dissection and blood loss, and a trochanteric osteotomy with an inherently increased risk of nonunion (6). Due to these risks, as well as a lengthy postoperative recovery, arthroscopic techniques have become increasingly more common for addressing labral pathology. Arthroscopic labral surgery provides benefits of a minimally invasive approach, outpatient surgery, lower overall complication rates, and a shorter recovery period with more rapid return to activity (6,7).

ANATOMY

The acetabular labrum is a complex structure consisting of a fibrocartilaginous rim of circumferential collagen fibers spanning the entirety of the acetabulum, becoming contiguous with the transverse acetabular ligament (TAL) and anchored through a well-defined 1- to 2-mm transitional zone of calcified cartilage at the acetabular rim. The labral surface immediately adjacent to the articular cartilage of the femoral head becomes continuous with the hyaline articular cartilage of the acetabular surface through a similar transitional zone (4). Histologically, the labrum is composed of dense connective tissue divided into bundles at the peripheral rim and transitions to fibrocartilage at the inner surface.

The vascular supply is derived primarily from the joint capsule, originating from the medial and lateral circumflex, inferior and deep branch of the superior gluteal arteries (4,8,9). There is a relatively hypovascular zone within the internal substance of the labrum and extending to the distal margin that may predispose this area to injury from acute or repetitive trauma and lead to degenerative change. The peripheral attachment of the labrum near its bony attachment has been shown to have a robust vascular supply, and in conjunction with the highly vascularized synovium, there may exist the potential of labral neovascularization and healing in the setting of labral injury (4,9).

PHYSIOLOGY

The acetabular labrum serves multiple purposes in the hip, including limiting extreme range of motion (ROM) and deepening the acetabulum to enhance the stability of the hip joint. The labrum also serves to increase the articulating surface area of the acetabulum. Studies have shown that the labrum contributes approximately 22% of the articulating surface of the hip (4). This serves to distribute the large forces occurring in the hip with athletic activities across a greater surface area (10). In conjunction with the TAL, it contains an inherent elasticity that allows excellent conformity with the articular surfaces during ROM while compensating for minor joint incongruities. This allows the labrum to dissipate high contact forces encountered by the hip joint during activity and weight bearing (10).

In addition, due to its low permeability, the labrum functions to form a hip fluid seal, or suction seal, around the femoral-acetabular joint (11–13). Evidence has suggested that the hip fluid seal is important for intra-articular fluid pressurization and hip stability with distraction forces (12–16). Intra-articular fluid pressurization during compressive loads results in pressurization of intra-articular fluid and the interstitial fluid within articular cartilage. This pressurization has been reported to protect the cartilage matrix from as much as 90% of load and decreases the friction between the two surfaces (17,18). Furthermore, negative intra-articular pressure is generated with distraction forces on the hip. This negative intra-articular pressure (suction effect) resists displacement of the femoral head, providing a stabilizing force within the hip joint. Both of these functions of the hip fluid seal are currently theorized to be reliant on an intact acetabular labrum (11,14).

Once injured or torn, the role of the labrum is compromised and can lead to further damage to surrounding structures in the hip. As demonstrated by Philippon et al., labral tears are associated with significantly decreased intra-articular fluid pressurization, which can result in increased articular cartilage loading, delamination, and subchondral cyst formation (12,13,18,19). It has been shown that the loads across the femoral and acetabular articular cartilage in a labrum-deficient hip are up to 92% greater than those encountered with an intact labrum. Labral deficiency also imparts decreased constraint of the femoral head, allowing the center of joint contact to displace laterally toward the acetabular rim, creating this focal area of increased articular forces. Furthermore, the mechanical stability of the hip may also be compromised due to disruption of the hip fluid seal, resulting in reduced restraint to hip distraction forces. Such alterations in the kinematics of the native hip anatomy may contribute to the progression of hip osteoarthritis following labral injury (14,16,17). This was initially evidenced by the increased incidence of osteoarthritis in patients with developmental dysplasia of the hip, chronic labral tears, and full-thickness chondral lesions (20). Attempting to improve the symptoms of hip pain while potentially reducing the progression of osteoarthritic degeneration of the femoroacetabular joint have spurred significant interest in the operative management of labral tears and associated pathology.

CLINICAL PRESENTATION

As discussed, labral pathology can result from a variety of mechanisms, including trauma, FAI, capsular laxity, and hip dysplasia, among others. In addition, patients with labral pathology can present with a multitude of clinical signs, symptoms, and examination findings. As a result, a thorough history and physical examination is critical to clearly elucidating a patient's symptoms and exacerbating factors. Often, these findings can play an important role in guiding future diagnostic and treatment options. A careful history including any inciting trauma; onset, duration, and progression of symptoms; aggravating and mitigating factors; previous interventions; and activity-related consequences should routinely be obtained during the initial visit. It is frequently helpful to ask the patient to demonstrate the activities or extremity position that reproduces the symptoms, as this may assist in identifying the etiology of the complaint.

Often, patients with labral pathology will present with anterior groin pain. Keeney et al. and McCarthy and Busconi, respectively, reported that 96% and 100% of individuals with an arthroscopically identified labral tear reported anterior groin pain (20,21). However, McCarthy and Busconi also demonstrated that the overall prevalence of anterior groin pain for individuals with other sources of intra-articular hip pathology was 98% (21). Therefore, anterior groin pain may not be specific to labral tears but can be related to other intra-articular pathologies as well. Less commonly, hip labral pathology can refer pain to the lateral hip, posterior hip, and/or anterior thigh. Keeney et al. demonstrated that 34% of patients with diagnosed labral tears complained of anterior thigh pain, 38% complained of lateral hip pain, and 17% complained of buttock/posterior hip pain.

In addition to pain, labral tears can also cause mechanical symptoms such as clicking, giving way, locking, and catching. Keeney et al. documented that 58% of individuals with a labral tear reported hip locking or catching. McCarthy and Busconi found that painful inguinal clicking and giving way significantly correlated to labral tears ($r = 0.79$, $p = 0.0005$ and $r = 0.41$, $p = 0.002$, respectively) (21,22). Narvani et al. demonstrated that clicking had 100% sensitivity and 85% specificity for a labral tear identified by magnetic resonance arthrography (MRA) (23). In addition, they reported that patient endorsement of clicking had a positive likelihood ratio of 6.67 for the presence of a labral tear (23).

Other etiologies of the presenting symptoms must also be carefully considered to identify possible contributing sources. These include other sources of intra-articular hip pathology and extra-articular hip pathology such as iliopsoas tendonitis, urogenital problems, sacroiliac (SI) joint pain, spinal pain, abdominal symptoms, soft tissue contusions, and abdominal wall pain. If there is a suspicion for an extra-articular or nonmusculoskeletal component to the patient's complaint, the history and physical examination must be adjusted appropriately (24).

PHYSICAL EXAMINATION

The clinical evaluation of a patient with hip pain can be challenging and requires a systematic approach to the physical examination to aid the clinician in correctly identifying the source of the complaint. These symptoms may arise from both an intra-articular and an extra-articular source, and care must be taken to appropriately direct the diagnostic algorithm to successfully locate the source of the complaint and guide therapeutic interventions. After an appropriate history has been obtained, the physical examination can assist the physician in further narrowing the diagnosis (24).

A focused physical examination should include evaluation of the lumbar spine, SI joints, and the femoroacetabular joint. The examination of the hip can be complicated by the relatively common incidence of referred pain from genitourinary, visceral, and gynecologic etiologies to the area in question (24). These external sources of pain may masquerade as hip pathology and must be ruled out (3).

In patients with unilateral complaints, all objective examinations should be compared to the contralateral side. A gait examination, if able to be performed, is frequently the initial step in the evaluation. Particular attention should be placed on stride length, core balance, posture, and the duration of the stance phase of gait. One should also take care to notice evidence of scoliosis, limb-length discrepancy, muscular deficit, or joint contractures (25). The focused examination of the hip should include localizing areas of maximal pain or tenderness and any atrophic muscular changes identified with palpation. Intra-articular pathology will rarely be associated with external discomfort. Hip ROM is assessed with comparison to the contralateral extremity in the supine position with all deficiencies documented. This should include measurement of flexion, extension, internal and external rotation, and any associated deficit or discomfort. Increased passive external rotation of the leg with the hip in neutral extension may indicate the presence of capsular laxity. Provocative testing is used to functionally evaluate patient symptoms in various limb positions. Placing the hip into flexion/adduction/internal rotation places the anterolateral femoral head and neck into proximity with the anterior and lateral acetabular margin. This may cause compression of the labrum and associated pain in the presence of a labral tear. Ito et al. reported that 24 out of 25 individuals with arthroscopically confirmed labral tears had a positive flexion internal rotation impingement test (26). The FABER test consists of flexion/abduction/external rotation of the hip and places the iliopsoas tendon on stretch while stressing the SI joints. Mitchell et al. reported that hip pain during the FABER test was 88% sensitive for intra-articular hip pathology. This study, however, did not find a correlation between a positive FABER test and specific hip pathology (27). The Ober test assesses iliotibial (IT) band tightness with the patient in the lateral position with the symptomatic extremity placed superiorly. A positive result is when the leg remains abducted while the hip and the knee are passively extended. A flexion contracture of the hip can be assessed with the Thomas test as it minimizes the ability to compensate for decreased hip extension with excessive lumbar lordosis. The contralateral hip is flexed, reducing lumbar lordosis and assessing full hip extension in the supine position. Assessment of a "snapping" sensation should also be performed as this may be due to the IT band gliding across the greater trochanter or the iliopsoas tendon riding over the anterior margin of the superior pubic ramus.

IMAGING

Imaging of the hip is a routine part of the diagnostic algorithm for management of intra-articular pathology and includes plain radiographs, computed tomography (CT), magnetic resonance imaging (MRI), and MRA. First, plain radiographs of the pelvis should be obtained as the initial evaluation of hip pathology. Radiographs can identify fractures, dislocation, arthritic change, bony abnormalities including FAI and dysplasia, and identification of radio-opaque loose bodies. Although these radiographs do not allow for soft tissue visualization, certain radiographic findings can increase suspicion for labral pathology, or identify another etiology responsible for the patient's symptoms. These may include stress fractures, cam or pincer-type femoral acetabular impingement, excessive acetabular retroversion, joint space narrowing, subchondral sclerosis, osteophyte formation, or femoral head collapse associated with avascular necrosis (AVN).

Computed tomography offers the greatest spatial resolution for assessing bony abnormalities of the hip and pelvis. The most common uses for CT around the hip include trauma, congenital hip dysplasia, preoperative prosthesis planning, evaluation of neoplasms, and hip imaging in patients who have contraindications to MRI. Coronal and sagittal reformatted images as well as three-dimensional reconstructions can help in further defining the anatomy of the abnormality. The addition of intra-articular contrast material allows improved identification of labral pathology and resolution of the articular surface (28). Yamamoto et al. examined 21 hip joints with contrast-enhanced CT and hip arthroscopy and reported that contrast-enhanced CT had a sensitivity of 92.3%, specificity of 100%, and accuracy of 95.2% (29). This demonstrates the diagnostic efficacy of contrast-enhanced CT, making it a viable alternative for patients with contraindications to MRI. However, the relatively high dose of radiation of CT imaging compared with plain radiographs and MRI is a significant disadvantage of this modality.

MRI has become the most common modality for the evaluation of hip pain with concern for labral pathology. Its ability to provide detailed images of both soft tissue and osseous abnormalities makes it superior to other modalities employed in intra-articular hip imaging (28). However, as good as MRI is in demonstrating detailed soft tissue anatomy, it has been found to have poor accuracy and sensitivity in detecting hip articular surface/cartilage abnormalities, osteochondral loose bodies, and labral pathology (28,30). As a result, MRA of the hip has become the best imaging modality for the detection and diagnosis of capsulolabral and osteochondral pathology (28,31,32). MRA allows improved visualization of the labrum, articular surface, and capsule via the injection of gadolinium contrast directly into the joint (Fig. 48-1). A labral tear is identified by a linear defect through the substance of the labrum. Czerny et al. compared conventional MRI with MRA in the diagnosis of labral tears and reported a sensitivity and accuracy of 80% and 65%, respectively, for conventional MRI compared with 95% and 88% with MRA (32). Czerny et al. reported in a different study that MRA had a sensitivity of 91%, specificity of 71%, and an accuracy of 88% in the diagnosis and correct staging of labral lesions, including labral degeneration, tearing, or detachment. Results such as these suggest that MRA may have a significant advantage over conventional MRI for the evaluation of capsulolabral structures in the hip (28,31,32).

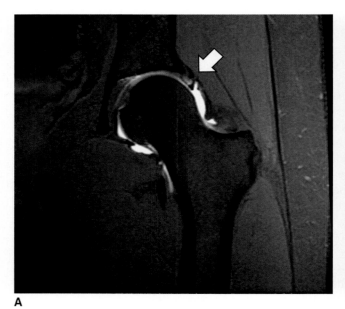 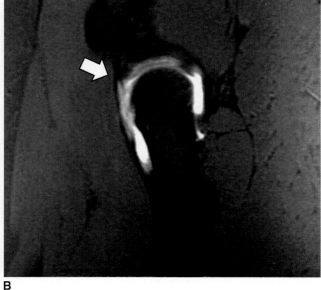

A   B

FIGURE 48-1

Coronal **(A)** and sagittal **(B)** views of MR arthrogram revealing a large labral tear of the left hip (*arrow*) (T1-weighted coronal image with fat suppression).

CLASSIFICATION

A classification of labral pathology identified during hip arthroscopy was described by Lage et al. in 1996. This classification of labral tears was divided into an etiologic classification and a morphological classification, each with four distinct subgroups. The etiologic classification includes traumatic, degenerative, idiopathic, and congenital groups. Traumatic tears were associated with an identifiable hip injury, degenerative tears are identified by the presence of degeneration of surrounding tissues, including the articular cartilage or the labrum itself, idiopathic tears have no identifiable cause and are not associated with degenerative changes, and congenital tears are associated with structurally normal but functionally abnormal labral tissue. The morphological classification describes the pattern of labral tearing and includes radial flap tears, radial fibrillated tears, longitudinal peripheral tears (i.e., bucket-handle tears), and unstable tears associated with congenital changes (33).

The American Academy of Orthopaedic Surgeons classification of labral tears is based on their appearance at arthroscopy. Stage 0 identifies a labral contusion with synovitis. Stage 1 signifies the presence of a discreet labral tear with normal articular cartilage. A stage 2 lesion contains focal articular damage of the femoral head without acetabular change. Stage 3 describes a labral tear with an adjacent focal acetabular lesion, with or without femoral head changes. These are further subclassified into a 3A lesion, involving <1 cm of the acetabular cartilage, and stage 3B lesions, involving >1 cm of articular cartilage. Stage 4 signifies extensive labral tearing with diffuse osteoarthritic changes throughout the joint (22,34).

Others have attempted to classify acetabular labral tears using MRA, but only moderate success has been found when compared to the gold standard of arthroscopic classification. Blankenbaker et al. examined 65 hip MRA studies with correlative hip arthroscopies. Each MRA was classified using the Czerny classification and Lage MRA modification, with each labral tear on hip arthroscopy being classified by the Lage classification. Blankenbaker et al. reported no correlation between the MRA Czerny and arthroscopic Lage classifications and only a borderline correlation ($p = 0.049$) between the MRA Lage classification and the arthroscopic Lage classification (31,34).

CONSERVATIVE MANAGEMENT

The ultimate success of nonsurgical management of labral pathology is often intimately related to the underlying etiology and the specific patient population. Intra-articular pathology occurring in the setting of bony abnormalities frequently encountered in FAI and dysplasia is unlikely to improve significantly with nonsurgical management, particularly in the athletically active patient. Groin pain that is reproduced with provocative maneuvers should raise concern for intra-articular pathology that may result in progressive joint damage if not recognized early. Conversely, a patient with radiographic FAI who is minimally symptomatic or an older patient with a prearthritic hip represents a different spectrum of hip pathology. These patients have demonstrated significant improvement in pain and function with conservative treatment alone, and therefore, an initial trial of nonoperative management is warranted (35).

Nonsurgical rehabilitation is best approached through a multimodal approach focusing initially on activity modification and physical therapy. Therapy is particularly useful for stretching and strengthening the dynamic stabilizers of the hip. Focused therapy on structures surrounding the hip such as the lumbopelvic musculature, iliopsoas, iliotibial band, and the trochanteric bursa can also be helpful. Overtime, directed therapy on improving ROM and sport-specific exercises can often return the patient to a more functional state. Athletic activity is gradually increased beginning with low-demand activities, such as cycling and the elliptical machine, and progressing to cutting and jumping activities.

An intra-articular injection with both local anesthetic and corticosteroid is often both diagnostic and therapeutic for patients with symptoms that are recalcitrant to nonoperative modalities. This can often be performed under ultrasound in the office. It is important to examine the patient prior to as well as following the injection. Immediate symptom relief following the injection, particularly with provocative maneuvers often localizes the pathology to the hip joint and provides the patient an idea of the potential symptom relief that can be achieved with operative intervention.

OPERATIVE MANAGEMENT

Operative management of labral pathology due to trauma was first described by Altenberg, who reported on two patients successfully treated with open labral excision (36). This is one of the earliest reports implicating the traumatic injury to the acetabular labrum as a source of hip pain. Since that time, several studies have been published describing multiple techniques for the evaluation and management of labral pathology (37). As hip arthroscopy has developed over the last several decades, most lesions of the acetabular labrum can be managed with this technique.

Hip arthroscopy is preferably performed under general anesthesia with appropriate muscular relaxation to allow adequate distraction of the hip joint. The patient is positioned supine with both extremities secured on a standard fracture table or using a commercially available device/table for hip distraction with placement of a well-padded perineal post. A thorough exam under anesthesia must be performed to determine the passive range of hip flexion, internal rotation, and external rotation.

The operative hip is then positioned in 10 degrees of flexion, 15 degrees of internal rotation, and neutral abduction. A minimum amount of traction is then applied to the operative extremity to obtain 6 to 8 mm of joint distraction to allow intra-articular instrument placement. Fluoroscopic image intensification is used to confirm joint distraction and procedural assistance and is also used to arrange to match preoperative imaging to compare the actual and planned procedures to help avoid iatrogenic overresection, potentially leading to hip instability, or underresection, particularly of posterosuperior pincer-type lesions (38–40).

A standard anterolateral portal for placement of the arthroscope is initially established under fluoroscopic guidance, typically located approximately 1 to 2 cm anterior and 1 to 2 cm proximal to the anterosuperior aspect of the greater trochanter. Placement of an anterior portal and other accessory portals are performed as necessary under direct visualization. The typical anterior portal is accessed at the intersection between a line from the anterior superior iliac spine (ASIS) down the shaft of the femur and a horizontal line at the level of the superior aspect of the greater trochanter. However, the authors prefer a modified anterior portal that is placed more laterally and distally to the standard anterior portal. This portal placement increases our distance from the lateral femoral cutaneous nerve (LFCN) and improves the trajectory for instrumentation of the labrum and acetabular rim. Once established, these portals allow excellent visualization and access for manipulation of the entire anterior, posterior, and lateral aspects of the labrum utilizing a combination of 30- and 70-degree arthroscopes. Evaluation of the femoroacetabular articular surfaces and management of concurrent pathology is also facilitated (38,39,41).

Access of the joint is performed utilizing a transverse interportal capsulotomy that is made using a beaver blade to preserve full-thickness capsular margins for later repair. Attention to remain between the labrum and femoral head to avoid iatrogenic labral or chondral injury is important. Initial arthroscopic evaluation of the labrum includes a thorough visual inspection followed by mechanical probing of the integrity of the structure. Careful attention should be paid to areas of tearing or fraying and associated degenerative changes. The location of the pathology within the substance of the labrum should also be considered as this can have implications for the likelihood of labral healing. Histological studies show that the distal third of the labral cartilage is relatively avascular and is likely to have poor healing potential. In contrast, the peripheral two thirds have been demonstrated histologically to contain a much more robust vascular supply with the added possibility of neovascularization from the neighboring synovium. This likely contributes to the ability of certain labral tears to be repaired primarily and preserve its protective function within the hip (9).

A thorough assessment of the labrum determines the management strategy that is employed. Current options for the majority of labral pathologies consist of debridement and repair. Recent studies have demonstrated that preservation and refixation of the labrum likely results in improved outcomes, but debridement may be necessary in the presence of significant intrasubstance cystic degeneration or ossification. If the labrum appears relatively normal with an intact chondrolabral junction, smaller areas of bony prominence of the acetabular rim may be resected via extracapsular exposure without formal detachment of the labrum. Labral debridement involves removing small, unstable radial and flap tears in the peripheral margin of the labrum that contribute to pain and mechanical symptoms. The goal is removal of abnormal tissue and any area potentially contributing to the patient's symptoms while preserving as much of the overall integrity as possible to minimize the deleterious effects of labral deficiency. This may be accomplished with a motorized shaver, a

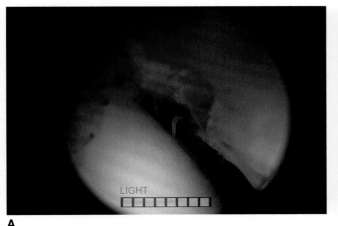
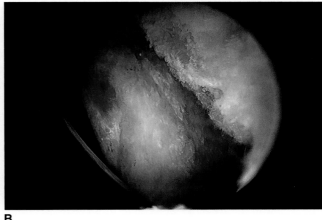

A   **B**

FIGURE 48-2

A: Degenerative tearing of the acetabular labrum, note the intrasubstance tearing of the labral tissue and the detachment of the labral base from the acetabular rim. **B:** Acetabular rim following debridement to a stable base for labral tissue reattachment.

flexible ligament chisel, or a monopolar radiofrequency ablation probe (42). The tissue should be gently debrided to a stable base (Fig. 48-2A and B). Attention must be paid to possible intra-articular sources of the labral tear including FAI, loose bodies, or other associated abnormalities. Direct arthroscopic observation of the labrum through a full ROM will help to identify contributing pathology that can subsequently be managed appropriately.

However, when more extensive bony resection is required, such as profunda deformities or significant focal rim resections, labral takedown, rim resection, and labral refixation are recommended. Once labral takedown and adequate rim resection is complete, labral refixation is indicated to reestablish femoral stability and maintain a physiologic joint seal (11,43). As previously discussed, the vascular supply at the base of the labrum is robust and can facilitate tissue healing. Reapproximation and preservation of the labral integrity manages to restore the native anatomy, provide relief of pain, and possibly slow the progression of degenerative osteoarthritis. This is accomplished through the maintenance of joint stability, fluid dynamics within the hip, and stress shielding of the femoroacetabular articular cartilage (44).

Following characterization of a labral tear through arthroscopic examination and probing, the extent of the labral tear must be determined through the mechanical debridement of surrounding nonviable tissue. This will often reveal the tear to be larger than initially appreciated on MRA or preliminary examination. Labral tears amenable to repair generally fall into one of two characteristic patterns.

The first pattern is a longitudinal detachment from the acetabular rim, analogous to a bucket-handle tear commonly encountered during management of meniscal tears. This longitudinal tearing generally occurs at the transition zone between the hyaline articular cartilage and the fibrocartilaginous labrum. On visual inspection, the labrum appears to have separated from the bony acetabular rim. The second characteristic tearing pattern is a midsubstance tear of the labrum oriented along the longitudinal fibers of the structure (4). If the labrum is detached from the bone, suture anchors are utilized to provide initial stabilization of the fibrocartilaginous rim to the acetabular margin. Preparation of the labrum and acetabulum may be completed with a motorized shaver and burr, respectively, to promote labral healing.

Suture anchors are then sequentially placed every 10 to 12 mm along the length of the tear in a distal-to-proximal trajectory to prevent intra-articular penetration. Fluoroscopy may be used for confirmation that the drill is superior to the acetabular sourcil. To avoid iatrogenic cartilage damage, the anchor should be placed slightly off the articular margin on the acetabular rim. During drilling and suture anchor placement, direct visualization of the articular surface is recommended to ensure that the articular surface is not penetrated. We occasionally utilize an accessory distal portal to assure a more favorable trajectory for anchor drilling and insertion that minimizes risk of joint penetration. Depending on anchor type, pretapping the anchor site may assist in preventing iatrogenic chondral injury due to subchondral fracture. Labral base fixation stitches are utilized when possible to minimize eversion and preserve the suction seal, but formal detachment of the labrum or marginal tissue quality may necessitate simple "loop around" stitch configuration (45). The authors prefer that knots be tied in a nonsliding fashion to avoid cutting through the labral tissue during the sliding of the abrasive braided suture material (Fig. 48-3A and B).

Operative management of pincer-type FAI and acetabular retroversion frequently involves elevating the labrum from its bony attachment prior to performing an osteoplasty. Following adequate resection of bony pathology, the labrum is then reattached via a technique similar to the one previously described for longitudinal labral tears occurring along the fibrocartilaginous rim.

Intrasubstance tears of the labrum oriented longitudinally are also amenable to arthroscopic repair. An interrupted suture technique involves utilizing arthroscopic instrumentation to place a suture through the peripheral margin of the tear between the articular surface and the proximal edge of the lesion. The suture is then passed distal to the tear and retrieved. The lesion is reapproximated as the suture is tied in an arthroscopic fashion with the knot placed extra-articular (1). Repair enhancement techniques, such as those used to augment red-white and white-white meniscal repair, may be of benefit in management of these intrasubstance longitudinal labral tears due to the decreased tissue vascularity in the more distal regions of the labrum. These include labral rasping, placement of a fibrin clot, growth factors, serum augmentation, and synovial abrasion. Such modalities may further assist with tissue regeneration as histological models have demonstrated a persistent superficial cleft located on the articular side of the labrum following repair and subsequent healing of an intrasubstance tear. This has been attributed to incomplete healing of intralabral portions of the tear (46).

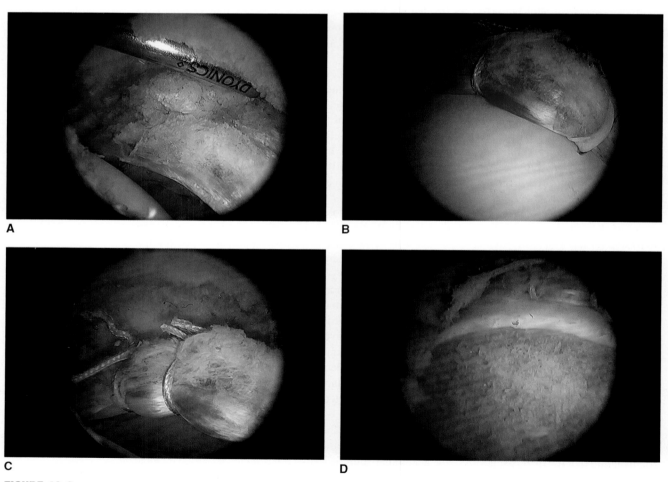

A   **B**

C   **D**

FIGURE 48-3

Repair of a longitudinal labral tear at the acetabular rim. The tear is debrided and probed **(A)**. The acetabular base is debrided, and suture anchors are sequentially placed at the rim along the length of the tear. Looped stitches are tied with knots facing away from the joint to secure the labrum to the base **(B–C)**. A femoral neck osteoplasty was performed to address the source of labral tearing and verified to not impinge arthroscopically with flexion, adduction, and internal rotation **(D)**.

Repair of radial tears with disruption of the longitudinal fibers is not well described, but this may provide some benefit due to the unique mechanical properties of the labrum. The continuous attachment of the labrum to the bony acetabular rim may provide partial continued stability in the presence of radial clefting. While the intra-articular seal is disrupted, the "bumper effect" of the labrum and contribution to the acetabular depth remain and may provide continued benefit.

The importance of diagnosing and treating pathology associated with the initial development of the labral tear at the time of debridement or repair cannot be stressed enough. This may include capsular plication for laxity, rim trim/acetabuloplasty for pincher FAI, or osteoplasty for cam FAI. Failure to manage these concomitant pathologies may lead to recurrence and poor postoperative results (7).

POSTOPERATIVE REHABILITATION

Rehabilitation following surgery is largely dependent on what is done intraoperatively to address the patient's hip pathology. Cheatham et al. performed a systematic review of six available literature in regard to postoperative rehabilitation and found that the available evidence supports a postoperative period of restricted weight bearing and mobility, which may result in improve efficacy for patient function, satisfaction, and return to competitive-level athletics (47). Additionally, another systematic review by Gzybowski et al. that included 18 studies consisting of 2,092 patients found that high heterogenicity in the current literature makes it difficult to determine any superiority of one program as compared to any other (48). Therefore, postoperative protocols are overall based on some fundamental principles but are dependent largely on physician preference and experience.

In general, the early phase of rehabilitation focuses largely on protecting the labrum through restricting specific positions of the hip while encouraging early motion. Early stationary bike riding without resistance along with a continuous passive motion machine (CPM) is helpful to help reduce postoperative stiffness. The CPM is also helpful in the immediate postoperative period to help maintain a neutral position of the hip during sleep. In cases where labral debridement is performed with or without minor recontouring of the acetabular rim, patients are able to resume weight bearing without restrictions postoperatively. Therapy for these patients is directed at restoring ROM and dynamic stabilizer strengthening. Hip flexion isotonic exercises are avoided early on and typically started after 4 weeks. The later phase of rehabilitation focuses on progressive lower extremity strengthen and ROM exercises, with sport-specific agility drills and plyometric after 3 months. Conversely, when a labral repair is performed, it is necessary to protect the repair postoperatively. Patients are limited to protected weight bearing on the operative extremity and are instructed to avoid deep flexion and external rotation > 20 degrees for the first month following surgery as this stresses the anterosuperior joint capsule. Progressive stretching and strengthening focusing on restoring muscle function, ROM, and neuromuscular control occurs over the next few months with sport-specific agility training beginning after 3 to 4 months.

COMPLICATIONS

Hip arthroscopy has a unique set of complications secondary to a steep learning curve coupled with challenging and often difficult to access anatomy. A brief overview of complications is presented in Table 48-1. Underresection of FAI pathology leading to reoperation is another complication associated with hip arthroscopy. Several authors have identified that persistent FAI or labral pathology is the most common reason for revision hip arthroscopy (49–51). To help ensure complete resection of all offending bony pathology, we will routinely use intraoperative fluoroscopy to evaluate the hip in various degrees of rotation.

A systematic review by Harris and colleagues consisting of over 6,000 patients reported the rate of major complications to be 0.58%, whereas the rate of minor complications was 7.5% (52). The most commonly reported complication was iatrogenic chondrolabral injury, which represented 57.6% of all reported complication. Nerve injuries were the second most commonly reported complication (17%) and with the exception of one case, all were transient neuropraxias. The most commonly involved nerves were the pudendal, LFCN, and sciatic nerve (in order of decreasing frequency) (52). The LFCN or its branches are always at risk with anterior portal placement. Proper padding of the perineal post and shorter traction times may help decrease the risk of pudendal neuropraxia.

TABLE 48-1 Complications Associated with Hip Arthroscopy

1. Iatrogenic chondrolabral injury
2. Neuropraxia (sciatic, lateral femoral cutaneous nerve and pudendal nerve)
3. Underresection of FAI
4. Direct neurovascular trauma
5. Osteonecrosis of the femoral head
6. Compression injury to the perineum
7. Fluid extravasation into the abdomen
8. Iatrogenic hip instability or fracture
9. DVT/PE

Weber et al. subsequently performed another systematic review of the complications following hip arthroscopy involving 53 studies and 8,189 hip arthroscopies performed in 8,071 subjects, finding that minor and major complication rates were 7.9% and 0.45%, respectively (53). Iatrogenic damage to the chondral surfaces or the labrum was the most common minor complication encountered, occurring in 4% of cases. Nerve injuries were rare, with pudendal nerve neuropraxia (0.79%) and LFCN neuropraxia (0.43%) as the two most common presentations. Major complications (fluid extravasations, hip dislocations, deep vein thrombosis (DVT)/pulmonary embolism (PE), septic arthrosis, AVN, femoral neck fracture, and death) were also rare, with fluid extravasation being the most frequent in 0.15% of case.

Duplantier et al. published a systematic review of hip dislocation or subluxation following hip arthroscopy, analyzing 10 articles consisting of 11 patients and determined that postarthroscopic hip instability was observed in patients with labral debridement, acetabular undercoverage (including iatrogenic resection), capsular insufficiency, or iliopsoas tenotomy (54). Additional rare, albeit catastrophic, complications have also been reported following hip arthroscopy (39,49,55–58). The rate of these complications is exceptionally low, however not insignificant. It is essential for physicians to be aware of these complications in an effort to not only improve surgical technique but to also appropriately inform patients regarding the risk of surgery.

RESULTS

Both labral debridement and repair have demonstrated significant improvements in pain and hip function postoperatively. Haddad et al. recently performed a systematic review of the literature reviewing debridement and reattachment of acetabular labral tears, including 28 studies representing a total of 1,609 patients (1,631 hips) (59). In their analysis, 12 studies were reviewed, which represented 506 patients (510 hips) who underwent labral debridement and found that the mean rate for good or excellent outcomes (modified Harris Hip Score [mHHS] > 80, pain improvement, satisfaction) was 82% in the absence of any observed OA. When examining the five available comparative studies at the time of publication, the authors determined that labral repair demonstrated good to excellent results, as well as superior satisfaction scores as compared to debridement cases.

Ayeni et al. subsequently performed the largest high-quality systematic review to date more specifically analyzing studies directly comparing patients undergoing labral debridement and those receiving labral repair, analyzing 490 subjects from six unique investigations reporting labral repair outcomes (60). Labral repair outcomes consistently and reliably outperformed labral debridement in a multitude of patient-reported outcome scores (mHHS, Hip Outcome Score (HOS), Non-Arthritic Hip Score, and Merle d'Aubigné score). The mHHS was pooled from three studies, which utilized the outcome in comparison of the two procedures and demonstrated that labral repair is associated with statistically significant clinically important difference in means between groups of 7.41 in favor of labral repair when compared to labral debridement. Methodological quality was rated individually as fair; however, GRADE recommendation was calculated to be low. However, it should be noted that a subsequent comparative study by Cetinkaya et al., which analyzed 34 patients who received labral debridement compared to 33 patients who received labral repair, found no significant difference in daily HOS between groups ($p > 0.05$) (61).

It is critical to understand that the presence of associated chondral lesions or preexisting osteoarthritis (OA) is likely one of the most critical prognostic factors when managing labral tears, regardless of technique. Farjo et al. reported that only 21% of patients with OA had a good to excellent result following labral debridement, and 42.9% went on to total hip arthroplasty (THA) at an average of 14 months postoperatively (62). Mftah et al. found that only 19% of patients with OA reported good to excellent results following labral debridement, with two case progressing to THA due to advancing arthritis (63). Arthritis had a significant correlation with low postoperative Harris Hip Scores and satisfaction (63). Byrd et al. reported that 88% (7 of 8) of patients who had evidence of degenerative change prior to hip arthroscopy were converted to THA at an average of 63 months (64). Philippon et al. found that patients with a joint space on radiographs of < 2 mm were 39 times more likely to progress to a THA at a mean time of 16 months following hip arthroscopy in a mixed group of labral repair and debridement cases (65).

CONCLUSIONS

The hip acetabular labrum is a critical structure in the appropriate function of the femoroacetabular joint. While it is most commonly injured in the setting of FAI, labral damage may also be a result of dysplasia, extra-articular impingement, and other pathology. Through evaluation of the objective and subjective findings is important for appropriate treatment recommendations. Initial conservative management may provide relief to some patients; however, when significant symptoms persist, hip arthroscopy has demonstrated superior results in alleviating pain. In addition to labrum, the underlying osseous deformity leading to pathology must be addressed. Several short-term and midterm comparative studies examining labral debridement and repair have been recently been published, providing a body of evidence for decision-making, which was previously unavailable. Intraoperatively, the literature supports labral refixation as the primary technique when available tissue allows a repair as opposed to debridement, demonstrating excellent short-term and midterm patient reported outcomes in nonarthritic patients.

REFERENCES

1. Kelly BT, Weiland DE, Schenker ML, et al. Arthroscopic labral repair in the hip: surgical technique and review of the literature. *Arthrosc J Arthrosc Relat Surg.* 2005;21:1496–1504.
2. Martin RL, Enseki KR, Draovitch P, et al. Acetabular labral tears of the hip: examination and diagnostic challenges. *J Orthop Sports Phys Ther.* 2006;36:503–515.
3. Philippon MJ. New frontiers in hip arthroscopy: the role of arthroscopic hip labral repair and capsulorrhaphy in the treatment of hip disorders. *Instr Course Lect.* 2006;55:309–316.
4. Seldes RM, Tan V, Hunt J, et al. Anatomy, histologic features, and vascularity of the adult acetabular labrum. *Clin Orthop.* 2001;232–240.
5. Harris WH, Bourne RB, Oh I. Intra-articular acetabular labrum: a possible etiological factor in certain cases of osteoarthritis of the hip. *J Bone Joint Surg Am.* 1979;61:510–514.
6. Botser IB, Smith TW, Nasser R, et al. Open surgical dislocation versus arthroscopy for femoroacetabular impingement: a comparison of clinical outcomes. *Arthrosc J Arthrosc Relat Surg Off Publ Arthrosc Assoc N Am Int Arthrosc Assoc.* 2011;27:270–278.
7. Larson CM, Giveans MR. Arthroscopic management of femoroacetabular impingement: early outcomes measures. *Arthrosc J Arthrosc Relat Surg.* 2008;24:540–546.
8. Kelly BT, Shapiro GS, Digiovanni CW, et al. Vascularity of the hip labrum: a cadaveric investigation. *Arthrosc J Arthrosc Relat Surg Off Publ Arthrosc Assoc N Am Int Arthrosc Assoc.* 2005;21:3–11.
9. Petersen W, Petersen F, Tillmann B. Structure and vascularization of the acetabular labrum with regard to the pathogenesis and healing of labral lesions. *Arch Orthop Trauma Surg.* 2003;123:283–288.
10. Nicholas J, Hershman E. *The Lower Extremity and Spine in Sports Medicine.* St. Louis, MO: Mosby Co; 1986.
11. Crawford MJ, Dy CJ, Alexander JW, et al. The 2007 Frank Stinchfield Award. The biomechanics of the hip labrum and the stability of the hip. *Clin Orthop.* 2007;465:16–22.
12. Nepple JJ, Philippon MJ, Campbell KJ, et al. The hip fluid seal—Part II: the effect of an acetabular labral tear, repair, resection, and reconstruction on hip stability to distraction. *Knee Surg Sports Traumatol Arthrosc Off J ESSKA.* 2014;22:730–736.
13. Philippon MJ, Nepple JJ, Campbell KJ, et al. The hip fluid seal—Part I: the effect of an acetabular labral tear, repair, resection, and reconstruction on hip fluid pressurization. *Knee Surg Sports Traumatol Arthrosc Off J ESSKA.* 2014;22:722–729.
14. Ferguson SJ, Bryant JT, Ganz R, et al. An in vitro investigation of the acetabular labral seal in hip joint mechanics. *J Biomech.* 2003;36:171–178.
15. Ferguson SJ, Bryant JT, Ganz R, et al. The acetabular labrum seal: a poroelastic finite element model. *Clin Biomech (Bristol, Avon).* 2000;15:463–468.
16. Ferguson SJ, Bryant JT, Ganz R, et al. The influence of the acetabular labrum on hip joint cartilage consolidation: a poroelastic finite element model. *J Biomech.* 2000;33:953–960.
17. Konrath GA, Hamel AJ, Olson SA, et al. The role of the acetabular labrum and the transverse acetabular ligament in load transmission in the hip. *J Bone Joint Surg Am.* 1998;80:1781–1788.
18. Soltz MA, Ateshian GA. Experimental verification and theoretical prediction of cartilage interstitial fluid pressurization at an impermeable contact interface in confined compression. *J Biomech.* 1998;31:927–934.

19. Song Y, Ito H, Kourtis L, et al. Articular cartilage friction increases in hip joints after the removal of acetabular labrum. *J Biomech.* 2012;45:524–530.

20. McCarthy JC, Noble PC, Schuck MR, et al. The watershed labral lesion: its relationship to early arthritis of the hip. *J Arthroplasty.* 2001;16:81–87.

21. McCarthy J, Busconi B. The role of hip arthroscopy in the diagnosis and treatment of hip disease. *Orthopedics.* 1995;18:753–756.

22. Keeney JA, Peelle MW, Jackson J, et al. Magnetic resonance arthrography versus arthroscopy in the evaluation of articular hip pathology. *Clin Orthop.* 2004;163–169.

23. Narvani AA, Tsiridis E, Kendall S, et al. A preliminary report on prevalence of acetabular labrum tears in sports patients with groin pain. *Knee Surg Sports Traumatol Arthrosc.* 2003;11:403–408.

24. Tibor LM, Sekiya JK. Differential diagnosis of pain around the hip joint. *Arthrosc J Arthrosc Relat Surg Off Publ Arthrosc Assoc N Am Int Arthrosc Assoc.* 2008;24:1407–1421.

25. Scopp JM, Moorman CT. The assessment of athletic hip injury. *Clin Sports Med.* 2001;20:647–659.

26. Ito K, Leunig M, Ganz R. Histopathologic features of the acetabular labrum in femoroacetabular impingement. *Clin Orthop* 2004;262–271.

27. Mitchell B, McCrory P, Brukner P, et al. Hip joint pathology: clinical presentation and correlation between magnetic resonance arthrography, ultrasound, and arthroscopic findings in 25 consecutive cases. *Clin J Sport Med Off J Can Acad Sport Med.* 2003;13:152–156.

28. Kelly BT, Williams RJ, Philippon MJ. Hip arthroscopy: current indications, treatment options, and management issues. *Am J Sports Med.* 2003;31:1020–1037.

29. Yamamoto Y, Tonotsuka H, Ueda T, et al. Usefulness of radial contrast-enhanced computed tomography for the diagnosis of acetabular labrum injury. *Arthrosc J Arthrosc Relat Surg Off Publ Arthrosc Assoc N Am Int Arthrosc Assoc.* 2007;23:1290–1294.

30. Edwards DJ, Lomas D, Villar RN. Diagnosis of the painful hip by magnetic resonance imaging and arthroscopy. *J Bone Joint Surg Br.* 1995;77:374–376.

31. Czerny C, Hofmann S, Urban M, et al. MR arthrography of the adult acetabular capsular-labral complex: correlation with surgery and anatomy. *AJR Am J Roentgenol.* 1999;173:345–349.

32. Czerny C, Kramer J, Neuhold A, et al. [Magnetic resonance imaging and magnetic resonance arthrography of the acetabular labrum: comparison with surgical findings]. *ROFO Fortschr Geb Rontgenstr Nuklearmed.* 2001;173:702–707.

33. Lage LA, Patel JV, Villar RN. The acetabular labral tear: an arthroscopic classification. *Arthroscopy.* 1996;12:269–272.

34. Blankenbaker DG, De Smet AA, Keene JS, et al. Classification and localization of acetabular labral tears. *Skeletal Radiol.* 2007;36:391–397.

35. Hunt D, Prather H, Harris Hayes M, et al. Clinical outcomes analysis of conservative and surgical treatment of patients with clinical indications of prearthritic, intra-articular hip disorders. *PM R.* 2012;4:479–487.

36. Altenberg AR. Acetabular labrum tears: a cause of hip pain and degenerative arthritis. *South Med J.* 1977;70:174–175.

37. Ikeda T, Awaya G, Suzuki S, et al. Torn acetabular labrum in young-patients—arthroscopic diagnosis and management. *J Bone Jt Surg Br Vol.* 1988;70:13–16.

38. Crawford K, Philippon MJ, Sekiya JK, et al. Microfracture of the hip in athletes. *Clin Sports Med.* 2006;25:327–335, x.

39. Ranawat AS, McClincy M, Sekiya JK. Anterior dislocation of the hip after arthroscopy in a patient with capsular laxity of the hip. A case report. *J Bone Jt Surg.* 2009;91:192–197.

40. Zumstein M, Hahn F, Sukthankar A, et al. How accurately can the acetabular rim be trimmed in hip arthroscopy for pincer-type femoral acetabular impingement: a cadaveric investigation. *Arthrosc J Arthrosc Relat Surg.* 2009;25:164–168.

41. Byrd JW. Hip arthroscopy. The supine position. *Clin Sports Med.* 2001;20:703–731.

42. Philippon MJ. Debridement of acetabular labral tears with associated thermal capsulorrhaphy. *Oper Tech Sports Med.* 2002;10:215–218.

43. Philippon MJ, Schenker ML. Arthroscopy for the treatment of femoroacetabular impingement in the athlete. *Clin Sports Med.* 2006;25:299–308, ix.

44. Dameron TB. Bucket-handle tear of acetabular labrum accompanying posterior dislocation of the hip. From J Bone Joint Surg 41A:131–134, 1959. *Clin Orthop.* 2003;8–10.

45. Larson CM. Arthroscopic management of pincer-type impingement. *Sports Med Arthrosc Rev.* 2010;18:100–107.

46. Philippon MJ, Arnoczky SP, Torrie A. Arthroscopic repair of the acetabular labrum: a histologic assessment of healing in an ovine model. *Arthrosc J Arthrosc Relat Surg Off Publ Arthrosc Assoc N Am Int Arthrosc Assoc.* 2007;23:376–380.

47. Cheatham SW, Enseki KR, Kolber MJ. Postoperative rehabilitation after hip arthroscopy: a search for the evidence. *J Sport Rehabil.* 2015;24:413–418.

48. Grzybowski JS, Malloy P, Stegemann C, et al. Rehabilitation following hip arthroscopy—a systematic review. *Front Surg.* 2015;2:21.

49. Clohisy JC, Nepple JJ, Larson CM, et al., Academic Network of Conservation Hip Outcome Research (ANCHOR) Members. Persistent structural disease is the most common cause of repeat hip preservation surgery. *Clin Orthop.* 2013;471:3788–3794.

50. Heyworth BE, Shindle MK, Voos JE, et al. Radiologic and intraoperative findings in revision hip arthroscopy. *Arthrosc J Arthrosc Relat Surg Off Publ Arthrosc Assoc N Am Int Arthrosc Assoc.* 2007;23:1295–1302.

51. Philippon MJ, Schenker ML, Briggs KK, et al. Revision hip arthroscopy. *Am J Sports Med.* 2007;35:1918–1921.

52. Harris JD, McCormick FM, Abrams GD, et al. Complications and reoperations during and after hip arthroscopy: a systematic review of 92 studies and more than 6,000 patients. *Arthrosc J Arthrosc Relat Surg Off Publ Arthrosc Assoc N Am Int Arthrosc Assoc.* 2013;29:589–595.

53. Weber AE, Harris JD, Nho SJ. Complications in hip arthroscopy: a systematic review and strategies for prevention. *Sports Med Arthrosc Rev.* 2015;23:187–193.

54. Duplantier NL, McCulloch PC, Nho SJ, et al. Hip dislocation or subluxation after hip arthroscopy: a systematic review. *Arthrosc J Arthrosc Relat Surg Off Publ Arthrosc Assoc N Am Int Arthrosc Assoc.* 2016;32:1428–1434.

55. Ayeni OR, Bedi A, Lorich DG, et al. Femoral neck fracture after arthroscopic management of femoroacetabular impingement: a case report. *J Bone Joint Surg Am.* 2011;93:e47.

56. Fowler J, Owens BD. Abdominal compartment syndrome after hip arthroscopy. *Arthrosc J Arthrosc Relat Surg Off Publ Arthrosc Assoc N Am Int Arthrosc Assoc.* 2010;26:128–130.

57. Matsuda DK. Acute iatrogenic dislocation following hip impingement arthroscopic surgery. *Arthrosc J Arthrosc Amp Relat Surg.* 2009;25:400–404.

58. Mei-Dan O, McConkey MO, Brick M. Catastrophic failure of hip arthroscopy due to iatrogenic instability: can partial division of the ligamentum teres and iliofemoral ligament cause subluxation? *Arthrosc J Arthrosc Relat Surg Off Publ Arthrosc Assoc N Am Int Arthrosc Assoc.* 2012;28:440–445.

59. Haddad B, Konan S, Haddad FS. Debridement versus re-attachment of acetabular labral tears. *Bone Jt J.* 2014;96-B:24–30.

60. Ayeni OR, Adamich J, Farrokhyar F, et al. Surgical management of labral tears during femoroacetabular impingement surgery: a systematic review. *Knee Surg Sports Traumatol Arthrosc.* 2014;22:756–762.

61. Cetinkaya S, Toker B, Ozden VE, et al. Arthroscopic labral repair versus labral debridement in patients with femoroacetabular impingement: a minimum 2.5 year follow-up study. *Hip Int J Clin Exp Res Hip Pathol Ther.* 2016;26:20–24.

62. Farjo LA, Glick JM, Sampson TG. Hip arthroscopy for acetabular labral tears. *Arthrosc J Arthrosc Relat Surg Off Publ Arthrosc Assoc N Am Int Arthrosc Assoc.* 1999;15:132–137.

63. Meftah M, Rodriguez JA, Panagopoulos G, et al. Long-term results of arthroscopic labral debridement: predictors of outcomes. *Orthopedics.* 2011;34:e588–e592.

64. Byrd JWT, Jones KS. Hip arthroscopy for labral pathology: prospective analysis with 10-year follow-up. *Arthrosc J Arthrosc Relat Surg Off Publ Arthrosc Assoc N Am Int Arthrosc Assoc.* 2009;25:365–368.

65. Philippon MJ, Briggs KK, Yen Y-M, et al. Outcomes following hip arthroscopy for femoroacetabular impingement with associated chondrolabral dysfunction: minimum two-year follow-up. *J Bone Joint Surg Br.* 2009;91:16–23.

49 Hip Arthroscopy, Femoroacetabular Impingement, and Instability of the Athlete's Hip

James B. Cowan, Zachary Vaughn, and Marc R. Safran

FEMOROACETABULAR IMPINGEMENT

Background

The pathology of femoroacetabular impingement (FAI) was formally described (1992) and published (1995) by Ganz, but first presented in the English literature in 1999 (1). Although FAI is a three-dimensional disorder with varying degrees and anatomic locations of pathologies, two main forms of impingement have been described. The first description was of an abnormality in acetabular overcoverage, known as pincer impingement. This results in crushing of the labrum and acetabular rim against the femoral head-neck junction, which can lead to complex degenerative labral tearing, edge loading of the acetabular rim, calcific changes to the labrum with possible labral ossification, and a "contrecoup" lesion of chondromalacia in the posterior aspect of the acetabulum and femoral head from subtle subluxation of the femoral head as it levers on the anterior acetabular rim (2–7).

The second form of FAI is cam impingement, resulting from a bony abnormality of the femoral head-neck junction with a loss of normal femoral head sphericity and femoral head-neck offset. This abnormal area of bone leads to labral-chondral separation and a delamination of articular cartilage at the acetabular periphery. Cam FAI anatomy is particularly prevalent in athletes, as it is thought the forces on the femoral head physis result in abnormal growth at the femoral head-neck junction (8,9). Additionally, cam anatomy may be seen in conjunction with dysplasia, as femoral head growth is not limited by the acetabulum, as well as with slipped capital femoral epiphysis (SCFE), which results in a deformity with loss of the femoral head-neck offset. Although characterized as separate entities, it is most common to have both types of FAI, although one form may predominate (2–7). The goal of treatment of FAI is to restore the normal anatomy of the acetabulum and the femoral head-neck junction, while also treating any associated pathology of the labrum and/or articular cartilage. Both open and arthroscopic techniques have been described for the treatment of FAI; however, recent advances in hip arthroscopy have made the arthroscopic treatment of intra-articular and extra-articular components of FAI a safe and reliable procedure in experienced hands.

A third, distinct, less-common, type of impingement between the pelvis and proximal femur is subspine impingement. This extra-articular pincer-type impingement was first described in 2011 and refers to impingement that occurs between the anterior inferior iliac spine (AIIS) and the distal femoral neck (10–12). Patients with subspine impingement may present quite similarly to patients with classic pincer impingement or acetabular retroversion, and AIIS morphology may even be responsible for a crossover sign seen on an appropriately positioned standard AP pelvis radiograph (13).

Recognition of this distinction is crucial, as performing an acetabuloplasty on a patient with sub-spine impingement could result in persistent symptoms or iatrogenic hip instability or dysplasia.

We believe that the labrum has several significant functions including increasing articular surface area, increasing acetabular volume, providing a fluid seal between the central and peripheral compartments, and providing a barrier to fluid flow from within articular cartilage (14,15). Thus, if a labral tear is reparable, then we will repair the labrum in conjunction with FAI surgery. If the labrum is damaged within its substance to the point of being irreparable, we will perform a partial labrectomy and, in situations of a shallow acetabulum and/or instability, a labral reconstruction with a free graft.

Indications and Contraindications

Indications

Hip arthroscopy has seen an increase in interest since the 1980s that has brought about a constant state of evolution with the advent of new instrumentation, improved knowledge of safety and techniques, and increasing surgeon experience, all of which have allowed for an expanding list of indications. Arthroscopic treatment for FAI is indicated only for patients with symptomatic FAI, with or without associated labral or chondral injury, as FAI morphology among asymptomatic individuals is not uncommon (16–19). Some authors believe that surgery for even asymptomatic FAI should be performed to prevent arthritis. Not everyone with FAI morphology will develop arthritis, and even though FAI may be a major cause of premature degenerative arthritis, there is no evidence that surgery for FAI will prevent arthritis (14). It is likely that the combination of this underlying anatomic morphology and various activities that require an extended range of motion (such as cycling, running, soccer, and martial arts) will result in the breakdown of soft tissues, resulting in symptomatic impingement. Therefore, we recommend that only the hip with symptoms that can be attributed to FAI should be treated surgically.

Contraindications

The arthroscopic treatment of FAI is contraindicated in any patient who has contraindications to general anesthesia or elective surgical interventions based on medical comorbidities or infections. Patients with evidence of significant degenerative changes on plain radiographs with joint space narrowing or a predominance of aching pain at rest due to arthritis are not likely to have significant benefit from arthroscopy (20–24). Surgical treatment of FAI should also be avoided in patients who do not obtain even temporary symptom relief with an intra-articular injection of local anesthetic and further evaluation should be directed at other diagnoses.

Preoperative Planning

History

Patients with symptomatic FAI generally present with an insidious onset of aching pain in the hip and groin. Common aggravating activities include putting on or taking off shoes and socks, motions that generate deep flexion of the hip joint, sitting for prolonged periods of time, arising from a seated position, ascending or descending stairs or steep hills, sudden starts and stops, or cutting and pivoting motions (25). The pain is typically worsened with impact activity and is described as originating from the groin, inguinal region, or deep within the joint (25). Patients may also note a gradual decrease in range of motion, particularly in flexion, adduction, and internal rotation (26). More abrupt onset of symptoms may be associated with a labral tear, labral-chondral separation, or a chondral flap, any of which can present with mechanical symptoms of painful locking, clicking, or catching.

Physical Examination

A complete review of the evaluation of the hip is beyond the scope of this chapter, but the reader is referred to references (27–29). A complete examination of the hip will include evaluating core and abdominal strength and ruling out pathology from the spine and knee. The initial examination begins with inspection of stance, gait, and the skin about the hip. Trendelenburg and Ober tests are utilized to evaluate weakness and tightness of the hip abductors, respectively. Hip range of motion must be carefully documented in the supine position and compared with the unaffected side. In patients with impingement, there is typically limited internal rotation, particularly when the hip is flexed to 90 degrees. A positive impingement test is elicited with pain generated when the hip is brought to 90 degrees of flexion, adducted across the midline, and internally rotated (Fig. 49-1). For the

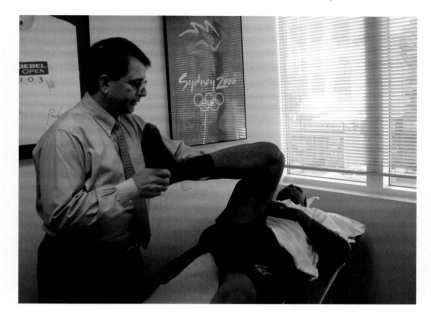

FIGURE 49-1

Impingement test. With the patient supine, the examiner brings the patient's hip to 90 degrees of flexion, adducts the hip, and then internally rotates the hip. Reproduction of groin pain is consistent with a positive impingement test, often associated with intra-articular hip pain. (Figure used by permission of Marc R. Safran, MD.)

subspine impingement test, the patient is supine and the thigh is passively brought into maximum flexion with neutral abduction and rotation. A positive test occurs when the patient's anterior pain is reproduced, often with limited flexion when compared to the contralateral side, indicating impingement between the AIIS and the distal anterolateral femoral neck (30). The patient with AIIS impingement may also have discomfort with rectus femoris stretching, assessed with the patient supine, the ipsilateral buttock at the edge of the examination table, and the symptomatic leg hyperextended over the edge of the table. Additionally, patients may have pain with a labral stress test, also known as the scour maneuver (passive circumduction of the hip from abduction and external rotation with flexion, to a flexed, adducted and internally rotated position with extension), or with a resisted straight leg raise generating groin pain. These tests are often positive in FAI, both cam and pincer types, and with other intra-articular pathology (27–29).

As previously noted, because FAI morphology is not uncommon in asymptomatic individuals, it is important to consider a broad differential diagnosis for patients who present with FAI morphology and hip symptoms. For example, patients may present with hip or groin pain due to disorders of the spine, peripheral nerves, abdomen, or genitourinary structures. Similarly, concomitant diagnoses such as core muscle injury do not occur infrequently with FAI (31–33).

Imaging Studies

Plain radiographs including an AP pelvis with the coccyx centered 1 to 3 cm above the pubic symphysis (Fig. 49-2A) and a true cross-table lateral (Fig. 49-2C) of the affected hip are essential to evaluating patients with hip pain consistent with FAI. The cross-table lateral, Dunn view, and modified Dunn view are true lateral views of the hip that provide information about the proximal femur and the acetabulum and are more useful than the frog-lateral projection (Fig. 49-2B), which provides limited evaluation of the acetabulum. On these images, the femoral head is generally symmetric and has a distinct femoral head-neck offset. The loss of this sphericity in the femoral head and neck region may be consistent with cam impingement (Fig. 49-2A–C) (34–36). This can be demonstrated by a lack of concavity to the femoral head-neck junction on the AP view, appearing that the femoral head is not centered over the femoral neck. In some cases, on the lateral view at the anterolateral femoral head-neck junction, a bony bump may project beyond the femoral head with a sharp transition or even a hook appearance. Pincer impingement can also be well evaluated on these routine radiographs, demonstrating coxa profunda, protrusio, acetabular retroversion, and evidence of developmental dysplasia and arthritic changes. Coxa profunda is demonstrated on the AP pelvis when the floor of medial acetabulum is at or beyond the ilioischial line and the center edge

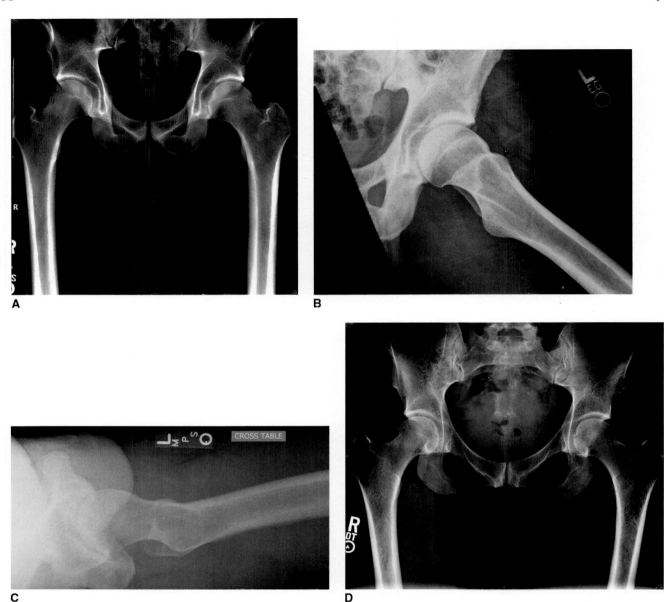

FIGURE 49-2

Combined Type Femoral Acetabular Impingement. **A:** AP pelvis radiograph of a 22-year-old collegiate basketball player that demonstrates the loss of femoral head-neck offset consistent with cam-type FAI. Note how the anterior wall of the acetabulum crosses the posterior wall, resulting in a figure-of-8 sign, indicative of cranial retroversion, seen with pincer impingement in both hips. Also, note the ossification of both hips, more clearly seen on the right hip. Thus, this patient has combined type FAI. **B, C:** Lateral radiographs—a frog lateral and a cross-table lateral radiograph, respectively, demonstrating the loss of femoral head-neck offset with an anterior bump. **D:** An AP pelvis radiograph of a 37-year-old elite female triathlete with bilateral coxa profunda, where the floor of the acetabulum extends beyond the ilioischial line. (Figures used by permission of Marc R. Safran, MD.)

angle is >35 degrees (Figs. 49-2D and 49-3). Protrusio is present when the most medial aspect of the femoral head is found to extend to or beyond the ilioischial line. The crossover sign is indicative of acetabular retroversion as the lines of the anterior wall and posterior wall are found to cross over one another on the properly positioned AP pelvis view (Fig. 49-2A). Dysplasia is evaluated with the lateral center edge angle of Wiberg measured on the AP view or the anterior center edge angle of Lequesne measured on the false profile view of the pelvis. With either measurement, a value of <25 degrees is considered abnormal and a sign of dysplasia (Fig. 49-3).

Additional imaging modalities include CT scans, particularly a 3D reconstruction series, and MRI sequences. The CT scan is helpful for demonstrating the bony anatomy involved in the impingement

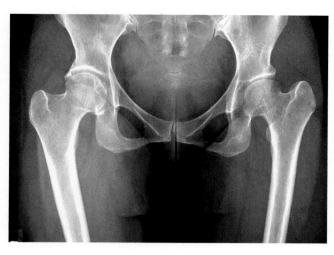

FIGURE 49-3

An AP radiograph of a 27-year-old woman with FAI on her right hip (coxa profunda and calcification of her labrum, functionally making her center edge angle 63 degrees) and dysplasia of her left hip, with a center edge angle of 24 degrees. (Figure used by permission of Marc R. Safran, MD.)

process, including evaluating the anatomy of the AIIS, while the MRI, particularly an MR arthrogram with a small field of view for the hip, is beneficial in alpha angle measurement, demonstrating the cam lesion, labral tears, chondral lesions, edema or cysts within the femoral neck, and femoral version. The alpha angle (Fig. 49-4) as described by Notzli to quantify the femoral head-neck junction offset is based upon measurements on a radially generated axial MRI sequence (37). Most surgeons use 55 degrees as a cutoff value for defining cam impingement; however, the accuracy and reproducibility of this measurement, and a positive correlation between correction of this measurement and surgical outcomes, have not been shown.

Our imaging protocol for the evaluation of FAI is to obtain a proper AP pelvis, cross-table lateral view, and a dedicated hip MR arthrogram utilizing a small field of view, with the use of intra-articular Gadolinium and local anesthetic. This injection helps confirm the intra-articular source of pain with the temporary relief of symptoms from the local anesthetic component (38).

Surgery

The goals of surgery for FAI are to relieve the abutment between the femoral head-neck junction and acetabular rim and to treat any associated pathologies such as labral tears and chondral lesions. While this may be done in the supine or lateral position, our preference is the supine position. The following describes our preferred arthroscopic technique for acetabuloplasty for pincer impingement and cheilectomy (or femoral osteoplasty) for cam impingement.

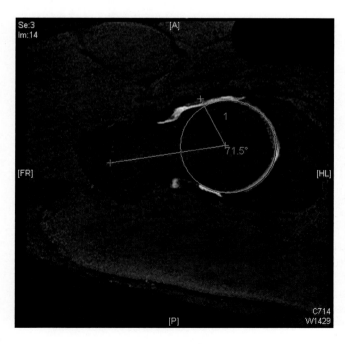

FIGURE 49-4

An example of an MRI from the basketball player in Figure 49-2, with the measurement of the alpha angle of 71 degrees. The alpha angle is measured as a line drawn perpendicular to the narrow part of the femoral neck. A circle is drawn that most closely approximates the head size. A line is drawn from the center of the head to the point where the anterolateral femoral head exceeds the radius of the circle. The angle made by these two lines is the alpha angle. An angle <50 or 55 degrees is considered normal. (Figure used by permission of Marc R. Safran, MD.)

Patient Positioning and Draping

The patient is anesthetized with a general anesthetic in the supine position on a traction or fracture table with the feet well padded in mobile spars for the legs. Paralysis is preferred to reduce the amount of force necessary to achieve adequate joint distraction, reducing the risk of pudendal nerve injury. The patient is brought into position against the padded perineal post and slightly lateralized away from the operative hip to allow for relief of pressure on the perineum and pudendal nerves and to allow for the appropriate direction of force for the traction (39). This places the perineal post against the proximal medial thigh of the operative hip. Gentle traction is applied to the contralateral leg in 45 to 60 degrees of abduction. The operative leg is placed in 10 degrees of abduction, with neutral rotation and neutral flexion-extension. Traction that is applied to the operative leg until 8 to 10 mm of joint space distraction is verified with fluoroscopy. The general room setup is depicted in Figure 49-5.

Operative Technique

The superior aspect of the greater trochanter is identified and the proposed anterolateral portal site is marked (39). This portal is created just anterior to the anterolateral margin of the superior aspect of the greater trochanter. Identification of this portal can be assisted with the use of a spinal needle placed superficially over the hip joint under fluoroscopy to identify the safe path of entry. The area is then prepped with betadine swabs, and an 18-gauge spinal needle is introduced at this site and into the hip joint under fluoroscopic guidance. Careful placement of the spinal needle will allow safe entry without damage to the chondral surfaces or labrum (39). Correct placement can be verified with removal of the stylet from the spinal needle, allowing air to enter the hip joint, creating an air-arthrogram, and relieving the intra-articular negative pressure seal. This verifies positioning and reduces the force necessary to achieve adequate distraction. To minimize total traction time, the needle is then removed and the traction released until after full prepping and draping is completed.

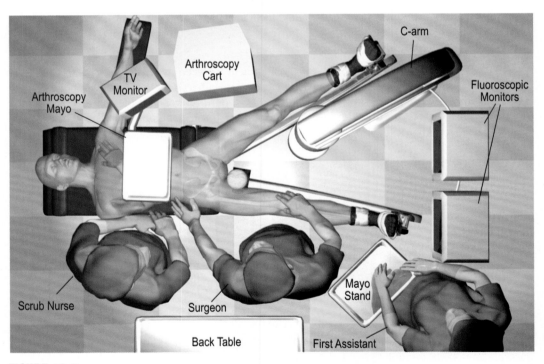

FIGURE 49-5

Typical operating room setup for supine hip arthroscopy utilized by the senior author. The patient is supine on a fracture table, with the perineal post lateralized toward the operative hip. The nonoperative leg is abducted 45 to 60 degrees and slight traction applied. The operative leg is abducted 10 degrees with neutral rotation and neutral flexion-extension. The surgeon, assistant, and scrub nurse are on the same side as the operative hip. The fluoroscopy machine is brought in between the patient's legs. The fluoroscopic monitor is at the foot of the table, while the arthroscopic monitor is across the patient from the surgeon. (Figure used by permission of Marc R. Safran, MD.)

Complete circumferential prepping of the leg to include the knee distally, the abdominal midline, and the iliac crest proximally is required. The sterile drape-covered fluoroscopy unit can be brought into position between the patient's legs and kept in position throughout the procedure (39). Once the patient is prepped and draped, traction is applied once again to the extremity. The anterolateral portal site is once again identified with the use of a spinal needle. Once within the hip joint, the stylet is removed and a guidewire is placed through the spinal needle. The needle is then removed and a superficial skin incision is made with an 11-blade scalpel over the guidewire. A blunt tipped, cannulated trocar is then introduced carefully over the guidewire and can be felt to penetrate the hip capsule and enter the joint (Fig. 49-6). The 70-degree arthroscope is then introduced and the remaining portals are created under arthroscopic visualization. The other described standard portals include a modified anterior portal and a posterolateral portal. The modified anterior portal is 5 to 7 cm distal and anterior-medial to the anterolateral portal at a 45-degree angle (Fig. 49-6). This portal has been used because it reduces the risk of injury to the lateral femoral cutaneous nerve, reduces the risk of postoperative rectus femoris tendinitis, and allows a better approach to the joint should a labral repair be warranted. The modified anterior portal is created in the same technique but augmented by arthroscopic guidance for placement of the spinal needle to avoid the labrum and chondral surfaces. Care should be taken to make the incision only through skin to reduce the risk to the lateral femoral cutaneous nerve. Once the portal and cannula are appropriately placed, the arthroscope can be placed into this modified anterior portal to visualize the anterolateral cannula to determine if it injured the labrum upon entry. The posterior portal is created off the posterolateral edge of the superior greater trochanter in identical fashion, typically posterior to but convergent with the trajectory of the anterolateral portal (Fig. 49-6B).

The evaluation of the central compartment of the hip will allow for treatment of labral and chondral lesions, the ligamentum teres, removal of loose bodies, and the treatment of pincer-type impingement. Seventy and 30-degree lenses are used for full evaluation of the hip joint. The 70-degree lens is useful to evaluate the periphery of the central compartment, allowing for effective treatment of labral, acetabular, and chondral lesions. The 30-degree arthroscope lens is most useful in evaluating the central area of the central compartment, the ligamentum teres, and for peripheral compartment treatment of cam-type impingement.

Surgical Treatment of Pincer FAI

After a complete evaluation of the central compartment of the hip, the offending area of the acetabular overcoverage can be addressed. As noted, with pincer type of pathology, the labrum may be ecchymotic, degenerative, and have cystic or calcific change, which may necessitate extensive

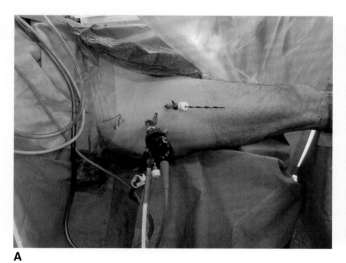
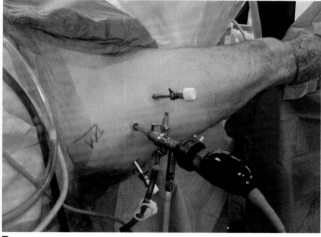

A **B**

FIGURE 49-6

Intraoperative photograph of a man undergoing central compartment arthroscopy of the right hip. **A:** The hip draped. The head is to the left and the feet (and knee as seen) to the right. The arthroscope is in the anterolateral portal, just anterior to the most proximal aspect of the greater trochanter. A probe is in a cannula in the modified anterior portal, approximately 7 cm anterior and medial to the anterolateral portal at a 45-degree angle. There is a cannula in the posterolateral cannula, seen better in **(B)**. (Figures used by permission of Marc R. Safran, MD.)

debridement or even resection. However, if we find that the overlaying labrum is healthy and intact, it can be carefully separated from the abnormal acetabular rim using an arthroscopic knife (banana blade), though some prefer to perform an acetabuloplasty while trying to keep the labrum intact. To detach the labrum, the arthroscopic knife is introduced typically through the anterior portal cannula, between the labrum and capsular reflection on the outer edge, and carefully between the labrum and articular cartilage, using the curvature of the blade to gently separate the labrum from the acetabular rim (Fig. 49-7), though an arthroscopic elevator can also be used to develop this plane of detachment. This must be delicately performed to avoid transection or damage to the labrum itself and avoiding undermining any healthy adjacent cartilage. After elevating the labrum, a nonabsorbable monofilament traction suture may be passed arthroscopically with a suture passer around the entire labrum to use as a traction device on the healthy labrum (Fig. 49-8). With the labrum detached, the underlying acetabular rim can be safely accessed for performing an acetabuloplasty. We utilize a hooded, round, high-speed burr to remove abnormal areas of bony overcoverage, removing the bone where the overcoverage exists, based on preoperative planning. We usually begin anteroinferiorly and progress laterally and posteriorly, when needed (Fig. 49-9). Typically, the anterior aspects of the acetabulum are addressed with the burr entering from the more anterior portal, while the superior (lateral) acetabulum is accessed via the anterolateral portal.

The amount of acetabular resection is typically 3 to 5 mm; however, this amount varies based on the degree of overcoverage and the extent of pathology. It can be estimated from preoperative imaging, verified with an intraoperative measurement with a laser-etched graduated probe, and examined with intraoperative fluoroscopy. Care should be taken not to overresect bone, causing iatrogenic dysplasia, which may result in hip instability and/or pain and early degenerative change. Using fluoroscopy, one can visualize the initial crossover sign and the initial anterior-inferior starting point just inferior to the start of the crossover sign and ultimately confirm the appropriate amount of resection once the line of the anterior wall is visible medial to the line of the posterior wall with a smooth gradual convergence of both lines as they meet superiorly. When this is confirmed, the appropriate version has been recreated. After the resection on the acetabular side, the labrum is repaired on the new acetabular rim with suture anchors (Fig. 49-10). After repair, the traction may be released and visualization from the peripheral compartment will verify restoration of the labral seal (Fig. 49-10C). Dynamic assessment can be performed to evaluate for residual areas of impingement.

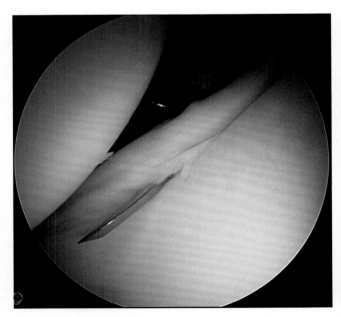

FIGURE 49-7

Arthroscopic view of a left hip of a 19-year-old female collegiate soccer player and sprinter, showing an arthroscopic knife between the labrum and acetabular cartilage. This knife is brought from behind the labrum to detach the labrum from the acetabular rim to allow for an acetabuloplasty. (Figure used by permission of Marc R. Safran, MD.)

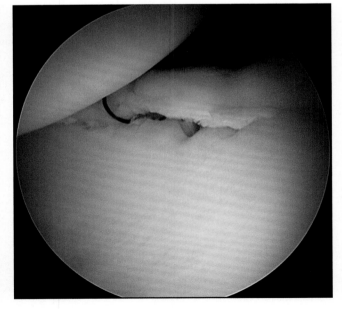

FIGURE 49-8

A nonabsorbable, monofilament suture is used to retract the detached labrum to enhance visualization of the acetabular rim to allow for acetabuloplasty and placement of the suture anchors. This is the same athlete as in Figure 49-7, without traction on suture. (Figure used by permission of Marc R. Safran, MD.)

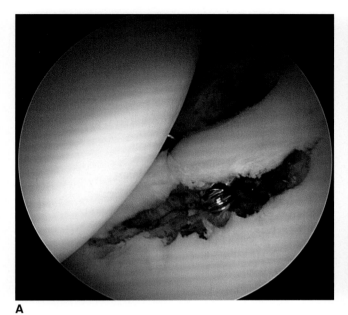
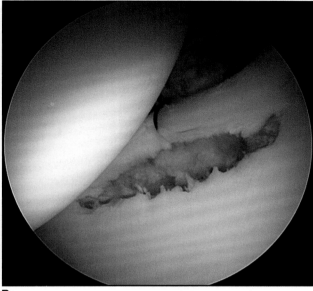

A   B

FIGURE 49-9

Arthroscopic view of an arthroscopic motorized burr being used to perform an acetabuloplasty. This is the same athlete as in Figures 49-7 and 49-8. **A:** Retraction of the labrum using the traction stitch. A chondroplasty has been performed and the burr is in place to perform the acetabuloplasty. **B:** The appearance after the acetabuloplasty has been completed. (Figures used by permission of Marc R. Safran, MD.)

It should be stressed that careful preoperative planning and intraoperative examination with fluoroscopy are vital to ensure that the level of resection is appropriate. An adequate AP projection of the pelvis should be obtained during patient positioning and may be adjusted by slight alteration to the plane of the traction table and rotation of the leg. This position should be maintained throughout the work in the central compartment.

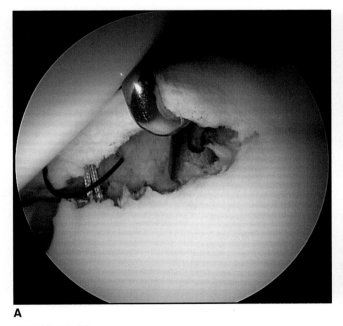
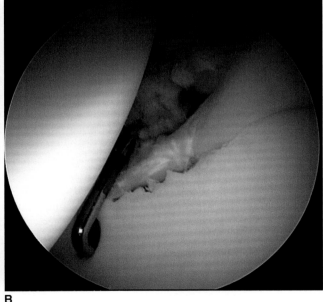

A   B

FIGURE 49-10

Arthroscopic labral repair. Same athlete as in Figures 49-7–49-9 undergoing the labral repair. **A:** Sutures placed in the labrum and the drill guide in place to drill and place another anchor. **B:** The labrum after the sutures has been tied. Note that the knots are behind the labrum, out of view, and out of potential contact with the femoral head.

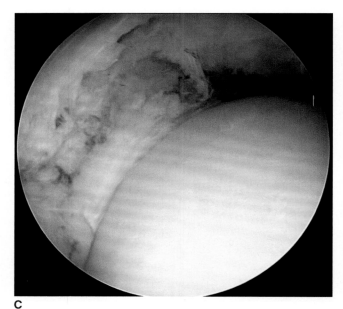

FIGURE 49-10 (*Continued*)

C: A 21-year-old collegiate rugby player demonstrating a cam lesion following acetabuloplasty and labral repair seen from the peripheral compartment. Again, note the suture knots away from the femoral head and the suction seal restored. (Figures used by permission of Marc R. Safran, MD.)

C

Surgical Treatment of Subspine Impingement

A diagnosis of subspine impingement may be confirmed by arthroscopic visualization of subspine impingement on dynamic arthroscopic examination and characteristic findings that may include anterior labral tearing or bruising at the level of the AIIS and anterosuperior chondral lesions (40,41). The rectus femoris tendon origin may be preserved by limiting the bony resection to the anterior and inferomedial aspect of the AIIS. Using a 5.5-mm arthroscopic burr, a resection of at least 11 mm should be performed to best create a normal morphologic relationship between the anteroinferior AIIS and anterior acetabular rim and allow for adequate clearance between the two (41,42).

Surgical Treatment of Cam FAI

Entering the peripheral compartment of the hip is required for treatment of cam type of impingement. This is performed by removing traction from the patient's leg with the preferred technique of keeping the foot in the traction boot with simple release of traction. This will allow for relaxation of the capsuloligamentous structures about the hip to improve maneuverability and still have control over the foot for dynamic evaluation. The space of the peripheral compartment can be further augmented by flexing the hip 20 to 45 degrees to further relax the capsule; however, this comes at the expense of altering the fluoroscopic image and may change the perception of the level of bone resection resulting in undercorrection or overresection of bone. Currently, we do not routinely place the hip in flexion and have found adequate space peripherally after performing our partial anterolateral capsulectomy.

To enter the peripheral compartment, the standard anterolateral portal and an accessory proximal anterolateral portal that made 3 to 4 cm proximal to and in line with the standard anterolateral portal are utilized (Fig. 49-11). The blunt trocar and sheath for the 30-degree arthroscope are placed through the anterolateral portal, onto the anterolateral aspect of the femoral head-neck junction, and at the apex of the deformity as visualized with fluoroscopy. The trocar is then exchanged for the arthroscope, keeping this position on the capsule and bone. An arthroscopic motorized 5.0-mm aggressive shaver is introduced through the accessory proximal anterolateral portal and, by using triangulation and fluoroscopy, is brought into position at the tip of the camera (Fig. 49-12). This maneuver places the shaver directly onto the overlying capsule. The shaver can then be utilized to clear away some of the soft tissue over the capsule, and as the shaver tip becomes visible, it is used to create a capsulotomy of the anterolateral capsule. This can then be enlarged to approximately 1.5 cm diameter as a partial capsulectomy to allow access to the peripheral compartment (Fig. 49-13). A radiofrequency wand may also be used to safely augment the partial capsulectomy as needed.

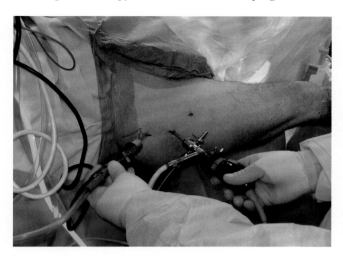

FIGURE 49-11

Portals utilized for peripheral compartment arthroscopy and decompression of the cam lesion. The right hip of this patient is exposed, with the feet to the right and the head to the left. The arthroscopic is in the standard anterolateral portal, just anterior to the most proximal aspect of the greater trochanter. The proximal anterolateral portal is 4 to 5 cm proximal to the standard anterolateral portal. (Figures used by permission of Marc R. Safran, MD.)

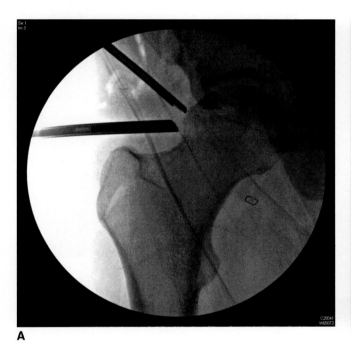

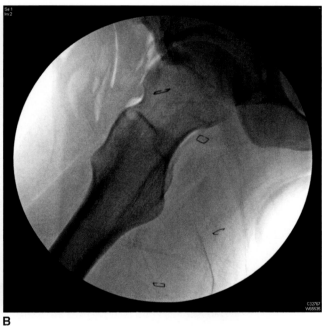

A **B**

FIGURE 49-12

Intraoperative fluoroscopic images of a 26-year-old male cricket player prior to cheilectomy. **A:** An intraoperative fluoroscopic AP view of the placement of the arthroscope and shaver to perform a partial capsulectomy to allow for visualization to perform a cheilectomy (femoral osteoplasty) for cam impingement. **B:** A frog leg lateral intraoperative fluoroscopic image of this same patient. (Figures used by permission of Marc R. Safran, MD.)

Once within the peripheral compartment, a partial synovectomy is performed to allow for adequate visualization of the femoral head-neck junction and the cam deformity (Figs. 49-13 to 49-15). Also, a previously performed acetabuloplasty and/or labral repair may be visualized, and verification of recreation of the labral seal (Fig. 49-10C) and evaluation for any residual areas of impingement with a dynamic assessment may be completed. Additionally, the lateral synovial fold, which is a marker for the retinacular vessels, the zona orbicularis, and medial synovial fold, which is a marker for the iliopsoas tendon on the other side of the capsule, can all be visualized.

The femoral head-neck junction in the presence of a cam lesion will often appear grossly abnormal simply from the surface but can be verified for location with fluoroscopy and dynamic evaluations (Fig. 49-14A and B). Using the motorized burr, the femoral head-neck offset is restored by removing

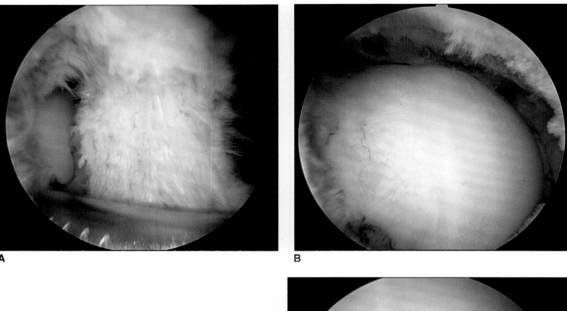

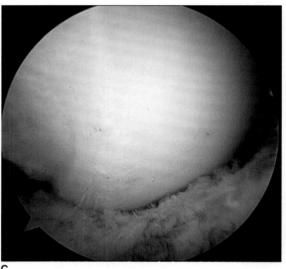

FIGURE 49-13

Arthroscopic view from a 21-year-old college basketball player of the capsular window and motorized shaver that allows access to the peripheral compartment without flexing the hip **(A)**. This allows visualization of the entire cam lesion anteriorly **(B)** and laterally **(C)**. This also allows a cheilectomy to be performed while watching arthroscopically and fluoroscopically without distortion that would occur as a result of having the femoral neck obliquely oriented to the fluoroscopic beam. (Figures used by permission of Marc R. Safran, MD.)

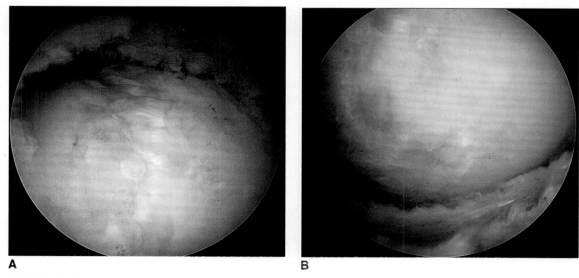

FIGURE 49-14

Arthroscopic view from the peripheral compartment for cam impingement of the left hip of a 21-year-old college football player. Note the cam lesion with irregularity and notching anteriorly **(A)** from the acetabulum and lateral wear from the impingement as well **(B)**.

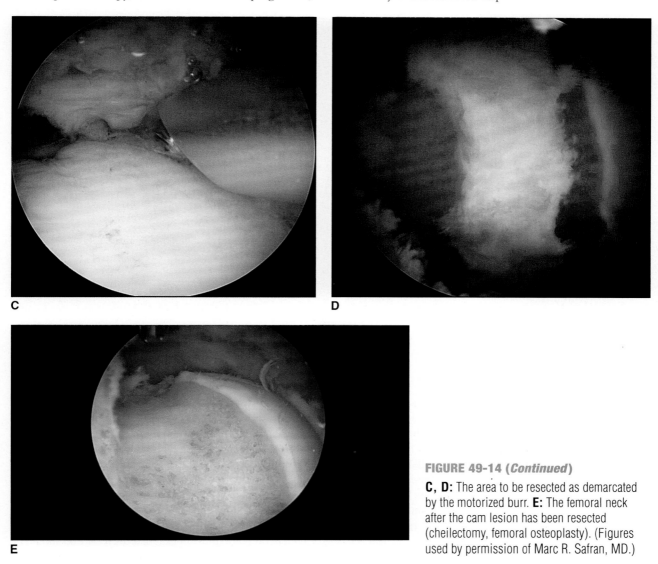

C

D

E

FIGURE 49-14 (*Continued*)

C, D: The area to be resected as demarcated by the motorized burr. **E:** The femoral neck after the cam lesion has been resected (cheilectomy, femoral osteoplasty). (Figures used by permission of Marc R. Safran, MD.)

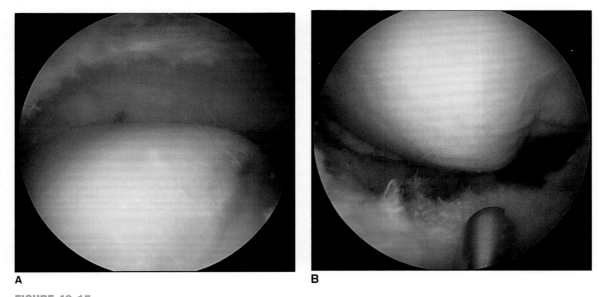

A

B

FIGURE 49-15

Arthroscopic view before and after a right hip cheilectomy of a 22-year-old professional basketball player. Note the elongated femoral head with loss of anterior **(A)** and lateral **(B)** offset.

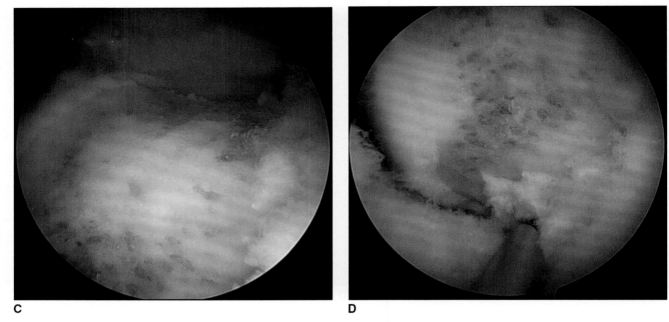

C   D

FIGURE 49-15 (*Continued*)
Restoration of the anterior **(C)** and lateral **(D)** head-neck junction offset following cheilectomy/femoral osteoplasty. (Figures used by permission of Marc R. Safran, MD.)

the area of excess bone (Fig. 49-14C–E). Depending on the specific location and size of the cam lesion, the hip may be rotated, flexed, abducted, or adducted to help reach different areas for bony resection. Also, the arthroscope and burr may be interchanged between these two portals as needed.

The ideal amount of bone to resect has not been determined. Some clinicians start their resection 7 to 10 mm from the labral edge and work distally. However, to restore the alpha angle, one must remove bone up to the labral edge. Yet, removal of bone to the labral edge can result in loss of the sealing function of the labrum. Furthermore, the clinical outcomes of decompression of the cam lesion have not been shown to correlate to restoration of the alpha angle to below 50 degrees.

The amount of bone removed is variable and should be individualized based on the pathology, with the goal of restoring normal head-neck offset. General guidelines suggest that the resection should be <1 cm deep, 8 mm from proximal to distal, and 15 mm medial to lateral, though again, this is a generalized starting point and the amount of resection needs to be customized to the degree of deformity. Mardones et al have determined that resection of over 30% of the femoral neck width increases the risk to fracture the femoral neck (43). Thus, resection is kept to <30% of the femoral neck width, and usually much less than that is necessary to eliminate the impingement. Sometimes, the cam lesion is well circumscribed and demarcated, while other times it is not. Thus, fluoroscopy can help identify the lesion, help assess how much bone is removed to avoid overresection and increase the risk of fracture, and help assure adequacy of resection (Fig. 49-16). The hip may be dynamically assessed under arthroscopic and fluoroscopic visualization to assure adequacy of bony resection.

After resection is complete, excess bone debris is removed with suction through an oscillating shaver to help minimize synovitis and heterotopic bone formation. Instruments are removed and portals closed. This allows for safe injection of local anesthetic into the operative site. Sterile bandages are applied. If a labral repair or capsulorrhaphy is performed, a hip abduction brace is applied with slight abduction and limited flexion, based on the location of the labral repair. A bunny boot is also placed on the patient's foot to limit external rotation.

Postoperative Management

There is little evidence or scientific investigation to guide postoperative rehabilitation following hip arthroscopy. Rehabilitation will also vary based on the procedure performed, whether a capsulotomy was performed and closed, surgeon experience of preference, and patient expectations. Our postoperative protocol has been developed in conjunction with physical therapists and has been modified over the years based on clinical experience and feedback from those physical therapists.

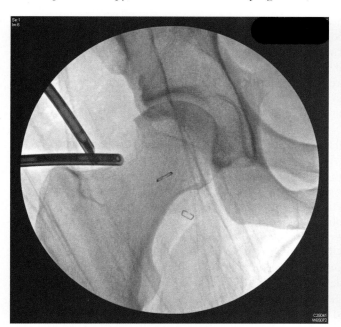
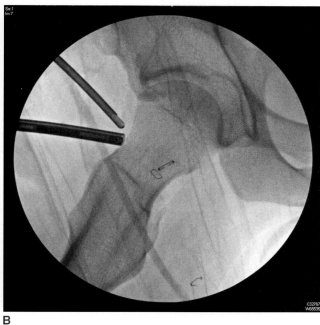

A   B

FIGURE 49-16

Intraoperative fluoroscopic images of the patient in Figure 49-9, following arthroscopic cheilectomy. **A, B:** AP and frog leg lateral postresection fluoroscopic images, confirming the adequacy of decompression. (Figures used by permission of Marc R. Safran, MD.)

Our protocol for postoperative rehabilitation after hip arthroscopy for the treatment of FAI includes flatfoot weight bearing to 20 lbs of pressure for 2 weeks assuming adequate bone quality. The duration of limited weight bearing is increased to 6 weeks if microfracture has been performed. Also, we add an extra week of limited weight bearing for every decade of age over age 39 for women and over age 49 for men following cam resection. This is to prevent femoral neck fractures and stress fractures, as reports have been noted with immediate full weight bearing. We reserve the use of a temporary abduction orthosis and a rotation limiting bunny boot for labral repairs and capsular plications to protect the repair. We encourage early motion, including the use of a continuous passive motion machine, passive circumduction exercises, and early physical therapy. Rehabilitation should ideally be performed with a physical therapist experienced in hip arthroscopy postoperative patients and includes stretching exercise as well as hip and core musculature strengthening. Proprioception exercises are also included in the early phases. Later phases of therapy (usually the 2nd and 3rd months) include balance progression, stationary cycling with resistance, strength training, side stepping, and elliptical training. By the 4th month, the rehabilitation progression includes plyometric exercises, agility drills, running, and side-to-side movements, anticipating a return to sports 4 to 6 months after surgery.

Results

The outcomes after arthroscopic treatment of FAI are increasingly reported in the literature. Although much of the literature on the arthroscopic treatment of FAI is level III or IV evidence, improvements in hip kinematics and range of motion, hip pain, quality of life, patient-reported outcome scores, activities of daily living, athletic function, hip kinematics, and patient satisfaction have been demonstrated in the literature (44–48). For athletes of all levels, hip arthroscopy has had favorable results with significant improvements in patient-reported outcomes scores (PROS) and a high rates of patient satisfaction and return to competitive sport (49–53). Results also demonstrate that despite various techniques used and pathologies encountered, the combined treatment of FAI and labral tears in the nonarthritic hip has good to excellent results in 75% to 95% of cases, with worse results in the presence of older patients, chondral damage, arthritic change, and incomplete treatment of FAI and associated pathologies (51,54–63). In fact, numerous studies report that incomplete arthroscopic correction of FAI morphology is a primary cause for revision procedures (20,64,65).

One review of the literature demonstrated that in over 800 cases of arthroscopically treated FAI, <3% progressed to hip arthroplasty compared with 18% among 179 cases of open hip dislocation (with trochanteric osteotomy) (66). The open dislocation requires an extensive approach, trochanteric osteotomy and refixation, limited weight bearing of up to 3 months, longer hospitalization, and the risk of significant blood loss and trochanteric nonunion, making the arthroscopic approach more desirable. Despite these differences, systematic reviews have found comparable outcomes between open and arthroscopic techniques with more complications related to trochanteric osteotomy in the open group (67–70).

Review of the literature confirms that the results are less predictably good when chondral damage is present and that the results of FAI surgery do not correlate with restoration of the alpha angle to <50 or 55 degrees (66). Results are significantly worse if the labral injury is addressed without also addressing any associated impingement pathology (65,71–73). One problem with assessing nonarthritic hip problems in the athletic patient is the lack of a methodologically sound, validated outcome measure (74). A research collaborative of clinically active hip arthroscopists (MAHORN group) completed a 5-year task of developing a methodologically sound, validated, hip outcomes score, the MAHORN Hip Outcomes Tool (MHOT), which has been published in 33 and 14 item forms, and called the iHOT (International Hip Outcomes Tool) (74,75). While much of the literature use outcome measures that were not designed or validated for young, active patients undergoing hip arthroscopy (such as the Harris Hip Score), currently there are other outcome measures available (such as iHOT (75), HAGOS (76), and HSAS (77)) that have been validated for a younger and more active patient population.

HIP MICROINSTABILITY

Indications and Contraindications

Background

Hip microinstability or atraumatic instability is an important and evolving diagnosis that must be included a differential diagnosis of hip or groin pain. The etiology of microinstability is likely multifactorial and patients may be categorized based on the underlying cause: bony abnormalities including developmental dysplasia of the hip, connective tissue disorders, trauma, repetitive microtrauma, iatrogenic, and idiopathic (78). One study reported that 35% of patients undergoing revision hip arthroscopy required capsular treatment due to instability (65). Hip stability is conferred by the bony acetabulum and soft tissue structures including the labrum, ligamentum teres, and capsuloligamentous complex (iliofemoral, ischiofemoral, and pubofemoral ligaments and the zona orbicularis). Normally, there is some translational motion between the femoral head and acetabulum. Subtle abnormalities in these stabilizing structures, in the setting of repetitive motions, can cause further damage to these structures or the chondral surfaces of the hip. This additional injury in turn results in further microinstability, further damage, and possibly subsequent pain, dysfunction, or disability. Further still, athletes involved in activities with extremes of motion may develop impingement with relatively normal femoral and acetabular bony anatomy (79). For example, dancers may forcefully try to gain external rotation ("turnout") while standing, which stretches the iliofemoral ligament, the strongest ligament in the body and part of the anterior hip capsule.

Indications

Arthroscopic treatment for hip microinstability is reserved for symptomatic patients who have failed nonoperative treatment including activity modification, oral anti-inflammatory medications, and physical therapy focusing on strengthening of the hip flexors, abductors, external rotators, and core muscles. While this treatment regimen is often successful, if 3 to 6 months of sustained nonoperative treatment has failed to provide adequate symptomatic relief, the risks and benefits of surgical intervention may be discussed with the patient.

Contraindications

The aforementioned contraindications to hip arthroscopy also apply to patients with hip microinstability: medical comorbidities or infection precluding general anesthesia or elective surgery, advanced degenerative changes of the hip, and patients who fail to experience relief from a local anesthetic intra-articular injection. The role of such injections is particularly important in this patient population because the sensitivity and specificity of physical examination tests for microinstability have not been reported and because, as noted above, imaging findings such as FAI and labral tears are not uncommon among asymptomatic individuals. It is mandatory to exclude bony morphologic causes for microinstability such as acetabular dysplasia or retroversion, as these patients may be made worse with hip arthroscopy may require open pelvis of proximal femur osteotomies to achieve symptomatic relief.

Preoperative Planning

History, Physical Examination, and Imaging

Patients with microinstability of the hip often present with vague hip or groin discomfort of insidious onset, with or without mechanical symptoms. In addition to some of the issues and questions mentioned above, when evaluating a patient for hip microinstability, history should focus on determining the presence or absence of risk factors such as developmental hip dysplasia, connective tissue disorders, previous hip subluxations or dislocations, prior hip surgery, and participation in activities requiring hypermobilities such as gymnastics, dance, and yoga.

In conjunction with the physical examination described above, patients suspected of hip microinstability should be evaluated for generalized ligamentous laxity and reproduction of symptoms (pain or apprehension) with certain additional physical examination tests. These tests include the anterior and posterior apprehension tests, the prone external rotation test, the dial test, and the abduction-extension-external rotation test (78,80,81). In a recently completed study pending publication, we found the hyperextension-external rotation test and the abduction-extension-external rotation test to be sensitive and specific for the diagnosis of hip instability. With the addition of the prone external rotation test, when all three tests were positive, 95% of patients had hip instability.

Imaging begins with plain radiographs as previously described. In patients suspected of having hip instability, it is particularly important to evaluate imaging for signs of acetabular dysplasia and retroversion, previous trauma, and femoral version. We recently identified a possible radiographic finding for instability, defined as the "cliff sign," in which the femoral head has a sudden drop off or flattening with a loss of sphericity (82). MRI or MRA is useful not only for evaluation of intra-articular structures, such as the labrum and articular cartilage, but also for assessment of the capsuloligamentous structures and hip joint recesses (83). A thin capsule (<3 mm) just distal to the zona orbicularis on axial view has been found to be consistent with hip instability (83), and we have found this to be particularly true in female patients. Despite a thorough and appropriate history, physical examination, and imaging, the diagnosis of hip microinstability may still be difficult. In such circumstances, dynamic fluoroscopic examination or traction fluoroscopy under anesthesia may be useful for evaluating hip stability and showing the "vacuum sign" indicative of abnormal hip distraction (Fig. 49-17) (84,85).

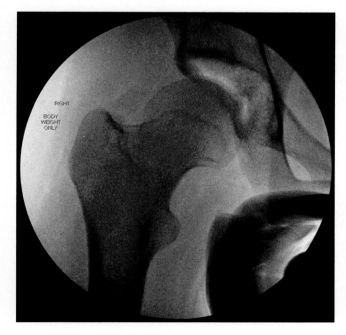

FIGURE 49-17

Fluoroscopic image of a right hip during dynamic examination under anesthesia. The presence of joint displacement along with a "vacuum sign" with only body weight traction is indicative of hip microinstability. (Figure used by permission of Marc R. Safran, MD.)

Surgery

Surgical Treatment of Microinstability

Patient positioning, draping, and the general arthroscopic approach to the hip are detailed above. In the setting of FAI with concomitant microinstability, after addressing all intra-articular pathology and completing the acetabuloplasty and/or femoral neck osteoplasty, capsular plication of the aforementioned partial capsulotomy is performed with a suture shuttling device. Although the patient size and degree of microinstability affect capsular management, often a motorized shaver is used to extend the capsulotomy to an anterolateral partial capsulectomy approximately 8 mm wide by 15 mm long. This capsulectomy is performed in the "bare area" between the iliofemoral and ischiofemoral ligaments to avoid overtightening one of the more discrete capsular ligaments (86). The capsulorrhaphy is performed by using a curved suture shuttling device to effectively close this interval with three to five interrupted sutures (Fig. 49-18).

Some surgeons prefer to make a capsulotomy between the anterior and anterolateral portals for access, avoiding the posterolateral portal. Other surgeons utilize this capsulotomy to perform a capsular shift via advancement of the iliofemoral ligament to tighten the hip. This type of interportal capsulotomy or T-capsulotomy results in transection of the iliofemoral ligament. Our preference is to avoid this technique in general, but especially in cases of symptomatic instability, as there is already a concern for inadequate hip stability and capsuloligamentous complex insufficiency in these patients. Cutting and repairing the iliofemoral ligament also comes with the concerns of overtightening the iliofemoral ligament (resulting in loss of hip external rotation), sutures pulling out (resulting in iliofemoral ligament insufficiency), and iatrogenic instability (87).

In addition to the postoperative instructions noted above, after the capsular closure, plication, or shift, the patient is placed in a hip abduction brace, which limits hip extension, abduction, and external rotation for 2 weeks.

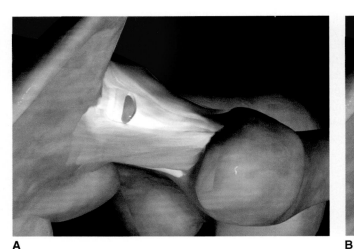

A

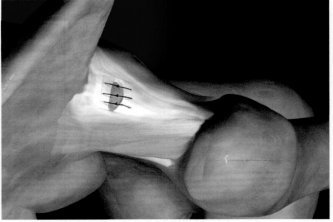

B

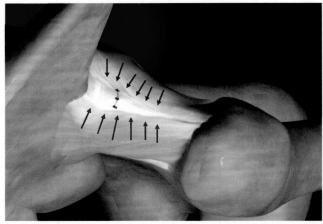

C

FIGURE 49-18

A: Interligamentous capsulotomy in the "bare area" between the iliofemoral (*blue*) and ischiofemoral (*green*) ligaments. **B:** Three to five sutures are passed across the capsulotomy site using a curved suture shuttling device. **C:** Capsular plication is achieved once the sutures are tied and the edges of the iliofemoral (*blue*) and ischiofemoral (*green*) ligaments are brought closer together, tightening the joint without overtightening any one specific ligament. (Figure used by permission of Marc R. Safran, MD.)

Results

Although the literature is limited for patients having primary hip arthroscopy for microinstability, in general, improved outcomes have been shown following arthroscopic hip capsular closure, plication, or shift. The first case series of isolated hip instability treated with capsular plication and labral surgery (no bony work) demonstrated excellent outcomes in 32 patients with a minimum of 1-year follow-up (88). The first case series of revision hip arthroscopy for capsular repair due to symptomatic instability was recently published and patient-reported outcome scores showed significant improvement at both 1- and 2-year follow-up (79). Similarly, capsular repair or plication has been shown to be a significant predictor of improved outcomes for revision hip arthroscopy (89). In a cohort study, patients with FAI who had a complete repair of their T-capsulotomy demonstrated significantly improved sport-specific outcome scores compared with individuals having only a partial capsular repair (90).

COMPLICATIONS

Complications related to hip arthroscopy are usually related to traction (too much or too little), patient positioning, and fluid management. Complication rates are between 1.4% and 6.1% and include inability to perform arthroscopy due to access issues; iatrogenic chondrolabral injury; skin or urogenital damage; instrument breakage; infection; abdominal compartment syndrome; heterotopic ossification; and neuropraxias of the sciatic, femoral, perineal, pudendal, or lateral femoral cutaneous nerves that often resolve spontaneously (91–93). A recent study using the PearlDiver database found that within 1 year of hip arthroscopy, the rates of minor complications, major complications, proximal femur fractures, and hip instability were 4.22%, 1.74%, 0.89%, and 0.58%, respectively (94). This increased rate of major complications compared with previous studies may be due to the use of the PearlDiver data, which is a general database that is not restricted to high-volume hip arthroscopists. The most commonly underreported complications are iatrogenic, including articular cartilage damage and labral injury.

Recent reports on the prevalence of asymptomatic deep vein thrombosis (DVT) and symptomatic DVT and PE following hip arthroscopy suggest that routine prophylaxis is not warranted, except in patients at increased risk (93,95–98). A prospective study using ultrasound to determine the incidence of DVT among low-risk patients undergoing hip arthroscopy found five DVT, four of which were symptomatic, among 115 patients (99). The authors did not identify any statistically significant patient or surgical factors associated with DVT.

Complications related to the arthroscopic treatment of FAI include femoral neck fracture related to overresection of the femoral neck when treating cam impingement and overresection of the acetabular rim leading to instability (100,101). Another risk is underresection of the femoral neck resulting in incomplete reshaping of the FAI deformity, although the exact amount and location to remove have yet to be defined (20,64,65). This is also likely underreported and may be the source of continued pain and dysfunction after surgery that results in revision procedures. The risk of avascular necrosis (AVN) after FAI surgery is a potential concern, although the area of resection is typically far away from the posterolateral femoral neck where the vessels are located. No cases of AVN have been reported after FAI surgery.

There have been several reports of instability after FAI surgery and hip arthroscopy (79,101–103). While catastrophic dislocations are apparent, there may also be more subtle instability that results after FAI surgery, as the senior author has been treating more patients for failed FAI surgery with instability.

ACKNOWLEDGEMENT

All intraoperative images and perioperative radiologic images are provided by Marc R. Safran, MD.

REFERENCES

1. Myers SR, Eijer H, Ganz R. Anterior femoroacetabular impingement after periacetabular osteotomy. *Clin Orthop Relat Res.* 1999;(363):93–99.
2. Beck M, Leunig M, Parvizi J, et al. Anterior femoroacetabular impingement: Part II. Midterm results of surgical treatment. *Clin Orthop Relat Res.* 2004;418:67–73.

3. Espinosa N, Rothenfluh DA, Beck M, et al. Treatment of femoroacetabular impingement: preliminary results of labral refixation. *J Bone Joint Surg Am.* 2006;88(5):925–935.

4. Ganz R, Parvizi J, Beck M, et al. Femoroacetabular impingement: a cause for osteoarthritis of the hip. *Clin Orthop Relat Res.* 2003;417:112–120.

5. Larson CM, Guanche CA, Kelly BT, et al. Advanced techniques in hip arthroscopy. *Instr Course Lect.* 2009;58:423–436.

6. Leunig M, Beck M, Dora C, et al. Femoroacetabular impingement: etiology and surgical concept. *Oper Tech Orthop.* 2005;15:247–255.

7. Philippon MJ, Stubbs AJ, Schenker ML, et al. Arthroscopic management of femoroacetabular impingement: osteoplasty technique and literature review. *Am J Sports Med.* 2007;35(9):1571–1580.

8. Agricola R, Bessems JH, Ginai AZ, et al. The development of cam-type deformity in adolescent and young male soccer players. *Am J Sports Med.* 2012;40:1099–1106.

9. Packer JD, Safran MR. The etiology of primary femoroacetabular impingement: genetics or acquired deformity? *J Hip Preserv Surg.* 2015;2(3):249–257.

10. Hetsroni I, Larson CM, Dela Torre K, et al. Anterior inferior iliac spine deformity as an extra-articular source for hip impingement: a series of 10 patients treated with arthroscopic decompression. *Arthroscopy.* 2012;28(11):1644–1653.

11. Hetsroni I, Poultsides L, Bedi A, et al. Anterior inferior iliac spine morphology correlates with hip range of motion: a classification system and dynamic model. *Clin Orthop Relat Res.* 2013;471(8):2497–2503.

12. Larson CM, Kelly BT, Stone RM. Making a case for anterior inferior iliac spine/subspine hip impingement: three representative case reports and proposed concept. *Arthroscopy.* 2011;27(12):1732–1737.

13. Zaltz I, Kelly BT, Hetsroni I, et al. The crossover sign overestimates acetabular retroversion. *Clin Orthop Relat Res.* 2013;471(8):2463–2470.

14. Hariri S, Eijer H, Safran MR. Labral tears. In: Bhandari M, ed. *Evidence Based Orthopaedics.* Oxford, UK: Wiley-Blackwell; 2011.

15. Safran MR. The acetabular labrum: anatomic and functional characteristics and rationale for surgical intervention. *J Am Acad Orthop Surg.* 2010;18(6):338–345.

16. Frank JM, Harris JD, Erickson BJ, et al. Prevalence of femoroacetabular impingement imaging findings in asymptomatic volunteers: a systematic review. *Arthroscopy.* 2015;31(6):1199–1204.

17. Hack K, Di Primio G, Rakhra K, et al. Prevalence of cam-type femoroacetabular impingement morphology in asymptomatic volunteers. *J Bone Joint Surg Am.* 2010;92(14):2436–2444.

18. Jung KA, Restrepo C, Hellman M, et al. The prevalence of cam-type femoroacetabular deformity in asymptomatic adults. *J Bone Joint Surg Br.* 2011;93(10):1303–1307.

19. Li Y, Helvie P, Mead M, et al. Prevalence of femoroacetabular impingement morphology in asymptomatic adolescents. *J Pediatr Orthop.* 2017;37:121–126.

20. Bogunovic L, Gottlieb M, Pashos G, et al. Why do hip arthroscopy procedures fail? *Clin Orthop Relat Res.* 2013;471(8):2523–2529.

21. Harris JD, McCormick FM, Abrams GD, et al. Complications and reoperations during and after hip arthroscopy: a systematic review of 92 studies and more than 6,000 patients. *Arthroscopy.* 2013;29(3):589–595.

22. Horisberger M, Brunner A, Herzog RF. Arthroscopic treatment of femoral acetabular impingement in patients with preoperative generalized degenerative changes. *Arthroscopy.* 2010;26(5):623–629.

23. Larson CM, Giveans MR, Taylor M. Does arthroscopic FAI correction improve function with radiographic arthritis? *Clin Orthop Relat Res.* 2011;469:1667–1676.

24. Philippon MJ, Briggs KK, Carlisle JC, et al. Joint space predicts THA after hip arthroscopy in patients 50 years and older. *Clin Orthop Relat Res.* 2013;471(8):2492–2496.

25. Philippon MJ, Maxwell RB, Johnston TL, et al. Clinical presentation of femoroacetabular impingement. *Knee Surg Sports Traumatol Arthrosc.* 2007;15(8):1041–1047.

26. Wyss TF, Clark JM, Weishaupt D, et al. Correlation between internal rotation and bony anatomy in the hip. *Clin Orthop Relat Res.* 2007;460:152–158.

27. Martin HD, Kelly BT, Leunig M, et al. The pattern and technique in the clinical evaluation of the adult hip: the common physical examination tests of hip specialists. *Arthroscopy.* 2010;26(2):161–172.

28. Martin RL, Kelly BT, Leunig M, et al. Reliability of clinical diagnosis in intraarticular hip diseases. *Knee Surg Sports Traumatol Arthrosc.* 2010;18(5):685–690.

29. Safran MR. Evaluation of the hip: history, physical examination, and imaging. *Oper Tech Sports Med.* 2005;13(1):2–12.

30. Poultsides LA, Bedi A, Kelly BT. An algorithmic approach to mechanical hip pain. *HSS J.* 2012;8(3):213–224.

31. Hammoud S, Bedi A, Magennis E, et al. High incidence of athletic pubalgia symptoms in professional athletes with symptomatic femoroacetabular impingement. *Arthroscopy.* 2012;28(10):1388–1395.

32. Hammoud S, Bedi A, Voos JE, et al. The recognition and evaluation of patterns of compensatory injury in patients with mechanical hip pain. *Sports Health.* 2014;6(2):108–118.

33. Larson CM, Pierce BR, Giveans MR. Treatment of athletes with symptomatic intra-articular hip pathology and athletic pubalgia/sports hernia: a case series. *Arthroscopy.* 2011;27(6):768–775.

34. Beck M, Kalhor M, Leunig M, et al. Hip morphology influences the pattern of damage to the acetabular cartilage: femoroacetabular impingement as a cause of early osteoarthritis of the hip. *J Bone Joint Surg Br.* 2005;87(7):1012–1018.

35. Lavigne M, Parvizi J, Beck M, et al. Anterior femoroacetabular impingement: part I. Techniques of joint preserving surgery. *Clin Orthop Relat Res.* 2004;(418):61–66.

36. Leunig M, Podeszwa D, Beck M, et al. Magnetic resonance arthrography of labral disorders in hips with dysplasia and impingement. *Clin Orthop Relat Res.* 2004;(418):74–80.

37. Notzli HP, Wyss TF, Stoecklin CH, et al. The contour of the femoral head-neck junction as a predictor for the risk of anterior impingement. *J Bone Joint Surg Br.* 2002;84(4):556–560.

38. Byrd JW, Jones KS. Diagnostic accuracy of clinical assessment, magnetic resonance imaging, magnetic resonance arthrography, and intra-articular injection in hip arthroscopy patients. *Am J Sports Med.* 2004;32(7):1668–1674.

39. Vaughn ZD, Safran MR. Supine approach to hip arthroscopy. In: Sekiya JK, Safran MR, Ranawat AS, et al., eds. *Techniques in Hip Arthroscopy and Joint Preservation Surgery.* Philadelphia, PA: Elsevier Science; 2010:88–94.

40. Amar E, Warschawski Y, Sharfman ZT, et al. Pathological findings in patients with low anterior inferior iliac spine impingement. *Surg Radiol Anat.* 2016;38(5):569–575.

41. Sharfman ZT, Grundshtein A, Paret M, et al. Surgical technique: arthroscopic osteoplasty of anterior inferior iliac spine for femoroacetabular impingement. *Arthrosc Tech.* 2016;5(3):e601–e606.

42. Amar E, Druckmann I, Flusser G, et al. The anterior inferior iliac spine: size, position, and location. An anthropometric and sex survey. *Arthroscopy.* 2013;29(5):874–881.

43. Mardones RM, Gonzalez C, Chen Q, et al. Surgical treatment of femoroacetabular impingement: evaluation of the effect of the size of the resection. *J Bone Joint Surg Am.* 2005;87(2):273–279.

44. Kierkegaard S, Langeskov-Christensen M, Lund B, et al. Pain, activities of daily living and sport function at different time points after hip arthroscopy in patients with femoroacetabular impingement: a systematic review with meta-analysis. *Br J Sports Med.* 2017;51(7):572–579.

45. Bedi A, Dolan M, Hetsroni I, et al. Surgical treatment of femoroacetabular impingement improves hip kinematics: a computer-assisted model. *Am J Sports Med.* 2011;29(1):43S–49S.

46. Malviya A, Stafford GH, Villar RN. Impact of arthroscopy of the hip for femoroacetabular impingement on quality of life at a mean follow-up of 3.2 years. *J Bone Joint Surg Br.* 2012;94(4):466–470.

47. Khan M, Habib A, de Sa D, et al. Arthroscopy up to date: hip femoroacetabular impingement. *Arthroscopy.* 2016;32(1):177–189.

48. Rylander JH, Shu B, Andriacchi TP, et al. Preoperative and postoperative sagittal plane hip kinematics in patients with femoroacetabular impingement during level walking. *Am J Sports Med.* 2011;39(suppl):36S–42S.

49. Byrd JW, Jones KS. Arthroscopic management of femoroacetabular impingement in athletes. *Am J Sports Med.* 2011;39(Suppl):7S–13S.

50. Nho SJ, Magennis EM, Singh CK, et al. Outcomes after the arthroscopic treatment of femoroacetabular impingement in a mixed group of high-level athletes. *Am J Sports Med.* 2011;39(1):14S–9S.

51. Philippon M, Schenker M, Briggs K, et al. Femoroacetabular impingement in 45 professional athletes: associated pathologies and return to sport following arthroscopic decompression. *Knee Surg Sports Traumatol Arthrosc.* 2007;15:908–914.

52. Sansone M, Ahlden M, Jonasson P, et al. Good results after hip arthroscopy for femoroacetabular impingement in top-level athletes. *Orthop J Sports Med.* 2015;3(2):2325967115569691.

53. Shibata K, Matsuda S, Safran MR. Arthroscopic hip surgery in the elite athlete: comparison of female and male competitive athletes. *Am J Sports Med.* 2017;45:1730–1739.

54. Byrd JW, Jones KS. Arthroscopic femoroplasty in the management of cam-type femoroacetabular impingement. *Clin Orthop Relat Res.* 2009;467(3):739–746.

55. Guanche CA, Bare AA. Arthroscopic treatment of femoroacetabular impingement. *Arthroscopy.* 2006;22(1):95–106.

56. Ilizaliturri VM Jr, Nossa-Barrera JM, Acosta-Rodriguez E, et al. Arthroscopic treatment of femoroacetabular impingement secondary to paediatric hip disorders. *J Bone Joint Surg Br.* 2007;89(8):1025–1030.

57. Ilizaliturri VM Jr, Orozco-Rodriguez L, Acosta-Rodriguez E, et al. Arthroscopic treatment of cam-type femoroacetabular impingement: preliminary report at 2 years minimum follow-up. *J Arthroplasty.* 2008;23(2):226–234.

58. Larson CM, Giveans MR. Arthroscopic management of femoroacetabular impingement: early outcomes measures. *Arthroscopy.* 2008;24(5):540–546.

59. Larson CM, Giveans MR. Arthroscopic debridement versus refixation of the acetabular labrum associated with femoroacetabular impingement. *Arthroscopy.* 2009;25(4):369–376.

60. Philippon MJ, Briggs KK, Yen YM, et al. Outcomes following hip arthroscopy for femoroacetabular impingement with associated chondrolabral dysfunction: minimum two-year follow-up. *J Bone Joint Surg Br.* 2009;91(1):16–23.

61. Sampson TG. Arthroscopic treatment of femoroacetabular impingement: a proposed technique with clinical experience. *Instr Course Lect.* 2006;55:337–346.

62. Stahelin L, Stahelin T, Jolles BM, et al. Arthroscopic offset restoration in femoroacetabular cam impingement: accuracy and early clinical outcome. *Arthroscopy.* 2008;24(1):51.e1–57.e1.

63. Frank RM, Lee S, Bush-Joseph CA, et al. Outcomes for hip arthroscopy according to sex and age: a comparative matched-group analysis. *J Bone Joint Surg Am.* 2016;98(10):797–804.

64. Clohisy JC, Nepple JJ, Larson CM, et al. Persistent structural disease is the most common cause of repeat hip preservation surgery. *Clin Orthop Relat Res.* 2013;471(12):3788–3794.

65. Philippon MJ, Schenker ML, Briggs KK, et al. Revision hip arthroscopy. *Am J Sports Med.* 2007;35(11):1918–1921.

66. Vaughn ZD, Safran MR. Arthroscopic femoral osteoplasty/cheilectomy for cam-type femoroacetabular impingement in the athlete. *Sports Med Arthrosc Rev.* 2010;18(2):90–99.

67. Botser IB, Smith TW, Nasser R, et al. Open surgical dislocation versus arthroscopy for femoroacetabular impingement: a comparison of clinical outcomes. *Arthroscopy.* 2011;27(2):270–278.

68. Matsuda DK, Carlisle JC, Arthurs SC, et al. Comparative systematic review of the open dislocation, mini-open, and arthroscopic surgeries for femoroacetabular impingement. *Arthroscopy.* 2011;27(2):252–269.

69. Ng VY, Arora N, Best TM, et al. Efficacy of surgery for femoroacetabular impingement: a systematic review. *Am J Sports Med.* 2010;38(11):2337–2345.

70. Papalia R, Del Buono A, Franceschi F, et al. Femoroacetabular impingement syndrome management: arthroscopy or open surgery? *Int Orthop.* 2012;36:903–914.

71. Bardakos NV, Vasconcelos JC, Villar RN. Early outcome of hip arthroscopy for femoroacetabular impingement: the role of femoral osteoplasty in symptomatic improvement. *J Bone Joint Surg Br.* 2008;90(12):1570–1575.

72. Brunner A, Horisberger M, Herzog RF. Evaluation of a computed tomography-based navigation system prototype for hip arthroscopy in the treatment of femoroacetabular cam impingement. *Arthroscopy.* 2009;25(4):382–391.

73. Heyworth BE, Shindle MK, Voos JE, et al. Radiologic and intraoperative findings in revision hip arthroscopy. *Arthroscopy.* 2007;23(12):1295–1302.

74. Hariri S, Safran MR. Hip arthroscopy assessment tools and outcomes. *Oper Tech Orthop.* 2010;20(4):264–277.

75. Mohtadi NG, Griffin DR, Pedersen ME, et al. The development and validation of a self-administered quality-of-life outcome measure for young, active patients with symptomatic hip disease: the International Hip Outcome Tool (iHOT-33). *Arthroscopy.* 2012;28(5):595–605; quiz 6.e1–10.e1.

76. Thorborg K, Holmich P, Christensen R, et al. The Copenhagen Hip and Groin Outcome Score (HAGOS): development and validation according to the COSMIN checklist. *Br J Sports Med.* 2011;45(6):478–491.

77. Naal FD, Miozzari HH, Kelly BT, et al. The Hip Sports Activity Scale (HSAS) for patients with femoroacetabular impingement. *Hip Int.* 2013;23(2):204–211.

78. Kalisvaart MM, Safran MR. Microinstability of the hip-it does exist: etiology, diagnosis and treatment. *J Hip Preserv Surg.* 2015;2(2):123–135.

79. Wylie JD, Beckmann JT, Maak TG, et al. Arthroscopic capsular repair for symptomatic hip instability after previous hip arthroscopic surgery. *Am J Sports Med.* 2016;44(1):39–45.

80. Philippon MJ, Zehms CT, Briggs KK, et al. Hip instability in the athlete. *Oper Tech Sports Med.* 2007;15(4):189–194.
81. Domb BG, Stake CE, Lindner D, et al. Arthroscopic capsular plication and labral preservation in borderline hip dysplasia: two-year clinical outcomes of a surgical approach to a challenging problem. *Am J Sports Med.* 2013;41(11):2591–2598.
82. Packer JD, Cowan JB, Rebolledo B, et al. "The Cliff Sign" — A New Radiographic Sign of Hip Instability. *International Society for Hip Arthroscopy Annual Meeting*; September 17, 2016; San Francisco, CA.
83. Magerkurth O, Jacobson JA, Morag Y, et al. Capsular laxity of the hip: findings at magnetic resonance arthrography. *Arthroscopy.* 2013;29(10):1615–1622.
84. Bellabarba C, Sheinkop MB, Kuo KN. Idiopathic hip instability. An unrecognized cause of coxa saltans in the adult. *Clin Orthop Relat Res.* 1998;(355):261–271.
85. Smith MV, Sekiya JK. Hip instability. *Sports Med Arthrosc Rev.* 2010;18(2):108–112.
86. Shu B, Safran MR. Hip instability: anatomic and clinical considerations of traumatic and atraumatic instability. *Clin Sports Med.* 2011;30(2):349–367.
87. Weber AE, Kuhns BD, Cvetanovich GL, et al. Does the hip capsule remain closed after hip arthroscopy with routine capsular closure for femoroacetabular impingement? a magnetic resonance imaging analysis in symptomatic postoperative patients. *Arthroscopy.* 2017;33(1):108–115.
88. Kalisvaart MM, Safran MR. Hip instability treated with arthroscopic capsular plication. *Knee Surg Sports Traumatol Arthrosc.* 2017;25(1):24–30.
89. Larson CM, Giveans MR, Samuelson KM, et al. Arthroscopic hip revision surgery for residual Femoroacetabular Impingement (FAI): surgical outcomes compared with a matched cohort after primary arthroscopic FAI correction. *Am J Sports Med.* 2014;42(8):1785–1790.
90. Frank RM, Lee S, Bush-Joseph CA, et al. Improved outcomes after hip arthroscopic surgery in patients undergoing T-capsulotomy with complete repair versus partial repair for femoroacetabular impingement: a comparative matched-pair analysis. *Am J Sports Med.* 2014;42(11):2634–2642.
91. Clarke MT, Arora A, Villar RN. Hip arthroscopy: complications in 1054 cases. *Clin Orthop Relat Res* 2003;(406):84–88.
92. Burrus MT, Cowan JB, Bedi A. Avoiding failure in hip arthroscopy: complications, pearls, and pitfalls. *Clin Sports Med.* 2016;35(3):487–501.
93. Weber AE, Harris JD, Nho SJ. Complications in hip arthroscopy: a systematic review and strategies for prevention. *Sports Med Arthrosc Rev.* 2015;23(4):187–193.
94. Truntzer JN, Hoppe DJ, Shapiro LM, et al. Complication rates for hip arthroscopy are underestimated: a population-based study. *Arthroscopy.* 2017;33:1194–1201.
95. Alaia MJ, Patel D, Levy A, et al. The incidence of venous thromboembolism (VTE)—after hip arthroscopy. *Bull Hosp Jt Dis (2013).* 2014;72(2):154–158.
96. Fukushima K, Takahira N, Uchiyama K, et al. The incidence of deep vein thrombosis (DVT) during hip arthroscopic surgery. *Arch Orthop Trauma Surg.* 2016;136(10):1431–1435.
97. Malviya A, Raza A, Jameson S, et al. Complications and survival analyses of hip arthroscopies performed in the national health service in England: a review of 6,395 cases. *Arthroscopy.* 2015;31(5):836–842.
98. Kowalczuk M, Bhandari M, Farrokhyar F, et al. Complications following hip arthroscopy: a systematic review and meta-analysis. *Knee Surg Sports Traumatol Arthrosc.* 2013;21(7):1669–1675.
99. Mohtadi NG, Johnston K, Gaudelli C, et al. The incidence of proximal deep vein thrombosis after elective hip arthroscopy: a prospective cohort study in low risk patients. *J Hip Preserv Surg.* 2016;3(4):295–303.
100. Ilizaliturri VM Jr. Complications of arthroscopic femoroacetabular impingement treatment: a review. *Clin Orthop Relat Res.* 2009;467(3):760–768.
101. Matsuda DK. Acute iatrogenic dislocation following hip impingement arthroscopic surgery. *Arthroscopy.* 2009;25(4):400–404.
102. Benali Y, Katthagen BD. Hip subluxation as a complication of arthroscopic debridement. *Arthroscopy.* 2009;25(4):405–407.
103. Ranawat AS, McClincy M, Sekiya JK. Anterior dislocation of the hip after arthroscopy in a patient with capsular laxity of the hip. A case report. *J Bone Joint Surg Am.* 2009;91(1):192–197.

50 Labral Reconstruction of the Hip

James R. Ross, Christopher M. Larson, and Asheesh Bedi

INTRODUCTION

Femoroacetabular impingement (FAI) and labral tears have been well described in the past decade with most literature characterizing the evaluation, diagnosis, and treatment of cam- and pincer-type FAI (1–7). Originally, the surgical treatment of labral tears of the hip primarily involved selective debridement of the diseased and damaged tissue (8). However, with the advent of modern-day procedures, labral tissue has been able to be preserved with reparative techniques, which have demonstrated superior results in regard to pain reduction, improved function, and return to activities (6). Labral reconstruction has also been developed and is increasingly utilized in the setting of irreparable labral tears. This technique utilizes a graft to reconstruct the native labrum, and has recently been shown to demonstrate promising early outcomes (9). This chapter reviews the indications for labral reconstruction, graft options, as well as the outcomes that are currently reported. Additionally, we outline the treatment algorithm, including a description of our arthroscopic technique for labral reconstruction.

Indications

The acetabular labrum has recently been recognized as a source of hip pain and mechanical symptoms. Injury to the labrum can occur due to trauma, FAI, hip dysplasia/instability, or it may be idiopathic (10–12). Surgical techniques to manage labral pathology have advanced substantially from initial access via surgical hip dislocation with labral debridement. Hip arthroscopy has allowed for improved visualization of the labral pathology, and advancements in this technique have permitted labral repair and even labral reconstruction when indicated. The acetabular labrum consists of fibrocartilaginous tissue that has circumferential collagen fibers that span the entire length of the acetabulum, eventually transitioning contiguously with the transverse acetabular ligament. In addition to being anchored via a transitional zone of calcified cartilage, the labrum is contiguous with the hyaline cartilage of the adjacent acetabulum. The labrum is composed of dense connective tissue at the peripheral rim and transitions to a fibrocartilage inner surface. The vascular supply is predominant via the capsular side of the labrum with perforating and circumferential vessels (10).

The labrum has an important role in the maintenance of normal hip function, via deepening of the acetabular socket, providing a suction-seal effect, and regulating fluid production. Previous cadaveric studies have demonstrated the importance of the acetabular labrum. Partial labral debridement has been shown to result in the loss of normal fluid pressurization and a loss of the normal hip seal (13). Labral reconstruction has been shown to improve fluid pressurization and reestablish the suction-seal effect of the hip (13), while also improving the stability to distractive forces when compared to partial labral debridement (14). Finally, labral reconstruction has demonstrated a reduction in contact pressure of the hip when compared to labral resection (15). These studies suggest that reconstruction of the labrum improves hip function, rather than treatment with a partial labral resection alone.

The indications for labral reconstruction continue to evolve. Arthroscopic labral repair has demonstrated superior patient-reported outcomes when compared to labral debridement (6). However, there are instances in which the labral tissue is deemed irreparable. Controversy exists in regard to treatment with either selective labral debridement or primary labral reconstruction. Currently, the most common indication for labral reconstruction is labral deficiency from previous labral debridement or resection, in which the patient continues to experience hip pain. Additionally, in revision settings with significant adhesions, it may not be possible to resect the adhesive tissues while preserving the labral tissue. Some surgeons, however, advocate for labral reconstruction in the setting of an irreparable labral tear or in the setting of insufficient labral tissue, which in the current author's experience is uncommon. In these situations, there may not be adequate tissue to restore the normal biomechanics and the suction-seal effect of the labrum.

Labral reconstruction may also be performed in a variety of other situations, such as labral degeneration with intrasubstance cystic changes, but in most of these cases, the labrum remains salvageable and reconstruction is not necessarily required. A labrum that is <2 to 3 mm may also be considered an indication for primary labral reconstruction, as there may not be sufficient tissue for repair or to maintain labral function when damaged (16). Finally, labral ossification may occur in select patients, is considered to be a cause of pincer-type FAI and may be the most common indication or consideration in the primary setting. These lesions may occur as small areas of ossification within the labral substance or may be as severe as circumferential ossification that encases the entire peripheral acetabular rim. In cases of complete ossification, there is no labral tissue that remains after resection of the ossification, and thus, a circumferential labral reconstruction may be performed to restore the labral function. Additionally, patients with global overcoverage and pincer FAI may have a diminutive labrum due to the repetitive crush injury secondary to the impaction injury that occurs. Currently, it is not clear whether treatment with selective debridement or labral reconstruction will impart superior outcomes within this patient population. The authors prefer to evaluate the hip seal intraoperatively when the labrum is not salvageable in order to determine the need for labral reconstruction. In some cases, the hip has a degree of congruency that provides a seal in the absence of a circumferential labrum. With the hip in full extension, traction is gradually applied, and if a seal is present (sudden fluid/blood egress or sudden release of the femoral head), a labral reconstruction might not be necessary unless mild dysplastic findings are present. If a seal is not present with this maneuver, then labral reconstruction should be considered.

Contraindications

- Age > 60 years
- Joint space <2 mm or <50% of the contralateral joint space
- Any bipolar grade 3 and 4 chondral changes
- Loss of joint space on MRI/CT
- Significant acetabular or femoral head cysts on MRI

PREOPERATIVE PREPARATION

A thorough history and physical examination, in addition to a standardized set of radiographs, are essential for the diagnosis and subsequent preoperative planning of patients with labral pathology. Patients with labral tears typically have a history of anterior hip pain, which is aggravated by hip flexion and internal rotation activities. Physical examination findings may reveal restricted range of motion and reproducible pain with anterior impingement testing. Initial radiographic evaluation should include well-positioned anteroposterior pelvis, false-profile, and Dunn lateral radiographs. The acetabular rim is evaluated for any pincer-type FAI, labral ossification, or acetabular rim fractures. A computed tomography (CT) scan with three-dimensional (3D) reconstructions can be helpful in further assessing acetabular rim morphology preoperatively and assist with surgical decision-making. The axial and 3D reconstructions may be helpful to identify the presence and extent of labral ossification. Proper evaluation and assessment is important, not only diagnostically but also for surgical preparation and treatment.

TECHNIQUE

Sierra and Trousdale first described labral reconstruction of the hip; however, this was performed in the setting of an open surgical dislocation of the hip and involved the use of ligamentum teres autograft (17). Labral reconstruction was eventually described as an arthroscopic technique by Philippon, utilizing iliotibial band autograft (18). This technique has been further refined, including segmental and circumferential reconstructions (19). We prefer to reconstruct the tissue that is deficient, rather than perform circumferential reconstructions in all patients.

Hip arthroscopy is performed in a standardized position and setup and adequate hip joint distraction. Three arthroscopic portals are established for labral reconstruction, including the anterolateral (AL), mid-anterior (MAP), and distal anterolateral (DALA) portals. Three portals are required in order to performing the shuttling of the labral reconstruction graft and facilitate suture management. These portals should be spaced adequately apart to avoid instrument crowding. After the creation of an interportal capsulotomy, the hip is inspected for any labral and/or chondral disease. Specifically with regard to the acetabular labrum, we assess for any intrasubstance degeneration, calcification, or insufficiency. Once the decision is made to proceed with labral reconstruction, the labrum is removed in the area of the tear and disease using a combination of arthroscopic biters and shaver, and in some cases, a small but healthy remnant of labrum can be left intact with the graft placed behind the remnant to assist with appropriate positioning anatomically. The resection continues both anteriorly and posteriorly until normal labral tissue is encountered. Once the diseased labral tissue is resected, the acetabular rim is decorticated using an arthroscopic bur, to create a bleeding surface for graft incorporation. Additionally, any acetabular overcoverage/pincer-type FAI is resected as templated preoperatively.

In the preparation of graft creation, the labral defect is measured. In order to do so, a labral anchor is inserted at the anterior border of the labral deficiency, at the junction with normal labral tissue. This is drilled and inserted through the MAP portal. Both sutures from this anchor are brought out through the DALA portal. The suture tails from this single anchor are then evened up, and both passed through the eyelet of a knot pusher. The knot pusher is then advanced along the sutures to the acetabular rim, at the hole of the anchor (Fig. 50-1A). Outside the hip, the sutures are both gripped together, and a snap is placed at the end of the knot pusher (Fig. 50-1B). The knot pusher is the advanced toward the posterior border of the labral deficiency, at the edge of the normal posterior labral tissue. As the knot pusher is advanced toward this location, the two suture tails from the anterior anchor are laid along the acetabular rim (Fig. 50-1C). Outside the hip, the sutures are again gripped together, and a second snap is placed at the end of the knot pusher (Fig. 50-1D). The distance between the two snaps is then measured, thus corresponding to the length of the labral deficiency (Fig. 50-1E). The authors prefer to add an additional 5 to 10 mm to the measured length, representing approximately 5 mm extra that will be on each end of the graft, where the future sutures will be passed.

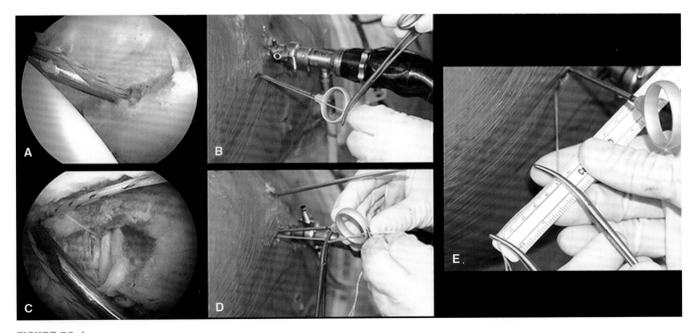

FIGURE 50-1

A: The knot pusher is advanced along the anterior anchor sutures to the acetabular rim. **B:** A snap is grasped at the end of the knot pusher to mark the first location on the sutures. **C:** The sutures are placed along the edge of the acetabular rim toward the junction of the posterior labral tissue. **D:** Another snap is grasped on the sutures at the end of the knot pusher to mark the distance of the labral deficiency. **E:** The distance between the snaps is measured.

Prior to the creation of the graft, the second labral anchor is placed at the posterior border of the labral deficiency, at the junction with the normal labral tissue. This anchor is drilled and inserted via the anterolateral or posterolateral portal depending on the location along the acetabular rim. The traction is released and attention is turned toward the creation of the labral graft.

The authors prefer to use iliotibial band allograft or autograft; however, longer grafts may necessitate the use of allograft as there may not be enough autograft tissue length available. Current literature does not support allograft or autograft as superior in regard to incorporation or clinical outcomes. If allograft is utilized, we prefer frozen or freeze-dried fascia lata. The graft is first prepared by soaking in 250 cc of normal saline with bacitracin and polymyxin. Once thawed, the graft is folded into thirds, so that the width measures approximately 12 to 15 mm. The ends are then cut in order to create a length in accordance with the labral deficiency, with the addition of 10 mm as described above. The graft is then tubularized with undyed, 2-0 Vicryl suture. We prefer to place an individual stay suture on each end of the graft and leave length to the suture in order to secure the graft within a Graftmaster. Once this is positioned, the 2-0 Vicryl suture is then run up and down the length of the graft to compact and tubularize the graft. The graft is then kept under tension on the Graftmaster, wrapped in a moist Ray-Tec.

At this point, the authors prefer to enter the peripheral compartment and perform the proximal femoral osteoplasty. We prefer to perform this prior to the placement of the labral graft to allow a period of rest from traction of the hip. Additionally, this sequence avoids any potential inadvertent injury to the graft during the femoral correction and also avoids any potential graft swelling with any prolonged time with continued arthroscopic fluid lavage.

Once femoral correction is achieved, traction is reapplied to the hip, and the arthroscope is then placed into the DALA portal. An 8.5 × 100 mm arthroscopic cannula is then inserted in both the MAP and the AL portals. One of the sutures from the anterior anchor is retrieved out the MAP portal and clamped to the drape, while the second suture from the anterior anchor is retrieved out the AL portal. One of the sutures from the most lateral/posterior anchor is also retrieved out the AL portal, through the cannula. The second suture from the posterior anchor remains in the AL portal, however, outside the cannula (Figs. 50-2 and 50-3).

A free needle is then used in order to pass the sutures from the AL portal cannula through the respective ends of the graft. The anterior anchor suture is passed through the planned anterior aspect of the graft, while the posterior anchor suture is passed through the planned posterior aspect of the graft. The sutures are passed approximately 5 mm from the edge of the graft, in order to allow good approximation to the native labral tissues. A suture claw grasper is the positioned in the MAP portal. With tension applied to each suture, the knot pusher is then placed over the anterior suture from the AL portal and is used to slide the graft down the anterior suture and through the cannula (Fig. 50-3).

Once the graft has partially entered the joint, the suture-retrieving device is used to pull the anterior suture out the MAP portal. Care is taken not to twist the graft or tangle the sutures. The suture

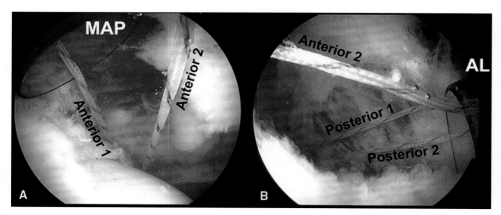

FIGURE 50-2

A: The view of the *MAP*, with the camera in the DALA portal. One suture from the anterior anchor is shuttled out the *MAP*, while the other suture is taken out the AL portal. **B:** The view of the *AL* portal. One suture from the anterior anchor and one suture from the posterior anchor are grasped out the *AL* portal.

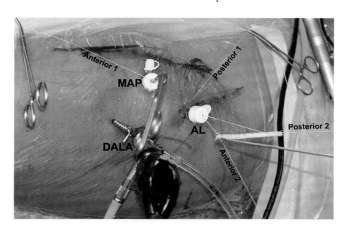

FIGURE 50-3

The setup of the sutures prior to shuttling of the labral reconstruction graft.

is grabbed in between the graft and the knot pusher (Fig. 50-4A). The knot pusher is then placed on the posterior anchor suture that remains within the AL portal. With tension applied to the suture, the knot pusher is used to push the remainder of the graft into the joint (Fig. 50-4B). This allows for slack within the graft and initial approximation of the graft anteriorly.

The anterior anchor is tied first by identifying the postsuture and tying an appropriate arthroscopic knot. The postanchor from the posterior anchor, which remains outside the AL cannula, is then grasped with a claw grasper and delivered through the AL cannula. The postsuture is again identified, and an arthroscopic knot is tied appropriately for the posterior anchor. At this point, the authors prefer to remove the AL cannula and place the arthroscope in the AL portal. Additional suture anchors are drilled and inserted through the DALA portal. The suture is first passed between the acetabular rim and the labral graft into the central aspect of the acetabulum. A piercing suture grasper is the passed through the labral graft, and the suture is grasped and delivered out the MAP cannula. A suture claw grasper is used to also retrieve the postsuture out the MAP cannula. An arthroscopic knot is again tied further securing the graft to the acetabular rim. This process is repeated placing anchors every 5 to 7 mm. A free no. 2 Ultrabraid (Smith & Nephew, Andover, MA) suture is then passed through the anterior end of the graft and retrieved with a piercing suture grasper through the mid-substance of the native labrum. The suture is then tied, completing a side-to-side repair between the native labrum and the graft. This is repeated for the posterior junction between the graft and native labrum. Traction is released, and the graft is inspected to ensure that there is adequate seal between the graft and the femoral head (Fig. 50-5).

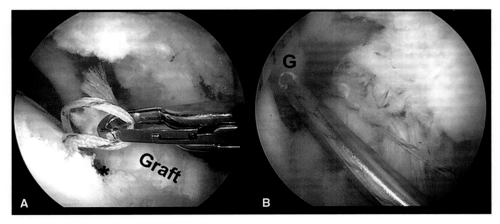

FIGURE 50-4

A: The graft is shuttled into the joint through the AL portal, using the knot pusher (*asterisk*). A suture grasper is placed through the MAP and used to retrieve the suture between the graft and the knot pusher (*asterisk*).
B: The knot pusher is then placed on the posterior anchor suture that is within AL portal and used to push the remainder of the graft (*G*) within the joint.

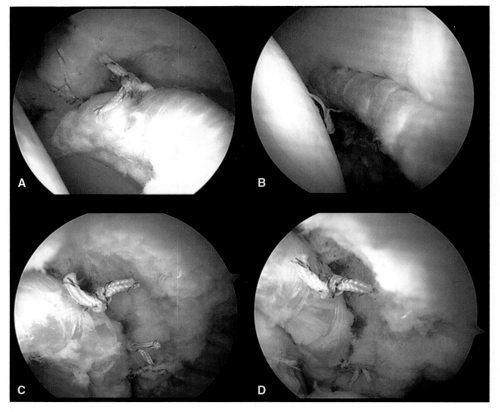

FIGURE 50-5

A: View of the anterior aspect of the graft from the AL portal. **B:** View of the posterior aspect of the graft from the MAP. **C:** View of the mid-portion of the graft from the MAP. **D:** Release of traction demonstrates the restoration of the labral seal.

PEARLS AND PITFALLS

- Three portals are required for optimum graft placement.
- Measurement of the labral defect with the suture technique is performed to ensure adequate graft length. An additional 10 mm is added to ensure for graft/native labrum apposition.
- Allow for a period of rest from traction by performing peripheral compartment correction prior to placement of the labral graft.
- Drill and place anchors from the DALA portal as close to the acetabular rim as possible without intra-articular penetration. This will avoid graft eversion.
- A side-to-side suture can further ensure labral continuity.

POSTOPERATIVE MANAGEMENT

Rehabilitation for labral reconstruction is similar to that for labral repair; however, patients are educated about the aneural nature of the labral graft. Patients remain toe-touch weight bearing for approximately 4 weeks. A continuous passive motion (CPM) machine can be started on the day of surgery, and physical therapy is initiated within 5 days from surgery. Heterotopic ossification prophylaxis in the form of nonsteroidal anti-inflammatory medications is prescribed for 2 to 4 weeks postoperatively. External rotation is limited for the first 2 weeks to protect the capsular repair. Active hip flexion or isometrics is also avoided for the first 4 weeks postoperatively to avoid hip flexor tendinitis. In our experience, full recovery takes approximately 6 months postoperatively.

COMPLICATIONS

Given the additional time that is required for hip distraction during labral reconstruction, the risk of traction-related injuries may be increased; however, multiple studies have documented no significant difference when compared to arthroscopic labral repair (20–22). Additionally, there exists a potential for intra-abdominal fluid extravasation given the occasional need to extend the capsulotomy anteriorly and given the increased length of surgery. Therefore, it is important for the surgeon and the anesthesiologist to be aware of this potential and know the signs of intra-abdominal compartment syndrome, such as a decrease in the core body temperature and an increase in abdominal pressure. Finally, if allograft tissue is used for the labral reconstruction, there is a very small risk of disease transmission that should be discussed with the patients prior to surgery (23).

RESULTS

Two initial studies evaluated the outcomes of labral reconstruction that was performed during open surgical dislocation. These studies were performed at the same institution, with the second study investigating 20 patients with a minimum of 1-year follow-up. Sixty-five percent of the patients underwent a subsequent surgery, with fifteen percent converting to a total hip arthroplasty (24). There has been an abundance of studies that have investigated the results of arthroscopic labral reconstruction since its initial description of the technique. The original report of labral reconstruction using fascia lata autograft in 2010 demonstrated a mean 23-point improvement in the Modified Harris Hip Score (mHHS) at a minimum of 2 years, with an 80% patient satisfaction. Nine percent of the patients had progression to total hip arthroplasty at a mean of 18 months (18). At a mean of 49-month follow-up (minimum 3 years), 24% of the patients had undergone conversion to THA. This was associated with increased age and joint space ≤2 mm. However, there remained a mean 24-point improvement in the mHHS (25). A study investigating 21 elite athletes demonstrated an 86% return to play when undergoing labral reconstruction using iliotibial band autograft (26). The HOS-Sport subscale improved a mean of 21 points among these patients.

Recently, there has been an interest in circumferential labral reconstructions rather than segmental reconstructions, in order to provide initial structural continuity through the entire labrum. A minimum 2-year study investigating 131 hips, demonstrated a mean improvement of 34 points on the mHHS and a 90% patient satisfaction (27). Fourteen percent of the hips underwent revision procedure at a mean of 17 months. The author also compared the results of labral reconstruction ($N = 98$) and labral repairs ($N = 15$) during the revision hip arthroscopy setting. Failure was defined by subsequent intra-articular hip surgery. Fifty percent of labral repairs were considered to have failed, compared to 12% of labral reconstructions. Patients who underwent revision labral repair were 2.6 times more likely to fail than patients who underwent labral reconstruction (28). However, other studies have not necessarily noted this difference, and further investigations are required (20).

CONCLUSIONS

Labral reconstruction has recently gained popularity as an alternative treatment option for labral pathology. Current indications include irreparable labral tears, insufficient labral tissue, labral ossification, and revision hip arthroscopy. Labral reconstruction has demonstrated restoration of fluid pressurization, stabilization of the hip to distraction, and reduced contact pressures when compared to labral deficiency (13–15). Although several surgical techniques and graft choices have been described and documented improvement in clinical outcomes, no technique has been accepted as superior. Further research is required to determine the optimal indications and technique(s) for labral reconstruction.

REFERENCES

1. Beck M, Leunig M, Parvizi J, et al. Anterior femoroacetabular impingement: part II. Midterm results of surgical treatment. *Clin Orthop Relat Res.* 2004;418:67–73.
2. Ganz R, Parvizi J, Beck M, et al. Femoroacetabular impingement: a cause for osteoarthritis of the hip. *Clin Orthop Relat Res.* 2003;417:112–120.
3. Larson CM. Arthroscopic management of pincer-type impingement. *Sports Med Arthrosc Rev.* 2010;18(2):100–107.
4. Notzli HP, Wyss TF, Stoecklin CH, et al. The contour of the femoral head-neck junction as a predictor for the risk of anterior impingement. *J Bone Joint Surg Br.* 2002;84(4):556–560.
5. Larson CM, Giveans MR. Arthroscopic management of femoroacetabular impingement: early outcomes measures. *Arthroscopy.* 2008;24(5):540–546.
6. Larson CM, Giveans MR. Arthroscopic debridement versus refixation of the acetabular labrum associated with femoroacetabular impingement. *Arthroscopy.* 2009;25(4):369–376.

7. Byrd JW, Jones KS. Arthroscopic femoroplasty in the management of cam-type femoroacetabular impingement. *Clin Orthop Relat Res.* 2009;467(3):739–746.

8. Byrd JW, Jones KS. Arthroscopic management of femoroacetabular impingement: minimum 2-year follow-up. *Arthroscopy.* 2010;27(10):1379–1388.

9. Ayeni OR, Alradwan H, de Sa D, et al. The hip labrum reconstruction: indications and outcomes—a systemic review. *Knee Surg Sports Traumatol Arthrosc.* 2014;22(4):737–743.

10. Seldes RM, Tan V, Hunt J, et al. Anatomy, histologic features, and vascularity of the adult acetabular labrum. *Clin Orthop Relat Res.* 2001;382:232–240.

11. Beck M, Kalhor M, Leunig M, et al. Hip morphology influences the pattern of damage to the acetabular cartilage: femoroacetabular impingement as a cause of early osteoarthritis of the hip. *J Bone Joint Surg Br.* 2005;87(7):1012–1018.

12. Klaue K, Dumin CW, Ganz R. The acetabular rim syndrome. A clinical presentation of dysplasia of the hip. *J Bone Joint Surg Br.* 1991;73(3):423–429.

13. Philippon MJ, Nepple JJ, Campbell KJ, et al. The hip fluid seal—part I: the effect of an acetabular labral tear, repair, resection, and reconstruction on hip fluid pressurization. *Knee Surg Sports Traumatol Arthrosc.* 2014;22(4):722–729.

14. Nepple JJ, Philippon MJ, Campbell KJ, et al. The hip fluid seal—part II: the effect of an acetabular labral tear, repair, resection, and reconstruction on hip stability to distraction. *Knee Surg Sports Traumatol Arthrosc.* 2014;22(4):730–736.

15. Lee S, Wuerz TH, Shewman E, et al. Labral reconstruction with iliotibial band autografts and semitendinosus allografts improve hip joint contact area and contact pressure: an in vitro analysis. *Am J Sports Med.* 2015;43(1):98–104.

16. Ejnisman L, Philippon MJ, Lertwanich P. Acetabular labral tears: diagnosis, repair, and a method for labral reconstruction. *Clin Sports Med.* 2011;30:317–329.

17. Sierra RJ, Trousdale RT. Labral reconstruction using the ligamentum teres capitis: report of a new technique. *Clin Orthop Relat Res.* 2009;467:753–759.

18. Philippon MJ, Briggs KK, Hay CJ, et al. Arthroscopic labral reconstruction in the hip using iliotibial band autograft: technique and early outcomes. *Arthroscopy.* 2010;26:750–756.

19. White BJ, Herzog MM. Arthroscopic labral reconstruction of the hip using iliotibial band allograft and front-to-back fixation technique. *Arthrosc Tech.* 2016;5(1):89–97.

20. Chandesakran S, Darwish N, Mu BH, et al. Arthroscopic reconstruction of the irreparable acetabular labrum: a match-controlled study. *Arthroscopy.* 2019;35(2):480–488.

21. Matsuda DK, Burchette RJ. Arthroscopic hip labral reconstruction with a gracilis autograft versus labral refixation: 2-year minimum outcomes. *Am J Sports Med.* 2013;41(5):980–987.

22. Kowalczuk M, Bhandari M, Farrokhyar F, et al. Complications following hip arthroscopy: a systematic review and meta-analysis. *Knee Surg Sports Traumatol Arthrosc.* 2013;21(7):1669–1675.

23. Hinsenkamp M, Muylle L, Eastlund T, et al. Adverse reactions and events related to musculoskeletal allograft: reviewed by the World Health Organisation Projection NOTIFY. *Int Orthop.* 2012;36(3):633–641.

24. Walker JA, Pagnotto M, Trousdale RT, et al. Preliminary pain and function after labral reconstruction during femoroacetabular impingement surgery. *Clin Orthop Relat Res.* 2012;470(12):3414–3420.

25. Geyer MR, Philippon MJ, Fagrelius TS, et al. Acetabular labral reconstruction with an iliotibial band autograft: outcome and survivorship analysis at minimum 3-year follow-up. *Am J Sports Med.* 2013;41(8):1750–1756.

26. Boykin RE, Patterson D, Briggs KK, et al. Results of arthroscopic labral reconstruction of the hip in elite athletes. *Am J Sports Med.* 2013;41(10):2296–2301.

27. White BJ, Stapleford AB, Hawkes TK, et al. Allograft use in arthroscopic labral reconstruction of the hip with front-to-back fixation technique: minimum 2-year follow-up. *Arthroscopy.* 2016;32(1):26–32.

28. White BJ, Patterson J, Herzog MM. Revision arthroscopic acetabular labral treatment: repair or reconstruct? *Arthroscopy.* 2016;32(12):2513–2520.

51 Subspine Impingement of the Hip

Jonathan E. Campbell, James R. Ross, and Christopher M. Larson

INTRODUCTION

Femoroacetabular impingement (FAI) has been well described in the past decade with most literature characterizing the evaluation, diagnosis, and treatment of cam- and pincer-type FAI (1–8). Recently, there has been an increased awareness of extra-articular sources of impingement such as trochanteric-pelvic, ischiofemoral, and anterior inferior iliac spine (AIIS) or subspine hip impingement (9–15). Subspine impingement occurs in a subset of patients as a result of pathologic contact between the AIIS and the distal femoral neck during hip flexion. There is also likely a soft tissue component with the rectus and or capsule being compressed between the AIIS and femoral neck. AIIS impingement can also be a source of unaddressed osseous impingement and failure after hip arthroscopy with a subsequent need for revision surgery. This chapter describes the pertinent anatomical structures that are implicated in subspine impingement as well as the identification of this unique source of hip pain. Additionally, we outline a treatment algorithm, including a description of the arthroscopic treatment.

INDICATIONS

The AIIS is a bony eminence located on the anterior and inferior aspect of the ilium, which is typically located proximal to the acetabular rim. This pelvic eminence begins as a separate apophysis, and typically begins ossification between the ages of 13 and 14 years. Fusion with the remainder of the ilium usually occurs between the ages of 16 and 18 years (16). The most cranial aspect of the AIIS is thought to give rise to the direct head of the rectus femoris, whereas the inferior aspect of the AIIS gives rise to a portion of the iliofemoral ligament.

Subspine impingement can result from a variety of etiologies. Apophyseal avulsion fractures at the AIIS can occur in adolescents resulting in acute pain and loss of function. After the avulsion, ossification and closure of the physis can lead to a distal extension of AIIS. Additionally, the rectus tendon may become fully or partially avulsed off the AIIS and heterotopic bone can form in the area of the avulsion in continuity with the AIIS, also leading to extra-articular impingement. Treatment of acetabular dysplasia with a periacetabular osteotomy (PAO), may also result in subspine impingement as the AIIS is flexed forward with the acetabular fragment. Finally, developmental abnormalities, such as acetabular retroversion, may predispose to subspine impingement during hip flexion along the head-neck junction or further distally.

PREOPERATIVE PREPARATION

A thorough history and physical examination, in addition to a standardized set of radiographs, is essential for the diagnosis and subsequent preoperative planning of a patient with subspinous impingement. Patients with subspine impingement typically have a history of anterior hip pain, which is aggravated by hip flexion activities such as prolonged sitting, squatting, sprinting, and kicking. Some patients may describe a "grinding" sensation anteriorly with flexion and lateral movements. Physical examination findings may reveal tenderness to palpation over the AIIS. Generally, there may also be a limitation in passive straight hip flexion, with pain anteriorly at the terminal range of flexion, with or without positive impingement signs (17). There may also be persistence of anterior hip pain elicited at the end range of straight hip flexion within 1 hour of an intra-articular injection of a local anesthetic (under fluoroscopic or ultrasound guidance), given that these injections are intra-articular and thus do not reach the area of extra-articular impingement (14).

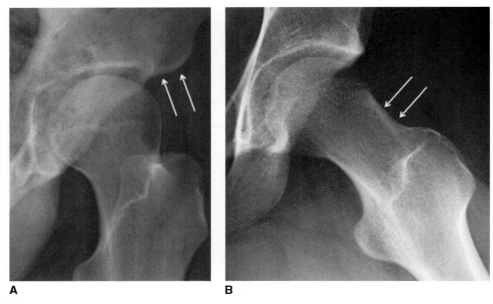

A **B**

FIGURE 51-1

Radiographic findings of subspine impingement. **A:** False-profile radiograph demonstrated cortical thickening (*arrows*) along the interior aspect of a Type II AIIS. **B:** Dunn lateral radiograph demonstrates distal femoral head-neck junction sclerosis (*arrows*).

Initial radiographic evaluation should include well-positioned anteroposterior pelvis, false-profile, and Dunn lateral radiographs. A low-lying AIIS may be mistaken for a positive cross-over sign, a surrogate marker for acetabular retroversion, and thus scrutiny of all the radiographic views is essential (18). Sclerosis on the inferior aspect of the AIIS on the false-profile view as well as at the distal head-neck junction on Dunn lateral view can be seen with subspine impingement. Impingement cysts can be seen along the distal femoral neck on the Dunn lateral view, which is typically more distal than with impingement at the acetabular rim (Fig. 51-1).

A computed tomography (CT) scan with three-dimensional (3D) reconstructions can be helpful in further assessing AIIS morphology preoperatively, and assist with surgical decision-making. A classification system developed by Hetsroni et al. (15) based on 3D CT scans, illustrates the prominence of the AIIS in relation to the acetabular rim. Using the head-on and ischium view of the 3D CT reconstruction, the AIIS is characterized based on a horizontal line drawn on the ischium view at the most inferior aspect of the junction of AIIS and ischium wall. In type I, the AIIS does not cross inferior to this line. In type II, a portion of the AIIS crosses inferior to the horizontal line but does not extend inferior to the superior acetabular rim. In type III, a portion of the AIIS crosses inferior to the horizontal line and the superior acetabular rim (Fig. 51-2). Proper classification and assessment is important, not only diagnostically, but also for surgical preparation and treatment. There is also a variable anterior extent of the AIIS which has not been well defined but can certainly predispose to subspine impingement.

TECHNIQUE

Hip arthroscopy is performed in a standardized position and set-up. Arthroscopic portals are established routinely with adequate hip joint distraction. After the creation of an interportal capsulotomy, the hip is inspected for any secondary signs of extra-articular impingement, specifically with regards to the AIIS. Focal ecchymosis of the labrum and/or the capsule in the region of the AIIS is a good indicator of subspinous impingement (Fig. 51-3). Once the diagnosis of subspinous impingement is confirmed, the authors prefer to treat this form of extra-articular impingement, prior to any labral repair or osteoplasty of the femoral head-neck junction but the decompression can be performed at any point during the case and with or without traction.

The AIIS can be located by placing the arthroscopic burr proximal to the acetabular rim with direct palpation, or via fluoroscopic assistance (Fig. 51-4). Once the AIIS is identified, the proximal capsular leaflet is reflected proximally off the acetabular rim and thus away from the labrum. This will often begin to expose the most caudal aspect of the AIIS. This is often best performed with

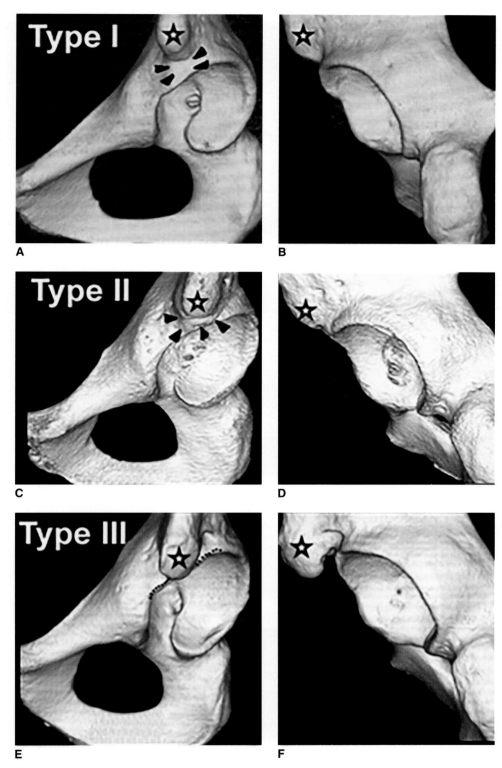

FIGURE 51-2

AIIS (*asterisk*) classification system with use of 3D reconstruction CT scans, with the use of the "head-on" **(A)**, **(C)**, and **(E)** and ischium **(B)**, **(D)** and **(F)** views. *Arrowheads* note a smooth **(A)** and bony prominences **(C)** on the ilium wall between the caudad level of the AIIS and the acetabular rim. (Adapted from Hetsroni I, Poultsides L, Bedi A, et al. Anterior inferior iliac spine morphology correlates with hip range of motion: a classification system and dynamic model. *Clin Orthop Relat Res.* 2013;471(8):2497–2503, with permission.)

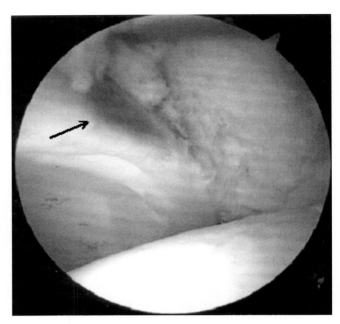

FIGURE 51-3

Focal ecchymosis of the labrum and capsule seen in the region of the AIIS is a good indicator of subspinous impingement (*arrow*).

a radiofrequency device, however, can also be performed using an arthroscopic shaver. The working instrument can either be used in the anterolateral or the mid-anterior portal. We prefer to view from the anterolateral portal, and use the instrument through the mid-anterior portal. A 5.5-mm round burr is then used to decompress and remove the AIIS prominence, from distal to proximal. Bony resection is begun at the acetabular rim, which coincides with the bare area of the AIIS. As the resection

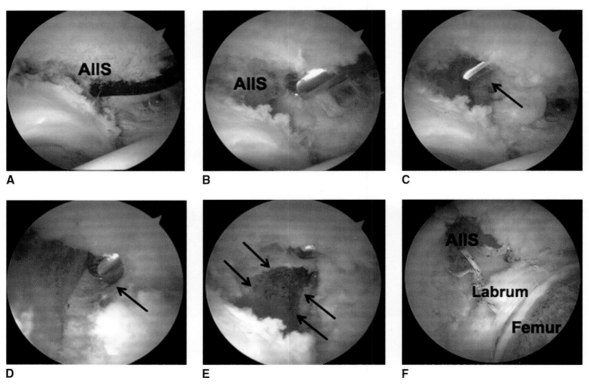

FIGURE 51-4

A: A radiofrequency device can be used to reflect the proximal capsular leaflet anteriorly exposing the AIIS. **B:** Arthroscopic burr is used to palpate the AIIS and begin the subspine decompression through the mid anterior portal. **C:** To gain further proximal access, a beaver blade (*arrow*) can be used to make longitudinal split in the rectus tendon. **D:** The decompression is carried further proximal with the burr inserted through this window (*arrow*). **E:** The completed AIIS decompression (*arrows*) is seen with preservation of the anterior and superior attachments of the rectus femoris. **F:** With traction released the AIIS decompression, labral repair, and femoral neck osteotomy can be seen.

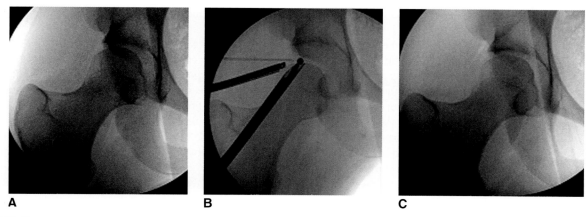

FIGURE 51-5

A: Preoperative AP fluoroscopic image prior to AIIS decompression. **B:** Intraoperative fluoroscopic image with burr palpating AIIS. **C:** Intraoperative fluoroscopic image depicting AIIS decompression to the level of the sourcil.

continues proximal, it may be helpful to release the traction of the hip in order to relieve tension from the rectus femoris and thus improve access to the AIIS. Additionally, this allows for diminished traction time and thus any traction-related side effects.

Intra-operative fluoroscopy can also be very helpful to ensure adequate decompression. An AP pelvis fluoroscopic radiograph may be used with the burr on the most caudal aspect of the AIIS resection. Decompression to the level of the acetabular sourcil is ideal in order to ensure adequate bony resection (Figs. 51-5 and 51-6). Additionally, the C-arm can be directed with a 45-degree

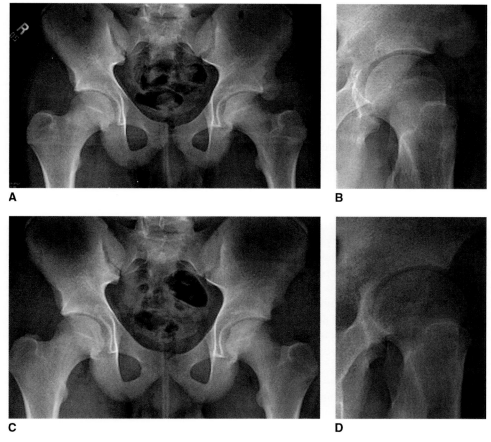

FIGURE 51-6

(A) AP and **(B)** false-profile radiographs show a left-sided post-traumatic type 3 AIIS deformity in a soccer player with prior AIIS avulsion injury. Post-operative **(C)** AP and **(D)** false-profile radiographs show decompression of AIIS deformity.

tilt, thus mimicking a false profile radiograph, further assisting with performing the planned decompression.

Occasionally, the tendon of the direct head of the rectus femoris may inhibit further proximal resection of the AIIS. In this situation, a beaver blade can be used to create a longitudinal window through the rectus tendon (Fig. 51-4). A slotted cannula is then placed in this window and used to deliver the bur into the desired position. This technique may help to avoid excessive capsular resection and also iatrogenic damage to the rectus tendon fibers. Hapa et al. (19) have shown that there is an anatomic "safe zone" devoid of rectus tendon on the AIIS. In their cadaver study, they showed that there is a consistent bare spot of approximately 0.5 by 1.5 cm devoid of rectus tendon footprint at the anterior and inferomedial aspect of the AIIS. Knowledge of this can help to avoid injury to the rectus tendon during decompression.

After decompression of the AIIS is complete, the labrum is reassessed for any tears. After treatment of the central compartment, the traction is released and the peripheral compartment is inspected for any femoral head-beck junction offset pathomorphology. In the setting of subspine impingement, the surgeon should pay particular attention to the anterior-inferior distal femoral head-neck junction along the medial synovial fold, which will often demonstrate sclerosis and hardening or sometimes very thick soft tissue build up. After completion of the bony decompression, the capsulotomy is closed using a suture passing device and No. 2 absorbable or nonabsorbable sutures.

PEARLS AND PITFALLS

- Three-Dimensional (3D) CT scan and False Profile plain radiographs can be utilized to classify the subspinous impingement and assist with surgical resection templating
- Traction may be released to limit traction time and also allow for relaxation of the rectus femoris tendon to assist with proximal AIIS resection
- A window can be created within the rectus femoris tendon to avoid tendon injury and detachment and minimize capsular resection
- Intra-operative fluoroscopy should be utilized to confirm appropriate decompression

POST-OPERATIVE MANAGEMENT

Heterotopic ossification prophylaxis in the form of nonsteroidal anti-inflammatory medications is prescribed for 3 to 4 weeks postoperatively. Weight bearing is determined by any other procedures that are performed. External rotation is limited for the first 2 weeks to protect the capsular repair. Active hip flexion or isometrics are also avoided for the first 4 weeks post-operatively to avoid hip flexor tendinitis.

COMPLICATIONS

There does exist a theoretical potential for hip flexion weakness in the setting of overly aggressive resection of the AIIS. However, we have not noted this clinically in patients who have undergone subspinous decompression, nor any documented cases of rectus femoris detachment. Given the proximity of the AIIS to the retroperitoneal space, there does exist a potential for intra-abdominal fluid extravasation. Therefore, it is important for the surgeon and the anesthesiologist to be aware of this potential, and know the signs of intra-abdominal compartment syndrome, such as a decrease in the core body temperature and an increase in abdominal pressure. We have also not seen symptomatic intra-abdominal fluid extravasation during cases that have underwent AIIS decompression.

RESULTS

A recent systematic review of arthroscopic treatment of subspine impingement by de Sa et al. (20) showed consistently good outcomes. The primary indications for surgical treatment of subspine impingement included persistent pain after intra-articular anesthetic injection with deep hip flexion and either pain with palpation of the AIIS and/or imaging showing a prominent AIIS. There were no reported contraindications to surgery. Hetsroni et al. (14) showed good outcomes with modified Harris Hip score (mHHS) improving 34.2 ± 18.0 points with a mean follow-up of 14.7 months.

They also showed a mean range of motion improvement of 18.5 degrees from a mean of 98.5 ± 6.7 degrees preoperatively to 117.0 ± 7.5 degrees postoperatively after arthroscopic AIIS decompression. The largest study in this review, by Hapa et al. (19) reported 22.2-point postoperative increase in the mHHS and a 3.0-point reduction in postoperative pain measured on the visual analog scale at a mean follow up of 11 months. There were only two reports of asymptomatic heterotopic ossification formation in all studies.

CONCLUSIONS

Arthroscopic decompression of AIIS deformities that are responsible for subspine impingement can result in improved range of motion and patient reported outcome measures. AIIS deformities can be iatrogenic, developmental, secondary to rectus femoris avulsions, or due to an adolescent injury with an apophyseal avulsion. A thorough physical examination and radiographic evaluation are necessary to formulate appropriate indications and achieve successful outcomes with surgical treatment.

REFERENCES

1. Beck M, Leunig M, Parvizi J, et al. Anterior femoroacetabular impingement: Part II. Midterm results of surgical treatment. *Clin Orthop Relat Res.* 2004;418:67–73.
2. Ganz R, Parvizi J, Beck M, et al. Femoroacetabular impingement: a cause for osteoarthritis of the hip. *Clin Orthop Relat Res.* 2003;417:112–120.
3. Larson CM. Arthroscopic management of pincer-type impingement. *Sports Med Arthrosc Rev.* 2010;18(2):100–107.
4. Notzli HP, Wyss TF, Stoecklin CH, et al. The contour of the femoral head-neck junction as a predictor for the risk of anterior impingement. *J Bone Joint Surg Br.* 2002;84(4):556–560.
5. Larson CM, Giveans MR. Arthroscopic management of femoroacetabular impingement: early outcomes measures. *Arthroscopy.* 2008;24(5):540–546.
6. Larson CM, Giveans MR. Arthroscopic debridement versus refixation of the acetabular labrum associated with femoroacetabular impingement. *Arthroscopy.* 2009;25(4):369–376.
7. Byrd JW, Jones KS. Arthroscopic femoroplasty in the management of cam-type femoroacetabular impingement. *Clin Orthop Relat Res.* 2009;467(3):739–746.
8. Philippon MJ, Briggs KK, Yen YM, et al: Outcomes following hip arthroscopy for femoroacetabular impingement with associated chondro-labral dysfunction: minimum two-year follow-up. *J Bone Joint Surg.* 2009;91(1):16–23.
9. Taneha AK, Bredella MA, Torriani M. Ischiofemoral impingement. *Magn Reson Imaging Clin N Am.* 2013;21(1):65–73.
10. Stafford GH, Villar RN. Ischiofemoral impingement. *J Bone Joint Surg Br.* 2011;93(10):1300–1302.
11. Macnicol MF, Makris D. Distal transfer of the greater trochanter. *J Bone Joint Surg Br.* 1991;73(5):838–841.
12. Leunig M, Ganz R. Relative neck lengthening and intracapital osteotomy for severe Perthes and Perthes-like deformities. *Bull NYU Hosp Jt Dis.* 2011;69(suppl 1):S62–S67.
13. Larson CM, Kelly BT, Stone RM. Making a case for anterior inferior iliac spine/subspine hip impingement: three representative case reports and proposed concept. *Arthroscopy.* 2011;27(12):1732–1737.
14. Hetsroni I, Larson CM, De la Torre K, et al. Anterior inferior iliac spine deformity as an extra-articular source of hip impingement: a series of 10 patients treated with arthroscopic decompression. *Arthroscopy.* 2012;28(11):1644–1653.
15. Hetsroni I, Poultsides L, Bedi A, et al. Anterior inferior iliac spine morphology correlates with hip range of motion: a classification system and dynamic model. *Clin Orthop Relat Res.* 2013;471(8):2497–2503.
16. Freyschmidt J, Brossmann J, Wiens J, et al. *Freyschmidt's "Koehler/Zimmer" Borderlands of Normal and Early Pathological Findings in Skeletal Radiology.* 5th Ed. New York: Thieme; 2003.
17. Klaue K, Durnin CW, Ganz R. The acetabular rim syndrome: a clinical presentation of dysplasia of the hip. *J Bone Joint Surg Br.* 1991;73:423–429.
18. Zaltz I, Kelly BT, Hetsroni I, et al. The crossover sign overestimates acetabular retroversion. *Clin Orthop Relat Res.* 2013;471(8):2463–2470.
19. Hapa O, Bedi A, Gursan O, et al. Anatomic footprint of the direct head of the rectus femoris origin: cadaveric study and clinical series of hips after arthroscopic anterior inferior iliac spine/subspine decompression. *Arthroscopy.* 2013;29:1932–1940.
20. de Sa D, Alradwan H, Cargnelli S, et al. Extra-articular hip impingement: a systematic review examining operative treatment of psoas, subspine, ischiofemoral, and greater trochanteric/pelvic impingement. *Arthroscopy.* 2014;30(8): 1026–1041.

52 Proximal Hamstring Avulsions

Philip N. Collis and Lee D. Kaplan

BACKGROUND/ETIOLOGY

Rupture of the proximal hamstring tendons from the ischial tuberosity was first reported in the literature in 1988, as a case report of two patients by Ishikawa et al. Both patients were treated with direct surgical repair and returned to sports (1). Prior reports of avulsion all included bony fracture of the ischial apophysis in the skeletally immature patient. The majority of hamstring injuries occur at the myotendinous junction and are classified as strains or tears to varying degrees (2–4). These are common injuries seen in athletes of multiple sports, especially those requiring rapid acceleration such as sprinters. True avulsions of proximal hamstrings account for only 3% to 11% of these injuries (5–7). In the younger population, these are often a result of high-level athletic participation, while in the older population, a slip or fall is commonly reported.

In 1990, Blasier and Morawa described a case report of hamstring rupture caused by a water skiing injury. The patient had direct repair and at 7-year follow-up, returned to sports despite having a 9% residual hamstring strength deficit (8). Water skiing has traditionally been a culprit for proximal hamstring injuries, as a result of forced hip flexion and knee extension while the hamstring musculature is engaged and contracted. Sallay et al. reported a case series of 12 patients who sustained proximal hamstring injuries as a result of water skiing. Six patients were considered novice skiers and six were experienced. All were repaired surgically. Ten of the twelve reported residual cramping in the posterior thigh with vigorous activity, seven returned to most of preinjury sports, and three resumed water skiing on a regular basis (9).

HISTORY AND PHYSICAL EXAMINATION

Diagnosis of a proximal hamstring avulsion is best delineated by a history and physical examination. Patients will describe a mechanism that caused a combination of eccentric hip flexion and knee extension. This is commonly a result of indirect trauma such as a slip and fall. They will often report a sudden "pulling" or "grabbing" sensation in the posterior thigh and in some cases an audible "pop." Patients will often complain of difficulty walking, difficulty arising from a chair, and significant bruising in the posterior thigh and lower buttocks region (2,4,10–13).

On presentation, patients may walk with a "stiff-legged" gait. Depending on the acuity of the injury, varying degrees of ecchymosis is seen from the proximal posterior thigh to the middle and distal thigh. A palpable defect proximally with a distal bulge from the retracted tendons is often felt. Patients will have hamstring weakness with functional testing in the prone position. This can be done at varying angles of knee flexion. Thorough neurovascular examination is important to delineate sciatic nerve injury or neuropraxia (2,4,10–13).

IMAGING

Plain radiographs including AP pelvis and lateral of the hip are often negative but can rule out other injuries such as avulsions or fractures. Magnetic resonance imaging is the most accurate in diagnosing injury to the hamstring origin (6). Normal appearing proximal hamstring tendons will appear with a homogenously low signal in continuity with the cortical bone of the ischial tuberosity. Acute avulsions will appear on T2 imaging as hyperintense signal between the tendon-bone

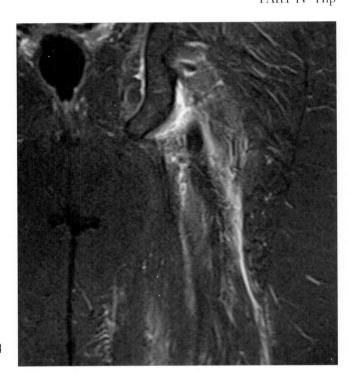

FIGURE 52-1

Coronal T2 MRI with an acute hamstring avulsion.

interface with discontinuity, representing fluid at the level of injury (3,6,7). Figures 52-1–52-8 show coronal and axial T2 cuts of a patient with an acute hamstring avulsion. The degree of retraction may correlate with the amount of fluid collection and signal at the tendon edge. Fluid signal may often track distally within the hamstring investing fascia and muscle. Chronic avulsions of the hamstring tendons in comparison will lack a distinct fluid collection. Other findings include fatty infiltration, decreased muscle volume, and scarring of the tendon to surroundings structures (3,6,7).

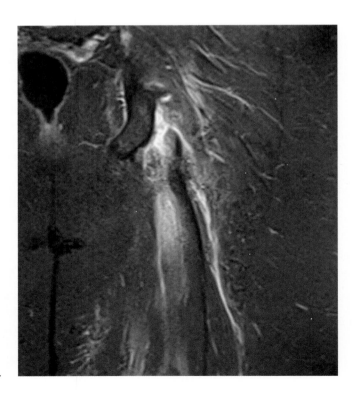

FIGURE 52-2

Coronal T2 MRI with acute hamstring avulsion with minimal tendon retraction.

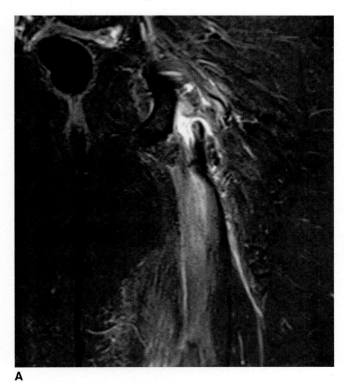

A

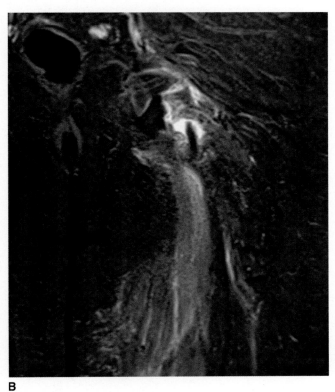

B

FIGURE 52-3

A and B: Coronal T2 MRI showing fluid tracking distally within the hamstring investing fascia and muscle.

Partial tears of the proximal hamstring origin will display hyperintense linear signal at the tendon-bone interface with a portion of the tendon still in continuity with the bone. This has been coined as the "sickle-sign" as the signal often appears crescent shaped on coronal and axial T2 sequences (10) as seen in Figure 52-9.

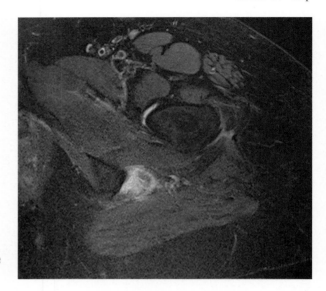

FIGURE 52-4

Axial T2 MRI showing high signal intensity at the site of hamstring tendon avulsion from the ischial tuberosity.

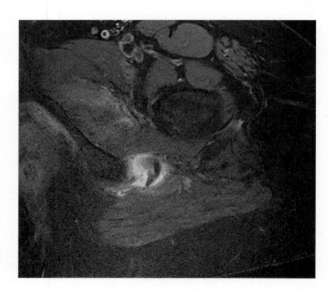

FIGURE 52-5

Axial T2 MRI showing fluid surrounding a torn hamstring tendon.

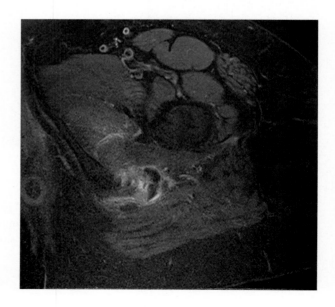

FIGURE 52-6

Axial T2 MRI high signal intensity seen around avulsed hamstring tendon.

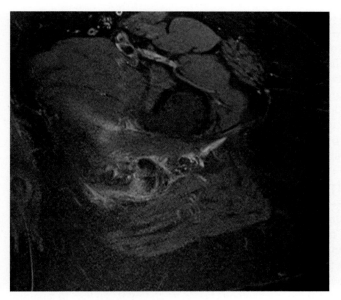

FIGURE 52-7
Axial T2 MRI fluid tracking distally within the posterior compartment.

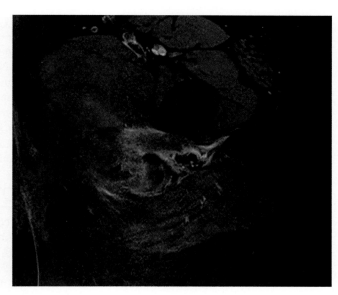

FIGURE 52-8
Soft tissue edema about the hamstring tendons.

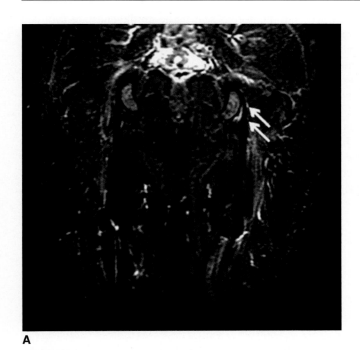

A

B

FIGURE 52-9
Coronal **(A)** and axial **(B)** axial T2 MRI. Partial hamstring tear showing the sickle sign. Hyperintense linear signal at the tendon-bone interface with a portion of the tendon still in continuity with the bone.

DIAGNOSIS AND DECISION-MAKING

It is important to differentiate hamstring strains from a complete or partial avulsion from the musculotendinous origin, as strains are predominantly treated conservatively. It is then important to distinguish between single-tendon, two-tendon, and three-tendon tears, as the treatment options can vary significantly. Surgical treatment of single tendon ruptures is not recommended as these typically will scar in to the intact tendons, and patients can return to their full strength. Two-tendon ruptures with >2 cm of retraction, or complete three-tendon ruptures, should be repaired primarily (4,5,7,10–12,14). A patient's prior activity level, age, expectations, chronicity of the injury, all need to be taken into account when deciding a treatment plan.

SURGICAL TECHNIQUE

The posterior approach to the ischium and proximal hamstring requires the patient is be placed in a prone position on the operating table. A transverse incision in line with the gluteal crease is most commonly used (Fig. 52-10). In chronic ruptures, or if the tendons are severely retracted, a longitudinal incision may be needed for adequate exposure. Dissection through the subcutaneous tissue is taken down to the gluteal fascia (Fig. 52-11), which is incised transversely. Care should be taken to identify and protect the posterior femoral cutaneous nerve, as cutting it can lead to a painful neuroma and numbness in the posterior thigh. The gluteus maximus muscle will need to be elevated and retracted superiorly for exposure to the ischium and hamstring tendons. Incising the hamstring fascia longitudinally will often release a large hematoma, which will need to be evacuated. Care should be made to identify and protect the sciatic nerve as it courses 1.2 cm laterally (15) from the hamstring origin on the ischial tuberosity (Fig. 52-12).

The hamstring tendons are then identified, and the fibrous scar tissue on the ends are debrided to healthy tendon. Excessive debridement, however, can lead to shortening of the tendon and make repair to the ischium technically difficult. The tendon ends are tagged with heavy, nonabsorbable suture and can be mobilized with blunt, finger-dissection (Fig. 52-13).

Preparation of the ischial tuberosity is critical to remove remaining fibrous tissue from the bone to create a bed for healing tendon to bone. This can be done with a periosteal elevator and rongeur, and the surface prepared with a rasp. Then, placement of three to five 4.5-mm PEEK SwiveLock (Arthrex, Naples, FL) suture anchors are placed in the native footprint of the hamstring origin (Fig. 52-14). This can be placed in a linear, "V," square or "X" formation depending on the quality and amount of bone surface area present. One limb from the preloaded suture anchor is passed down and up the semimembranosus and/or conjoint tendon in a Krackow fashion, while the second limb is passed a single time through the proximal tendon. This allows the ends to be tied down in a sliding

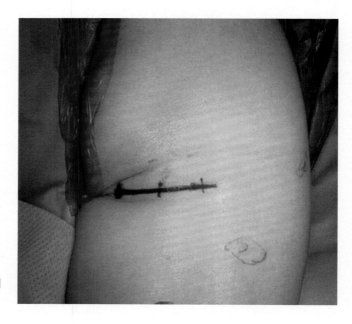

FIGURE 52-10

Transverse incision in line with the gluteal crease.

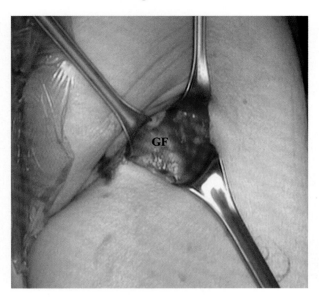

FIGURE 52-11

Dissection through the subcutaneous tissue is taken down to the gluteal fascia (*GF*).

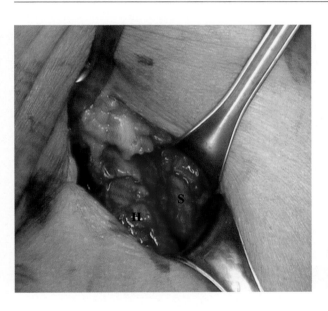

FIGURE 52-12

Avulsed hamstring tendon (*H*) and coursing lateral to it is the sciatic nerve (*S*).

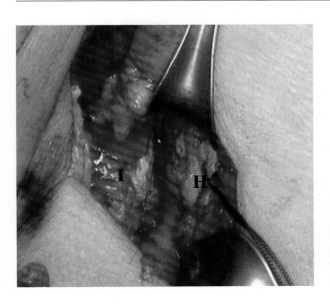

FIGURE 52-13

Fibrous scar on the avulsed hamstring tendon end (*H*) in proximity to the ischial tuberosity (*I*).

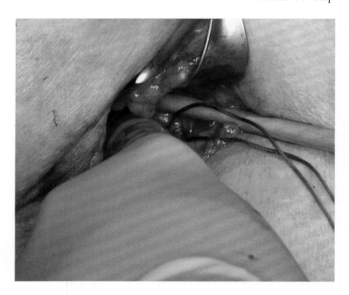

FIGURE 52-14

Suture anchor placed in the native footprint of the hamstring origin.

fashion, bringing the tendon to the ischial tuberosity. If there is little or no retraction, the suture limbs can be passed in a horizontal mattress fashion and tied down sequentially (Fig. 52-15). After repair (Fig. 52-16), a layered closure with absorbable suture to reapproximate the gluteal fascia and eliminate dead space is performed (Fig. 52-17). A subcuticular Monocryl closure is performed for cosmesis (Fig. 52-18).

POSTOPERATIVE

Postoperative measures may vary depending on the amount of tension on the repaired hamstring tendons. Placement in a hip orthosis to limit hip flexion from 30 to 40 degrees is advocated for up to 6 to 8 weeks (11). A hinged knee brace locked anywhere from 30 to 90 degrees is typically placed in the immediate postoperative period to prevent knee extension. This is kept in place for up to 6 to 8 weeks. Protected "toe-touch" weight bearing with crutches is initiated for the first 4 to 6 weeks. Physical therapy is delayed until 2 weeks, and the patient is begun on passive hip motion. Active hip flexion is begun at 4 weeks and stretching program at 6 weeks. By 6 weeks, the patient is progressed to full weight bearing as tolerated and transitioned out of their brace. Isokinetic closed

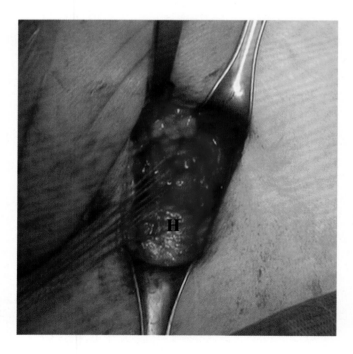

FIGURE 52-15

Core sutures from anchor on ischial tuberosity and passing through avulsed hamstring tendon (*H*).

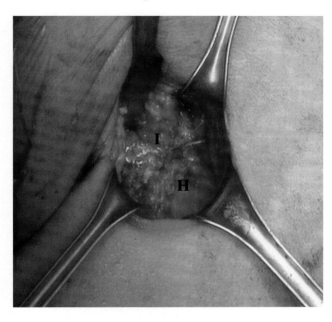

FIGURE 52-16

Repaired hamstring tendon (*H*) avulsion on ischial tuberosity (*I*).

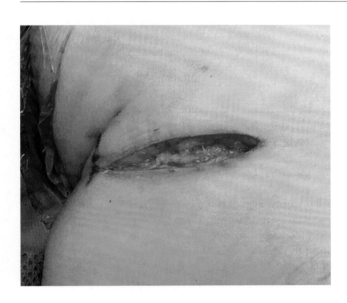

FIGURE 52-17

Closure with absorbable suture to reapproximate the gluteal fascia and eliminate dead space is performed.

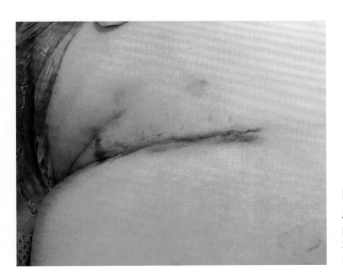

FIGURE 52-18

A subcuticular Monocryl closure is performed for cosmesis. GF, gluteal fascia; S, sciatic nerve; I, ischial tuberosity; H, hamstring tendons.

chain exercises are begun anywhere between 8 and 12 weeks postoperative. Sports-specific training progression is begun at approximately the 12-week mark (10,11).

Risk factors for venous thromboembolism should be taken into account when prescribing prophylaxis. Patients with low risk are given daily aspirin for 4 weeks postoperative, while those with increased risk should be started on oral and/or subcutaneous factor Xa inhibitors.

COMPLICATIONS

As with any surgical procedure, there are several complications that can be avoided with careful planning and surgical technique. Nerve complications have been reported in up to 9% of cases. Injury or damage to the posterior femoral cutaneous nerve can result in a painful neuroma if cut, posterior thigh numbness, and burning sensations in the back of the leg. The inferior gluteal nerve and artery can be at risk with gluteal muscle retraction, as it is approximately 5.0 cm proximal to the inferior border of the gluteus maximus (15). Neuropraxia to the sciatic nerve due to over-retraction or manipulation can lead to nerve palsy and foot drop, as well as paresthesias down the back of the leg (21).

Appropriate hemostasis and closure of potential dead space can help prevent complications of seroma or hematoma formation postoperatively. Standard sterile technique is crucial to reduce potential complications of infection, which has been reported in 3% of cases (21). Perioperative antibiotics should be administered. Given the proximity of the incision to the perineal region, proper patient education on wound care and daily dressing changes can help prevent contamination.

Protection of the repair in the early postoperative period is crucial to prevent rerupture and the need for revision surgery. Reoperation rates have been reported in up to 3% of cases. Deep venous thrombosis has been documented in 1% of patients, and standard mechanical and chemoprophylaxis is indicated (21).

OUTCOMES

Nonsurgical management of complete proximal hamstring avulsions has been shown to yield noticeable subjective and functional strength deficits. In a study by Hofmann et al., patients elected to be treated without surgery for complete avulsions and found at 31-month follow-up, an average hamstring strength of 62% to 66% compared to the contralateral leg. Half of these patients stated they regretted not undergoing surgical management (2).

Operative repair of complete proximal hamstring avulsions has shown more promising results. In a review of 72 proximal hamstring repairs at 24-month follow-up, Wood et al. found the mean postoperative hamstring strength to be 84% and endurance to be 89% compared to the contralateral side. They found a 79% rate of return to sport by 6 months, including all professional level athletes returning to their selective sport (22). Cohen et al. reviewed 52 patients after proximal hamstring repair with an average 33-month follow-up and measured subjective functional outcome scores with excellent overall results and 98% patient satisfaction. Seventy percent of their patients returned to the same sporting activity by which they injured their hamstring initially (5). Repair of incomplete avulsions has also been reported with success by Aldridge et al., who looked at 23 patients at 2-year follow-up, and average strength increase from 64% to 88% (16). Timing of surgical intervention has been evaluated by Subbu et al. They retrospectively evaluated 112 patients with surgical repair within 6 weeks, 6 months, and after 6 months from time of injury. While there was a high return to sport rate among all groups at 96.4%, they found athletes within the acute repair group returned to sport 9 weeks earlier than the delayed repair group and 13 weeks faster than the late repair group (17). Rust et al. also compared acute versus chronic repair of hamstring avulsions in 72 patients and found superior satisfaction and return to play in patients undergoing acute repairs (18).

REFERENCES

1. Ishikawa K, Kai K, Mizuta H. Avulsion of the hamstring muscles from the ischial tuberosity. *Clin Orthop Relat Res.* 1988;(232):153–155.
2. Klingele KE, Sallay PI. Surgical repair of complete proximal hamstring tendon rupture. *Am J Sports Med.* 2002;30(5):742–747.
3. Linklater JM, Hamilton B, Carmichael J, et al. Hamstring injuries: anatomy, imaging, and intervention. *Semin Musculoskelet Radiol.* 2010;14(2):131–161.

4. Wood DG, Packham I, Trikha SP, et al. Avulsion of the proximal hamstring origin. *J Bone Joint Surg Am.* 2008;38(12):754–760.
5. Hofmann KJ, Paggi A, Connors D, et al. Complete avulsion of the proximal hamstring insertion: functional outcomes after nonsurgical treatment. *J Bone Joint Surg Am.* 2014;96(12):1022–1025.
6. Koulouris G, Connell D. Evaluation of the hamstring muscle complex following acute injury. *Skeletal Radiol.* 2003;32(10):582–589.
7. Van Der Made AD, Reurink G, Gouttebarge V, et al. Outcome after surgical repair of proximal Hamstring avulsions: a systematic review. *Am J Sports Med.* 2015;43(11):2841051.
8. Blasier RB, Morawa LG. Complete rupture of the hamstring origin from a water skiing injury. *Am J Sports Med.* 1990;18(4):425–427.
9. Sallay PI, Friedman RL, Coogan PG, et al. Hamstring muscle injuries among water skiers. *Am J Sports Med.* 1996;24(2):130–136.
10. Bowman KF Jr, Cohen SB, Bradley JP. Operative management of partial-thickness tears of the proximal hamstring muscles in athletes. *Am J Sports Med.* 2013;41(6):1363–1371.
11. Cohen SB, Rangavajjula A, Vyas D, et al. Functional results and outcomes after repair of proximal hamstring avulsions. *Am J Sports Med.* 2012;40(9):2092–2098.
12. Orava S, Kujala UM. Rupture of the ischial origin of the hamstring muscles. *Am J Sports Med.* 1995;23(6):702–705.
13. Skaara HE, Moksnes H, Frihagen F, et al. Self-reported and performance-based functional outcomes after surgical repair of proximal hamstring avulsions. *Am J Sports Med.* 2013;41(11):2577–2584.
14. Cohen S, Bradley J. Acute proximal hamstring rupture. *J Am Acad Orthop Surg.* 2007;15(6):350–355.
15. Miller SL, Webb GR. The proximal origin of the hamstrings and surrounding anatomy encountered during repair. Surgical technique. *J Bone Joint Surg Am.* 2008;90(suppl 2 Pt 1):108–116.
16. Aldridge SE, Heilpern GN, Carmichael JR, et al. Incomplete avulsion of the proximal insertion of the hamstring: outcome two years following surgical repair. *J Bone Joint Surg Br.* 2012;94(5):660–662.
17. Subbu R, Benjamin-Laing H, Haddad F. Timing of surgery for complete proximal hamstring avulsion injuries: successful clinical outcomes at 6 weeks, 6 months, and after 6 months of injury. *Am J Sports Med.* 2015;43(2):385–391.
18. Rust DA, Giveans MR, Stone RM, et al. Functional outcomes and return to sports after acute repair, chronic repair, and allograft reconstruction for proximal hamstring ruptures. *Am J Sports Med.* 2014;42(6):1377–1383.
19. Orava S, Hetsroni I, Marom N, et al. Surgical excision of posttraumatic ossifications at the proximal hamstrings in young athletes: technique and outcomes. *Am J Sports Med.* 2015;43(6):1331–1336.
20. Sarimo J, Lempainen L, Mattila K, et al. Complete proximal hamstring avulsions: a series of 41 patients with operative treatment. *Am J Sports Med.* 2008;36(6):1110–1115.

53 Anterior Ankle Arthroscopy: Indications and Surgical Technique

Conor I. Murphy, Taylor Cabe, and Mark C. Drakos

INTRODUCTION

Anterior ankle arthroscopy is a surgical technique used to treat a variety of intra-articular pathologies while avoiding the morbidity of an arthrotomy or osteotomy to gain access to the ankle joint. Advances in technology, smaller instrumentation, and expanded indications have increased the demand and utilization of ankle arthroscopy. With these improvements in the treatment of foot and ankle pathology, ankle arthroscopy has become a necessary skill to be a complete foot and ankle orthopaedic surgeon.

OVERVIEW

Ankle arthroscopy is a well-established procedure to diagnose and treat a number of foot and ankle disorders. Ease of access and direct visualization of intra-articular structures allows for the focused assessment of articular cartilage, ligaments, and capsular or synovial tissues. It also has become an evolving tool to evaluate syndesmotic stability and accuracy of reduction in fracture cases (1–5). The equipment necessary for ankle arthroscopy is very similar compared to shoulder and knee arthroscopy. However, the joint is smaller and tighter making it technically more challenging than some of the larger joints. As such, noninvasive distraction is frequently used to aid in visualization. The thin soft tissue envelope around the ankle joint allows for direct palpation of bony landmarks and topographical orientation for access to the joint. Overall morbidity of ankle arthroscopy is relatively low, thus making this procedure a safe and multipurpose tool.

TECHNIQUE

Equipment

Necessary equipment for ankle arthroscopy includes a noninvasive distraction system, spinal needle, 3.5- or 2.0-mm 30-degree arthroscope, pressure inflow or gravity inflow fluid delivery system, arthroscopy shaver, arthroscopic burr, and small joint arthroscopy instruments such as probe, grasper, curette, and awl.

A leg holder placed under the knee is required to provide countertraction as well as flex the knee to allow ankle joint accessibility and mobility during the procedure. Ideally, the knee will be bent at approximately 90 degrees so that axial traction can be pulled from the foot along the

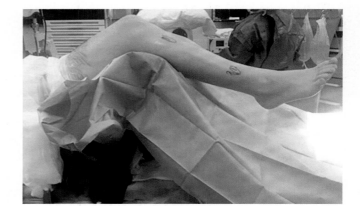

FIGURE 53-1

Proper positioning of the operative leg in the leg holder with the hip flexed and the knee flexed to approximately 45 degrees to allow for ankle access, mobility, and distraction during the procedure.

axis of the tibia. The back of the knee must be well padded with a gel roll or soft foam to prevent peroneal nerve palsy at the level of the fibular head. A tourniquet can be used but is not often necessary (6,7).

Positioning

The patient is placed supine on the table with the well leg flat on the table. The operative leg is placed in the leg holder with the hip flexed approximately 45 to 60 degrees and the knee flexed approximately 90 degrees depending on the size of the patient's leg (Fig. 53-1). Proper positioning of the operative leg must be confirmed prior to skin sterilization to allow for adequate distraction of the ankle joint as well as height of the leg holder. If a tourniquet is to be used, it should be placed at the level of the thigh to avoid alteration in tension of the Achilles tendon and gastrocnemius-soleus complex.

The skin is prepped and the leg is draped in the usual sterile fashion. The noninvasive ankle distractor strap is then placed around the ankle (Figs. 53-2 and 53-3; Arthrex Inc., Naples, FL). Distraction is applied manually to the desired tension of the surgeon. Studies have demonstrated that neurologic change of the tibial nerve does not occur until 30 lb of tension, which is beyond the threshold of the ankle distractor strap (8). This should provide approximately 4 to 5 mm of distraction at the level of the ankle joint, which is ample space to allow a 2.7-mm arthroscope access. If the patient has ankle instability, the distraction is improved and the arthroscopic examination is facilitated. In revision cases, specifically those with arthrofibrosis or patients who have had prior ankle or pilon fractures, the surgeon may have to clear a space in the anterior aspect of the ankle to expose the joint. Moreover, distraction may be more difficult in these cases, and one must be prepared to open if visualization is not able to be attained.

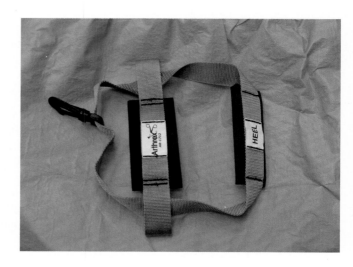

FIGURE 53-2

Noninvasive distraction strap. (This image provided courtesy of: Arthrex®, Naples, FL, 2019.)

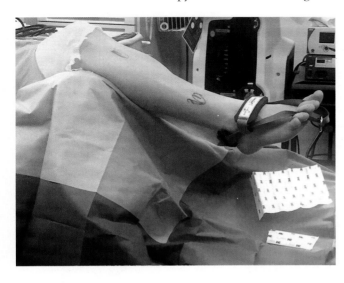

FIGURE 53-3

Positioning of the operative leg after sterilization with the noninvasive distraction strap in place prior to application of distraction.

Portal Placement

Anterior ankle arthroscopy is performed through two anterior portals, the anteromedial and anterolateral portals. Location and orientation of these portals is determined by palpable anatomic structures and their known relationship to underlying neurovascular structures (Fig. 53-4). Blunt dissection after superficial skin incision is preferred to avoid damage to these neurovascular structures.

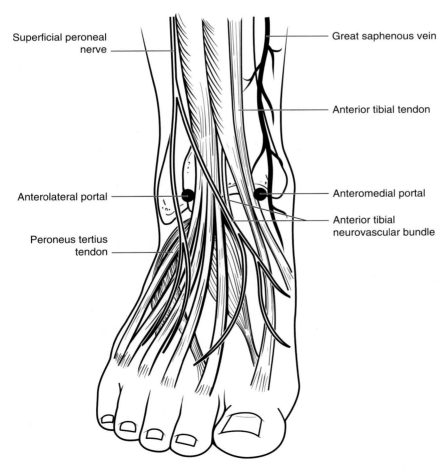

FIGURE 53-4

Portal anatomy for ankle arthroscopy.

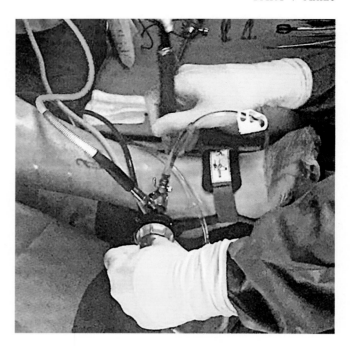

FIGURE 53-5

Anteromedial and anterolateral portal placement.

The anteromedial portal is placed at the level of the tibiotalar joint just medial to the anterior tibialis tendon and lateral to the saphenous vein and nerve, which overlies the anterior border of the medial malleolus. The height should be at the level of the shoulder of the talus. The ideal location is within the notch of Harty, a medial notch within the convex-shaped anterior tibial plafond at the junction with the medial malleolus. Furthermore, we recommend staying on the low side of the anteromedial soft spot given the upslope of the anterior talus. This portal is accessed first as it provides the easiest access with the least risk of damage to neurovascular structures. Next, the arthroscope is used to illuminate the lateral portal. A superficial skin incision with a no. 15-blade scalpel is made followed by blunt dissection with a hemostat. The intermediate branch of the superficial peroneal nerve often runs in line with this portal. Therefore, it is critical to use sharp dissection for skin only and then a blunt hemostat to develop the portal. A blunt trocar is used to penetrate the anterior joint capsule and avoid damage to the articular cartilage. Then, the 30-degree, 2.7-mm arthroscope is introduced through the trocar.

The anterolateral portal is created just lateral to the peroneus tertius at the level of the tibiotalar joint between the articulation of the fibula and tibia. Special care must be taken to avoid injuring the superficial peroneal nerve as it crosses the tibiotalar joint in this vicinity. The cutaneous branches of this nerve course along the inferior extensor retinaculum, crossing anterior to the fourth and fifth toe extensor tendons, and run toward the third webspace. The skin can be transilluminated with the arthroscope through the anteromedial portal to assist with visualization of these cutaneous nerve branches. The spinal needle is placed under direct intra-articular visualization with confirmation that adequate accessibility of the ankle joint can be achieved through its location. After confirming that the cutaneous branches of the superficial peroneal nerve are not overlying the portal and adequate access to the joint can be achieved, a superficial skin incision is made followed by blunt dissection through the joint capsule with a hemostat (Fig. 53-5).

Diagnostic Ankle Arthroscopy

Diagnostic anterior ankle arthroscopy should include an 8-point examination of the central talus, lateral talus, medial talus, medal and lateral gutters, tibiofibular syndesmosis, deltoid ligament, and anterior process of the talus (Fig. 53-6). Furthermore, the articular cartilage of the tibial plafond, that anterior border of the tibial plafond, and the lateral ankle ligaments must be inspected. Visualization is achieved through the anteromedial portal while the anterolateral portal primarily serves as the working portal for instruments.

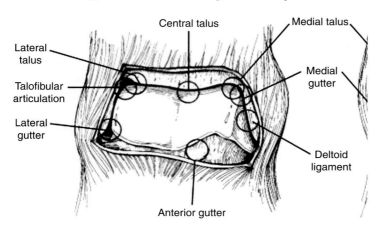

FIGURE 53-6

Eight-point anterior examination of the ankle.

SPECIAL CONSIDERATIONS

Anterior Ankle Impingement

Anterior ankle impingement may exist secondary to a variety of etiologies, both soft tissue and bony. Identifying the exact source of the patient's symptomatology may not always be possible in the clinical setting. Plain films will often identify anterior bony spurs across either the anterior tibial plafond or talar neck that result in limited ankle range of motion and pain (Fig. 53-7). Magnetic resonance imaging (MRI) can elucidate soft tissue pathology such as congenital bands, scar tissue, synovial hypertrophy, and loose body. In certain instances where both pathologies are concomitant, diagnostic arthroscopy and treatment can be of high yield.

Successful removal of anterior bony spurs of the tibial plafond or talar neck can be performed arthroscopically with a 4-mm burr, eliminating the need for open arthrotomy. It can be difficult to assess when adequate resection down to the native anterior tibial margin or talar neck has been achieved. Intraoperative fluoroscopy is utilized to localize these bony spurs and avoid over- or underresection. Resection of bony spurs should be reserved until the end of the case to avoid decreased visualization secondary to bleeding. Of note, running the burr on reverse can minimize the chances of overaggressive resection or assist with refining jagged edges or uneven surfaces.

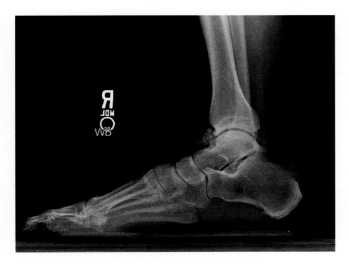

FIGURE 53-7

Lateral radiograph of a right ankle with anterior distal tibial osteophytes.

Osteochondral Lesions of the Talus

First-line management for an osteochondral lesion of the talus (OLT) is arthroscopic evaluation and treatment. Arthroscopy allows for a variety of treatment options for managing an OLT including removal of loose body or unstable lesion, primary repair, microfracture, or other novel treatment options for cartilage rejuvenation. These injuries are typically identified by patient history followed by plain films (Fig. 53-8) and MRI (Fig. 53-9).

Initial treatment is composed of curettage and debridement of any unstable OLT. The simplest intervention and standard of care for small, superficial lesions with intact subchondral bone entails debridement of any injured cartilage to a surrounding healthy and stable rim of cartilage followed by microfracture using an awl (9). This technique stimulates bleeding from the subchondral bone marrow and release of mesenchymal stem cells and growth factors to form a fibrocartilage layer to fill the defect. Research has demonstrated that the utility of this technique is limited to OLTs smaller than 150 mm^2 in surface area (10–12).

In the setting of larger OLTs (those larger than 150 mm^2) with a subchondral bone defect, autograft or allograft bone can be morselized and deposited through the trocar into the bony defect and then covered with an osteochondral allograft cartilage layer. This technique is still being researched with a variety of graft options, but initial results are promising.

Arthroscopic-Assisted Arthrodesis

In the appropriate patient population, arthroscopic-assisted ankle fusion yields high fusion rates and low complication rates. Patients with excessive angular deformities, significant bone loss, poor vascular circulation, and prior failed fusion may not qualify for arthroscopic ankle arthrodesis. Results have demonstrated comparable fusion rates to open procedures, quicker healing time, reduced narcotic use, improved cosmesis, and shorter hospital admissions (13).

Debridement of the tibiotalar articular cartilage, the medial and lateral gutters of the ankle, and the superficial subchondral bone is achieved through the use of curettes, arthroscopic shavers, and a burr. Resection of anterior tibial osteophytes is also necessary to achieve proper joint visualization and anatomic reduction for proper fusion. Excessive debridement of the underlying bone disrupts the topography of the tibiotalar joint, which naturally imparts stability through its bony morphology. Intraoperative fluoroscopy must be used to ensure reduction and proper position of the ankle for fusion. Fixation is achieved with percutaneous transarticular cannulated 6.5-mm or 7.0-mm screws.

Trauma

There is an increasing body of evidence to suggest that ankle arthroscopy can be a useful adjuvant tool in the management of ankle fractures and associated traumatic injuries to the articular cartilage and tibiofibular syndesmosis (2). The literature supports that a large volume of syndesmotic injuries is malreduced at the time of fixation (4). Direct visualization of the syndesmosis with ankle arthroscopy may assist with more anatomic reduction. It may also assist with diagnosis of syndesmotic injury and clarification between stable and unstable injuries (5).

Furthermore, acute full-thickness talar cartilage lesions can be present in up to 78% of ankle fractures, especially when the patient sustains an ankle dislocation or syndesmotic disruption and instability (14). Diagnosis of these cartilage lesions at the time of surgical management of the ankle fracture can assist with postoperative activity and follow-up protocols. In addition, with newer grafting techniques, acute full-thickness cartilage injuries can be addressed at the index procedure, which may improve outcomes. It is still unknown if acute surgical management of a traumatic OLT affects clinical outcome versus nonoperative management.

Infection

Similar to arthroscopic management of septic arthritis in the shoulder and knee, the ankle is also amenable to irrigation and debridement of septic arthritis. Adequate exposure and visualization of the ankle joint can be achieved arthroscopically thus obviating the need for an arthrotomy in the setting of septic arthritis. Arthroscopic irrigation of infectious material combined with synovial debridement is effective in the treatment of septic ankle arthritis.

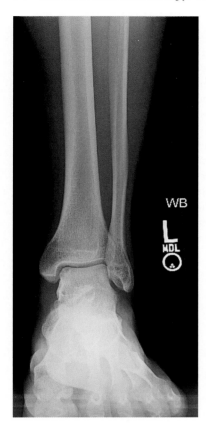

FIGURE 53-8

AP radiograph of a left ankle with medial talar dome osteochondral lesion.

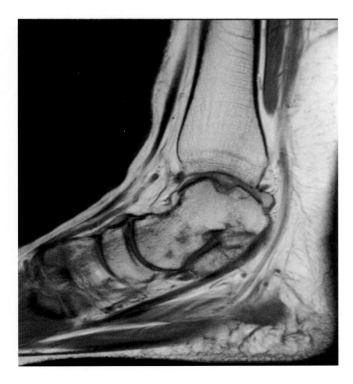

FIGURE 53-9

MRI of a left ankle with medial talar dome osteochondral lesion.

COMPLICATIONS

Complications unique to ankle arthroscopy are primarily related to neurologic injury during antero-lateral portal placement. Care must be taken to avoid damage to the cutaneous branches of the superficial peroneal nerve by properly transilluminating the skin and identifying palpable anatomic landmarks when choosing portal location. Careful incision through the skin followed by blunt dissection thereafter is the safest method of accessing the ankle joint.

Damage to the deep peroneal nerve or dorsalis pedis artery is rare and easily avoided prior to placement of the anteromedial portal placement by properly identifying the tibialis anterior tendon and extensor hallucis longus tendon with palpation. Also, care must be taken to avoid debridement into the anterior synovium over the ankle as the neurovascular bundle and extensor tendons may be violated. Occasionally, the saphenous nerve or vein can be injured if the anteromedial portal is placed too far medially along the border of the medial malleolus. Again, this is rare and can easily be avoided with a detailed knowledge of the topographical anatomy of the anterior ankle joint and understanding its relation to the underlying neurovascular structures.

REFERENCES

1. Schairer WW, Nwachukwu BU, Dare DM, et al. Arthroscopically assisted open reduction-internal fixation of ankle fractures: significance of the arthroscopic ankle drive-through sign. *Arthrosc Tech.* 2016;5(2):e407–e412. doi:10.1016/j.eats.2016.01.018.
2. Chan KB, Lui TH. Role of ankle arthroscopy in management of acute ankle fracture. *Arthroscopy.* 2016;32(11): 2373–2380. doi:10.1016/j.arthro.2016.08.016.
3. Chen XZ, Chen Y, Liu CG, et al. Arthroscopy-assisted surgery for acute ankle fractures: a systematic review. *Arthroscopy.* 2015;31(11):2224–2231. doi:10.1016/j.arthro.2015.03.043.
4. Gardner MJ, Demetrakopoulos D, Briggs SM, et al. Malreduction of the tibiofibular syndesmosis in ankle fractures. *Foot Ankle Int.* 2006;27(10):788–792. doi:10.1177/107110070602701005.
5. Lubberts B, Guss D, Vopat BG, et al. The arthroscopic syndesmotic assessment tool can differentiate between stable and unstable ankle syndesmoses. *Knee Surg Sports Traumatol Arthrosc.* 2018. doi:10.1007/s00167-018-5229-3.
6. Zaidi R, Hasan K, Sharma A, et al. Ankle arthroscopy: a study of tourniquet versus no tourniquet. *Foot Ankle Int.* 2014;35(5):478–482. doi:10.1177/1071100713518504.
7. Amendola N. Not using a tourniquet during anterior ankle arthroscopy did not affect postoperative intra-articular bleeding or function at six months. *J Bone Joint Surg Am.* 2018;100(4):344. doi:10.2106/jbjs.17.01433.
8. Dowdy PA, Watson BV, Amendola A, et al. Noninvasive ankle distraction: relationship between force, magnitude of distraction, and nerve conduction abnormalities. *Arthroscopy.* 1996;12(1):64–69.
9. Tol JL, Struijs PA, Bossuyt PM, et al. Treatment strategies in osteochondral defects of the talar dome: a systematic review. *Foot Ankle Int.* 2000;21(2):119–126.
10. Chuckpaiwong B, Berkson EM, Theodore GH. Microfracture for osteochondral lesions of the ankle: outcome analysis and outcome predictors of 105 cases. *Arthroscopy.* 2008;24(1):106–112. doi:10.1016/j.arthro.2007.07.022.
11. Ramponi L, Yasui Y, Murawski CD, et al. Lesion size is a predictor of clinical outcomes after bone marrow stimulation for osteochondral lesions of the talus: a systematic review. *Am J Sports Med.* 2017;45(7):1698–1705. doi:10.1177/0363546516668292.
12. Choi WJ, Park KK, Kim BS, et al. Osteochondral lesion of the talus: is there a critical defect size for poor outcome? *Am J Sports Med.* 2009;37(10):1974–1980. doi:10.1177/0363546509335765.
13. Park JH, Kim HJ, Suh DH, et al. Arthroscopic versus open ankle arthrodesis: a systematic review. *Arthroscopy.* 2018;34(3):988–997. doi:10.1016/j.arthro.2017.08.284.
14. Da Cunha RJ, Karnovsky SC, Schairer W, et al. Ankle arthroscopy for diagnosis of full-thickness talar cartilage lesions in the setting of acute ankle fractures. *Arthroscopy.* 2018;34(6):1950–1957. doi:10.1016/j.arthro.2017.12.003.

54 Posterior Ankle Arthroscopy and Tendoscopy

Mikel L. Reilingh, Peter A. J. de Leeuw, Maayke van Sterkenburg, and C. Niek van Dijk

INTRODUCTION

Ankle arthroscopy has been developed and improved over the last 40 years. Nowadays, this minimal invasive technique is increasingly used for dealing with a wide range of ankle pathologies. In 1931, Burman was the first orthopedic surgeon attempting ankle joint arthroscopy in vivo and concluded that the ankle joint was unsuitable for arthroscopy, because of its narrow interarticular access (1). Technical improvements, such as smaller diameter arthroscopes and joint distraction methods, made it possible for Watanabe in 1972 to report on a series of 28 ankle arthroscopies (2).

Van Dijk et al. (3) were the first to describe endoscopic access to the tendons by tendoscopy. These included tendoscopy of the posterior tibial tendon, the peroneal tendons (4,5), and of the Achilles tendon (6), which was followed by endoscopic treatment for retrocalcaneal bursitis, called endoscopic calcaneoplasty (7,8). In 2000, a two-portal endoscopic hindfoot approach was introduced (9). In 2008, the results of 55 consecutive patients with posterior ankle impingement were reported on with a good to excellent outcome in 74% of patients (10). This minimal invasive technique provides excellent access to the posterior aspect of the ankle and subtalar joint. Furthermore, extra-articular structures of the hindfoot such as the os trigonum, flexor hallucis longus (FHL), and the deep portion of the deltoid ligament can be assessed (9).

INDICATIONS AND CONTRAINDICATIONS OF THE PROCEDURES

Contraindications for endoscopic/arthroscopic procedures are few but important. Relative contraindications include severe edema and a tenuous vascular status. More absolute contraindications include localized soft tissue infection and severe degenerative joint disease in arthroscopic procedures. Obesity, although not a contraindication, significantly contributes to a prolonged intraoperative surgical time and postoperative morbidity (11).

The different indications can be categorized according to the location of the pathology.

ARTICULAR PATHOLOGY

Posterior Compartment Ankle Joint

The main indications include both soft tissue and/or bony pathology. Soft tissue pathology mainly includes chronic synovitis, chondromatosis, and excessive scar tissue. Bony pathology includes loose bodies, ossicles, posttraumatic calcifications, avulsion fragments, and osteophytes of the posterior tibial rim. An osteochondral defect (OCD) in the ankle joint that cannot be approached by means of anterior ankle arthroscopy with the ankle in maximum plantar flexion can be assessed through posterior ankle arthroscopy.

Osteochondral Defects

A traumatic insult is widely accepted as the most important etiologic factor of an OCD of the talus. In 93% to 98% of the lateral talar lesions, trauma has been described and for medial lesions in 61% to 70% (12,13). OCDs can either heal and remain asymptomatic or progress to deep ankle pain on weight bearing, prolonged joint swelling, recurrent synovitis, diminished range of motion, and formation of subchondral bone cysts. However, absence of swelling and diminished range of motion does not rule out an OCD.

Routine radiographs of the ankle should be obtained after careful history taking and physical examination of the ankle. These consist of weight-bearing anteroposterior (AP) (mortise) and lateral views of both ankles (Fig. 54-1A and B). Initially, the damage may be too small to be visualized on a routine radiograph. The OCD sometimes becomes apparent on radiographs at a later stage. A posteromedial or posterolateral defect may be revealed by a heel rise mortise view with the ankle in plantar flexion (14) (Fig. 54-2). Additionally, computer tomography can be performed to confirm diagnosis and to plan arthroscopic treatment (15) (Fig. 54-1C and D).

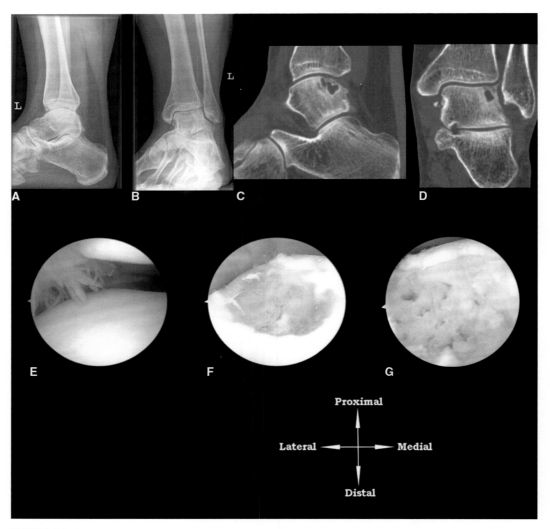

FIGURE 54-1

A 28-year-old female patient presenting with deep left ankle pain after an inversion trauma 1 year before. Physical examination revealed mild ankle swelling, no recognizable pain on palpation, and a normal range of motion. In this case, the OD is too small to be visualized on standard weight-bearing lateral **(A)** and anteroposterior **(B)** radiographs of the left ankle. On a sagittal **(C)** and coronal **(D)** computed tomography, a posterolateral OD of the talus, with cyst formation is visible. **E:** By posterior ankle arthroscopy, the OD can be identified. **F:** All unstable cartilage including the underlying necrotic bone is removed with a shaver. **G:** Arthroscopic view of the microfractured lesion.

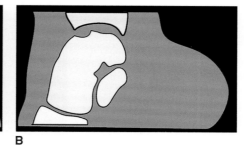

FIGURE 54-2

Talar ODs can most frequently be addressed through anterior ankle arthroscopy; nevertheless, posteriorly located ODs could sometimes be approached through a posterior ankle arthroscopy more easily. To determine which arthroscopic procedure is most suited, the ankle is forced in maximum plantar flexion. **A:** Posteriorly located talar OD with the foot in neutral position. **B:** By forcing the foot in maximum plantar flexion the OD moves anteriorly. In this case, the OD can be reached via anterior ankle.

In case of a symptomatic OCD, arthroscopic débridement and bone marrow stimulation remain the best treatment that is currently available for defects up to 15 mm in diameter (13,16). With this technique, all unstable cartilage including the underlying necrotic bone is removed. Any cysts underlying the defect are opened and curetted. After débridement, multiple connections with the subchondral bone are created by drilling or microfracturing. The objective is to partially destroy the calcified zone that is most often present and to create multiple openings into the subchondral bone (Fig. 54-1). Intraosseous blood vessels are disrupted, and the release of growth factors leads to the formation of a fibrin clot. The growth of local new blood vessels is stimulated, marrow cells are introduced in the OCD, and fibrocartilaginous tissue is formed (17).

Posterior Compartment Subtalar Joint

The main indications are removal of osteophytes; treatment of degenerative changes in the subtalar joint, including talar cystic lesions; loose body removal; and a subtalar arthrodesis in case of osteoarthritis (18–21). Intraosseous talar ganglions can also be treated arthroscopically (22).

PERIARTICULAR PATHOLOGY

Posterior Ankle Impingement

Posterior ankle impingement syndrome encompasses a group of pathologies that are characterized by posterior ankle pain in plantar flexion. The mechanism can be caused by overuse or trauma. It is important to differentiate between these two groups, because posterior impingement from overuse has a better prognosis (23) and patients are more satisfied after arthroscopic treatment (10).

The overuse group mainly exists from ballet dancers, downhill runners, and soccer players (23–25). In professional ballet, the specific dancing maneuvers force the ankle in hyperplantar flexion. The anatomical structures in between the calcaneus and the posterior part of the distal tibia thereby become compressed. Through exercise, the dancer will attempt to increase the range of motion and joint mobility, ultimately decreasing the distance between the calcaneus and the talus. The anatomical structures at the back of the ankle joint hereby become compressed. Running with more pronounced plantar flexion, such as downhill running, imposes repetitive stresses on the anatomical structures of the posterior ankle area (26). Kicking with the foot in plantar flexion results in high forces on the anatomical structures in the hindfoot. These repetitive high forces can eventually cause posterior ankle impingement.

An isolated or combined hyperplantar flexion—and supination—trauma can damage these structures and may finally lead to a chronic posterior ankle impingement syndrome. Congenital anatomic anomalies such as a prominent posterior talar process, os trigonum, or talus bipartitus (27) could facilitate the occurrence of the syndrome, especially in combination with overuse injury (28–30). An os trigonum is estimated to be present in 1.7% to 30% and occurs bilaterally in 1.4% of the people (28,31,32). During plantar flexion, the soft tissue structures such as synovium, posterior ankle

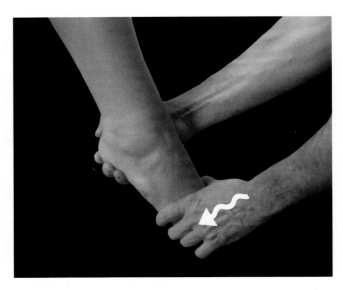

FIGURE 54-3

The forced hyperplantar flexion test is performed with the patient sitting with the knee flexed in 90 degrees. The test should be performed with repetitive, quick, passive hyperplantar flexion movements (*arrow*). The test can be repeated in slight external rotation or slight internal rotation of the foot relative to the tibia. The investigator can apply this rotational movement on the point of maximal plantar flexion, thereby "grinding" the (enlarged) posterior talar process/os trigonum in between tibia and calcaneus.

capsule, or one of the posterior ligamentous structures can get pinched and compressed, eventually resulting in swelling, partial rupture, or fibrosis.

The diagnosis is made by means of physical examination. The forced passive hyperplantar flexion test is positive when the patient complains of recognizable pain during the test (Fig. 54-3). A negative test rules out the posterior ankle impingement syndrome. A positive test is followed by a diagnostic infiltration with Xylocaine. Disappearance of pain following infiltration confirms the diagnosis. For radiographic detection of posterior impingement, the AP ankle view typically does not show abnormalities. On a lateral view, the posterolateral part of the talus is often superimposed on the medial talar process. Therefore, detection of a posterolateral talar process or os trigonum is often not possible. We recommend lateral radiographs with the foot in 25 degrees of external rotation in relation to the standard lateral radiographs (29).

In case conservative treatment fails, excision of soft tissue overgrowth and osteophytes results in good functional and clinical outcome in symptomatic posterior ankle impingement (10,33).

Deep Portion of the Deltoid Ligament/Cedell Fracture

Hyperdorsiflexion or eversion trauma can result in avulsion of the posterior talotibial ligament at its insertion into the medial tubercle of the talus. This may result in posttraumatic calcifications or ossicles in the deep portion of the deltoid ligament. These patients typically present with posteromedial ankle pain that is aggravated by running and walking on uneven grounds. Cedell was the first to report four cases of young athletes with ligament avulsion of the deep portion from the posteromedial talar process of the deltoid ligament (34).

Flexor Hallucis Longus Tendon Pathology

Posterior ankle impingement syndrome is often accompanied by tenosynovitis or degeneration of the FHL, especially in ballet dancers (30,35,36). The patient experiences pain in the posteromedial part of the ankle (30). On physical examination, the tendon can be palpated behind the medial malleolus. By asking the patient to repetitively flex the big toe, while the ankle is in 10 to 20 degree plantar flexion, the FHL tendon can be identified in its gliding channel, in between the medial and the lateral talar process. In case of tendinitis or chronic inflammation, crepitus and recognizable pain can be provoked by the examiner putting the palpating/compressing finger just behind the medial malleolus. In some cases, a painful nodule in the tendon exists. Arthroscopic treatment can be considered when nonoperative treatment fails to improve symptoms. Débridement of the FHL and release of the flexor retinaculum and tendon sheath up to the level of the sustentaculum tali can be performed in order to achieve unrestricted movement of the tendon.

Peroneal Tendon Pathology

Peroneal tendon pathology frequently coexists with or is secondary to chronic lateral ankle instability. These disorders often cause chronic ankle pain in runners and ballet dancers (37). Posttraumatic lateral ankle pain is seen frequently, but peroneal tendon pathology is not always recognized as a cause of these symptoms. In a study by Dombek et al. (38), only 60% of peroneal tendon disorders were accurately diagnosed at first clinical evaluation. Because the peroneal tendons act as lateral ankle stabilizers, in chronic instability of the ankle more strain is put on these tendons, resulting in hypertrophic tendinopathy, tenosynovitis, and ultimately in tendon tears (4).

Pathology consists of tenosynovitis, tendon dislocation or subluxation, and (subtotal) rupture or snapping of one or both of the peroneal tendons. It accounts for the majority of symptoms at the posterolateral aspect of the ankle (39). Other causes of posterolateral ankle pain are rheumatoid synovitis, bony spurs, calcifications or ossicles, pathology to the posterior talofibular ligament, or disorders of the posterior compartment of the subtalar joint. Posterior ankle impingement can present as posterolateral ankle pain. On clinical examination, there is recognizable tenderness over the tendons on palpation. Swelling, tendon dislocation, and signs of tenosynovitis can be found in peroneal tendon pathology.

The diagnosis of peroneal tendon pathology can be difficult in a patient with lateral ankle pain. A detailed history should include the presence of associated conditions such as rheumatoid arthritis, psoriasis, hyperparathyroidism, diabetic neuropathy, calcaneal fracture, fluoroquinolone use, and local steroid injections. These can all increase the prevalence of peroneal tendon dysfunction (40). A diagnostic differentiation must be made with fatigue fractures or fractures of the fibula, posterior impingement of the ankle, and lesions of the lateral ligament complex.

Additional investigation such as magnetic resonance imaging (MRI) and ultrasonography may be helpful in confirming the diagnosis in (partial) tears of the tendon of peroneus brevis or longus (41,42). Posttraumatic or postsurgical adhesions and irregularities of the posterior aspect of the fibula (peroneal groove) can also be responsible for symptoms in this region.

In case of recurrent peroneal tendon dislocation, the primary indication for treatment is pain. After several months of conservative treatment without improvement, open or nowadays endoscopic/tendoscopic treatment options are available (4,43). An endoscopic fibular groove–deepening technique, based on the posterior ankle arthroscopic portals (9), with one additional portal 4 cm proximal to the posterolateral portal (44) was recently introduced. Other peroneal tendon pathologies such as synovitis, adhesion, and exostosis can safely be assessed through tendoscopy, resulting in good to excellent clinical outcome (4).

Posterior Tibial Tendon Pathology

In the absence of intra-articular ankle pathology, posteromedial ankle pain is most often caused by disorders of the posterior tibial tendon.

Inactivity of the posterior tibial tendon gives midtarsal instability and is the commonest cause of adult onset flatfoot deformity. The relative strength of this tendon is more than twice that of its primary antagonist, the peroneus brevis tendon. Without the activity of the posterior tibial tendon, there is no stability at the midtarsal joint, and the forward propulsive force of the gastrocnemius-soleus complex acts at the midfoot instead of at the midtarsal heads. Total dysfunction eventually leads to a flatfoot deformity.

These disorders can be divided into two groups: the younger group of patients with dysfunction of the tendon, caused by some form of systemic inflammatory disease (e.g., rheumatoid arthritis), and an older group of patients whose tendon dysfunction is mostly caused by chronic overuse (45).

Following trauma, surgery, and fractures, adhesions and irregularity of the posterior aspect of the tibia can be responsible for symptoms in this region.

Mostly, a dysfunctional posterior tibial tendon evolves into a painful tenosynovitis. Tenosynovitis is also a common extra-articular manifestation of rheumatoid arthritis, where hindfoot problems are a significant cause of disability. Tenosynovitis in rheumatoid patients eventually leads to a ruptured tendon (46).

Although the precise etiology is unknown, the condition is classified on the basis of clinical and radiographic findings. In the early stage of dysfunction, patients complain of persisting ankle pain medially along the course of the tendon, in addition to fatigue and aching on the plantar medial aspect of the ankle. When a tenosynovitis is present, swelling is common. On clinical examination, valgus angulation of the hindfoot is frequently seen, with accompanying abduction of the forefoot, the "too many toes" sign (47). This sign is positive when the examiner inspects the patient's foot from behind: in case of significant forefoot abduction, three or more toes are visible lateral to the calcaneus, where normally only one or two toes are seen.

Intra-articular lesions such as a posteromedial impingement syndrome, subtalar pathology, calcifications in the dorsal capsule of the ankle joint, loose bodies, or OCDs should be excluded. Entrapment of the posterior tibial nerve in the tarsal canal is commonly known as a tarsal tunnel syndrome. Clinical examination is normally sufficient to adequately differentiate these disorders from an isolated posterior tibia tendon disorder.

For additional investigation, MRI is the best method to assess a tendon rupture (48). Also, ultrasound imaging is known as a cost-effective and accurate method to evaluate disorders of the tendon (49).

Initially, conservative management is indicated, with rest combined with nonsteroidal anti-inflammatory drugs (NSAIDs), and immobilization using a plaster cast or tape. There is no consensus whether to use corticosteroid injections; some cases of tendon rupture following corticosteroid injections have recently been described (50).

After failure of 3 to 6 months of conservative management, surgery is indicated (51). This can be performed open or endoscopically. An open synovectomy is performed by sharp dissection of the inflamed synovium, while preserving blood supply to the tendon. Postoperative management consists of plaster cast immobilization for 3 weeks with the possible disadvantage of new formation of adhesions, followed by wearing a functional brace with controlled ankle movement for another 3 weeks, and physical therapy (52).

Johnson and Strom classified tenosynovitis of the posterior tibial tendon into three stages (53): stage I, tenosynovitis where the tendon length is normal; stage II, elongated tendon with mobile hindfoot deformity; and stage III, elongated tendon with fixed hindfoot deformity. Myerson modified the classification by adding stage IV: a valgus angulation of the talus and early degeneration of the ankle joint (45). Endoscopic synovectomy is our surgical modality of choice for stage I when access allows radical removal of inflamed synovium (54). Several studies have been described previously in which endoscopic synovectomy was successfully performed, offering the advantages that are related to minimally invasive surgery (3,5).

Achilles Tendon Pathology

Pathology of the Achilles tendon can be divided into noninsertional and insertional problems (55,56). The first type can present as local degeneration of the tendon that can be combined with paratendinopathy. Insertional problems are related to abnormalities at the insertion of the Achilles tendon, including the posterior aspect of the calcaneus and the retrocalcaneal bursa. The noninsertional tendinopathy can be divided into three entities: tendinopathy, paratendinopathy, and a combination of both. Isolated tendinopathy seldom occurs (6,57). General symptoms include painful swelling typically 4 to 6 cm proximal to the insertion, and stiffness especially when getting up after a period of rest.

Patients with tendinopathy can present with three patterns: diffuse thickening of the tendon, local degeneration of the tendon that is mechanically intact, or insufficiency of the tendon with a partial tear. In paratendinopathy, there is local thickening or inflammation of the paratendon. Clinically, a differentiation between tendinopathy and paratendinopathy can be made. Maffulli et al. describe the Royal London Hospital test, which is found to be positive in patients with isolated tendinopathy of the main body of the tendon: the portion of the tendon originally found to be tender on palpation shows little or no pain with the ankle in maximum dorsiflexion (57,58). In paratendinopathy, the area of swelling does not move with dorsiflexion and plantar flexion of the ankle, where it does in tendinopathy (6,58). Paratendinopathy can be acute or chronic. Differential diagnoses are pathology of the tendons of the peroneus longus and brevis, intra-articular pathology of the ankle joint and subtalar joint, degenerative changes of the posterior tibial tendon, and tendinopathy of the FHL muscle; these must be ruled out. MRI and ultrasound can be used to differentiate between the various forms of tendinopathy (59).

We normally initiate conservative management. Modification of the activity level of the patient is advised together with avoidance of strenuous activities in case of paratendinopathy. Shoe modifications and inlays can be given. Physical therapy includes an extensive eccentric exercise program, which can be combined with icing and NSAIDs (60,61). Shockwave treatment, a night splint, and cast immobilization are alternative conservative methods. Sclerosing injections of neovascularization and accompanying nerves around the Achilles tendon have initially shown promising results and are based on the observation that neovascularization is seen in the vast majority of patients with Achilles tendinopathy but not in pain-free normal tendons (62,63).

If these conservative measures fail, surgery must be considered. The percentage of patients requiring surgery is around 25% (64,65). The technique used for operative management of tendinopathy depends on the stage of the disease. Local degeneration and thickening are usually treated by open excision and curettage. An insufficient Achilles tendon due to extensive degeneration can be reconstructed. Isolated paratendinopathy can be treated by excision of the diseased paratendon.

Open surgery produces a guarded prognosis and is associated with a higher risk of complications than endoscopy (23,66,67). Open techniques are also associated with an extensive rehabilitation period of 4 to 12 months. Therefore, recently minimally invasive techniques were developed. Percutaneous needling of the tendon has been described, but until now no results have been published. Testa et al. described a minimally invasive technique consisting of percutaneous longitudinal tenotomies (68,69), which was later optimized by adding ultrasound control. Eighty-three percent of patients reported symptomatic benefit at the time of their best outcome; however, the median time to return to sports was 6.5 months (70).

In combined tendinopathy and paratendinopathy, the question is whether both pathologies contribute to the complaints. An anatomic cadaver study described degenerative changes of the Achilles tendon in as much as 34% of subjects with no complaints (71). Khan et al. (72) found abnormal morphology not only in 65% (37 of 57) of symptomatic tendons but also in 32% (9 of 28) of asymptomatic Achilles tendons assessed by using ultrasound. Therefore, it is questionable whether degeneration of the tendon itself is the main cause of the pain. The authors focus mainly on management of the paratendinopathy leaving the tendinopathy untouched. The current approach for patients with tendinopathy of the Achilles tendon is an endoscopic release of the paratendon at the level of the nodule in the tendon. In the presence of the plantaris tendon, this tendon is resected, since we believe it has a part in the maintenance of medially located symptoms. Good functional and clinical outcome of patients treated with an endoscopic release for noninsertional tendinopathy combined with a paratendinopathy are described (73).

OPERATIVE TECHNIQUES

Posterior Ankle Arthroscopy

The procedure is carried out as outpatient surgery under general anesthesia or spinal anesthesia. The patient is placed prone. The involved leg is marked to avoid wrong-side surgery, with a tourniquet inflated around the thigh. The patient's ankle is placed slightly over the distal edge of the table, and a small support is placed under the lower leg, making it possible to move the ankle freely. A support is placed at the ipsilateral side of the pelvis to safely rotate the table when needed (Fig. 54-4). A 4-mm arthroscope with an inclination angle of 30 degrees is routinely used.

For irrigation, normal saline is used, and flow is obtained by using gravity. Apart from the standard excisional and motorized instruments for treatment of osteophytes and ossicles, a 4-mm chisel and periosteal elevator can be useful.

The anatomical landmarks on the ankle are the lateral malleolus, medial and lateral border of the Achilles tendon, and the sole of the foot. The ankle is kept in a 90-degree position. A straight line is drawn from the tip of the lateral malleolus to the Achilles tendon, parallel to the sole of the foot (Fig. 54-5).

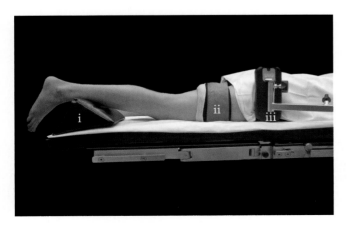

FIGURE 54-4

The patient is placed in the prone position with a tourniquet inflated around the thigh (*ii*). The affected heel is positioned slightly over the edge of the operation table and is raised with a triangular-shaped cushion (*i*) allowing free ankle movement. The ipsilateral hip is supported for safe operation table rotation (*iii*).

FIGURE 54-5

For marking the anatomical landmarks that are needed for portal placement, the ankle is kept in a neutral position. A hook can be useful to determine the plane in which the portal must be positioned. A straight line is drawn from the tip of the lateral malleolus to the Achilles tendon, parallel to the foot sole. The posterolateral portal (*arrow*) is made just above the line from the tip of the lateral malleolus to the interception with the Achilles tendon. The posteromedial portal is located at the same level of the posterolateral portal, medially to the Achilles tendon.

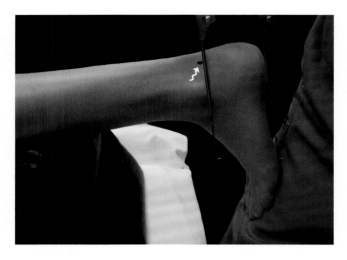

The posterolateral portal is made directly in front of the Achilles tendon just proximal of this line. After making a vertical stab incision, the subcutaneous layer is split by a mosquito clamp. The mosquito clamp is directed toward the first interdigital webspace. When the tip of the clamp touches the bone, it is exchanged for a 4.5-mm arthroscopic shaft with the blunt trocar pointing in the same direction. By palpating the bone in the sagittal plane, the level of the ankle joint and subtalar joint can often be distinguished since the prominent posterior talar process or os trigonum can be felt as a posterior prominence in between the two joints. The trocar is situated extra-articularly at the level of the ankle joint. The trocar will be exchanged for the 4-mm arthroscope with the standard direction of view 30 degrees to the lateral side.

The posteromedial portal is made medially to the Achilles tendon, at the same level as the posterolateral portal, medially to the lateral malleolus. After making a vertical stab incision, a mosquito clamp is pointed into the direction of the arthroscopic shaft in a 90-degree angle. When the mosquito clamp touches the shaft of the arthroscope, the shaft is used as a guide to "travel" anteriorly in the direction of the ankle joint, all the way down while contacting the arthroscope shaft until it reaches the bone. The arthroscopic shaft is subsequently pulled slightly backward and is lifted until the tip of the mosquito clamp becomes visible. The clamp is used to spread the extra-articular soft tissue in front of the tip of the lens. After exchanging the mosquito clamp for a 5-mm full radius resector, the fatty tissue overlying the posterior ankle capsule, lateral to the FHL tendon, is resected. The tip of the shaver is directed in a lateral and slightly plantar direction toward the lateral aspect of the subtalar joint.

Once this tissue is débrided, the ankle and subtalar joints can be entered easily by penetrating the very thin joint capsule. At the level of the ankle joint, the superficial and deep component (transverse ligament) of the posterior tibiofibular ligament is recognized as well as the posterior talofibular ligament. The posterior talar process can be freed from scar tissue, and the FHL tendon is identified. This tendon should be located first, before addressing the pathology. The FHL tendon is an important safety landmark, since the neurovascular bundle runs just medial to this tendon. After removal of the thin joint capsule of the ankle joint, the intermalleolar and transverse ligaments need to be lifted in order to enter and inspect the ankle joint.

On the medial side, the tip of the medial malleolus can be visualized as well as the deep portion of the deltoid ligament. By opening the joint capsule from inside out at the level of the medial malleolus, the tendon sheath of the posterior tibial tendon and the FHL tendon can be opened when desired, and the arthroscope may now be introduced into the tendon sheath. Inspection of both tendons is now possible.

By applying manual distraction to the calcaneus, the posterior compartment of the ankle opens up, and the shaver can be introduced into the posterior ankle compartment. We prefer to apply a soft tissue distractor at this point (8). A synovectomy and/or capsulectomy can be performed. Inspection of the talar dome is possible over almost its entire surface as well as the complete tibial plafond. Identification of an OCD or subchondral cystic lesion may lead to débridement and drilling. The posterior syndesmotic ligaments are inspected and débrided if fibrotic or ruptured.

Removal of a symptomatic os trigonum, a nonunion of a fracture of the posterior talar process, or a symptomatic large posterior talar prominence involves partial detachment of the posterior talofibular ligament and release of the flexor retinaculum, which both attach to the posterior talar prominence. Release of the FHL tendon involves detachment of the flexor retinaculum from the posterior talar process. The tendon sheath can now be entered with the scope, following the tendon under the medial malleolus and a further release is performed.

Bleeding is controlled by electrocautery at the end of the procedure. Wound closure and dressing are performed as in anterior ankle arthroscopy. Prophylactic antibiotics are not routinely given. After surgery, patients are instructed to weight bear as tolerated.

Posterior ankle arthroscopy is an advanced endoscopic procedure. Surgeons are advised to train themselves in cadaveric sessions to adapt the technique before treating their patients (74).

Peroneal Tendoscopy

The patient is placed in the lateral decubitus position, with the operative side up. Before anesthesia is administered, the patient is asked to actively evert the affected foot. In this way, the tendon can be palpated, and the location of the portals is drawn onto the skin (Fig. 54-6). The surgery can be performed under local, regional, epidural, or general anesthesia. A support is placed under the affected leg making it possible to move the ankle freely. After exsanguination, a tourniquet is inflated around the thigh of the affected leg.

A distal portal is made first, 2 to 2.5 cm distal to the posterior edge of the lateral malleolus. An incision is made through the skin, and the tendon sheath is penetrated with an arthroscopic shaft with a blunt trocar. After this, a 2.7-mm, 30-degree arthroscope is introduced.

The inspection starts approximately 6 cm proximal to the posterior tip of the fibula, where a thin membrane splits the tendon compartment into two separate tendon chambers. More distally, the tendons lie in one compartment. A second portal is made 2 to 2.5 cm proximal to the posterior edge of the lateral malleolus under direct vision by placing a spinal needle, producing a portal directly over the tendons. Through the distal portal, a complete overview of both tendons can be obtained.

By rotating the arthroscope over and in between both tendons, the whole compartment can be inspected. When a total synovectomy of the tendon sheath has to be performed, it is advisable to make a third portal more distal or more proximal than the portals described previously.

When a rupture of one of the tendons is seen, endoscopic synovectomy is performed, and the rupture is repaired through a mini-open approach.

In patients with recurrent dislocation of the peroneal tendon, endoscopic fibular groove deepening can be performed through this tendoscopic approach. It is a time-consuming procedure because of the limited working area. Groove deepening is performed from within the tendon sheath with the risk of iatrogenic damage to the tendons. We therefore prefer an approach, based on the 2-portal hindfoot technique, with an additional portal located 4 cm proximal to the posterolateral portal (44).

At the end of the procedure, the portals are sutured to prevent sinus formation, and a compressive dressing is applied. Antibiotics are not routinely given.

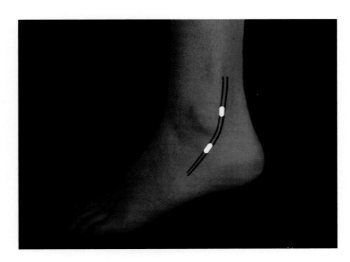

FIGURE 54-6

The patient is placed in the lateral decubitus position. Alternatively, the patient can also be placed in the supine position with the foot in endorotation. A support can be placed under the leg, being able to move the ankle freely. The patient is asked to evert the foot; thereby the peroneal tendons can usually be visualized clearly. Its course is drawn on the skin (in *black*), and the location of the portals is marked (in *white*).

Posterior Tibial Tendoscopy

The procedure can be performed on an outpatient basis under local, regional, or general anesthesia. The patient is placed in the supine position. A tourniquet is placed around the upper leg. Before anesthesia, the patient is asked to actively invert the foot, so that the posterior tibial tendon can be palpated and the portals can be marked. Access to the tendon can be obtained anywhere along its course.

We prefer to make the two main portals directly over the tendon 2 to 3 cm distal and 2 to 3 cm proximal to the posterior edge of the medial malleolus (Fig. 54-7). The distal portal is made first: the incision is made through the skin, and the tendon sheath is penetrated by the arthroscopic shaft with a blunt trocar. A 2.7-mm, 30-degree arthroscope is introduced, and the tendon sheath is filled with saline. Irrigation is performed using gravity flow.

Under direct vision, the proximal portal is made by introducing a spinal needle, and subsequently an incision is made into the tendon sheath. Instruments such as a retrograde knife, a shaver system, blunt probes, and scissors can be used. For synovectomy in patients with rheumatoid arthritis, a 3.5-mm shaver can be used. The complete tendon sheath can be inspected by rotating the arthroscope around the tendon.

Synovectomy can be performed with a complete overview of the tendon from the distal portal, over the insertion of the navicular bone to approximately 6 cm above the tip of the medial malleolus.

Special attention should be given while inspecting the tendon sheath, the posterior aspect of the medial malleolar surface, and the posterior ankle joint capsule. The tendon sheath between the posterior tibial tendon and the flexor digitorum longus is relatively thin: inspection of the correct tendon should always be checked. This can be accomplished by passively flexing and extending the toes; if the tendon sheath of the flexor digitorum longus tendon is entered, the tendon will move up and down.

When remaining in the posterior tibial tendon sheath, the neurovascular bundle is not in danger.

When a rupture of the posterior tibial tendon is seen, endoscopic synovectomy is performed, and the rupture is repaired through a mini-open approach. Magnifying the tendon endoscopically pronounces the localization and extent of the rupture, thereby minimizing the incision for repair. At the end of the procedure, the portals are sutured to prevent sinus formation.

Achilles Tendoscopy

Local, epidural, spinal, and general anesthesia can be used for this procedure, which can be performed on an outpatient basis. The patient is in prone position. A tourniquet is placed around the thigh of the affected leg, and a bolster is placed under the foot. Because the surgeon needs to be able to obtain full plantar and dorsiflexion, the foot is placed right over the end of the table.

The authors mostly use a 2.7-mm arthroscope for endoscopy of a combined tendinopathy and paratendinopathy. This small-diameter short arthroscope yields an excellent picture comparable to the standard 4-mm arthroscope; however, it cannot deliver the same amount of irrigation fluid per time as the 4-mm sheath can. This is important in procedures in which a large-diameter shaver is

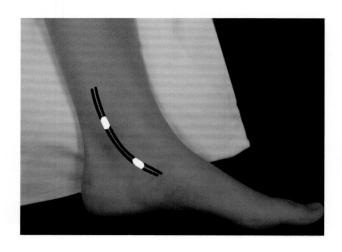

FIGURE 54-7

The patient is in the supine position. The two main portals (indicated in *white*) are made directly over the posterior tibial tendon (indicated with *black lines*) 2 to 3 cm distal and 2 to 3 cm proximal to the posterior edge of the medial malleolus.

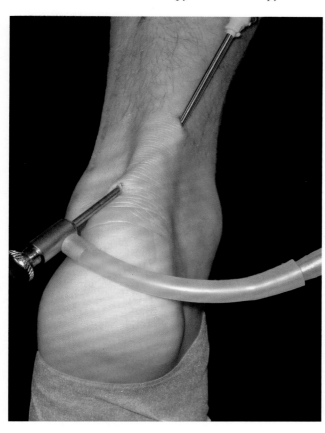

FIGURE 54-8

In case of peritendinitis of the Achilles tendon, the portals are created 2 to 3 cm proximal and 2 to 4 cm distal of the lesion. The distal portal is made first through the skin only. After introduction of a spinal needle under direct vision, an incision is made at the location of the proximal portal. Instruments like a probe or a small shaver can be introduced.

used (e.g., in endoscopic calcaneoplasty). When a 4-mm arthroscope is used, gravity inflow of irrigation fluid is usually sufficient. A pressurized bag or pump device sometimes is used with the 2.7-mm arthroscope.

The distal portal is located on the lateral border of the Achilles tendon, 2 to 3 cm distal to the pathologic nodule. The proximal portal is located medial to the border of the Achilles tendon, 2 to 4 cm above the nodule (Fig. 54-8). When the portals are placed this way, it is usually possible to visualize and work around the whole surface of the tendon, over a length of approximately 10 cm.

The distal portal is made first. After making the skin incision, the mosquito clamp is introduced, followed by the blunt 2.7-mm trocar in a craniomedial direction. With this blunt trocar, the paratendon is approached and is blindly released from the tendon by moving around it. Subsequently, the 2.7-mm, 30-degree arthroscope is introduced. To minimize the risk of iatrogenic damage, the arthroscope should be kept on the tendon. At this moment, it can be confirmed whether the surgeon is in the right layer between paratendon and Achilles tendon. If not, now it can be identified, and a further release can be performed.

The proximal portal is made by introducing a spinal needle, followed by a mosquito clamp and probe. The plantaris tendon can be identified at the anteromedial border of the Achilles tendon. In a typical case of local paratendinopathy, the plantaris tendon, the Achilles tendon, and the paratendon are tight together in the process. Removal of the local thickened paratendon on the anteromedial side of the Achilles tendon at the level of the nodule, and release of the plantaris tendon are the goals of this procedure. In cases where the fibrotic paratendon is firmly attached to the lateral or posterior border of the tendon, a release in these areas is performed. Neovessels accompanied by small nerve fibers can be found in this area and are removed with a 2.7-mm bone cutter shaver. The tendon proper remains untouched.

Changing portals can be helpful. At the end of the procedure, it must be possible to move the arthroscope over the complete symptomatic area of the Achilles tendon.

After the procedure, the portals are sutured.

Aftercare consists of a compressive dressing for 2 to 3 days. Patients are encouraged to actively perform range of motion exercises. Full weight bearing is allowed as tolerated. Initially, the foot must be elevated when not walking.

POSTOPERATIVE MANAGEMENT AND REHABILITATION

In all indications as described in this chapter, the patient can be discharged the same day of surgery. The patient is instructed to elevate the foot when not walking to prevent edema. In most cases, postoperative management consists of a pressure bandage and partial weight bearing for 2 to 3 days. Full weight bearing is allowed as tolerated, and active range of motion exercises for at least three times a day for 10 minutes is advised starting immediately post surgery.

If an OCD is the indication for operation, the patient is kept non–weight bearing and placed in a well-padded short leg cast during the immediate postoperative period. At 2 weeks postoperatively, the patient is placed in a controlled action motion (CAM) walker boot. Partial weight bearing and gentle ankle range of motion exercises are permitted. Weight bearing is advanced based on radiographic evidence of osteotomy healing. At 6 weeks, the patient can discontinue the use of the CAM walker. Repetitive impact activities, such as jogging and aerobics, can be resumed after 6 to 8 months. Return to high-level sports is permitted after 12 months.

In case of an endoscopic groove deepening in order to treat recurrent peroneal tendon dislocation, partial weight bearing is advised for 5 days. A soft brace is applied for 4 to 6 weeks with the permission to fully bear weight. With satisfaction of the surgeon and the patient, no further outpatient department contact is necessary. Patients with limited range of motion are directed to a physiotherapist.

TECHNICAL ALTERNATIVES AND PITFALLS

Posterior Ankle Arthroscopy/Endoscopic Groove Deepening Technique

In the hindfoot, the crural fascia can be quite thick. This local thickening is called the Rouvière ligament (75). This ligament needs to be at least partially excised or sectioned, using arthroscopic punch or scissors, to reach the level of the ankle and the subtalar joint. The position of the arthroscope is important; the view should always be to the lateral side. At introduction, the arthroscope must be pointed in the direction between the first and the second toe to remain in a safe area. The FHL tendon is an important landmark. The working area is laterally with respect to the FHL tendon. The FHL tendon can safely be identified by shaving on top of the posterior talar process while the opening of the shaver is pointing toward the bone. While staying in contact with the bone, the tip of the shaver should be moved slowly and slightly twisted to the medial side. The shaver must be twisted approximately 45 degrees so that the opening of the shaver is directed 45 degrees distally and 45 degrees to the lateral side, and thus the blunt back of the shaver blade is turned toward the FHL tendon. The contour of the posterior talar process is followed until the shaver can be pushed in between the posterior talar process and the FHL tendon. Shaving should be stopped at this moment and the FHL tendon must be identified. The opening of the shaver should always be directed away from the tendon at this point. In case of a posterior tarsal tunnel syndrome, release of the neurovascular bundle can be performed. The FHL tendon should then be passed medially with a mosquito clamp and with caution to the neurovascular bundle. If a hypertrophic posterior talar process is removed by using a chisel, care must be taken not to place the chisel too far anteriorly. Only the inferoposterior part of the process should be removed with the chisel. The remnant of the process can be taken away with a bone cutter shaver. If initially the chisel is placed too much anteriorly, it is hard to avoid taking away too much bone at the level of the subtalar joint.

Loose bony particles can easily be created with the microfracture awl in case of puncturing the subchondral plate in ODs. They can become detached upon withdrawal of the awl. If the particles are not taken out properly, they may act as loose bodies and should therefore be removed (76).

During endoscopic groove deepening for recurrent peroneal tendon dislocation, the posterior ankle ligament is potentially at risk. Medial from the fibular groove the posterior syndesmotic ligaments and the posterior talofibular ligament are located. The contour of the groove must be followed from proximal to distal. The calcaneofibular ligament inserts more anteriorly in the most distal part of the lateral malleolus. The fibular groove must be deepened anteriorly and distally, while the shaver is directed medial from the calcaneofibular ligament insertion (44).

The depth of the fibular groove needs to be sufficient in order to prevent redislocation of the peroneal tendons and should approximately be 5 mm. At the end of the procedure, the ankle is manipulated to check whether sufficient bone is excised. Removing too much fibular bone could induce weakening, which could eventually result in a fracture of the remaining lateral rim. It is important to smoothen the created lateral edge of the groove in order to prevent it from causing peroneal tendon (length) ruptures. In fact, this is the most important pitfall and should therefore always be carefully checked.

The advantage of a two-portal procedure (9) and also of the three-portal endoscopic groove deepening technique (44) with the patient in the prone position is the working space that can be created in between the Achilles tendon and the back of the ankle and subtalar joint. The position is ergonomic for the orthopaedic surgeon. Soft tissue distraction can easily be applied (77).

DISCUSSION/CONSIDERATION

Arthroscopy has become an important operative technique in treating a wide variety of ankle pathology. It provides a minimally invasive approach as a good alternative to the already-existing open surgical techniques. The surgeon must be familiar with the anatomy and must try to use routine portals in ankle arthroscopy (78). Ideally, these routine portals can be used to treat the vast majority of pathology, without the need for additional portals.

The authors feel that the posteromedial and lateral portal, as described in 2000, possess the criteria (9). Also, portals must provide a safe access, as is anatomically demonstrated to be the case for these posterior endoscopic portals (79).

Recently, a retrospective study was published in which 16 posterior ankle arthroscopies were evaluated (33). The patients all had a good functional and clinical outcome at a mean follow-up of 32 months. One patient had a temporary numbness in the region of the scar. Similar results were published in a prospective study of the senior author (10). In total, 55 posterior ankle arthroscopies were assessed. All patients had a posterior ankle impingement syndrome. Good to excellent functional and clinical outcome was reported on in 74% of the cases. One complication occurred, being a temporary sensational loss of the posteromedial heel. The two-portal endoscopic hindfoot approach compares favorably to open surgery with regard to less morbidity and a quicker recovery (10).

The technique is now expanding to other areas in the hindfoot. The endoscopic groove deepening technique for recurrent peroneal tendon dislocation, as described in this chapter, is one of these new possibilities (44). Also, subtalar arthrodesis can be successfully performed with this technique in patients who have primary degenerative joint disease of the subtalar joint without gross deformity or bone loss (21).

REFERENCES

1. Burman MS. Arthroscopy of direct visualization of joints. An experimental cadaver study. *J Bone Joint Surg.* 1931;13:669–695.
2. Watanabe M. *Selfoc-Arthroscope (Watanabe no. 24 arthroscope). Monograph.* Tokyo: Teishin Hospital; 1972.
3. van Dijk CN, Kort N, Scholten PE. Tendoscopy of the posterior tibial tendon. *Arthroscopy.* 1997;13(6):692–698.
4. Scholten PE, van Dijk CN. Tendoscopy of the peroneal tendons. *Foot Ankle Clin.* 2006;11(2):415–420, vii.
5. van Dijk CN, Kort N. Tendoscopy of the peroneal tendons. *Arthroscopy.* 1998;14(5):471–478.
6. Steenstra F, van Dijk CN. Achilles tendoscopy. *Foot Ankle Clin.* 2006;11(2):429–438, viii.
7. Scholten PE, van Dijk CN. Endoscopic calcaneoplasty. *Foot Ankle Clin.* 2006;11(2):439–446, viii.
8. van Dijk CN, van Dyk GE, Scholten PE, et al. Endoscopic calcaneoplasty. *Am J Sports Med.* 2001;29(2):185–189.
9. van Dijk CN, Scholten PE, Krips R. A 2-portal endoscopic approach for diagnosis and treatment of posterior ankle pathology. *Arthroscopy.* 2000;16(8):871–876.
10. Scholten PE, Sierevelt IN, van Dijk CN. Hindfoot endoscopy for posterior ankle impingement. *J Bone Joint Surg Am.* 2008;90(12):2665–2672.
11. Japour C, Vohra P, Giorgini R, et al. Ankle arthroscopy: follow-up study of 33 ankles–effect of physical therapy and obesity. *J Foot Ankle Surg.* 1996;35(3):199–209.
12. Flick AB, Gould N. Osteochondritis dissecans of the talus (transchondral fractures of the talus): review of the literature and new surgical approach for medial dome lesions. *Foot Ankle.* 1985;5(4):165–185.
13. Dahmen J, Lambers KT, Reilingh ML, et al. No superior treatment for primary osteochondral defects of the talus. *Knee Surg Sports Traumatol Arthrosc.* 2018;26(7):2177–2182.
14. Verhagen RA, Maas M, Dijkgraaf MG, et al. Prospective study on diagnostic strategies in osteochondral lesions of the talus. Is MRI superior to helical CT? *J Bone Joint Surg Br.* 2005;87(1):41–46.
15. Reis ND, Zinman C, Besser MI, et al. High-resolution computerised tomography in clinical orthopaedics. *J Bone Joint Surg Br.* 1982;64(1):20–24.
16. Tol JL, Struijs PA, Bossuyt PM, et al. Treatment strategies in osteochondral defects of the talar dome: a systematic review. *Foot Ankle Int.* 2000;21(2):119–126.
17. O'Driscoll SW. The healing and regeneration of articular cartilage. *J Bone Joint Surg Am.* 1998;80(12):1795–1812.
18. Amendola A, Lee KB, Saltzman CL, et al. Technique and early experience with posterior arthroscopic subtalar arthrodesis. *Foot Ankle Int.* 2007;28(3):298–302.

19. Glanzmann MC, Sanhueza-Hernandez R. Arthroscopic subtalar arthrodesis for symptomatic osteoarthritis of the hind-foot: a prospective study of 41 cases. *Foot Ankle Int.* 2007;28(1):2–7.
20. Carro LP, Golano P, Vega J. Arthroscopic subtalar arthrodesis: the posterior approach in the prone position. *Arthroscopy.* 2007;23(4):445.e1–445.e4.
21. Beimers L, de Leeuw PA, van Dijk CN. A 3-portal approach for arthroscopic subtalar arthrodesis. *Knee Surg Sports Traumatol Arthrosc.* 2009;17:830–834.
22. Scholten PE, Altena MC, Krips R, et al. Treatment of a large intraosseous talar ganglion by means of hindfoot endoscopy. *Arthroscopy.* 2003;19(1):96–100.
23. Hamilton WG, Geppert MJ, Thompson FM. Pain in the posterior aspect of the ankle in dancers. Differential diagnosis and operative treatment. *J Bone Joint Surg Am.* 1996;78(10):1491–1500.
24. van Dijk CN, Lim LS, Poortman A, et al. Degenerative joint disease in female ballet dancers. *Am J Sports Med.* 1995;23(3):295–300.
25. Hedrick MR, McBryde AM. Posterior ankle impingement. *Foot Ankle Int.* 1994;15(1):2–8.
26. Maquirriain J. Posterior ankle impingement syndrome. *J Am Acad Orthop Surg.* 2005;13(6):365–371.
27. Weinstein SL, Bonfiglio M. Unusual accessory (bipartite) talus simulating fracture. A case report. *J Bone Joint Surg Am.* 1975;57(8):1161–1163.
28. Lapidus PW. A note on the fracture of os trigonum syndrome. Report of a case. *Bull Hosp Jt Dis.* 1972;33(2):150–154.
29. van Dijk CN. Anterior and posterior ankle impingement. *Foot Ankle Clin.* 2006;11(3):663–683.
30. Hamilton WG. Tendonitis about the ankle joint in classical ballet dancers. *Am J Sports Med.* 1977;5(2):84–88.
31. Zwiers R, Baltes TPA, Opdam KTM, et al. Prevalence of os trigonum on CT imaging. *Foot Ankle Int.* 2018;39(3):338–342.
32. Bizarro AH. On sesamoid and supernumerary bones of the limbs. *J Anat.* 1921;55:256–268.
33. Willits K, Sonneveld H, Amendola A, et al. Outcome of posterior ankle arthroscopy for hindfoot impingement. *Arthroscopy.* 2008;24(2):196–202.
34. Cedell CA. Rupture of the posterior talotibial ligament with the avulsion of a bone fragment from the talus. *Acta Orthop Scand.* 1974;45(3):454–461.
35. Gould N. Stenosing tenosynovitis of the flexor hallucis longus tendon at the great toe. *Foot Ankle.* 1981;2(1):46–48.
36. Krackow KA. Acute, traumatic rupture of a flexor hallucis longus tendon: a case report. *Clin Orthop Relat Res.* 1980;(150):261–262.
37. Bassett FH III, Speer KP. Longitudinal rupture of the peroneal tendons. *Am J Sports Med.* 1993;21(3):354–357.
38. Dombek MF, Lamm BM, Saltrick K, et al. Peroneal tendon tears: a retrospective review. *J Foot Ankle Surg.* 2003;42(5):250–258.
39. Schweitzer GJ. Stenosing peroneal tenovaginitis. Case reports. *S Afr Med J.* 1982;61(14):521–523.
40. Heckman DS, Reddy S, Pedowitz D, et al. Operative treatment for peroneal tendon disorders. *J Bone Joint Surg Am.* 2008;90(2):404–418.
41. Rosenberg ZS, Bencardino J, Astion D, et al. MRI features of chronic injuries of the superior peroneal retinaculum. *Am J Roentgenol.* 2003;181(6):1551–1557.
42. Yao L, Tong DJ, Cracchiolo A, et al. MR findings in peroneal tendonopathy. *J Comput Assist Tomogr.* 1995;19(3):460–464.
43. Lui TH. Endoscopic peroneal retinaculum reconstruction. *Knee Surg Sports Traumatol Arthrosc.* 2006;14(5):478–481.
44. de Leeuw PAJ, Golano P, van Dijk CN. A 3-portal endoscopic groove deepening technique for recurrent peroneal tendon dislocation. *Tech Foot Ankle Surg.* 2008;7(4):250–256.
45. Myerson MS. Adult acquired flatfoot deformity: treatment of dysfunction of the posterior tibial tendon. *Instr Course Lect.* 1997;46:393–405.
46. Michelson J, Easley M, Wigley FM, et al. Posterior tibial tendon dysfunction in rheumatoid arthritis. *Foot Ankle Int.* 1995;16(3):156–161.
47. Trnka HJ. Dysfunction of the tendon of tibialis posterior. *J Bone Joint Surg Br.* 2004;86(7):939–946.
48. Kong A, Van der V. Imaging of tibialis posterior dysfunction. *Br J Radiol.* 2008;81(970):826–836.
49. Miller SD, Van HM, Boruta PM, et al. Ultrasound in the diagnosis of posterior tibial tendon pathology. *Foot Ankle Int.* 1996;17(9):555–558.
50. Porter DA, Baxter DE, Clanton TO, et al. Posterior tibial tendon tears in young competitive athletes: two case reports. *Foot Ankle Int.* 1998;19(9):627–630.
51. Lui TH. Endoscopic assisted posterior tibial tendon reconstruction for stage 2 posterior tibial tendon insufficiency. *Knee Surg Sports Traumatol Arthrosc.* 2007;15(10):1228–1234.
52. Bare AA, Haddad SL. Tenosynovitis of the posterior tibial tendon. *Foot Ankle Clin.* 2001;6(1):37–66.
53. Johnson KA, Strom DE. Tibialis posterior tendon dysfunction. *Clin Orthop Relat Res.* 1989;(239):196–206.
54. Paus AC. Arthroscopic synovectomy. When, which diseases and which joints. *Z Rheumatol.* 1996;55(6):394–400.
55. Clain MR, Baxter DE. Achilles tendinitis. *Foot Ankle.* 1992;13(8):482–487.
56. Saltzman CL, Tearse DS. Achilles tendon injuries. *J Am Acad Orthop Surg.* 1998;6(5):316–325.
57. Maffulli N, Kenward MG, Testa V, et al. Clinical diagnosis of Achilles tendinopathy with tendinosis. *Clin J Sport Med.* 2003;13(1):11–15.
58. Maffulli N, Walley G, Sayana MK, et al. Eccentric calf muscle training in athletic patients with Achilles tendinopathy. *Disabil Rehabil.* 2008;30(20–22):1677–1684.
59. Ko R, Porter M. *Interactive Foot and Ankle 2.* London: Primal Pictures; 2000.
60. Woodley BL, Newsham-West RJ, Baxter GD. Chronic tendinopathy: effectiveness of eccentric exercise. *Br J Sports Med.* 2007;41(4):188–198.
61. Mafi N, Lorentzon R, Alfredson H. Superior short-term results with eccentric calf muscle training compared to concentric training in a randomized prospective multicenter study on patients with chronic Achilles tendinosis. *Knee Surg Sports Traumatol Arthrosc.* 2001;9(1):42–47.
62. Andersson G, Danielson P, Alfredson H, et al. Nerve-related characteristics of ventral paratendinous tissue in chronic Achilles tendinosis. *Knee Surg Sports Traumatol Arthrosc.* 2007;15(10):1272–1279.
63. Willberg L, Sunding K, Ohberg L, et al. Sclerosing injections to treat midportion Achilles tendinosis: a randomised controlled study evaluating two different concentrations of Polidocanol. *Knee Surg Sports Traumatol Arthrosc.* 2008;16(9):859–864.
64. Kvist M. Achilles tendon injuries in athletes. *Ann Chir Gynaecol.* 1991;80(2):188–201.
65. Maffulli N. Augmented repair of acute Achilles tendon ruptures using gastrocnemius-soleus fascia. *Int Orthop.* 2005;29(2):134.

66. Marotta JJ, Micheli LJ. Os trigonum impingement in dancers. *Am J Sports Med.* 1992;20(5):533–536.
67. Abramowitz Y, Wollstein R, Barzilay Y, et al. Outcome of resection of a symptomatic os trigonum. *J Bone Joint Surg Am.* 2003;85-A(6):1051–1057.
68. Maffulli N, Testa V, Capasso G, et al. Results of percutaneous longitudinal tenotomy for Achilles tendinopathy in middle- and long-distance runners. *Am J Sports Med.* 1997;25(6):835–840.
69. Testa V, Maffulli N, Capasso G, et al. Percutaneous longitudinal tenotomy in chronic Achilles tendonitis. *Bull Hosp Jt Dis.* 1996;54(4):241–244.
70. Testa V, Capasso G, Benazzo F, et al. Management of Achilles tendinopathy by ultrasound-guided percutaneous tenotomy. *Med Sci Sports Exerc.* 2002;34(4):573–580.
71. Kannus P, Jozsa L. Histopathological changes preceding spontaneous rupture of a tendon. A controlled study of 891 patients. *J Bone Joint Surg Am.* 1991;73(10):1507–1525.
72. Khan KM, Forster BB, Robinson J, et al. Are ultrasound and magnetic resonance imaging of value in assessment of Achilles tendon disorders? A two year prospective study. *Br J Sports Med.* 2003;37(2):149–153.
73. Opdam KTM, Baltes TPA, Zwiers R, et al. Endoscopic treatment of mid-portion Achilles tendinopathy: a retrospective case series of patient satisfaction and functional outcome at a 2- to 8-year follow-up. *Arthroscopy.* 2018;34(1):264–269.
74. Amsterdam Foot and Ankle Platform. 2009. Ref Type: Internet Communication. Available at: www.ankleplatform.com.
75. Rouviere H, Canela Lazaro M. Le ligament Peroneo-Astragalo-Calcaneen. *Annales Dánatomie Pathologique.* 1932;7(9):745–750.
76. van Bergen CJ, de Leeuw PA, van Dijk CN. Potential pitfall in the microfracturing technique during the arthroscopic treatment of an osteochondral lesion. *Knee Surg Sports Traumatol Arthrosc.* 2009;17(2):184–187.
77. van Dijk CN, de Leeuw PA. Imaging from an orthopaedic point of view. What the orthopaedic surgeon expects from the radiologist? *Eur J Radiol.* 2007;62(1):2–5.
78. Barber FA, Click J, Britt BT. Complications of ankle arthroscopy. *Foot Ankle.* 1990;10(5):263–266.
79. Lijoi F, Lughi M, Baccarani G. Posterior arthroscopic approach to the ankle: an anatomic study. *Arthroscopy.* 2003;19(1):62–67.

55 Lateral Ankle Instability: Modified Broström, Suture Tape Augmentation, Reconstruction, and Arthroscopy

Alexander S. Kuczmarski, Samuel I. Rosenberg, and C. Thomas Haytmanek Jr

INTRODUCTION

Lateral ankle ligament sprains are one of the most common injuries in sports (1–6). Most of these injuries respond to conservative treatment with a physical therapy program emphasizing proprioceptive training, range of motion, and strength training of the supportive musculature (5,7,8). Surgical correction in the patient with persistent lateral ankle instability and dysfunction has been described utilizing a number of anatomic and nonanatomic operations (9–13). Many of the historic methods of ankle stabilization sacrificed some or all of an often-normal peroneal tendon (11–13). Disadvantages of such procedures include large exposures with increased risk of nerve injury, sacrificing a peroneal tendon, increased operative time, and reduced range of motion from nonanatomic tunnel positions (14).

Lennart Broström published the first in a series of articles on the operative treatment of lateral ankle ligament sprains (7,9,10,15–17). Broström proposed direct primary repair of the lateral ligaments in patients with chronic lateral ankle instability. The operation he described was an anatomic repair formulated on the premise that the anterior talofibular ligament (ATFL) is contained in a portion of the anterolateral ankle capsule (9,15). He also proposed repair of the calcaneofibular ligament (CFL) when indicated. This operation restored the normal length of the lateral ligaments and respected their normal anatomic locations (10). The Broström repair was recommended for the treatment of both acute ruptures and chronic instability (9,10).

Several modifications of Broström's original procedure have been described, the most popular being reinforcement of the primary ligament repair using a portion of the inferior extensor retinaculum, which is sutured to the periosteum of the distal fibula (18). This modification is referred to as the Broström-Gould procedure or the modified Broström and adds stability to the repair, limits inversion, and helps address subtalar instability (19).

Indications for primary lateral ankle ligament repair include chronic instability leading to dysfunction unresolved after an aggressive rehabilitation program. Carefully selected professional and elite athletes may benefit from the procedure in the setting of an acute sprain with complete rupture of the lateral ligamentous complex. This chapter will focus on the patient with chronic lateral ankle instability.

PREOPERATIVE PLANNING

Patients being considered for lateral ankle ligament repair should have severe functional limitation from lateral ankle instability. This dysfunction persists despite completion of a standard rehabilitation and proprioception training program. Athletes describe giving way, frequent sprains, and an inability to perform at their prior level of competition. Pain may be present but is less of a consideration than is instability. If pain is the major complaint, other sources of pain should be investigated, such as osteochondral lesions, peroneal tendon pathology, occult fracture, or nerve injury. Among the most frequent presentations is the athlete with a severe acute lateral ankle sprain who relates that this happens with unnatural frequency or ease, suggesting an acute or chronic presentation. In these situations, anatomic repair of the ligaments is an excellent choice because it does not restrict subtalar motion and spares the peroneal tendons.

Ankle instability can be evaluated by physical examination with the anterior drawer and talar tilt tests. Both tests stress both lateral ankle ligaments, with the anterior drawer test focusing more on the ATFL and the talar tilt test focusing more on the CFL (Fig. 55-1). Comparison with the contralateral side gives the examiner an idea of the degree of increased laxity of the affected ankle. The motion of the hindfoot should be carefully evaluated during these examinations. Decreased motion of the tibiotalar or subtalar joints could indicate a tarsal coalition, which should be concurrently addressed as it predisposes to recurrent ankle sprains and chronic instability.

A thorough evaluation of the posture of the foot and ankle with the patient standing is required before proceeding with surgery. A patient with a cavus foot (Fig. 55-2) or hindfoot varus can be predisposed to lateral ankle ligament injury. These patients may require realignment of the foot's posture to prevent lateral ligament repair failure. Tarsal coalitions can also present as recurrent sprains due to increased hindfoot rigidity and may be a source of ongoing difficulty after a lateral ligament repair if not addressed appropriately. These underlying anatomic abnormalities can be associated with additional soft tissue pathology, such as peroneal tendon subluxations or tears, lateral impingement, synovitis, or sinus tarsi syndrome.

Plain radiographs should be evaluated for fractures, osteochondral lesions, loose bodies, cavus deformity, and tarsal coalitions. Stress views can be used to measure anterior drawer and talar tilt gapping, including side-to-side differences, using either fluoroscopy with a mini c-arm or plain radiography (Figs. 55-3 and 55-4). There is still controversy as to the exact degree of opening or side-to-side difference that indicates the need for surgical intervention, but providers must account for patient symptoms regardless of the threshold value used. Magnetic resonance imaging (MRI) provides a precise view of the ligament injury (Figs. 55-5 and 55-6) and is sensitive for concomitant pathology. Peroneal tendon tears, tarsal coalitions, osteochondral lesions, and loose bodies are readily apparent on MRI. All of these imaging studies should be evaluated in the context of the patient's history and physical examination.

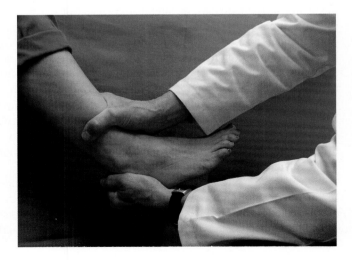

FIGURE 55-1

The talar tilt test is performed by stabilizing the distal tibia and exerting a varus force on the hindfoot.

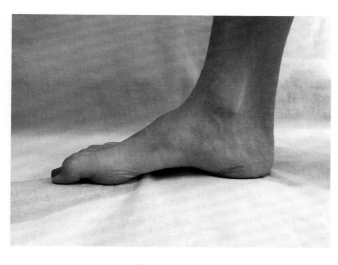

FIGURE 55-2

Medial view of a cavus deformity. This patient is predisposed to recurrent lateral ankle sprains.

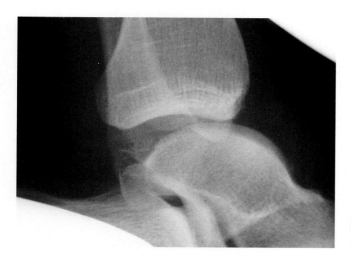

FIGURE 55-3

Positive anterior drawer stress x-ray.

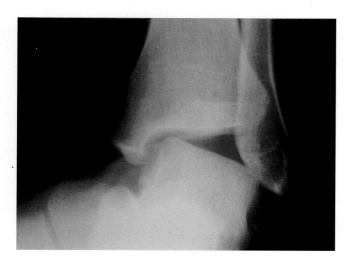

FIGURE 55-4

Positive talar tilt stress x-ray.

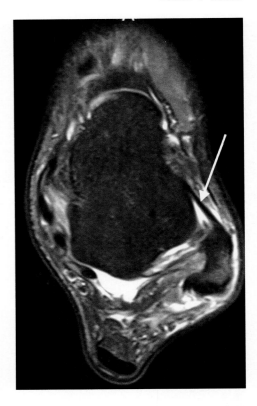

FIGURE 55-5

Axial view of an MRI showing an intact ATFL (indicated by *arrow*).

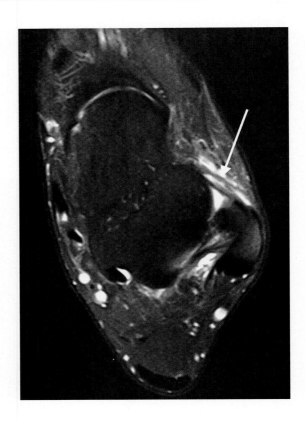

FIGURE 55-6

Axial view of an MRI revealing an injured ATFL (indicated by *arrow*).

SURGERY

Lateral ankle ligament repair is typically performed as an outpatient surgery. The patient is placed supine on the operating table with a bump under the ipsilateral hip to slightly internally rotate the extremity. Placing a small stack of towels under the distal tibia allows the heel to float freely in order to avoid anterior displacement caused by the operating table during repair. The lower leg is exsanguinated, and a thigh tourniquet is inflated. Alternatively, the patient can be placed laterally on the operating table and the foot and ankle can be exsanguinated before a calf tourniquet is inflated. A calf tourniquet should be avoided if peroneal tendon work is indicated because inflation can shorten the peroneal tendons.

The typical incision is started at the level of the tibial plafond along the anterior border of the distal fibula, curving in a J shape posteriorly and stopping at the level of the peroneal tendons (Fig. 55-7). Alternative incisions can be used if concomitant pathology is to be addressed. For example, an incision can be made along the course of the peroneal tendons if peroneal tendon pathology is to be addressed concurrently. Care is taken to avoid damage to the lateral branch of the superficial peroneal nerve anteriorly and the sural nerve posteriorly. An anterior branch of the sural nerve can sometimes cross over the distal fibula in the middle of the incision.

The dissection proceeds through the subcutaneous layer to the anterolateral ankle joint capsule. The anterior inferior tibiofibular ligament can be a useful landmark because it attaches to the anterior fibula proximal to the ATFL origin. The inferior extensor retinaculum is superficial to the capsule and is composed of ligaments coursing from the dorsal ankle and foot, which combine and insert at the sinus tarsi. The lax ATFL fibers are seen running within the anterolateral capsule (Fig. 55-8).

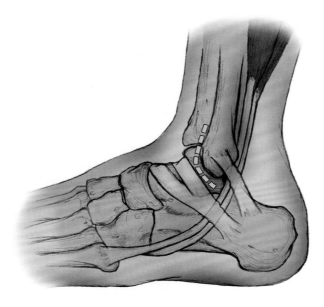

FIGURE 55-7

The typical incision is started at the level of the tibial plafond along the anterior border of the distal fibula, curving in a J shape posteriorly and ending at the level of the peroneal tendons.

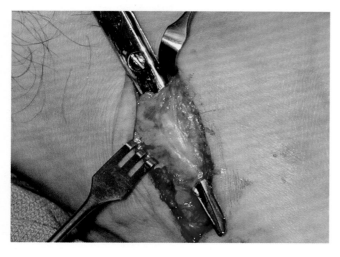

FIGURE 55-8

The lax ATFL fibers are seen running within the anterolateral capsule.

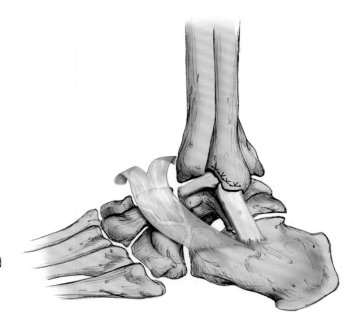

FIGURE 55-9

The ATFL and capsule can be transected directly off the bone and repaired through drill holes or with suture anchors.

The ATFL and capsule are then divided with a small cuff of tissue attached to the lateral malleolus left to repair the imbricated ligament. Alternatively, the ATFL and capsule can be transected directly off the bone and repaired through drill holes or with suture anchors (Fig. 55-9). This type of repair should be performed in the setting of an avulsion injury.

The CFL can be identified by retracting the peroneal tendons below the fibula. From its origin on the distal fibula, the CFL runs posteriorly and inferiorly to insert on the calcaneus. If it appears stretched, it can be divided and imbricated. The CFL can also be completely avulsed. If the CFL is avulsed from the calcaneus, the injury can be repaired with suture anchors. We prefer bioabsorbable or all-suture anchors to avoid imaging, hardware removal, and reconstruction problems from metallic anchors or poorly placed tunnels.

The CFL should be repaired first, since it is the more difficult ligament to visualize. The ligaments are repaired in their anatomic positions and under tension, specifically in neutral dorsiflexion and slight inversion, preserving a normal range of motion (Fig. 55-10). After the ligaments are sutured, redundant tissue can be excised or used as reinforcement over the substance of the repair.

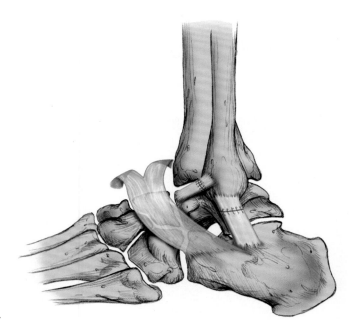

FIGURE 55-10

The ligaments are repaired in their anatomic positions under tension, preserving a normal range of motion.

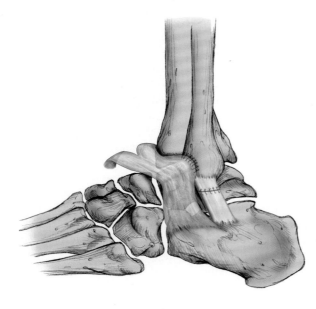

FIGURE 55-11

The previously identified inferior extensor retinaculum can be imbricated and sutured over the ATFL repair with absorbable sutures to the periosteum of the distal fibula.

The previously identified inferior extensor retinaculum can then be imbricated and sutured over the ATFL repair to the periosteum of the distal fibula with absorbable sutures (18) (Fig. 55-11). This reinforces the primary repair and is referred to as the Broström-Gould procedure or the modified Broström (19). The stability of the ankle is carefully examined, and the incision is closed in layers.

Direct repair of the ATFL has recently been augmented with suture tape. The InternalBrace (Arthrex, Naples, FL) includes BioComposite SwiveLock (Arthrex, Naples, FL) anchors and FiberTape (Arthrex, Naples, FL) suture. Suture anchors are placed at the origin and insertion of the ATFL, protecting the primary repair during healing (20). Care is taken to not overtighten the suture, as it is designed to be a checkrein or seat belt, not an artificial ligament.

When there is a paucity of quality ligamentous tissue, the patient is a high-level athlete, the patient is heavy, or the direct repair fails, reconstruction may be indicated. We prefer the use of a semitendinosus tendon allograft to prevent donor site morbidity in the patient and to reduce operative time, especially for surgeons unfamiliar with graft harvest techniques (21). Anatomic tunnels are drilled in the talus, calcaneus, and fibula. Reconstruction of both lateral ligaments is accomplished with a single allograft. Bioabsorbable screws are used to fix the allograft in the tunnels (22). The strength and stiffness of this reconstruction are not significantly different from the intact ATFL (21).

Patients undergoing lateral ankle ligament repair have a high incidence of associated intra-articular pathology (23,24). Ankle arthroscopy is a useful adjunct to lateral ligament repair as it allows evaluation and treatment of the full spectrum of concomitant intra-articular pathology (25). Loose bodies, synovitis, impingement, osteochondral lesions, and osteophytes can all be addressed with arthroscopy at the time of surgery. The procedure has the disadvantage of fluid extravasation into the soft tissues, making dissection more challenging when trying to find and repair torn lateral ligaments that are contiguous with the capsule.

Arthroscopy is also being utilized for the repair (26). Most arthroscopic techniques only repair the ATFL, leading some authors to recommend arthroscopic repair when only mild to moderate ankle instability (<15 degrees of talar tilt) is present. Stress radiographs can be helpful in this determination (26,27). Standard anteromedial and anterolateral portals are created (26–29). If more working area is needed, a third portal can be utilized (30–32). First, the joint is inspected, and any intra-articular pathology is addressed (26,27,29–32). Most commonly, a modified Broström procedure using two suture anchors is chosen to anatomically secure the ATFL, inferior extensor retinaculum, and capsule to the fibula (26,27,29,30). A biomechanical study found the arthroscopic modified Broström procedure using suture anchors to provide ankle stability similar to the open procedure (33).

POSTOPERATIVE MANAGEMENT

The patient is sent home in a splint for 10 to 14 days, which is followed by 2 weeks of weight-bearing progression. Once at full weight bearing, a 2-week boot wean is commenced. The patients work with physical therapy and limit passive inversion for the first 6 weeks postoperatively. After 6 weeks, we progress to an outcomes-based therapy program as the patient strengthens.

RESULTS

A systematic review reported an average American Orthopaedic Foot and Ankle Society (AOFAS) score of 90.1 and a satisfaction rate of 91.7% at an average follow-up of 73.4 months after open Broström ATFL repair (34). The modified Broström procedure has stood the test of time. Hamilton reported 93% successful results after surgical repair of the lateral ankle ligaments, with athletes and dancers returning to previous competitive levels (19). Review studies of the modified Broström typically show an 85% to 95% success rate (35). The modified Broström procedure produces excellent clinical outcomes regardless of when the patient presents. In one study, patients who presented more than 4 years after their initial injury all had excellent clinical outcomes, were satisfied with their surgery, and were stable at final physical examination (36). A systematic review of outcomes after the modified Broström procedure reported a revision rate of 1.2% after a weighted mean follow-up of 8.4 years. The sole reason for revision was overconstraint of the joint (37).

Cho reported no differences in clinical outcomes between the modified Broström procedure and the InternalBrace (Arthrex, Naples, FL) (38). Coetzee reported minimal pain, high satisfaction, excellent clinical outcomes, and an average return to sport of 84.1 days after suture-augmented Broström repair (39).

Good to excellent clinical outcomes and significant reductions in anterior drawer and talar tilt gapping are seen after anatomic reconstruction of both lateral ankle ligaments using a semitendinosus tendon allograft. This is accompanied by high rates of stability, return to full activity, and satisfaction as well as a low rate of complications (40–42).

Excellent clinical outcomes are seen after arthroscopic repair of the lateral ankle ligaments. A systematic review reported an average AOFAS score of 92.48 and a satisfaction rate of 96.4% at an average of 37.2 months of follow-up (34). Short-term clinical outcomes scores following arthroscopy are significantly better than those after open procedures, including an earlier return to activity (29,34,43). There are no significant differences in long-term clinical outcome scores between the arthroscopic and open procedures (29,43).

COMPLICATIONS

Nerve injury, although rare, is the most common complication of lateral ankle ligament repair. Hypersensitivity or hyposensitivity has an incidence of 7% to 19%. Most of these nerve injuries occur during outdated tenodesis procedures, with the sural nerve at highest risk. The superficial peroneal nerve can be harmed with an incision either too proximal along the fibula or too distal over the dorsum of the foot. The sural nerve can be injured if the incision extends too far beyond the margin of the peroneal tendons. Recurrence of instability, delayed wound healing, superficial infection, deep infection, stiffness, and deep venous thrombosis have also been reported (38,39,44).

REFERENCES

1. Garrick JG. The frequency of injury, mechanism of injury, and epidemiology of ankle sprains. *Am J Sports Med.* 1977;5:241–242.
2. Elmslie RC. Recurrent subluxation of the ankle-joint. *Ann Surg.* 1934;100:364–367.
3. Hennrikus WL, Mapes RC, Lyons PM, et al. Outcomes of the Chrisman-Snook and modified Broström procedures for chronic lateral ankle instability. *Am J Sports Med.* 1996;24:400–404.
4. Gould N, Seligson D, Gassman J. Early and late repair of the lateral ligament of the ankle. *Foot Ankle.* 1980;1:84–89.
5. Krips R, van Dijk N, Halasi T, et al. Long-term outcome of anatomical reconstruction versus tenodesis for the treatment of chronic anterolateral instability of the ankle joint: a multicenter study. *Foot Ankle.* 2001;22:415–421.
6. Sammarco JS. Complications of lateral ankle ligament reconstruction. *Clin Orthop.* 2001;391:123–132.
7. Broström L. Sprained ankles. I. Anatomic lesions in recent sprains. *Acta Chir Scand.* 1964;128:483–495.
8. Broström L. Sprained ankles. V. Treatment and prognosis in recent ligament ruptures. *Acta Chir Scand.* 1966;132:537–550.
9. Glasgow M, Jackson A, Jamieson AM. Instability of the ankle after injury to the lateral ligament. *J Bone Joint Surg Br.* 1980;62:196–200.
10. Broström L, Liljedahl S, Lindvall N. Sprained ankles. II. Arthrographic diagnosis of recent ligament ruptures. *Acta Chir Scand.* 1965;129:485–499.
11. Broström L. Sprained ankles. III. Clinical observations in recent ligament ruptures. *Acta Chir Scand.* 1965;130:560–569.
12. Evans DL. Recurrent instability of the ankle: a method of surgical treatment. *Proc R Soc Med.* 1953;46:343–344.
13. Chrisman OD, Snook GA. Reconstruction of lateral ligament tears of the ankle: an experimental study and clinical evaluation of seven patients treated by a modification of the Elmslie procedure. *J Bone Joint Surg Am.* 1969;51:904–912.

14. Taga I, Shino K, Inoue M, et al. Articular cartilage lesions in ankles with lateral ligament injury. An arthroscopic study. *Am J Sports Med*. 1993;21:120–127.
15. Smith RW, Reischl SF. Treatment of ankle sprains in young athletes. *Am J Sports Med*. 1986;14:465–471.
16. Lassiter TE Jr, Malone TR, Garrett WE Jr. Injury to the lateral ligaments of the ankle. *Orthop Clin North Am*. 1989;20:629–640.
17. Colville MR. Surgical treatment of the unstable ankle. *J Am Acad Orthop Surg*. 1998;6:368–377.
18. Girard P, Anderson RB, Davis WH, et al. Clinical evaluation of the modified Broström-Evans procedure to restore ankle stability. *Foot Ankle*. 1999;20:246–252.
19. Sammarco JS, Carrasquillo HA. Surgical revision after failed lateral ankle reconstruction. *Foot Ankle*. 1995;16:748–753.
20. Viens NA, Wijdicks CA, Campbell KJ, et al. Anterior talofibular ligament ruptures, part 1: Biomechanical comparison of augmented Broström repair techniques with the intact anterior talofibular ligament. *Am J Sports Med*. 2014;42:405–411.
21. Clanton TO, Viens NA, Campbell KJ, et al. Anterior talofibular ligament ruptures, part 2: Biomechanical comparison of anterior talofibular ligament reconstruction using semitendinosus allografts with the intact ligament. *Am J Sports Med*. 2014;42:412–416.
22. Hua Y, Chen S, Jin Y, et al. Anatomical reconstruction of the lateral ligaments of the ankle with semitendinosus allograft. *Int Orthop*. 2012;36:2027–2031.
23. Cooper PS, Murray TF. Arthroscopy of the foot and ankle in the athlete. *Clin Sports Med*. 1996;15:805–824.
24. Clanton TO. Failed lateral ankle ligament reconstruction. In: Nunley JA, Pfeffer GB, Sanders RW, Trepman E, eds. *Advanced Reconstruction: Foot and Ankle*. Rosemont, IL: American Academy of Orthopaedic Surgeons; 2004:267–271.
25. Broström L. Sprained ankles. VI. Surgical treatment of "chronic" ligament ruptures. *Acta Chir Scand*. 1966;132:551–565.
26. Acevedo JI, Mangone PG. Arthroscopic lateral ankle ligament reconstruction. *Tech Foot Ankle Surg*. 2011;10:111.
27. Labib SA, Slone HS. Ankle arthroscopy for lateral ankle instability. *Tech Foot Ankle Surg*. 2015;14:25–27.
28. Golano P, Vega J, Pérez-Carro L, et al. Ankle anatomy for the arthroscopist. Part I: The portals. *Foot Ankle Clin*. 2006;11(2):253–273, v.
29. Matsui K, Takao M, Miyamoto W, et al. Early recovery after arthroscopic repair compared to open repair of the anterior talofibular ligament for lateral instability of the ankle. *Arch Orthop Trauma Surg*. 2016;136:93–100.
30. Cottom JM, Rigby RB. The "all inside" arthroscopic Broström procedure: a prospective study of 40 consecutive patients. *J Foot Ankle Surg*. 2013;52:568–574.
31. Lui TH. Arthroscopic-assisted lateral ligamentous reconstruction in combined ankle and subtalar instability. *Arthroscopy*. 2007;23:554.
32. Nery C, Raduan F, Del Buono A, et al. Arthroscopic-assisted Broström-Gould for chronic ankle instability: a long-term follow-up. *Am J Sports Med*. 2011;39:2381–2388.
33. Giza E, Whitlow SR, Williams BT, et al. Biomechanical analysis of an arthroscopic Broström ankle ligament repair and a suture anchor-augmented repair. *Foot Ankle Int*. 2015;36:836–841.
34. Guelfi M, Zamperetti M, Pantalone A, et al. Open and arthroscopic lateral ligament repair for treatment of chronic ankle instability: a systematic review. *Foot Ankle Surg*. 2018;24:11–18.
35. Brand RL, Collins MDF. Operative management of ligamentous injuries to the ankle. *Clin Sports Med*. 1982;1:117–130.
36. Hassan S, Thurston D, Sian T, et al. Clinical outcomes of the modified Broström technique in the management of chronic ankle instability after early, intermediate, and delayed presentation. *J Foot Ankle Surg*. 2018;57:685–688.
37. So E, Preston N, Holmes T. Intermediate- to long-term longevity and incidence of revision of the modified Broström-Gould procedure for lateral ankle ligament repair: a systematic review. *J Foot Ankle Surg*. 2017;56:1076–1080.
38. Cho BK, Park JK, Choi SM, et al. A randomized comparison between lateral ligaments augmentation using suture-tape and modified Broström repair in young female patients with chronic ankle instability. *Foot Ankle Surg*. 2017;18:S1268–S7731.
39. Coetzee JC, Ellington JK, Ronan JA, et al. Functional results of open Broström ankle ligament repair augmented with a suture tape. *Foot Ankle Int*. 2018;39:304–310.
40. Jung HG, Kim TH, Park JY, et al. Anatomic reconstruction of the anterior talofibular and calcaneofibular ligaments using a semitendinosus tendon allograft and interference screws. *Knee Surg Sports Traumatol Arthrosc*. 2012;20:1432–1437.
41. Wang W, Xu GH. Allograft tendon reconstruction of the anterior talofibular ligament and calcaneofibular ligament in the treatment of chronic ankle instability. *BMC Musculoskelet Disord*. 2017;18:150.
42. Jung HG, Shin MH, Park JT, et al. Anatomical reconstruction of lateral ankle ligaments using free tendon allografts and biotenodesis screws. *Foot Ankle Int*. 2015;36:1064–1071.
43. Brown AJ, Shimozono Y, Hurley ET, et al. Arthroscopic versus open repair of lateral ankle ligament for chronic lateral ankle instability: a meta-analysis. *Knee Surg Sports Traumatol Arthrosc*. 2018. Available at: https://link.springer.com/article/10.1007%2Fs00167-018-5100-6
44. Karlsson J, Eriksson B, Bergsten T, et al. Comparison of two anatomic reconstructions for chronic lateral instability of the ankle joint. *Am J Sports Med*. 1997;25:48–53.

56 Posterior Tibial Tendon Release and Stabilization

Monique C. Chambers, Stephanie M. Jones, Justin J. Hicks,
Arthur R. McDowell, Alan Yong Yan, and MaCalus V. Hogan

INTRODUCTION

Posterior tibial tendon insufficiency (PTTI) and/or dysfunction (PTTD) is a chronic, degenerative disease of the posterior tibialis tendon. The posterior tibialis tendon functions to plantarflex the ankle and provides essential support to the arch of the foot (1–3). Dysfunction of the posterior tibial tendon leads to collapse of the medial longitudinal arch and formation of an acquired flatfoot deformity (3,4). Patients develop compromised gait mechanics and abnormal plantar loading resulting in debilitating foot and ankle pain as well as progressive joint degeneration (5).

PTTI commonly presents in middle-aged and elderly women. Overall risk of PTTI increases for patients with obesity, hypertension, diabetes, seronegative arthropathies, inflammatory arthritis, chronic corticosteroid use, congenital flatfoot deformity, and/or a family history of flat feet (2,3,5–8).

Rarely, however, PTTD may also occur in young adults, adolescents, and athletes. The athletic population may, in fact, demonstrate a susceptibility to PTTI, as chronic overuse leads to repetitive overload, inflammation, and progressive degeneration of the tendon (9,10). Athletes who engage in soccer, basketball, running, gymnastics, and ballet appear to be at an increased risk due to the repetitive plantarflexion motion and excessive loading of the midfoot associated with these sports (3).

In athletes, PTTI often initially presents as tendinitis and/or tenosynovitis, which may be adequately managed nonoperatively (3,9). However, chronic PTTD may require extensive surgical intervention to address severe tendon degeneration and worsening deformity. Thus, in athletes, prompt diagnosis and treatment of PTTD can avoid prolonged time away from sports; and ultimately, prevent long-term disability, pain, and deformity (7).

ANATOMY

The posterior tibialis tendon originates from the posterior tibia, fibula, and interosseous membrane and courses through the tarsal tunnel at the posteromedial border of the distal tibia. The posterior tibial tendon has its primary insertion on the medial aspect of the navicular (2,3). The posterior tibial tendon structurally elevates the medial longitudinal arch of the foot and functions to plantarflex the ankle as well as adduct and invert the subtalar joint (1–3). The posterior tibial tendon also contributes a vital role in the gait cycle. During midstance, the posterior tibial tendon locks the transverse tarsal joints in place to provide a rigid lever for the midfoot and facilitates the push-off phase (4). In this sense, the posterior tibial tendon acts as the primary dynamic stabilizer of the midfoot (2,3).

ETIOLOGY

The precise mechanism of PTTD is unknown; however, chronic, rather than acute, tendon injury has been demonstrated as a key factor in the process. Progressive degeneration of the posterior tibial tendon commonly occurs where the tendon courses posterior to the distal tip of the medial malleolus (4). The posterior tibial tendon acutely changes direction at this location, resulting in a hypovascular, or "watershed," region about 3-cm proximal to the level of tendon insertion on the navicular (2,4,6). Chronic tendon ischemia in this area and repetitive loading of the posteromedial foot and ankle, as in the athlete, predisposes to tendonitis, tenosynovitis, and tendinosis. Chronic inflammation also decreases the elastic properties of the tissue resulting in elongation and attenuation of the tendon (3,6). Dysfunction of the posterior tibial tendon leads to collapse of the medial column of the midfoot and abnormal joint loading throughout the hindfoot, ultimately resulting in the characteristic planovalgus, or flatfoot, deformity (2,3). Failure of the posterior tibial tendon results in unopposed eversion of the subtalar joint causes abduction of the midfoot and valgus alignment of the heel (2–4).

While the posterior tibial tendon is the key contributor to the development of flat foot deformity, failure of the surrounding anatomic structures enhances the severity and progression of the disease. The spring ligament complex, plantar fascia, plantar ligaments, talonavicular capsule, and deltoid ligament often contribute to PTTI to some extent (2–4). For example, in the late stages of PTTI, failure of the deltoid ligament is responsible for valgus deformity of the ankle mortise (4). As a result of this anatomic interplay, PTTI is now often referred to as acquired flat foot deformity (AAFD) due to the appreciation that the pathology encompasses more than just the posterior tibial tendon itself (5).

CLINICAL PRESENTATION

Approximately 50% of posterior tibial tendon injuries are initially misdiagnosed as an ankle sprain, leading to delayed presentation (11). A proper understanding of the presenting symptoms and classic examination findings may ensure prompt diagnosis and treatment. A thorough patient history is important, as clinical presentation can vary broadly depending on the extent of tendon degeneration and foot deformity.

In the early phases of PTTI, patients often complain of plantar medial aching and fatigue and/or posteromedial ankle pain and swelling (5). Pain symptoms in PTTI are usually exacerbated with prolonged standing or walking, and patients will often report difficulty with climbing stairs and walking on uneven ground (6). Patients will also note dysfunction in the push-off phase of their gait, stating that they are unable to run or have difficulty taking long strides. Most characteristically, patients will state that they are "weak" and unable to perform a single-leg heel raise (3,5).

As PTTI becomes more severe, planovalgus deformity will develop and medial pain will often migrate laterally (3,6,10). Lateral ankle pain occurs as worsening valgus deformity of the hindfoot results in compression of the lateral ankle structures and development of subfibular impingement syndrome (6,10). Patients may note that standing with the foot slightly inverted or walking on the outside of their foot may alleviate their pain (2). Patients will often complain that their "arch is flattening" and that it is increasingly difficult to wear regular shoes (4,12). Some may report irregular wear on the sole of their shoes, noting that the inside of the heel wears faster than the outside.

End-stage chronic PTTI may rarely result in acute rupture of the posterior tibial tendon. In this case, the patient may counterintuitively present with temporary resolution of pain symptoms (3).

CLINICAL EVALUATION

Physical Examination

A detailed physical examination of the foot and ankle is necessary to characterize the severity of tendon dysfunction and stage the level of flatfoot deformity. It is essential to examine the bilateral feet and ankles, regularly comparing the affected extremity to the unaffected side.

Patients will often present with pathognomonic swelling of the posteromedial ankle, along the anatomic course of the posterior tibial tendon (5,6,13,14). Additionally, the medial longitudinal arch may be collapsed, and/or the heel may be in a valgus alignment (13,14). Careful examination of the foot posteriorly may reveal the "too many toes sign," in which appearance of the third, second, and even the great toe may be appreciated (7,13) (Fig. 56-1). Palpation of the posteromedial ankle may elicit pain, and patients may also demonstrate tenderness of the medial longitudinal arch. Passive and active range of motion may reveal pain and/or weakness with plantarflexion and inversion. Patients should be asked to perform a single-leg heel rise to assess the integrity and strength of the posterior tibial tendon (14). Inability to perform a single-leg heel raise should raise suspicion for PTTD (13,14).

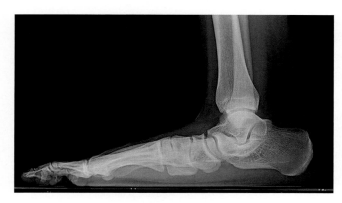

FIGURE 56-1

Lateral plain radiograph of the foot depicting acquired flatfoot deformity due to chronic posterior tibial tendon insufficiency.

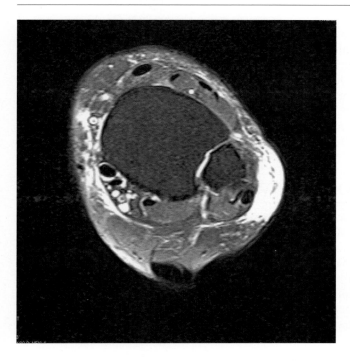

FIGURE 56-2

T2 axial MRI depicting edema and tenosynovitis of the posterior tibial tendon.

Imaging

Imaging is an additional component of the clinical assessment. Weight-bearing radiographs of the foot and ankle should be obtained to assess alignment of the bony anatomy and evaluate for degenerative changes such as joint space narrowing and subchondral sclerosis (14) (Fig. 56-1). Advanced imaging such as magnetic resonance imaging (MRI) and ultrasound are particularly useful to evaluate the posterior tibial tendon and identify tenosynovitis or tendon tears (15) (Fig. 56-2). Furthermore, advanced imaging may provide valuable information for preoperative planning.

CLASSIFICATION

Johnson and Strom first described staging of PTTD in 1989; however, the original classification system has since been modified and revised. Current classification of PTTI is based on a combination of characteristic clinical and radiographic findings (Table 56-1).

Classification of PTTD can be categorized into four stages. Stage I PTTD is tenosynovitis of the posterior tibial tendon. Patients typically present with medial ankle pain without deformity. Patients are still able to perform a single-leg heel raise; however, they may experience pain with repetitive heel raises (15,16). Radiographs at this stage are typically normal. Stage II PTTD is the most common presentation of acquired flatfoot deformity (14,16). Patients have worsened medial ankle pain, flattening of the medial arch, and are unable to perform a single-leg heel raise. The heel develops a valgus alignment; however, the hindfoot remains flexible. Stage III PTTD occurs when the

Stage	Clinical Presentation	Radiographic Findings
I	• Pain and/or swelling of PTT • No deformity	• Normal
II	• Pain and/or swelling of PTT • Flexible hindfoot valgus deformity	• Hindfoot valgus • Forefoot abduction
III	• Pain and/or swelling of PTT • Rigid hindfoot valgus deformity • Lateral ankle impingement	• Hindfoot valgus • Forefoot abduction • Subtalar arthritis
IV	• Pain and/or swelling of PTT • Flexible/rigid hindfoot valgus deformity • Lateral ankle impingement • Rigid tibiotalar valgus deformity	• Hindfoot valgus • Forefoot abduction • Subtalar arthritis • Tibiotalar valgus

TABLE 56-1 Radiographic Findings Based on Classification of PTTI

hindfoot is fixed in a rigid valgus alignment (17). Often at this stage, patients develop arthritis of the subtalar joint and hindfoot, which can be seen on radiographs (8,16). Stage IV is characterized by deformity of the ankle joint. As such, hindfoot deformity in Stage IV can be either flexible or rigid. Long-standing hindfoot valgus alignment causes attenuation of the deltoid ligament and results in valgus alignment of the tibiotalar joint (8). Valgus alignment, as well as degenerative changes of the tibiotalar joint, can commonly be seen on plain radiographs, as dorsolateral peritalar subluxation, increased talo-first metatarsal angle, increased tibiotalar tilt, decreased calcaneal pitch, and loss of talar head coverage of the navicular (7,15,16).

NONOPERATIVE AND OPERATIVE MANAGEMENT

Both nonoperative and operative treatment options exist for PTTD; however; the indication for each varies based on the stage of tendon dysfunction (Table 56-2). As such, accurate staging is crucial for proper management of PTTD (8).

Approximately 80% of PTTI responds to nonoperative management (14). However, nonoperative management is indicated primarily for Stage I PTTD. Nonoperative treatment typically includes pain control and management of swelling, as well as rest and off-loading of the posterior tibial tendon using a plaster cast, controlled-ankle movement (CAM) boot, and/or foot-ankle orthoses (8). However, Stage I PTTD may be treated with open or endoscopic tendon debridement, if nonoperative management has failed.

Surgical management is usually employed for Stage II PTTD and aims to correct the flexible hindfoot deformity and dynamically stabilize the medial longitudinal arch of the foot (8). Operative

TABLE 56-2 Management of Posterior Tibial Dysfunction by Classification

Stage	Treatment
I	• Cast • Tall CAM boot • Orthotics • Open or endoscopic tendon debridement
II	• Tendon transfer • Medial displacement calcaneal osteotomy (MDCO) • Gastrocnemius release/recession • Spring ligament repair • Deltoid ligament repair
III	• Hindfoot arthrodesis • Subtalar • Calcaneocuboid • Talonavicular
IV	• Hindfoot arthrodesis • Subtalar • Calcaneocuboid • Talonavicular • Ankle arthrodesis

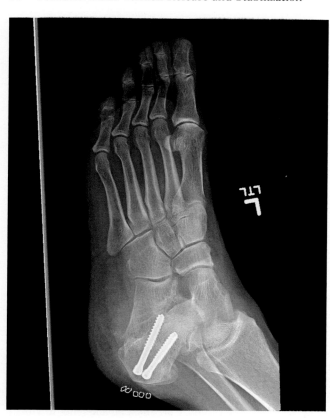

FIGURE 56-3

Oblique plain radiograph of the foot after medial displacement calcaneal osteotomy (MDCO).

management for Stage II PTTD may be more challenging than debridement, as the posterior tibial tendon is often elongated or ruptured. A tendon transfer is a frequently used technique for operative management of Stage II PTTD; and flexor digitorum longus (FDL), flexor hallucis longus (FHL), and tibialis anterior have all been used (15). Medial displacement calcaneal osteotomy (MDCO) is often performed in conjunction with tendon transfer, in order to restore the shape of the medial longitudinal arch (5,17) (Figs. 56-3 and 56-4). Attention to the surrounding soft-tissue stabilizers may also be considered at this stage, such as repair of the spring ligament and gastrocnemius lengthening procedures.

Operative management of Stage III and Stage IV PTTI is more complex, as these stages characteristically involve advanced deformity, attenuation of the soft-tissue structures, and joint degeneration (15). Stages III and IV PTTD are often treated with arthrodesis procedures. In Stage III PTTD, single, double, or triple arthrodesis may be performed on the subtalar, calcaneocuboid, and/or talonavicular joints (8,18). Stage IV PTTD requires a combination of operative techniques to address both hindfoot and tibiotalar deformity. Hindfoot valgus, whether flexible or rigid, can be addressed using the same techniques as indicated for the lesser stages. Early-stage ankle valgus is

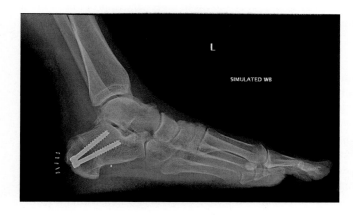

FIGURE 56-4

Lateral plain radiograph of the foot after medial displacement calcaneal osteotomy (MDCO).

often corrected with deltoid ligament reconstruction in an attempt to preserve integrity of the ankle joint (18,19). However, as ankle valgus continues to progress, extensive damage and degeneration of the tibiotalar joint may be best managed with ankle arthrodesis (8).

OPERATIVE TECHNIQUES

FDL Transfer

The patient should be positioned supine on the operating table. A bump should be placed under the ipsilateral buttock in order to internally rotate the leg. The operative extremity should be prepped and draped in a sterile fashion. Under tourniquet control, a 5-cm incision should be made over the medial aspect of the navicular bone and the navicular-cuneiform joint. Sharp and blunt dissection may be performed to adequately expose the FDL tendon. Once the FDL has been identified, examine the tendon for any gross defect. If the integrity of the FDL tendon is intact, debride and cut the tendon. Measure the diameter of the FDL, and prepare the navicular for tenodesis. It is recommended to use a reamer that is 0.5 to 1 mm larger than the diameter of the tendon. Whipstitch the end of the FDL tendon, and prepare for insertion into the navicular using a tenodesis screw. It is important to maintain appropriate tension on the tendon during insertion. Skin and soft tissues should be closed in layers and appropriate wound dressings should be placed; the operative extremity should be placed in a neutral splint.

Medial Displacement Calcaneal Osteotomy

The patient should be positioned supine on the operating table. A bump should be placed under the ipsilateral buttock in order to internally rotate the leg. The operative extremity should be prepped and draped in a sterile fashion. Under tourniquet control, an oblique lateral incision is made over the calcaneus. If necessary, perform blunt dissection down to bone, while being mindful of the sural nerve and its branches. Using a sagittal saw, begin the osteotomy. Care must be taken not to violate the medial cortex. An osteotome should be used to complete the osteotomy of the medial cortex. A lamina spreader may be used to open the osteotomy and create space for medial translation. Shift the calcaneus medially until appropriate hindfoot alignment is achieved. Using fluoroscopic guidance, attention should turn to fixation of the calcaneal osteotomy. An additional 2-cm incision may be made at the posterior calcaneus. Provisional fixation of the "heel slide" may be maintained using Kirschner (K) wires. Rigid fixation should be achieved with partially threaded (lag) screws (Figs. 56-3 and 56-4). Final plain radiographs are recommended to ensure adequate reconstruction of the hindfoot. Skin and soft tissues should be closed in layers and appropriate wound dressings should be placed; the operative extremity should be placed in a neutral splint (20).

Gastrocnemius Lengthening

The patient should be positioned prone on the operating table. The operative extremity should be prepped and draped in a sterile fashion. Under tourniquet control, a small incision should be made over the gastrocnemius, slightly medial to the midline. Blunt and sharp dissection should be performed to expose the gastrocnemius sheath. Care must be taken to avoid injury to the deep posterior neurovascular bundle. Once identified, the gastrocnemius sheath should be cut along the horizontal plane. The ipsilateral ankle should be cycled through plantarflexion-dorsiflexion to ensure an increase in range of motion. Skin and soft tissues should be closed in layers and appropriate wound dressings should be placed; the operative extremity should be placed in a mildly plantarflexed splint.

Subtalar Arthrodesis

The patient should be positioned supine on the operating table. A bump should be placed under the ipsilateral buttock in order to internally rotate the leg. The operative extremity should be prepped and draped in a sterile fashion. Under tourniquet control, incise distally from 1 cm below the lateral malleolus to the base of the fourth metatarsal. Blunt and sharp dissection should be performed, taking care not to injure the sural nerve and its branches. Identify the surrounding anatomic structures: peroneal tendon sheath, extensor digitorum brevis (EDB), sinus tarsi fat pad, and talocalcaneal ligament. Do not disrupt the peroneal tendon sheath; however, create a flap with the EDB and the sinus tarsi fat pad, and release the talocalcaneal ligament. At this point, the lateral subtalar joint may be visualized. Use a lamina spreader to open the joint, and remove the articular cartilage from the subtalar joint with a curette. Ensure that the medial articular cartilage is removed. Once all articular cartilage has been removed, use small osteotomes or a 2.0-mm drill to create bleeding of the subchondral bone, as these vascular channels will aid in fusion. At this point, local autograft bone or cellular bone matrix may be used to pack the subtalar joint. Under fluoroscopic guidance, place the ankle in 7 degrees of valgus, and K-wires may be used to achieve provisional fixation. Large and small fragment cannulated lag screws may be used for rigid fixation. Hardware position should be confirmed with final fluoroscopic images. Skin and soft tissues should be closed in layers, and appropriate wound dressings should be placed; the operative extremity should be placed in a neutral splint.

POSTOPERATIVE MANAGEMENT

Postoperative management and the recovery time course vary depending on the type of procedure performed.

Following posterior tibial tendon debridement and tenosynovectomy, patients are initially placed in a plaster splint for 2 weeks postoperatively and transitioned into a CAM boot for 4 weeks thereafter. Early range of motion exercises and physical therapy is highly recommended, especially in the elite, competitive athlete. Return to full daily activity is typically allowed between 6 and 8 weeks postoperatively with use of a lace-up ankle brace, and full return to competitive sports can be expected around 3 to 4 months postoperatively.

Following flatfoot reconstruction, with MDCO the patient is placed in a plaster splint with the foot inverted and plantarflexed for 2 weeks postoperatively. After 2 weeks, the patient is transitioned into a short-leg cast and remains non–weight bearing for 4 weeks. At around 4 to 6 weeks, the short-leg cast is removed, and the patient is allowed to progressively weight bear in a CAM boot. Physical therapy can began around 8 to 10 weeks postoperatively, and full return to sports usually occurs between 6 and 9 months following surgery with the use of a lace-up ankle brace and/or an over-the-counter orthotic. Full-length arch supports are recommended, as they have been shown to reduce recurrence.

COMPLICATIONS

Complications of operative management for PTTI commonly include infection, nerve and vessel injury, deep vein thrombosis (DVT), nonunion, malunion, and symptomatic hardware. Symptomatic hardware is a common complaint for patients, and many will require a second procedure for the removal of hardware (5). Procedure-specific complications may include failure of tendon transfer, undercorrection, overcorrection, failed arthrodesis, and damage to surrounding structures based on the surgical approach (5,21). However, the risk for postoperative complication is influenced by patient factors such as previous surgery, age, diabetes, peripheral vascular disease, tobacco use, and chronic steroid use, among others (5).

NONOPERATIVE OUTCOMES

Non-operative management has been indicated for early PTTD, and demonstrates reasonable outcomes. After 4 months of nonoperative treatment for Stages I and II PTTD, 87% of patients reported improved subjective and functional outcomes (21,22). Kulig et al. (23) examined the influence of footwear on patients with symptomatic flatfoot deformity. Activation of the posterior tibial tendon was improved with use of a shoe orthosis when compared to barefoot. Thus, Kulig et al. indicate a role for orthosis in the nonoperative management of PTTD and flatfoot deformity.

Similarly, Chao et al. (24) treated 37 with PTTD using molded foot-ankle orthoses and found that at a mean follow-up of 20.3 months 67% of patients had good or excellent results based on assessments of pain, function, use of an assistive device, distance of ambulation. and satisfaction. Four patients responded poorly to management with the molded orthosis and required surgery.

Alvarez et al. (22) used a structures non-operative mangment protocol of orthotics and physical to treat patients with Stage I and Stage II. Alvarez et al. reported that after a median of 10 physical therapy visits over a median 4 month period, 83% of patients had improved subjectve and functional outcomes scores and 89% of patients were satisfied. However, 11% of patients required surgery after failed non-operative management.

Overall, non-operative management has good outcomes when implemented early in the disease course of PTTD. However, a subset of these patients may still require operative intervention.

OPERATIVE OUTCOMES

Outcomes following the various operative techniques employed at each of the different stages of PTTD are varied, but overall reassuring. Teasdall and Johnson treated 19 patients with synovectomy and debridement for Stage I PTTD. Complete relief of pain was observed in 74% of patients, while 16% reported minor pain, 5% moderate pain, and 5% continued pain. Only two patients did not perceive any improvement in pain and subsequently received subtalar fusion (25). McCormack et al. reported on a series of tenosynovectomies in eight young competitive athletes at an average follow-up of 22 months. Seven athletes returned to full sports participation without difficulty, but one patient had periodic pain and was unable to continue participation in sports (26). Also in an international systemic review, Lohrer and Nauck identified 61 published cases of posterior tibial tendon dislocations. Among the cases identified, 58% were induced by sports, and surgery was performed for 83% of the cases using a variety of operative techniques. Treatment outcomes were favorable, as 80% were reported as asymptomatic, 12% were reported as good, and 8% were reported as fair/moderate (11). Myerson et al. (21) specifically examined treatment of PTTD with FDL transfer and calcaneal osteotomy and found positive outcomes at a mean follow-up of 5.2 years postoperatively. The mean American Orthopaedic Foot and Ankle Society (AOFAS) score at follow-up was 79 points out of 100 total points and subtalar joint motion was evaluated as normal in 44% of patients. Additionally, 91.5% of patients were entirely satisfied with the procedure at the time of follow-up. Additionally, 97% experienced pain relief, 94% reported improved function, 87% demonstrated higher foot arches, and 84% could comfortably wear regular shoes without orthoses or shoe modifications. Overall, operative management of PTTD can yield excellent results if the appropriate procedural technique is employed for the stage of PTT disease.

CONCLUSION

PTTD is a progressively, debilitating disease that should be considered in the athlete who presents with medial ankle pain and flatfoot deformity. A thorough history and physical examination are needed to promptly diagnose and treat PTTD effectively. If identified early, many athletes may be adequately treated nonoperatively; thus, decreasing time away from sport. However, if the PTT disease is advanced and deformity is severe, many athletes will require operative management to improve pain, alignment, and function. However, postoperative recovery and return to sport vary based on the surgical procedure performed. Nonetheless, both nonoperative management and operative management for PTTI have demonstrated reassuring outcomes, when implemented at the appropriate stage of dysfunction.

REFERENCES

1. Johnson K, Strom D. Tibialis posterior tendon dysfunction. *Clin Orthop Relat Res*. 1989;(239):196–206. doi:10.1046/j.1460-9584.1999.00161.x.
2. Myerson MS. Adult acquired flatfoot deformity: treatment of dysfunction of the posterior tibial tendon. *J Bone Joint Surg Am*. 1997;79(9):1434.
3. Soliman SB, Spicer PJ, van Holsbeeck MT. Sonographic and radiographic findings of posterior tibial tendon dysfunction: a practical step forward. *Skeletal Radiol*. 2019;48(1):11–27. doi:10.1007/s00256-018-2976-7.
4. Smyth NA, Aiyer AA, Kaplan JR, et al. Adult-acquired flatfoot deformity. *Eur J Orthop Surg Traumatol*. 2017;27(4):433–439. doi:10.1007/s00590-017-1945-5.
5. Pinney SJ, Lin SS. Current concept review: acquired adult flatfoot deformity. *Foot Ankle Int*. 2006;27(1):66–75. doi:10.1177/107110070602700113.
6. Wukich DK, Tuason DA. Diagnosis and treatment of chronic ankle pain. *J Bone Jt Surg*. 2010;92-A(10):2002–2016. doi:10.1016/j.mporth.2012.04.006.
7. Fu FH. *Master Techniques in Orthopaedic Surgery: Sports Medicine*. Lippincott Williams & Wilkins; 2012.
8. Bubra PS, Keighley G, Rateesh S, et al. Posterior tibial tendon dysfunction: an overlooked cause of foot deformity. *J Family Med Prim Care*. 2015;4(1):26–29.
9. Vanderhave KL, Miller D. Foot and ankle problems in the adolescent athlete. *Curr Opin Orthop*. 2005;16:45–49. doi:10.1097/01.bco.0000157074.54110.43.
10. DeOrio JK, Shapiro SA, McNeil RB, et al. Validity of the posterior tibial edema sign in posterior tibial tendon dysfunction. *Foot Ankle Int*. 2011;32(2):189–192. doi:10.3113/FAI.2011.0189.
11. Lohrer H, Nauck T. Posterior tibial tendon dislocation: a systematic review of the literature and presentation of a case. *Br J Sports Med*. 2010;44(6):398–406. doi:10.1136/bjsm.2007.040204.
12. Mccormick JJ, Johnson JE. Medial column procedures in the correction of adult acquired flatfoot deformity. *Foot Ankle Clin*. 2012;17:283–298. doi:10.1016/j.fcl.2012.03.003.
13. Geideman WM, Johnson JE. Posterior tibial tendon dysfunction. *J Orthop Sports Phys Ther*. 2000;30(2):68–77.

14. Zaw H, Calder JD. Operative management options for symptomatic flexible adult acquired flatfoot deformity: a review. *Knee Surg Sports Traumatol Arthrosc.* 2010;18(2):135–142. doi:10.1007/s00167-009-1015-6.

15. Ling SK, Lui TH. Posterior tibial tendon dysfunction: an overview. *Open Orthop J.* 2017;11:714–723. doi:10.2174/1874325001711010714.

16. DiPaola, M, Raikin, SM. Tendon transfers and realignment osteotomies for treatment of stage II posterior tibial tendon dysfunction. *Foot Ankle Clin.* 2007;12:273–285.

17. Deland JT. Adult-acquired flatfoot deformity. *J Am Acad Orthop Surg.* 2008;16(7):399–406. doi:10.5435/00124635-200807000-00005.

18. Maskill MP, Loveland JD, Mendicino RW, et al. Triple arthrodesis for the adult-acquired flatfoot deformity. *Clin Podiatr Med Surg.* 2007;24(4):765–778. doi:10.1016/j.cpm.2007.07.005.

19. Lui TH, Chan LK. Safety and efficacy of talonavicular arthroscopy in arthroscopic triple arthrodesis. A cadaveric study. *Knee Surg Sports Traumatol Arthrosc.* 2010;18(5):607–611. doi:10.1007/s00167-010-1098-0.

20. Haddad SL, Myerson MS, Younger A, et al. Symposium: adult acquired flatfoot deformity. *Foot Ankle Int.* 2011;32(1):95–111. doi:10.3113/FAI.2011.0095.

21. Myerson MS, Badekas A, Schon LC. Treatment of stage II posterior tibial tendon deficiency with flexor digitorum longus tendon transfer and calcaneal osteotomy. *Foot Ankle Int.* 2004;25(7):445–450. doi:10.1177/107110070402500701.

22. Alvarez RG, Marini A, Schmitt C, et al. Stage I and II posterior tibial tendon dysfunction treated by a structured nonoperative management protocol: an orthosis and exercise program. *Foot Ankle Int.* 2006;27(1):2–8.

23. Kulig K, Burnfield JM, Reischl S, et al. Effect of foot orthoses on tibialis posterior activation in persons with pes planus. *Med Sci Sports Exerc.* 2005;37(1):24–29.

24. Chao W, Wapner KL, Lee TH, et al. Nonoperative management of posterior tibial tendon dysfunction. *Foot Ankle Int.* 1996;17(12):736–741. doi:10.1177/107110079601701204.

25. Teasdall RD, Johnson KA. Surgical treatment of stage I posterior tibial tendon dysfunction. *Foot Ankle Int.* 1994;15(12):646–648. doi:10.1177/107110079401501203.

26. McCormack AP, Varner KE, Marymont J V. Surgical treatment for posterior tibial tendonitis in young competitive athletes. *Foot Ankle Int.* 2003;24(7):535–538.

57 Indications for the Operative Management of Peroneal Tendon Injuries

Monique C. Chambers, Joseph J. Kromka, Justin J. Hicks, Arthur R. McDowell, Stephanie M. Jones, Alan Yong Yan, and MaCalus V. Hogan

INTRODUCTION

The lateral ankle ligaments contribute to the primary stability of the ankle and are supported by the intact peroneal tendons. The peroneal tendons include the peroneus brevis, the peroneus longus, and the peroneus tertius. These tendons function to prevent excessive supination and eversion of the ankle. However, the peroneal tendons can undergo repetitive stress in athletes who frequently perform cutting or pivoting movements that place forced or excessive tension on the lateral ankle structures. As a result, pathology such as tenosynovitis, tendinopathy, subluxation, and/or tears of the peroneal tendons may develop and prevent optimal athletic performance. Early peroneal tendon pathology may be managed nonoperatively. However, advanced, chronic tendon disease and acute tendon ruptures may be best managed with operative intervention. When operative management has failed to provide symptomatic relief operative management may be the best option to restore ankle stability, improve functional performance, and return confidence to the athlete.

INDICATIONS/CONTRAINDICATIONS

In the athletic population, peroneal tendon pathology may include tenosynovitis, tendinopathy, subluxation, tear, and/or a ganglion cyst formation (Fig. 57-1). Peroneal tendinitis or tenosynovitis is caused by inflammation within the tendon sheath of the peroneus longus or brevis, usually the result of chronic repetitive activity. As a result, peroneal tenosynovitis or tendinitis often develops in athletes such as runners, dancers, or skiers. Patients with peroneal tendinitis report pain and swelling of the lateral ankle with concurrent feelings of instability, which leads to a lack of confidence in performing athletic activities. Initial management involves nonsteroidal anti-inflammatory medications, rest, and activity modifications. In particular, patients with a varus hindfoot may benefit significantly from orthotics with a lateral heel wedge. If patients fail initial nonoperative management, a trial of immobilization is appropriate with a short leg cast or controlled ankle movement (CAM) boot. Steroid injections are generally avoided for peroneal tendon pathology due to the increased risk of tendon rupture (1). Peroneal tendinitis or tenosynovitis recalcitrant to nonoperative management may be considered for surgical intervention. Contraindications for surgery include comorbid medical conditions that may impact the patient's ability to tolerate anesthesia.

Acute peroneal tendon tears or traumatic subluxation are relatively rare. An acute longitudinal tear of the peroneal longus or brevis (Fig. 57-2) may occur with sudden inversion injuries. Subluxations, on the other hand, are usually the result of sudden dorsiflexion and inversion of the ankle with concomitant peroneal muscle contraction (2). These injuries may be initially managed nonoperatively. However, there is a high failure rate for nonoperative management of peroneal tendon tears and/or subluxation in the athletic population (2). Thus, if the peroneal tendon tear or subluxation

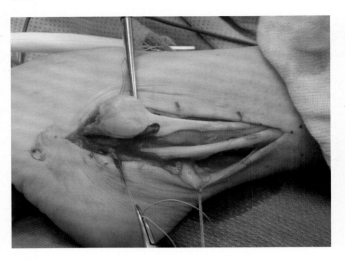

FIGURE 57-1

Ganglion cyst formation from a torn peroneal tendon.

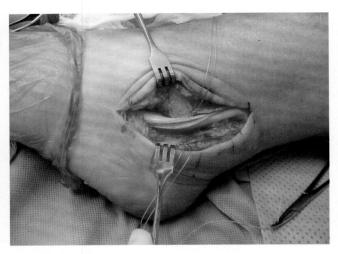

FIGURE 57-2

Longitudinal tear of the peroneus brevis.

significantly compromises the athlete's ability to return to a high level of competitive performance, primary operative intervention may be best indicated.

PREOPERATIVE EVALUATION

In addition to a detailed history and a thorough physical examination, imaging modalities are used to assess the patient's anatomy and identify any potential causes for the presenting symptoms. Foot and ankle radiographs are routinely used to assess for fractures or joint degeneration. Additionally, radiographs may reveal underlying contributors to the peroneal tendon pathoogy and ankle instability, such as an os peroneum, a prominent peroneal tubercle, or even an occult syndesmotic injury. While radiographs may provide useful information, magnetic resonance imaging (MRI) is the most sensitive diagnostic imaging study for peroneal tendon tears. The MRI may assist the surgeon in assessing the degree of tendon disruption and planning the best surgical approach to address the pathology (3).

POSITIONING

The patient is placed in a supine position with a bump placed under the ipsilateral hip. This allows for internal rotation at the lower extremity, which provides better visibility of the lateral ankle to easily access the peroneal tendons. A thigh tourniquet is used to control blood flow to the distal limb. Once the patient has been prepped, a sterile bump is placed under the ipsilateral distal tibia to allow the ankle to move freely.

PROCEDURE

For procedures involving the peroneal tendons, local, regional, epidural, or general anesthesia can be used. A saphenous/popliteal nerve block allows for better pain control in the immediate postoperative period. The peroneal tendon sheath can be accessed via an open incision or tenoscopically. For an open approach, an incision is made just posterior to the fibula and parallel to the tendons. The incision should be large enough to visualize and access all areas of anticipated pathology. Incise through the subcutaneous tissue and adipose. Care must be taken to avoid damage to the superficial peroneal and sural nerves during proximal and distal dissection, respectively. The peroneal tendon sheath should be incised in a linear fashion far enough posterior to the fibula so that closure of the sheath is possible (4).

With a tenoscopic approach, the patient should actively evert the affected foot prior to undergoing anesthesia in order to palpate the tendons to mark the appropriate portal sites on the skin as seen in Figure 57-3. The distal port is created first, 2 to 2.5 cm distal to the posterior edge of the lateral malleolus. An incision is made through the skin, and the tendon sheath is penetrated with

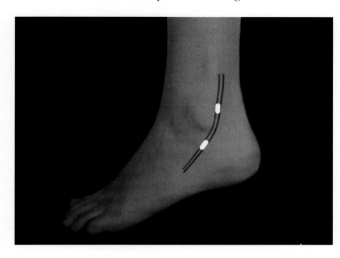

FIGURE 57-3

The course of the peroneal tendons is drawn on the skin (*black*), and the location of the tenoscopic portals is marked (*white*).

an arthroscopic sheath with a blunt trocar. Next, a 2.7-mm arthroscope is introduced. A diagnostic inspection begins approximately 6 cm proximal to the posterior tip of the fibula, where a thin membrane splits the tendon compartment into two separate tendon chambers. Distally, the tendons lie in one compartment, so this portal allows a complete overview of both tendons. A second portal is then created 2 to 2.5 cm proximal to the posterior edge of the lateral malleolus under direct visualization by placing a spinal needle and producing a portal directly over the tendons (Fig. 57-4). By rotating the arthroscope between both tendons, the entire compartment can be inspected.

The extent of tendon damage guides the optimal surgical technique and is summarized in Table 57-1. For tears involving <50% of the cross-sectional area of the tendon, an excision of the degenerative regions along with areas of tenosynovitis followed by tubularization of the remaining tendon is recommended (5).

If more than 50% of the cross-sectional area is involved, the tendons are repaired via tenodesis, graft reconstruction, autogenous tendon transfer, or acellular matrix allograft (5–9). Tenodesis of the two units both proximally and distally is recommended. The proximal tenodesis should occur 3 to 4 cm above the tip of the fibular malleolus, and the distal tenodesis should occur 5 to 6 cm below the tip of the fibular malleolus to avoid impingement (2,5,7,10–12).

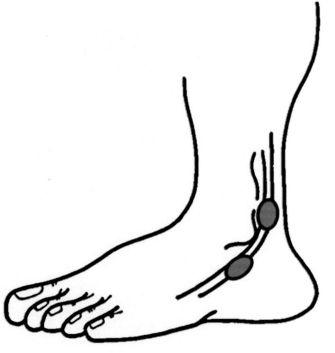

FIGURE 57-4

Course of the peroneal tendons posterior to the lateral malleolus (*black*) and the location of the distal and proximal tenoscopic portal sites (*red*). (Original artwork contribtued by Stephanie M. Jones, BA; Pittsburgh, PA.)

TABLE 57-1 Indications for Peroneal Tendon Repair

Cross-Sectional Area of Involvement	Peroneal Tendons	Surgical Technique		Comments
<50%	Both intact	• Tubularization		Minimizes the suture footprint and restores a smooth external surface to the peroneal tendon
>50%	One intact	• Tenodesis		Care must be taken to avoid excessive scarring and subfibular impingement
	None intact	• No, proximal muscle excursion	Tendon transfer • *Flexor hallucis longus* • *Flexor digitorum longus* • *Plantaris*	May be used to provide reinforcement of the superior peroneal retinaculum
		• Yes, proximal muscle excursion	Tendon reconstruction • *Silicone rod* • *Hamstring allograft*	Staged reconstruction may be favorable in cases of chronic peroneal tendinopathy

Graft reconstruction may be performed using a peroneal or semitendinosus allograft anchored to the native distal stump of the tendon with a Pulvertaft weave or to the fifth metatarsal using 3.5-mm suture anchors. Adequate muscle length should be left before proximal fixation, which can be assessed by placing the foot in a neutral position (8). Autogenous tendon transfers include transfer of the flexor digitorum longus (FDL) or flexor hallucis longus (FHL) (6,10,13). The use of acellular dermal matrix allograft to augment tendon defects have been reported as well but has limited use compared to other techniques (14,15).

For recurrent peroneal tendon subluxation, anatomic reattachment of the retinaculum with potential for reinforcement with tissue transfer and groove deepening is often effective (Table 57-2). Tendon rerouting behind the calcaneofibular ligament and bone-block procedures with a fibular osteotomy followed by the posterior displacement of the lateral fragment can serve as mechanical restraints to the peroneal tendons (16). However, these are less commonly utilized approaches. The preferred treatment is to restore the native anatomy by anatomic reattachment of the retinaculum and

TABLE 57-2 Techniques for Recurrent Peroneal Tendon Subluxation/Dislocations

Surgical Technique	Comments
Retinaculum repair	Aims to anatomically restore the native physical restraint of the peroneal tendons
Bone-block procedures • *Partial sagittal fibular osteotomy* • *Complete sagittal fibular osteotomy*	Aims to provide a physical block to prevent subluxation/dislocation the peroneal tendons
Retinacular reinforcement via local tissue transfer • *Plantaris* • *Peroneus brevis* • *Achilles tendon* • *Peroneus quartus* • *Periosteal flap*	Aims to physically buttress the native, anatomic restraint of the peroneal tendons
Tendon rerouting • *Calcaneofibular ligament*	Aims to change the course of the peroneal tendons and use existing anatomic structures as a physical restraint of the peroneal tendons
Retromalleolar groove-deepening procedures • *Direct* • *Indirect*	Aims to deepen the retrofibular sulcus/peroneal groove and prevent subluxation/dislocation of the peroneal tendons Often used in conjunction with repair and/or reinforcement of the superior peroneal retinaculum

deepening of the retromalleolar groove (17). An osseous trough is created along the posterolateral aspect of the fibula with an osteotome, and three or four lateral to medial drill holes are made along the trough. The retinaculum is attached to the trough with nonabsorbable suture. Alternatively, the edge of the retinaculum can be secured deep to the inferior edge of the fibular trough to additionally reduce the space available for the tendons and further secure them in the retromalleolar groove (17). However, patients with recurrent subluxation may have insufficiency of the peroneal retinaculum; thus, the existing retinaculum can be augmented with transfers of Achilles tendon, periosteum, plantaris, or peroneus brevis (18–21).

Groove-deepening procedures involve incising the superior peroneal retinaculum (SPR), dislocating the peroneal tendons anteriorly, and then raising an osseous flap from the posterolateral fibula. This is deepened to a depth of 5 mm with a burr, the tendons are relocated, and the retinaculum is repaired (17,22). Groove deepening can be performed from within the tendon sheath, but this risks iatrogenic damage to the tendons. Portal sites are sutured to prevent sinus formation, and a compressive dressing is applied.

PEARLS/PITFALLS

During repair of peroneal tendon tears, both tendons should be inspected circumferentially so that pathology is not missed. Of note, brevis pathology is usually more common and extensive than longus pathology (23). When tubularizing a tendon, it is preferable to perform an inside-out technique to minimize the amount of nonabsorbable suture on the external surface of the tendon (24). If the retromalleolar groove is crowded as with a low-lying brevis muscle belly, the brevis muscle can be excised to provide room for movement of the peroneal tendons (4).

For endoscopic groove-deepening procedures, awareness of the surrounding ligaments is important, as they are at risk for injury (Fig. 57-5). The posterior syndesmotic ligaments and the posterior talofibular ligaments are located medial to the fibular groove, which require following the contour of the groove proximally to distally. The calcaneofibular ligament inserts more anteriorly in the most distal part of the lateral malleolus. The fibular groove must be deepened anteriorly and distally while keeping the shaver directed medial to the calcaneofibular ligament insertion (25). The depth of the fibular groove should be deep enough, approximately 5 mm, to prevent recurrent dislocation of the peroneal tendons (26). It is essential to smoothen the lateral edge of the groove because sharp edges could cause peroneal tendon ruptures. At the end of the procedure, the ankle should be manipulated to see if enough bone has been removed. However, removing too much bone could result in fracture of the remaining lateral rim.

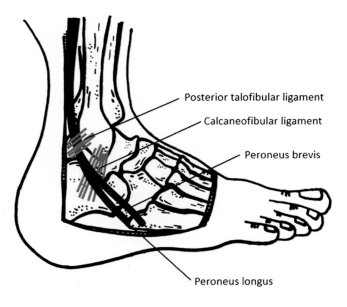

Posterior talofibular ligament

Calcaneofibular ligament

Peroneus brevis

Peroneus longus

FIGURE 57-5

The peroneal tendons pass in close proximity to the posterior talofibular ligament and calcaneofibular ligament, which are at risk for injury during groove-deepening procedures. (Original artwork contribtued by Stephanie M. Jones, BA; Pittsburgh, PA.)

POSTOPERATIVE MANAGEMENT

For repair of peroneal tendon tears the patient can be discharged the same day as surgery. The patient is placed in a lower leg plaster splint immediately postoperatively. The patient remains non–weight beating (NWB) in a splint for 1-2 weeks. Stitches may be removed at around 2 weeks postoperatively and the patient may be transitioned into a short-leg cast or CAM boot. Based on the performed procedure and surgeon preferences, the patient may begin a partial weight-bearing protocol between 2 and 4 weeks postoperatively. At 6 weeks postoperative, the patient should be full weight bearing and the CAM boot may be discontinued. Physical therapy can begin and the patient should work to regain ankle range of motion (ROM) and strength of the peroneal tendons. Initially, active ROM, strength, and low stress proprioception exercises can be performed in physical therapy. Between 8 and 12 weeks, eccentric, concentric, and isotonic exercises can be added. At 12 weeks, patients may progress to running, but more advanced provocation of the peroneal tendons and sports-specific training should not begin until at least 24 weeks postoperatively (27).

For recurrent peroneal dislocations treated with groove deepening, patients are placed in a lower leg splint and are partial WB for 5 days. Patients are allowed to progressively bear more weight over the next 4 to 6 weeks. Physical therapy can be initiated at this time and activities gradually resumed. Patients with isolated peroneal dislocations may return to full activities in 3 to 5 months (28).

COMPLICATIONS

Common complications in repair of peroneal tendon tears include infection, dehiscence, weakness, sural neuritis, and recurrent tendon pathology (29). For primary tears, the rates of these complications are not well characterized in the literature. However, in recurrent dislocations, wound dehiscence has been reported at 2.3% to 2.6% with reoperation rates from 2.8% to 3.4% (30). Bone-block procedures have been associated with nonunion, tendon irritation, and tendon adherence to the underlying bone (17,21,31).

RESULTS

Current outcomes for peroneal tendon repairs are largely reported in case reports and retrospective reviews. In a recent study, Guillo and Calder reported outcomes of five high-level male athletes with an average follow-up of 21.8 months. Each athlete was able to return to sporting activities at the same level prior to injury, although time to return to sport was not reported (32). Bassett and Speer reported the outcomes of eight college-level athletes who sustained longitudinal tears to either the peroneus brevis ($n = 3$) or peroneus longus ($n = 5$); all were able to return to full activity following repair (33). Porter et al. demonstrated return to sport by 3 months following surgery in 13 high-level athletes who underwent peroneal tendon repair and SPR reconstruction for symptomatic peroneal tendon subluxation with no recurrent subluxation or dislocation at 35 months' follow-up (16). Steel et al., however, reported that only 46% of their patients were able to successfully return to sports at 31 months follow-up.

Moreover, patients with tears <50% thickness and treated operatively with debridement and primary operative repair have excellent long-term functional outcomes, and the majority of patients return to their previous level of activity without need for reoperation (12,34). For patients with tears >50%, treatment with tenodesis is a simple procedure with good functional results, but almost 50% of patients may not resume full activities and almost two-thirds of patients have activity-related pain (5). Allograft bridging with peroneal or semitendinosus allografts is a more demanding procedure but is associated with increased return to preinjury activity levels and functional scores (8). Patients treated with tendon transfers have been reported to have some persistent strength and balance deficits in the operative extremity, but this does not seem to affect patient satisfaction with the procedure or patient activity levels (35).

Surgical treatment for recurrent dislocations provides improvement in the postoperative American Orthopaedic Foot and Ankle Society (AOFAS) score and high satisfaction rates. The redislocation rate is <1.5% at long-term follow-up. Patients treated with both groove deepening and SPR repair have higher rates of return to sports than patients treated with SPR repair alone (28). Overall, studies demonstrate good or excellent outcomes in 90% of cases with high rates of return to sports and improved AOFAS scores.

CONCLUSION

The peroneal tendons help to provide stability to the ankle by preventing excessive supination and eversion. In the athlete, chronic overuse and repetitive stress of the peroneal tendons can result in tenosynovitis, tears, subluxation, and/or ganglion cyst formation. While most of these pathologies may be treated nonoperatively, acute peroneal tendon tears and traumatic subluxation should be treated surgically. However, care must be taken to determine whether primary operative intervention may be necessary in the athlete, particulalry if the peroneal tendon pathology compromises the athletes' ability to perform in competition. Various approaches and techniques are available to treat peroneal tendon pathology, such as, tendon transfers, and reconstruction. Overall, operative management of athletes with peroneal tendon injuries and/or pathology has been associated with ability to return to full athletic activity and improvement in patient-reported functional outcome scores and satisfaction.

REFERENCES

1. Borland S, Jung S, Hugh IA. Complete rupture of the peroneus longus tendon secondary to injection. *Foot (Edinb).* 2009;19(4):229–231. doi:10.1016/j.foot.2009.07.001.
2. Heckman DS, et al. Operative treatment for peroneal tendon disorders. *J Bone Joint Surg Am.* 2008;90(2):404–418.
3. Sobel M, Bohne WH, Levy ME. Longitudinal attrition of the peroneus brevis tendon in the fibular groove: an anatomic study. *Foot Ankle.* 1990;11(3):124–128.
4. Cass AD, Camasta CA, Smith SE. *Peroneal Tendon Disorders: Preoperative and Intraoperative Decision Making.* The Podiatry Institute; 2009:1–8.
5. Krause JO, Brodsky JW. Peroneus brevis tendon tears: pathophysiology, surgical reconstruction, and clinical results. *Foot Ankle Int.* 1998;19(5):271–279.
6. Redfern D, Myerson M. The management of concomitant tears of the peroneus longus and brevis tendons. *Foot Ankle Int.* 2004;25(10):695–707.
7. Stamatis, ED, Karaoglanis GC, Salvage options for peroneal tendon ruptures. *Foot Ankle Clin.* 2014;19(1):87–95.
8. Mook WR, Parekh SG, Nunley JA. Allograft reconstruction of peroneal tendons: operative technique and clinical outcomes. *Foot Ankle Int.* 2013;34(9):1212–1220.
9. Drew GM, Gower AJ, Marriott AS. Pharmacological characterization of alpha-adrenoceptors which mediate clonidine-induced sedation [proceedings]. *Br J Pharmacol.* 1977;61(3):468P.
10. Squires N, Myerson MS, Gamba C. Surgical treatment of peroneal tendon tears. *Foot Ankle Clin.* 2007;12(4):675–695, vii.
11. Zgonis T, et al. Peroneal tendon pathology. *Clin Podiatr Med Surg.* 2005;22(1):79–85.
12. Demetracopoulos CA, et al. Long-term results of debridement and primary repair of peroneal tendon tears. *Foot Ankle Int.* 2014;35(3):252–257.
13. Jockel JR, Brodsky JW. Single-stage flexor tendon transfer for the treatment of severe concomitant peroneus longus and brevis tendon tears. *Foot Ankle Int.* 2013;34(5):666–672.
14. Rapley JH, Crates J, Barber A. Mid-substance peroneal tendon defects augmented with an acellular dermal matrix allograft. *Foot Ankle Int.* 2010;31(2):136–140.
15. Branch JP. A tendon graft weave using an acellular dermal matrix for repair of the Achilles tendon and other foot and ankle tendons. *J Foot Ankle Surg.* 2011;50(2):257–265.
16. Porter D, et al. Peroneal tendon subluxation in athletes: fibular groove deepening and retinacular reconstruction. *Foot Ankle Int.* 2005;26(6):436–441.
17. Maffulli N, et al. Recurrent subluxation of the peroneal tendons. *Am J Sports Med.* 2006;34(6):986–992.
18. Jones E. Operative treatment of chronic dislocation of the peroneal tendons. *J Bone Joint Surg Am.* 1932;14:574–576.
19. Tan V, Lin SS, Okereke E. Superior peroneal retinaculoplasty: a surgical technique for peroneal subluxation. *Clin Orthop Relat Res.* 2003;(410):320–325.
20. Adachi N, et al. Superior retinaculoplasty for recurrent dislocation of peroneal tendons. *Foot Ankle Int.* 2006;27(12):1074–1078.
21. Selmani E, Gjata V, Gjika E. Current concepts review: peroneal tendon disorders. *Foot Ankle Int.* 2006;27(3):221–228.
22. Kollias SL, Ferkel RD. Fibular grooving for recurrent peroneal tendon subluxation. *Am J Sports Med.* 1997;25(3):329–335.
23. Dombek MF, et al. Peroneal tendon tears: a retrospective review. *J Foot Ankle Surg.* 2003;42(5):250–258.
24. Schwartz JM, Giakoumis M, Banks AS. A simple technique for repair of chronic tendinopathy. *J Foot Ankle Surg.* 2015;54(1):143–144.
25. de Leeuw PAJ, van Dijk CN, Golanó P. A 3-portal endoscopic groove deepening technique for recurrent peroneal tendon dislocation. *Tech Foot Ankle Surg.* 2008;7(4):250–256.
26. Saragas NP, et al. Peroneal tendon dislocation/subluxation—case series and review of the literature. *Foot Ankle Surg.* 2016;22(2):125–130.
27. van Dijk PA, et al. Rehabilitation after surgical treatment of peroneal tendon tears and ruptures. *Knee Surg Sports Traumatol Arthrosc.* 2016;24(4):1165–1174.
28. van Dijk PA, et al. Return to sports and clinical outcomes in patients treated for peroneal tendon dislocation: a systematic review. *Knee Surg Sports Traumatol Arthrosc.* 2016;24(4):1155–1164.
29. Barp EA, Erickson JG. Complications of tendon surgery in the foot and ankle. *Clin Podiatr Med Surg.* 2016;33(1):163–175.
30. Yasui Y, et al. Incidence of reoperation and wound dehiscence in patients treated for peroneal tendon dislocations: comparison between osteotomy versus soft tissue procedures. *Knee Surg Sports Traumatol Arthrosc.* 2018;26(3):897–902.
31. Kelly RE. An operation for chronic dislocation of the peroneal tendons. *Br J Surg.* 2005;7(28):502–504.
32. Guillo S, Calder JD. Treatment of recurring peroneal tendon subluxation in athletes: endoscopic repair of the retinaculum. *Foot Ankle Clin.* 2013;18(2):293–300. doi:10.1016/j.fcl.2013.02.007.
33. Bassett FH III, Speer KP. Longitudinal rupture of the peroneal tendons. *Am J Sports Med.* 1993;21(3):354–357.
34. Steginsky B, et al. Patient-reported outcomes and return to activity after peroneus brevis repair. *Foot Ankle Int.* 2016;37(2):178–185.
35. Seybold JD, et al. Outcome of lateral transfer of the FHL or FDL for concomitant peroneal tendon tears. *Foot Ankle Int.* 2016;37(6):576–581.

58 Achilles Tendon Injury and Surgical Repair

Megan Walters, Monique C. Chambers, Malcolm E. Dombrowski, Stephanie M. Jones, Alan Yong Yan, and MaCalus V. Hogan

INTRODUCTION

Achilles tendon injuries are one of the most common foot and ankle pathologies in sports medicine. Overuse injuries such as chronic tendinopathy, retrocalcaneal bursitis, or Achilles tendon rupture may result in pain or irritation. For active patients who want to return to their previous activities, an Achilles tendon repair is often pursued to achieve the optimal possibility of return to a high level of athletic performance.

INDICATIONS/CONTRAINDICATIONS

The decision between operative and nonoperative management for acute Achilles tendon ruptures remains controversial. The best treatment should be individualized for the specific patient's characteristics, expectations, and goals. Age, activity level, smoking status, and medical comorbidities help guide treatment recommendations. Patients should be educated on the risks and benefits of all treatment options in order to make an informed decision that is realistic and optimized for the patient's goals.

Historically, nonsurgical management has been reserved for individuals with poor wound healing potential, sedentary lifestyles, heavy tobacco use, and other medical comorbidities that potentiate wound healing complications (e.g., diabetic neuropathy, protein deficiency). Nonoperative management decreases the risks inherent to surgery, such as wound complications and infection. However, there have also been reports of a higher overall risk of rerupture when immobilization techniques alone are used (1). Traditionally, nonoperative management included immobilization in a plaster cast for 6 to 8 weeks. However, recent literature reports a decrease in the rerupture rate when an early functional rehabilitation protocol is used with expedited range of motion exercises (2) and has become the preferred treatment in some countries (2). Additional benefits to nonoperative management include significantly decreased direct and indirect costs to the patient.

Operative management offers potential benefits of decreased rerupture risk, restoration of the length and tension of the muscle-tendon unit, possible earlier return to sport or activity, and ultimately an increase in muscular strength and endurance (3–8). However, surgical management can increase the risk of minor complications when compared to nonoperative management (9). Surgery is recommended for active patients with good wound healing potential. Surgery may also prove beneficial for symptomatic patients with chronic Achilles tendon tears that have failed conservative management.

PREOPERATIVE EVALUATION

Acute Achilles tendon ruptures are commonly due to attempted plantar flexion of a well-planted, dorsiflexed foot or rapidly forced dorsiflexion of a plantar flexed foot (10). Such injuries occur when quickly stepping to pivot, landing from a jump, slamming on a brake pedal in a motor vehicle collision, or falling from a height. Chronic Achilles tendon ruptures typically present with persistent plantar flexion weakness and a history of a prior painful event that was considered inconsequential (11).

In the immediate postinjury period, ecchymosis and calf swelling are often present. The majority of patients will not tolerate flat foot weight bearing, and those who do will demonstrate weakness with a heel rise on the affected limb. The presence of increased passive dorsiflexion (Matles test), a palpable defect in the tendon, and lack of plantar flexion response to the Thompson test has been shown to have 100% sensitivity in diagnosing acute Achilles tendon ruptures (12,13). Some patients do continue to have limited plantar flexion strength and/or reactive plantar flexion with the Thompson test due to secondary plantarflexors remaining intact. In a patient who provides a good history, two of the above findings are sufficient to establish the diagnosis of Achilles tendon rupture, and imaging is not typically required (12,14,15).

There are no absolute contraindications to operative management of acute Achilles tendon ruptures, and it should be considered as a treatment option for all patients. Therefore, when making a recommendation, it is important to consider patient factors that may increase the risk of postoperative complications and comorbidity such as diabetes, neuropathy, immunocompromised states, age above 65 years, tobacco use, sedentary lifestyle, obesity (body mass index [BMI] > 30), peripheral vascular disease, or local/systemic dermatologic disorders (14).

POSITIONING

The patient should be positioned prone on the operating table. Beware of pressure on the eyes, as this has been associated with a risk of residual blindness due to prone positioning. All bony prominences should be well padded, and chest rolls should be placed longitudinally along the patient's torso. The arms should be abducted with the shoulders and elbows flexed less than 90 degrees and the arms anterior to the chest. The patient should be positioned such that the feet hang off the bed distally, or a towel bump can be used to place under the patient's ankle to elevate the foot off the OR table and allow for passive dorsiflexion during the procedure. A tourniquet is placed on the proximal thigh, and the operative extremity is prepped and draped up to the tourniquet. Preoperative antibiotics should be administered within 1 hour of incision.

SURGICAL TECHNIQUE

An approximately 8-cm longitudinal incision is made just medial to the border of the palpable Achilles tendon (Fig. 58-1). Placing the incision in this location prevents the incision from lying directly over the repair and is more cosmetically pleasing. This incision can safely be extended, if needed, to adequately view the proximal and distal tendon stumps. Dissection is carried through the subcutaneous tissue to the level of the superficial fascia. Care should be taken to identify and protect the sural nerve and lesser saphenous vein. The sural nerve is located along the lateral border of the Achilles tendon approximately 10 cm proximal to its calcaneal insertion and continues distally running parallel to the tendon. Incise the fascia in line with the skin incision. At this time, an assistant

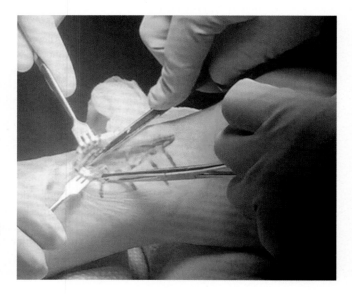

FIGURE 58-1

Posteromedial incision along the medial border of the Achilles tendon to identify the proximal and distal ends of the ruptured Achilles tendon.

should hold retractors deep to the fascia to expose the full width of the tendon. Self-retaining retractors are effective but have a higher propensity for iatrogenic soft tissue injury compared to manual retractors.

The paratenon is then identified. Carefully incise the paratenon longitudinally along the midline of the tendon. Then, develop the plane between the paratenon and the Achilles tendon until the medial and lateral tendon borders can clearly be seen at least 4 cm proximal and distal to the rupture. The paratenon not only serves as a vascular supply but also allows for smooth gliding of the tendon with ankle motion (16). Thus, it is important to maintain the paratenon as an intact layer, as it will be closed at the end of the procedure. It is not uncommon for the paratenon to be disrupted at the level of the rupture; however, remnants capable of covering the repair are often identifiable.

Next, irrigate the hematoma and debride the rupture site until the two tendon stumps are clearly identified. Utilizing Allis tissue forceps, gather the proximal stump at its distal end. Biomechanical testing has shown that polyblend sutures have a smaller gap formation and increased load to failure when compared to polyester sutures (17). Therefore, utilizing a no. 2 or 5 polyblend suture, enter the tendon in its torn end and throw at least three locking-loop stitches along the medial and lateral borders of the tendon. The locking-loop stitch, introduced by Krackow in 1986 (Fig. 58-2), has demonstrated superior mechanical properties to the Kessler, Bunnell, and other suture techniques for tendon and ligament repairs (18–20).

Although the number of core strands has demonstrated superior strength properties in the lab, in clinical practice, no difference in outcomes or complication rates between the traditional two-stranded single Krackow and a four-stranded double Krackow have been demonstrated (21). Another factor that leads to an improved biomechanical strength profile is to increase the suture caliber (22). However, this fact has to be balanced with the need for a low-profile repair due to the superficial location and potential for irritation. Recently, multiple modifications of the Krackow stitch and other suture configurations have been developed to further improve the strength profile of the tendon repair (23,24). Ultimately, determination of the exact stitch configuration is based upon surgeon clinical experience and comfort with the technique.

Regardless of selected suture configuration, repeat the same process for the distal stump and tie the core strands together, allowing the foot to reach up to 30 degrees of plantar flexion to achieve contact between the tendon ends. Complete the repair with a running epitendinous stitch that incorporates approximately 2.5 cm of the tendon proximal and distal to the primary repair site to improve strength and decrease gap formation (25). It is important to avoid piercing the suture used for the

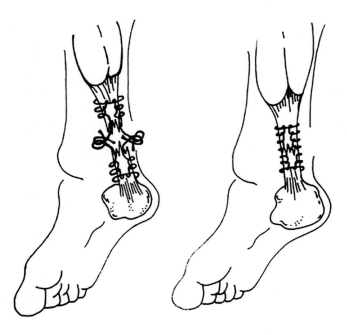

FIGURE 58-2

The suture pattern of the Krackow stitch, along with the final position of the Achilles tendon repair once completed and tied. (Original artwork contributed by Stephanie M. Jones, BA; Pittsburgh, PA.)

locking-loop stitch with the needle for the epitendinous stitch to prevent weakening the repair. Close the paratenon over the tendon and repair utilizing a 2-0 absorbable stitch.

Once the primary repair is complete, reapproximate the subcutaneous tissue with interrupted deep dermal stitches. Finally, close the skin with a running subcuticular stitch. Place Steri-Strips across the incision without tensioning to avoid blisters, and cover with a sterile dressing. While the patient is in the prone position, flex the knee 90 degrees to place a well-padded, posterior splint with the ankle positioned in a resting plantar flexed state.

In chronic Achilles tendon ruptures, in which retraction has occurred and a persistent gap exists between tendon ends even after maximal plantar flexion, multiple techniques have been described for local tendon transfer, autograft, and allograft. Flexor hallucis longus (FHL) transfer has demonstrated good to excellent results in multiple clinical studies (26–28). This is performed by making a medial incision to localize the FHL at the knot of Henry. Tendon transection is then performed as distally as possible; the remaining distal stump is sutured to the flexor digitorum longus (FDL) tendon. The FHL tendon is then retracted into the posteromedial surgical wound overlying the Achilles tendon defect. The FHL is then attached to the calcaneus through osseous tunnels or to the distal stump through a soft tissue attachment with the foot in neutral dorsiflexion. Peroneus brevis transfer, semitendinosus autograft, V-Y fascial turndown, and many other reconstruction options are also described in the literature with favorable results (29–31).

PEARLS/PITFALLS

- Longitudinal incision should be placed over the medial aspect of the tendon for improved cosmesis and wound healing.
- Manual retraction is safer on soft tissues than self-retainers.
- Preserve the paratenon layer for closure.
- Polyblend has a superior biomechanical profile than a polyester stitch material.
- Running, locking-loop stitch configuration has shown superior biomechanical properties.
- Reinforcement with adjunct procedures of acute ruptures is unnecessary.
- Reconstruction with local tendon transfer, autograft, and allograft are all viable options for chronic ruptures.

POSTOPERATIVE MANAGEMENT

The optimal postoperative protocol is determined largely based on the need for augmentation during the procedure and progress in the postoperative period. The literature has demonstrated a benefit in functional outcomes and patient satisfaction with early weight bearing and functional rehabilitation protocols (1,32–35). Therefore, the following protocol is an accelerated rehabilitation approach to the postoperative management following the repair of an acute Achilles tendon rupture.

Initially, the patient is immobilized in the lower leg splint placed postoperatively and should be non–weight bearing for 2 weeks to allow wound healing. The splint is removed at the first postoperative visit, and the incision is evaluated for any signs of infection. The patient is then placed into a cast or controlled ankle movement (CAM) boot with a heel wedge that limits dorsiflexion to neutral, and remains non–weight bearing until the stitches have been removed. A progressive weight-bearing protocol is started at 4 weeks postoperatively. A home exercise program should include range of motion with the goal of passive plantar flexion and active dorsiflexion to neutral. When the patient returns at 6 weeks follow-up, progression to full weight-bearing status is allowed with the foot in neutral dorsiflexion and the incision should be fully healed. Physical therapy with stretching and strengthening is initiated at 8 to 10 weeks postoperatively. Return to running and jumping activity is initiated when the patient is able to perform 15 single-leg heel raises on the operative extremity.

COMPLICATIONS

Acute Achilles tendon ruptures are at risk of rerupture regardless of whether operative or nonoperative treatment is selected. However, surgical repair is associated with a lower rerupture rate reported in multiple studies with current estimates around 5% (36–38). Thromboembolic disease can also affect patients treated surgically and nonsurgically. Currently, the evidence regarding the use of pharmacologic prophylaxis is lacking and inconsistent.

Wound complications, such as issues with healing and infection, and sural neuritis are much more likely with operative treatment than conservative management. Careful soft tissue handling during the procedure and placing a well-padded splint postoperatively are important technical considerations to minimize this risk. Diabetes and smoking status are critical patient factors that are associated with delayed wound healing and an increased risk of infection. Current estimates of infection rates following surgical repair of acute Achilles tendon ruptures range from 0.2% to 3.6% (39). The management of a postoperative wound infection ranges from oral antibiotics with weekly follow-up to surgical debridement and delayed reconstruction as a result of tissue loss.

RESULTS

The results of management of Achilles tendon ruptures depend on the specific treatment. Surgical repairs may be open, minimally invasive, or percutaneous, with or without biologic augmentation. Nonsurgical management may involve cast immobilization or functional rehabilitation with early range of motion.

The results of surgical management and nonoperative management of acute Achilles tendon ruptures are similar in terms of rerupture rate with the advent of early functional rehabilitation protocols (40). However, a recent systematic review comparing surgical versus nonsurgical management showed that operative management may result in a decreased overall rerupture rate. Nonetheless, there is an increased rate of minor complications, with an additional benefit of early return to work (36). In terms of functional outcomes, a randomized study of 100 patients compared surgical repair with accelerated postoperative functional rehabilitation to patients with functional rehabilitation alone (1). This study showed better performance on all functional tests after surgery, although the only parameters that were statistically significant were the hop and jump tests. In the same study, there were no reruptures in the surgical group compared to 5 in the nonoperative group, although this was not statistically significant (1). Surgical management not only offers a faster return to work and sport but also offers an increase in plantar flexion strength (41), which is an important consideration for athletes. Overall, larger studies are necessary to further elucidate any functional differences in surgical versus nonsurgical repair with early functional rehabilitation.

When comparing open versus percutaneous minimally invasive surgical repair of the Achilles tendon, McMahon et al. showed that there was no difference in the rerupture rates, tissue adhesion formation, and deep infections (42). However, there was a significantly lower rate of superficial infections in the percutaneous repair group (42), as an alternative to open management.

In a recent prospective randomized trial, comparison between gastrocnemius fascial augmented repairs and nonaugmented Achilles tendon repairs, there was no difference in clinical outcomes, tendon elongation, strength, rerupture, or complication rates at 14 years of follow-up (43). This is consistent with previous studies comparing augmented versus nonaugmented repair of the Achilles tendon (44,45). In general, end-to-end repair as described above is sufficient without a routine need for augmentation.

Finally, biologic augmentation with platelet-rich plasma (PRP) or bone marrow aspirate concentrate (BMAC) has become more widely used as an adjunct to operative management. In a study of 12 athletes comparing open repair with and without PRP, there was a quicker return to sport and faster recovery for range of motion with the use of PRP (46). However, another study investigating the use of PRP showed no difference in functional outcomes or mechanical tendon properties at 1-year follow-up between PRP and the control group. BMAC has been increasingly used, although there are no clinical studies published. There are, however, promising animal studies that show the potential for benefit. In a rat model by Okamoto et al., Achilles tendon repair with and without BMAC showed an increase in overall strength to tendon failure in the BMAC group at postoperative days 7, 14, and 28 (47). Further clinical studies are needed to investigate the benefits of biologic augmentation in surgical repair of the Achilles tendon.

REFERENCES

1. Olsson N, Silbernagel KG, Eriksson BI, et al. Stable surgical repair with accelerated rehabilitation versus nonsurgical treatment for acute Achilles tendon ruptures: a randomized controlled study. *Am J Sports Med.* 2013;41(12):2867–2876.
2. Kadakia AR, Dekker RG II, Ho BS. Acute Achilles tendon ruptures: an update on treatment. *J Am Acad Orthop Surg.* 2017;25(1):23–31.
3. Bhandari M, Guyatt GH, Siddiqui F, et al. Treatment of acute Achilles tendon ruptures: a systematic overview and metaanalysis. *Clin Orthop Relat Res.* 2002(400):190–200.

4. Cetti R, Christensen SE, Ejsted R, et al. Operative versus nonoperative treatment of Achilles tendon rupture. A prospective randomized study and review of the literature. *Am J Sports Med.* 1993;21(6):791–799.

5. Habusta SF. Bilateral simultaneous rupture of the Achilles tendon. A rare traumatic injury. *Clin Orthop Relat Res.* 1995;(320):231–234.

6. Leppilahti J, Orava S. Total Achilles tendon rupture. A review. *Sports Med.* 1998;25(2):79–100.

7. Maffulli N. Rupture of the Achilles tendon. *J Bone Joint Surg Am.* 1999;81(7):1019–1036.

8. Strauss EJ, Ishak C, Jazrawi L, et al. Operative treatment of acute Achilles tendon ruptures: an institutional review of clinical outcomes. *Injury.* 2007;38(7):832–838.

9. Khan RJ, Fick D, Keogh A, et al. Treatment of acute Achilles tendon ruptures. A meta-analysis of randomized, controlled trials. *J Bone Joint Surg Am.* 2005;87(10):2202–2210.

10. Arner O, Lindholm A. Subcutaneous rupture of the Achilles tendon; a study of 92 cases. *Acta Chir Scand Suppl.* 1959;116(suppl 239):1–51.

11. Hattrup SJ, Johnson KA. A review of ruptures of the Achilles tendon. *Foot Ankle.* 1985;6(1):34–38.

12. Garras DN, Raikin SM, Bhat SB, et al. MRI is unnecessary for diagnosing acute Achilles tendon ruptures: clinical diagnostic criteria. *Clin Orthop Relat Res.* 2012;470(8):2268–2273.

13. Thompson TC, Doherty JH. Spontaneous rupture of tendon of Achilles: a new clinical diagnostic test. *J Trauma.* 1962;2:126–129.

14. Chiodo CP, Glazebrook M, Bluman EM, et al. Diagnosis and treatment of acute Achilles tendon rupture. *J Am Acad Orthop Surg.* 2010;18(8):503–510.

15. Gross CE, Nunley JA II. Acute Achilles tendon ruptures. *Foot Ankle Int.* 2016;37(2):233–239.

16. Lohrer H, Arentz S, Nauck T, et al. The Achilles tendon insertion is crescent-shaped: an in vitro anatomic investigation. *Clin Orthop Relat Res.* 2008;466(9):2230–2237.

17. Benthien RA, Aronow MS, Doran-Diaz V, et al. Cyclic loading of Achilles tendon repairs: a comparison of polyester and polyblend suture. *Foot Ankle Int.* 2006;27(7):512–518.

18. Hahn JM, Inceoglu S, Wongworawat MD. Biomechanical comparison of Krackow locking stitch versus nonlocking loop stitch with varying number of throws. *Am J Sports Med.* 2014;42(12):3003–3008.

19. Krackow KA, Thomas SC, Jones LC. A new stitch for ligament-tendon fixation. Brief note. *J Bone Joint Surg Am.* 1986;68(5):764–766.

20. Watson TW, Jurist KA, Yang KH, et al. The strength of Achilles tendon repair: an in vitro study of the biomechanical behavior in human cadaver tendons. *Foot Ankle Int.* 1995;16(4):191–195.

21. Choi GW, Kim HJ, Lee TH, et al. Clinical comparison of the two-stranded single and four-stranded double Krackow techniques for acute Achilles tendon ruptures. *Knee Surg Sports Traumatol Arthrosc.* 2017;25(6):1878–1883.

22. Hapa O, Erduran M, Havitcioglu H, et al. Strength of different Krackow stitch configurations using high-strength suture. *J Foot Ankle Surg.* 2013;52(4):448–450.

23. Hong CK, Kuo TH, Yeh ML, et al. Do needleless knots have similar strength as the Krackow suture? An in vitro Porcine Tendon Study. *Clin Orthop Relat Res.* 2017;475(2):552–557.

24. Labib SA, Hoffler CE II, Shah JN, et al. The gift box open Achilles tendon repair method: a retrospective clinical series. *J Foot Ankle Surg.* 2016;55(1):39–44.

25. Lee SJ, Goldsmith S, Nicholas SJ, et al. Optimizing Achilles tendon repair: effect of epitendinous suture augmentation on the strength of Achilles tendon repairs. *Foot Ankle Int.* 2008;29(4):427–432.

26. Ahmad J, Jones K, Raikin SM. Treatment of chronic Achilles tendon ruptures with large defects. *Foot Ankle Spec.* 2016;9(5):400–408.

27. Mahajan RH, Dalal RB. Flexor hallucis longus tendon transfer for reconstruction of chronically ruptured Achilles tendons. *J Orthop Surg (Hong Kong).* 2009;17(2):194–198.

28. Rahm S, Spross C, Gerber F, et al. Operative treatment of chronic irreparable Achilles tendon ruptures with large flexor hallucis longus tendon transfers. *Foot Ankle Int.* 2013;34(8):1100–1110.

29. Maffulli N, Spiezia F, Longo UG, et al. Less-invasive reconstruction of chronic Achilles tendon ruptures using a peroneus brevis tendon transfer. *Am J Sports Med.* 2010;38(11):2304–2312.

30. Singh A, Nag K, Roy SP, et al. Repair of Achilles tendon ruptures with peroneus brevis tendon augmentation. *J Orthop Surg (Hong Kong).* 2014;22(1):52–55.

31. Dumbre Patil SS, Dumbre Patil VS, Basa VR, et al. Semitendinosus tendon autograft for reconstruction of large defects in chronic Achilles tendon ruptures. *Foot Ankle Int.* 2014;35(7):699–705.

32. Brumann M, Baumbach SF, Mutschler W, et al. Accelerated rehabilitation following Achilles tendon repair after acute rupture—development of an evidence-based treatment protocol. *Injury.* 2014;45(11):1782–1790.

33. Carter TR, Fowler PJ, Blokker C. Functional postoperative treatment of Achilles tendon repair. *Am J Sports Med.* 1992;20(4):459–462.

34. Suchak AA, Bostick GP, Beaupre LA, et al. The influence of early weight-bearing compared with non-weight-bearing after surgical repair of the Achilles tendon. *J Bone Joint Surg Am.* 2008;90(9):1876–1883.

35. Zhao JG, Meng XH, Liu L, et al. Early functional rehabilitation versus traditional immobilization for surgical Achilles tendon repair after acute rupture: a systematic review of overlapping meta-analyses. *Sci Rep.* 2017;7:39871.

36. Erickson BJ, Mascarenhas R, Saltzman BM, et al. Is operative treatment of Achilles tendon ruptures superior to nonoperative treatment? A systematic review of overlapping meta-analyses. *Orthop J Sports Med.* 2015;3(4):2325967115579188.

37. Lantto I, Heikkinen J, Flinkkila T, et al. A prospective randomized trial comparing surgical and nonsurgical treatments of acute Achilles tendon ruptures. *Am J Sports Med.* 2016;44(9):2406–2414.

38. van der Eng DM, Schepers T, Goslings JC, et al. Rerupture rate after early weightbearing in operative versus conservative treatment of Achilles tendon ruptures: a meta-analysis. *J Foot Ankle Surg.* 2013;52(5):622–628.

39. Fourniols E, Lazennec JY, Rousseau MA. Salvage technique for postoperative infection and necrosis of the Achilles tendon. *Orthop Traumatol Surg Res.* 2012;98(8):915–920.

40. Soroceanu A, Sidhwa F, Aarabi S, et al. Surgical versus nonsurgical treatment of acute Achilles tendon rupture: a meta-analysis of randomized trials. *J Bone Joint Surg Am.* 2012;94(23):2136-2143.

41. Willits K, Amendola A, Bryant D, et al. Operative versus nonoperative treatment of acute Achilles tendon ruptures: a multicenter randomized trial using accelerated functional rehabilitation. *J Bone Joint Surg Am.* 2010;92(17):2767–2775.

42. McMahon SE, Smith TO, Hing CB. A meta-analysis of randomised controlled trials comparing conventional to minimally invasive approaches for repair of an Achilles tendon rupture. *Foot Ankle Surg.* 2011;17(4):211–217.

43. Heikkinen J, Lantto I, Flinkkila T, et al. Augmented compared with nonaugmented surgical repair after total Achilles rupture: results of a prospective randomized trial with thirteen or more years of follow-up. *J Bone Joint Surg Am.* 2016;98(2):85–92.
44. Nyyssonen T, Saarikoski H, Kaukonen JP, et al. Simple end-to-end suture versus augmented repair in acute Achilles tendon ruptures: a retrospective comparison in 98 patients. *Acta Orthop Scand.* 2003;74(2):206–208.
45. Zell RA, Santoro VM. Augmented repair of acute Achilles tendon ruptures. *Foot Ankle Int.* 2000;21(6):469–474.
46. Sanchez M, Anitua E, Azofra J, et al. Comparison of surgically repaired Achilles tendon tears using platelet-rich fibrin matrices. *Am J Sports Med.* 2007;35(2):245–251.
47. Okamoto N, Kushida T, Oe K, et al. Treating Achilles tendon rupture in rats with bone-marrow-cell transplantation therapy. *J Bone Joint Surg Am.* 2010;92(17):2776–2784.

59 Treatment of Osteochondral Lesions of the Talar Dome: Surgical Options

Kyle R. Duchman and Annunziato Amendola

INTRODUCTION

Osteochondral lesions of the talar dome are being increasingly recognized as a source of persistent ankle pain and disability. Increased recognition of osteochondral lesions of the talus is secondary to a combination of factors, including increased awareness of the high likelihood of lesions in patients with acute ankle sprains (1), rotational ankle fractures (2,3), and chronic instability, as well as improved imaging modalities (4–7). As the recognition of osteochondral lesions of the talus has improved, treatment strategies and techniques have evolved significantly. While treatment strategies range from nonoperative management with or without casting or immobilization to surgical management with fragment excision, bone marrow stimulation, autologous or allograft osteochondral transfer, or newer biologic interventions, the relatively recent improvements and increased feasibility of ankle arthroscopy have undoubtedly aided in the diagnosis and surgical management of osteochondral lesions of the talar dome (8–10). As our understanding of these lesions continues to improve, outcomes following surgical management have shown consistently favorable long-term results (9,11,12). The following will discuss the surgical options available for treatment of osteochondral lesions of the talar dome, focusing on more recent surgical options and indications while briefly discussing historical surgical treatment options during the evolving management of these lesions.

ETIOLOGY

The majority of osteochondral lesions of the talar dome occur following a traumatic event, either isolated or recurrent in nature. Upwards of 80% of patients recall a history of trauma to their ankle (9,13,14), although metabolic, vascular, and genetic causes have also been implicated (15,16). Investigations on the incidence of osteochondral lesions of the talus following common ankle injuries, including isolated ankle sprains and rotational ankle fractures, suggest that these lesions occur in approximately 50% of ankle sprains and more than 70% of ankle fractures (1–3). Given the relatively high rate of ankle sprains in the active US population, it is not surprising that osteochondral lesions of the talar dome remain a common source of prolonged pain.

Historically, osteochondral lesions of the talar dome associated with trauma were thought to most frequently involve the anterolateral portion of the articular surface of the talar dome, while more chronic lesions associated with microinstability were thought to occur posteromedially, frequently associated with cystic changes (13,17). According to the original descriptions by Berndt and Harty (14), it was thought that anterolateral lesions were the result of a shear force across the lateral talar dome during inversion ankle injuries, while posteromedial lesions were the result of repetitive microtrauma and exacerbated by collateral ligament insufficiency. More recent studies, however, have questioned the classic bimodal anterolateral and posteromedial distribution of these lesions. These studies, aided by magnetic resonance imaging (MRI), reported that osteochondral lesions of the talar dome most frequently occurred in the centromedial and centrolateral region when using the popularized sagittal-coronal grid system, with relatively few lesions reported in the classic anterolateral or posteromedial locations (18,19). Interestingly, in the study by Orr et al., which restricted evaluation to only symptomatic patients, centrolateral lesions were noted to be twice as common as centromedial lesions, with lateral lesions almost always related to a specific traumatic event (18). Regardless of the exact lesion location, a traumatic incident or history remains the most consistent etiology.

HISTORY AND PHYSICAL EXAMINATION

Osteochondral lesions of the talar dome are most frequently the result of trauma (20), and as such, patients frequently recall a history of trauma, as either an isolated or a recurrent event. However, the time to presentation relative to the index event may vary substantially. As osteochondral lesions of the talus are frequently not recognized with routine radiographs during screening of acute ankle injuries (21,22), patients rarely present acutely. Rather, patients typically describe a course of persistent ankle pain and disability that may last as long as 3 to 6 months after their initial injury despite multiple attempts at treatment, which often includes a period of immobilization or bracing, rest, anti-inflammatory medications, or physical therapy. Additionally, patients may note persistent swelling of the ankle made worse by weight bearing while rarely reporting mechanical symptoms associated with ankle range of motion, including catching, clicking, or locking. In patients who present with this clinical scenario, there should be a high level of clinical suspicion for an osteochondral lesion of the talus or other elusive diagnoses, including a fracture of the lateral process of the talus or subtle instability of the tibiofibular syndesmosis (23,24). While there is not a single symptom or sign specific to osteochondral lesions of the talus that will be reported by patients, the constellation of a history of ankle trauma that fails to improve with persistent pain after 3 to 6 months of appropriate treatment should elicit further workup.

As a relatively superficial joint, there are a variety of nonspecific physical examination findings that, together with the history, often point toward the presence of an osteochondral lesion of the talar dome. Inspection may reveal a mild effusion, which can be best visualized as fullness in the lateral gutter. Additionally, it is important to inspect the overall alignment of the patient's lower extremity during weight-bearing stance, as this may guide further orthotic or surgical management. Palpation of the lateral and medial dome of the talus in neutral as well as maximal plantar flexion may illicit localized pain with more anterior lesions, although significant synovitis may result in relatively diffuse pain to palpation along the entire joint line. With posteromedial lesions, maximal dorsiflexion will bring the lesion posterior to the medial malleolus, allowing palpation directly on the posteromedial talar body. Both active and passive range of motion should be assessed, as patients with osteochondral lesions of the talus often have limitations in range of motion. Special ankle tests, including assessment of the lateral ligamentous complex, which can be assessed using the anterior or anterolateral drawer test (25,26), may suggest the possibility of osteochondral lesions of the talus. The external rotation stress examination can be used to help identify injury to the deltoid ligament or syndesmosis, which may be an independent cause of pain or a finding occurring in association with an osteochondral lesion of the talus that may need to be concomitantly addressed (27). Just like the history, while there is not a test or examination maneuver specific to osteochondral lesions of the talar dome, so having a systematic approach to the examination and a heightened awareness for lesions in the appropriate clinical setting will aid in both diagnosis and future treatment of these lesions.

IMAGING STUDIES

While standard radiographic studies, including anteroposterior, lateral, and mortise standing views of the ankle, lack sensitivity for detection of symptomatic osteochondral lesions of the talar dome, they are important for preoperative planning (Fig. 59-1). Additionally, a Canale view is useful to assess the talar profile (28), which is important when preparing for larger autograft or allograft transplantation procedures. If there is clinical concern for malalignment or planned concomitant realignment procedure, long-leg alignment radiographs and standing hindfoot alignment views should be obtained (29). While historically relevant, there is little utility for dedicated plantar flexion views to assess posteromedial lesions due largely to the improved access to advanced imaging techniques, including MRI and computed tomography (CT), which have superior diagnostic sensitivity and specificity (21,30).

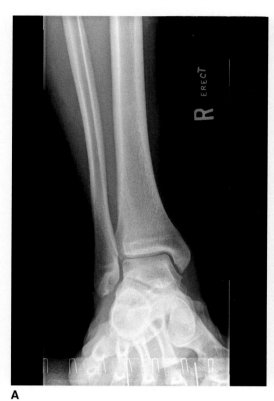
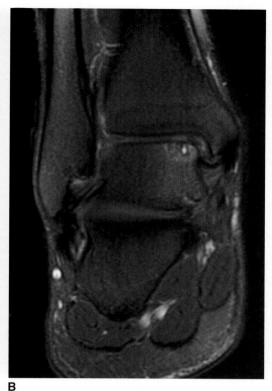

A   **B**

FIGURE 59-1

A: Anteroposterior radiograph of the right ankle in a patient with persistent pain after an ankle sprain. Radiographic findings do not indicate the presence of an osteochondral lesion. **B:** Magnetic resonance imaging (MRI) in the same patient reveals a cystic lesion within the posteromedial aspect of the talar dome with small amount of surrounding bone edema on coronal T2 images.

In the setting of negative plain radiographs, MRI and CT provide high sensitivity and specificity, with reported sensitivity and specificity for both modalities ranging from 70% to 100% (5,7,21). MRI, while serving as a slightly more sensitive diagnostic tool, can also detect bony edema, which may serve as a surrogate for stability of a detected lesion while also providing valuable information on the surrounding soft tissues. However, MRI does tend to overestimate the size of detected lesions due to the surrounding bony edema. Due to the fact that lesion size is often used to guide surgical decision-making algorithms (31) and, in some scenarios, may predict treatment success or failures (32,33), CT continues to play an important role in preoperative planning. Additionally, when osteochondral allograft resurfacing procedures are being considered for treatment of large lesions of the talar dome, CT scan is often a prerequisite to obtain an appropriately sized bulk talar allograft. With this in mind, MRI remains a useful tool for detection of occult lesions given its high sensitivity, while CT provides additional information for operative decision-making and preoperative planning.

CLASSIFICATION

A variety of classification systems for osteochondral lesions of the talar dome have been proposed. An ideal classification system allows for critical components of a diagnosis or disease process to be clearly communicated and understood between two knowledgeable parties while also serving to guide treatment decisions. Most classification systems for osteochondral lesions of the talus, however, have evolved alongside imaging modalities. The Berndt and Harty classification provided the first image-based classification of osteochondral lesions of the talar dome (14). Their classification system was based on plain radiographs and described stage 1 lesions as a small area of trabecular compression; stage 2 as a partial or incompletely detached fragment; stage 3 as a completely detached, nondisplaced fragment; and stage 4 as completely detached and displaced (Table 59-1). Nearly 30 years after the original classification proposed by Berndt and Harty, Anderson and

TABLE 59-1 Image-Based Classifications for Osteochondral Lesions of the Talar Dome

	Berndt and Harty Classification	**Imaging Modality**
Stage 1	Trabecular compression	Radiographs
Stage 2	Incompletely detached fragment	Radiographs
Stage 3	Completely detached, nondisplaced fragment	Radiographs
Stage 4	Completely detached, displaced fragment	Radiographs
Stage 5[a]	Radiolucent "fibrous" defect	CT[b]
MODIFIED STAGING SYSTEM OF BERNDT AND HARTY		
Stage I	Subchondral trabecular compression	CT/MRI[c]
Stage II	Incomplete separation of the fragment	CT/MRI
Stage IIA	Formation of a subchondral cyst	CT/MRI
Stage III	Unattached, undisplaced fragment	CT/MRI
Stage IV	Displaced fragment	CT/MRI
REVISED CLASSIFICATION OF BERNDT AND HARTY		
Stage 1	Articular cartilage damage only	MRI
Stage 2a	Cartilage injury with underlying fracture, edema	MRI
Stage 2b	Cartilage injury with underlying fracture, no edema	MRI
Stage 3	Detached but undisplaced fragment	MRI
Stage 4	Detached and displaced fragment	MRI
Stage 5	Subchondral cyst	MRI

[a]Addition by Loomer R, Fisher C, Lloyd-Smith R, et al. Osteochondral lesions of the talus. *Am J Sports Med.* 1993;21:13–19.
[b]Computed Tomography.
[c]Magnetic Resonance Imaging.

colleagues proposed a modified staging system based on MRI and CT findings, adding a "stage IIA" to the system, which described an incompletely detached fragment with an underlying cystic component (34). An addition to the original Berndt and Harty classification was later proposed by Loomer et al., which included a stage 5 lesion described as a radiolucent "fibrous" defect with intact overlying cartilage on CT scan (17). Hepple et al. would later propose a completely MRI-based revised classification system using the framework of the original Berndt and Harty classification while also acknowledging previous modifications (22). While other classification systems exist (5,35), the Berndt and Harty classification, with modifications included, remains the most consistently cited and recognized image-based classification for osteochondral defects of the talar dome (9). Additionally, the classification and subsequent modifications do provide some guidance as to specific treatment options, including the use of retrograde drilling for lesions with an intact articular surface (36) and bone marrow stimulation or replacement of the entire osteochondral unit in lesions with significant bone marrow edema or cystic changes (37,38).

INDICATIONS

Given the relatively benign natural history and limited progression of asymptomatic osteochondral lesions of the talus (39), surgical intervention is limited to symptomatic individuals. Why nondisplaced lesions remain asymptomatic in some individuals while causing significant symptoms and disability in others is likely due to multifactorial mechanical and biologic factors that continue to be investigated (40). Patients with nondisplaced lesions should undergo a trial of nonoperative treatment, including a period of immobilization followed by progressive range of motion, weight bearing, and physical therapy focused on strengthening. If flexible malalignment is an issue, orthotics to shift loads should also be considered. In lieu of absolute or consistently reported indications in the literature, patients who fail a 3- to 6-month trial of appropriate nonoperative treatment are candidates for surgical intervention, as are symptomatic patients with displaced lesions who, in our experience, respond less favorably to trials of nonoperative management. Additionally, when considering surgical management, assessment of contributing factors, including malalignment, instability, and bony impingement, is essential during preoperative evaluation in order to optimize outcomes. In general, failed nonoperative management in a symptomatic patient with an osteochondral lesion of the talus is considered an indication for surgery.

Contraindications to surgical intervention include active infection, malignancy, chronic regional pain syndrome, malalignment or instability that is not correctable with a staged or concomitant procedure, or tibial plafond cartilage lesions that articulate with the osteochondral lesion of the talus, creating a "bipolar" lesion. Additionally, depending on the planned intervention, skeletal immaturity may be a relative contraindication to surgery, particularly if an osteotomy is required in the setting of open physes.

A vast array of surgical procedures have been described for a wide variety of osteochondral lesions of the talar dome. Despite classifications that have attempted to guide surgical management, the indications and decision-making for specific surgical procedures are largely limited to retrospective reports, case series, and expert opinion, without clear superiority for any specific procedure. A systematic review identified a single randomized trial that compared chondroplasty, microfracture, and osteochondral autograft transplantation with no differences noted at minimum 2-year follow-up (41). The systematic review itself concluded that treatment with bone marrow stimulation, including microfracture or drilling, provided the most effective treatment for symptomatic osteochondral lesions based on the best available evidence (9). In general, the primary method of treatment is arthroscopic debridement and marrow stimulation. More recent studies have confirmed the speculation that certain procedures may be better suited for larger lesions given the deteriorating outcomes of microfracture on lesions measuring >1 cm^2 (32,33). Even prior to these studies, many surgeons factored lesion size into their treatment algorithm, with donor site morbidity limiting the applicability of osteochondral autograft transplantation procedures in very large lesions (Fig. 59-2). In this setting, autologous chondrocyte implantation (ACI), fresh osteochondral allograft, or particulate allograft articular cartilage procedures may provide benefits that cannot be provided by other procedures. Additional factors, including cystic components of the lesion or a previously failed bone marrow stimulation procedure, may guide treatment decisions. However, there is little to no strong evidence to support rigid indications for specific procedures in specific clinical settings. Relative indications, as well as a discussion of the risks and benefits associated with specific procedures routinely used to address osteochondral lesions of the talar dome, will be discussed further in the following section on surgical techniques.

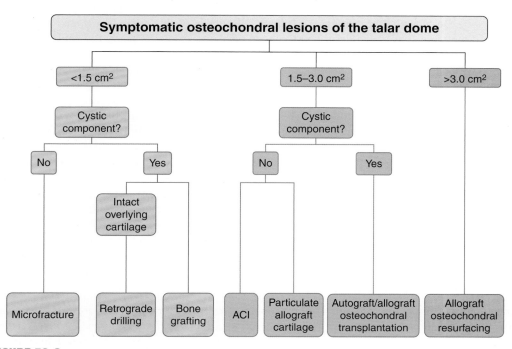

FIGURE 59-2

Size-based treatment algorithm for symptomatic, osteochondral lesions of the talar dome that have not undergone previous surgery.

SURGICAL TECHNIQUES

Multiple surgical procedures have been proposed to address osteochondral lesions of the talar dome. While there remains insufficient evidence to recommend a specific procedure, each procedure provides unique advantages and disadvantages. Since the talar dome is contained within the ankle mortise, the approach for each procedure must be thoughtfully considered. Fortunately, advances in ankle arthroscopy have provided a relatively noninvasive approach to access nearly the entire surface of the talar dome for bone marrow stimulation techniques using thoughtful positioning and noninvasive distraction techniques. Where applicable, posterior ankle arthroscopy can provide improved access for lesions that have proved difficult to reach with standard approaches (42). Because of the improved access, expedited recovery, limited morbidity, and sufficient clinical outcomes provided by treatment techniques amenable to arthroscopic means, including the majority of bone marrow stimulation procedures, some have suggested that these procedures be used as the first-line treatment for those presenting with osteochondral lesions of the talar dome.

In some scenarios, however, lesions may be better addressed by open as opposed to arthroscopic techniques. This is often the case for relatively large lesions (>1.5 cm^2), lesions that have failed a primary bone marrow stimulation procedure, lesions being addressed by techniques that require perpendicular access to the surface of the talar dome, or lesions with a significant cystic component underlying a cartilage defect that requires replacement of the entire osteochondral unit. Open procedures are specific to the region of the involved talar dome, making thoughtful preoperative planning essential. Up to 75% of the talar dome surface can be accessed via anteromedial, anterolateral, posteromedial, or posterolateral arthrotomies (43). Access can often be improved through limited soft tissue releases, including release of the anterolateral tibiofibular ligament, allowing improved access to lateral lesions with inversion and plantar flexion of the ankle. The soft tissue releases are easily repaired primarily at the conclusion of the procedure. Additionally, an extensile anterior or classic "total ankle" approach between the extensor hallucis longus and tibialis anterior can be used for very large lesions requiring allograft transplantation (44).

Lesions that extend into the central portion of the talar dome and posteromedially have historically provided the greatest challenge. A variety of osteotomies have been described to access these difficult lesions. Muir et al. found that even with the laterally based Chaput osteotomy and medial malleolus osteotomy, the central and posterior two thirds of the talar surface remains difficult to access (43). Fortunately, the majority of lesions fall outside of this area (18,19), and an array of unique osteotomies have been described to obtain adequate access to nearly the entire surface of the talar dome (45–50). While providing improved access, many osteotomies require additional fixation with the possibility for symptomatic hardware and delayed rehabilitation to optimize union, although the rate of nonunion with adequate fixation remains low (51–53).

The following will expand upon the techniques and specific indications for each procedure in the authors' experience given the limited high-level evidence currently available. Modern treatments that will be discussed in more detail include bone marrow stimulation, ACI, autograft osteochondral transplantation, allograft osteochondral resurfacing, particulate allograft cartilage therapies, and, briefly, biologic and other cell-based therapies. While historically relevant (54–56), isolated excision of osteochondral defects without bone marrow stimulation (microfracture or drilling) or other associated procedures will not be discussed. Additionally, treatment of large, acute osteochondral fragments that are amenable to open reduction internal fixation techniques will not be discussed. In the authors' experience, open reduction internal fixation of lesions should only be considered in clearly acute cases with intact cartilage over an osteochondral fragment that involves greater than one third of the talar dome.

Bone Marrow Stimulation

Bone marrow stimulation techniques are the most frequently performed procedures for osteochondral lesions of the talar dome and include microfracture and drilling techniques. Microfracture, which was popularized by Dr. J. Richard Steadman in the 1990s for osteochondral defects in the knee, aims to gain access to mesenchymal stem cells below the subchondral plate, allowing organized formation of a type I fibrocartilage layer when given appropriate biomechanical and biologic conditions (57). For osteochondral lesions of the talar dome, the procedure is most frequently performed using minimally invasive, arthroscopic techniques, which allows nearly universal access to the talar dome (42). Bone marrow stimulation techniques are ideal for patients with Berndt and Harty stage 1 and 2 lesions that have failed conservative treatment or stage 3 and 4 lesions with symptomatic loose or free fragments that measure <1 to 1.5 cm^2. While some aggregate data suggest that bone marrow stimulation techniques should be considered for all primary osteochondral lesions of the talar dome (9), outcomes for larger lesions are not as promising (32,33).

After diagnostic arthroscopy, the damaged cartilage overlying the defect is debrided with a curette or mechanical shaver. It is important to debride the lesion back to a circumferential stable rim of cartilage to allow a base for eventual clot formation. This can prove to be a challenge on some areas of the talus, including the medial and lateral shoulder of the talus, and in these areas, other techniques that provide more structural support, such as autologous osteochondral transplantation or allograft osteochondral resurfacing, may be considered. After achieving a stable circumferential cartilaginous rim, the calcified cartilage layer is removed using a curette or mechanical shaver. If there is a significant cystic component underlying the lesion, as is the case with stage IIA lesions using the modified staging of Berndt and Harty described by Anderson et al. (34), care should be taken to thoroughly debride all cystic components and necrotic bone. Depending on the size of the defect after debridement, autologous cancellous bone grafting can prove useful (Fig. 59-3). After completing these steps, microfracture awls are introduced and subchondral channels 3 to 4 mm in depth are created, spacing the channels 3 to 4 mm apart across the entire surface of the lesion. Microfracture awls were originally favored over drilling, as they were less likely to produce heat, reducing the risk for adjacent bone necrosis. However, more recent studies suggest that equivalent clinical outcomes can be achieved with subchondral drilling using Kirschner wires in the setting of a water-cooled, arthroscopic medium (58). After creation of the subchondral channels with awls or drilling, arthroscopic fluid inflow should be shut off to visualize blood or fat droplets eluting from the channels, confirming adequate access to the bone marrow and mesenchymal stem cells.

Falling into the bone marrow stimulation category, retrograde drilling of subchondral cystic lesions with normal overlying articular cartilage, including stage 5 radiolucent "fibrous" defects as described by Loomer et al. (17) and in the revised classification of Berndt and Harty by Hepple et al. (22), has been described. In the authors' experience, these are relatively rare lesions, and arthroscopic assessment is required to confirm intact cartilage overlying the cystic component. Using intraoperative fluoroscopy, wires can be targeted to cystic areas through the sinus tarsi or off the lateral border of the fibula for posteromedial and posterolateral lesions, respectively (36,59). A cannulated drill can then be placed over the guidewire to drill and decompress the cystic lesion. Using fluoroscopic and arthroscopic techniques simultaneously, care is taken to drill the underlying cystic lesion while avoiding iatrogenic injury to the intact overlying cartilage. While the indications for this technique are limited, it does provide a useful strategy for very specific lesions with reported clinical efficacy.

In general, microfracture and drilling can serve to address nearly all osteochondral lesions of the talar dome. However, other procedures should be considered for patients that have previously failed a bone marrow stimulation procedure, for lesions measuring >1.5 cm^2, and for lesions where a stable circumferential cartilaginous rim cannot be obtained.

Autologous Chondrocyte Implantation

Since bone marrow stimulation techniques can only yield fibrocartilage, other techniques have evolved to recreate the hyaline cartilage articular surface. Originally described for use in the knee (60), ACI has been applied to the treatment of osteochondral lesions of the talar dome (61–65). While recreating the hyaline cartilage articular surface has remained elusive, ACI has shown the ability to produce "hyaline-like" cartilage over relatively large areas (66). ACI is a two-stage procedure. The first stage of the procedure includes an articular cartilage biopsy, which is typically performed arthroscopically, and tissue is obtained from healthy cartilage areas of the involved talus (61) or intercondylar notch of the knee (65). Although cartilage cells from the involved or detached osteochondral fragment may be viable (67), we typically do not harvest cells from this area. Following biopsy, the chondrocytes are isolated and expanded by proprietary means. During the second stage of the procedure, the expanded chondrocytes are implanted into the prepared defect.

ACI is indicated for patients with large lesions measuring >1.5 cm^2 and for those patients who have previously failed a bone marrow stimulation procedure. The second stage of ACI procedures is typically performed through an arthrotomy or osteotomy, depending on the location of the lesion. Typically, an arthrotomy suffices for exposure, as newer generation ACI techniques do not require

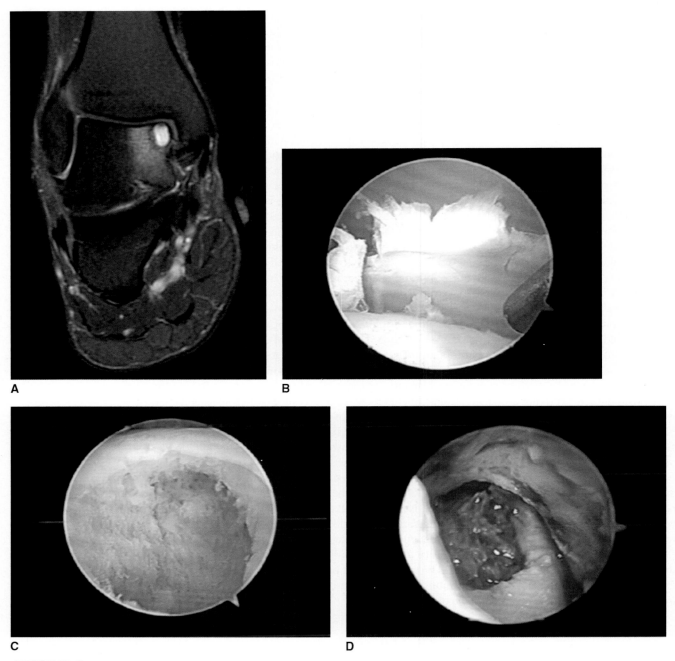

FIGURE 59-3

A: Osteochondral lesion of the medial talar dome with a large, fluid-filled cystic component as seen on coronal T2 MRI. **B:** Arthroscopic image viewing through the anterolateral portal with probe through the anteromedial portal reveals a large cartilage flap overlying the cystic component posteromedially. **C:** Arthroscopic image viewing the debrided cyst through the anteromedial portal. A stable cartilaginous rim and debridement of all underlying necrotic bone were achieved arthroscopically using a mechanical shaver and curettes. **D:** Autologous cancellous bone grafting of the cyst using bone from the ipsilateral iliac crest was performed through a 3-cm miniarthrotomy via extension of the anteromedial arthroscopic portal.

perpendicular access. ACI has gone through several iterations since its inception. Many of the limitations of the first- and second-generation techniques have been at least in part alleviated by the development of third-generation ACI techniques, also known as matrix-induced ACI or MACI (Vericel Corporation, Cambridge, MA). During the chondrocyte isolation and expansion process, cells are embedded in a type I/III collagen matrix, thus negating the need for a watertight patch or seal over the expanded chondrocytes (68). Instead, the lesion is simply measured and the collagen matrix cut to size and implanted, with a fibrin glue placed over the matrix and lesion. Further advances in embedded chondrocyte collagenous scaffolds and concomitant bone grafting procedures may serve to further expand the indications for future generations of ACI where increased structural support is needed (69,70).

ACI is a viable option for large, osteochondral lesions of the talar dome. However, negative aspects of the procedure, including the need for two surgical interventions, cost, and concern for donor site morbidity, limit its widespread use. At the time of this publication, MACI is the only form of ACI available in the United States. While it has recently been approved for use in the knee for US patients, its use in the ankle for treatment of osteochondral lesions of the talar dome remains off label. The procedure is not frequently covered by third-party payers, limiting its application in this area. While newer generations of ACI with imbedded chondrocyte scaffolds have improved significantly upon first- and second-generation ACI techniques, other procedures should be considered in lesions with inadequate structural support secondary to location or subchondral bone loss.

Autograft Osteochondral Transplantation

Autograft osteochondral transplantation provides a structural graft material with an overlying hyaline cartilage layer. Because of the structural properties of the harvested osteochondral plugs, autograft osteochondral transplantation is an ideal procedure for lesions with large cystic components or bony edema on MRI that are best treated with replacement of the osteochondral unit, lesions with significant bone loss or limited structural support, and lesions that have failed a primary bone marrow stimulation procedure. Autograft osteochondral transplantation procedures can be performed on lesions larger than 1.5 cm^2, although donor site morbidity must be considered as lesions get larger (71–73).

The first step of an autograft osteochondral transplantation procedure, which can be performed as a single stage unlike ACI, is preparation of the osteochondral talar defect. We typically begin with a standard diagnostic ankle arthroscopy to gain a better understanding of the size of the defect. The defect is debrided arthroscopically to a stable cartilaginous rim and measurements are made with a probe to confirm that autograft osteochondral transplantation remains a viable option. Due to the need for perpendicular access to the defect, further preparation of the osteochondral defect and subsequent graft transfer are typically performed open and may necessitate an osteotomy to obtain perpendicular access. For many anterior lesions, a small arthrotomy in line with the standard anterolateral or anteromedial anterior ankle arthroscopy portal will suffice when coupled with ankle plantar flexion to gain access to the lesion. With the lesion identified and prepared back to a stable base, sizing templates are used to plan both the size and number of osteochondral autograft plugs needed. Templating should plan to completely fill the defect while abutting the healthy neighboring cartilage, without unnecessarily removing healthy adjacent tissue. For smaller lesions, a larger, single plug may suffice. For larger lesions, multiple smaller plugs, so-called mosaicplasty, are often needed. After templating, a cylindrical chisel is introduced at the osteochondral defect or recipient site. The surface of the cylindrical chisel should remain perpendicular to the recipient site and impacted to a depth of 12 to 15 mm depending on the depth of the cystic component. Attention is then turned to the donor site for autograft harvest. For treatment of osteochondral defects of the talar dome, harvest from the talus itself or the ipsilateral knee are viable options, although the knee typically is more appropriate for larger lesions (74,75). Harvest from the knee may be performed via a miniarthrotomy or arthroscopic techniques. For larger lesions, harvest along the medial or lateral femoral condyles proximal to the sulcus terminalis is the preferred location, although harvest from the intercondylar notch is an option for smaller lesions. The cylindrical harvest chisel at the donor site is typically 1 mm larger in diameter than the prepared recipient site and driven to a depth of 1 to 2 mm beyond the prepared donor site as well. By slightly oversizing the harvested plug, good interference fit can be achieved. Again, it is important to maintain the chisel perpendicular to the donor cartilage. The harvested osteochondral plug is then carefully placed at the recipient site and gently tapped into place to achieve a flush surface with the surrounding cartilage, which is necessary to restore normal contact pressures, as both elevated and recessed graft placement can lead to increased contact pressures on the graft itself and the adjacent cartilage, respectively (76). If a mosaicplasty is planned, we prefer to prepare the recipient site and then harvest from the donor site in a sequential fashion for each plug, as this allows us to fine-tune the fit of the plugs at every step—in order to achieve adequate interference fit and appropriate contour. The donor site(s) are typically backfilled with cancellous autograft taken from the plugs during preparation of the recipient site, although prefabricated osteochondral allograft plugs can be used to fill the defects, typically with a plug that measures 1 mm larger in diameter than the cylindrical chisel used to harvest.

Autologous osteochondral transplantation provides a variety of advantages, including the ability to transfer hyaline cartilage to the osteochondral defect while also replacing the entire osteochondral unit in lesions with large cystic components, such as stage IIA (34) or stage 5 lesions (22). Autologous osteochondral transfer can also be used for relatively large lesions, although one must plan and discuss with the patient the location of the donor site depending on the amount of autograft tissue anticipated. The primary disadvantage of autologous osteochondral transfer is donor site morbidity. Harvest from the ipsilateral knee is not without consequence for patients undergoing autologous osteochondral transfer (72,73), while harvest options from the talus are limited. Despite transplanting hyaline cartilage, the local mechanical properties of transplanted plugs from the knee do not necessarily replicate the local mechanical properties of the talus (77). Additionally, successful transplantation relies upon healing of the transferred bone plugs and, when necessary, union of osteotomies about the ankle. Because of the unique advantages and disadvantages of autologous osteochondral transplantation, careful selection of appropriate lesions, namely, those with a large cystic component or lack of structural support, as well as a thoughtful conversation with patients regarding donor site morbidity, is required.

Allograft Osteochondral Resurfacing

Allograft osteochondral resurfacing of the talus has recently gained popularity. Allograft osteochondral resurfacing affords several advantages to other resurfacing procedures, including the fact that it is a single-stage procedure without donor site morbidity. However, allograft transplantation does raise some concerns, including the potential for transmission of infectious disease, immune-mediated failures, lack of chondrocyte viability, and failure of incorporation of the graft. The potential effect of chondrocyte viability, or lack thereof, should not be understated as an important factor influencing clinical outcomes (78). Fresh osteochondral allografts are preferred and testing of fresh allografts takes 14 days prior to release of the graft for implantation. Previous studies have indicated that prolonged storage, particularly storage beyond 28 days from harvest, may significantly decrease chondrocyte viability of the fresh allograft (79). Because of this, flexibility in a patient's and surgeon's schedule is important, as surgery should be scheduled as soon as possible once an appropriately sized graft has become available. Additionally, storage medium and storage techniques may influence chondrocyte viability (78,80,81), and because of this, surgeons should have a sound understanding of the processing and storage techniques used by the companies that provide them allograft tissues.

Allograft osteochondral resurfacing proceeds similarly to an autograft osteochondral transplantation. Prior to surgery, a contralateral CT of the ankle is typically required to obtain an appropriately sized graft. Additionally, a Canale view of the contralateral ankle can be useful, as it provides a comparison to guide contouring intraoperatively. Allograft osteochondral resurfacing is typically performed for larger lesions of the talus that require an arthrotomy or osteotomy. Still, a thorough diagnostic arthroscopy is useful, as it can serve to better define the lesion and guide the approach. After determining the extent of the osteochondral defect and performing the appropriate open approach, the lesion is thoroughly debrided or excised. Typically, osteochondral resurfacing is performed with one of two techniques. The first is similar to autograft osteochondral transplantation and includes preparation of the donor site with cylindrical recipient chisels, followed by harvesting of a slightly oversized plug to achieve interference fit from the same area on the allograft on the back table. Being able to harvest from the same region on a size-matched allograft talus provides the advantage of better matching the contour of the native talus. The second technique includes more extensive resection of the lesion, using either saws or larger, cannulated coring reamers to prepare the recipient site as well as the donor allograft on the back table (31,82). Careful measurements and markings are critical to obtain an appropriately sized allograft segment from corresponding regions of the talus. If a circumferential core is planned, these can sometimes be interference fit without additional fixation. However, fixation of segmental graft with headless compression screws or countersunk screw head is often required. As with autograft osteochondral transplantation plugs, it is important to achieve a flush interface between the graft and adjacent native tissue in order to avoid increased contact pressure on the graft itself or neighboring tissue.

Osteochondral allograft resurfacing is an evolving treatment for large osteochondral lesions of the talar dome. The primary advantage of osteochondral allograft resurfacing is that it negates the need for autograft donor tissue, thus eliminating donor site morbidity. Additionally, osteochondral allograft resurfacing can address very large structural defects, including defects of the medial and lateral talar shoulder, which proves challenging with techniques that require a relatively well-contained defect. However, osteochondral allograft resurfacing techniques require a great deal of preoperative planning, and maintenance of chondrocyte viability remains a concern. While the technique can provide significant clinical improvement for patients with large, difficult to treat lesions, the need for reoperation following these procedures approaches 25% (51), which should be discussed preoperatively with patients. As storage techniques continue to improve and the effect of chondrocyte viability on clinical outcomes is more closely followed, this continues to be an exciting treatment area to address osteochondral lesions of the talar dome moving forward.

Particulate Allograft Cartilage

Particulate allograft cartilage is a relatively new treatment option for osteochondral lesions of the talar dome. Particulate allograft cartilage is essentially minced allograft cartilage that contains viable chondrocytes. Compared to other allograft tissues, particulate allograft cartilage does not theoretically elicit an immune response, as it contains only chondrocytes and extracellular matrix proteins and not subchondral bone. Additionally, as an allograft tissue, there is no donor site morbidity associated with the procedure. *DeNovo* NT (Zimmer Inc., Warsaw, IN) is an example of a particulate allograft cartilage, and one package can cover a defect measuring up to 2.0 cm². While examples of its use for osteochondral lesions of the talar dome are limited, it has shown early promise (83,84).

A diagnostic arthroscopy is typically performed to better appreciate the chondral defect. The defect can be prepared by arthroscopic or open techniques, and preparation includes curettage of the lesion to produce a stable cartilaginous rim. The calcified cartilage layer is removed carefully with a curette, but care is taken not to penetrate the underlying subchondral bone. If there is a large cystic component, the cyst can be debrided with a curette. However, as the particulate allograft cartilage is not a structural graft, bone grafting with autograft or allograft cancellous chips may be necessary (84). After preparation of the defect, the defect must be dried of any blood or residual arthroscopic fluid. Because of this, particulate cartilage treatments were historically completed using open techniques. However, several creative ways to perform the procedure arthroscopically, using dry arthroscopic techniques after preparation of the defect, have been described (85,86). A thin layer of fibrin glue is applied to the base of the lesion, and while still in its liquid state, particulate allograft cartilage is placed within the lesion on top of the fibrin glue. A final layer of fibrin glue is then placed on top of the particulate allograft cartilage chips and allowed to dry (Fig. 59-4). Enough particulate allograft cartilage should be placed to create a flush surface with the surrounding native cartilage.

There remains much to be learned about the role of particulate allograft cartilage for osteochondral lesions of the talus. Currently, the indications for particulate allograft cartilage seem to overlap with bone marrow stimulation techniques. The potential advantages of particulate allograft cartilage, including the fact that it is a single-stage procedure without donor site morbidity and the potential to yield hyaline cartilage, make it an exciting new option for the treatment of osteochondral lesions of the talar dome. However, as a new therapy, the clinical outcomes will need to be closely followed and indications better defined.

Biologic and Other Cell-Based Therapies

While biologic and cell-based therapies as a stand-alone therapy, such as platelet-rich plasma (PRP) or mesenchymal stem cell injection, have limited support from the literature (87), their role as adjuncts during operative management of patients with osteochondral lesions of the talar dome has been better explored (88). The most studied biologic agents in this area include PRP, concentrated bone marrow aspirate (CBMA), and hyaluronic acid (HA). PRP is prepared from whole blood, while CBMA is prepared from marrow aspirates, most commonly from the iliac crest. HA is commercially available in several forms. Typically, these agents are used at the end of microfracture procedures. If performed arthroscopically, as much fluid as possible is removed from the joint prior to injecting the PRP or CBMA into the base of the prepared lesion as well as the surrounding joint. Several randomized studies and retrospective series have shown promising clinical and image-based results for both PRP and CBMA when compared to microfracture alone (89–91). HA, on the other hand, may be best utilized postoperatively to improve results compared to microfracture alone (92). Another application for these agents, specifically CBMA, may be to aid integration of autologous and allograft bone plugs during autologous osteochondral transplantation or allograft resurfacing

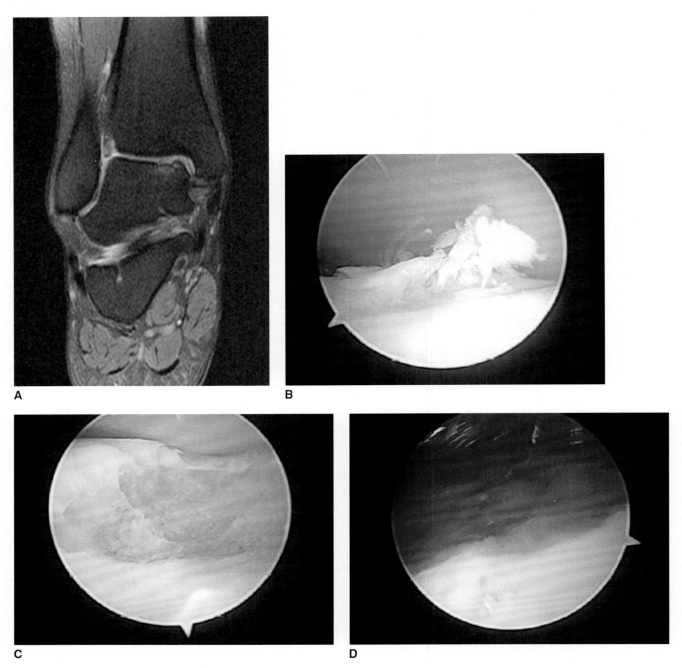

FIGURE 59-4

A: Osteochondral lesion of the posteromedial talar dome without significant cystic component of edema on coronal T2 images. **B:** Arthroscopic image viewing through the anterolateral portal reveals fibrillated cartilage overlying the posteromedial talar dome. **C:** Arthroscopic image viewing from the anteromedial portal after debridement of the fibrillated cartilage to the level of subchondral bone using a mechanical shaver. The calcified cartilage layer is debrided while leaving the subchondral bone intact. **D:** Fibrin glue overlying particulate allograft cartilage. Particulate allograft cartilage and fibrin glue applied through a 3-cm arthrotomy in line with the anteromedial arthroscopic portal.

procedures. While not specifically examined for osteochondral lesions of the talar dome, CBMA has displayed promising results for allograft resurfacing in the knee (93). In addition to these suspensions, a variety of biologic matrices have been described in conjunction with bone marrow stimulation techniques, theoretically creating a local environment to promote chondrogenesis (70,94–96). As biologic and cell-based therapies continue to evolve, further follow-up is warranted in order to determine the specific clinical situations where their application will improve outcomes for treatment of osteochondral lesions of the talus.

POSTOPERATIVE REHABILITATION

Postoperative rehabilitation is dependent on the specific procedure performed, including whether an osteotomy was needed in order to access and treat the osteochondral lesion of the talar dome. Additionally, if a concomitant procedure is performed, rehabilitation goals and timelines may have to be altered. We believe that it is important to initiate active ankle range of motion early after cartilage procedures for the talus. Because of this, concomitant procedures should be completed with adequate fixation to allow early active range of motion.

Patients undergoing bone marrow stimulation procedures, including microfracture, drilling, or retrograde drilling of osteochondral lesions of the talar dome without osteotomy, are placed in a below-knee walking boot postoperatively and kept non–weight bearing for the first 2 weeks while encouraging active ankle range of motion exercises. Touchdown weight bearing is initiated at 2 weeks postoperatively, with the goal of achieving full weight bearing by 6 weeks postoperatively. If the area undergoing bone marrow stimulation was large (>1.5 cm^2) or involved the medial or lateral shoulder of the talus without a circumferential cartilage rim, full weight bearing is delayed until 6 weeks postoperatively. At 6 weeks postoperatively, formal physical therapy is initiated, focusing on ankle range of motion, gait training, and strengthening exercises. As strength improves, proprioceptive exercises are initiated. Patients typically achieve full return to sport by 12 weeks postoperatively.

If a resurfacing procedure was performed without an osteotomy, including ACI, autograft osteochondral transplantation, allograft cartilage resurfacing, or particulated allograft cartilage procedures, the patient is placed in a below-knee walking boot and kept non–weight bearing for the first 6 weeks while encouraging immediate active ankle range of motion exercises. Transition to full weight bearing is started at 6 weeks postoperatively. At that time, formal physical therapy is initiated as described previously, with return to sport activities started at 12 weeks postoperatively.

When an osteotomy is performed, regardless of the technique used to address the osteochondral lesion of talar dome, the patient is placed in a rigid splint for 2 weeks and then transitioned to a below-knee walking boot. At 2 weeks postoperatively, the patient is encouraged to begin active ankle range of motion exercises while remaining non–weight bearing on the operative extremity. Transition to full weight bearing is started at 6 weeks postoperatively, and the postoperative course then remains unchanged from previously described rehabilitation protocols. Clinically, patients are followed with radiographs to confirm bony union of the osteotomy site. If there is concern for delayed union of the osteotomy or delayed autograft/allograft osteochondral plug incorporation, CT can be a useful tool. In our experience, healing of the autograft/allograft osteochondral plug typically mirrors that of the osteotomy, which is often easier to assess clinically with radiographs than osteochondral plug incorporation.

PEARLS AND PITFALLS

In the majority of clinical scenarios, bone marrow stimulation techniques should be the primary treatment option for patients with symptomatic lesions of the talar dome who have not previously undergone surgery (Table 59-2). From a technical perspective, maintaining perpendicular access to the lesion is essential for a variety of techniques. For bone marrow stimulation techniques, this may be achieved by angle microfracture awls or percutaneous incisions to allow access with drills or wires. For osteochondral autograft or allograft procedures, achieving perpendicularity may require more extensile exposures or osteotomies that are specific to the area of the lesion.

In general, many clinical and technical failures can be avoided with appropriate preoperative planning. Advanced imaging is an essential tool preoperatively and, where available, should be used routinely. Additionally, failure to create a stable, neutral mechanical environment will unnecessarily lead to failure. Particularly when considering larger restorative or resurfacing procedures, the mechanical axis and stability of the ankle joint should be considered. Ligamentous laxity is usually easily addressed in the same stage as the resurfacing procedure, whereas realignment procedures, including osteotomies, may be performed concomitantly or in a staged fashion.

TABLE 59-2 Pearls and Pitfalls	
Pearls	**Pitfalls**
• Consider operative intervention in patients with truly symptomatic lesions, not incidental findings • Obtain appropriate preoperative imaging • Understand whether the lesion is primarily a surface lesion or if the subchondral bone is significantly involved • Bone marrow stimulation techniques should remain the primary treatment for the majority of lesions • Address concomitant ligamentous instability or malalignment when performing restorative or resurfacing procedures • When performing concomitant procedures or osteotomies for access, utilize adequate fixation to allow early range of motion	• Failure to address concomitant ligamentous laxity or malalignment • Inadequate debridement of necrotic bone • Failure to achieve perpendicular lesion access when performing bone marrow stimulation techniques or cylindrical osteochondral autograft or allograft plugs • Prolonged postoperative immobilization

RESULTS

Given the diversity of osteochondral lesions of the talus and wide array of procedures designed to address those lesions, few randomized comparative studies exist. Gobbi et al. randomized patients to chondroplasty, microfracture, and autograft osteochondral transplantation and found no significant clinical differences up to 2 years postoperatively (41). Similarly, several systematic reviews have analyzed a variety of surgical techniques without clear superiority of one technique compared to the other (9,97). The nebulous outcomes reported by systematic reviews are frequently the result of heterogenous cohorts, a lack of clearly reported indications, and, most notably, inconsistencies in reporting of patient outcomes (98). Still, there is information to be garnered from these studies. The most commonly studied procedures for osteochondral defects of the talar dome include bone marrow stimulation techniques, excision and curettage, ACI, and osteochondral autograft transplantation. While the range of good or excellent outcomes for each individual treatment was relatively wide, weighted rates for all treatments identified successful outcomes in 75% to 85% of patients undergoing operative treatment (9).

Limited randomized studies and a lack of clear superiority for treatments make it difficult to better define indications for treatment of osteochondral defects of the talar dome, but there is value in looking at more specific subgroups of patients and lesions. For example, a retrospective case report and systematic review found that patients with lesions >1.0 to 1.5 cm^2 undergoing bone marrow stimulation achieve inferior outcomes to those with smaller lesions treated with bone marrow stimulation techniques (32,33). Another comparative study investigated the outcomes of autograft osteochondral transplantation and allograft cartilage resurfacing for similarly sized lesions. Ahmad and Jones found that allograft cartilage resurfacing provided similar results to autograft osteochondral transplantation with autograft from the knee while avoiding donor site morbidity (99). Lastly, Lee et al. found that lesions measuring <1 cm^2 treated with bone marrow stimulation achieved consistently good results regardless of whether a cystic component was or was not present under the lesions (38). Such studies are important, as they help better define indications and outcomes for a diverse population of patients and lesions. While good and excellent outcomes can be achieved with a variety of treatment techniques for osteochondral lesions of the talar dome, future research should focus on clear reporting of surgical indications, granular data presentation, and the consistent use of validated clinical outcomes in order to improve our understanding of these lesions while improving patient outcomes.

COMPLICATIONS

Complications during and following surgical intervention for treatment of osteochondral lesions of the talar dome are specific to the surgical procedure itself. Unique complications for each procedure will be discussed, but the list of complications should not be considered complete. As ankle arthroscopy is becoming a more common diagnostic and therapeutic technique for treatment of these lesions, it is important to understand complications associated with the use of the technique. While the morbidity of these complications is small, complications may occur in as many as 4% to 9% of patients and were most frequently noted to be transient neurologic deficits related to portal placement

(100,101). Outside of reoperation, complications following bone marrow stimulation procedures are consistent with those reported for ankle arthroscopy alone, with bone marrow stimulation itself adding very little morbidity to the procedure. Graft hypertrophy is a unique complication of ACI that was most significant with the use of first-generation periosteal patches. With the advent of second- and third-generation techniques, this has in large part resolved, although soft tissue hypertrophy can still occur (102,103). Donor site morbidity following autologous osteochondral transplantation using autologous graft from the knee can be a significant source of morbidity, although obtaining knee-specific outcomes is not routinely performed following treatment of osteochondral lesions of the talar dome (73). Patients with a body mass index >25 kg/m^2 may be at particular risk for persistent knee pain and symptoms after autograft harvest, and other options may want to be considered in these patients (72). Although avoiding donor site issues, osteochondral allograft resurfacing procedures are often performed for large lesions that frequently require more extensive approaches and osteotomies. Because of this, complications following osteochondral allograft resurfacing are more frequent than other procedures. A recent systematic review evaluated outcomes, including complications, following osteochondral allograft resurfacing (51). The most common complication was noted to be progression of degenerative changes requiring reoperation followed by subsequent reoperation for hardware removal. Overall, reoperation rates approached 25%. Less commonly noted complications requiring reoperation were nonunion of the osteotomy site or graft collapse, which occurred in 1% and 3% of cases, respectively. It should be noted that a small amount of graft collapse or subsidence identified radiographically is not uncommon following osteochondral allograft resurfacing, particularly for larger grafts (104). These radiographic findings must be correlated clinically, as the majority of patients remain asymptomatic. When determining treatment plans and discussing potential surgical options with patients, it is important to discuss the unique complications associated with each procedure while weighing the potential benefits that each technique provides.

CONCLUSION

Osteochondral lesions of the talar dome are being increasingly recognized as a source of pain and disability and often occur in patients with a history of an isolated or recurrent traumatic injury to the ankle. In patients who have failed to improve with a period of nonoperative treatment, a variety of surgical options exist to treat these lesions with consistently good to excellent outcomes reported in 80% to 85% of patients regardless of which modern treatment technique is utilized. While a single surgical technique has failed to show clinical superiority for treatment of osteochondral lesions of the talar dome, this is due in large part to the heterogeneity of lesions as well as the diverse population of patients that sustain these injuries with variable demands and treatment goals. Several studies have helped identify particular lesions and patient populations that may be more or less suitable for a given treatment technique, thus helping to better define indications while aiding in clinical decision-making. Further studies like this will only aid to improve our understanding of these difficult to treat lesions. In general, it is important to note the shortcomings in the currently available literature, and moving forward, efforts to improve research methodology, including stratification of analysis based on clinically relevant patient and disease factors while obtaining mid- and long-term outcomes, will be critical to improve patient outcomes in the evolving treatment of osteochondral lesions of the talar dome.

REFERENCES

1. Saxena A, Eakin C. Articular talar injuries in athletes. *Am J Sports Med.* 2007;35:1680–1687.
2. Hintermann B, Regazzoni P, Lampert C, et al. Arthroscopic findings in acute fractures of the ankle. *J Bone Joint Surg Br.* 2000;82:345–351.
3. Leontaritis N, Hinojosa L, Panchbhavi VK. Arthroscopically detected intra-articular lesions associated with acute ankle fractures. *J Bone Joint Surg Am.* 2009;91:333–339.
4. Tan TC, Wilcox DM, Frank L, et al. MR imaging of articular cartilage in the ankle: comparison of available imaging sequences and methods of measurement in cadavers. *Skeletal Radiol.* 1996;25:749–755.
5. Mintz DN, Tashjian GS, Connell DA, et al. Osteochondral lesions of the talus: a new magnetic resonance grading system with arthroscopic correlation. *Arthroscopy.* 2003;19:353–359.
6. Leumann A, Valderrabano V, Plaass C, et al. A novel imaging method for osteochondral lesions of the talus—comparison of SPECT-CT with MRI. *Am J Sports Med.* 2011;39:1095–1101.
7. Gatlin CC, Matheny LM, Ho CP, et al. Diagnostic accuracy of 3.0 Tesla magnetic resonance imaging for the detection of articular cartilage lesions of the talus. *Foot Ankle Int.* 2015;36:288–292.
8. Kraeutler MJ, Chahla J, Dean CS, et al. Current concepts review update: osteochondral lesions of the talus. *Foot Ankle Int.* 2017;38:331–342.

9. Zengerink M, Struijs PA, Tol JL, et al. Treatment of osteochondral lesions of the talus: a systematic review. *Knee Surg Sports Traumatol Arthrosc.* 2010;18:238–246.

10. Murawski CD, Kennedy JG. Operative treatment of osteochondral lesions of the talus. *J Bone Joint Surg Am.* 2013;95:1045–1054.

11. van Eekeren I, van Bergen C, Sierevelt I, et al. Return to sports after arthroscopic debridement and bone marrow stimulation of osteochondral talar defects: a 5- to 24-year follow-up study. *Knee Surg Sports Traumatol Arthrosc.* 2016;24:1311–1315.

12. van Bergen CJ, Kox LS, Maas M, et al. Arthroscopic treatment of osteochondral defects of the talus: outcomes at eight to twenty years of follow-up. *J Bone Joint Surg Am.* 2013;95:519–525.

13. Canale ST, Belding R. Osteochondral lesions of the talus. *J Bone Joint Surg Am.* 1980;62:97–102.

14. Berndt AL, Harty M. Transchondral fractures (osteochondritis dissecans) of the talus. *J Bone Joint Surg Am.* 1959;41-A:988–1020.

15. Stougaard J. Familial occurrence of osteochondritis dissecans. *J Bone Joint Surg Br.* 1964;46:542–543.

16. Carlson C, Meuten D, Richardson D. Ischemic necrosis of cartilage in spontaneous and experimental lesions of osteochondrosis. *J Orthop Res.* 1991;9:317–329.

17. Loomer R, Fisher C, Lloyd-Smith R, et al. Osteochondral lesions of the talus. *Am J Sports Med.* 1993;21:13–19.

18. Orr JD, Dutton JR, Fowler JT. Anatomic location and morphology of symptomatic, operatively treated osteochondral lesions of the talus. *Foot Ankle Int.* 2012;33:1051–1057.

19. Raikin SM, Elias I, Zoga AC, et al. Osteochondral lesions of the talus: localization and morphologic data from 424 patients using a novel anatomical grid scheme. *Foot Ankle Int.* 2007;28:154–161.

20. Tol J, Struijs P, Bossuyt P, et al. Treatment strategies in osteochondral defects of the talar dome: a systematic review. *Foot Ankle Int.* 2000;21:119–126.

21. Verhagen R, Maas M, Dijkgraaf M, et al. Prospective study on diagnostic strategies in osteochondral lesions of the talus. *J Bone Joint Surg Br.* 2005;87:41–46.

22. Hepple S, Winson IG, Glew D. Osteochondral lesions of the talus: a revised classification. *Foot Ankle Int.* 1999;20:789–793.

23. Bonvin F, Montet X, Copercini M, et al. Imaging of fractures of the lateral process of the talus, a frequently missed diagnosis. *Eur J Radiol.* 2003;47:64–70.

24. Williams GN, Jones MH, Amendola A. Syndesmotic ankle sprains in athletes. *Am J Sports Med.* 2007;35:1197–1207.

25. van Dijk CN, Mol BWJ, Lim LS, et al. Diagnosis of ligament rupture of the ankle joint: physical examination, arthrography, stress radiography and sonography compared in 160 patients after inversion trauma. *Acta Orthop Scand.* 1996;67:566–570.

26. Vaseenon T, Gao Y, Phisitkul P. Comparison of two manual tests for ankle laxity due to rupture of the lateral ankle ligaments. *Iowa Orthop J.* 2012;32:9.

27. Femino JE, Vaseenon T, Phistkul P, et al. Varus external rotation stress test for radiographic detection of deep deltoid ligament disruption with and without syndesmotic disruption: a cadaveric study. *Foot Ankle Int.* 2013;34:251–260.

28. Canale ST, Kelly F Jr. Fractures of the neck of the talus. Long-term evaluation of seventy-one cases. *J Bone Joint Surg Am.* 1978;60:143–156.

29. Saltzman CL, El-Khoury GY. The hindfoot alignment view. *Foot Ankle Int.* 1995;16:572–576.

30. Thompson JP, Loomer RL. Osteochondral lesions of the talus in a sports medicine clinic: a new radiographic technique and surgical approach. *Am J Sports Med.* 1984;12:460–463.

31. Dragoni M, Bonasia DE, Amendola A. Osteochondral talar allograft for large osteochondral defects: technique tip. *Foot Ankle Int.* 2011;32:910–916.

32. Cuttica DJ, Smith WB, Hyer CF, et al. Osteochondral lesions of the talus: predictors of clinical outcome. *Foot Ankle Int.* 2011;32:1045–1051.

33. Ramponi L, Yasui Y, Murawski CD, et al. Lesion size is a predictor of clinical outcomes after bone marrow stimulation for osteochondral lesions of the talus: a systematic review. *Am J Sports Med.* 2017;45:1698–1705.

34. Anderson I, Crichton K, Grattan-Smith T, et al. Osteochondral fractures of the dome of the talus. *J Bone Joint Surg Am.* 1989;71:1143–1152.

35. Griffith JF, Lau DTY, Yeung DKW, et al. High-resolution MR imaging of talar osteochondral lesions with new classification. *Skeletal Radiol.* 2012;41:387–399.

36. Kono M, Takao M, Naito K, et al. Retrograde drilling for osteochondral lesions of the talar dome. *Am J Sports Med.* 2006;34:1450–1456.

37. Scranton P, Frey C, Feder K. Outcome of osteochondral autograft transplantation for type-V cystic osteochondral lesions of the talus. *J Bone Joint Surg Br.* 2006;88:614–619.

38. Lee KB, Park HW, Cho HJ, et al. Comparison of arthroscopic microfracture for osteochondral lesions of the talus with and without subchondral cyst. *Am J Sports Med.* 2015;43:1951–1956.

39. Klammer G, Maquieira GJ, Spahn S, et al. Natural history of nonoperatively treated osteochondral lesions of the talus. *Foot Ankle Int.* 2015;36:24–31.

40. Van Dijk CN, Reilingh ML, Zengerink M, et al. Osteochondral defects in the ankle: why painful? *Knee Surg Sports Traumatol Arthrosc.* 2010;18:570–580.

41. Gobbi A, Francisco RA, Lubowitz JH, et al. Osteochondral lesions of the talus: randomized controlled trial comparing chondroplasty, microfracture, and osteochondral autograft transplantation. *Arthroscopy.* 2006;22:1085–1092.

42. Phisitkul P, Akoh CC, Rungprai C, et al. Optimizing arthroscopy for osteochondral lesions of the talus: the effect of ankle positions and distraction during anterior and posterior arthroscopy in a cadaveric model. *Arthroscopy.* 2017;33:2238–2245.

43. Muir D, Saltzman CL, Tochigi Y, et al. Talar dome access for osteochondral lesions. *Am J Sports Med.* 2006;34:1457–1463.

44. Bugbee WD, Khanna G, Cavallo M, et al. Bipolar fresh osteochondral allografting of the tibiotalar joint. *J Bone Joint Surg Am.* 2013;95:426–432.

45. Alexander IJ, Watson JT. Step-cut osteotomy of the medial malleolus for exposure of the medial ankle joint space. *Foot Ankle.* 1991;11:242–243.

46. Gianakos AL, Hannon CP, Ross KA, et al. Anterolateral tibial osteotomy for accessing osteochondral lesions of the talus in autologous osteochondral transplantation: functional and t2 MRI analysis. *Foot Ankle Int.* 2015;36:531–538.

47. Lee K-B, Yang H-K, Moon E-S, et al. Modified step-cut medial malleolar osteotomy for osteochondral grafting of the talus. *Foot Ankle Int.* 2008;29:1107–1110.

48. Siegel SJ, Mount AC. Step-cut medial malleolar osteotomy: literature review and case reports. *J Foot Ankle Surg.* 2012;51:226–233.

49. Tochigi Y, Amendola A, Muir D, et al. Surgical approach for centrolateral talar osteochondral lesions with an anterolateral osteotomy. *Foot Ankle Int.* 2002;23:1038–1039.

50. Garras DN, Santangelo JA, Wang DW, et al. A quantitative comparison of surgical approaches for posterolateral osteochondral lesions of the talus. *Foot Ankle Int.* 2008;29:6.

51. VanTienderen RJ, Dunn JC, Kusnezov N, et al. Osteochondral allograft transfer for treatment of osteochondral lesions of the talus: a systematic review. *Arthroscopy.* 2017;33:217–222.

52. Lamb J, Murawski CD, Deyer TW, et al. Chevron-type medial malleolar osteotomy: a functional, radiographic and quantitative T2-mapping MRI analysis. *Knee Surg Sports Traumatol Arthrosc.* 2013;21:1283–1288.

53. Leumann A, Horisberger M, Buettner O, et al. Medial malleolar osteotomy for the treatment of talar osteochondral lesions: anatomical and morbidity considerations. *Knee Surg Sports Traumatol Arthrosc.* 2016;24:2133–2139.

54. Kelbérine F, Frank A. Arthroscopic treatment of osteochondral lesions of the talar dome: a retrospective study of 48 cases. *Arthroscopy.* 1999;15:77–84.

55. O'Farrell T, Costello B. Osteochondritis dissecans of the talus. The late results of surgical treatment. *J Bone Joint Surg Br.* 1982;64:494–497.

56. Ray RB, Coughlin EJ Jr. Osteochondritis dissecans of the talus. *J Bone Joint Surg Am.* 1947;29:697–710.

57. Steadman JR, Rodkey WG, Briggs KK. Microfracture: its history and experience of the developing surgeon. *Cartilage.* 2010;1:78–86.

58. Choi J-I, Lee K-B. Comparison of clinical outcomes between arthroscopic subchondral drilling and microfracture for osteochondral lesions of the talus. *Knee Surg Sports Traumatol Arthrosc.* 2016;24:2140–2147.

59. Taranow WS, Bisignani GA, Towers JD, et al. Retrograde drilling of osteochondral lesions of the medial talar dome. *Foot Ankle Int.* 1999;20:474–480.

60. Brittberg M, Lindahl A, Nilsson A, et al. Treatment of deep cartilage defects in the knee with autologous chondrocyte transplantation. *N Engl J Med.* 1994;331:889–895.

61. Baums M, Heidrich G, Schultz W, et al. Autologous chondrocyte transplantation for treating cartilage defects of the talus. *J Bone Joint Surg Am.* 2006;88:303–308.

62. Niemeyer P, Salzmann G, Schmal H, et al. Autologous chondrocyte implantation for the treatment of chondral and osteochondral defects of the talus: a meta-analysis of available evidence. *Knee Surg Sports Traumatol Arthrosc.* 2012;20:1696–1703.

63. Petersen L, Brittberg M, Lindahl A. Autologous chondrocyte transplantation of the ankle. *Foot Ankle Clin.* 2003;8:291–303.

64. Whittaker J-P, Smith G, Makwana N, et al. Early results of autologous chondrocyte implantation in the talus. *J Bone Joint Surg Br.* 2005;87:179–183.

65. Kwak SK, Kern BS, Ferkel RD, et al. Autologous chondrocyte implantation of the ankle: 2-to 10-year results. *Am J Sports Med.* 2014;42:2156–2164.

66. Desando G, Bartolotti I, Vannini F, et al. Repair potential of matrix-induced bone marrow aspirate concentrate and matrix-induced autologous chondrocyte implantation for talar osteochondral repair: patterns of some catabolic, inflammatory, and pain mediators. *Cartilage.* 2017;8:50–60.

67. Giannini S, Buda R, Grigolo B, et al. The detached osteochondral fragment as a source of cells for autologous chondrocyte implantation (ACI) in the ankle joint. *Osteoarthritis Cartilage.* 2005;13:601–607.

68. Kreulen C, Giza E, Walton J, et al. Seven-year follow-up of matrix-induced autologous implantation in talus articular defects. *Foot Ankle Spec.* 2018;11:133–137.

69. Middendorf JM, Griffin DJ, Shortkroff S, et al. Mechanical properties and structure-function relationships of human chondrocyte-seeded cartilage constructs after in vitro culture. *J Orthop Res.* 2017;35:2298–2306.

70. Valderrabano V, Miska M, Leumann A, et al. Reconstruction of osteochondral lesions of the talus with autologous spongiosa grafts and autologous matrix-induced chondrogenesis. *Am J Sports Med.* 2013;41:519–527.

71. LaPrade RF, Botker JC. Donor-site morbidity after osteochondral autograft transfer procedures. *Arthroscopy.* 2004;20:e69–e73.

72. Paul J, Sagstetter A, Kriner M, et al. Donor-site morbidity after osteochondral autologous transplantation for lesions of the talus. *J Bone Joint Surg Am.* 2009;91:1683–1688.

73. Reddy S, Pedowitz DI, Parekh SG, et al. The morbidity associated with osteochondral harvest from asymptomatic knees for the treatment of osteochondral lesions of the talus. *Am J Sports Med.* 2007;35:80–85.

74. Lee C-H, Chao K-H, Huang G-S, et al. Osteochondral autografts for osteochondritis dissecans of the talus. *Foot Ankle Int.* 2003;24:815–822.

75. Kreuz PC, Steinwachs M, Erggelet C, et al. Mosaicplasty with autogenous talar autograft for osteochondral lesions of the talus after failed primary arthroscopic management. *Am J Sports Med.* 2006;34:55–63.

76. Latt LD, Glisson RR, Montijo HE, et al. Effect of graft height mismatch on contact pressures with osteochondral grafting of the talus. *Am J Sports Med.* 2011;39:2662–2669.

77. Henak CR, Ross KA, Bonnevie ED, et al. Human talar and femoral cartilage have distinct mechanical properties near the articular surface. *J Biomech.* 2016;49:3320–3327.

78. Cook JL, Stannard JP, Stoker AM, et al. Importance of donor chondrocyte viability for osteochondral allografts. *Am J Sports Med.* 2016;44:1260–1268.

79. Williams SK, Amiel D, Ball ST, et al. Prolonged storage effects on the articular cartilage of fresh human osteochondral allografts. *J Bone Joint Surg Am.* 2003;85:2111–2120.

80. Qi J, Hu Z, Song H, et al. Cartilage storage at 4°C with regular culture medium replacement benefits chondrocyte viability of osteochondral grafts in vitro. *Cell Tissue Bank.* 2016;17:473–479.

81. Cook JL, Stoker AM, Stannard JP, et al. A novel system improves preservation of osteochondral allografts. *Clin Orthop Relat Res.* 2014;472:3404–3414.

82. Adams SB Jr, Viens NA, Easley ME, et al. Midterm results of osteochondral lesions of the talar shoulder treated with fresh osteochondral allograft transplantation. *J Bone Joint Surg Am.* 2011;93:648–654.

83. Saltzman BM, Lin J, Lee S. Particulated juvenile articular cartilage allograft transplantation for osteochondral talar lesions. *Cartilage.* 2017;8:61–72.

84. Coetzee JC, Giza E, Schon LC, et al. Treatment of osteochondral lesions of the talus with particulated juvenile cartilage. *Foot Ankle Int.* 2013;34:1205–1211.

85. Giza E, Delman C, Coetzee JC, et al. Arthroscopic treatment of talus osteochondral lesions with particulated juvenile allograft cartilage. *Foot Ankle Int.* 2014;35:1087–1094.

86. Adams SB, Demetracopoulos CA, Parekh SG, et al. Arthroscopic particulated juvenile cartilage allograft transplantation for the treatment of osteochondral lesions of the talus. *Arthrosc Tech.* 2014;3:e533–e537.

87. Mei-Dan O, Carmont MR, Laver L, et al. Platelet-rich plasma or hyaluronate in the management of osteochondral lesions of the talus. *Am J Sports Med.* 2012;40:534–541.

88. Yasui Y, Ross AW, Kennedy JG. Platelet-rich plasma and concentrated bone marrow aspirate in surgical treatment for osteochondral lesions of the talus. *Foot Ankle Clin.* 2016;21:869–884.

89. Görmeli G, Karakaplan M, Görmeli CA, et al. Clinical effects of platelet-rich plasma and hyaluronic acid as an additional therapy for talar osteochondral lesions treated with microfracture surgery: a prospective randomized clinical trial. *Foot Ankle Int.* 2015;36:891–900.

90. Guney A, Akar M, Karaman I, et al. Clinical outcomes of platelet rich plasma (PRP) as an adjunct to microfracture surgery in osteochondral lesions of the talus. *Knee Surg Sports Traumatol Arthrosc.* 2015;23:2384–2389.

91. Hannon CP, Ross KA, Murawski CD, et al. Arthroscopic bone marrow stimulation and concentrated bone marrow aspirate for osteochondral lesions of the talus: a case-control study of functional and magnetic resonance observation of cartilage repair tissue outcomes. *Arthroscopy.* 2016;32:339–347.

92. Doral M, Bilge O, Batmaz G, et al. Treatment of osteochondral lesions of the talus with microfracture technique and postoperative hyaluronan injection. *Knee Surg Sports Traumatol Arthrosc.* 2012;20:1398–1403.

93. Oladeji LO, Stannard JP, Cook CR, et al. Effects of autogenous bone marrow aspirate concentrate on radiographic integration of femoral condylar osteochondral allografts. *Am J Sports Med.* 2017;45:2797–2803.

94. Usuelli FG, de Girolamo L, Grassi M, et al. All-arthroscopic autologous matrix-induced chondrogenesis for the treatment of osteochondral lesions of the talus. *Arthrosc Tech.* 2015;4:e255–e259.

95. Gottschalk O, Altenberger S, Baumbach S, et al. Functional medium-term results after autologous matrix-induced chondrogenesis for osteochondral lesions of the talus: a 5-year prospective cohort study. *J Foot Ankle Surg.* 2017;56:930–936.

96. Wiewiorski M, Barg A, Valderrabano V. Autologous matrix-induced chondrogenesis in osteochondral lesions of the talus. *Foot Ankle Clin.* 2013;18:151–158.

97. Dahmen J, Lambers KT, Reilingh ML, et al. No superior treatment for primary osteochondral defects of the talus. *Knee Surg Sports Traumatol Arthrosc.* 2018;26:2142–2157.

98. Hannon CP, Murawski CD, Fansa AM, et al. Microfracture for osteochondral lesions of the talus: a systematic review of reporting of outcome data. *Am J Sports Med.* 2013;41:689–695.

99. Ahmad J, Jones K. Comparison of osteochondral autografts and allografts for treatment of recurrent or large talar osteochondral lesions. *Foot Ankle Int.* 2016;37:40–50.

100. Ferkel RD, Small HN, Gittins JE. Complications in foot and ankle arthroscopy. *Clin Orthop Relat Res.* 2001;391:89–104.

101. Zwiers R, Wiegerinck JI, Murawski CD, et al. Arthroscopic treatment for anterior ankle impingement: a systematic review of the current literature. *Arthroscopy.* 2015;31:1585–1596.

102. Kreuz P, Steinwachs M, Erggelet C, et al. Classification of graft hypertrophy after autologous chondrocyte implantation of full-thickness chondral defects in the knee. *Osteoarthritis Cartilage.* 2007;15:1339–1347.

103. Gomoll AH, Probst C, Farr J, et al. Use of a type I/III bilayer collagen membrane decreases reoperation rates for symptomatic hypertrophy after autologous chondrocyte implantation. *Am J Sports Med.* 2009;37:20S–23S.

104. Raikin SM. Fresh osteochondral allografts for large-volume cystic osteochondral defects of the talus. *J Bone Joint Surg Am.* 2009;91:2818–2826.

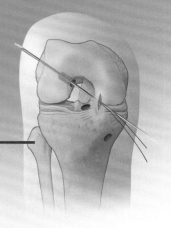

Index

Note: Page numbers followed by *f* indicate figure. Page numbers followed by *t* indicate table.